THE

CHAUKHAMBA AYURVIJNAN STUDIES

37

Studies on Medicinal Plants & Drugs in

DHANVANTARI-NIGHAṆṬU

Commented by Late Vd. D. K. Kamat upto Chapter V. Further enlarged and commented up to the end with complete Sanskrit Text and English translation, different readings, notes, comments etc. by

Dr. S. D. Kamat

M.F.A.M. (Mah.)

ज्ञाने सर्वं प्रतिष्ठितम्

CHAUKHAMBA SANSKRIT PRATISHTHAN

DELHI

Published by :
CHAUKHAMBA SANSKRIT PRATISHTHAN
38 U. A. Bungalow Road, Jawahar Nagar,
Post Box No. 2113, Delhi-110007
Phone : 3956391

Also available at :
CHOWKHAMBA VIDYABHAWAN
Chowk, Post Box No. 1069
Varanasi-221001
Tele : 320404

•

CHAUKHAMBA SURBHARATI PRAKASHAN
K 37/117, Gopal Mandir Lane,
Post Box No. 1129
Varanasi-221001
Tele : 335263

First Published : 2002
Price :

ISBN : 81-7084-179-7

Printed at :
A.K. Lithographer
Delhi

Contents

Sr. No.		Page No.
1)	Preface.	I-XIII
2)	Forward to the vol. I by Pdt.Shivsharma.	XIV
3)	Preface to the vol. I by Kamat & Mahajan.	XV-XVII
4)	Introduction to vol. 1 by Dr. G.S.Pendse.	XVIII
5)	Introduction to vol. 2 by Prof. P.V.Sharma.	XXX-XXXV
6)	The treatise and it's Constitution.	
	i) The treatise.	XXXVI-XLVII
	ii) The constitution.	XLVIII-LVI
	iii) Study of Ayurvedic Nighaṇṭus.	LVII--LXIV
7)	Proforma & System of Transliteration.	LXV-LXVII
8)	Index of Heading names.	*A-1 -A-20*
9)	द्रव्यावलिः Dravyāvali, मंगलाचरणम् Mangalācaraṇam, ग्रन्थस्य कारणम् Purpose of the treatise.	*B-1 - B-4*
10)	गणद्रव्यावलिः Gaṇadravyāvalih.	*C-1 - C-20*
11)	Study of plants in Guḍūcyādi Chapter I गुडूच्यादि वर्ग :- १.	1-119
12)	Study of plants - Śatapuṣpādi Chapter II शतपुष्पादि वर्ग :- २.	121-190
13)	Study of plants - Candanādi Chapter III चंदनादि वर्ग :- ३.	191-273
14)	Study of plants - Karavīradi Chapter IV करवीरादि वर्ग :- ४.	275-384
15)	Study of plants - Āmrādi Chapter V आम्रादि वर्ग :- ५.	385-522
16)	Study of drugs - Suvarṇādi Chapter VI सुवर्णादि वर्ग :- ६.	523-644
17)	Study of drugs - Miśrakādi Chapter VII मिश्रकादि वर्ग :- ७	645-669
18)	Bibliography.	670-681
19)	Index	
	Index A-Botanical names, synonyms and other drugs.	682-716
	Index B-Sanskṛt names, synonyms etc.	717-858

Preface

The first volume of the studies on medicinal plants in Dhanvantarīya Nighaṇṭu. गुडूच्यादि वर्ग Guḍucyādi chapter was written and published by my Late father Vd. D.K.Kamat and Prof. S.D.Mahajan in 1972. The second volume शतपुष्पादि वर्ग Śatapuṣpādi chapter was published by me in 1979. Out of the remaining five chapters viz. चंदनादि तृतीय वर्ग 3rd Candanādi chapter, करवीरादि चतुर्थ वर्ग 4th Karavīrādi chapter and the आम्रादि पञ्चम वर्ग 5th Āmrādi chapter which consist most of the herbal drugs of this Dhanvantari Nighaṇṭu were commented upon by Late Vd. D.K.Kamat and the Mṣṣ in his own hand writing was ready in different files. After the publication of the Vol. II; I was very eager to complete and publish the remaining 5 volumes, but I could not do so for various reasons. I am now happy in completing the remaining work of my Late father and publishing the निघण्टु Nighaṇṭu - with its full text for the benefit of scholars. Here in this present book I have made certain additions and insertions without doing any harm to the original substance of the comments of Mṣṣ. The additions or insertions are as noted below :

1) As stated earlier the Mṣṣ of the above mentioned Dhn.Ni. was ready only upto the V th Chapter i.e आम्रादि वर्ग *Āmrādi Chapter;* the remaining chapters i.e.सुवर्णादि वर्ग VIth the *Suvarṇādi Chapter* and the मिश्रकादि वर्ग VII th *Miśrakādi Chapter* were not commented upon, but to complete the work I have myself commented upon in the same style and proforma. It is up to the scholars to decide to what extent I have been succeeded in this attempt.

2) As the published volumes and also unpublilshed Mss did not contain the Sanskrit text, the reader has to depend on other books containing the text. The edition published by आनन्दाश्रम मुद्रणालय Ānandāśrama mudraṇālaya was referred by Late Vd. D.K.Kamat. It is out of print for a long time. Therefore I have included the text in संस्कृत Sanskrit. As the text is added and also all the Chapters brought together, made it necessary to rearrange the contents, index etc.

3) Two editions of this Nighaṇṭu are published recently. One is commented by Dr. Guruprasadji Sharma, edited by Prof. Priyavratji Sharma and published by Chaukhamba Publishers (Sometimes I have mentioned as Chaukhamba edition) and the second by Dr. Jharkhande Ojha.

In the meantime Prof. Priyavratji Sharma, the great scholar of Ayurveda has edited a number Nighaṇṭus, the important one from the point of Dhanvantari Nighaṇṭu is शोढलनिघण्टु Soḍhala Nighaṇṭu. I have also obtained 3 other Mṣṣ of Dh.Ni. from the University of Mumbai.and 2MṢṢ from Bhandarakar oriental library Pune. All these have been referred for the present edition of Dhn.Ni.

The commentators of अमरकोश Amarkosh ,- क्षीरस्वामी Ksiraswāmi - and श्रीवल्लभ उपाध्याय Shrivallabha Upadhyaya - the commentator of Nighantusesha[1] had quoted Dhanvantari Nighaṇṭu very often. There are some different readings mentioned in Anandasram edition. Such different readings which I felt important are mentioned in the foot notes of this book.

The commentators interpret or comment on the basis of the original text, therefore, it is necessary to have the correct text. I have tried to provide the correct text in the light of all these available Nighaṇṭus, Mṣṣ and other works mentioned above. Some of the verses of this Nighaṇṭu are taken from the classical texts, (i.e. Samhitās) the references of the same are also mentioned in this book.

4) *The properties, medicinal uses etc. of the drugs are not commented here, because the aim of the study is limited only to the correct identification and confirmation of the plants in this Nighaṇṭu,* though it is true that the final confirmation requires further substantiation by pharmacological, clinical experimental and other methods of studies.

However, for the purpose of completion of the work I have translated the properties and actions of the drugs which are mentioned in the text.

For the purpose of comments on pharmacological actions the correct and authentic terminology in modern languages for the original sanskrit terms is also necessary. Without this the exact meanings cannot be understood. Let us take an example of the term वृष्य - *Vrsya.* It is usually termed as aphrodisiac[2]. The term वृष्य *vrṣya* according to Ayurvedic terminology includes various factors and shades of meaning, involving different sites of actions as mentioned below :-

1) यत्किंचित् मधुरं स्निग्धं बृंहणं बलवर्धनम् ।
मनसो हर्षणं यच्च तत्सर्वं वृष्यमुच्यते ॥ A.H.U.40.35

2) यस्माच्छुक्रस्य वृद्धिः स्यात् शुक्रलं हि तदुच्यते ।
यथा नागबलाद्याः स्युर्बीजं च कपिकच्छुजम् ॥
यस्मात् द्रव्यात् भवेत्स्त्रीषु हर्षो वाजीकरं हि तत् ।
यथाऽश्वगन्धा मुशली शर्करा च शतावरी ॥ Sarng.

---

१ निघण्टुशेष - published by Lalbhai Dalpatbhai Ahamadabad - 9. June 1968.

२ "aphrodisiac - exciting sexual desires" Gloss. of Bot.terms by R.L.Heing.1899.
वृष्या (कपिकच्छु) - promotes virility , कपिकच्छु बीज (seeds of Kapikachu-aphrodisiac, Treatise on Indian Medicinal Plants-Asima Chatterjee Vol.II-p.102,03.)

3) ... ... तत्र जनकं मांसघृतादिकं यत् रसादिधातुक्रमेण
परिणतं प्रधान-धातुपुष्टिं करोति ।प्रवर्तकं उच्चटा चूर्णादिकं
शुक्रविरेचनकरम् । ... जनकप्रवर्तकं तु क्षीरगव्यघृतगोधूममाषकाकाण्डफलादिकम् ।
डल्हण (सु.चि. २६.)

4) प्रवर्तनी स्त्री शुक्रस्य रेचनं बृहतीफलम् ।
जातीफलं स्तंम्भकं च शोषणी च हरीतकी ॥
दुग्धं माषाश्च भल्लातफलमज्जाऽमलानि च ।
प्रवर्तकानि कथ्यन्ते जनकानि च रेतसः ॥ शार्ङ्ग.खं. १

It can be appreciated from the above that all the different shades of meanings of the term वृष्य-*Vṛṣya* cannot be explained by the term 'aphrodisiac' alone.

There are also other books available, written by eminent scholars on this subject, as well as the translations of the classical books which may be referred by the interested readers to understand the properties, medicinal uses etc. of the drugs included in this निघण्टु Nighaṇṭu.

5) The title of the book of the first two volumes is given as "Studies on medicinal plants in *"Dhanvantarīya Nighaṇṭu"* as the study is limited to the plants only and no text was provided, but in this present work all the drugs, all the chapters including the text with English translation have been provided and is titled as "Studies on the medicinal plants in "Dhanvantari Nighaṇṭu"

I have retained the old name धन्वन्तरि निघण्टु Dhanvantari Nighaṇṭu which is accepted by the old scholars. Late. Vd. Purandare has accepted the name धन्वन्तरीय निघण्टु Dhanvantarīya Nighaṇṭu which is mentioned by the compiler of Raj. ni for the purpose of metrical arrangement of the verse.

6) ***Since what time the title "Dhanvantari Nighaṇṭu" is prevailing ?***

"From the introductary verses it appears that the actual title of the original work was *Dravyāvali* and not *Dhanvantari Nighaṇṭu*...."The composition of Nighaṇṭus having description of properties and actions of drugs along with synonyms is a later development. The original text Dravyāvali consisted of synonyms only... ... Thus the existing text of *Dhanvantari Nighaṇṭu* is *Dravyāvali* added with descriptions of properties and actions....

On the basis of internal evidences it may be said that the process continued till the 13th Cent. A.D. It appears, after addition having com-

---

Note :- "Aphrodisiac - stimulating or increasing the sexual apetite, passion and virile power, eg. strychnine, Damiana, Canabis indica. They act on the genital centre of the cord and brain. They may also act indirectly by irritating the bladder and urethra as cantherdis.
Nadkarni. Mat. Medi.II P.512.

वृष्य – Spermatogenic - Bhisagratna sen

वृष्य – Spermatopoetic - Treatise on Indi med. plants Vol. II P.185- Asima chaterjee.

pleted in Dravyāvali it began to be known by the new title of Dhanvantari Nighaṇṭu ...."

(Prof. P.V.Sharma. Preface to the 2nd Vol. of Dhn.Ni.of Vd.D.K.Kamat.P.6-7)

(1) The *Dravyāvali* and the Dhanvantari Nighaṇṭu are of two different authors and written at different periods.

(2) From external and internal evidences the *Dravyāvali* may be placed in the 10th Cent. A.D. as it is quoted by Kṣ́iraswāmi (11 Cent. A.D.) and the *Dhanvantari Nighaṇṭu* in the 13th Cent. A.D."

(Intro. to Dravyaguna by Prof. P.V.Sharma 1976)

Whether the original work consisted of synonyms only or not is very difficult to decide, but Ksīraswāmī (whose period is accepted as 11th Cent.A.D) has mentioned the name of this Nighaṇṭu as *Dhanvantari Nighaṇṭu* on the following pages 56 (twice), 59,62,67,74,77,80,82,110, 111 (Amarakośa - Kṣ́īraswāmī Comm.). He has not mentioned *Dravyāvali* anywhere. Therefore the name of this Nighaṇṭu was prevailing as *Dhanvantari Nighaṇṭu* since the time of Kṣ́iraswāmi i.e. from 11th cent.A.D. In the classical books (i.e. संहिता) the properties and actions of the drugs are mentioned but the compilation with synonyms with different classification of groups (गण) is the most important practical aspect of this Nighaṇṭu.

Another important evidence is obtained from 'Śoḍhala Nighaṇṭu'. He clearly stated that he had mentioned the same drugs and Dravyāvali which had been mentioned by Dhanvantari and actually, by comparison it seems to be true. I have made use of this Śoḍhala Nighaṇṭu in deciding the correct readings (पाठशोधन) of the *Gaṇcvadrāvyavali* of the present Dhn. Ni. and the same are mentioned in foot notes.

धन्वन्तरिमतादेष स्वल्पसंक्षेपविस्तरः ।
सोढलेन सतार्थोऽयं ग्रथ्यते नामसंग्रहः ॥

तान्येवौषधनामानि धन्वन्तर्युदितानि च ।
द्रव्यावली तथा सैव संक्षेपाय नवाकृतिः ॥ (Śodhal p.1.)

At this stage it will not be improper to mention a discrepancy found in the 6th Chapter i.e. सुवर्णादि वर्ग Suvarṇādi varga of the present Dhanvantari Nighaṇṭu and the *Suvarṇādi varga* of Śoḍhala Nighaṇṭu. The VIth Chapter of the present Dhn.Ni. contains various drugs like metals, gems, food substances and many others, while Śoḍhala has mentioned only the metals mentioned in the 1st Stanza (verse) of the present Dhn.Ni.

i.e.

सुवर्णरौप्यताम्राणि त्रपुरीतिश्च सीसकम् ।
कांस्यं लौहं च योज्यानि गरदोषप्रशान्तये ॥

(Dhn. Ni. & Śodhala) Chapter VI-1

This may perhaps suggest that the original द्रव्यावली – Dravyāvali was consisting this much portion only. (that means the Nighaṇṭu ends there only). Because after this portion there is a significant difference between the drugs mentioned in the present Dhn.Ni. and those of the Śoḍhala. Up to this i.e upto the आम्रादि वर्ग Āmrādi Chapter- Śoḍhalaś statement that he had followed the Dhn. Ni. had been so much meticulously observed that I was inclined to infer that whatever portion mentioned after this verse and the whole Miśrakadi Chapter of the present Dhn.Ni. is a later addition.

But क्षीरस्वामी - Kśiraswāmī on अमरकोश - Amarakośa (11th Cent. A.D.) has mentioned certain readings from the *Suvarṇādi* and *Miśrakādi* Chapters of the present Dhn. Ni. eg.

"धन्वन्तरिस्तु - कुंकुमागरुकस्तूरी कर्पूरं चन्दनं तथा ।
महासुगन्धमित्युक्तं नामतो यक्षकर्दमः ॥"

(Kśiraswāmi Amar P.111, Dhn.Ni G.P.Sharma P. 267)

"यद्धन्वन्तरिः
हरितालं च गोदन्तं पीतकं नटमण्डनम् ।
आलं च तालं गौरं च पिञ्जरं विस्रगंधिकम् ॥"

(Kśiraswāmi Amar P.156, Dhn. Ni. G.P.Sharma P. 276)

"आह च (धन्वन्तरिः)
काञ्चिकं काञ्जिकं वीरं कुल्माषाभिषुतं तथा ।
अवन्तिसोमं धान्याम्लमारनालं महारसम् ॥
सौवीरकं सुवीराम्लं तथा शुक्तं तुषोदकम् । "

(Kśiraswāmī Amar P. 146, Dhn.Ni.G.P.Sharma P.220)

"द्विगुणाम्बु श्वेतरस ... केवलं मथितं स्मृतम् । इति धन्वन्तरिः ।

(Kśiraswāmī Amar P.148; Dhn. Ni.G.P.Sharma P.214)

These quotations of Kśiraswāmi clearly suggest that there was a Mss of Dhn.Ni. corroborating with the text of the present Dhn.Ni.up to the मिश्रकादि वर्ग - Miśrakādi Chapter. This pobably also suggests that Śodhala and Kśiraswāmī had different Mss of Dhn.Ni. for reference before them.

7) ***Why the Nighaṇṭu is titled as Dhanvantari Nighaṇṭu***. The question has been discussed to some extent in 'Treatise and its Constitution' (P. XXXVII). Some scholars had raised doubts about the statement - 'द्रव्यावलिः समादिष्टा धन्वन्तरिमुखोद्गता'. This Dravyāvali has been compiled as narrated by Dhanvantari. To understand this statement the basic concepts of the old Indian Scholars has to be taken into consideration. To them the *name was not important, but the contents were important. The new trea-

---

* "नात्मार्थं नापि कामार्थं अथ भूतदयां प्रति ।" Caraka.
"नामूलं लिख्यते किञ्चित" A.Sangraha.
"एतद् ब्रह्मा भाषते ब्रह्मजो वा" Vagbhat.
"पुराणमित्येव न साधु सर्वं... ... सन्तः परीक्ष्यान्यतरत् भजन्ते" कालिदास. These are some of the statements which suggest the basic concepts of old Indian Scholars.

tise would not have been accepted unless it is consistant with the classical books.

Royalty, Patents, Rights, Economic gains etc. are very recent ideas to our scholors.

I have provided the list of verses taken from the classical books i.e. Samhitās. It is evident from the list of verses that the *maximum references have been taken from सुश्रुत संहिता Suśruta Samhitā. This Samhitā is "as narrated by the Lord Dhanvantari" 'धन्वन्तरिमुखोद्गता' is an accepted truth. Therefore, this Nighaṇṭu also becomes indirectly narrated by Lord Dhanvantari.

8) ***The list of verses or portions from the various books.***
(The references are mentioned under appropriate headings.)

Suśruta - सुश्रुतसंहिता (Arranged according to the chapters in Dhn.Ni.)

1)	Bilvaphala	बिल्वफल S.S. 46.174
2)	Ṭaṅkaṇa Kśāraḥ	टंकणक्षारः S.S.46,325
3)	Biḍalavaṇam	बिडलवणम् S.S.46,316
4)	Sauvarcalam	सौवर्चलम् S.S.46,317
5)	Audbhidam	औद्भिदम् S.S. 46,319
6)	Sāmudram	सामुद्रम् S.S.46,315
7)	Ārdrā Kustumbarī	आर्द्रा कुस्तुम्बरी S.S.46,230
8)	Ārdrakam	आर्द्रकम् S.S.46,227
9)	Sita maricam	सितमरिचम् S.S.46,225
10)	Kapittham	कपित्थम् S.S.46,147-48
11)	Mūlakam	मूलकम् S.S.46,241-42.
12)	Rasonaḥ	रसोनः S.S.46,244-45
13)	Taṇḍulīyaḥ	तण्डुलीयः S.S.46.258
14)	Kāsamardaḥ	कासमर्दः S.S. 46.236
15)	Properties of Ikśuḥ	इक्षुगुणाः S.S.45.155
16)	Bisam	बिसम् S.S.46.303
17)	Āmraḥ	आम्रः S.S.46.153-54
18)	Jambīraḥ	जम्बीरः S.S.46.162-62.
19)	Airāvatam	ऐरावतम् S.S.46.161
20)	Mātuluṅgam	मातुलुङ्गम् S.S.46.149-52
21)	Cāṅgerī	चांगेरी S.S.46.273
22)	Tindukam	तिन्दुकम् S.S.46.168
23)	Madhūka Kusumam	मधूकं कुसुमम् S.S.46.186
24)	Pīlu phalam	पीलुफलम् S.S.46.

* व्यपदेशस्तु भूयसा । अ.ह.

25)	Tālaḥ	तालः S.S.46.179
26)	Priyālaḥ	प्रियालः S.S.46.156 & S.S.46.205
27)	Nārikelaḥ	नारिकेलः S.S.46.180
28)	Jambūphalam	जम्बूफलम् S.S.46.166
29)	Rajādanam	राजादनम् S.S.46.166
30)	Karkandhu Kolādi	कर्कन्धुकोलादि S.S.46.145-46.
31)	Bakula phalam	बकुल फलम् S.S.46.145-46
32)	Kulatthaḥ	कुलत्थः S.S.46.36-38
33)	Tila tailam	तिलतैलम् S.S.45-113
34)	Atasī tailam	अतसी तैलम् S.S.45.116
35)	Sarṣapa tailam	सर्षप तैलम् S.S.45.117
36)	Eraṇḍa tailam	एरण्डतैलम् S.S.45.117
37)	Goghṛtam	गोघृतम् S.S.45.97
38)	Mahiṣī ghṛtam	महिषीघृतम् S.S.45.98
39)	Ajā ghṛtam	अजा घृतम् S.S.45.98.
40)	Āvika ghṛtam	आविक घृतम् S.S.45.101
41)	Uṣṭrī ghṛtam	उष्ट्री घृतम् S.S.45.100
42)	Hastinī ghṛtam	हस्तिनीघृतम् S.S.45.104
43)	Strī ghṛtam	स्त्री घृतम् S.S.45.103
44)	Purāṇa ghṛtam	पुराणघृतम् S.S.45.108
45)	Dugdham	दुग्धम् S.S.45.48
46)	Gokśiram	गोक्षीरम् S.S.45.52.53
47)	Ajāpayaḥ	अजापयः S.S.45.52.53
48)	Aurabhra payaḥ	औरभ्रपयः 45.54
49)	Mahiṣī payaḥ	महिषीपयः S.S.45.58
50)	Hastinī Payaḥ	हस्तिनी पयः S.S.45.58
51)	General properties of Milk	सामान्य दुग्धगुणाः S.S.45.64
52)	Godadhi	गोदधि S.S.45.67.68
53)	Ajādadhi	अजादधि S.S.45.68.69
54)	Āvika dadhi	आविक दधि S.S.45.71
55)	Mahiṣī dadhi	महिषी दधि S.S.45.70
56)	Uṣṭrī dadhi	उष्ट्री दधि S.S.45.70.71
57)	Aśvā dadhi	अश्वा दधि S.S.45.72.73
58)	Hastinī dadhi	हस्तिनी दधि S.S.45.74-75
59)	Strī dadhi	स्त्री दधि S.S.45.73
60)	General properties of curds	दधि सामान्य गुणाः S.S.45.79
61)	Seasonal uses of curds-properties	ऋतुविशेषेण दध्नो गुणाः S.S.45.80-75
62)	Contraindications for the use of Buttermilk	तक्रनिषेधः S.S.45.86
63)	Indications for the use of Buttermilk	तक्रसेवनम् S.S.45.87
64)	Properties of Buttermilk according to Doṣās	दोष विशेषेण तक्रगुणाः S.S.45.87
65)	Takra Kurcikā	तक्रकूर्चिका S.S.45.90
66)	Takra-maṇḍaḥ	तक्रमण्डः S.S.45.90

67) Kilātaḥ किलाटः S.S.45.91
68) Moraṭaḥ मोरटः S.S.45.91
69) Types of Honey मधुजातयः S.S.45.133
70) Kṡaudra madhu क्षौद्रमधु S.S.45.135
71) Mākṡika madhu माक्षिक मधु S.S.54.45.136
72) Honey not to be heated etc. मधुनः ऊष्णैर्विरोधः S.S.45.144-45
73) Ṡukta (Properties) शुक्तगुणाः S.S.45.210-211
74) Prasannā प्रसन्ना S.S.45.178-78
75) Yava Surā यव सुरा S.S.45.178-79
76) Ākṡikī surā आक्षिकी सुरा S.S.45.179
77) Madhūka sīdhuḥ मधूक सीधुः S.S.45.191
78) Kohalaḥ Jagalaṣca कोहलः जगलश्च S.S.45-180
79) Bakkasaḥ बक्कसः S.S.45..180
80) Gauda sīdhuḥ गौडसीधुः S.S.45.182-83
81) Ṡītarasikaḥ शीतरसिकः S.S.45.185
82) Maireyaḥ मैरेयः S.S.45.189
83) Ākṡika Sīdhuḥ आक्षिक सीधुः S.S.45.186
84) Jāmbava sīdhuḥ जाम्बव सीधुः S.S.45.187
85) Ariṣṭaḥ अरिष्टः S.S.45.194-98
86) Alcoholic beverages to be avoided वर्ज्यमद्यम् S.S.45.198-209
87) Gaganāmbu गगनाम्बु S.S.45.26
88) CandrakāntaVāri चंद्रकान्त वारि S.S.45.26
89) Properties of Nādeya Jala etc. नादेयादि जलगुणाः S.S.45.31.37
90) Water-Ṡimilar to Gaganāmbu गगनाम्बु सदृशं जलम् S.S.45.40
91) Conditions where water should be used less पानीयं मन्दमाचरेत् S.S.45.46
92) Properties of river water according to regions स्थानादिभेदेन नदीजलगुणाः S.S.45.22.23
93) Properties of cow's urine गोमूत्रम् S.S.220-28
94) Manthaḥ मन्थः S.S.46.385

Verses borrowed from Caraka samhitā - चरकसंहिता

1) Synonyms for Koṡātakī कोशातकी पर्यायाः C.Kalp. 6.3-4
2) Dravantī द्रवन्ती C.Kalp. 12.3
3) Ṡnuhī स्नुही C.Kalp.11
4) Ṡyāmā श्यामा C.Kalp. 7..4
5) Ṡuklabhāṇḍī शुक्लभाण्डी C.Kalp.7.5
6) Ṡāli vrīhi - properties शाली व्रीही गुणाः C.Su.27.14
7) Yavaḥ यवः C.Su.27.19
8) Rājamāṣaḥ राजमाषः C.Su.27.25
9) Āḍhakī आढकी C.Su.27.33
10) Tailam तैलम् C.Su.27.286
11) Contraindications for curds दधि निषेधः C.S.8.61-62
12) Types of Honey मधुप्रकाराः C.S.Su.27.244
13) Kāñjikam- काञ्जिकम C.S.Su.27.192

14) Sauvīram- Tuṣodakam सौवीरं-तुषोदकम् C.S.Su. 27.191
15) Properties of water of various rivers विविध नदीजलगुणाः C.S.Su.27.209-11

Verses borrowed from Aṣṭānga Saṃgraha (अष्टाङ्गसंग्रह)

1) Jīvantī	जीवन्ती A.S.Su 7.129
2) Twakśirī	त्वक्क्षीरी A.S.su 12.
3) Prapauṇḍarīkam	प्रपौण्डरीकम् A.S.Su12.74
4) Kākamācī	काकमाची A.S.Su.7.193
5) Āmraḥ	आम्रः A.S.su.7.186
6) Sahakāra rasaḥ	सहकार रसः A.S.su. 7.188
7) Yavaḥ	यवः A.S.Su.18.19
8) Certain types of Taila	तैल विशेषाः A.S.Su.6.99-101,104-15
9) Curds	दधि A.S.Su.6.62
10) Mārdwikam	मार्द्वीकम् A.S.Su.6
11) Khārjūram	खार्जूरम् A.S.Su.6.120

Verses from Aṣṭāngahṛdayam अष्टाङ्गहृदयम्

1) Madanaḥ	मदनः A.H.Kalp.1.9
2) Kaṭukālāmbunī	कटुकालाम्बुनी A.H.Kalp 1.27 (Carak.Kalp. 3.4)
3) Jīmūtakaḥ	जीमूतकः A.H.Kalp. 1.19
4) Kūṣmāṇḍaḥ	कूष्माण्डः A.H.Kalp. 6.88
5) Dhāmārgavaḥ	धामार्गवः A.H.Kalp. 1.41
6) Kośātakī	कोशातकी A.H.Kalp. 1.41
7) Śuklabhāṇḍī	शुक्लभाण्डी A.H.Su.2.1
8) Godhūmaḥ-	गोधूमः A.H.Su.6.15
9) Goghṛtam	गोघृतम् A.H.Su.5.37-38
10) General properties of butter milk	तक्रसामान्य गुणाः A.H.Su.5.33-34
11) Proeprties of alco. beverages	मद्यगुणाः A.H.Su-5.62-64
12) Khārjūram	खार्जूरम् A.H.Su.5-73
13) Madhvāsavaḥ	मध्वासवः A.H.Su.5.75

Verses possibly taken from Rājanighaṇṭu

Raj Ni. is a later work and he has followed Dhn.Ni. However, it appears that someone afterwards might have added some more plant names or synonyms in the Dhn.Ni. This assumption is based on the peculiar style of Raj.Ni. In this Nighaṇṭu the synonyms are restricted by mentioning their total number at the end. This peculiar style might have been adopted, to avoid more additions by any person or copywriters. Therefore it can be presumed undoubtedly that whenever such type of arrangement of mentioning the total number of synonyms is found in the present Dhn.Ni. those stanzas or verses might have been copied down partly or wholely from the Raj.Ni.

This can be seen in the following places:-

1) Under the heading 50) त्रपुसम् Trapusam त्रपुसा तोयफला चैव हस्तिदन्तफला मुनिः ॥
2) Under the same heading
डङ्गरी नागशुण्डी च गजदन्तफला मुनिः ॥
3) माडः under the heading (19) Tālaḥ तालः
4) Under the heading अश्वत्थः Aśvathaḥ-chapter V (Raj.Ni.Chapter11)
चैत्यद्रुमो धर्मवृक्षः चन्द्रकरमिताह्वयः ।

(This reading is found in Raj Ni.Sahito Dhn.Ni. of Anandaśram Edi. only.)

5) Under the heading Amṛtam अमृतम् Chapter VII
गरलं स्थावराद्यं स्यात् प्रोक्तं चैकादशाह्वयम् ॥

9) *Whether the additional plants in the Gaṇadravyāvali are mentioned by someone else other than the compiler of Gaṇadravyāvali* गणद्रव्यावलि *or Paryāyanāmadravyāvali* पर्यायनाम द्रव्यावलि ?

It is seen in this Nighaṇṭu that there are certain drugs other than those which are mentioned in *Gaṇadravyāvali* गणद्रव्यावलि. These additional drugs are either consistant in certain respects of the original *Gaṇadravyāvali* plants or are inconsistant with them eg. भङ्गा Canabis with *Medā* मेदा, खस्तिलः (poppy seeds) with तिल (sesamum) etc. These may be called as unauthentic (or misfits) additions. It is very difficult to sort out such misfits (unauthentic) additions.But all the additional plants are not unauthentic additions. eg.Somavalka- सोमवल्क is an additional plant under the heading Khadira- खदिर. Somavalka सोमवल्क has got some pharmacologial and morphological similarity with खदिर Khadira. While commenting on 'कदरः खदिरः सिते । सोमवल्कोऽपि... Amar II-IV (Page 62) Kśiraswāmi had qnoted Dhn.Ni. as "आह च - कदरः (खदिरः) श्वेतसारोऽन्यः सोमवल्कः पथिद्रुमः ।". This shows that Kśiraswāmi had a Mss of Dhn. Ni. in which this additional plant of सोमवल्क - Somavalka was mentioned. Therefore, all the additional plants are not unauthentic and many of them might have been mentioned by the compiler of the Dhn.Ni.

10) ***Whether Dhn.Ni. had followed Aṣṭānga Nighaṇṭu ?***

Contrary to the common belief that Dhn.Ni. is the oldest of all the available Nighaṇṭus (See appendix "Some opinions" of vol I) Prof. Priya Vratji Sharma believes that Aṣṭānga Ni.might have been the available oldest Nighaṇṭu......

"Thus it has to be decided whether Aṣṭānga Nighaṇṭu followed Dhanvantari Nighaṇṭu or vice-versa or both have derived their information from some common source. As we shall discuss later, the facts described in Astāng Ni. are different from those in Dhn.Ni. to a great extent, the descriptions in the latter are more in a advanced stage and lastly the verses quoted from Rasa-ratna samuccaya are found in the Dhn.Ni...

It appears that the Aṣṭānga Nighaṇṭu was followed by Dhanvantari Nighaṇṭu" (Introduction to Ast.Ni. by Prof. Sharmaji).

Prof. Sharmaji has raised 3 points here 1) facts described in Aṣt. Ni are different. Ast. Ni. has mainly restricted himself to the Gaṇās of Vagbhat, while Dhn.Ni. has recorded separate Gaṇas and a Gaṇadravyāvali. It can be seen that the advanced descriptive method does not always suggest the posteriority eg. if we see varieties of Ikśu mentioned in Suśruta Samhitā and compare them with those of Dhn.Ni. we find an advanced description in Suśruta Samhita. It is true that there are certain portions taken from *Rasaratna Samuccaya* - रसरत्न समुच्चय. This is a later addition, but who has done it and when is difficult to sort out unless further study is done. Therefore, a further substantive evidence is required to prove the posteriority of Dhn.Ni. to Astānga Nighaṇṭu. Further, if Ast. Ni. is the first Nighaṇṭu of this kind it would have been definitely mentioned & referred by the subsequent workers who wrote on this subject. The Mṣṣ of Dhn.Ni. are scattered all over India (and successively abroad) and referred, respected and mentioned by subsequent workers like Śoḍhala, Raj.Ni and commentators like Kśiraswāmī, Shrivallabha Upadhyaya, Shivkosh etc. Though this is not a very sound or undisputable evidence, it has got some significance in the traditional belief that Dhn.Ni. is the oldest available Nighaṇṭu.

11) ***Whether the classification of Dhn.Ni. is unscientific. ?***

Ach. Bapalalji Vaidya in the introduction to Nighaṇṭuśeṣa निघण्टु शेष had mentioned

"Most of the Nighaṇtus give the classes or groups like Haritakyādi, Guḍūcyādi, Āmrādi etc. But this classification has no scientific basis. The classification done by Caraka and Suśuṛta is according to the principles of common function. The classes like *Urdhvabhāgahara, Śirovircana*,.... .... are formed on the basis of common functions. Even the class *Daśemāni* (the name given by Carak to a group or class of ten medicinal substances) is formed according to the same principle. The classess recognised by Suśruta are also based on this very principle. Vāgbhaṭa follows Caraka and hence he imitates Caraka in this matter. But he has left out Daśemāni of Caraka which is really very important. This classification or grouping which is based on the principle of common function could be regarded as scientific.But the groupings like Guḍūcyādi, Haritakyādi, etc. given in Dhanvantari Nighaṇṭu, Rāja Nighaṇṭu, Kaiyadeva Nighaṇṭu and other later Nighaṇṭus could not be called scientific.

Āch. Hemacandra has not accepted the classifications recognised by his ancient predecessors. He has divided his Nighaṇṭu into six Kāṇḍas viz. Vṛksa, Gulma, Latā,Śākā, Tṛṇa and Dhānya. This is the special feature of this Nighaṇṭu. This type of classification is not found in any other Nighaṇṭu." (Intro. to Ni. śeṣa Page-11)

Āch. Bapalaljis contention is not correct as the Gaṇas mentioned in

Dhn.Ni. eg. Kafajwarahara, Pittajwarahara, Vata jwarahara, Sannipātahara, Jīvanīya, Vāmakgaṇa, Virecana etc. are based on similar functions (Rājnighaṇṭu has also mentioned the morphological classification like Latā, Gulma, Vṛkṣa etc) and hence the classification mentioned in Dhn.Ni. cannot be called as unscientific.

12) ***Acknowledgement by Late Vd.D.K.Kamat***

Late Vd.D.K.Kamat has written few words of aknowledgement for the volume II. As the hand written paper was not available at the time of publication of Vol II; I could not produce it then. I feel it will be proper to mention it here.

"For the studies of medicinal plants in Dhanvantarīya Nighaṇṭu a number of books, periodicals, etc. have been used by us and these have been mentioned in the Bibliography of the volume I. Those referred subsequently or thereafter have been mentioned wherever necessary. We are grateful to all of them. A special mention must be made of Th. Balwantsimhaji and Dr. Chunekar for their 'Glossary of Vegetable drugs in Bṛhattrayī, for the sake of abbreviation mentioned as 'Balvantji' only. we have quoted the references of classical books (Samhitās) from this Glossary. We have also quoted some discussions from this Glossary because either these agree with or differ from our opinions. We have also referred the Hindi Commentary on Bhavaprakash by Dr.K.C.Chunekar and his Vānaspatika Anusandhān Darshikā. Similarly, many references are also taken from Dravyaguṇavigñyān of Ach.Priyavratji Sharma. We are grateful to all of them.

13) In the absence of definite terminology it is a difficult task to translate the Sanskrit text into English, however for the completion of the work I have translated the same with the terminology used by the old scholars in this field. It is to be gratfully mentioned here that Prof. Priyavratji Sharma has published his 'Drvyaguṇa Koṣa' (1997) which has remained very useful to me.

While translating the text *Rasa, Vīrya, Vipāka* and *Guṇas* have been mentioned first, because on the basis of these the Ayurvedic conceptions of pharmacological action is explained. It is followed by the uses in various disorders.

The first volume of the book was published in 1972 and the second volume in 1979. I have included these volumes here except the appendixes especially to the volume I. Therefore whenever references from these are mentioned especially in the introduction these should be understood from the vol. I. However, I have included appendix c.2 under the heading 'Bibliography.'

Many persons have helped me in completing the work. It is not possible to mention all of them. I am extremely grateful to Dr. K.C. Chunekar who has constantly encouraged and guided me in various ways. He has also gone through the final copy of this book. My elder brother

Late Vd. V.D. Kamat, has gone through the earlier portion of *Gaṇadravyāvali* and had given his critical suggestions. His sad demise in the month of March 1998 is constantly felt by me, while editing the remaining portion of this book. I am also grateful to Vd. B.K. Padhye Gurjar for his experienced and valuable suggestions and going through the prefinal copy of this book very carefully. Mention must be made of Prof. S.D. Mahajan, who was the coauthor of the 1st volume of this book. Prof. Ramanbhai Mistry of K.G. Mittal college has gone through the prefinal copy and given me his valuable suggestions.

I am grateful to Vd. Nalini Karuṇākaran and Mr. Rāmanathan and his daughter in law Vd. Mrs. Chitrā K. for the transliteration of Malyalam names from *Abhidhānamañjari*.

I am also thankful to Mr. Dnyanesh Rege & Mr. Vijay Rege of Veena Prniters for their untired efforts in bringing out this work for publication.

Inspite of our honest efforts; printing and other mistakes might have remained in this publication. However, I shall be highly gratified if this publication proves useful to the students, lovers and workers in this branch of Ayurveda.

Dr. S.D. Kamat.
M.F.A.M. (Bom), D.S.A.C. (Bom) Ayurvedacarya
'Prasad' S.N. Road, Mulund . Mumbai-400 080.
Date

FORWARD TO THE VOLUME I

- By Late Pandit Shiv Sharma

Vaidya D.K.Kamat,the author of this treatise 'Studies on Medicinal plants in ***'Dhanwantariya Nighantu'*** is a veteran Ayurvedic vaidya of Konkan, a coastal area of Maharashtra, characterised by small hills and forests rich in vegetation. His zeal for study of Ayurvedic medicinal plants must have been greatly stimulated and fed by the abundance of the herbal wealth around him in the land of his birth. Dr. G. S. Pendse, who appears to have followed the research career of the author intimately has in the preface,(introduction) given a fascinating account of the trials and tribulations undergone by the author and the obstacles overcome by him in order to complete the task of acquring first-hand knowledge of the medicinal plants of the region. In this mission he has been ably assisted by his botanist collaborator, Prof. S.D. Mahajan. This happy collaboration has resulted in the preparation and publication of the present useful work in English. The choice of language will carry the utility of the book to parts of India beyond the frontier of Kokan and Maharashtra. This will enable the scholars and scientists all over the country to reap the benefits of Vaidya Kamat's laudable effort.

I have to concede seniority to Vaidya Kamat not only in the matter of age (he is in his eighties), but also in the knowledge of the subject treated in this book. Against this background, his desire to have the Foreword written by me constitutes more an honour to me than to him. However, since my long association with the All India Ayurvedic Congress, the Central and Sate Councils and Committees and various University Faculties has kept me in close touch with the Ayurvedic profession and scholarships of the entire country, my assessment of Vaidya Kamat's work may help a large number of people in India to make use of the knowledge collected and recorded by Vaidya Kamat in this excellent publication . This appears to me to be the only justification for my writing this Foreword.

'Dhanwantariya Nighantu' is a treatise on Ayurvedic herbs and drugs with its main portion, Guduchyadi Varga, dealing with medicinal plants exclusively. Vaidya Kamat has dealt with this portion, i.e., the medicinal plants, only. He has done an excllent job of identifying the plants and their variants which will go a long way in removing confusion with regard to the identity of a large number of plants prevalent among the Ayurvedic physicians and suppliers of Ayurvedic herbs. Prof. S.D. Mahajan has greatly helped in fixing the identities of these plants by supplying their botanical names.

The publication should prove of considerable practical use to the students and practitioners of Ayurveda and to research scholars requiring contact with medicinal plants for intiating research in them. I welcome the addition of this book to the existing lierature on this subject.

Shiv Sharma

February : 14, 1972

PREFACE TO THE VOLUME I*

("Naturalists are born and made; that the sacred fire cannot be extinguished by poverty nor lighted from a college taper. That the men whose work is now classical and whose devotion is our privilege to honour, owed less to education in any sense than they did to self denial steadfastness, energy, a passion for seeking out the truth and an innate love of nature. These are the qualities which enabled them to gather fruit of the tree of knowledge.")

William Healey Dall
The Bibliography, Published
by The Smithisonia Institution,
Washington1946.

We are very much gratified to publish this work on the studies on Dhanvantari's medicinal plants. As Dr. G. S. Pendse, in his scholarly introduction, has exnlicitly explained the background and objects of this work, it is not necessary to say much about the same.

It should be made clear at the outset that the author and the editor did not start this work with the predetermined aim of publishing anything. But only as a specimen the accumulated data and the compilation of some Marathi notes were sent to several authorities in the field, who appreciated the direction of work and encouraged us to prepare the manuscript (vide p.125). The draft manuscript prepared by the author in Marathi was brought to the notice of Dr. G. S. Pendse, Poona. After the perusal of the same, with full appreciation and encourgement, he kindly suggested to translate it in English and insisted that it was worth publishing and should be published. The English version of the manuscript was prepared by the author according to the plan and Proforma suggested by Dr. Pendse.

It was a very difficult problem to seek a publisher to such a work especially when neither financial assistance for a promising market was deemed to be available. In this situation, we decided to publish at least the Guḍūchyādi Chapter that too in a concise form ourselves, in 1970. We prepared the second manuscript accordingly by omitting many details and explanations.

Since then, in search of a suitable printer, as we were completely new in this field. we contacted several printing presses at Mumbai, Poona and Kolhapur. One printer in Poona accepted the work in 1971, but expressed his inability to carry it in May 1971. Finally it was another fortunate event that we came across the Manager of Veda-Vidya

* Vol. I. Published in 1972. The appendixes are not included in this book.

Mudranalaya, Poona, who readily and gladly accepted the work in May 1971 and completed the same in June 1972.

It may kindly be noted that we do not claim in any way that this work is all-exhaustive and fool-proof. On the contrary it is an humble effort of spade-work type, and there is much scope in this field for future workers.

The extent and scope of the work will be evident from the Contents, while the plan and pattern can be understood by going through the Proforma. The author has given different pertinent references from various sources; and tried to confirm the botanical names of plants after considering the suitable ones by taking an overall judgement, in each case. We accept that it was quite necessary to provide the reasoning and explanation to substantiate the selection of particular plants at many places. Moreover, illustrations of plants, at least the controversial ones, would have definitely increased the clarity and utility of the treatise.We were actually keenly desirous to include not only these things,but also the morphological descriptions, floral formulāe and floral diagrams of all the confirmed plants. It would have naturally increased the size and consequently the printing cost of the book at least doubly if not trebly. It is only the financial aspect that prevented us in doing so.

We have tried to provide some references and articles from some of the referred books, but in some cases we could not furnish the details like place, pages or stanzas etc., due to some difficulties in obtaining the same books. Similarly, we beg an apology of the readers for the printing mistakes which have crept in, even after several Proof reading, for which we are responsible and not the Printer. The readers are requsted to kindly refer to the errata for the corrections of mistakes already noticed, and bring to our notice, additional ones if there are any.

We are greatly indebted to honourable Paṇdit Shiv Sharma and Dr.C.Dwarakanath for their favour of providing Foreward and opinions to this work. We take these words of appreciation and encouragement as our greatest honour. It is beyond the power of our expression to offer them a vote of thanks in appropriate words. May their kind words and guidance inspire us to complete this work in an elaborate and sophisticated manner.

We want to express our deep sense of gratitude and respect to Dr.G.S.Pendse,Honorary Director, Indian Drug Research Association, Poona for the favour of his scholarly Introduction of this work, and for guidance and encouragement given from time to time.

We gratefully acknowledge the encouragement and facilities given by Dr.T.S.Mahabale M.Sc.;Ph.D.etc.,formerly Head of Dept. of Botany University of Poona;. Prin. C.M.R.Desai, B.A.,L.L.B,M.Ed.,G.K.Gokhale,

College Kolhapur; Authorities of Ayurved Seva Sangha; the Authorities who have encouraged us by giving their worthy opinions (vide App.D) on marathi work and Dr.G.S.Puri M.Sc.,Ph.D.etc. formerly regional Botanist B.S.I. at Poona and Allahabad.

Dr.N.K.Bhide of All India Institute of Medical Sciences, New Delhi, has enlighted us by way of provoking discussion on this subject and kindly made valuable suggestions particularly regarding our preface. Thanks are due to him.

We offer a vote of thanks to Dr.A.V.Sathe, M.Sc.Ph.D.,Poona for arranging the opportunity of acquainting us with Dr.Bhide

We also offer vote of thanks to Dr.S.D.Kamat, M. F. A. M.; D.S.A.C.,*'Ayurvedacharya'* for his help in preparing the English version of the 'Treatise and its Constitution'.

The Manager Shree Vinod Shroff, and the staff of Veda-Vidya Mudranalaya, have taken keen interest and great efforts in the execution of the printing of this work. They have completed this complicated work in a commendable manner and calculated period. We admit without hesitation that much of the credit of this publication goes to their kind co-operation. Many thanks to all of them.

This work is dedicated to the unknown power which inspired us and got it done through us and to all the previous compilers of revered Ayurvedic books and modern writers whose minds and hands were engaged in the field to Ayurvedic Medicine.

Suggestions of all kinds are most cordially welcome.

POONA **D.K.K.**
15th June 1972 **S.D.M.**

INTRODUCTION TO VOLUME I

- Dr. G.S.Pendse

It is really a pleasure to write an introduction to this treatise,which is a sheer labour of love of a single man with an occasional help from his younger associate. The chief author, Vaidya D.K.Kamat belongs to Konkan and has now reached a ripe age of eighty, when he is completing this treatise. For a number of years, he was after his cherished ideal. Born and brought up in Chiplun taluka in the district of Ratnagiri in Konkan a middle class poor family, his early life was passed in the midst of the poor population of cultivators and inhabitants of Taḷa-Konkan, under fairly hard circumstances. Curiousity is the basis of any research enquiry. It must also be accompanied by a desire and full effort to satisfy that curiosity or else, it becomes only an idle inquisitiveness. Vaidya Kamat is endowed with these rare and singular qualities. His curiosity regarding the habits and practices of these poor-hilly populations, made him start his work, when he was ,on vegetable materials locally available and used as foods and medicinal plants. He did neither wait for a wealthy man to support him, nor did he enquire whether the Government budget is available to get some grant for this work. Even though, he was not a trained botanist, he started the study of systematics of Botany with a single idea of identification of the plant materials, he was collecting so labouriously from the local populations. He took the help from the Botanical Suvey of India on one side and eminent Kavirajas on the other, such as Vaidya late A.R.Kalawari of Ratnagiri. It was a fortunate event that a young man like Shri S.D.Mahajan, who was a trained Botanist joined him actively at this stage and Vaidya Kamat could secure an active help from this young scientist. Some areas were surveyed by Vaidya Kamat and Shri Mahajan jointly and it was very beneficial to both of them. Both of them surveyed the area of Baramati in addition to Konkan areas. The officer-in-charge of the Botanical Survey of India, Poona, Shri Puri gave them a good co-operation in the matter of identification of the collected specimens. An excellent opportunity arose for these scientists, when they got an invitation from *'Sarvodaya Yojana'* and *'Ayurveda Seva Sangh'* of Nasik for the survey of 'Adivasis' in Nasik district for the medicinal and food plants they used. They jointly completed this work, resulting in a collction of some 250 interesting specimens, which were given to the Ayurveda Seva Sangh of Nasik and also to the Poona University.

It is also worth noting that Vaidya Kamat was engaged in a trade from 1945 onwards for a few years, which was intimately related to forest products, although he happened to serve as a draftsman during some earlier years. This is again a point to illustrate the principle, that his low economic status, or his struggle for bread and butter did not come in the way of his pursuit of knowledge. In fact, this is what is known as ardent desire and internal urge of the pursuit of knowledge or *'Antarvedana'* in the language of Yoga-Vasistha, which is responsible for any *'Siddhi'* or achievement. In the absense of this, mere qualifications, pays, emoluments, vehicles and facilities will not be of much use to bring out a performance and achievement in any undertaking. It is a pity to note that Govt. has been emphasising these values more than the actual output of work and also trying to judge the performance on the criterion of the expenditure of money. It is easy to realise that the performance does require an expenditure but the expenditure cannot be correct criterion of performance. Once the false values are propogated, it is but natural that there is a race for expenditure of budgets. It is necessary to emphasize here that all the schemes should be 'Man-oriented' and not merely 'Money - oriented'. Unless this principal is recognised and practised and the planning shaped accordingly, there are few chances of success in any scheme which may appear very promising on paper.

Somehow Vaidya Kamat did not remain in service for a long time. He was not deterred by this event. On the contrary, he engaged himself in a trade, which was based on the knowledge he gained during his forest work. There are a number of trades related to the forest products. He picked up one of them. *Acacia sundra* is a common tree in the western and Southern forest. The economic aspect of this tree is well-known. The total export of Catechu was valued at Rs. 3696186 as early as in 1895-96, which has been fluctuating since then. The process of obtaining **'Kata'** (Catechu) is a traditional process practised by villagers. The commerce of Catechu is not small. A good quality also yields a good return. Shri Kamat took to this trade, secured all the know-how of the work and started a forest industry, which satisfied his wants and also gave him a good opportunity to keep up his pursuit of plant-knowledge.

It is after all such hard labour and pursuit of pure knowledge for years together, in spite of all sorts of difficulties, Vaidya Kamat started writing some articles on topics of identificaion of plant materials mentioned in 'Dhanvantariya Nighantu' and 'Raj Nighantu'. These articles appeared in *'Ayurved Patrika'* Nasik and were not contradicted by anybody even now. He was then encouraged to take up a full work of preparing a glossary of medicinal plants in *'Dhanvantariya Nighantu'*, which is the work of his life-time. I have particularly touched the relevent points in the life of Vaidya Kamat to show how curiousity, hard work and perseverance to follow the ideal irrespective of odd circumstances, are the necessary qualities for a research worker to achieve something worth the trouble during one's life-time.

The treatise, which goes under the title, ***Dhanvantariya Nighantu'*** is attributed to Dhanvantari. The only critically edited copy available, is printed by **'Anandasharm'** in its Sanskrit series in 1925 by late Shri M.V.Purandare and published by late Shri V.G.Apte. The number of this treatise is 33 and it is a matter of great service done by **'Anandashram'** and Shri V.G.Apate to have carried out such task of critically editing this valuable treatise,as well as some other interesting Sanskrit manuscripts in that period. In the absense of this effort, many important works would simply not have been available today. This book is edited on the basis of fifteen manuscripts obtained from various sources. All of them are obtained in Maharashtra except one, which belongs to Sondur outside Maharashtra. This is also the oldest amongst all dated Saka (1536) (1414 A.D.). In many of them metalic preparations are not given. The Sondur manuscript also does not contain any description of metals or their preparations.

The term, Nighantu means only a vocabulary or a glossary of terms. It was originally applied to the glossary of Vedic terms prepared by **'Yaska'**.The terms **'Kosha'** and **'Nighanta'** are also not quite identical. 'Kosha' is mere dictionary of words to help the writers. But Nighantu gives more desriptions of the terms used in any text. Thus, the Ayurvedic Nighantus are mainly compiled with an object to compile terms in Ayurvedic texts and also to furnish some more important information about the terms or even their definitions. It is but natural that the Nighantu literature came into existence after the Ayurvedic texts. Nighantus have, therefore, served a very useful purpose of collecting all the available information of the time, when a particular Nighantu was written. This compilation usually tries to collect all the relevant information, such as names of drugs from various sources, vegetable, mineral and animal; their synonyms, their actions and uses. The other terms occuring in the texts related to Anatomy, Physiology and Pharmacodynamics are also compiled in many Nighantus. In spite of several lexicons existing today, published and unpublished, **Dhanvantariya Nighantu'** still remains a standard text to study the source materials of drugs. The main part of this Nighantu consists of the vegetable kingdom. The entire wealth of drugs is classified into several categories, in which the sixth category, mentions the vegetable, mineral and animal drugs. The seventh category is known as 'Mishra' and contains many subjects unerlated to each other. This part is really miscellaneous in nature. The first 'Guduchyadi' chapter only contains the information of important drugs of vegetable kingdom.

It is but natural that this treatise,which is supposed to be the earliest available Nighantu, consists mainly of vegetable drugs if it is realised that the early Ayurvedic texts during the **'Ārsha'** period, as it is called, contain mainly vegetable drugs. These early texts of Ayurveda from Caraka upto Vagbhata are **'Ārsha'** treatises and vegetable drugs were mostly used in that period. A few mineral and animal drugs were, no doubt, used and they are also mentioned in Nighantus. But the chief source materials belonged to vegetable kingdom.

Nighantu, by its very nature, is a reflection of the various practices of the period in which it is compiled. **'Dhanvantariya Nighantu',** being the earliest; naturally contains many vegetable drugs and a manuscript used by **'Anandashram'** belonging to Sondur and dated Sake 1536, does not contain any description of the metals and their preparations. It is, therefore, very likely that the later copyists of the 'Nighantus' must have added many new practices and terms to the original texts unless all the manuscripts all over India are collected, studied and effort is made to find out the orginal work and interpolations of the later dates. A fairly exhaustive list of Ayurvedic Nighantus as they exist in the various oriental libraries of India and mentioned in different catalogues is given in the **'Laghu Nighanta'**,a critically published manuscript by the Indian Drugs Research Association, Poona. This list mentions 14 Nighantus as **'Dhanvantariya Nighantus'.** Aufrecht's catalogue mentions about five manuscipts. Many of these manuscripts are widely distributed from Bikaner and Ujjain in the North to Madras in the South. Quite likely that some of them are in other countries. In addition, there are likely to be many manuscripts in different languages of India, which are not mentioned here in the catalogues of the Oriental Libraries. It is a great task to bring all these manuscripts and critically edit 'Dhanvantariya Nighantu'. In the absence of such all-pervading attempt, the present manuscript published by the **'Anandashram'** serves a good purpose as a basic material on which one can work further.

The authorship of **'Dhanvantariya Nighantu'** is a controversial matter as is the case with many sanskrit texts. Vaidya D.K.Kamat has given some valuable references here, which show that this treatise is possibly written by some one, who belongs to a school of Dhanvantari and this view seems to be quite reasonable. There are many other treatises on medical subjects, which are attributed to Dhanvantari. All of them are possibly written by different writers and are attributed to Dhanvantari.

The period of this **'Nighantu'** is also an unknown factor. This Dhanvantariya Nighantu is certainly written after the period of Vagbhata, which is now taken to be about the 4th century A.D. It is rather strange that **'the Dhanvantariya Nighantu** does not mention any previous works from which the writer has been benefitted. The writer however, mentions that he has collated this Nighantu from a number of already existing Nighantus from the innumerable treasury of lexicons exsisting in Sanskrit and vernacular in different states. The internal evidence does not help us further than this. Hardly, there is much external evidence available to judge this period. A poet by name Dhanvantari, is mentioned in the court of Vikramaditya amongst the nine gems of the king. All this can be only a fiction and cannot be taken as historical evidence. There is a salutation to **'Kamakshi'** in the beginning. The famous 'Kamakshi' temple is in the South and it is likely that the author belongs to South India. There is also a salutation to God Dhanvantari, who need not be understood as the author of this treatise. The beginning also mentions the name as **'Dhanvantariya Nighantu'.** The other terms used in some manuscripts is **'Guduchyadi Nighantu'.** It is likely that the original Nighantu might have been restricted to the first part **'Ganadravyavali'** of the present seven parts of **'Paryayanamadravyawali'.** Since not only it consists mostly of the vegetable drugs but more than about 75% of the vegetable drugs in the whole of **'Dhanvantariya Nighantu'** are included in the first part **'Ganadravyavali'.** The first part has, therefore assumed an importance from the point of view of covering the bulk of the important vegetable drugs used by the Ayurvedists. It is, therefore, also in the fitness of things that Vaidya Kamat has covered the 1st Guduchyadi chapter of the present seven parts (Paryayanamadravyavali) in which Guduchyadi chapter of the first part of Ganadravyavali is also included.

The critical edition of the ancient texts and the proper identification of plant materials mentioned in them are highly important steps even in modern research of Medicianl plants. This part is not much appreciated by medical practitioners of any system and needs some elaboration.

Whenever one starts reading these ancient texts, first point that strikes immediately as a common point all over, mentioned by most of the authors, whenever writing about the vegetable drugs is mentioned in the following quotation. Caraka, in **Sūtra-sthana'** makes a clear mention of this point as follows:-

ओषधिर्नामरूपाभ्यां जानतेह्यजपावने ।
अविपाश्चैव गोपाश्च ये चान्ये वनवासिनः ॥

Cha. Su. 1-120

The **'Nama'** and **'Rupa'** of the plants is better understood by the cow-boys and other inhabitants of the forest areas and it is necessary to acquire that knowledge from them. **Dhanvantariya Nighantu'** also mentions in the beginning:-

किरातगोपालकतापसाद्या वनेचरास्तत्कुशलास्तथाऽन्ये ॥
विदन्ति नानाविधभेषजानां प्रमाणवर्णाकृतिनामजातीः ॥ ६ ॥
प्रायो जनाः सन्ति वनेचरास्ते गोपादयः प्राक्तननामसंज्ञाः ॥ ८ ॥

Dhn. Ni. P.1,

The wandering tribes of the forests such as **'Kirata'**, **'Gopalaka'**,

Tapasas' and others have the knowledge of the various materials used as drugs with their dosage, colour, appearances, names and also kinds or species. Usually these nomadic forest tribes know very well the vernacular names.

The above references from **'Caraka'** to the present **'Nighantu'** are more than enough to show that most of the plants and other materials,which have found a place in Ayurveda, were originally observed in the actual practices of these forest primitive nomads. The branch of this knowledge goes under the title **'Folk-medicine'**, which is not related and can be related to any system of scientific medicine.

Folk-medicine consists of the independent traditional practices of primitive nomadic tribes anywhere on the face of this earth. These practices are older than any civilisation. They exist now, they existed before, and they will exist forever, as long as such tribes inhabit the face of the earth in any part of the world. In fact, the folk-medicine is the birth-place of many medicines, which have found their proper place in the scientific medicine. This principle can be illustrated by a number of examples from all over the world.

The use of Cinchona by a few Jesuits in South America in the 17th century is a good example. Having obtained that knowledge from the nomads the bark was then exported by those Jesuits to Europe and was called as a Jesuit-powder'. Louis the XIVth had brought this secret from Dr. Tabot and it became a common drug in Europe. Few medicinal plants have been subjected to a more intensive scientific study as Cinchona. The further scientific progress is now wellknown. Isolation of alkaloids and synthetic anti-malarials on the chemical side, breeding experiments to increase the active constituents in the plants, cultivation studies to introduce useful species in the different parts of the world, are some of the many aspects of scientific work to which this plant was subjected.

Digitalis, another important cardiac drug was detected by William Withering in England from a Gipsy woman, who used to prescribe it in combination with several crude drugs in cases of dropsy. After a great labour, extending over a period of several years, he published his account of the foxglove in 1785. It was only after this, that the scientific medicine picked it up for further work. It was after several decades that an eminent chemist Stoll succeeded in separating the glycosides and even now digitalis leaf is standardised and used as such.

Centuries ago, **'tropine'** drugs were used as pain-killers in tooth-ache. Greek physicians used **'Mandrake'** in operations also. White squill, which grows in the sandy soils round about the Mediterranean shore, was used as a cardiotonic and has been mentioned in Eber's Papyrus about the 18th Century B.C. Red Squill was used in the 13th century as a rat-poision by the Arabs. Cod liver oil has been picked up in scientific medicine from the practices of Cod-fisheries in Norway and other countries.

Even the most common practices practically of Cathartics are copied from the folk-medicine. Early practices in all the countries were revolving round the use of Cathartics and Emetics. Most of the Greek advances were copied from the still earlier civilisation like Egypticians and Minoan on the coastal lands of the Mediterranean and Mesapotemian. The well-known remedy of aloes, now in B.P. was mentioned in Egyptian Papyrus along with many others, such as Castor oil, Caraway, Dill and Coriander. Eating dates and drinking olive oil to aid evacuation of bowels was recommended from early times. Different drugs used as Cathartics today have the origin in different countries. Cascara was originally used by the Indians of California. Senna originates mainly from Arabia and Rhubarb from China. The leaves of Aloes are from Africa, while Podophyllum is an old drug of the American Indians. The purgative drugs used in this country centuries ago, are quite different from these. Fifteen plants have been mentioned in Caraka as purgatives, out of which 'Trivrut' त्रिवृत् is mentioned as a very useful and convenient.

त्रिवृत सुख विरेचनानाम । *Carak Su. 25-40*

Another plant mentioned is **'Danti'** (दन्ती). Both of them are identified as Ipomea turpethum and Baliospermum montanum respectively. These are the special purgatives used in India and not in any other country in the world. Ayurveda obviously copied these from the folk-medicine, in the period of Carak as they are not mentioned earlier in Buddhistic medicine. Ayurveda, being the scientific medicine, developing in this country, at that time it can be stated that those remedies were copied by the then existing scientific medicine in India from *Folk-medicine.*

A good deal of interest is shown in all civilzations regarding the drugs used for rejuvenation. Ayurveda mentions some with this property. But one actual story*, which took place in this century, is worth noting here. In 1932 there was a report from an Englishman in Siam (now Thailand) that the Thai natives got a new lease of life by eating the root of **'Kwao'**, vine, a creeper of the bean family. In 1948, Australian researchers mounted an expedition in Thailand, being interested in such type of drugs. With the aid of local botanists, they brought back a good load of **'Kwao'** root from Thailand. The report of the Englishman was based again on the ancient Burmese Medical treatise, inscribed on palm tree leaves,

(*Example quoted from 'Drugs' life Science Library)

which had been found in a temple wrecked by lightening. **'Kwao'** was well known in both Burma and Thailand and was reported to make old people young. Research work of these Australian scientists, showed that it was quite potent and showed activity both on ' in -vitro' and in 'in-vivo'. When the compound was isolated, it was thoroughly worked out as regards its chemical structure etc. It was found that it was chemically and pharmacologically a known group of drugs, which go under a common title, 'Estrogens'. The investigation in folk-medicine, thus, has resulted in a discovery of a new plant material yielding a known valuable compound. Stone in 1937 happened to learn from the country folk of the region, where his parish was located that they treated fevers with a decoction made from the bark of Willow, a common tree in that area. Stone treated fifty patients with Willow bark and in almost all cases, he found that the fever was reduced, he wrote a letter to the Royal Society of London. This is the origin of 'Salicilates' used in the scientific medicine. The term is derived from the Latin word 'Salix' (Willow).

Folk-medicine, is thus, a birth place of many great discoveries of new materials, which can be used as drugs in scientific medicine.This approach to the study of medicinal plants is being systematically followed by many scientific organisations, such as World Life Reasearch Institute of Colton, California, many Research and Development departments of the Pharmaceutical companies in different countries, such as Smith Cline and French of Philadelphia and even the *University Departments*. Dr. H. W. Halstead, Director of the *World Life Research Institute* spent many months in journerys through the South American jungles, studying the *remedies of Indian Witch doctors*. Medical Missionaries of South America helped him actively in this search. Amongst the potentially useful substances turned up in this manner, is one oral contracepetive and also a digitalis- like drug. Halsted respects the *sharp observations of the Witch doctors* and feel that *pharmacologist, who neglects this information may miss,* very valuable hints. Even the Indian *snake root* was laughed out in the offices of the scientific laboratories. But one company took the hint and made millions of dollars by marketing reserpine. *Dr. R. A. Ruffauf* of Philadelphia carefully screens every report on alkaloids and starts with a search in the forest where he tests the alkaloid on the spot. The hunt of new drugs from plant and animal kingdoms, involves hundreds of pharmacologists and field explorers, Not that these efforts always succeed, Not that there are few failures in this approach. But it must be emphasized that this approach of the *systematic study of folk-medicine does yield a very valuable information,* which sometimes yields very interesting and promising results.

Folk-medicine existed since the advent of man on earth. It is in existence now and not likely to disappear any time in future. It has been exploited by all scientific systems of medicine including Ayurveda in our country and it is no doubt, a very valuable approach in the hunt for new drugs.

In addition to this aspect, it is necessary to realise that plant chemistry gives valuable clues for new compounds with physiological activity. The isolation of a new compound for a chemist is like the birth of a son in the family for a common man and many such new clues are obtained by the chemist from the new plant kingdom. *Opium, Cinchona. Digitalis, Rauwolfia serpentina, Belladona, Vinca rosea* and a host of other plants have not only yielded in the past valuable chemical compounds, but it is through their study that new clues were obtained by the synthetic chemist to produce new compounds with similar and new physiological actions. Thus the study of plants is highly important, not only from the point of view of the development of new compounds but also for the knowledge *related to chemical processes going on in the* living organisations.

There is also another consideration in the study of folk-medicine practices. The relationship between poisons and drugs is very interesting. Caraka has ably pointed out.

यथा विषं यथा शस्त्रं यथाग्निरशनिर्यथा ॥१२४
तथौषधमविज्ञातं विज्ञातममृतं यथा । Cha. Su. 1.124, 25
योगादपि विषं तीक्ष्णमुत्तमं भेषजं भवेत् ।
भेषजं चापि दुर्युक्तंतीक्ष्णं संपद्यते विषम् ॥ Cha. Su . 1.126

A deadly poison can become a good drug and a drug misused can become a deadly posion. This principle of a relationship between a drug and a posion was thus well recognised since the very early period. Opium, Belladona, *Curare* and most of the many potent drugs used today in scientific medicine, were used as poisons once and can also act as poisons if misused.

' Dhanvantariya Nighantu ' also states very clearly the same principle in brief as follows :-

अमृतं स्याद्वत्सनाभो विषमुग्रं महौषधम् ।
-Dhn. Ni, Vii-28 p. 316

A deadly poison can be a good drug. The author gives an example of ' Vatsnabha ' or aconite, which can be used as a good drug and is known as a bad poison. The usual ' Shuddhi ' of this poisonous material is carried out by keeping it in cow's urine for three days.

Folk-practices have been observed also from the point of view of the use of poisonous materials. The Peruvian Indian used to dip his arrows in *Curare,* when he prepared them for hunting a deadly poison, which gives rise to paralysis and used to kill humans as well. The Roman Emperor Claudius was poisoned with *Belladona,* Hamlet's father with *henbane* and Romeo with *aconite.* The poisonous roots of *Dioscoreas* or *Mexican yams* have yielded *diosgenine,* which is a useful material for preparing modern *oral contraceptives.*

The scientific curiosity of men, has not leftout the animal poisons as well. For example, poisonous creatures in the depth of oceans are also searched in this efforts. The waters along the coast of Australia, have already shown some promise. Toxin from the toad fish has been used to assist brain surgery, some sponges manufacture a substance, which destroys bacteria and the toxin of Starfish may inhibit a tumour. The Australian zoologist has made reef-dwellers as his speciality, who tries to develop useful drugs from the deadly creatures of reef-dwellers.

Thus, it will be seen that the scientist study ancient medicines, poisons, comb the jungles and study the sea creatures and other animal kingdom as well, for valuable source-materials of new drugs. The eminent pharmaceutical companies, scientific societies and other academic bodies spend large amounts in this quest, which sometimes yield valuable information from nature for the human brain to work further. Millions of dollors spent every year on such projects are not taken as a waste.

Apart from the claim of Ayurveda that it is a self contained sceintific system of diagnosis and treatment by itself,. the study of *folk-medicine* is a recognised approach not only by the scientific world but *also by Ayurveda.* Before the advance of experimental medicine, Ayurveda and Unani were the only systems of medical practice in India. Ayurveda has also developed on this soil as a separate and distinct method of thought and action. Unani system was brought to India in the 8th Century A. D. by Arab invaders. This is also based on many folk medicines and it also flourished in the soil of India. With this contact, Ayurveda also absorbed many good practices and there was no quarrel. However, with the advent of experimental medicine in India, which has shown great advances during the last century, the old systems of Unani and Ayurved are now in melting pot. The duty of every *scientist in India is to try hard to pick up the best practices and conceptions available in these systems, which did work for several centuries,* subject them to a scientific method with all the zeal of an *unbiased* scientific worker and bring it to the notice of the scientific world. The Western scientists are likely to reduce both these systems, *now to a status of folk-medicine in India.*

No doubt, that the ancient systems do recognise the importance of folk - medicine and its study. But there is something more, Dhanvantariya Nighantu puts it, as follows :-

तेभ्यः सकाशादुपलभ्य वैद्यः पश्चाच्च शास्त्रेषु विमृश्य बुद्ध्या ।
विकल्पयेद्द्रव्यरसप्रभावान्विपाकवीर्याणि तथा प्रयोगात् ॥

Dhn. Ni. Stanza 7, p. 1,

Thus a thinking vaidya, after obtaining these remedies in a crude form from the folk-medicine, tries to put them to scientific investigations and thinking by proper understanding of its 'Rasa-Virya-Vipak (रस,वीर्य, विपाक) and Prabhava' (प्रभाव) uses it after proper experimentation. The process of scientific thought of this ancient Vaidya was of a kind, *which the modern scientist cannot appreciate for obvious reasons.* There is hardly any demonstration in this matter to show that an entirely unknown substance can be taken for experiment by this *ancient method* and used as a drug in this way. They now have to take the aid of the modern scientific method and disciplines to study that unknown substance. In spite of this, *astute* observations of ancients do remain as facts. नास्तिद्रव्यमनौषधम् ।

There is no material which cannot be used as a drug. The search is wide, deep and continuous, pervades all nature, whether mineral. animal or vegetable kingdoms. And again Caraka makes another remark :

न आयुर्वेदस्य परं पारं तस्मात् शश्वदभियोगं कुर्यात् ॥

There is no end to the knowledge of Ayurveda, it is, therefore, necessary to take it as a life pursuit !

The modern scintific thinker therefore should serve as an important medium between the ancient lore and the modern world. The more they render service to the ancient lore in this way, the more they will render the proper service to the ancients as well as to the modern science. Vaidya Kamat has served *as an unbiased scientist by elucidating the correct identities of the basic vegeable source materials used as drugs by our ancients. In fact, this is the first step towards further complicated steps in science,* and Vaidya Kamat has admittedly discharged this basic duty in the best way possible. The author of this work has given some valuable suggestions as to the interpretaions of nomenclatures. The synonyms given by the author of **'Dhanvantariya Nighantu'** are some times enough suggestive of the habit of the plant. The same name may indicate different plants in the different provinces of India. Vaidya Kamat has made valuable suggestions for the study of this subject by any person and has given important references to the literature on the topic.

The authours have mentioned about 17 plants as plants of doubtful identity. The Glossary of Vegetable drugs in Vagbhat gives twenty-three. A little comparison will show that the plants like **'Kshirakakoli'** are the plants of doubtful identity all over. Some plants of doubtful identity existing in Vagbhata are not mentioned by **'Dhanvantariya Nighantu'.** In the absence of adequate descriptions of these doubtful plants, their identification, has been a great problem to every body. The traditions in this matter also seem to have been vanished. Another possible approach is to collect the'so called' genuine bazaar materials and apply a number of modern techniques to find out their sources. It may then be possible to say something in the matter of these unknown drugs.

Shri Kamat and his colleague Prof. Mahajan have published only the first chapter **'Guduchyādi'** chapter of the **'Dhanvantariya Nighantu'** so far. It is true that most of the vegetable drugs are covered by this chapter. However, it is necessary to undertake the other parts also to complete the work and it is necessary that these authors should get the necessary financial support, either from the Govt. or a patron in this matter. A good publisher should also be able to undertake such publications as they are of a great value in both, research and practice of Ayurveda.

I wish Vaidya Kamat and Prof. Mahajan every success in their undertaking so that they will follow up this line of important work in future.

G. S. Pendse
Honorary Director,
Drugs Research Laboratory,
I. D. R. A.
561/B. Shivajinagar, Poona 5

Poona :
1-1-1972

INTRODUCTION TO VOL. II

by Prof. P. V. Sharma

Vaidya D.K.Kamat published his studies on Medicinal Plants in Dhanvantarīya Nihaṇtu (Vol. I) in 1972. Now Vol. II is coming out. Vaidya Kamat is no more but he completed this work before he left this world which is being published by his son Shri S.D.Kamat. I pay my respectful regards to the departed soul. His contributions in the field of Dravyaguṇa have been historical for which he will be ever remembered by the coming generations.

Dhanvantari Nighaṇtu because of its association with the Divine name 'Dhanvantari ' has been regarded in some circle as the oldest among the Nighaṇtus but this does not hold correct because of the following facts:-

1. In introductary verses it is mentioned that the work is composed by taking a portion of the ocean like literature of Nighaṇtus"[1]. This indicates that there was a large number of Nighaṇtus previously on which Dhanvntari Nighaṇtu is based.
2. Though the text starts with salutation to Dhanvantari, there is no mention of his authorship in introductary verses. Only at the end of the *Suvarṇādi Varga* in *Gaṇadavyavali* there is one line which says "thus Dravyāvali is read as emanated from Dhanvantri's mouth"[2] but this line is quite doubtful because of the following reasons :-
   - (a) The verse is not complete being only a half of the Anuṣṭubh meter.
   - (b) The line is quite detached with the context and looks unwarranted.
   - (c) If at all it was to be inserted, it should have come at the end of the *Miśrakādi varga* (7th Chapter) rather than after the *suvarṇādi varga* (6th Ch.).

This shows that probably Dhnvantari is not connected with the authorship of this work nor this is the earliest Nighaṇtu. The word 'Dhanvantari' in later period became as an epithet of a great Ayurvedic Scholar and it is not improbable that the word has been used here in this sense, In several manuscripts. Mahendra Bhogika, Son of Krṣṇabhogika and resident of Sthānvīśwara (Thaneswar)[3], has been said as the author of this work.

---

१. तथा निघण्टाम्बुनिधेरनन्ताद् गृहणाम्यहं किंचिदिहैकदेशम्

२. द्रव्यावलिः समादिष्टा धन्वन्तरिमुखोद्गता ।

३. कृष्णभोगिकपुत्रेण स्थाण्वीश्वरनिवासिना ।

Another important fact is that Dhnvantari Nighaṇṭu, though a very valuable Nighaṇṭu. has not been quoted by any author or commentator in Ayurvedic field before Aruna Datta, the commentator on Vagbhata's Aṣṭānga-Hṛday. Jejjata, Cakrapani and even Dalhaṇa does not refer to him who has given detailed interpretation on drugs. In another field, Kṡiraswami (11th cent. A.D.), Jejjata (9th cent. A.D.) does not refer to him. Hence this may be placed conveniently between 9th and 11 th Cent. A.D, e.g. 10th Cent. A.D.

From introductory verses it appears that the actual title of the original work was 'Dravyāvalî[1] and not 'Dhanvantari Nighaṇṭu' which is not mentioned at all in this context. The earlier Nighaṇṭu followed the style of the vedic Nighaṇṭu which consisted of only synonyms and no discription of substances. The composition of Nighaṇṭus having descsription of properties and actions of drugs alongwith synonyms is a later development. The original text Dravyāvali consisted of synonyms only as evident from the author's statement in introductions[2] Description of properties and actions was added to it later on as appears from the second salutary verse[3]. Thus the exsiting text of Dhanvantari Nighaṇṭu is Dravyavali added with description of properties and actions.This addition, of course, was not outcome of a day, instead it must have taken a long time during which Dravyāvali in its original form was current[4], on the basis of internal evidences it may be said that the process continued till 13 th Cent. A.D[5] . It appers that after addition having completed in Dravyāvali, it began to be known by the new title of Dhanvantari Nighaṇṭu. In the form of

---

महेंद्रभोगिकेनेयं कृता द्रव्यावली शुभा ॥ -Des. Cat. Sams. Mss.,
B.O.R.I.Poona, Vol. XVI, Pt. I,S1. 105-111.

१. ' द्रव्यावलिं विना वैद्यास्ते वैद्या हास्यभाजनम् ।'
' द्रव्यावल्यभिधानानां तृतीयमपि लोचनम् ।'
' द्रव्यावलिनिविष्टानां द्रव्याणां नामनिर्णयम् ।'
' लोक-प्रसिद्धं वक्ष्यामि यथागमपरिस्फुटम् ॥'
' शतत्रयं च द्रव्याणां त्रिसप्तत्यधिकोत्तरम् ।
हिताय वैद्यपुत्राणां द्रव्यावल्यां प्रकाशितम् ॥'

२. गणद्रव्यावलि ह्युक्ता सयोगा सहमात्रया ।
पर्यायनामान्युच्यंते गुडूच्यादेर्यथाक्रमम् ।

३. धन्वन्तरिपदद्वंद्वं नत्वा लोकहितार्थिनाम् ।
रसवीर्यविपाकादि द्रव्याणां कथ्यते मया ॥

४. There are several Mss. of Dravyavali in oriental libraries. I have located two Mss. Mithila Research Institute, Darbhanga (Bihar) and one in B.H.U.Library.

५. P.V.Sharma; The date of Dhanvantari Nighaṇṭu, I.J.H.S. Vol.5, No.2.1970

६. Hardatt Shrama (ed.)- Nāmalingānuśāna, with the commentary Amarakoṣodghatana by Ksiraṣwami & N.G.Sardesai, Poona Oriental Book Agency, 1942. Introduction p. Vii-viii-

७. T.Ganapatī Shastri (ed.)-The Nāmaliṅgānusasana of Amarasimha, Pt.I. Trivandrum Sanskrit Series No. XXXIII, 1914 Preface.

Dravyāvali, it may not be the first Nighaṇṭu but as the Dhanavantari Nighaṇṭu it sems to be the first Nighaṇṭu having description of properties and actions of drugs. This was followed by later authors like Śoḍhala, Madanpāla, Kaiyadeva and Bhāvamiśhra.

Kśiraswāmi's contention that Dhanvantari Nighaṇṭu preceded the Amarakosa and that the Vanauṣadhi varga of the latter is based on the former[7] does not hold correct. The date of the Amarakoṣa is fixed as in 4th Cent. A.D.[1] during Gupta period because Amara Simha preceded Candrogāmin, a Buddhist Grammerian of Bengal and teacher of Vasurāta (450 A.D.) The Amarakosa was translated into Chinese by Guṇarāta of Ujjayani in 6th Cent. A.D. and as such it must be prior to this. Accordingly if the above contention of Kśiraswāmi is accepted, the Dhanvatari Nighaṇṭu will have to be placed even earlier to that.

Main argument in his favour put forth by Kśiraswāmi is that in certain places the author of the Amarakoṣa, though tried to follow to Dhanvantarī Nighaṇṭu sincerely was confused in certain readings and that is why he proposed changed versions. The following examples are given by him :-

1. The Dhanvantari Nighaṇṭu reads 'Bālapatra' for Yavāsā and Khadira but Amarasimha mistaking it as 'Bālaputra' made the synonym 'Bālatanaya' for Khadira.
2. The word 'Upacitrā' is for Dantî and pṛśniprṇī but in the Amarakosa Dravantī is confused with Dantī and as such the synonym 'Upacitrā' is mentioned for the same.
3. Dhanvantari reads 'Padmavarṇa' a synonym for Puṣkramūla but Amarasimha confusing it as Padmaparṇa has given it as a synonym for the same.
4. Dhanvantari has given 'Śitalaivātaka' as a synonym for Śaṇaparṇī but Amara simha taking it as a compound has split it into two-Sītala and Vātala.
5. 'Mahauṣadha' is a synonym for Viṣa and and not for Ativiṣa but Amarasimha taking 'Viṣā' as 'Viṣa' has used this synonym for Ativiṣa.
6. 'Nādeyī' once already used has again been used due to similar confusion.
7. Citrā' is a synonym for Viśālā and Dravantī. Amarasimha by confusion has used this synonym for Gavākśī.
8. 'Sevya' is used for Lāmajjak and Uśira but Amarasimha confusing them as one has mentioned both 'Sevya' and 'Amṛṇāla' as synonyms for 'Uśira' itself.

By these examples Kśiraswāmi has tried to show that the text of

Dhanvantari Nighaṇṭu was always before Amara-Simha when he was composing the Vanauṣadhi varga though under confusion he has changed some of the readings.

Let us examine critically the above examples one by one.

1.'Bālapatra' as a synonym for Khadira has not been used only in the Dhanvantri Nighaṇṭu but also in other earlier Nighaṇṭus like the Aṣṭāṅga Nighaṇṭu of Vahata. Secondly, the word ' Tanaya' (Prasava) means offshoots from the main body of the plant such as leaves flowers as well as fruits. Here the author used it for leaves. As Bhanuji Dīkṣita say, it is also possible that the original reading 'Balapatra' might have been changed to 'Bālaputra' due to transcriptional error. This however, does not preclude the antecedence of the Dhanvantari Nighaṇṭu because the synonym of Bālaputra is also seen in the Aṣṭāṅga Hṛdaya which might be the common source for all the after works.

2. In use of the synonym 'Citrā and Upacitrā' there has not been any hard and fast rule. In the Aṣṭāṅga Nighaṇṭu, Citrā and Upacitrā have been used for Dantī and Nāgadantī respectively. In Paryāyaratr amālā, both the words have been used for Dantī. Hence it should not be surprising if Amarasimha also used both these words as synonyms for Dravantī. On this ground to allege mistake on the part of the author of the Amarakoṣa in following the Dhanvantari Nighaṇṭu is a far-fetched imagination.

3. The word 'Padmavarṇa' is not found in synonyms of Puṣkaramula in the present edition (Anadashram; Poona,2nd ed.,1925). It is possible that the manuscript before Kṣiraswāmi might be having this version due to transcriptional error. Secondly, 'Padmavarṇa' is not at all a fitting synonym. Instead 'Padmapatra' is the correct synonym denoting the size and shape of the leaves of the plant. Moreover, this synonym has been accepted by almost all the Nighaṇṭus.

4. As regards 'Sītalavātaka' it is not found in the present edition of the Dhanavantari Nighaṇṭu. In the Amarakoṣa, Bhānuujī Dīkṣita has supported both the versions 'Sītalah' Vātakah and 'Sitalavātakaḥ' naturally there is no diference between these two.

5. 'Mahauṣadha' in fact, means 'great remedy' (or panacea) which may be applicable to any popular drug. (Ativiṣa' being a very popular drug particutarly for children's disorders, deserves this epithet quite well. Amarasimha being such a great all round scholar could not distinguish between 'Viṣa' and 'Viṣā' is not at all acceptable. Instead he has used this synonym quite knowingly. This has also been used for 'Laśuna' which again supports the above idea.

6. Nādeyī Bhumijmbukā' has come twice in the Amarakoṣa

(11- 4, 38 and 118) but in different contexts. In the first context they denote 'Nāraṅga' while in the other they are for 'Bhujambu'. It is to be noted that the word 'Nādeyī', has been used for four different plants in the Amarkoṣa-Jalavetasa, Nāgraṅga, Tarkāri and Bhujambu. In Dhn. Nighaṇṭu it is used similarly except for Nāgaraṅga. Dhanvantari acted judiciously and left the synonym in case of Nāraṅga.

7. It is no mistake if the synonym 'Citrā' is used for Gavāk'si as explained above (item 2). K'siraswmi himself satisfies himsef by saying that Vi'sāla being only a type of Gavak'sī there is no any mistake. In Dhanvantari Nighaṇṭu, Citrā has been used as a synonym for several drugs like Durvā, Bilva, Manjiṣṭhā, Dravantī etc..

8. There has been confusion regarding identity of Lāmajjaka and U'sira since long. Hence it was but natural for Amarasimha too to mention the synonyms like that.

The internal evidence also do not support the view of K'siraswāmi about antecedence of the Dhanvantari Nighaṇṭu. The contents of the Dhanvantari Nighaṇṭu are much more in developed state which show its posteriority. The following examples would suffice :-

1. Some drugs which found entrance during medieval period such as Agnijāra (Ambara) which are described in the Dhanvantari Nighaṇṭu but are absent in the Amarakoṣa.

2. Some of the drugs such as Kaṁkuṣṭha (latex of Swarṇak'sirī) is described in the Dhanvantari Nighaṇṭu but are absent in the Amarakoṣa. Had the Dhanvantari Nighaṇṭu been before Amarasimha, he must have utilised this important material.

3. The type of Karañja are two in ancient texts, five in the Amarakoṣa and six in the Dhanvantari Nighaṇṭu. It shows the developed state of classificition in the Dhanvantari Nighaṇṭu and consequently its posteriority.

4. Gajapippalī has been said as the fruit of Cavya in the Dhanvantari Nighaṇṭu but this fact is conspicuously absent in the Amarako'sa. This ieda is certainly a later one which places the Dhanvantari Nighaṇṭu posterior to the Amarakoṣa.

Thus, the Amarakoṣa is posterior to Vāgbhaṭa but anterior to the Dhanvantari Nighaṇṭu. There is no doubt that some Nighaṇṭu was certainly before Amarasimha on the basis of which he has been able to compile the Vanauṣadhi varga which is unique in respect of material as well as

1. P. V. Sharma : The Vanausadhi Varga of Amarakoṣa and its Historical implications; Paper presented at the International Congress of Human Sciences, August, 1976.

presentation but certainly that was not the Dhanvantari Nighaṇṭu but its predecessors the existence of which is mentioned in the introductory verses.

The value of the Dhanvantari Nighaṇṭu can't be overemphasized because being the first nighaṇṭu in the descriptive style provided model for later works. But , at the same time, it needs critical scrutiny because of having been developed at the juncture of the ancient and medieval periods which was actually a transition phase as regards the knowledge and identity of drugs.

I am glad that such important study has been done by Vaidya D.K. Kamat in the present series which may be able to solve mysteries and controversies current since long.

The Ayurvedic community should be grateful to him for this valuable work. Shri S.D.Kamat, his devoted son, is enagaged in publishing the work done by his father for which he deserves thanks and congratulations, from scholars. I hope, he will continue his efforts in this direction and would publish all the volumes in series so that a complete picture of the critical study of the Dhanvantari Nighaṇṭu is presented before the world of scholars.

Banaras Hindu University, **P. V. Sharma**
Varanasi. 30-5-79

THE TREATISE AND ITS CONSTITUTION

Abbreviations occurring under the heading subjects.

EPP-- Editor Purandare's Prastāvikā's (प्रस्ताविका) page.

CDP-- Prastāvanā (प्रस्तावना introduction) of the compiler of the treatise page.

PLB-- Purandare's list of collected MSS. page.

DP-- Dhanvantarīya Nighaṇṭu page.

CHAPTER I

THE TREATISE

(i) *Dhanvantarīyas and Dhanvantarīya Nighaṇṭu.*

(ii) *Controversy regarding the compilers and the Treatise.*

(iii) *The Edition and its editor Purandare's Prastāvikā.*

(iv) *Purpose of the Treatise* (ग्रन्थस्य कारणम्)

(i) ***Dhanvantarīās and Dhanvantarīya Nighaṇṭu.***

The name of the compiler and the period of the compilation is not mentioned in this book. The term Dhanvantari (धन्वन्तरि) is mentioned in this book at two occasions. At the very beginning the complier has prayed the God Ādi Deva Dhanvantarī (a) (आदि देव धन्वन्तरि), and at the end of Suvarṇādi Chapter in Ganadravyāvali (b) (सुवर्णादि वर्ग गणद्रव्यावलि). He mentions that this Nighaṇṭu (निघण्टु) is written as it was told by Dhanvantari (धन्वन्तरि मुखोद्गता). These are the only places where the term Dhanvantari (धन्वन्तरि) is used.

Out of these, the first occasion is merely for the sake of prayer, and not for the compilers own sake, is very clear. The other mentioned reference ' Dhanvantarī' mukhodgatā, (धन्वन्तरि मुखोद्गता), has been discussed in later chapters. According to that and as it does not correlate with the traditional beginning and end of a book (उपक्रमोपसंहार),to what extent we should trust it, is doubtful.

In spite of our opinion, 'Dhanvantariya' (धन्वन्तरीय) references have been given by (1)Kshiraswami (क्षीरस्वामि) the commentator of Amarakoṣa (अमरकोष) in the eleventh century A.D.,(2) and Aruṇadutta (अरुणदत्त) (3)

---

a. CDP 1 b. - CDP - 7

1. Vide Oak's introduction to Amarakosha, p. 62
2. Vide Gode Vol. I. p. 160 etc.
3. Ashta. hr. pp. 118, 232, 234 etc

the commentator of Aṣṭānigahṛdaya (अष्टांग हृदय) in the 13th century (4) A.D. and by the author of Shivakosh (5) flourished in 1677. (6) A.D. These references correlate with the present text of Dhanvantatīya Nighaṇṭu (धन्वन्तरीय निघण्टु). It, therefore, seems that this Nighaṇṭu is known as 'Dhanvantarīya Nighaṇṭu traditionally for a long time.

In some books this Nighaṇṭu has been mentioned as 'Guḍūchyādi Nighaṇṭu, (गुडूच्यादि निघण्टु). or 'Dravyāvali Dhanvantarīya (द्रव्यावलि धन्वन्तरीया) (7). These names have been mentioned because the description of plants in this book commences with Guḍūchyādi Chapter (गुडूच्यादि वर्ग) while 'Gaṇadravyāvali' (गणद्रव्यावलि) appears as in Sushrut Samhitā (सुश्रुत संहिता) (8) and because traditionally it is known to be Dhanvantari, it is called as 'Dravyāvali Dhanvantarīyā'(द्रव्यावलि धन्वन्तरीया)

One of the following reasons also might have been responsible for the name 'Dhanvantarīya Nighaṇṭu'(धन्वन्तरीय निघण्टु) : –

(1) At the beginning of the book the compiler has mentioned the name of Dhanvantari.

(2) There were two schools of Ayurveda, viz. -Atreya school of clinical method (आत्रेय संप्रदाय कायचिकित्सा) and Dhanvantariya school of surgical method (9) (धन्वन्तरीय संप्रदाय शस्त्रचिकित्सा). The compiler might have been a follower of the Dhanvantari school (धन्वन्तरि संप्रदाय) The commentators might have known this traditionally, therefore the name Dhanvantarīya Nighaṇṭu was adopted.

(3) There was also a Dhanvantari lineage (गोत्र) (10) in the Sārswata (सारस्वत) brāhmins (ब्राह्मण) who had followed the study of Ayurveda. Dr.Gananath Sen has mentioned that he has known the traditional Ayurvedic physicians of this lineage in Sindh and Bengal. One of the Physicians (वैद्याचार्य) of this Gotra (गोत्र) might have compiled this book.

---

4. Vide Gode, Vol. I. p. 121
5. Vide Harshe. Index to authors, app. p. 167 (धन्वन्तरि)
6. Harshe, intro. p.ii.
7. Vide F.N.DP. 1.
8. Su. Su. 38.

9.a सोऽयं द्विविधः संप्रदायस्तत्राद्यः धन्वन्तरि सम्प्रदायः सुश्रुत सम्प्रदायो वेति द्वितीयस्तु भरद्वाज आत्रेयसम्प्रदायो वेति। Gananath Sen, Sharira p. ख.

9-b. तथाचोक्तः धन्वन्तरे। Aruna, Kunte, Su. 5-44.

c. धन्वन्तरिस्तु। ....। Aruna, Kunte, Su. 19-23.

d. श्रावणी श्रावितापूर्वं ......इति धान्वन्तरीयाः। Harshe p. 100.

e. तत्रैव पिण्डिते शूले संपक्वं गुल्ममादिशेत्। तत्र धान्वन्तरीयाणामधिकारः क्रियाविधौ। Ca. Ci. 5-43, 44.

f. शल्यविषयस्य परतन्त्रीयत्वेनोपादानमपि धान्वन्तरं सम्प्रदायमुपस्थापयति। आत्रेयसंहिताम् इति धन्वन्तरिः धान्वन्तरमतम् इति बहुशो धन्वन्तरेस्तत्सांम्प्रदायिकानां च पूर्वाचार्यत्वेन संसमानं निर्देशनमस्ति - इति धन्वन्तरि सम्प्रदायस्य बहुलि भावे सति। Acharya Yadavaji Su.Sa. p. 9.

10. अस्ति चापरोऽपि धन्वन्तरिनाम ऋषिः केषाञ्चिद् विप्राणां गोत्रप्रवर्तकः सोऽपि वैद्याचार्यः इत्यनुमीयते। यस्तद्गोत्रीया वैद्याख्य सारस्वत ब्राह्मणा अद्यापि पञ्चनदेषु वंगेषु दृष्यन्ते। *Gananath, Bhanumati teeka, Indroduction.*

We feel that the above given reasons (especially the second one) might have been known to the commentators by tradition, *and that tradition has been follwed up to this time.* Moreover, it can also be inferred that the first part i.e.' *Gaṇadravyāvali'* (गणद्रव्यावलि) was compiled by one of the disciples of Dhanvartarīya school; and later on another follower of the same school might have supplemented it by the addition of *'Paryāyanām Dravyāvali'* (पर्यायनामद्रव्यावलि). Any way, it seems to be quite certain that both of these parts are not compiled by the same author.

This history of the compiler and his period has not been completely unveiled. Over and above all this, the subsequent copy-writers have done many differences of readings (पाठभेद) and interpolations, (प्रक्षिप्त) to the original text, adding to the controversies about the book and its compiler. General idea of the same can be summarised as follows :-

(ii) ***Controversy regarding the compilers and the Treatise.***

The controversy of the book is a very complex subject, because there are several differences of readings.

(1) In some manuscripts 'Gaṇadravyāvali' (गणद्रव्यावलि) itself is not included (10a). In some other readings (पाठ) have been included. (11).

(2) There is a difference of opinion among the scholars as to whether the first part-- ' Gaṇadravyāvali ' (गणद्रव्यावलि) should be considered to be the part of this book or not. (12).

(3) Some believe that the compiler was a learned physician in the court of *Vikramaditya Chandragupta II* (13) *Sahasanka* (विक्रमादित्य, चंद्रगुप्त, 2, साहसांक).

(4) Some others believe that the compiler was with the *Shakari Vikramaditya* (14) (शकारि विक्रमादित्य) by whose name the Vikram Samvat (विक्रम संवत) is going on.

(5) According to some others there is no mention of Dhanvantari as a physician in the Navaratna legend (नवरत्न कथा) (15) but as a mathematician and poet.

(6) Some hold that this book was compiled by a disciple of Dhanvantari - the teacher of Sushrutacharya (सुश्रुताचार्य) (16)

On what basis these inferences are concluded is not clear but probably on the basis of edition published by Anandashram Press Poona आनन्दाश्रम मुद्रणालय, पुणे) (17) and the famous worthless legend of Kāvyasangraha (काव्यसंग्रह).

10-a. Vide PLB. ग.ञ.
11. Vide PLB. ख.च, छ.
12. Vide App. B-1-8.
13. Vide App. B-1-9
14. Vide App. B-1-10
15. Vide App. B-1-11
16. Vide App. B-1-12
17. Vide App. 2-9

In such controversy it is a problem which edition should be taken as authorised. It goes without saying that different editions will have different inversions and different subject described therein, subsequently changing our discussion, interpretation and inferences based on them. If the version from Kavyasangraha (18) (काव्यसंग्रह) is taken for decision, how much importance it deserves as a historical document is uncertain and even debatable. Whether the learned persons mentioned in this version are contemporary (19). Morevover, between the period of Panini (पाणिनि)and Chandragupta (चंद्रगुप्त) there were four or five kings having the name of Vikramaditya (विक्रमादित्य).(20)

If the whole book lincluding ' Gaṇadravyāvali ' (गणद्रव्यावलि) is compiled by one person, the heading names and the pharmacological properities of the medicinal plants described in ' Gaṇadravyāvali,' (गणद्रव्यावलि) and ' Paryāyanām dravyāvali ' (पर्यायनाम द्रव्यावलि) should be similar. (21) On the other hand if the compilers are two, who were they and what was their period?

(7) In Gaṇadravyāvali (गणद्रव्यावलि)at the end of Suvarṇādi chapter (सुवर्णादि वर्ग) it has been mentioned that 'this Dravyāvali has been compiled as told by Dhanvantari' (द्रव्यावलिः समादिष्टा धन्वन्तरि मुखोद्गता) (22) To what extent the statement is pervading ? If it is implied for the whole

---

18. Vide App. B-1-10 foot note.

19.a. Vararuchi (वररुचि) contemporary to Panini (पाणिनि) Ketkar p. 315

b.According to Rajawade, Prakritprakasha (प्राकृतप्रकाश) of Vararuchi may have come into existence before Buddha i.e. B.C.600. Ketkar, p. 322.

c. Vararuchi two. One of them is Katyayan the compiler of ' Vartikas' (बार्तिक), and the next the eldest son of the brahman Chandragupt (चन्द्रगुप्त) disciple of Patanlali.

--Patanjali, p. 29.

d. Katyayan B.C. 500-350. Ketkar p. 446.

e. Panini (पाणिनि) B.C. 750-700, Ketkar p. 446.

f. Varahamihira 505 A.D. Gode 1- 103.

g. Kshapanaka (क्षपणक) 925 A. D. ibid, p. 111

h. Kalidas as two. The period of one about B.C. - 30 A.D. and probably another Kalidasa. lived during the Gupta period.

Kalidasa by Prof. R. D. Karmarkar,

Review by Pusalkar, Bhand. Oriental Re-Institute, Annals, 1959.

20. The kings noted under the name Vikramaditya (विक्रमादित्य).

a. Vikramaditya the king of Pataliputra 300 years anterior to Naravahan (नरवाहन son of काशीराज उदयन of कौशांबी). Ketkar , pp. 50-51.

Vishamashil Vikramaditya of Avanti- Ujjain, anterior to Udaan -ibid pp.50,107,112.

c.Trivikram Vikramaditya, ibid p. 31.

d.Shakari Vikramaditya by whose name the Samvat (संवत्) year began. vide App. B-1-10.

e. Sahasanka Vikramaditya Chandragupta II (son of Samudragupta), about 400-503 A.D. -vide Ayur. Patrika 15-9-69, p. 76.

21 . Vide Dhn. N. p. 7. 22. ibid. p. 7.

book, why it should appear at the end of the 6th chapter ?Why it has not mentioned in the beginning (उपक्रम) or at the end (उपसंहार) ? If the verse is limited only to the 6th chapter, who is this Dhanvantari? Then who has (or have) written the other chapters? This verse is included in Anandashram edition but not in some other editions. (23) These are some of the questions which have remained unanswered so far.

Though there are these controversies regarding the compiler and his period they do not and should not interfere with and devaluate the importance of the contents of this great work. It is a work on the medicinal plants, and their pharmacological actions on the human body, studied at about the beginning of Christ era. The compiler has collected the information about medicinal plants and their properties right from the time of Atharvaved (अथर्ववेद) to the Samhitā grantha (संहिता ग्रंथ) period.

There is no controversy regarding the practical experience and usefulness of the drugs mentioned in Ayurvedic texts (संहिता ग्रंथ).

The same tradition has been followed in this treatise. But in addition, the compiler has overcome the practical diffiiculty in identification and confirmation of medicinal plants by providing the morphological descriptions which are not given in the original Ayurvedic texts and in the Vedic literature. Thus giving the description of plants, their names and synonyms occuring in the Ayurvedic texts, the complier has opened the path of knowledge of the traditional Ayurvedic plants. Hence the importance of the treatise cannot be underestimated.

Many more Nighaṇṭus were compiled after this, mainly based on this pioneer work, but the accuracy and extensiveness of morphologlical descriptions of plants are not found in many other Nighaṇṭus. To some extent these qualities are found in Rajanighaṇṭu (राजनिघंट्ट), mainly because, it is based on this Nighaṇṭu or is rather its commentary in poetical arrangement.

The very facts that the medicinal plants in traditional Ayurvedic texts (संहिता ग्रंथ) are incorporated in it, and Rajanighaṇṭu (राजनिघंट्ट), is also based on it, clearly establish the paramount importance of Dhanvantarīya Nighaṇṭu in the study of Ayurveda and Ayurvedic medicinal plants. But the present state of affairs seems to be otherwise. It seems to have been neglected in the curriculi and syllabi of the course of Ayurvedic medicine in our country. Ayurvedic students, unfortunately, do not study it. We suspect with fear that some may not be knowing even its name. There are about half a dozen commentaries in regional languages on Bhāva Prakasha Nighaṇṭu (भाव-प्रकाश निघंट्ट)compiled by Bhava Mishra (भाव-मिश्र) which is generally studied today by Ayurvedic students. Neither Dhanvantarīya Nighaṇṭu nor Raj Nighaṇṭu has been studied in this manner. These works, therefore , for want of any detailed study or a

23. Vide App. B-2 p. 97 MS 3831.

commentary; could not have come into light upto this date. In case of Rāj Nighaṇṭu the situation is somewhat better, as its printed edition is available, but the matter was still worse about Dhanvantarīya Nighaṇṭu due to non-availability of the same. Therefore, if the Anandāshram Press (आनन्दाश्रम मुद्रणालय) would not have published this book, the very existence of this Nighaṇṭu would have been in danger. In this situation, the students and lovers of Ayurveda should and will remain grateful to the publishers of Anandashram Press, for ever.

It seems that there was a commentary on Dhanvantari Nighaṇṭu in Sanskrit. But it is nowhere available today. It is also learned that a few manuscripts of this Nighaṇṭu are preserved (संरक्षित) (24), but they are spread all over the country, and are not easily available to the common student. As there is no edition available but for that published by Anandāshram Press, we have taken the same as authentic for our study.

(iii) ***The Edition and its editor Purandare's Prastavikā*** (प्रस्ताविका)

This edition is published by the Late Vinayak Ganesh Apte (विनायक गणेश आपटे) and printed at Ānandāshram Press, Poona, for the first time in 1897. It is edited by the late Vaidya Narayan Vitthal Purandare (नारायण विट्ठल पुरंदरे). Its publiction No. is 33 of Anandashram Sanskrit Series.(आनंदाश्रम संस्कृत ग्रंथावलि कमांक ३३.) The second reprinted edition was published in 1925.

In the introduction of the book, the editor (N.V. Purandare) has given the justification of the addition of Rajanighaṇṭu (25) in this edition. According to him, Dhanvantarīya Nighaṇṭu being very old, the addition of Rājanighaṇṭu will facilitate its understanding, *The main subject of his study is, however,* Dhanvantarīya Nighaṇṭu' (26) based on the manuscript which he studied, and used to read very often. Besides this 'base-manuscript' in his own collection, he had procured about a dozen (27) other manuscripts for comparative study and reference work, the differences of readings (पाठभेद) have been given in the foot-notes.

In the Prastavikā the editor has clarified the purpose of the numbers given before and after the plant names(28). The same shall be discussed at length in the following pages. (chapter II).

He has further added the Ekartha Dvyarthadi Kosh (एकार्थ द्वयर्थादि कोश) according to the available manuscripts. It is also mentioned that the index of synonyms occurring in both the Nighaṇṭus as well as the index of

24. Vide App. B-2, p. 94,96
25. Vide EPP. 1,2.
26. Vide EPP. 2-6.
27. Vide PLB. 1,2,
28. Vide EPP. 3,7.

names in regional languages, have been supplied. But the latter is, however, not found in the book. (29) After the regards to the learned men, the Prastavikā has been concluded by the contents of Dhanvantarīya Nighaṇṭu and Rājnighaṇṭu.

(iv) ***Purpose of the Treatise*** (ग्रन्थस्य कारणम्).

The original book (subject matter) starts after the editor's Prastavikā. Following the usual traditional practice, the compiler begins with a prayer to the deity 'Kamākṣi ' (कामाक्षी) and Vighnarāj' (विघ्नराज Gaṇesh गणेश) and a stanza of salutation to Dhanvantari (धन्वन्तरि). (30) In the heading he has mentioned that hereafter starts the 'Dhanvantarīya Nighaṇṭu'. It is noted in the foot-note by the editor Purandare that in some manuscripts the book is called as Guḍūchyādi Nighaṇṭu (गुडूच्यादि निघण्टु) or Dravyāvali Dhanvantariyā (द्रव्यावलि धन्वन्तरीया).(31) Then the purpose of the book (ग्रन्थस्य कारणम्) has been explained upto 19th stanza.

While explaining the purpose of the book the compiler has given the idea of difficulty in identification of medicinal plants even at that time. (32) He further gives the ways and means of their identification and practical application; and emphasizes the importance of the study of Nighaṇṭu.

The compiler then states that some medicinal plants recognized by Ayurvedic texts as well as famous in public are not dealt with in detail in this book, (33) to avoid repetitions (न गृह्य.... श्लोक ४) He mentions some such plants and explains how to use them. (34)

He admits in the very beginning the difficulties in compiling this Nighaṇṭu due to the vast number of plants in various current regional languages and descrepancies in the names of medicinal plants noted in Sanskrit and regional (प्राकृत) languages. Moreover he says that several Nighaṇṭus compiled previously were present at that time.

We should pay attention here to the noteworthy point that the compiler was conversant with the other literature on this subject in various, regional (प्राकृतनामसंज्ञाः) and folk language from different regions. (34a).

For identification of plants, he advises to obtain the knowledge of plants from Kirāt (किरात),Gopāl (गोपाल),Vanachara (वनचर) [People of aboriginal tribes](35) and others proficient in this subject. *Such knowledge should not be underetimated nor discarded only because it is in the regional or folk language* (जन भाषा), *because the 'speech' is meant for action. Information, therefore, should be collected from all the possible* (36) *sources, irrespective of languages and regions. This piece of advice given*

---

29. Vide EPP, 1-9. 30. Vide CDP. 1. 31. Vide CDP. 1.
32. Vide CDP. 1,2 stanzas 2,9, 10. 33. Vide CDP. 1-4; 2-1 6.
34. Vide CDP. 1-6 34-a Vide CDP.1-2.

by the compiler is of prime importance to the students and lovers of this subject. Its sense should be carefully understood. It is a great blunder in research work to neglect and disgrace any knowledge only because it is available through regional or folk languages.

The research mind is high above the limitations of country, religion, casts and sects. It seeks help and evidences from whatever sections they are available for purpose of advancement of science. The science of medicine has not sprung from a few 'brains',-- it is an ocean of knowledge collected through vast experiences from the time immemorial (37). The ways and means of obtaining such knowledge were various. The man in those days studied nature. He keenly observed natural phenomena and their consequences. They learned many things from animals(38) which they observed and studied in their natural habitat and activities. They experienced seasonal changes and their effects on human being as well as other creatures. All such things have been recorded in Atharvaveda (अथर्ववेद) -where we find the mention of even the germs, their different types, habits and even their pathogenic activities ! (39).Some of the names of medicinal plants, recorded in Ayurvedic litreature clearly indicate that Vedic people had come in contact with other people like

---

35. Vide CDP. 1-6, 7, 8, 2-11. 12.

36-a. अत्रापि फलानामप्रसिद्धानां च येषां नामानि नोक्तानि तानि नानादेश कुलेभ्योऽपभ्रंश संस्कारादिनाधिगन्तव्यानि ।

Indu. Ashta. San. vide Gode Vol. I, p. 158.

b. परतन्त्र प्रत्ययानाम् । (p.951)
यस्यार्थस्य प्रसिद्धितो न स्वकीयमुदाहरणं शक्यमभिधातुं नापि अन्येभ्यो भिषक् तनुध्य : । ततस्तस्मिन् द्वये परतंत्रादुदाहरणं कल्प्यते । यथा (ह. सू.अ. १-१९)
कालार्थ कर्मणां योगो इत्युक्तम् । ...... तत्र बौद्धतन्त्रप्रत्ययेन निश्चीयते ।

Ashta. hr. Vajikarana.

c. But as long as those applications remain understood, a travelling physician who should wish to procure an Arabin or Indian plant, and without asking for it for its learned or vulger name, should hunt for it in the woods by its botanical character, would remember as a geoghrapher who desiring to inquire by name for a street or a Town, but waits with tables and instruments for a proper occasion to deterrmine in longitudes and latitudes.

Sir William Jone's work
Vol. II page 47, London 17, 9.

37-a. How long man has existed is matter of speculation but there existed men-like creatures, relics of which have been in many places. Since disease and ill-health must accompany living flesh, blood and health, speculation to relieve these must have been there since the dawn of human life on the earth, and medicine can therefore be as old as the human race.

B. Sen, M.D.M.R.C.P ele
The Indian Practitioner Jan. 1964, page 145.

b. Doubtless he will then be convinced that no scientific progress can be regarded as a sudden and autonomous formation but that each our achievements is closely allied to the past without knowledge of which it cannot be understood.

History of Medicine, page 9

Sumerians(सुमेरियन), Chaldians (40) (खाल्डियन), Turushkas (तुरुष्क), Balhiks (बाल्हिक), Persians (पारसिक), Greeks (यवन), Arabians (म्लेच्छ), Barbars (बर्बर), Shakas (शक),(41), etc. Some of the authorities even believe that the study of medicinal plants was started in the Mediterranean region.(42). We do not fully agree with this view, as this is a subject of study of human migration and spread of civilization, which we feel, has not reached its perfection to draw any definite conclusion. This belief is rather contradistinctive

---

c. Notable progress in the field of rhinoplasty which derives evidently from a long evolution of ancient concepts how the medicinal thoughts of India for the most part has developed according to the interest and traditions of that country, rigid fidelity to ancestral teaching. History of Medicine Page 86.

d. He (Flliozat) possibly regards (Vedic) literature was fully developed on the Indian soil which may not be a fact. It has its origin in the hoary past and some elements of its ancient traditions will have to be examined more closely and co-ordinated with similar traditions in other ancient records now available.

Dr. Harshe, p. xxv.

38.a. भेषज्यविद्या गुरवो पशुपक्षिणः ।

Ayurvediya Histopdasha by. Ranajitraya Desai, 1925 p. 305.

b. या सुपर्णा अङ्गिरसी दिव्या (हुवे)

Pt. Saravlekar, AV. viii-7.

c. The eagle digests the poison like food.

Dr. Shende,p. 34, AV.vi-4-3.

39-a ओतो मे इन्द्रश्चाग्निश्च क्रिमिं जम्भयतां ।
यो अक्षौपरिसर्पति यो नासे परिसर्पति ।
दन्तां ये मध्ये गच्छति तं क्रिमिं जम्भ. ॥ ३ AV. v-23.

b. ये क्रिमयः पर्वतेषु वनेष्वोषधीषु पशुष्वप्स्व १ न्तः॥ + ॥५॥ AV. ii-31

c. अप्सु मे सोमोऽब्रवीदन्तर्विश्वानि भेषजा ॥ RV.i-23

d. याओषधिः पूर्वाजाता देवेभ्यस्त्रियुगं पुरा ॥ RV.X-9.

40-a. **Chaldians' trade with Dravidians** before Vedic languages found its way into India before 1500 B.C. -Ayangar,p. 137.

b. Our attention was first invited to the Summarian element in the AV, by the Late Mr. B.G. Tilak.

Thus AV, V-13 is a charm against snake poison-

षैमातस्य बभ्रोरपोदकस्य च । आलगी च बिलगी च उरुगुलाया ॥

Now, how such foreign words and ideas could creep into the AV. Samhita is a matter of discussion. Tilak thought that the Vedic people, prior to the second millenium before Christ might have come into contact with the Assayrians as neighbours or traders. The Summerian Element in the Atharvaveda. Karambelkar, App -C.

41-a. Origin of culltivated plants.

The Aryan tribes who dwelt originally to the North of Mesopotamia, it spread west-ward and south-ward driving out or subjugating Turanian and Dravidian nations. Then their speech and those which are derived from it in Europe and Hindustan, show that they 'knew and transported several species'.

De Candolle, p.19.

b. Vide Pt.Hemraj Sharma, pp. 71,76,83,84,86,96,104,114

c. Vide Harshe, intro.pp.xlvii-liii.

(43). Dr. Max Muller the eminent philologist of the East and the west has laid down as a rule which is nearer the truth and acceptable (44). Suffice it to say that the Vedic people had definitely come in contact with other civilizations both in and outside Indian continent, and there was a free exchange of thoughts and ideas. This is an established historical fact substantiated by some of the names of medicinal plants too. (44d) Is it then possible that such endeavouring society might have discarded or neglected the knowledge from the original inhabitants of this country ? Ne. On the other hand they utilised and assimilated such knowledge and incorporated the plant names after their sanskritization (45), for example :- 'Kshauma' (क्षौम) (46) has been mentioned in Samhitas (47) (संहिता) where it has been recommended for bandaging purpose. The critics of these books call

---

42. A fine net work. then, runs through the history of medicine from the thought of our most ancient ancestors upto the present time, a thought truly which I have indicated, exhibits truly interesting cycle. We know for instance, to cite one among many, eloquent examples, that throughout the first great period of civilization medicine was essentially ***Mediterranean*** cultivated almost exclusively in the countries that touched this sea. **History of Medi. pp. 7-8.**

43. Vide History of Medicine, pp. 84-85.

44. Max Muller is probably nearer the truth in saying that both Indian and Greek philosophies were autochthonic, and that neither of the two nations borrowed their thoughts from the other (Thomsons's Law of thought App. p. 285). As the human mind is alike everywhere. Introduction to Tarkasangraha of Annambhatta Published by Dr. S.K.Belwalkar,B.O.R.I. Poona 4.

44-a. The distinctive features of Ayurveda naturally have been developed on this soil by ancients, based on their own observations and the typical philosophies they had, as regards evolution and analysis of the universe and existence. Dwarkanath (110 Dwarkanath C. Intro. to Kayacikitsta, preface p. xiii.) observes- "It must be stated, that the basic Doctrines and concepts of this system, represented by 'Dosa-Dhatu-Mala Siddhanta' offers itself as existing conceptual scheme of medical science to the world."
Studies in Indian Medicinal Plants Used in Ayurveda Cathartics,
by G.S. Pendse and M.A. Ayengar, I.D.R.A. Poona, p. 35.

b. Some scholars like F.E. Pargiter have shown that 'the Aryas ' went out of India and settled in different parts of the earth, they are the originators of all early civilizations,

c. Ancient History and Culture, by C,M, Kulkurni Karnataka Publishing House Bombay 3. 1969 p. 36.

d. Vide F.N. 54-. p. ixl.

45-a. The Dravidian names of things connected with all the these arts are natives and not foreign (i.e. borrowed from Sanskrit). .....it will be most probably turn out that many Sanskrit words connected with these arts were borrowed from the Dravidian. Ayangar pp. 220-21.

(b). *Ghosha* (घोशा Santala) - Kosha, Koshataki (कोशातकी :) Dhn. Ni. p.96.
(c). *Banda* (बंदा Santala) Vanda, Vandaka (वन्दका) Dhn. Ni. p.153.
(d). *Haladika* (Dhn. Ni. p.17)Haridra.
(e). *Ranakadali*(रानकदली) Dhn. Ni. p. 149) Kashthakadali. (काष्ठकदली)
(f). *Nihidunga* (निहिडुंग) Dhn. Ni. p.57) Sunk (स्नुक).

Kshauma' as **'Atasi'** (48), (अतसी) but in the texts, both are mentioned differently as separate plants. According to Dhanvantarīya Nighaṇṭu also Kshauma and Atasī are not synonymous. (Dhn. ni. p.231).

In China, durable silk-like fibres are extracted from the plant Kshauma '(49) (क्षौम Botanical name -*Boehmeria nivea* Gaud) were known as 'Kshau -ma' (क्षौ- Kshau name of the plant and म Ma name of the extracted fibre). This Chinese name was sanskritized (modified in Sanskrit) as 'Kshauma' (क्षौम)- 'Kshuma' (क्षुमा)-Uma (उमा, the wife of the Lord Shiva). In course of time *'Kshauma'* was replaced for bandage purpose, by the plants *'Atasi* (अतसी), *'Nilika'* (नीलिका), *'Saṇa'* (शण) etc. This is why *'Atasi'* is given as an alernative name (or synonym) to *Kshauma* in later works. The original workers however, as evidenced from the texts were knowing that these are two separate plants.(49)a,

The history of' Aphukam' (अफुकम्) is also similar. This substance extracted by Greeks from the capsules of 'Khaskhas' plant *(Papaver somniferum* L), seems to have brought to India by Arabs in 2nd or 3rd century A.D. (50). It seems to be the 'horrible gum' described in the Bombay Gazeteers. (50). 'Aphu-am'(अफुअम्)in original Semetic (Hebrew?) (51)

(g). *Eranda* (एरंड) Rubu, Rubuka (Raj-Ni. pp.67, 68, Ca- Su. 4-4 Harshe, Intro. pp.xxxi; xiviii).

(h). *Alabu* (अलाबु) Gorakshatumbi (Dhn. Ni. p.40; Harshe xlviii)

(i) *Kuetimbari* - Dhanyakam (Dhn. Ni. p 82;) Kothamaticn. (Tam.), Kothumbari (Kan.), Grain plant. (Assyrian Vide Harshe, p. xiviii).

rj) *Asuri* (आसुरी) सर्षप (Dhn. Ni. p.146) Ca; Su, 27-101.

(k) *Taru* (तरु) Sumerian and Sanskrit the same name. (Harshe p. xlix).

(l) *Neema* (नीम) as above (ibid).

(m) *Arimeda* (अरिमेद) as above (ibid).

46-a. ' Kshuma ' (क्षौम). Su. Su. 18-16; 45-116, (Ghanekar).

b. ' Kshauma ' (क्षौम वसाना)Maitreya Sam. SKS. p. 24.

47 - ' Atasi ' (अतसी) Su. Su. 45-115.

47-a. कौशेयमुष्णं, क्षौमं तु शीतलम् ॥ Ashta, hr, Su, 29-57.

48. सतिला सातसी वीजा... । उमाऽयो (गुग्गुलु :...॥ उमा -अतसी ।
Cakra, Ca-Ci-25-51. 53.

48-b. क्षौमेत्यादि । क्षौमम् अतसीतन्तु ॥ Dulhan Su, Su, 18-16.

c. Besides cotton-cloth it was made also from fiberlike resham (रेशम silk) Bhashyakara (भाष्यकार) has called (named) it ' Kshaumavastra ' (क्षौमवस्त्र),It was prepared from ' Kshauma ' (क्षौम).Cloth was also made fcom 'Kausheya' (कौशेय The cocoon of a silk-worm-Apte).

It is difficult to tell that, when the cloth of ' Kshaum' (क्षौम) was begun in.
(Translated from Hindi). -Patanjli, p.319.

49-a. Vide Watt. Dict 'B' p. 472.

b. Vide Boehmeria nivea Gaud. -Uphof.

c. China-grass silk, vide De Candolle, pp. 146-148.

was modifided in Sanskrit as Aphukam (अफुकम्); and became the part of Indian medicine. (52) Many such examples can be cited, but we restrain from doing so as it would be out of scope of the present treatise. These(53) examples have been furnished only to substantiate and confirm the compiler's statement that knowledge about medicinal plants can be obtained and should be entertained even from cow-man and from every possible source (54).

Thus after explaining the purpose of this book, the main subject-matter starts with Ganadravyāvali (गणद्रव्यावलि).

---

50. Import.-Wine; like horrible gum; corol etc.etc.
The periplus of the Erythrean sea (AD. 240-260).
Bom. Gaz. Vol. I, p. i, App. p. 543.

51. Vide Watt. Dict. 'P' p. 24.

52. Vide Dhan. Ni. Chapter 6p. 232.

53. Vide Fote note 45 a, b supra.

54. Vide F.N. 36-a, b, c supra.

54-a. Example (Vide Dhn. Ni.) (Continued from p.xxxvi).
b. बाल्हीकम्- कुङ्कुमम (p. 95),हिङ्गु (77).
c. रोमकम् -उद्भिदम् (74). लोहम् (210).
d. तुरुष्क : -सिल्हक : (98).(Shilarasa),
e. पारशवम् - लोहम् (210).
f. बर्बरम - वोलम् (108).
g, दरदम्- हिङ्गुलम् (214).
h. चीनकम्-लोहम् (210). चीनक; प्रियङ्गु (225).corn.

CHAPTER II
THE CONSTITUTION

(i) *Ganadravyāvali.* (गणद्रव्यावलि).
(ii) *Paryāyanamadravyāvali.* (पर्यायनाम द्रव्यावलि).
(iii) *Relation of Rājanighanṭu with Dhanvantarīya Nighanṭu.*
(iv) *Dhavantariya Nighanṭu along with Rājanighanṭu.*
(v) *Ayurvedic Nighanṭus.*
(vi) *Similative terms and terms of Pharmacological actions.*
(vii) *Compiler's Method of Describing Plants.*

(i) *Gaṇadravyāvali.*

Ganadravyāvali (गणद्रव्यावलि) [has been divided into] consists of seven chapters (वर्ग महागण), These chapters are further divided into classes (गण) each comprising of several medicinal plants. Every class is recognised by and named after the first plant mentioned in it; e.g. Guḍūcyādi (गुडूच्यादि)- Guḍūcī and others, (Guḍūcī being the first mentioned plant),Śatapuṣpādī class (शतपुष्पादि वर्ग), etc, This portion of 7 chapters continues upto the page 19. [in the edition of Anandasharm Press, 1925].

The Gaṇadrvyāvalī (गणद्रव्यावलि) begins with the Guḍūcyādī chapter (गुडूच्यादि वर्ग, गुडूच्यादि महागण) (55) consisting of ten classes (गण) described in twelve stanzas (श्लोक). Each class contains medicinal plants having similar properties. The same system is followed in the remaining chapters.

The general plan and the method of describing the *classes* (गण) here, shows striking similarity with that of '*Suśruta Samhitā* (56) (सुश्रुत संहिता) (56)

(ii) ***Paryāyanāma Dravyāvali*** (पर्यायनाम द्रव्यावलि)

After the completion of 'Gaṇadravyāvalị (गणद्रव्यावलि) the compiler has taken again to write the ' Guḍūcyādī chapters' in the same order.

---

55. Vide Dhn. ni. p. 2.

56. Vide Su. Su. 38,

५६-a. परं मत्सकाशस्थे ६३३ नेवार संवल्लिखिते ताडपत्रीये सुश्रुत पुस्तके पुष्पिकाया पूर्वभागे सुश्रुते शल्यतन्त्रे इति उत्तरतन्त्रान्ते इति सौश्रुते म (स) होत्तरतन्त्रे चतुःषष्टितमोऽध्यायः अतो निघण्टुर्भविष्यति तदुत्तरगते निघण्टुभागे समाप्ते सौश्रुत्यां संहितायां म (स) होत्तरायां निघण्टु : समाप्तः इति लेखो दृश्यते ।
तेन सुश्रुतस्य वंशेन सांप्रदायिकेन वा सुश्रुताचार्येण सुश्रुतस्य पूर्वतन्त्रं संस्कृतमुत्तरतन्त्रं निघण्टु भागश्च योजितेत्यनुमीयते ॥ Acharya Yadavji, Su Su. Introduction p. 19.

Note :- From this reference quoted by A. Yadavji, it seems that there is included also a Nighanṭu in Newar (नेवार- नेपाल) MS of Suśruta (सुश्रुत).This Nighanṭu may be perhaps similar to Gaṇadravyāvali ' (गणद्रव्यावलि),the first part of Dhn. Ni. But as the MS. referred above is not before us we cannot come on any definite point of opinion.

This seemingly unreasonable repetition he clearly states at the end of ' Miśrakādi' (मिश्रकादि) chapter.

......For the benefit of the learned Vaidyas I write again the Gaṇadravyāvali with Paryāyanāma Dravyāvali ' (57).

Further he states "For the benefit of the people I write (कथ्यते मया) the Rasa, Vīrya and Vipāka (रस, वीर्य, विपाक) (58). In such wording the compiler of the further new arrangement has explained the reason of the repetition and this new arrangement of compiler was necessarily required here.

For though the broad outline of therapeutics is given in the 'Gaṇadravyāvli', it is not sufficient for the complete understanding and identification of medicinal plants. Pharmacological properties as well as alternative names (पर्यायनाम) are absolutely essential for that purpose. The *Paryāyanāma dravyāvali* (पर्यायनाम द्रव्यावलि) has been added to overcome these shortcomings of 'Gaṇadravyāvali'. The classes, sub-classes and plants (with their morphological and pharmacological properties) occur here in the same order as in 'Gaṇadravyāvali'. This compilation, however, is not entitled by a separate heading; suggesting that it is merely a supplement of 'Gaṇadravyāvali'. *We have coined the name 'Paryāyanāma dravyāvali'* (पर्यायनाम द्रव्यावलि), for this compilation to distinguish it from *'Gaṇadravyāvali'* (गणद्रव्यावलि), and to faciliate the reference work. These two words - *'Ganadravyāvali'* and *'Paryāyanāma dravyāvali'* have been freely used in the present treatise, as also mentioned in our *proforma* (ग्रंथरचना पद्धति).

'Paryāyanāma dravyāvali' is thus the compilers' own compilation. He has described the morphology and pharmacology of plants in stanzas which are serially numbered,. Although the term Paryāyanāmadravyāvali is not used, the compiler has differentiated the plants included in it by adopting a peculiar numbering system. There are two sets of serial numbers (59). The plants in 'Gaṇadravyāvāli' have serial numbers before the heading names, as 1. Guḍūcī (गुड्ची). 2. Ativiṣā (अतिविषा), 3. Mūrvā (मूर्वा), 10. Kaṭukā (कटुका) 25. Śāliparṇi (शालिपर्णी), 86. Balā (बला), etc; while the plants in 'Paryāyanamadravyāvali ' have serial numbers after their name, as- Moraṭā (1), Yāsaḥ (2), Somavalkaḥ (3), Kapaṭam. (14)Vijayā (24) Rāsnā (82), etc. These serial numbers can be called as *pre-numbers*

57. हितायवैद्य विदुषां द्रव्यावल्यां प्रकाशितम् । गणद्रव्यावलि ह्युक्ता सं (स) योगा सहमात्रया ॥ पर्यायनामान्युच्यन्ते गुडूच्यादेर्यथाक्रमम् ॥ ४ ॥ Dhn. Ni. P. 7

57-a. Vide FN. 65 infra.

58. रसवीर्यविपाकादि द्रव्याणां कथ्यते मया ॥ Dhn. Ni. p. 7 v.D. 3

59. Vide EPP. 3-7.

(Gaṇadravyāvali) and *Post numbers* (Paryāyanāmadravyāvali) respectively, the same system being adhered to, in the pages of this treatise.

One more thing, however, should be taken into account in this respect. The editor [Purandare] has incorporated the additional plants from Raja-Nighaṇṭu along with *'Paryāyanāma dravyavāli.'* These plants have been fitted in the second series bearing post-name serial numbers (post-numbers). This is evidently not the compilers arangement and will be discussed at length in following pages. (vide iv infra).

(iii) ***Relation of Rājanighaṇṭu with Dhanvantarīya nighaṇṭu.***

To make this ancient treatise more comprehensive and useful and perhaps to facilitate easy understanding, the editor (Purandare) has incorporated selectd medicinal plants from Rāj-Nighaṇṭu showing similalrity to those of 'Dhanvantarīya Nighaṇṭu '. While making these additions due precaution has been taken to avoid any confusion by quoting the references of plant names. Moreover, these plants do not bear separate heading names nor serial numbers.

An instance can be taken from 'Guḍūcyādi' chapter I (गुडूच्यादि प्रथमो वर्गः). After the completion of the original description (Dhanvantari's) of 'Guḍūchī ' (गुडूची) there is a verse - 'Guḍūcyādi III chapter of Rajanighaṇṭu' (राजनिघण्टौ गुडूच्यादि तृतीयो वर्गः) - followed by the Rajanighaṇṭu's description of 'Gūḍūcī' (60). In this fashion Rājanighaṇṭu's plants have been recorded and described under each heading. There are only few instances e.g. Vijayā (विजया)(P. 31) where Rājanighaṇṭu's descriptions are not added in this manner.

'Paryāyanāmadravyāvali' relating to 'Guḍūcyādi' chapter. (गुडूच्यादि वर्ग) terminates by 'Earṇḍa' (एरंड) on page (67). Below this the plant 'Vrisamedhā'; (वृषमेधा) is described. This, being out of the (Guḍūcyādi) chapter, is designated as 'Vargetara' (वर्गेतर) (61).

'Miśrakadi' (मिश्रकादि) seven chapters are dealt with in the same manner and are completed on page 317. Finally, the pages 435-441 are concerned with 'Dhanvantariya Nighaṇṭu's' Ekarth, Dvyartha koṣa (एकार्थ द्व्यर्थ कोश),

(iv) ***Dhanvantarīya Nighaṇṭu along with Rājanighaṇṭu.***

The Plants of 'Rāja-nighaṇṭu' not occurred in 'Dhanvantạrīya nighaṇṭu'.

(Non-Dhanvantarīya plants).

We have already discussed why and how the 'Rājanighaṇṭu's plants are incorporated along with those of 'Dhanvantariya nighaṇṭu'. Besides

60. Vide Dhn. Ni. p. 8.
61. Vide Dhn. ni. p..68.

this, the editor (Purandare) has also included 'Rāja-nighaṇṭu's plants, which are not in accordance with the headings of 'Dhanvantarīya nighaṇṭu'. *with separate headings.* While doing so, however, he has taken the precaution of including only such plants having some similalrity -Morphological or pharmacological - to the original plants of Dhanvantari. For example , Somavalka (सोमवल्क 3) has been given under Dhanvantarīya's heading 'Khadira' (खदिर 7). The post-number (3) of the Somavalka clearly denotes that it belongs to *Paryāyanāmadravyāvali;* there is also Rāja-nighaṇṭu's reference of plant accomodated along with Dhanvantari's heading. It is indicated by mentioning the name and chapter of Rājnighaṇṭu [Page 12]. After this there are four more plants bearing different headings and separate serial numbers, namely, Tāmrakanṭaka (ताम्रकंटक,8), Viṭkhadira (विट्खदिर 9), Ari (अरि 10) and Khadira (खदिर Catachu 11). These don't belong to Dhanvantari's, Paryāyanāmadravyāvali', but are *solely of Rāja-nighaṇṭu.* These are clearly distinguished from both the 'Dravyāvalis' by separate heading and different serial numbers.

Now the question arises as to why these plants are incorporated here, especially when they are not related to the heading of 'Dhanvantarīya Nighaṇṭu'. But the arrangement is not totally useless or unreasonable. They have been included probably with two objects, viz, (1) Similarity in morphology and (2) Similarity in pharmacology. Thus these four plants described under the heading 'Khadira' (खदिर) are of similar morpholigical characters while those included under the heading 'Pāṣānabheda' (पाषाणभेद) [page 36] may be similar in pharmacological action.

Probably 'Pāṣāṇabhed' (पाषाणभेद) is a medicinal stone* similar to that of Opal (ओपल). We had occasions to see such stones named as 'Ahira' (अहिरा) in Marathi and Yunani -which were used in the diseases of the eye like corneal ulcers. Dhanvantarīya Nighaṇṭu and Raja Nighaṇṭu describe it by the terms 'Nagabhid' (नगभिद्) and 'Śilāgarbhajā' (शिलगर्भजा).Chemically, it is mainly the Carbonate of Iron and Calcium. [Abhi. Bu. D.,page 153]. But 'Vaṭapatrī' (वटपत्री) given under this heading is plant-the leaves of which somewhat resemble to those of Banyan (वट), *Ficus bengalensis* L.

A kind of wood (root) is available in the market under the name 'Pāṣaṇabheda' (पाषाणभेद) . Some writers have identified it as *Bergenia ligulata* Engle., syn. *Saxifraga ligulata* Wall.

In this way the editor (Purandare) has incorported Rāja Nighaṇṭu's additional plants under different headings at some places. Their different headings (and Sr. number) clearly indicate that they don't belong to 'Paryāyanāmadravyāvali' .This arrangement, we feel, is useful (and reasonable also) in overcoming the controversy regarding some medicinal plants.

* Presently, *saxifraga ligulata* Wall. is accepted as Pāṣāṇbabheda. S. D. Kamat.

As the plants of 'Rajnighaṇṭu' have been incorporated along with those of 'Dhanvantarīya Nighaṇṭu', the book is aptly named 'Rājanighaṇṭu sahita Dhanvantarīya Nighaṇṭu' (राज निघण्टु सहित धन्वन्तरीय निघण्टु) (62). After such inclusion the remaining portion of Rājnighaṇṭu has been added in the form of appendix under the heading of 'Pariśiṣṭam'(परिशिष्टम्, pages 319 - 434), which terminates by the 23rd chapter of Rājanighaṇṭu with Ekārtha, Dvyartha Koṣās (एकार्थ, द्वयर्थ कोश).

We have restricted our study only to the Dhanvantari's Medicinal plants. The plants of Rājanighaṇṭu not occuring in 'Paryāyanāmadravyāvali' are not considered in this treatise.

So far we have discussed the Editor's (Purandare) arrangment of the treatise, now let us see what scheme and method Dhanvantariya Nighaṇṭu has adopted in the description of medicinal plants.

(V) ***Ayurvedic Nighaṇṭu*** (आयुर्वेदिक निघण्टु).

Ayurvedic Nighaṇṭu (निघण्टु) is not merely a dictionary. Some authorities use the term 'lexicon' as its synonym. The term may be appropriate for the compilations like Amarakoṣa (अमरकोश), Hālayudha (हलायुध), Śivakośa (शिवकोश), etc.,but it falls short to understand the construction of Nighaṇṭus. Dr Dymocks 'Pharmacographia Indica', having an arrangment nearly similar to that of Nighaṇṭus, is some times named as 'Materia medica' this term too, seems to be unfit to describe the particular patterm of Nighaṇṭus compilation.In Materia Medica prime importance is attributed to the pharmacological properties of drugs(63). To understand the arrangement in the Nighaṇṭus, we have to follow the meaning as denoted by the arrangment in 'Yāska's Nirukta' (यास्क निरुक्त). It is, therefore, necessary to coin a new term in English, perfectly and completely appropriating the term 'Nighaṇṭu'.

Ayurvedic Nighaṇṭu (निघण्टु) is a compilation of drugs with their pharmacological actions on the body according to "Tridoṣa system" (त्रिदोष पध्दति, order or disorder of three humours) and a short account of their therapeutics known from the continuous ancient tradition. It consists of description of the drugs in morphological terms followed by its properties and pharmacological actions. Such a compilation, based on the traditional doctrine is known as Ayurvedic Nighaṇṭu.

vi. *Similative terms and terms of Pharmacological Action*
(रुपम्, उपमा, गुणज्ञापक पदानि च)

The compilers of Nighaṇṭus describe a drug by similative terms followed by the terms of pharmacological actions. The use of similative terms in describing the morphology of herbs(रुप,उपमाज्ञापक पद) is a special feature of Nighaṇṭus. The nature of this terminology and its utility in identification and confirmation of medicinal plants, is explained

62. Vide EPP. 1,2

63. Materia medica is the science which deals with the sourcses descriptions and preparation of drugs -Dr. Ghosh, p.2.

elsewhere in this treatise (Vide Appx. B-4).

Once the plant is introduced by similative terms, the Nighaṇṭus describe their pharmacological actions according to the 'tridosh system'(त्रिदोष पध्दति), tastes of saps (मधुरादि रस), active principle (वीर्य), change after complete digestion (विपाक) and the pharmacological qualities (गुण- उष्ण, शीत, गुरु, लघु इ.). This is followed by the specific diseases and disorders on which a particular drug is effective.

In this manner every drug is described by the similative and the pharmacological terms

The question here arises - 'What is the necessity of giving the pharmacological actions after describing the drug in morphological and similative terms ? The question apparently seems to be resonable, but the situation is quite differeent. The modern science of botany has reached much perfection as compared to that in the ancient times, for easy understanding and identification of any plant. Today any plant can be identified with help of various disciplines like morphology, taxonomy and anatomy, without considering its pharmacological action. It was not so at that time. It therefore seems likely that the similative terms and pharmacological actions, etc. have been suppliemented to facilitate the understanding and identification of plants. Many centuries have passed after the compilation of these Nighaṇṭus. At present we do not understand the method and terminology in its full and exact sense(64). Perhaps due to interrupted tradition or otherwise, many technical terms might have lost their original meaning and sense.

These difficulties are not completely removed as yet. Consequently, we have to take a longer course in identification and confirmation of plant. We have to determine any plant with certainty only after correlating the similative and morphological terms in the texts, the traditional information available from the eminent Ayurvedic physicians and the implied meanings of the names and descriptive terms. Not only etymological interpretation is necessary, but sometimes we have to read between the lines. And this is not all. Before drawing any definite conclusions, we must consider the desired pharmacological action of a drug as indicated by the compiler. To sum up an overall judgement free from any bias, is absolutely essential for the correct identification and confirmation of Ayurvedic plants.

We hope the couple of examples given below would make the point clear.

---

64. I am very solicious to give Indian plants there true Indian application because I am fully persued that Linnaeous himself would have adopted them, had he been known the learned and the ancient languages of this country. For I am doubting the great importance, for languages expire as nation decay, and the true sense of many apilative in every dead language must be lost in the course of ages.

Sir W. Jone's Work Vol.II. P.47, London 1799

(1) *'Yavatiktā'* (यवतिक्ता) - The herb Yavatikatā mentioned in *Caraka Samhitā* चरक संहिता, कल्प 11) has been identified by some authorities as *Ipomea hederacea* (Linn.) Jacq. The *Bhāṣyakāra* (भाष्यकार), however, suggest that it is the same drug as *' Kālamegha* (कालमेघ; अ. हृ. को. सू. 15) But *Kālamegha* has been botanically confirmed as *Andrographis paniculata* Nees. The two plants are entirely different from each other belonging to different plant families (कुल)- *Convolvulaceae* and *Aacnthaceae* respectively. Here arises the difficulty which of these two plants is *'Yavatiktā'* of *Carakācārya* (चरकाचार्य). In this situation, we have to take into consideration the pharmacological properties and action of the drug. Caraka (चरक) has described it as purgative (विरेचक) while that of Bhāṣyakar is not purgative. It is antipyretic (ज्वरहारक).As *Ipomea hederacea* is purgative and not *Andrographis paniculata;* the former plant should be accepted as 'Yavatiktā' of Caraka.

2) *Tilvaka* (तिल्वक) Tilvaka has been described by Susruta (सुश्रुत) as purgative (रेचक, तिल्वक, अधोभाग हराणि. Su. Su. 39-3). In Dhanvantariya Nighaṇṭu it has been mentioned as *'Kaṣāya'* (कषाय). *'Rūkṣa'* (रूक्ष) and *'grāhī'* (ग्राही astringent.) The botanical name of Tilvaka of Dhanvantarīya has been confirmed as *Symplocos racemosa* Roxb., which is not having purgative properties. Now the question ariees - *'which is the 'Tilvaka' having the purgative property ? desired by Suśrut ?'* Not only that Dhanvantari's Tilvaka' is non-purgative, but on the contrary, it is used in diarrhoea (अतिसार भेषजम्). The Editor of Abhidhan mañjarī (अभिधानमञ्जरी). has pointed out that 'Tilvaka-lodhra' (तिल्वकलोध्र) is not desired here, but another plant having 'similar leaves (लोध्रपत्रकाकार), vide Abhi. Manj., p. 19). Prof. Balavansingji has suggested *Wendlandia exserta* DC. for Tilka mentioning that its bark has purgative properties. (Balvantsingji Bihar (247). In Śrauta Sutra (श्रौत सूत्र) also 'Tilaka' (तिलक) and 'Tilvaka' are separately mentioned. (श्रौ. को. सं. page 792).

(vii) ***Compiler's Method of Description :***

(1) The compiler has described the medicinal plants one by one in serial order. The principle drug-names have been used for heading (heading names) in the Ānandāśram edition, e.g., Guḍūcī (गुड़ूची), Mūrvā (मूर्वा),etc. This is followed by the morphological and similative terms. Moreover, the suitable names (synonyms) from other Ayurvedic texts (Samhitās) and Vedic literature have been provided. Finally the properties and pharmacological actions are described. This method of description greatlyfacilitates the identification and understanding of the traditional plants.

(2) Sometimes under one heading two or three plants are included with their pharmacological actions. This is clearly indicated by the

terms like अन्या (other) e.g. 'Guḍūchī' and 'Kandaguḍūcī' (गुडूची, कन्दगुडूची). In some cases, however, two plants have been noted giving the pharmacological properties of only one e.g., among Syonāka (स्योनाक) and Ṭiṇṭuka (टिण्टुक), the compiler has given the pharmacological action of : 'Ṭiṇṭuka' only.

(3) At some places, out of two plants given under one heading, only one is described in pharmacological terms as in (2) above, but the other plant has been dealt with under separate heading. For instance, under 'Dhanvayāsa' (धन्वयास), 'Yāsa' (यास) has been mentioned without giving its pharmcological properties. Further 'Yāsa' (यास) has been treated separately giving its pharmacological action. The same way 'Mūrvā' and 'Moraṭa' are mentioned together giving the action of only 'Mūrvā', followed' by this 'Moraṭā' which is described once again.

(4) In certain cases, two plants are not compiled under one heading, but according to tradition and practice it seems that there are two separate plants in actual usage; e.g. 'Aśmantakā' and 'Amlapatraka' (अम्लपत्रक). We have included such plants at suitable places.

(5) Description of a plant, frequently, consists of contradictory terms, indicating that there are two or three separate plants. In 'Mūrvā'(मूर्वा), for example, two terms are used 'Madhurasā' (मधुरसा) and 'Tejanī' (तेजनी) which are contradictory. Etymologically, 'Mūrvā' means that the fiber which is used for binding purpose and for making girdle of Kśatriyās.(मूर्वा-बंधने). In different regions different plants are used for the preparation of strings and are locally called as Mūrvā. 'Corasnāyu' (चोरस्नायु) of Dalhaṇa (डल्हण) (*Sansiviera* sp. family Liliaceae) is utilised for binding all over the world. In Maharashtra 'Moravela' (मोरवेल) Marathi; (*Clematis* spp. family *Ranunculaceae)* is generally known as Mūrvā. Thus, Mūrvā itself is a debatable plant, which has been cited here as an instance. There are other contradictory plants too.

(6) The names of Gods and Goddesses many times denote the extraordinary qualities of those plants. e.g. 'Suvarcalā' (सुवर्चला, वर्चस-तेज), 'Sūryakāntā' (सूर्यकान्ता), 'Sarasvatī (सरस्वती, Goddess of speech), 'Swayambhuvā (स्वयंभुवा) self-grown etc.

(7) Sometimes the plant names are suggestive of their flowering time : e.g. 'Mādhaveṣṭa' (माधवेष्टा),Vasanta dūtī (वसंतदूती)-flowering in the spring season; Śāradā (शारदा) -flowering in the 'Śarada' season (September - October), etc.

(8) Occasionally, the names of plants denote the supposed affinity or liking of deities; e.g. 'Gaṇeśakusumam'(गणेशकुसुमम्)-the Lord Gaṇeśa is very fond of these flowers;.'Caṇḍīkusumam' (चण्डीकुसुमम्) the flowers are used for worshiping the Goddess Chaṇḍi (चण्डी).

(9) In certain descriptions some symbolic names of Gods and Goddesses are used. This is so in the cases of Spṛkka' (स्पृक्का, Dhn ni. p. 108) and Murā (मुरा. 3.27, p. 109) where all the terms are the names of Gods. Here, the morpholocical terms are not adequate or enough for the identification of the plants. In such cases one has to rely mainly on the traditional knowledge and usage of the plants concerned. Such plants might be non-Indian.

(10) There are a few instances in which the exact meaning of the descriptive terms (or names) cannot be understood. Under 'Śāliparṇī' (शालिपर्णी) there is a verse- (आलकं, पालकं, दग्धं, सबलं + बोटं)- the meaning of which is beyond the power of our interpretation and understanding. Moreover this 'Śāliparṇī' (शालिपर्णी) seems to be quite different from the generally accepted 'Sāliparni' namely *Desmodium* sp., *(*fam.). *Leguminosae)*

(11) Rājanighaṇṭu's plants recorded under Dhanvantarī's heading names (by the editor Purandare) are not always the same or even similar. For example Rājanighaṇṭu's 'Pṛsniparṇī ' (पृश्निपर्णी) has been correlated with and included under the heading name 'Pṛṣhṭiparṇī' (पृष्टिपर्णी), but 'Dhanvantari's Pṛṣṭiparṇī is altogether different from the former. Both these plants, however,are recorded in the original Ayurvedic texts and Vedic literature (संहिता ग्रंथ) (66).

(12) Rarely, the compiler has included the plants of different species under one heading, perhaps indicating the difference of opinion regarding the included plants. In such cases, he has made it clear by using the term 'anyacca' (अन्यच्च) before such plant names. Thus, under the heading -Pratarirka Kšauma (प्रतरिर्क-क्षौम), the term अन्यच्च is used followed by 'Atasi' (अतसी), which is altogether different from the former (Dhanvantari Nighaṇṭu, p. 231).

(13) It is also found at places that Rājanighaṇṭu's plants are not recorded under some heading names of Dhanvantari, e.g. Vijayā (विजया,Dhanvantari Nighaṇṭu, p.31) and Kusumbham (कुसुम्भम् Dhanvantari Nighaṇṭu p. 232).

We hope this discussion and clarification would suffice to give a general idea of the compiler's method of dealing with the medicinal plants.

The original book comprises nonbotanical drugs like 'salts from the second chapter (शतपुष्पादि वर्ग) onwards. Suvarṇādi chapter (सुवर्णादि वर्ग) consists of drugs derived from metals, minerals, urine, liquids, oils, etc. As our study is restricted to the botanical drugs and that too of the 'Guḍūcyādi' chapter (गुडूच्यादि वर्ग), only the medicinal plants are treated here, excluding the above mentioned non-botanical drugs. The main object of the present study is the *botanical confirmation* of Dhanvantari's medicinal plants.

CHAPTER III

STUDY OF AYURVEDIC NIGHANṬUS

(i) *Method of Studying The Nighanṭus.*

(ii) *Assistance of Modern Botany.*

(i) *Method of Studying the Nighanṭus.*

The study of Nighanṭus necessitates the understanding of its peculiar method and terminology -particularly the similtive and pharmacological terms. We have already referred to this point earlier; and the readers are advised to see Appendix B-4 for morphological and similtive terms.

A working knowledge of Ayurvedic texts (आयुर्वेदीय संहिता ग्रंथ) would be much useful to understand the pharmacological terms. The beginners in the subject are recommended to aquaint themselves with the commentary of Suśruta Samhitā (सुश्रुत संहिता) in Hindi by Dr. Ghanekar. The chapters 38 to 43 and 46 of Susṛuta Samhitā are especially useful to understand, the Tridoṣa theory (त्रिदोष पद्धति), the terms of pharmacological actions used in Ayurveda and the names of diseases.

For the correct and traditional meaning of morphological terms, other Nighaṇṭus (65) and Sanskṛit Koshas (संस्कृत कोश) will be helpful. Out of the various Sanskrit Koshas, the Amarakosha (अमरकोश) should be given the prime importance, as, according to its critic- Sarvānanda (शर्वानंद) it has followed the traditions of Vararuci (वररुचि) (66) and Vyāḍī (व्याडी) hence preserving the old traditions and notions in a better way.

There are about half a dozen commentaries on Amarakośha (67), but that of Kśiraswāmī (क्षीरस्वामी) serves our purpose the best. It is nearer

---

६५-a पर्यायाः निघण्टुज्ञानात् देशभाषासंस्काराच्च किञ्चित् ज्ञायन्ते ।

b. The other Nighantuas are :-

1-Paryāyaratnamālā (पर्यायरत्नमाला) or Ratnamālā (रत्नमाला) of Mādhavakara, author of Rugvinscaya (रुग्विनिश्चय) 8th or 9th century.

2. Paryāyamuktāvalī (पर्यायमुक्तावली) or Muktāvalī (मुक्तावली).

3. Nighaṇṭuseṣa (निघण्टुशेष) of Hemachandra.

4. Abhidhānaratnamālā (अभिधानरत्नमाला)

5. Madanavinoda (मदनविनोद) 1374 A.D.

6. Sabdachandrikā (शब्दचंद्रिका) of Carkrapāṇidutta.

7. Dakśināmūrti Nighaṇṭu. 8- Dravyamuktāvali (द्रव्यमुक्तावली).

9. Paryāyārṇava (पर्यायार्णव).

The above references are collected from Gode Vol. I, p. 158.

c-Harshe Shivakosha Introduction , p. xv.

d. Laghu Nighaṇṭu App, C.

66. Dr. Ketkar p. 314.

to and correlating with Dhanvantarīya Nighaṇṭu as evidenced by the references of the latter in the former. Of the other commentaries those of Bhānujī Dīkśit (भानुजी दीक्षित) and Maheśwara (महेश्वर) are noteworthy. Bhānujī Dīkśit has provided the etymology of plant names while Maheśwara has incorporated the synonyms of plants in Indian languages. Śivakoś (शिवकोश) edited by Dr. Harshe and especially its preface is also valuable for the correlation and confirmation of plants. 'Dr.Pendse's Glossary of Vagbhatta's plants and M.K. Vaidya's Aṣṭ.hr.kośa are also useful for confirmation of plants. In Vaidya's kośa and in Aur. O. Ni. are included regional names of plants. Many a medical plants have been mentioned in Atharva veda (अथर्व वेद), in Sūtra book (सूत्र ग्रंथ), Samskāra book (संस्कार ग्रंथ) etc. (67a) All these are more or less useful. The utility of the Śounakīya Sākha (शौनकीय शाखा) of Atharvaveda with its Kauśika Sūtra (कौशिक सूत्र) with Sāyaṇa (सायण) in the comparative study of Athervavedic and Ayurvedic medicinal plants cannot be over emphasized.

Various commentaries and Ayurvedic texts especially those of Dalhaṇa (डल्हण) on Suśruta Samhitā (सुश्रुत संहिता), Dipikā (दीपिका) on Sārṅgadhara Samhitā (शार्ङगधर संहिता) and commentay of Rasa paddhati (रसपध्दति) are useful in this subject. From these commentaries we get current regional names of traditional plants in use.

'Abhidhānmañjarī' (अभिधानमञ्जरी) is very useful for the knowledge of plants in South India. This seems to have been compiled before 14th century. This great work as well as commentaries on Aṣṭaṅg hriadaya (अष्टांग हृदय) by Dāspandit (दासपण्डित) and Sivasena (शिवसेन) have been written in Devanāgari (देवनागरी) script, but the regional plant names are given in Malyālam (मल्यालम्) script. We have got some of these names in Abhidhana Mañjari transliterated into roman and Devanāgarī script. More work in this line would be a boon to future workers.

Among the modern works in English, the books written by Dr.Mukherji, Dr.Chopra and Handa, Mr.Hill and Mr.Nelson are very

67. Some commentaries on Amarakośa (अमरकोश).

a. Bhānuji Dīkśita 1630 A.D. son of Bhaṭṭojī Dīkṣita (1575 - 1650 A.D.) Gode I pp. 49,52-53.

b. Subhūtichandra, a commentator Amarkoṣa, Gode I-217 1062-1172,

c. Kśīraswāmī Second half of the eleventh century. Gode I. 160

d. Sarvananda. Tikāsarvaswa on Amarkoṣa He used 10 previous commentaries on Amarkosa in A.D.1159. Gode I 184, 219.

e. Lingabhatta. Commentrator on Amarkośa. Gode I 220.

f. Padāratha candrikā of Bṛhaspatī (बृहस्पती) surname Rāyamukuṭamanī (रायमुकुटमणि) was composed in 1431 A.D. it is based on 16 earlier commentaries on Amarkosa - Gode I, 49.

g. Maheśwara-- Tīkā on Amarakośa.

67 a. Vide FN. 36- a p. xxxiii.

useful. Special mention must be made here of Dr.Roxburgh and Dr.Dymock, as plants descibed by them are much similar to those in Ayurvedic nighaṇṭus. A Great and voluminous work by Dr. Watt, namely, 'Dictionary of Economic products of India' is extreemly valuable as a reference of work. Dr. Watt has given modern, regional, tribal names of plants and the references of the plants available at that time. Moreover he has tried to confirm the plants with historical and philological background. He has also incorporated the opinions, experiments and experiences of other eminent authorities in various fields. Another noteworthy work is that by Kirtikar and Basu (Indian Medicinal Plants) its special featuttre being the botanical illustrations of medicinal plants, appealing to the biginners in this subject. There are sevaral other illustrted books published by the Europeans, but those are not easily available to the common reader.

Paṇḍit Bhagīrath's work is important from the point of view of correlating Ayurvedic plant names with those in regional languages. Other praiseworthy workers in the field are Vd. Bapalalji (बापालालजी), Dr. V.G. Desai (डॉ. देसाई), Dr. Priyavrat Sharma (प्रियव्रत शर्मा), Dr. Dwivedi and Dr.Balwant Sinhaji (बलवंत सिंहजी).Balwant Simhaji has discussed some controversial and unidentifiable plants, suggesting names for them. Abhinava Būtī Darpan (अभिनव बूटी दर्पण) comprises several articles by different contributors on one and the same plant with some of the figures. The students and workers in this field are requested and advised to refer to the comprehensive bibliography furnished at the end of this treatise. What is intended here in the last few pages is to give the general idea and guidelines of methodology and references to the biginners.

For the overall and resonable judgement in the identification as well as confirmation of plants, one has to take into account many other coniderations and evidences from the related fields of knowledge(68) The plants described in Ayurvedic Nighaṇṭus are not all from the Indian subcontinent. As Nighaṇṭus have incorporated medicinal plants right from the time of Vedas, it is but natural that some of these are non Indian(69) occuring in the non Indian regions and people with whom the Vedic people came in contact either as neighbours or traders(70), it is quite resonable to believe that knowledge of medicinal plants in these regions and of those people was incorporated in the Vedic and nonvedic literature(71)

The collection of the Nighaṇṭus might have been enriched by the

68. De Candole, pp. 23,25, 27.
69. Vide F.N. 54-a supra p.xxxix.
70. Vide F.N. 40,41 supra p.xxxv.
71-a. सुपर्णो जातः ...। तदासुरी युधा जीता ... ।२। AV.i-2; i-24.
b. ..Āsuri or Śyāma ... This remedy was in possession of an Asura woman.
-Dr.Shende. AV. vi -108; iii-2, 3.
c. पिप्पली ... । असुरास्त्वाऽन्यखनन ...३ ॥ असुरः पूर्वेदेवाः ।
Sāyaṇa (सायण) AV. vi - 109

other way also. According to historical and anthropological evidences, it is a well established fact that ancient Indian people had come in close contact with Assyrians (असुर) Egyptians (इजिप्त), Israilis (इस्रायल) etc. The latter had established not only commercial but also cultural relations with India. We have sufficient ground to state that some of them had setteled in India. There was a confluence of different people and cultures, so much so that some Assyrians (असुर) had aquired the position of 'Devas' (देव) in the Indian culture(72).

We have already discussed this point earlier. It is but natural that during that period under such circumstances there was a great flux of exchange of thoughts, knowledge and experiences. The literature on this subject, therefore proves useful in the confirmation of some plants; from this view point the preface to Śivakośa by Dr. Harshe (शिवकोश - हर्षे), "Atharva vedic civilization" by Dr. Karambelkar, "Religon and Philosophy of Athrvaveda' by Dr.Shende and the preface of Kāsyapa samhitā (in Sanskrit) by Paṇḍit Hemraj Sharma are very useful. This vast literary province abounds with innumerable manuals, treatises and compiled by Indian and western authorities. It is advisable to avail of such literature, wherever pertinent to remove the controversies regarding the identification of plants.

Uptill now we have explained the nature, methods and direction of literary research. Howsoever important and necessary it may be, the literary knowledge alone will not suffice. For understanding, identification and confirmation of plants, practical study is absolutely necessary. It necessitates the study of botanical sciences.

(ii) *Assistance of modern Botany.*

Botany is a tremendously vast science of nature. It is divided and further subdivided into several branches. But the more important to our purpose are Morphology, Taxonomy and Phyto-geography.

1. MORPHOLOGY : Deals with the structure and form of plants and plant organs.

2. TAXONOMY : This is a science of identification, classification and nomenclature of plants. All the known plants in the world are named and arranged according to a system of classification. There are

72-a. कौरव्य माण्डुक्याभ्यां च कौरव्य माण्डुकयोरासुरेरुपसंख्यानं कर्तव्यम् ॥
आसूरीयः कल्पः 4-1-19 वा. पं 44 Patanjali, p. 442

b. Hymns in Rv., where in Asura is used , not in the sense of demons but in the sense of god or superior god. Asura deites must have been the deities of India at one time. Otherwise the name 'Purva deva' for the older gods of the Asuras cannot be explained.

Resume page 48, Ketakar

several systems of classification, out of which that of *Bentham* and *Hooker* is of great practical value - it is followed in the countries of British Commonwealth including India and is followed in this treatise also.

Herbarium (plural herbaria) is the collection of herbarium specimens.

A flora is a book comprising a list of all known plants in a particular area, arranged in a classified way.

Botanical gardens are another source of plant study, where you can observe and study living plants.

3. ECOLOGY : Is the branch of Biology dealing with interrelationship between oraganisms and their environment

4. PHYTOGEOGRAPHY or *Plant geography* : It comprises the study of geographical distribution of plants their original homes and endemism.

Our basic books of Ayurvedic study are the original Ayurvedic texts. (classical books).

These basic books mainly composed in the region of Uttar Pradesh ,(73) Punjab and Sindh, are not compiled by single author in a particular period(74). On the contrary it is a collection of knowledge by a number of persons, a traditional inheritage assembled during a considerable long span of time.

The compiler of Nighaṇṭus were inhabitants of the Indo gangetic plains. They were followers of the traditional culture and had collected the knowledge of plants known to them traditionally along with the plants which were in their surroundings. As this society spread out in other parts of the country, book - described traditional plants became unavailable and hence to some extent forgotten (75). To overcome this difficulty they discovered plants from their surroundings, having similar medicinal properties. Though these plants were not exactly similar to the original plants they had to subsitute them due to unaviodable circumstances. This is one of the reason why the different varieties and species of plants are used in different regions of India.

In such diverse conditions, there arises a difficulty of how to obtain the knowledge of, and to confirm the book descibed plant.

In such multiliguistic nation like India the situation becomes still worse. It is therefore obvious that most of the plants have many local and regional names. This is a great barrier in collecting informationa about

73-a. तदाभूतेष्वनुक्रोशं पुरस्कृत्य महर्षयः । समेताः पुण्यकर्माणा पार्श्वे हिमवतः शुभे ॥ Ca. Su. 1-7.

b. औषधीनां पराभूमि हिमावाञ्शैलसत्तमः । Ca.Ci.1-38

74. Vide FN.(17). p.xxxiv.

75. Vide Ayur. Patrika 10-1968.p.513.

5

the desired plants. Let us examplify by citing a concrete example of Guḍūcī (गुड्ची) of the compiler. It is known as 'Guḷavela' (गुळवेल) in Marathi and 'Giloya' (गिलोय) in Hindi. We have actually observed and studied the plant of Maharashtra and confirmed it as Guḍūcī of the compiler. But if we go to a Bengali Ādivāsī (aboriginal people) and ask him to bring Guḍūcī. he will bring a different plant known to him as Guḍūcī. Morphologically it will not exactly correlate or match with our Guḍūcī.. This is because another plant from the same genus (गोत्र) is used as Gūḍucī in that region. In Madras state (Tamilnadu) we come across third variety of Guḍūcī ! (See Guḍūcī.).

The only way out to overcome these and such other difficulties is to take the assistance of Botany. There should be some arrangement so that any plant should have only one authentic name all over the world. This problem can be solved only by taxonomy. with the help of botanical names.

The following points will emphasize the importance and utility of botanical sciences in this subject :-

(1) There is one and only one botanical name for each plant. This name is understood by the botanical world.

(2) Once the botanical name is understood, the characters, uses, geographical distribution, localities of the plant and regional names can be rapidly obtained by referring suitable 'floras'.

(3)In many cases if a regional name of the plant is known its botanical eqiuivallent can be determined.

(4) With the help of botanical names we are in a position to understand the history of the plants and their geographical distribution at present as well in the past.

(5) Certain drugs, being quite similar in their gross (macroscopic) morphology, have been mentioned as one and the same plant by some compilers; while the others treat them as different plants. According to some botanists this controversy can be ended with the help of anatomy, by studying the internal microscopic structure of the plants concerned. This method is often practised in pharmacognosy.

A. It is, however advisable to bear in mind the following points while seeking help from botany or botanists :-

(1) As the botanists may not be and usually do not understand the Ayurvedic terminology and plant names, it is always advisable to procure actual plant specimens for identification.

(2) The classification of flowering plants is primarily based on the characters of flowers, fruits and seeds which are more stable, i.e. less variables. The characters of roots, stem, and leaves are of secondary importance. Thus according to botany flower colour, leaf size , plant juice

etc. may not be considered as distinguishing characters for the differantiation of species, e.g. the four o'clock plant (Gulabaski- गुलाबक्षी) having different colurs of the flowers are treated as only one species namely *Mirabilis jalapa* Linn.

(3) *Vatsanābha* (वत्सनाभ)-- Bacanāg (बचनाग) :- *Aconitium* species. There are two varieties - toxic and non toxic according to the character of the juices. Some of the plants belonging to both the varieties grow together and are morphologically very similar. Botanists have not differentiated these two varieties but the local people dig (76) and eat it.

(4) *Bahāvā* (बहावा) : there are two kinds of bahāvā one with fruit pulp having sweet taste (*Cassia fistula* -आरग्वध) while the other having the bitter taste (*Cassia rhombifolia* Roxb- कर्णिकार). Both the species are however given as synonymous in Cooke. Fl.

Several such examples can be furnished to show that such plants are used for different purposes, but they perhaps might have been neglected to differntiate with means of other botanical branches. But as the aims and objects of Botany and Ayurveda are different, the characters of plants which may be important from botanical standpoint but may be unimportant in Ayurved and vice-versa. The student of this subject, therefore should take into consideration the trend of experience, Pharmacological action ,tradition and text along with the botanical knowledge of plants.

B. We had a passing remark on plant geography, distribution of plants and particularly the original home of plant species in earlier pages. These points need further explanation and clarification.

According to the basic tenets of plant geography, plant species originates in a particular area and then spreads over other parts of the world. The migration and ultimate distribution of the species being determined and delimited by various factors like geographical barriers, dispersal mechanisms and climatic tolerance. If this principle is accepted in toto, it is rather difficult to explain the discontinuous distribution of some plant species and occurance of some others in both the hemispheres - Eastern and Western.

A. Wegner has put forward a "**Theory of Continental Drift** ", also known as '**Wegners Theory**' [The origin of continents and ocean - by Wegner]. According to him all the present day continents were at one time (million of years ago) joined together in a continuous landmass which he called '**Pangaea**'. Modification of this theory has been proposed by Du Toit (1937) who postulates that there were two initial continents, the northern '**Laurasia**' and the southern - '**Gondwana**' seperated by the sea of '**Tethys**' The origin of continents from the originally continuous landmasses certainly explains many of the problems of the present day plant

76. Vide Watt Dict Vol. 'Datura', p.30.

distribution.

This topic is concerned with the confirmation of some Ayurvedic plants which are present in old and new world and supposed to be of American origin. If the American home of these plants is accepted, a question is raised - 'how and when they have migrated to India? If they are believed to be migrated before the formation of the continents in the geological antiquity there is no harm in treating them as Indian or oriental plants. But some believe that these have been introduced to India in the recent past by Dutch and Portuguese colonists (77). Although many plants have been introduced by such colonists to India without any doubt, as far as Ayurvedic plants are concerned, this hypothesis is of little value. The Ayurvedic literature is unquestionably much ancient than the arrival of the Portuguese or other colonists in India.

Another point worth of mention here is about the recent hypothesis of Viviloe, who postulates the multiple origin of plant species in space and time. According to him plants belonging to one species might have originated independently in different parts of the world simultanously, or at different times, due to similar environmental conditions. This postulation though not widely accepted, seems to be more reasonable and understandable for the natural disposition of plants.

Without going into this vast and much debatable domain of plant geography, we can safely state that the American origin of many plants is not universally accepted (78). Further it is suggested by many authorities that when the decision about the origin of plants cannot be taken by botanical and plant geographical tenets and evidences, it should be taken with the help of history and philology (79). We have supplimented a list of such plants whose botanical origin is supposed to be American but which are occuring in India from the unknown time and are historically and philologically of Indian origin.

It therefore seems to be more reasonable as well as safer to consider such American plants which are prevalent in India or in the old world before the arrival of Portuguese (1494 A.D.)to be common plants of the old and new world.

We shall be highly gratified if this work proves useful to the students, lovers and workers in this branch of Ayurveda.

77-a. Reply from Birbal Sahni Institute. Lucknow, dated 7th October 1961.

b. Reply from Prof.T.S.Mahabale, Department of Botany Ganeshkhind, Poona dated 27-10-61

78. Reply from Botanical Office Calcutta. Dated 11-1-1962. Vide App. B 3(b) p.99

79-a Vide Watt Dict. Vol.'R' p. 519.

b. Vide De Candolle, pp. 16,23,25.27.

Proforma and system of transliteration

Proforma

The serial numbers coming prior to the heading (prenumbers) correspond to the serial order of plants in Gaṇadravyāvali (गणद्रव्यावली) the first part (Dhn.ni..p2). The number following the heading (post-number) indicates the serial number in the same chapter of Paryāyanāmadravyāvali (पर्यायनामद्रव्यावलि) (the second part Dhn.ni.p.7)only for plants not treated in Gaṇadravyavali i.e. in the first part.

I-a- Accepted valid botanical name and its synonym (if any).

b- Name of the person by whom the plant is confirmed.

c- Locality and distribution.

d- Reference of figures (if any).

II-a- **Important Synonyms occuring under the heading of Dhanvantari Nighaṇṭu and Raj. ni.**

b- **Names in Modern Ayurvedic and scientific literature**

Eng. - English; S. or Sans.or Sk.. - Sanskrit; Ben.or B.- Bengali
Bom. - Bombay; Mar. - Marathi; H. Hindi Konkan; Goa;
Guj. - Gujarati; M. - Madras; Tel. - Telagu; Tam. - Tamil;
Mal. - Malayalam; Kan. - Kannada; Ker. - Kerala.

III. **References in Ayurvedic and Vedic Literature.**

a- Charaka, Sushruta, Ashtangahridaya, Ashtangasangraha and Vedic Literature.

b- Other Nighaṇṭus and Kosha books.

c- Commentators on Charaka, Sushruta, Ashtangahridaya and Rasagranthas etc.

d- Watt Dictionary.

e- Chopra.

f- Roxburgh.

g- Dymock.

IV. **Other references from Literature in English and Modern Indian Languages.**

V **Names of plants found in some modern writings irrelevant to the accepted name.**

GENERAL :

(1) Abbreviations :

Ashta. hr.	...	Ashtangahridaya.(अष्टांगहृदय).
Ashta. San.	...	Ashtanga Sangraha. (अष्टांग संग्रह).
A.V.	...	Atharva Veda. (अथर्व वेद).
Ca.	...	Charaka (चरक)
Ci.	...	Chikitsasthana. (चिकित्सास्थान).
Dhn. ni.	...	Dhanvantariya Nighantu.(धन्वन्तरीय निघण्टु).
Kal.	...	Kalpasthan. (कल्पस्थान).
Raj. ni.	...	Raja Nighantu. (राज निघण्टु).
Rg.	...	Rigveda (ऋग्वेद).
Sharn. M.	...	Sharngadhara Samhita, Madhyam Khanda.(शार्ङ्गधर संहिता मध्यम खंड).
Sa.	...	Sharirasthana (शारीरस्थान).
Su.	...	Sushruta. (सुश्रुत).
Sū. or Su.	...	Sutrasthana. (सूत्रस्थान).
U.	...	Uttarasthana or Uttaratantra. (उत्तरस्थान अथवा उत्तरतंत्र).
FN	...	Foot note.

(2) For abbreviations of referred books see Bibliography.

(3) The figures noted after the references-the former denotes-Canto, chapter, part, act, mandal, adhyaya etc. and the later denotes-the number, verse, shloka, (श्लोक) mantra, stanza, etc.

(4) Reference quoted from books in Modern Indian languages translated summarily into English, keeping the spelling of Botanical names of plants as occurring there.In many of these books authorities of Botanical names of plants are not mentioned.

Abbreviations used by the present editor.

Dhn. Ni. - Dhanvantari nighaṇṭu.

Raj. ni. - Rājnighaṇṭu.

Gloss. Chopra, A Glossary of Indian Medicinal plants.

U.P.I. Useful plants of India. 1986. C.C.I.R.

नि.शे. टीका – निघण्टुशेष टीका.

क्षी., क्षीर. – क्षीरस्वामी.

Comp., Comp. to Gloss. - Companion to Chopra's Gloss. By Meharotra et al. 1987.

System of Transliteration

अ	a	ढ्	ḍh
आ	ā	ण्	ṇ
इ	i	त्	t
ई	ī	थ्	th
उ	u	द्	d
ऊ	ū	ध्	dh
ऋ	ṛ	न्	n
		प्	p
ए	e	फ्	ph /(f)
ऐ	ai	ब्	b
ओ	o	भ्	bh
औ	au	म्	m
क्	k	य्	y
ख्	kh	र्	r
ग्	g	ल्	l
घ्	gh	व्	v/(w)
ङ्	ṅ	श्	ś
च्	c	ष्	ṣ
छ्	ch	स्	s
ज्	j	ह्	h
झ्	jh	ळ	ḷ
ञ्	ñ	क्ष	kś
ट्	ṭ	ज्ञ	jñ
ठ्	ṭh	(Visargaḥ):	ḥ
ड्	ḍ	(Anuswaraḥ)	m&ṅ
		as appropriate	

(**Note '-'** (dash) above the alphabet may be replaced at some places by '^'(carat) especially on (i.). This system is optionally followed in previous pages and in quotations from other books in further portion of this book.)

Index of Heading Names

Sr. No.			Page No.

Gudūcyādi Chapter 1 गुडूच्यादिः प्रथमो वर्गः

1.	(१)	Gudūcī- गुडूची	1
2.	(२)	Ativiṣā अतिविषा	4
3.	(३)	Mūrvā मूर्वा	5
		Moraṭaḥ मोरटः (१)	6
4.	(४)	Mañjiṣṭhā मंजिष्ठा	6
5.	(५)	Dhanvayāsaḥ धन्वयासः	7
		Yāsaḥ यासः (२)	8
6.	(६)	Vāsakaḥ वासकः	9
7.	(७)	Khadiraḥ खदिरः	9
		Somavalkaḥ सोमवल्कः (३)	10
8.	(८)	Nimbaḥ - निम्बः	11
		Mahānimbaḥ महानिम्बः	12
9.	(९)	Kirātatiktaḥ किराततिक्तः	13
10.	(१०)	Kaṭukā कटुका	14
11.	(११)	Mustā मुस्ता	15
		Jalamustam जलमुस्तम् (१०)	16
12.	(१२)	Parpaṭaḥ पर्पटः	17
13.	(१३)	Vālakam वालकम्	17
14.	(१४)	Paṭolaḥ पटोलः	18
		Swādupatrafalā स्वादुपत्रफला (11)	19
15.	(१५)	Niśādwayam निशाद्वयम्	19
		Haridrā – हरिद्रा	19
16.		Dāruharidrā – दारुहरिद्रा	20
17.	(१६)	Śaṭhī शठी	21
		Gandhapalāśī गन्धपलाशी (12)	22
18.	(१७)	Puṣkaramūlam पुष्करमूलम् (मूलं Mūlam)	23
19.	(१८)	Bhārngī भार्ङ्गी	24
		Śwāsāriḥ श्वासारिः (13)	25
20.	(१९)	Pāṭhā पाठा	25
21.	(२०)	Kaṭfalaḥ कट्फलः	26
22.	(२१)	Devadāru देवदारु	27

* Pre numbers in English show the plants mentioned in *Paryāyanāmadravyāvalī* - *पर्याय नाम द्रव्यावली* adopted by Late Vd. D.K.Kamat while the bracketed pre nos.in Devanāgarī- देवनागरी show the heading names as per *Gaṇadravyāvalī* accepted by me. (S.D. Kamat)

* Post numbers are given as per Ānandās'ram edition in which plants from Raj. Ni. are also included by the Editior Vd. Purandare. This edition has been followed by Late Vd.D.K.Kamat.

Sr. No.			Page No.
23.	(२२)	Kattṛṇam कत्तृणम्	28
		Kapaṭam कपटम् (14)	29
		Guṇṭhaḥ गुण्ठः (15)	29
24.	(२३)	Śṛṅgī शृङ्गी	30
		Ajaśṛṅgi अजशृङ्गी (16)	
	(२४)	Parṇinīdvayam पर्णिनीद्वयम्	32
25.		Śāliparṇī शालिपर्णी	32
26.		Pṛṣṭiparṇī पृष्टिपर्णी	33
	(२५)	Bṛhatidwayam बृहतीद्वयम	34
27.		Bṛhatī - बृहती	34-35
28.		Kaṇṭakārī कण्टकारी	35
		Lakśmaṇā -लक्ष्मणा (19)	36
		Kāsaghnī कासघ्नी (20)	37
		Vṛntākī वृन्ताकी (21)	37
29.	(२६)	Gokśurah गोक्षुरः	38
30.	(२७)	Bilvaḥ बिल्वः	39
31.	(२८)	Agnimanthaḥ अग्निमंथः	40
32.	(२९)	Śyonākaḥ श्योनाकः	41
		Araluḥ अरलुः	41
33.	(३०)	Kāśmaryaḥ काश्मर्यः	42
34.	(३१)	Pāṭalā पाटला	43
		Kāṣṭhapāṭalā काष्ठपाटला (23)	44
35.	(३२)	Jīvakaḥ जीवकः	44
36.	(३३)	Ṛṣabhakaḥ ऋषभकः	45
	(३४)	मेदे Mede	45
37.		Medā - मेदा & Mahāmedā – महामेदा	45
		Vijayā विजया (24)	46
	(३५)	Kākolidwayam काकोलीद्वयम्	47
38.		Kākolī काकोली	47
39.		Kśīrakākolī क्षीरकाकोली	47
	(३६)	Parṇiṇīdwayam –पर्णिनीद्वयम्	48
40.		Māṣaparṇī- माषपर्णी	48
41.		Mudgaparṇī - मुद्गपर्णी	48
42.	(३७)	Jīvantī जीवन्ती	49
43.	(३८)	Madhuyaṣṭī मधुयष्टी	52
		Klītanakam क्लीतनकम् (25)	52
44.	(३९)	Ṛddhiḥ ऋद्धिः	53
45.	(४०)	Vidārī विदारी	53
		Kśīravidārī क्षीरविदारी	54
46.	(४१)	Ātmaguptā आत्मगुप्ता	55
		Dadhipuṣpī दधिपुष्पी	55

Sr. No.			Page No.
47.	(४२)	Śitivāraḥ शितिवारः	56
48.	(४३)	Pāṣāṇabhedakaḥ पाषाणभेदकः	57
	(४४)	Śrāvaṇyau - श्रावण्यौ	58
		Śrāvaṇī श्रावणी	58
	(४५)	Śārive सारिवे	59
50.		Sārivā सारिवा	59
51.		Kṛṣṇamūlī कृष्णमूली	60
52.	(४६)	Bākucī बाकुची	61
53.	(४७)	Madanaḥ मदनः	62
54.	(४८)	Kaṭukālāmbunī कटुकालाम्बुनी (Ikśvākuḥ) (इक्ष्वाकुः)	62-63
55.	(४९)	Jīmutaḥ जीमूतः	63
56.	(५०)	Trapusam त्रपुसम्	64
		Urvāruḥ उर्वारुः (34)	65
		Vālukam - वालुकम् (35)	66
		Śīrṇavṛntam शीर्णवृन्तम् (38)	66
		Cirbhaṭam चिर्भटम् (41)	66
		Daṅgarī डङ्गरी (43)	67
		Kūṣmāṇḍikā कूष्माण्डिका (44)	68
		Vandhyākarkoṭakī - वंध्याकर्कोटकी (46)	68
		Karkoṭakī - कर्कोटकी (47)	69
57.	(५२)	Dhāmārgavaḥ धामार्गवः	69
	*(५१)	Kṛtavedhanam - कृतवेधनम्	70
		Kośātakī कोशातकी (50)	70
58.	(५३)	Aśmantakaḥ अश्मन्तकः	72
59.	(५४)	Kovidāraḥ कोविदारः	73
60.	(५५)	Viṣāṇikaḥ (विषाणिकः) (Āvartakī - आवर्तकी)	74
61.	(५६)	Śaṇapuṣpī शणपुष्पी	75
62.	(५७)	Bimbī - बिम्बी	76
	(५८)	Trifalā.- त्रिफला	76
63.		Harītakī हरीतकी	76
64.		Bibhītakaḥ बिभीतकः	78
65.		Vayasthā - वयस्था (Āmalakī - आमलकी)	79
		Pracīnāmalakam प्राचीनामलकम् (52)	80
66.	(५९)	Āragvadhaḥ आरग्वधः	80
		Karṇikāraḥ कर्णिकारः (55)	81
67.	(६०)	Dantī दन्ती	84
		Araṇī अरणी (56)	85
		Recakaḥ रेचकः (57)	85

* Serial no. mentioned in Gaṇadravyāvali गणद्रव्यावली is as above, while Late Vd. D.K. Kamat has follwed the serial no. of Ānandāśrama Edition. (S.D.K.)

Sr. No.			Page No.
68.	(६१)	Dravantī द्रवन्ती	86
69.	(६२)	Nîlinī नीलिनी	87
70.	(६३)	Snuk स्नुक्	88
71.	(६४)	Sātalā सातला	89
	(६५)	Kāñcanaksīrī कांचनक्षीरी	90
72.		Ksīriṇī क्षीरिणी	90
		Sarvaksīrī सर्वक्षीरी (59)	91
73.	(६६)	Syāmātrivṛt श्यामात्रिवृत्	92
		Suklabhaṇḍī शुक्लभण्डी (60)	94
74.	(६७)	Indravāruṇī - इन्द्रवारुणी (Aindrī-ऐन्द्री)	95
75.	(६८)	Vīsālā - विशाला	95
		Swetapuspī श्वेतपुष्पी (61)	96
76.	(६९)	Trāyamāṇā - त्रायमाणा	96
77.	(७०)	Saṅkhinī - शंखिनी (Yavatiktā - यवतिक्ता)	98
78.	(७१)	Aṅkoṭaḥ - अङ्कोटः	99
79.	(७२)	Apāmargaḥ अपामार्गः	100
		Raktapuspaḥ रक्तपुष्पः (62)	101
80.	(७३)	Tejovatī - तेजोवती (तेजस्विनी –Tejasvinī)	101
81.	(७४)	Jyotiṣmatī ज्योतिष्मती	103
82.	(७५)	Rāsnā - रास्ना	104
83.	(७६)	Asvagandhā - अश्वगंधा	105
84.	(७७)	Varsābhūḥ वर्षाभूः	106
		(Punarnavā - पुनर्नवा)	106
		Krūraḥ क्रूरः (63)	108
85.	(७८)	Sahacaraḥ सहचरः	109
		(Saireyakaḥ) (सैरेयकः)	109
86.	(७९)	Balā बला	110
		Mahābalā महाबला (65)	110
		Gāṅgerukī - गांगेरुकी (66).	112
		Balikā - बलिका (67)	113
		Balā pañcaka - बलापञ्चक (68)	113
87.	(८०)	Prasāraṇi - प्रसारणी	114
	(८१)	Satāvaryau –शतावर्यौ	115
88.		Satāvarī- शतावरी	115
		Sahasravīryā -.सहस्त्रवीर्या (69)	116
89.	(८२)	Eraṇḍaḥ - एरण्डः	117
		Vṛsanedhā - वृषमेधा	118

Sr. No.			Page No.

Śatapuṣpādi Chapter II. शतपुष्पादिर्द्वितीयो वर्गः ।

1	(१)	Śatapuṣpā - शतपुष्पा	121
2	(२)	Miśreyā - मिश्रेया	122
3	(३)	Vacā - वचा	125
		Medhyā - मेध्या (1)	126
4	(४)	Hapuṣā - हपुषा	127
5	(५)	Viḍaṅgam - विडङ्गम्	130
6	(६)	Kuṭajaḥ कुटजः	131
7	(७)	Indrayavaḥ - इन्द्रयवः	132
	(८)	Trikśārāḥ - त्रिक्षाराः	133
8		Yavakśaraḥ यवक्षारः	133
9		Swarjikākśaraḥ स्वर्जिकाक्षारः	133-134
10		Ṭaṅkaṇakśāraḥ टंकणक्षारः	134
	(९)	Lavaṇāni - लवणानि	134
11		Saindhavam - सैंधवम्	134-35
12		Biḍalavaṇam - बिडलवणम्	135
13		Sauvarcalam - सौवर्चलम्	135-36
14		Audbhidam - औद्भिदम्	136
15		Sāmudram - सामुद्रम्	136
16	(१०)	Hiṅgu - हिंगु	137
17		Hiṅgupatrī - हिंगुपत्री (2)	138
18	(११)	Hiṅguśivāṭī - हिंगुशिवाटी	139
19	(१२)	Tumbaru - तुम्बरु	140
20	(१३)	Sukśmailā - सूक्ष्मैला	141
		Bhadrailā - भद्रैला (10)	142
21	(१४)	Kesaram-Nāgapuṣpam केसरम्-नागपुष्पम्	143
22	(१५)	Twak (Cocam) त्वक् (चोचम्)	145
23	(१६)	Patram (Tamālapatram) पत्रम् , (तमालपत्रम्)	146
24	(१७)	Tālīsakam - तालीसकम्	147
25	(१८)	Tugā-Vamśarocanā तुगा-वंशरोचना	150
		Palāśagandhā-पलाशगंधा (11)	150
26	(१९)	Pṛthvikā (Upakuñcī) पृथ्वीका (उपकुञ्ची)	153
27	(२०)	Dāḍimam - दाडिमम्	155
28	(२१)	Dhānyakam - धान्यकम्	155-56
29	(२२)	Jīrakam - जीरकम्	156
		Śuklaḥ - (12) शुक्लः	157
		Kṛṣṇjīrakam - (13) कृष्णजीरकम्	158
		Bṛhatpālī (14) बृहत्पाली	159
30	(२३)	Pippalī - पिप्पली	160
31	(२४)	Pippalīmūlam - पिप्पलीमूलम्	161

Sr. No.			Page No.
32	(२५)	Cavyam - चव्यम्	161
		(Gajapippalī) (गजपिप्पली)	
		Śreyasī (श्रेयसी) (15)	162
33.	(२६)	Citrakaḥ - चित्रकः	164f-165
34.	(२७)	Nāgaram - Ārdrakam नागरम् - आर्द्रकम्	167
35	(२८)	Maricam - मरिचम्	168
		Śvetamaricam - श्वेतमरिचम् (20)	168
36	(२९)	Dīpyakam - दीप्यकम्	169
		(Yavānī)-(यवानी)	169
		Yavānikā (21) यवानिका	171
		Yāvanī Yavānī यावनी यवानी (22)	172
37	(३०)	Vṛkśāmlam - वृक्षाम्लम्	173
38	(३१)	Amlavetasaḥ (Amlaḥ) अम्लवेतसः (अम्लः)	177
39	(३२)	Ajmodā - अजमोदा	183
40	(३३)	Ajagandhā अजगन्धा	184
41	(३४)	Kapitthaḥ कपित्थः	187
42	(३५)	Śarkarā शर्करा	188
		Madhuśarkarā - मधुशर्करा (23)	188
		Yavāsa śarkarā - यवासशर्करा	189

Candanādi Chapter III चन्दनादिस्तृतीयो वर्गः

1	*Candanam चन्दनम्	191
	Raktacandanam रक्तचंदनम् (1)	193
	Kucandanam कुचन्दनम् (2)	193-94
	Kālīyakam - कालीयकम् (3)	194
	Barbarikam - बर्बरिकम् (4)	195
	Haricandanam - हरिचंदनम् (5)	195
2	Kumkumam - कुंकुमम्	197
3	Uśīram - उशीरम्	198
4	Priyaṅguḥ - प्रियंगुः	200-01
5	Tūṇiḥ - तूणिः	202
6	Rocanā - रोचना	203
7	Turuṣkaḥ - तुरुष्कः	204
8	Agaruḥ अगरुः	206
	Kāleyakam कालेयकम् (5)	207
9	Kastūrī - कस्तूरी	208
10	Karpūraḥ कर्पूरः	208-09
11	Jātipatrī - जातिपत्री	211

* Pre numbers given by Late Vd. D.K.Kamat correspond exactly with the heading names in Gaṇadravyāvali therefore Devanāgarī numbers are not given. S.D.Kamat

Sr. No.		Page No.
12	Jātifalam - जातीफलम्	211
13	Kamkolam - कंकोलम्	213
14	Pūgaḥ - पूगः (पूगफलम् –Pugaphalam)	213
15	Lavaṅgam लवङ्गम्	214
16	Nalikā नलिका	216
17	Naladam (Māmsī) नलदम् (मांसी)	217
	Gandha māmsi - गंधमांसी (12)	217
18	Kuṣṭham - कुष्टम्	218-19
19	Hareṇuḥ (Reṇukā) हरेणुः (रेणुका)	220
20	Tagaram - तगरम्	221
21	Plavam - (Paripelavam) - प्लवम (परिपेलवम)	222
22	Nakham - नखम्	223
23	Vyāghranakham - व्याघ्रनखम्	223
24	Spṛkkā - स्पृक्का	224
25	Bolaḥ - बोलः (बोलम् –Bolam)	226
26	Damanakaḥ - दमनकः	228
	Damaḥ - दमः (14)	229
27	Murā - मुरा	229
28	Sthauṇeyakam - स्थौणेयकम्	230
29	Çorakaḥ - चोरकः	232
30	Śaileyam - शैलेयम्	234-35
31	Elavālukam - एलवालुकम्	236
32	Saralaḥ - सरलः	237
33	Saptaparṇaḥ - सप्तपर्णः	238
34	Lākśā - लाक्षा	239
35	Tāmalakī - तामलकी	240
36	Lāmajjakam - लामज्जकम्	241
37	Padmakam - पद्मकम्	242
38	Dhātakī - धातकी	242
39	Prapauṇḍarīkam - प्रपौण्डरीकम्	243
40	Karcūraḥ - कर्चूरः	244
41	Manaḥśilā - मनःशिला	245
42	Sindūraḥ - सिन्दूरः	246
	Girisindūraḥ - गिरिसिन्दूरः (15)	246
43	Saurāṣṭrī - सौराष्ट्री	247
44	Gandhakaḥ - गंधकः (गन्धकद्वयम् Gandhak dwayam)	247
	Vaṭasaugandhikaḥ - वटसौगंधिकः (16)	248
45	Mācikā (Ambikā)माचिका -(अम्बष्टा -Ambaṣṭhā)	248
46	Sikthakam (सिक्थकम्)	249
47	Rālaḥ (Sarjarasaḥ) रालः (सर्जरसः)	250
48	Kāsīsam कासीसम	251

Sr. No.			Page No.
49		Puraḥ - (Gugguluḥ) – पुरः (गुग्गुलुः)	252
50		Kundaruḥ - कुन्दरुः	254
51		Śryāhvaḥ - Śrīveṣṭakaḥ – श्याह्वः – श्रीवेष्टकः	252 -55
52		Sallakī - शल्लकी	256
53		Kampillaḥ - कंपिल्लः	257
54		Kaṅkuṣṭham - कंकुष्ठम्	258
55		Aruṣkaram - अरुष्करम् (भल्लातक –Bhallātakaḥ)	259
56		Tuttham - तुत्थम्	260
57		Tāpyam - ताप्यम् – हेममाक्षिकम्	261
58		Añjanam - अंजनम्	261
59		(Gairika) Dhātuḥ -(गैरिक) धातुः	262
		Suvarṇagairikam - सुवर्णगैरिकम् (24)	262-63
60		(Samudra) fenam - समुद्रफेनम्	263
61		Cakśuṣyā - चक्षुष्या	263-64
		Rasāñjanam - रसाञ्जनम् (20)	264-65
62		Rītijam (Puṣpāñjanam) –रीतिजम (पुष्पाञ्जनम)	265
		Śilājatuḥ - (शिलाजतुः) (22)	266
63		Katakam - कतकम्:	266-67
64		Lodhraḥ - लोध्रः	267
		Kramukaḥ - क्रमुकः	270
65		Śaṅkhaḥ - शङ्खः (25)	271
		Vargetarāṇi . (Plants out of the Chapter.) वर्गेतराणि	
		Jiṅgiṇī- जिंगिणी	272
		Bahulā - बहुला (Tāmbūlī - ताम्बूली)	273

Karvīrādiḥ Chapter IV - करवीरादिश्चतुर्थो वर्गः

1	(१)	Karavīraḥ - करवीरः	275
2	(२)	Cakramardah - चक्रमर्दः	277
		(Eḍagajaḥ - एडगजः)	
3	(३)	Dhattūraḥ - धत्तूरः	278
4	(४)	Lāṅgalī - लाङ्गली	
		Kalikarī -कलिकारी	280
5	(५)	Bhṛṅgarājaḥ - भृङ्गराजः	280
6	(६)	Arkaḥ - अर्कः	282
		Rājārkaḥ - राजार्कः (1)	282
		Svetārkaḥ - श्वेतार्कः (2)	282
		Svetamandāraḥ - श्वेतमन्दारः (3)	283
7	(७)	Būkaḥ बूकः	284
8		Kākamācī - काकमाची	285
		Kākajaṅghā - काकजङ्घा (4)	287
		Kākanāsā - काकनासा (5)	288-89

Sr. No.			Page No.
		Kākādanī - काकादनी (6)	290
		Cūḍāmaṇiḥ - चूडामणिः (7)	291
		Svetakāmbhojī - श्वेतकाम्भोजी (8)	292
9	(९)	Mūlakam - मूलकम्	292-93
		Cāṇākhyamūlakam- चाणाख्यमूलकम् (9)	293
		Gṛñjanam - गृञ्जनम् (10)	294
		Piṇḍamūlam - पिण्डमूलम् (11)	294
10	(१०)	Śigruḥ - शिग्रुः	295
11	(११)	Sarṣapaḥ - सर्षपः	297
		Rājakṡavakaḥ राजक्षवकः (12)	298-299
12	(१२)	Bhūtika-Bhūtṛṇa (Bhūstṛṇa) भूतीक -भूतृण (भूस्तृण)	299-300
13	(१३)	Surasā सुरसा	301
14	(१४)	Jambīraḥ - जम्बीरः	302
15	(१५)	Kuṭherakaḥ - कुठेरकः	303
		Śālukaḥ - शालुकः (13)	304
16	(१६)	Sumukhaḥ - सुमुखः	305
17	(१७)	Āsurī - आसुरी	305
18	(१८)	Kāṇḍīraḥ - काण्डीरः	308-09
19	(१९)	Jalapippalī - जलपिप्पली	310
20	(२०)	Rasonaḥ - रसोनः	311
21	(२१)	(Gṛñjanaḥ) - (गृञ्जनः)	314
		Gṛñjaram- गृञ्जरम्	
22	(२२)	Palāṇḍuḥ - पलाण्डुः	315
	(२३)	Durdrumaḥ - दुर्द्रुमः	315
23	(२४)	Kadalī - कदली	316
		Kāṣṭhakadalī - काष्ठकदली (14)	317
		Girikadalī - गिरिकदली (15)	317
		Suvarṇakadalī - सुवर्णकदली (16)	317
24	(२५)	Sinduvāraḥ सिन्दुवारः	318-19
25	(२६)	Śephālikā - शेफालिका (Nirguṇḍī) निर्गुण्डी	321
26	(२७)	Aśvakṡurakaḥ-अश्वक्षुरकः (Girikarṇikā-गिरिकर्णिका)	323
27	(२८)	Jantukārī - जन्तुकारी	324
28	(२९)	Padmā - (Padmacāriṇī) पद्मा (पद्मचारिणी)	325
29	(३०)	Gṛṣṭiḥ (Vārāhī) गृष्टिः (वाराही)	326
30	(३१)	Māṁsarohiṇī - मांसरोहिणी	329-30
31	(३२)	Vandakā - वन्दका	331
32	(३३)	Suvarcalā - सुवर्चला	333
		Brāhmī - ब्राम्ही (18)	336
		Kṡudrapatrā - क्षुद्रपत्रा (19)	336
	(३४)	Nākulyau नाकुल्यौ	339
33		Nākulī नाकुली	339
34		Mahāsugandhā - महासुगंधा	342

Sr. No.			Page No.
35		Vṛddhadārkaḥ - वृद्धदारुकः	342
	(३६)	Raktapādyau - रक्तपाद्यौ	344
36		Raktapādī - रक्तपादी	344
37		Viśvagranthiḥ - विश्वग्रंथिः	347
38	(३७)	Saṅkhapuṣpī - शंङ्खपुष्पी	349
		Viṣṇukrāntā - विष्णुक्रान्ता (20)	352
39	(३८)	Taṇḍulīyakaḥ - तण्डुलीयकः	355
40	(३९)	Kāsamardaḥ - कासमर्दः	356
41	(४०)	Ikśavaḥ इक्षवः	357
		Guḍaḥ गुडः (21)	357
42	(४१)	Kāśaḥ काशः	359
	(४२)	Darbhau दर्भौ	360
43		Muñjaḥ - मुञ्जः	360
44		Mṛdudarbhaḥ - मृदुदर्भः (कुशः -Kuśaḥ)	361
45	(४३)	Śaradwayam - शरद्वयम्	363
		Śaraḥ - शरः	363
46	(४४)	Vaṁśaḥ - वंशः	364
		Vaṁśāgram वंशाग्रम् (22)	365
47	(४५)	Nalaḥ - नलः	366
		Mahānalaḥ - महानलः (23)	367
48	(४६)	Durvā दूर्वा	367-68
	(४७)	Śvetanīlāruṇotpalam श्वेतनीलारुणोत्पलम्	369
49		Puṇḍarīkam - पुण्डरीकम्	369
50		Saugandhikam - सौगन्धिकम्	371
51		Raktapadmam रक्तपद्मम्	372
		Kumudam कुमुदम् (24)	373
		Kśudramutpalam क्षुद्रमुत्पलम् (25)	374
52	(४८)	Padminī पद्मिनी	374
53		Padmabījam पद्मबीजम्	375
54		Mṛṇālam - मृणालम् (Bisam) बिसम	376
55		Padmamūlam पद्ममूलम्	376-77
56		Padmakesaram पद्मकेसरम्	377
	(१)	Balāmoṭā - बलामोटा	378
	(२)	Somavalli - सोमवल्ली	380
	(३)	Potaki - पोतकी	382
	(४)	Arsoghnah - अर्शोघ्नः (Suranah - सूरणः)	383

Āmrādiḥ Chapter V -आम्रादिः पञ्चमो वर्गः

1		Āmraḥ - आम्रः	385
		Kśudrāmraḥ - क्षुद्राम्रः (1)	387
		Rājāmraḥ - राजाम्रः (2)	388
2		Āmrātakaḥ - आम्रातकः	388

Sr. No.		Page No.
3	Jambīraḥ – जम्बीरः	389
	Madhu Jambīraḥ - मधुजम्बीरः (4)	390
4	Nārangaḥ - नारङ्गः	391
5	Bījapūrakaḥ - बीजपूरकः (बीजपूर्णः –Bijapūrṇaḥ)	395
	Madhukarkaṭī - मधुकर्कटी	397
6	Amlikā - अम्लिका	398
	Ksudrāmlikā - क्षुद्राम्लिका (7)	399
7	Ārukam - आरुकम्	399
8	Bhavyam - भव्यम् (भवम् - Bhavam)	401
9	Tindukaḥ - तिन्दुकः	401-02
10	Vikaṅkataḥ - विकंकतः	404
11	Madhūkaḥ - मधूकः	406
	Jaladaḥ - जलदः (8)	408
12	Pīluḥ - पीलुः	409
	Bṛhatpīluḥ - बृहत्पीलुः	410
13	Kharjūraḥ - खर्जूरः (Kharjūrī - खर्जूरी)	411
	Dīpyā - दीप्या (9)	412
14	Drākśā - द्राक्षा	413
	Uttarāpathikā - उत्तरापथिका (10)	413-14
15	Akśoṭaḥ - अक्षोटः (Akśoḍaḥ- अक्षोडः)	414
16	Parūṣakaḥ - परूषकः	416
17	Tūdaḥ - तूदः	416-17
18	Pālevatam - पालेवतम्	418
19	Tālaḥ - तालः	421
	Māḍaḥ - माडः (13)	422
20	Priyālaḥ - प्रियालः	423
21	Nārikelaḥ – नारिकेलः	424
22	Vaṭaḥ - वटः	426
23	Aśvatthaḥ - अश्वत्थः (पिप्पलः – Pippalaḥ)	427
24	Plakśaḥ - प्लक्षः	428
25	Jambūḥ - जम्बूः	433
26	Udumbaraḥ - उदुम्बरः	435-436
27	Falguḥ - फल्गुः (काकोदुम्बरिका–Kākodumbarikā)	437
28	Kśīrī - क्षीरी	439
29	Śleṣmātakaḥ - श्लेष्मातकः	440
30	Śamī - शमी	442
31	Kolam - कोलम् (बदरम् –Badaram)	445
32	Karīrḥ - करीरः	448
33	Karamardakam - करमर्दकम्	449

Separate heading numbers in Devanāgrī are not given as they correspond with the pre-numbers exactly given by Late Vd. D.K. Kamat (S.D.Kamat.)

Sr. No.			Page No.
34		Kadambau - कदम्बौ	451
35		Karañjau - करञ्जौ	455
		Udakīryaḥ - उदकीर्यः (15)	461
		Angāravallikā - अंगारवल्लिका (16)	462
36		Sirīṣaḥ - शिरीषः	462-63
37		Arjunaḥ - अर्जुनः	464
38		Vetasaḥ - वेतसः	467
39		Varuṇaḥ - वरुणः	472
40		Śimśapā - शिंशपा	473
41		Sarjaḥ - सर्जः	476
		Aśanaḥ - अशनः (19)	479
42		Śālmalī - शाल्मली	481
43		Muṣkakaḥ - मुष्ककः	483
		Rohitakaḥ - रोहितकः (21)	485
44		Arimaḥ - अरिमः (इरिमेद –Irimedaḥ)	489
45		Mallikā - मल्लिका	492-93
46		Vārṣikī - वार्षिकी	495
47		Jātī - जाती	496
48		Vāsantī - वासन्ती	498
49		Graiṣmī - ग्रैष्मी	498
50		Campakaḥ - चम्पकः	499-500
51		Taruṇyau - तरुण्यौ	501
52		Kubjakaḥ - कुब्जकः	502
53	(५२)	Yūthikā - यूथिका	504
54	(५३)	Kundaḥ - कुन्दः	505-06
55	(५४)	Śatapatrī- शतपत्रीः	507
56	(५५)	Atimuktaḥ - अतिमुक्तः	509
57	(५६)	Bakulaḥ - बकुलः	510
58	(५७)	Kiṅkirātaḥ - किंकिरातः	511
59	(५८)	Tilakaḥ - तिलकः	513
60	(५९)	Aśokaḥ - अशोकः	516
61	(६०)	Kimśukaḥ - किंशुकः	517-18
		Ketakīdwayam - केतकी द्वयम्	520
		Gaṇeruka - गणेरुका	521
		Sāgaḥ - सागः	521
		Dhavaḥ - धवः	522

Suvarnādiḥ Chapter VI - सुवर्णादिः षष्ठो वर्गः ।

1	Suvarṇam - सुवर्णम्	523
2	Raupyam - रौप्यम्	523
3	Tāmram - ताम्रम्	524

Sr. No.		Page No.
4	Trapu - त्रपु	525
5	Rītiḥ - रीतिः (रीतिका - Rītikā)	525-26
6	Sīsakam - सीसकम्	526
7	Kāmsyam - कांस्यम्	526-27
8	Loham - लोहम्	527
	Vartaloham - वर्तलोहम् (1)	528
	Lohocchiṣṭam - लोहोच्छिष्टम् (2)	529
9	Pāradaḥ - पारदः	529
	Hiṅgulaḥ - हिंगुलः (3)	530
10	Vaikrāntam - वैक्रान्तम्	530-31
11	Gārutmatam - गारुत्मतम्	531
12	Hīrakam - हीरकम्	532
	Rājāvartaḥ - राजावर्तः (4)	533
13	Muktā - मुक्ता (मौत्तिक्कम् -Mauktikam)	533
14	Pravālam - प्रवालम्	533
	Dhānyavargaḥ - धान्यवर्गः	534
15	Śāliḥ - शालिः	534
16	Vrīhiḥ - व्रीहिः	537-38
17	Yavaḥ - यवः	538
18	Mudgaḥ - मुद्गः	540
19	Rājamāṣaḥ - राजमाषः	542
20	Kodravaḥ - कोद्रवः	543
21	Nivāraḥ - नीवारः	544
22	Śyāmākaḥ - श्यामाकः	545
23	Kaṅguḥ - कङ्गुः	546
24	Vanamudgaḥ - वनमुद्गः	548
25	Āḍhakī- आढकी	549
26	Masūrikā - मसूरिका	550
27	Godhūmaḥ - गोधूमः	551
28	Dhānyamāṣaḥ - धान्यमाषः	552
29	Caṇakaḥ - चणकः	553
30	Vartulaḥ - वर्तुलः	554
31	Kulatthaḥ - कुलत्थः	556-57
	Jūrṇā - जूर्णा (7)	558
	Karaṭaḥ - करटः (8)	560
	Niṣpāvaḥ - निष्पावः (9)	561
	Methikā - मेथिका (14)	562
	Vanamethikā - वनमेथिका (15)	563
	Atasī - अतसी (16)	564
	Kusumbham - कुसुम्भमः (17)	566
	Khastilaḥ - खस्तिलः (18)	567

Sr. No.		Page No.
	Khastila Valkalaḥ - खस्तिलवल्कलः (19)	567
	Afūkam - अफूकम् (20)	567
	Tilaḥ - तिलः (21)	568
	Dravadravyāni- द्रवद्रव्याणि	569
32	Tailam - तैलम्	569
	Tilatailam - तिलतैलम् (22)	570
	Atasītailam - अतसीतैलम् (23)	570
	Sarṣapatailam - सर्षपतैलम् (24)	571
	Eraṇḍatailam - एरण्डतैलम् (25)	571
	Kusumbhatailam - कुसुम्भतैलम् (26)	571
	Kośāmratailam - कोशाम्रतैलम् (27)	572
	Ātmaguptā tailam - आत्मगुप्तातैलम् (28)	572
	Nimba tailam - निम्बतैलम् (29)	572
	Akśatailam - अक्षतैलम् (30)	572
	Taila Viśeṣāḥ - तैल विशेषाः	572-73
33	Sarpiḥ (Ghṛtam) - सर्पिः (घृतम्)	574
	Goghṛtam - गोघृतम् (32)	574
	Mahiṣīghṛtam - महिषीघृतम् (33)	574
	Ajāghṛtam - अजाघृतम् (34)	575
	Āvikam ghṛtam - आविकं घृतम् (35)	575
	Uṣṭrīghṛtam - उष्ट्रीघृतम् (36)	575
	Aśvāghṛtam - अश्वाघृतम् (37)	575
	Gardabhī ghṛtam - गर्दभी घृतम् (38)	576
	Hastinī ghṛtam - हस्तिनीघृतम् (40)	576
	Strī (Mānuṣam) ghṛtam - स्त्री(मानुषं) घृतम् (41)	576
	Purānaghṛtam - पुराणघृतम् (42)	576-77
34	Payaḥ (Ksīram) - पयः (क्षीरम्) (दुग्धं –Dugdham)	577
	Gokśīram - गोक्षीरम् (43)	578
	Ajāpayaḥ- अजापयः (44)	578
	Aurabhrapayaḥ - औरभ्रपयः	579
	Mahiṣīpayaḥ - महिषीपयः (46)	579
	Uṣṭrīpayaḥ - उष्ट्रीपयः (47)	579
	Aśvāpayaḥ - अश्वापयः (48)	579
	Gardabhīpayaḥ - गर्दभीपयः (49)	580
	Mānuṣīpayaḥ - मानुषीपयः (51)	580
	Hastinīpayaḥ - हस्तिनीपयः (52)	580
35	*Takram - Dadhi* - तक्रम्–दधि	580
	Dadhi - दधि (53)	582
	Mathita dadhi - मथित दधि (54)	583
	Godadhi - गोदधि (55)	583
	Ajādadhi - अजादधि (56)	583
	Āvikadadhi - आविकदधि (57)	584

Sr. No.		Page No.
	Mahiṣī dadhi - महिषी दधि (58)	584
	Uṣṭrī dadhi - उष्ट्रीदधि (59)	584
	Aśvādadhi -अश्वादधि (60)	584
	Gardabhī dadhi - गर्दभी दधि (61)	584
	Hastinī dadhi - हस्तिनी दधि (62)	585
	Strī (Mānuṣa) dadhi - स्त्री(मानुष) दधि (63)	585
	Sāmānya dadhi gunāḥ - सामान्यदधिगुणाः	585
	Ṛtuviśeṣeṇa dadhiguṇāḥ - ऋतुविशेषेण दधिगुणाः	586
	Takaram - तक्रम् (तक्रवर्गः)	587
	Takrabhedāḥ - तक्रभेदाः	587
	Takra Sāmānyagunāḥ - तक्रसामान्यगुणाः	588
	Pakvā pakva takragunāḥ - पक्वापक्व तक्रगुणाः	588-89
	Takra niṣedhaḥ - तक्रनिषेधः	589
	Takra sevanam - तक्र सेवनम्	590
	Takra kūrcikā - तक्रकूर्चिका	590
	Maṇḍah - मण्डः	590
	Piyuṣmoraṭau - पीयूषमोरटौ	590
	Navanītam - नवनीतम् (64)	591
36	Madhu - मधु (Kśaudram - क्षौद्रम्)	591
	Madhu sāmānyaguṇāh - मधु सामान्यगुणाः	591
	Madhu viśiṣṭaguṇāḥ - मधु विशिष्टगुणाः	593
	Bhrāmara madhu - भ्रामर मधु	593
	Kśaudra madhu - क्षौद्रमधु	593
	Mākśika madhu - माक्षिक मधु	593
	Ṃādhvī Sitā - माध्वी सिता	594
37	Śuktam - शुक्तम्	594
38	Kāñjikam - काञ्जिकम्	595
	Sauvīrakam सौवीरकं Tuṣodakam तुषोदकं (65)	595
	Madyavargaḥ - मद्यवर्गः	
39	Surā (bhedāḥ) - सुरा (भेदाः)	596
	Madyasāmānyaguṇāḥ - मद्यसामान्यगुणाः	596-97
	Surā - सुरा	597
	Prasannā - प्रसन्ना	597
	Yavasurādayaḥ -यवसुरादयः	598
	Sīdhubhedāḥ - सीधुभेदाः	598
	Madhūkasīdhuḥ- मधूकसीधुः	598
	Rasāsavaḥ - रसासवः	598
	Kohalaḥ Jagalaḥsca- कोहलो जगलश्च	599
	Bakkasaḥ - बक्कसः	599
	Mārdwīkam - मार्द्वीकम्	599
	Khārjūram - खार्जूरम्	600

Sr. No.		Page No.
	Gauḍasīdhuḥ & Śārkara sīdhuḥ - गौडसीधुः शार्कर सीधुः	600
	Śītarasikaḥ शीतरसिकः	600
40	Āsavam -(types) - आसवम् - (तद्भेदाश्च)	600
	Śārkaraḥ & Mādhavaḥ - शार्करो माधवश्च	601
	Surāsavaḥ - सुरासवः	601
	Marieyaḥ - मैरेयः	601
	Ākṣika sīdhuḥ - आक्षिक सीधुः	601
	Jāmbava sīdhuḥ - जाम्बव सीधुः	601
	Ariṣṭaḥ - अरिष्टः	602
	Navajīrṇa madyaguṇāḥ-नवजीर्णमद्यगुणाः	602
	Varjya madyam - वर्ज्यमद्यम्	603
	Madyaprabhāvaḥ - मद्यप्रभावः	604
	Prakṛtyanusāreṇa Madyapariṇāmāḥ प्रकृत्यनुसारेण मद्यपरिणामाः	604
41	Marjikā - मर्जिका	605
	Jalavargaḥ - जलवर्गः	
42	Jalam- जलम्	
	Jalasādharaṇa gunākarmāṇi - जलसाधारण गुणकर्माणि	
	Gaganāmbu - गगनाम्बु	606
	Anārtavadibhedāḥ - अनार्तवादिभेदाः	606
	Amśūdakam- अंशुदकम्	607
	Candrakānta Jalam -चन्द्रकान्त जलम्	607
	Nādeyādi Jalagunāḥ - नादेयादिजल गुणाः	607-08
	Ānūpādi deśabhedena Jalabhedaḥ आनूपादि देशभेदेन जलभेदाः	609
	Grāhyāgrāhya Jalaswarūpāṇi ग्राहया ग्राह्य जलस्वरूपाणि	610
	Śṛtādijalabhedena guṇakarmāṇi - श्रृतादि जलभेदेन गुणकर्माणि	610
	Varjya Jalam - वर्ज्यजलम्	612
	Pañcavidha bhauma jalam - पञ्चविध भौमजलम्	613
	Nārikelodakam - नारिकेलोदकम्	614
	Māmsadravyāni - *मांसद्रव्याणि*	614
43	*Śarīravargaḥ* - शरीरवर्गः (पुरुषः) (Puruṣaḥ)	614
	Mānuṣaḥ - मानुषः	614
	Strī - स्त्री	615
	Śarīram - शरीरम्	615
	Vācā - वाचा	615
	Vāyuḥ - वायुः	616
	Pittam - पित्तम्	616
	Śleṣmā - श्लेष्मा	617

Sr. No.		Page No.
	Mohaḥ - मोहः	617
	Prakṛtayaḥ - प्रकृतयः	617
44	*Śarīra dhātavāḥ* - शारीर धातवः	618
	Asthi - अस्थि	618
	Māmsam - मांसम्	618
	Vasā - वसा	618
	Raktam - रक्तम्	619
	Śukram - शुक्रं	619
	Majjā - मज्जा	619
	Rasaḥ - रसः	619
	Saptadhatu Janikramaḥ - सप्तधातुजनिक्रमः	620
	Prāṇivargaḥ - प्राणीवर्गः	620
45	Hastī - हस्ती	620
46	Aśvaḥ - अश्वः	620-21
47	Uṣṭraḥ - उष्ट्रः	621
48	Gardabhaḥ (Kharaḥ) - गर्दभः (खरः)	621
	Aśvataraḥ अश्वतरः (66)	622
49	Ajaḥ - अजः	622
50	Aviḥ - अविः	622-23
51	Vṛkaḥ - वृकः	623
52	Vyāghraḥ - व्याघ्रः	623
	Śarabhaḥ - शरभः (67)	623
53	Kesarī - केसरी	624
54	Varāhaḥ - वराहः (Sūkraḥ - सूकरः)	624
55	Mṛgaḥ - मृगः	624
56	Mahiṣaḥ - महिषः	625
57	Balīvardaḥ - बलीवर्दः	625
	Matsyaḥ Vargaḥ - *मत्स्य वर्गः*	
	Matsyaḥ - मत्स्यः	626
	Viśiṣṭa Matsyānām Guṇakarmāṇi - विशिष्ट मत्स्यानां गुणकर्माणि	626
	Matsyabhedāḥ - मत्स्यभेदाः	627
	Rohitaḥ - रोहितः	628
	Pāṭhīnaḥ - पाठीनः	628
	Śafari, Proṣṭhī, Cilicimaśca - शफरी, प्रोष्टी चिलिचिमश्च	628
	Nadeyādi matsyāḥ - नादेयादि मत्स्याः	629
	Śiśumārādīnām Guṇakarmāṇi - शिशुमारादीनां गुणकर्माणि	629
59	Kacchapaḥ - कच्छपः	630
60	Āmūṣikā - आमूषिका	630
	Mūṣakaḥ - मूषकः (68)	630

Sr. No.		Page No.
	Mahāmūṣakaḥ - महामूषकः (69)	630
61	Biḍālaḥ - बिडालः	631
	Biḍāla Viśeṣāḥ - बिडाल विशेषाः (70)	631
62	Śṛgālaḥ - शृगालः	632
	Tarakśuḥ - तरक्षुः (71)	632
	Kukkuraḥ - कुक्कुरः (72)	632
63	Markaṭaḥ - मर्कटः	632
64	Barhiḥ - बर्हिः	633
65	Śilīmukhaḥ - शिलीमुखः (श्रमरः –Bhramaraḥ)	633
66	Śukaḥ - शुकः	634
67	Sārikā - सारिका	634
68	Cakravākaḥ - चक्रवाकः	634-35
69	Hamsaḥ - हंसः	635
70	Kukkuṭaḥ - कुक्कुटः	635
71	Lāvaḥ - लावः	636
72	Kokilaḥ - कोकिलः	636-37
	Kākaḥ - काकः (73)	637
73	Ulūkaḥ - उलूकः	638
74	Sarpaḥ - सर्पः	638
	Sarpaviśeṣāḥ - सर्पविशेषाः	639
75	Maṇḍūkaḥ - मण्डूकः	640
76	Malam - मलम्	640
	Gomayam - गोमयम्	641
77	Mūtram - मूत्रम्	641
	Gomūtram - गोमूत्रम्	641
	Ajā mūtram - अजामूत्रम्	641
	Meṣīmūtram - मेषीमूत्रम्	642
	Mahiṣīmūtram - महिषीमूत्रम्	642
	Gajamūtram - गजमूत्रम्	642
	Aśvamūtram - अश्वमूत्रम्	642
	Ūṣṭramūtram - ऊष्ट्रमूत्रम्	643
	Gardabha mūtram - गर्दभमूत्रम्	643
	Mānuṣa mūtram - मानुषमूत्रम्	643
78	Medaḥ - मेदः	643
79	Twak - त्वक्	643
80	Roma - रोम	644

Miśrakādi Chapter VII - मिश्रकादिः सप्तमोवर्गः

	Trifalā - त्रिफला	645
	Swādutrifalā - स्वादुत्रिफला	645
	Sugandhi trifalā - सुगंधि त्रिफला	645
	Trikaṭukam - त्रिकटुकम्	646

Sr. No.		Page No.
	Cātutbhadrakam - चातुर्भद्रकम्	646
	Dwitiyam Cāturbhadrakam - द्वितीयं चातुर्भद्रकम्	646
	Tṛtiyam Cāturbhadrakam - तृतीयं चातुर्भद्रकम्	647
	Pañcakolakam - पञ्चकोलकम्	647
	Pañcavalkalam - पञ्चवल्कलम्	647
	Pañcabhṛṅgam - पञ्चभृङ्गम्	648
	Madhyama Pañcamūlam - मध्यम पञ्चमूलम्	648
	Laghu Pañcamūlam - लघु पञ्चमूलम्	648
	Bṛhat-Pañcamūlam - बृहत् -पञ्चमूलम्	649
	Tṛṇa Pañcamūlam - तृणपञ्चमूलम्	649
	Jivana Pañcamūlam - जीवन पञ्चमूलम्	649
	Pañca Pañcamūlam - पञ्चपञ्चमूलम्	649-650
	Jivanaiya Gaṇaḥ - जीवनीयगणः	650
	Veśavāraḥ - वेशवारः	650
	Sambhāraḥ - संभारः	651
	Śikhariṇī - शिखरिणी	651
	Sarvauṣadhiḥ - सर्वौषधिः	652
	Sugandhāmalakam - सुगन्धामलकम्	652
	Pañcasugandhikam - पञ्चसुगन्धिकम्	652
	Parārdham - परार्धम्	653
	Vāṭyapuṣpam - वाट्यपुष्पम्	653
	Yakśakardamaḥ - यक्षकर्दमः	653
	Manthaḥ - मन्थः	653
	Santarpaṇam - संतर्पणम्	654
	Pañcamṛtam - पञ्चामृतम्	654
	Pañcāgavyam - पञ्चगव्यम्	654
	Pañcāmlakam - पञ्चाम्लकम्	654
	Dwitiyam Pañcāmlakam - द्वितीयं पञ्चाम्लकम्	655
	Pañca Nimbakam - पञ्चनिम्बकम्	655
	Lavaṇa pañcakam - लवणपञ्चकम्	655
	Pañcaśairiṣam - पञ्चशैरीषम	655
	Pañcāṅgam - पञ्चाङ्गम	655
	Pañca sārpakam - पञ्च सार्पकम्	656
	Pañca sūraṇam - पञ्चसूरणम्	656
	Pañca siddhauṣadhiḥ -पञ्चसिद्धौषधिः	656
	Raktavargaḥ - रक्तवर्गः	656
	Śuklavargah - शुक्लवर्गः	657
	Pañcagaṇaḥ - पञ्चगणः	657
	Mūtrāṣṭakam - मूत्राष्टकम्	657
	Kśāratrayam - क्षारत्रयम्	657
	Kśārapañcakam - क्षारपञ्चकम्	657
	Kśārāṣṭakam - क्षाराष्टकम्	657

Sr. No.		Page No.
	Kṣārasaṭkam - क्षारषट्कम्	658
	Trilavaṇam - त्रिलवणम्	658
	Lavaṇaṣaṭkam - लवणषट्कम्	658
	Trimadhuram - त्रिमधुरम्	658
	Ṣaḍrasāḥ - षड्रसाः	659
	Auṣadham - औषधम्	659
	Pathyam - पथ्यम्	660
	Ārogyam - आरोग्यम्	660
	Nīrogaḥ - नीरोगः	660
	Rogī - रोगी	660
	Vaidyaḥ - वैद्यः	660
	Āhāraḥ - आहारः	660
	Aṣtavidhamannam - अष्टविधमन्नम्	661
	Saptadhātavaḥ (Swarṇādi) - सप्तधातवः (स्वर्णादि)	661
	Upadhātavaḥ - उपधातवः	661
	Navaratnāni - नवरत्नानि	661
	Pañcaratnāni - पञ्चरत्नानि	662
	Uparatnāni - उपरत्नानि	662
	Uparasāḥ - उपरसाः	662
	Sādharaṇarasāḥ - साधारणरसाः	662
	Dhātavah -धातवः	663
1	Viṣāṇi - विषाणि	663
	Viṣam, Viṣabhedāḥ - विषं, विषभेदाः	663
	Sthāvaraviṣāṇi - स्थावर विषाणि	663
	Varjyaviṣāṇi - वर्ज्य विषाणि	663-64
	Kālakūṭah - कालकूटः	664
	Vatsanābhaḥ - वत्सनाभः	664
	Śṛngikaḥ - शृङ्गिकः	664
	Pradīpanaḥ - प्रदीपनः	665
	Hālāhalaḥ - हालाहलः	665
	Brahmaputraḥ - ब्रम्हपुत्र	665
	Hāridraḥ - हारिद्रः	665
	Saktukaḥ - सक्तुकः	665
	Saurāṣṭrikaḥ - सौराष्ट्रिकः	666
	Jaṅgama Viṣāsrayāḥ - जंगमविषाश्रयाः	666
	Viṣaguṇakarmmāṇi - विषगुणकर्माणिः	666
	Haritālam - हरितालम्	666
	Amṛtam-(Vatsanābhaḥ) - अमृतं -(वत्सनाभः)	667
2	Upaviṣāṇi - उपविषाणि	667
3	Viṣapraśamanānī- विषप्रशमनानि	667

अथ द्रव्यावलिः । Dravyāvalih

नमामि धन्वन्तरिमादिदेवं सुरासुरैर्वन्दितपादपद्मम् ।
लोके जरारुग्भयमृत्युनाशं धातारमीशं विविधौषधीनाम् ॥१॥

This is the salutary stanza in which compiler salutes the Ādideva Lord Dhanvantari whose lotus like feet are bowed to by *Suras & Asuras* alike and who holds various drugs within himself and destroys the fear of old age, diseases and death on this Earth.

ग्रन्थप्रयोजनम्

अनेकदेशान्तरभाषितेषु सर्वेष्वथ प्राकृतसंस्कृतेषु ।
गूढेष्वगूढेषु च नास्ति संख्या द्रव्याभिधानेषु तथौषधीषु ॥२॥

प्रयोजनं यस्य तु यावदेव तावत्स गृह्णाति यथाऽम्बुकूपात् ।
तथा निघण्टाम्बुनिधेरनन्ताद् गृह्णाम्यहं किञ्चिदिहैकदेशम् ॥३॥

There are innumerable drugs (medicinal plants either explicitly mentioned or otherwise) and their nomenclature either in Sanskṛta or in Prākṛta i.e. in regional languages is also innumerable.

However, according to one's own need an individual takes water from the well, similarly, I am also mentioning few drugs from the ocean like literature of the Nighaṇṭus. (It is suggested here that there were many Nighaṇṭus before the compilers work. But he has not mentioned their names.)

नामोक्तमेकस्य यदौषधस्य नामापरस्यापि तदेव चोक्तम् ।
शास्त्रेषु लोकेषु च यत्प्रसिद्धं न गृह्यतेऽसौ पुनरुक्तदोषः ॥४॥

It appears that one drug especially medicinal plant is known by a particular name. The other plant also be known by the same name. Because this practice is followed in the treatises and in the common usage therefore it cannot be called as repetition.

(The names which are famous in treatises and in public are not mentioned here to avoid repetition.) (see XLII)

तुल्याभिधानानि तु यानि शिष्टैर्द्रव्याणि योगे विनिवेशितानि ।
अर्थाधिकारागमसम्प्रदायैर्विभज्य तर्केण च तानि युञ्ज्यात् ॥५॥

When it is found that such different drugs having similar nomenclature are mentioned in a single formulation then the purpose, the reference (context), the treatise, and the reasoning should be taken into consideration for their proper usage.

किरात गोपालकतापसाद्या वनेचरास्तत्कुशलास्तथाऽन्ये ।
विदन्ति नानाविधभेषजानां प्रमाणवर्णाकृति नामजातीः ॥६॥

Kirātas - aboriginal tribes, shepherds (cowherds), hermits and other experts who are conversant (with the plants) know the size, shape, colour, name, habitat and types of various plants.
(They have a better knowledge of external morphology of the plants and their types, varieties etc.)

तेभ्यः सकाशादुपलभ्य वैद्यः पश्चाच्च शास्त्रेषु विमृश्य बुद्ध्या ।
विकल्पयेद् द्रव्यरसप्रभावान् विपाकवीर्याणि तथा प्रयोगात् ॥७॥

Therefore the physician (vaidya) should obtain the above mentioned knowledge and then comparing the same with the standard texts of the treatises with deep study and scientific reasoning and by pharmacological experimental work, should confirm (pharmacological) properties of the drug like rasa, vīrya, vipāka, prabhāva, etc.

प्रायो जनाः सन्ति वनेचरास्ते गोपादयः प्राकृतनामसंज्ञाः ।
प्रयोजनार्था वचनप्रवृत्तिर्यस्मात्ततः प्राकृतमित्यदोषः ॥८॥

Cowherds and the others who move in the forests use the names in *प्राकृत*-Prākṛta. Here it means the local languages, but since the language is meant to serve the purpose of extending the thoughts this cannot be called a drawback.

एकं तु नाम प्रथितं बहूनामेकस्य नामानि तथा बहूनि ।
द्रव्यस्य जात्याकृतिवर्णवीर्यरसप्रभावादि गुणैर्भवन्ति ॥९॥

One particular name is given to many drugs (plants) while one drug (plant) is known by many names. These names are given according to specificity (*जाती*), morphological characters (आकृति-वर्ण) and pharmacological properties like रस -rasa, वीर्य- vīrya, विपाक-vipāka and प्रभाव - prabhāva etc.

नाम श्रुतं केनचिदेकमेव तेनैव जानाति स भेषजं तु ।
अन्यस्तथाऽन्येन तु वेत्ति नाम्ना तदेव चान्योऽथ परेण कश्चित् ॥१०॥

Somebody might have heard a single name of a plant and he identifies the same plant by that particular name only. While the other person identifies it by some other name and the third one identifies the same plant which is known to himself and thus the names of plant vary in different regions.

बहून्यथ प्राकृतसंस्कृतानि नामानि विज्ञाय बहूंश्च पृष्ट्वा ।
दृष्ट्वा च संस्पृश्य च जातिलिंगैर्विद्यात् भिषग्भेषजमादरेण ॥११॥

Therefore one should identify the drug plants by collecting various regional as well as sanskṛta names in the texts and by integrating them with the names of the local people; by seeing (observation) by perception of the specificity and the morphological characters (लिंगैः) with utmost care.

गोपालास्तापसा व्याधा ये चान्ये वनचारिणः ।
मूलाहाराश्च ये तेभ्यो भेषजव्यक्तिरिष्यते ॥१२॥ Su.Su. 37.10

The plants should be identified with the help of cowherds, hermits, hunters and fowlers and others who move in the forests and who live on only by eating roots and tubers (of the plants).

अनामविन्मोहमुपैति वैद्यो न वेत्ति पश्यन्नपि भेषजानि ।
क्रियाक्रमो भेषजमूलमेव तद् भेषजं चापि निघण्टुमूलम् ॥१३॥

The physician gets confused without the knowledge of the names of drug plants and is unable to identify even on seeing them. The management of the diseases by various methods like purgation, emesis etc. depends upon the knowledge of the drug plants, and this knowledge of the drugs is based on Nighaṇṭus.

तस्मान्निघण्टुरित्येष नातिसंक्षेपविस्तरः ।
हिताय वैद्यपुत्राणां यथावत् संप्रकाश्यते ॥१४॥

Therefore this Nighaṇṭu neither too exhaustive nor too concise has been compiled for the benefit of the students of Ayurveda.

द्रव्यावलिं विना वैद्यास्ते वैद्या हास्यभाजनम् ।
द्रव्यावल्यभिधानानां तृतीयमिव लोचनम् ॥१५॥

द्रव्यावलिनिविष्टानां द्रव्याणां नामनिर्णयम् ।
लोकप्रसिद्धं वक्ष्यामि यथागमपरिस्फुटम् ॥१६॥

The vaidyas (physicians) who do not possess the knowledge of this Dravyāvalī (Nighaṇṭu) may be subjcted to ridicule and for those who possess this knowledge of the names of the plants mentioned in the text of this *द्रव्यावलि* - Dravyāvali - may help them like a third eye. I shall explain the names (nomenclature) of the drug plants mentioned in this *द्रव्यावलि* - Dravyāvali by their popular names as well as by the names deseribed in the text (of treatise).

अनन्तपारस्य निगृह्य किंचित्सारं चिकित्सागमसागरस्य ।
उक्तो मया संप्रति कल्पयोगाद् द्रव्यावलीनामसमुच्चयोऽयम् ॥१७॥

Taking a short extract of the endless ocean like text of the theraputics, I have prepared this compendium (treatise) *द्रव्यावलि नाम समुच्चय* (Dravyavali Nāma Samuccaya) by various formulations (*कल्पयोगात्*).

विचार्य दोषौषधदेशकालं वपुर्वयःसात्म्यबलाग्निमात्रम् ।
विकारहेत्वाकृतिसाध्यताश्च ततश्चिकित्सेद् भिषगामयार्तिम् ॥ १८

The physician after taking into consideration the various factors the *दोष* (Doṣas), *औषध* (drugs), the location (*देश*), time (*काल*) *वपुः* (Physical condition), *वयः* (age), *सात्म्य* (Sātmya), strength (*बल*), काल (time) *अग्निप्रमाण* (digestive and metabolic state), *हेतु* (Etiological factors), *आकृति* (external characters and pathology) and *साध्यासाध्यता* (Prognosis) should start the treatment.

ज्वराभिभूते षडहे व्यतीते विपक्वदोषे कृतलंघनाद्यैः ।
यद्भेषजं वैद्यवरप्रयुक्तं निःसंशयं हन्त्यचिरेण रोगान् ॥१९॥

e.g. if a person is having fever (*ज्वर* or *निजज्वर*), with the application of लंघन (*Langhana*) therapy for six days and when the offending *दोष* (*Doṣas*) are separated from the tissues *विपक्व दोषे*, or properly dealt with by the body, at that stage the properly selected medicine by the physician (Vaidya) will certainly cure the patient from the disease.

अथ गणद्रव्यावलिः
GAṆADRAVYĀVALIḤ

अथ गुडूच्यादिः प्रथमो वर्गः
GUḌŪCYĀDIḤ CHAPTER I.

गुडूच्यतिविषामूर्वा मञ्जिष्ठा धन्वयासकैः ।
वासाखदिरनिम्बैश्च पिबेत्क्वाथं कफज्वरे[1] ॥१॥

किराततिक्तकटुकामुस्तापर्पटकाम्बुभिः ।
पटोल द्विनिशाभ्यां च पिबेत्क्वाथं तु पैत्तिके ॥२

शठीपुष्करभार्गीभिः पाठा कट्फलदारुभिः ।
कट्तृणेनाथ शृङ्ग्या च पिबेत्क्वाथं तु वातिके ॥३॥

As already said that the drugs will be mentioned according to various formulations, useful in various diseases the *Gaṇadravyāvali* गणद्रव्यावली is stated below.

Since, ज्वर - *Jwara* is the foremost and most common amongst the diseases that affects the human beings and गुडूची - *Guḍūcī* is the most effective शमन - *Śamana* type of drug in the management of ज्वर - *Jwara,* the chapter begins with the plant गुडूची - *Guḍūcī* and the chapter is called as गुडूच्यादिवर्ग- Guḍūcyādi Chapter. The chapter is called by the name of the first plant of that particular chapter. eg. शतपुष्पादि Śatapuṣpādi, चंदनादि Candanādi etc.1) गुडूची-Guḍūcī 2) अतिविषा Ativiṣā 3) मूर्वा Mūrvā 4) मंजिष्ठा Mañjiṣṭhā 5) धन्वयास Dhanvayāsa 6) वासा Vāsā 7) खदिर Khadira 8) निम्ब Nimba. The decoction of these plants should be used in कफज्वर *kaphajwara.* 9) किराततिक्त Kirātatikta 10) कटुका Kaṭukā 11) मुस्ता Mustā 12) पर्पट Parpaṭa 13) अम्बु (वालक) Ambu (Vālaka) 14) पटोल Paṭola 15) द्विनिशा -(हरिद्रा, दारुहरिद्रा) - Dwiniśā - Haridrā & Dāruharidrā. The decoction of these plants should be used in पित्तज्वर *Pittajwara.* 16) शठी Śathī 17) पुष्कर (मूल) Puṣkaramūla 18) भार्ङ्गी Bhārṅgī 19) पाठा Pāṭhā 20) कट्फल Kaṭfala 21) दारु (देवदारु)
Dāru-(devadāru) & (22) कट्तृण Kaṭtṛṇa (23) शृंगी- कर्कटशृंगी Śṛṅgī Karkaṭśṛṅgī.

The decoction of these plants should be used in वातज्वर *Vātajwara.*

पर्ण्यौ बृहत्यौ गोकण्टो बिल्वोऽग्निमन्थनोऽरलुः ।
काश्मर्यः पाटला चेति संन्निपातहरो गणः ॥४॥

The reading 'पिबेत्क्वाथं तु वातिके' has been accepted by all the published as well as in most of the Mss. However, खदिर - *Khadira,* वासा - *Vāsā*, निंब - *Nimba* which are mentioned here are contraindicated in वातज्वर - *Vātajwara* therefore,the reading of शोढल - *Śodhala* is accepted here. S.D.K.

24) पर्ण्यौ Parṇyau i.e. Pṛsṇiparṇī- पृश्निपर्णी and śālaparṇī शालपर्णी 25) बृहत्यौ Bṛhatyau i.e.बृहती & क्षुद्रा कण्टकारी Bṛhatī and kśudrā kaṇṭa-kārī 26) गोकण्ट - Gokaṇṭa 27) बिल्व - Bilva 28) अग्निमन्थन Agnimanthana, 29) अरलु Aralu 30) काश्मर्यः Kāśmaryaḥ 31) पाटला Pātalā.

The decoction of the roots of these drug plants cure संनिपात ज्वर Sannipatajwara. It is called as संनिपातहर गण *Sannipātahara gaṇa.* The संनिपात *Sannipāta* is a condition caused by the vitiation of three *doṣas.*

It is the famous, combination of ten roots दशमूल *Daśamūla* of Ayurveda. It is again mentioned in the मिश्रकादि वर्ग Misrakādi chapter. But there the context is different and hence cannot be called as repetition there.

जीवकर्षभकौ मेदे काकोल्यौ द्वे च योजिते ।
द्वे [१] सुपर्ण्यौ च जीवन्ती मधुकं रक्तपित्तनुत् ॥५॥

32) जीवकः Jīvakaḥ 33) Ṛṣabhakaḥ ऋषभकः 34) मेदे Mede i.e. मेदा & महामेदा Medā & Mahāmedā 35) काकोल्यौ Kākolyau i.e. काकोलि Kākolī & क्षीर काकोलि KśiraKākoli 36) सुपर्ण्यौ Suparṇyau i.e. मुद्गपर्णी Mudgaparṇi & माषपर्णी Māṣaparṇī 37) जीवन्ती Jīvantī & 38) मधुकम् Madhukam. These plants should be used in रक्तपित्त विकार (Diseases caused by *Rakta and Pitta doṣas)* (Haemorrhagic disorders).

This is the well known जीवनीय Jīvanīya gaṇa of the classical books and also mentioned in Miśrakādi chapter - मिश्रकादि वर्ग.

ऋद्धिर्विदार्यात्मगुप्ता शितिवाराश्मभेदकौ ।
श्रावण्यौ सारिवे चोभे बाकुची रक्तवातनुत् ॥६॥

39) ऋद्धि Ṛddhi 40) विदारी Vidārī 41) आत्मगुप्ता Ātmaguptā 42) शितिवार Śitivāra 43) अश्मभेदक Aśmabhedaka 44) श्रावण्यौ Śrāvaṇyau i.e. two types of Sravanī 45) सारिवे (i.e. two types of sārivā) & 46) बाकुची Bākucī .

These drug plants are used in रक्त & वात विकार (i.e. diseases caused by *Rakta and Vāta doṣās.)*

मदनेक्ष्वाकुजीमूतस्त्रपुसं कृतवेधनम् ।
धामार्गवोऽश्मन्तकश्च कोविदारो विषाणिका[२]॥७॥

शणपुष्पी तथा बिम्बी स्नेहस्वेदवतां तथा ।
श्रेष्ठमेतत्प्रयोक्तव्यं वमनं श्लेष्मरोगिणाम् ॥८॥

---

१ "द्वे सूर्पपर्ण्यौ" इति पा.
२ "विषाणिका " as appeared in paryāya Nāmāvali.

47) मदनः Madanaḥ 48) इक्ष्वाकुः Ikśvākuḥ 49) जीमूतः Jīmūtaḥ 50) त्रपुसम् Trapusam 51) कृतवेधनम् Kṛtavedhanam 52) धामार्गवः Dhāmārgavaḥ 53) अश्मन्तकः Aśmantakaḥ 54) कोविदारः Kovidāraḥ 55) विषाणिकः Viṣāṇikaḥ 56) शणपुष्पी Śaṇapuṣpī 57) बिम्बी Bimbī

These drug plants are used for वमन चिकित्सा (therapy of Emesis) which is followed after the procedure of स्नेहन *Snehana* and स्वेदन *Svedana* therapy. This वमन *Vamana* therapy is the most effective (श्रेष्ठम) treatment for the disorders caused by कफदोष - *Kaphadoṣa.*

त्रिफलाऽऽरग्वधो दन्ती द्रवन्ती नीलिनी सुधा ।
सप्तला काञ्चनक्षीरी त्रिवृता चेन्द्रवारुणी ॥९

विशाला त्रायमाणा च शङ्खिन्यङ्कोल एव च ।
श्रेष्ठं पित्तविकारेषु योज्यमेतद् विरेचनम् ॥१०

58) त्रिफला Trifalā i.e. हरीतकी Harītakī, आमलकी Āmalakī & बिभीतक Bibhītaka 59) आरग्वध Āragvadha 60) दन्ती Dantī 61) द्रवन्ती Dravantī 62)नीलिनी Nīlinī 63) सुधा Sudhā 64) सप्तला Saptalā 65) कांचनक्षीरी Kañcanakśīrī 66) त्रिवृता Trivritā 67) इन्द्रवारुणी Indravāruṇī 68) विशाला Viśālā 69) त्रायमाणा Trāyamāṇā 70) शंखिनी Śaṅkhinī & 71) अंकोल Aṅkola.

These are the drug plants used for विरेचन - *Virecana* which is the most effective treatment of पित्तदोष - *Pittadoṣa.*

अपामार्गस्तेजवती तथा ज्योतिष्मतीफलम् ।
योज्यं नस्यं कृमिव्याधौ[१] शिरोरोगे च पीनसे ॥११॥

72) अपामार्ग Apāmārga 73) तेजवती Tejavatī 74) ज्योतिष्मती Jyotiṣmatī; fruits of these drug plants are to be used as नस्य - *Nasya* nasal medication in कृमिरोग Kṛmiroga, शिरोरोग - *Śiroroga.* (diseases of the head), diseases of ear, nose, throat, eyes and पीनस *Pinasa* (ch. sinusitis) etc.

रास्नाऽश्वगंधा वर्षाभूस्तथा सहचरो बला ।
प्रसारणी शतावर्याविरण्डश्चापि सर्वतः ॥१२॥

आस्थापनं कल्पमेतैस्तथा वातानुलोमनम्[२] ।
तैलं कषाय[३]पिष्टैश्च गोक्षीरैः[४] साधितं जयेत् ॥१३॥

---

१. "कृतिव्याधौ" इति आनन्दाश्रम मुद्रित पुस्तके पाठः । अत्र तु शोढल संमतः पाठः स्वीकृतः साधुत्वात् ।
२. "वातेऽनुवासनम्" इति शोढल पाठः ।
३. "कषाय पेष्यैस्तु" इति शोढलः ।
४. "सक्षीरं" शोढल संमतः पाठः ।

वातशोणितमर्शांसि ज्वरमुन्मादमर्दितम् ।
कट्यूरुपार्श्वपृष्ठार्ति शोषं शोफं सवेपथुम् ॥१४॥

75) रास्ना Rāsnā 76) अश्वगन्धा Aśvagandhā 77) वर्षाभू Varṣābhū 78) सहचरः Sahacaraḥ 79) बला Balā 80) प्रसारणी Prasāraṇī 81) शतावर्यौ Śatāvaryau & 82) एरण्डः Eraṇḍaḥ

आस्थापन कल्प - Āsthāpana Kalpa i.e. decoction of these plants is used for आस्थापन बस्ति Āsthāpana basti therapy. The oil prepared with the above mentioned plants (the decoction, paste etc. of these plants), cow milk, should be used for स्नेहबस्ती Snehabasti or अनुवासन बस्ति Anuvāsana basti therapy. आस्थापन बस्ति *Āsthāpana basti* therapy and अनुवासनबस्ति *Anuvāsana basti* therapy should be used in the treatment of वात शोणित - *Vātaśoṇita* (? Gout), अर्श Arśa. (Piles in ano), ज्वर (Jwara) (in certain stages and types of fevers, उन्माद - *Unmāda* - (certain psychological disorders), अर्दित - *Ardita* (facial palsy and some other types of palsies), कटि, ऊरु, पार्श्व, पृष्ठ – अर्ति, Kati, Uru, Pārśva, Pṛṣtha-arti (i.e. various types of pains and aches in the lumbosacral region, the thighs, the ribs and the back), शोष *Śoṣa* (disorders caused by atrophy, muscular weakness), शोफ *Śofa* - various types of inflammatory conditions, oedema, वेपथु - *Vepathu* - tremors (eg. Parkinson's disease.)

गुडूच्यादिरयं वर्गः प्रथमः परिकीर्तितः ।
ऊर्ध्वाधोदोषहरणः सर्वामयविनाशनः ॥

Thus has been told the first Guḍūcyādi Chapter in which the drugs are mentioned for removal of the *Doṣās* from both the routes upper and lower and generally for all the types of diseases.

अथ शतपुष्पादिर्द्वितीयो वर्गः ।
Śatapuṣpādiḥ Chapter II

शतपुष्पा मिशिर्वचा हपुषा कृमिहा तथा ।
सवत्सकश्चेन्द्रयवा त्रिक्षारा लवणानि च ॥१५॥

हिंगुर्हिंगुशिवाटी च तुम्बरुत्वक्फलानि च ।
एभिः सुसाधितं सर्पिः पयसा योनिदोषनुत् ॥१६॥

मूत्रकृच्छ्रार्तिशूलघ्नं वन्ध्यानामपि गर्भदम् ।
ग्रहण्यर्शःपाण्डुरोगप्लीहगुल्मोदरापहम् ॥१७॥

1) शतपुष्पा Śatapuṣpā 2) मिशि Miśi 3) वचा Vacā 4) हपुषा Hapuṣā 5) कृमिहा Kṛmihā (viḍangam), 6) वत्सकः (कुटजः) Vatsakaḥ (Kuṭajaḥ), 7) इन्द्रयवः Indrayavaḥ 8) त्रिक्षाराः Trikśārāḥ, 9) लवणानि (Lavaṇāni), 10) हिंगु Hingu 11) हिंगु शिवाटी Hinguśivāṭī 12) तुम्बरु Tumbaru.

The ghee prepared with milk and the bark & fruits of the above mentioned drugs is useful in योनी दोष (disorders of the female reproductive organs, स्त्रीवन्ध्यत्व(female sterility), disorders of ग्रहणी Grahaṇī, अर्श - Arśa- Piles in ano, पाण्डु *Panḍu* (certain types of anaemias), प्लीहा *Plīhā*- certain disorders of spleen, गुल्म -*Gulma* (certain intestinal disorders eg. diverticulae) उदर विकार - *Udara vikāra* (eg. Ascites), Pain due to मूत्रकृच्छ्र *Mutrakṛchra*, शूल *Śūla* (various types of colics).

सूक्ष्मैला केसरं त्वक् च पत्रं तालीसकं तुगा ।
पृथ्वीका दाडिमं धान्यं जीरकं च द्विकार्षिकम् ॥१८॥

पिप्पली पिप्पलीमूलं चव्यचित्रकनागरम् ।
मरीचं दीप्यकं चैव वृक्षाम्लं साम्लवेतसम् ॥१९॥

अजमोदाजगन्धे च दधित्थं चेति कार्षिकम् ।
प्रदेयमिह शुद्धायाः शर्करायाश्चतुष्पलम् ॥२०॥

चूर्णमग्निप्रदं नाम परमं रुचिवर्धनम् ।
प्लीहाकासामयार्शांसि श्वासं शूलं ज्वरं वमिम् ॥२१॥

निहन्ति दीपयत्यग्निं बलवर्णकरं परम् ।
वातानुलोमनं हृद्यं कण्ठजिव्हाविशोधनम् ॥२२॥

13) सूक्ष्मैला Sūkśmailā 14) केसर Kesara 15) त्वक् Twak 16) पत्रम् Patram 17) तालीसकम् Tālīsakam 18) तुगा Tugā 19) पृथ्वीका Pṛthvīkā 20) दाडिमम् Dāḍimam 21) धान्यम् Dhānyam 22) जीरकम् Jīrakam each measuring 2 Karṣas (2 tolas) 23) पिप्पली Pippalī, 24) पिप्पलीमूल Pippalīmūla 25) चव्यम्Cavyam 26) चित्रक Citraka 27) नागरम् Nāgaram 28) मरीचम् Marīcam29) दीप्यकम् Dīpyakam 30) वृक्षाम्लम् Vṛkśāmlam 31) अम्लवेतसम Amlavetasam 32) अजमोदा Ajamodā 33) अजगन्धा Ajagandhā 34) दधित्थम् Dadhittham (कपित्थम् Kapittham) each measuring 1 कर्ष Karṣa(1 Tola), and to this 35) शर्करा Śarkarā meausuring चतुःपलम् Catuḥpalam (16 tolas) should be mixed.

All these made into powders and mixed together. The mixture of all these powders is known as अग्निप्रद चूर्ण *Agniprada Chūrṇa*. This *chūrṇa* is very effective to improve the taste and is useful in the following conditions like प्लीहा *Plīhā* (disorders of spleen), कासामय *Kāsāmaya* (disorders of the respiratory passage), अर्श Arśa (Piles in ano) श्वास *Śwāsa* (Bronchial asthma, Bronchospasms), शूल *Śūla* (intestinal colic), ज्वर *Jwara*,(fevers), वमि *Vami* (Vomiting).

It stimulates the digestive (and assimilative) power, improves physical strength and the complexion of the body. It is carminative, cordial and clears the throat and the tongue.

शतपुष्पादिको वर्गः द्वितीयः परिकीर्तितः ।
कायाग्निदीपनो बल्यो वक्त्रसौगन्ध्य तीक्ष्णकृत् ॥

Thus has been described the शतपुष्पादि *Śatapuṣpādi* second chapter. The drugs mentioned in it stimulate and strengthen the digestive (and metabolic) capacity of the body. They also improve the taste and odour of the mouth.

अथ चन्दनादिस्तृतीयो वर्गः ।
Candanādiḥ Chapter III.

चन्दनं कुंकुमोशीरं प्रियङ्गुस्तुणिरोचना ।
तुरुष्कागरुकस्तूर्यः कर्पूरो जातिपत्रिका ॥ २३॥

जातिकंक्कोलपूगानां लवङ्गस्य फलानि च ।
नलिका नलदं कुष्टं हरेणुस्तगरं प्लवम् ॥ २४॥

नखं व्याघ्रनखं स्पृक्का बोलो दमनकं मुरा ।
स्थौणेयकं चोरकं च शैलेयं त्वेलवालुकम् ॥ २५॥

सरलं सप्तपर्णं च लाक्षा तामलकी तथा ।
लामज्जकं पद्मकं च धातक्याः कुसुमानि च ॥२६॥
प्रपौण्डरीकं कर्चूरं समांशैः सममात्रिकैः ॥
महासुगन्धमित्येतत् प्रस्थं तैलस्य साधयेत् ॥२७॥
प्रस्वेदमलदौर्गन्ध्य कण्डूकुष्टहरं परम् ॥
अनेनाभ्यक्तगात्रस्तु वृद्धः सप्ततिकोऽपि वा ॥२८॥

युवा भवति शुक्राढ्यः स्त्रीणामत्यन्तवल्लभः ।
सुभगो दर्शनीयश्च गच्छेच्च प्रमदाशतम् ॥२९॥
वन्ध्याऽपि लभते गर्भं षण्डोऽपि पुरुषायते ।
अपुत्रः पुत्रमाप्नोति जीवेच्च शरदां शतम् ॥३०॥

1) चंदन Candana 2) कुंकुम Kumkuma 3) उशीर Usīra 4) प्रियङ्गु Priyangu 5) तुणि Tuṇi 6) रोचना Rocanā 7) तुरुष्क Turuṣka 8) अगुरु Aguru 9) कस्तूरी

Kastūrī 10) कर्पूर Karpūra 11) जातिपत्रिका Jātipatrikā 12) जातीफल Jātiphala 13) कंकोल Kamkola 14) पूग Pūga and 15) लवङ्ग Lavanga (fruits of) 16) नलिका Nalikā 17)नलद Nalada 18) कुष्ठ Kuṣṭha 19) हरेणु Hareṇu 20) तगर Tagara 21) प्लव Plava 22) नख Nakha 23) व्याघ्रनख Vyāghranakha 24) स्पृक्का Spṛkkā 25) बोल Bola 26) दमनक Damanaka 27) मुरा Murā 28) स्थौणेयक Sthauṇeyaka 29) चोरक Coraka 30) शैलेय Śaileya 31) एलवालुक Elavāluka 32) सरल Sarala 33) सप्तपर्ण Saptaparṇa 34) लाक्षा Lākśā 35) तामलकी Tāmalakī 36) लामज्जक Lāmajjaka 37) पद्मक Padmaka 38) flowers of धातकी Dhātakī 39) प्रपौण्डरीक Prapauṇḍarīka 40) कर्चूर Karcūra.

All these drugs should be taken in equal proportion and one प्रस्थ - *Prastha* oil (sesamum oil) is prepared (as per procedure). This is called as महासुगन्ध तैल - *Mahāsugandha Taila.* It removes the bad odour of the body due to excessive sweating, and is very effective in pruritus, and skin disorders, with regular massage of this oil on the whole body, an old man of even seventy years old looks younger, and improves his rejuvinative capacity, is attracted by women, becomes fortunate, good looking and enjoys many women. Impotent man having no child gets the capacity to have a child and lives longer.

मनःशिला ससिन्दूरं सौराष्ट्री गन्धमाचिका[१] ।
ससिक्थकः सर्जरसः कासीसं पुरकुन्दरु ॥ ३१॥

श्याह्वः सल्लकि कम्पिल्लं सकंकुष्ठमरुष्करम् ।
एभिर्गोमूत्रसंसिद्धं कटुतैलं विपाचयेत् ॥ ३२॥

पामाविचर्चिकादद्रुकण्डुकुष्ठकृमिव्रणान् ।
अभ्यङ्गान्नाशयत्येव नाम्ना विद्रावणं मतम् ॥ ३३ ॥

41) मनःशिला Manaḥśilā - Realgar, 42) सिन्दूर - Sindūra - Red lead 43) सौराष्ट्री - Saurāṣṭrī - Alum. 44) गन्धक Gandhaka- sulphur 45) माचिका- Macikā 46) सिक्थक Sikthaka-wax 47) सर्जरस - Sarjarasa - gum resin of śala tree. 48) कासीस - Kāsīsa-ferrous sulphate 49) पुर -Pura-guggulu (gum resin of guggul tree.) 50) कुन्दुरु -Kunduru 51) श्याह्वः Śryāvhaḥ 52) सल्लकी - Sallakī 53) कम्पिल्ल Kampilla 54) कंकुष्ठ Kamkuṣṭha 55) अरुष्कर Aruṣkara.

कटुतैल - Kaṭutaila (Oil of mustard) is prepared with all the above drugs and cowurine. It is known as *Vidrāvaṇa Taila.* The massage of this oil cures skin disorders like पामा- *Pāmā* (Scabies), विचर्चिका *Vicarcikā,* दद्रु *Dadru,* कण्डू *Kaṇḍū* (Pruritus), कुष्ठ skin disorders कृमि *Kṛmi* (pathological microorganisms of the skin- parasites etc.) and व्रण *Vraṇa* (various ulcers and sores).

---

१ 'गन्धकद्वयम्' इति आनन्दा. पुस्तके पाठः । 'गन्धकोमची' इति शोढल पाठः । (see F. N. p. 247)

तुत्थं तु ताप्याञ्जन धातुफेनैश्चक्षुष्यरीतिकतरोध्रशङ्खैः ।
नेत्राञ्जनं काचमलार्तिकण्डूरुग्दाहतैमिर्यहरं परं च ॥३४॥

56) तुत्थ - Tuttha (Copper sulphate), 57) ताप्य Tāpya (copper pyrite) 58) अञ्जन Añjana (Galena) 59) धातु Dhātu (गैरिक - Gairika- ochre) 60) समुद्रफेन Samudrafena (os sepiae) 61) चक्षुष्या Cakśuṣyā 62) रीतीज Ritīja - पुष्पाञ्जन Puspāñjana (zinc oxide) 63) कतक Kataka 64) रोध्र Rodhra 65) शंख Sankha (Conch).

The नेत्राञ्जन *Netrāñjana* prepared from these drugs is useful in various opthalmic disorders like काच *(Kāca)*, irritation, pruritus, pain, burning and तिमिर *Timira.*

चन्दनादिरयं वर्गस्तृतीयः परिकीर्तितः ।
श्रीमतां भोगिनामर्हः प्रायो गन्धगुणाश्रयः ॥

Thus the third चंदनादि वर्ग Candanādi Chapter has been told. This chapter mainly consists of aromatic perfumery drugs which are mainly useful to the kings and wealthy people.

अथ करवीरादिश्चतुर्थो वर्गः ।

Karviradiḥ Chapter IV.

करवीरस्त्वेडगजो धत्तूरो लाङ्गली तथा ।
भृङ्गार्कबूक काकाह्वा मूलकं शिग्रुसर्षपौ ॥३५॥

भूतिः सुरसजम्बीरं कुठेरः सुमुखासुरी ।
एभिः सुतक्रसौवीरैर्दद्रुमण्डलतां जयेत् ॥३६॥

सिध्मातिपामापिटका कृमिकुष्ठानि नाशयेत् ।
एभिर्गोमूत्र संसिद्धं कटुतैलं विपाचयेत् ॥३७॥

1) करवीर Karavīra 2) एडगज Eḍagaja 3) धत्तूर Dhattūra 4) लांगली Lāngalī 5) भृङ्गराज Bhṛngarāja 6) अर्क Arka 7) बूक Būka 8) काकाह्वा Kākāhvā 9) मूलक Mūlaka 10) शिग्रु Sigru 11) सर्षप Sarṣapa 12) भूतिक Bhūtika 13) सुरस Surasa 14) जम्बीर Jambīra 15) कुठेर Kuṭhera 16) सुमुख Sumukha 17) आसुरी Āsurī.

With these drugs and buttermilk, Kāñjī, Cowurine, the mustard oil

1. "रेरङगमुद्वर्तनं भवेत" इति साधु पाठभेदः आनन्दा.पुस्तके ।
२. "दद्रुमुद्वर्तनं" इति शोढल पाठः । अस्मिन् स्थाने--- "सिध्मानि पामापिटकान् कृमींश्च कुष्ठान्यरुंषि प्रसुतान व्रणांश्च। गोमूत्र सिद्धं कटुतैलमेभिर्विनाशयेत् सर्व विचर्चिकाश्च ॥" इति शोढल पाठः ।

should be prepared as per procedure.This oil by external application is useful in Sidhma (fungal inf. of skin), scabies, boils, worms and skin disorders.

[1]काण्डीर जलपिप्पल्यौ रसोनो गृञ्जनं तथा ।
पलाण्डुदुर्द्रुमश्चैव योज्यं कृमिविनाशनम् ॥३८॥

18) काण्डीर Kāṇḍīra 19) जलपिप्पली Jala Pippalī 20) रसोन Rasona 21) गृञ्जन Gṛñjana 22) पलाण्डु Palāṇḍu 23) दुर्द्रुम Durdṛuma

These drugs should be used in कृमिविकार -*Kṛmivikāra* (intestinal worms ?).

कदली सिन्दुवारौ च निर्गुण्डी गिरिकर्णिका ।
जन्तुकारी च पद्मा च वाराही मांसरोहिणी ॥३९॥

वन्दकादित्यकान्ता च नाकुल्यौ वृद्धदारकः ।
रक्तपाद्यौ शङ्खपुष्पी तण्डुली कासमर्दकः ॥४०॥

पिष्टैस्तु बस्तमूत्रेण योज्यमेतद् गदे ज्वरे ।
नस्ये धूमप्रयोगेषु सर्वभूतग्रहापहम् ॥४१॥

उन्मादमोहज्वरकृच्छ्लूताजलाग्निचोरोरगवृश्चिकादीन् ।
उपद्रवानेष विषाणि हन्ति सकृत्रिमस्थावरजङ्गमानि ॥४२॥

24) कदली Kadalī 25) सिन्दुवार Sinduvāra 26) निर्गुण्डी Nirguṇḍī 27) गिरिकर्णिका Girikarṇikā 28) जन्तुकारी Jantukārī 29) पद्मा Padmā 30) वाराही Vārāhī 31) मांसरोहिणी Māmsarohiṇī 32) वन्दका Vandakā 33) आदित्यकान्ता Ādityakāntā 34) नाकुल्यौ Nākulyau 35) वृद्धदारक Vṛddhadāraka 36) रक्तपाद्यौ Raktapadyau 37) शंखपुष्पी Śaṅkhapuṣpī 38) तण्डुलीय Taṇḍulīya 39) कासमर्द Kāsamarda.

The paste of these drug plants should be treated in goat's urine (shegoat's) and can be used as नस्य (Nasya - *Avapīḍa Nasya.* अवपीडनस्य)and *Dhūma* therapy (धूम) as per the procedures laid down in the texts.

This therapy is useful in भूतग्रह *Bhūtagraha,* उन्माद *Unmāda,* अपस्मार *Apasmāra* etc. and also useful in certain fevers when associated with above mentioned conditions. This is also useful in poisonous effects caused by immovable (स्थावर) & movable - जंगम substances, as well as from natural and artificially prepared poisons.

[2]इक्षवस्त्रिविधाः काशो दर्भौ द्वौ च शरस्तथा ।
वंशो नलश्च दूर्वा च श्वेतनीलारुणोत्पलम् ॥४३॥

---

१. "गण्डीर गजपिप्पल्यौ" इति शोढल पाठः । पर्यायेषु तु (पृ.५५) "गजपिप्पली"स्थाने "जलपिप्पल्याः" पर्यायः शोढलेन लिखिताः । S.D.Kamat.}

२ "इक्षवो विविधाः" इति शोढल पाठः । "त्रिविधाः" इक्षवः इति मुद्रित निघण्टौ अपिच पर्यायनाम द्रव्यावल्यां स्पष्टीकृताः । स.दि.कामत.

पद्मिनी पद्मबीजं च मृणालं मूलकेसरम् ।
एतद्धि रक्तपित्तोत्थे विकारे परमं हितम् ॥४४॥

40) इक्षवः - त्रिविधाः Iks'avaḥ trividhāḥ 41) काशः Kāsaḥ 42) दर्भौ Darbhau 43) शरौ Sarau 44) वंशः Vamsaḥ 45) नलः Nalaḥ 46) दूर्वा Durvā 47) श्वेतनीलारुणोत्पलम् Svetanilāruṇotpalam 48) पद्मिनी-बीज - मृणालं - मूल - केसरम् - Padmini (its) bijam, mrṇālam, mūlam & kesaram.

These drug plants are useful in the disorders caused by रक्त-पित्तदोष Rakta and Pitta doṣas - bleeding disorders.

करवीरादिको वर्गश्चतुर्थः समुदाहृतः ।
नानाव्याधिप्रशमनो नानाद्रव्यसमाश्रयः॥

Thus has been said the Karavirādi IV th chapter in which various drugs have been mentioned. These cure various diseases.

अथ आम्रादिः पञ्चमो वर्गः ।
Āmrādiḥ Chapter V.

आम्राम्रातकजम्बीरंनारङ्गं बीजपूरकम् ।
अम्लिकारुकभव्यानि तिन्दुकश्च विकंकतम् ॥१॥

मधूकं पीलु खर्जूरं द्राक्षाक्षोडपरूषकम् ।
तूदं पालेवतं तालं प्रियालं नारिकेलकम् ॥२॥

वटाश्वत्थप्लक्षजम्बूदुम्बरं फल्गु क्षीरिणी ।
श्लेष्मातकः शमी कोलं करीरं करमर्दकम्* ॥३॥

एषां फलानि हृद्यानि यथाकालर्तुकानि च ।
समाहृत्य प्रयोज्यानि बलवर्णाग्निवृद्धये ॥४॥

1) आम्र Āmra 2) आम्रातक Āmrātaka 3) जम्बीर Jambira 4) नारङ्ग Nāranga 5) बीजपूरक Bijapūraka 6) अम्लिका Amlikā 7) आरुक Āruka 8) भव्य Bhavya 9) तिन्दुक Tinduka 10) विकंकत Vikankata 11) मधूक Madhūka 12) पीलु Pilu 13) खर्जूर Kharjūra 14) द्राक्षा Drāksā 15) अक्षोड Aksoḍa 16) परुषक Paruṣaka 17) तूद Tūda 18) पालेवत Pālevata 19) ताल Tāla 20) प्रियाल Priyāla 21) नारिकेल Nārikela 22) वट Vaṭa 23) अश्वत्थ Asvattha 24) प्लक्ष Plaksa 25) जम्बू Jambū 26) उदुम्बर Udumbara 27) फल्गु Falgu 28) क्षीरिणी Ksiriṇi 29) श्लेष्मातक Sleṣmātaka 30) शमी Sami 31) कोल Kola 32) करीर Karira 33) करमर्दक Karamardaka.

* संहिताग्रंथेषु निर्दिष्टफलवर्गस्य साम्यमत्र द्रष्टव्यम् । स.दि.कामत.

The fruits of these plants, being seasonal and of proper ripening times should be used for increasing the strength, वर्ण *Varṇa* -complexion - lustre and digestive capacity.

कदम्बौ द्वौ करञ्जौ च शिरीषार्जुनवेतसाः ।
वरुणः शिंशपा सर्जः शाल्मली मुष्ककोऽरिमः ॥५

एषां पयः प्रपिष्टानि वल्कलानि च योजयेत् ।
विसर्पव्रणरुग्दाहशोफार्तानां प्रशान्तये* ॥६॥

34) कदम्बौ Kadambau 35) करञ्जौ Karañjau 36) शिरीष Śirīṣa 37) अर्जुन Arjuna 38) वेतस Vetasa 39) वरुण Varuṇa 40) शिंशपा Śiṁśapā 41) सर्ज Sarja 42) शाल्मली Śālmalī 43) मुष्कक Muṣkaka 44) अरिम Arima

(Stem bark) containing sap (latex) of all these drug plants should be used in विसर्प - *Visarpa* (Erysipelas), abscess, wounds, and other painful, inflammatory and oedamatous conditions.

पुष्पवर्ग (Flowers)

मल्लिका वार्षिकी जाती वासन्तीग्रैष्मचम्पकाः ।
तरुण्यौ यूथिका कुन्दशतपत्रातिमुक्तकाः ॥७॥

बकुलः किंकिरातश्च तिलकाशोककिंशुकाः ।
पुष्पाण्येतानि धार्याणि हृद्यसौगन्ध्यमिच्छता ॥८॥

45) मल्लिका Mallikā 46) वार्षिकी Vārṣikī 47) जाती Jātī 48) वासन्ती Vāsantī 49) ग्रैष्मी Graiṣmī 50) चम्पक Campaka 51) तरुण्यौ Taruṇyau-2 types of तरुणी- *Taruṇī* 52) यूथिका Yūthikā 53) कुन्द Kunda 54) शतपत्र Śatapatrā 55) अतिमुक्तक Atimuktaka 56) बकुल Bakula 57) किंकिरात Kiṁkirāta 58) तिलक Tilaka 59) अशोक Aśoka & 60) किंशुक Kiṁśuka.

Those who like the pleasing fragrance should hold the flowers of these plants on the body.

आम्रादिरयमुद्दिष्टो वर्गः श्रेष्ठस्तु पञ्चमः ।
हर्षणो गन्धसौरभ्यफलत्वक्पुष्पसंश्रयः ॥

Thus the Āmrādi fifth and the most important chapter has been told. Here the plants having fruits with pleasing odour, क्षीरिवृक्ष latex or sap containing plants and flowers having fragrance are mentioned.

---

१) "प्रतिष्ठानि" इति शोढल पाठः । The stembark should contain sap i.e. these should be used in wet state and not the dried ones. S.D.Kamat.

* The fruits and sap containing stembarks are mentioned for the purpose of example. By this, many which are not mentioned here, and are in practical use should also be taken into consideration.

अथ सुवर्णादिः षष्ठो वर्गः ।
Suvarnadiḥ Chapter VI.

सुवर्णरौप्यताम्राणि त्रपु रीतिश्च सीसकम् ।
कांस्यं लौहं* च योज्यानि गरदोषप्रशान्तये ॥१॥

1) सुवर्ण Suvarṇa - Gold 2) रौप्य Raupya Silver 3) ताम्र Tāmra-Copper 4) त्रपु Trapu - Tin 5) रीतिः Ritiḥ - Pittala 6) सीसक Sīsaka-Lead 7) कांस्य Kāmsya - Bell metal 8) लोह Loha-iron are the metals which should be used in गरदोष *Gara doṣa* (artificially prepared poison).

रसवैक्रान्त गारुत्मं हीरमुक्तप्रवालकम् ।
क्षय पाण्डुमतीसारं गरलादि विषं जयेत् ॥२

9) रस-Rasa (Mercury) 10) वैक्रान्त Vaikrānta 11) गारुत्म-Gārutma 12) हीरक Hīrakā (Diamond) 13) मुक्ता Muktā (Pearl) 14) प्रवाल Prawāla. These gems should be used in क्षय *Ksaya,* -consumption, पांडु *Pāṇḍu* अतिसार *diarrhoea* and गरल *Garala.* (a type of poison).

शालिव्रीहियवा मुद्गा राजमाषाश्च कोद्रवाः ।
नीवारश्यामकौ कङ्गुर्वनमुद्गाढकी तथा ॥३॥

श्लेष्मपित्तहरा ह्येताः शीतलाः शुक्रला अपि ।
तद्वन्मसूरिका हन्ति मसूरीं ग्रहणीं तथा ॥४॥

15) शालि Śāli 16) व्रीहि Virīhī 17) यव Yava 18) मुद्ग Mudga 19) राजमाष Rājamāṣa 20) कोद्रव Kodrava 21) नीवार Nīvāra 22) श्यामाक Śyāmāka 23) कङ्गु Kangu 24) वनमुद्ग Vanamudga 25) आढकी Āḍhakī etc. are used in *Ślesma*-श्लेष्म and *Pitta* पित्त disorders. These are *Śītavīrya* and *Vṛṣya.* 26) मसूरिका Masūrikā has similar properties and is useful in ग्रहणी *Grahaṇī* and मसूरिका *Masūrikā* (Chicken pox).

गोधूमधान्यमाषाद्या विज्ञेया गुरुशीतलाः ।
वृष्या मलकराः प्रोक्ताः स्निग्धा वातविनाशनाः ॥५॥

चणका वर्तुलाः प्रोक्ता वातला रक्तपित्तहाः ।
कुलित्थाः श्वासहिक्कार्शःकफशुक्रानिलापहाः ॥६॥

27) गोधूम Godhūma 28) धान्यमाष Dhānyamāṣa etc. are गुरु *Guru,* शीतवीर्य *Śītavīrya,* वृष्य *Vṛṣya,* मलकर *Malakara* (increase faecal quantity), स्निग्ध *Snigdha* and useful in disorders of वात *Vāta.* 29) चणक Caṇaka 30)

---

* Śodhala mentions these 8 metals only. The drugs mentioned here onwards does not seem to be included by him. His Miśrakādi chapter also differs considerably. The reference of this is already done in the preface. S.D.Kamat.

वर्तुल Vartula aggravate वातदोष *Vātadoṣa* and cure रक्त *Rakta* and पित्तदोष *Pittadoṣa.* 31) कुलित्थ Kulittha is useful in श्वास-*Śwāsa,* हिक्का *Hiccā* (Hiccup) and *Arśa* - अर्श (Piles). It pacifies कफ *Kapha,* वात *Vāta* and शुक्र *Śukra* (dhātu).

तैलं सर्पिः पयस्तक्रं क्षौद्रं सूक्तं सकाञ्जिकम् ।
सुरासवं मर्जिका च जलं च विविधं शुभम् ॥७॥

पानाय परिषेकाय नस्यायालोडनाय च ।
भेषजानां प्रयोज्यं स्यात्प्रयोगेषु यथाविधि ॥८॥

32) तैलम् Tailam 33) सर्पिः Sarpiḥ (ghee), 34) पयः Payaḥ 35) तक्रम् Takram 36) क्षौद्रम् Kśaudram (Honey) 37) सूक्तम् Sūktam 38) काञ्जिकम् Kāñjikam 39) सुरा Surā 40) आसवम् Āsavam 41) मर्जिका Marjikā 42) जलम् (Jalam) Pure water from various sources.

These Liquid substances are useful for drinking, परिषेक *Pariṣeka* (bathing,either of the whole body or of the affected portions by various appliances), nasal medication, and also as a suitable vehicle for other medicines.

शरीरम् *Śarīram (पुरुष वर्ग)*

पुरुषः स्त्रीवपुर्वाचा वातपित्तकफास्तथा ।
मोहं प्रकृतिरेतानि शरीरं यैश्च तिष्ठति ॥९॥

The above mentioned drugs and those which will be mentioned herein afterwards are to be used on the living body. Therefore the important constituents of the living body i.e. 43) शरीरम् are mentioned here in short as पुरुषः,Puruṣaḥ, स्त्री Strī, वपुः Vapuḥ (Body), वाचा Vācā वातः Vātaḥ, पित्तम् Pittam, कफः Kafaḥ, मोहः Mohaḥ, प्रकृतिः- Prakṛtiḥ.

सप्तधातवः *Saptadhātavah*

अस्थि मांसं वसा रक्तं शुक्रं मज्जा तथा रसः ।
एते तु धातवः सप्त ज्ञातव्या हि भिषग्वरैः ॥१०॥

The above mentioned शारीरभाव *Śariabhāva* (Constituents) remain and perform their functions with the help of the tissues of the body i.e.44) धातवः

These are mentioned here as अस्थि *Asthi* (Bony tissue), मांसम् *Māmsam* (Muscular tissue), वसा *Vasā* (fatty tissue), मज्जा *Majjā* (tissues in the bony cavities), रस-रक्त *Rasa-Rakta* (Blood & other tissues in the fluid state), शुक्र *Śukra* (the constituent causing regeneration). These (seven) are called as सप्तधातवः *Saptadhātavaḥ* and the physician should know them thoroughly.

मांसवर्ग *Meat class.*

हस्त्यश्वोष्ट्रखराजाविवृकव्याघ्राश्च केसरी ।
वराहमृग इत्येषा मांसं योज्यं तु बृंहणम् ॥११॥

45) हस्ती Hastī, 46) अश्वः Aśvaḥ, 47) उष्ट्रः Ūṣṭraḥ, 48) खरः Kharaḥ 49) अजः Ajaḥ 50) अविः Aviḥ 51) वृकः Vṛkaḥ 52) व्याघ्रः Vyāghraḥ 53) केसरी Kesarī 54) वराहः Varāhaḥ 55) मृगः Mṛgaḥ. The meat of all these animals is बृंहण *Bṛmhaṇa*.

महिषोऽथ बलीवर्दो मत्स्यः कच्छप एव च ।
आमूषिका बिडालानां शृगालकपिबर्हिषाम् ॥१२॥
शिलीमुख शुकस्यापि सारिका चक्रवाकयोः ।
हंस कुक्कुटलावानां कोकिलोलूकभोगिनाम् ॥१३॥
भेकादीनां च विण्मूत्रैर्मेदस्त्वग्रोमसंयुतैः ।
धूपं दद्याज्ज्वरार्तेभ्यो उन्मत्तेभ्यो विशेषतः ॥१४॥
अपस्माराभिभूतेभ्यो ग्रहार्तेभ्यस्तथैव च ।
प्राप्नुयादायुरारोग्यं बलं वर्णं मनःस्थिरम् ॥१५॥
योगानेतान् समाश्रित्य मांसद्रव्यसमाश्रयान् ।
द्रव्यावलिः समादिष्टा धन्वन्तरिमुखोद्गता ॥१६॥

It is stated that the drugs are mentioned in compound formulations (योग). Here, though the animals can be used as बृंहण Bṛmhaṇa as mentioned in the above mentioned verse, the formulation-योग has given somewhat importance to विट्-*Viṭ*, मूत्र *Mūtra,* मल *Mala* etc. therefore these are mentioned under separate headings. 56) महिषः Mahiṣaḥ 57) बलीवर्दः Balivardaḥ 58) मत्स्यः Matsyaḥ 59) कच्छपः Kacchapaḥ 60) आमूषिका Āmūṣikā 61) बिडालः Biḍālaḥ 62) शृगालः Sṛgālaḥ 63) कपिः Kapiḥ 64) बर्हिः Barhiḥ 65) शिलीमुखः Śilīmukhaḥ, 66) शुकः Śukaḥ 67) सारिका Sārikā 68) चक्रवाकः Cakravākaḥ 69) हंसः Hamsaḥ 70) कुक्कुटः Kukkuṭaḥ 71) लावः Lāvaḥ 72) कोकिलः Kokilaḥ 73) उलूकः Ulūkaḥ 74) भोगी Bhogī 75) भेक Bheka. धूप *Dhūpa* prepared with 76) मलम् Malam (faeces) 77) मूत्रम् Mūtram (Urine) 78) मेदस् Medas 79) त्वक् Twak 80) रोम Roma (Hairs) of these animals can be used for धूपन कर्म *Dhūpan Karma* especially in fevers when the patient has become excited or violent and also in the conditions like vitiation by उन्माद *Unmāda*, अपस्मार *Apasmāra.* (Epilepsy), ग्रहार्त *Grahārta.* With this procedure the patient's mind becomes calm and is restored to normalcy, strength of the body is increased and the lustre of the body is improved.

Here the Dravyāvalī द्रव्यावली part is described as has been told by

धन्वन्तरि Dhanvantari by way of fomulations (योगान्) consisting (mainly) of मांसद्रव्याणि Māṃsadravyāṇi (Meat Substances).

सुवर्णादिरयं वर्गः षष्ठ उक्तो यथाक्रमम् ।
धातुद्रव्यद्रवद्रव्यमांसद्रव्यसमाश्रयः ॥

Thus the sixth सुवर्णादि Suvarṇādi chapter has been told as in order. It consists of धातुद्रव्य *Dhātudravya*. (metal substances,) द्रवद्रव्य *Dravadrvya*-fluid substances and मांसद्रव्य *Māṃsadravya* (Meat substances).

अथ मिश्रकादिः सप्तमो वर्गः ।

Miśrakādiḥ Chapter VII.

मिश्रको व्यस्तयोगाश्च विषाण्यष्टादशापि च ।
उपविषाणि सर्वाणि तथा प्रशमनानि च ॥१॥

एतत्सर्वं समासेन वक्षाम्यत्र यथाक्रमम् ।
योगानेतान् प्रयुञ्जीत पुरुषो नित्यमात्मवान् ॥२॥

सत्सु पूजामवाप्नोति परत्रेह च नन्दति ।

Miśrakādi chapter -मिश्रकादि वर्ग contains various formulations consisting of various drugs & 1) विषाणि अष्टादश - *Viṣāṇi Aṣṭādaśa*- Eighteen types of poisons 2) उपविषाणि सर्वाणि *Upaviṣāṇi Sarvāṇi* and 3) विषप्रशमनानि-*Viṣapraśamanāni* (Drugs for the treatment of poisons, may be called as antidotal drugs). All these will be told serially and in a concise form. आत्मवान् पुरुषः the restraintful person should use these formulations regularly (in his practice) and by doing so he will be (respected) by all and feel happy in his life.

शतत्रयं च द्रव्याणां त्रिसप्तत्त्यधिकोत्तरम् ॥३॥
हिताय वैद्यपुत्राणां द्रव्यावल्यां प्रकाशितम् ॥

गणद्रव्यावली ह्युक्ता सयोगा सहमात्रया ॥४॥
[1]पर्यायनामान्युच्यन्ते गुडूच्यादेर्यथाक्रमम् ॥

Three hundred and seventy three drugs are mentioned in this *Dravyāvali* द्रव्यावलि for the benefit of the students of Ayurveda. This *Gaṇadravyāvali* गणद्रव्यावलि is told with formulations (योग) and doses (मात्रा). Now the synonyms (with properties) of *Guḍūcī* गुडूची etc. will be mentioned serially.

---

* 'द्रव्यावलिः समादिष्टा' Dravyāvaliḥ Samadiṣṭā has been already discussed to some extent in the preface.

१) पर्याय नामानि – एकार्थवाचकाः शब्दाः पर्यायाः इत्युच्यन्ते । उपलक्षणात्मकं चेदम् । तेन गुणाकर्मादयोऽपि उक्ताः । S.D.Kamat.

इति मिश्रकादिः सप्तमो वर्गः ।

Thus ends the Miśrakādi seventh chapter

At the end of this *Miśrakādi* chapter the total number of drugs is mentioned as 373. This has a striking similarily with the verse in *Uttaratantra* of *Suśruta Samhitā.*

शतं च पञ्च द्रव्याणां त्रिसप्तत्यधिकोत्तरम् ।
व्यासतः कीर्तितं तद्धि .... // S.S.U.66.8

It has been already mentioned at the end of the sixth chapter that-

"द्रव्यावलिः समादिष्टा धन्वन्तरि मुखोद्गता ।"

This perhaps suggests that the *Gaṇadravyāvali* and the Nighaṇṭu ends there only. Again at the end of the seventh chapter, it is mentioned that the *Gaṇadravyāvali* is told. It apparently seems to be a repetition. Before, mentioning the synonyms, properties etc. there is again a salutation-

"धन्वन्तरिपदद्वंद्वं नत्वा लोकहितार्थिना ।
रसवीर्य विपाकादि द्रव्याणां कथ्यते मया ॥"

This suggests that the latter portion might have been compiled by someone else.

Śoḍhalanighaṇṭukāra शोढलनिघण्टुकार has mentioned that he has mentioned the same *Dravyāvali* द्रव्यावलि which is mentioned in *Dhn.Ni* ध.नि.

धन्वन्तरिमतादेष स्वल्पसंक्षेप विस्तरः ।
सोढलेन सतार्थोऽयं ग्रथ्यते नामसंग्रहः ॥६॥
तान्येवौषधनामानि धन्वन्तर्युदितानि च ।
द्रव्यावली तथा सैव संक्षेपाय नवाकृतिः ॥७॥ Sodhala p. 1

and by actual comparison of these two *Dravyāvalis* it seems that Śodhala has strictly followed Dhn.Ni.(except his own *Lakśmaṇādivarga.* लक्ष्मणादि वर्ग). But, in Śodhala Ni. only the metalic substances of Dhn.Ni. are mentioned and the sixth Suvarṇadi chapter ends there only.

सुवर्णरूप्यताम्राणि त्रपुरीतिश्च सीसकम् ।
कांस्यं लौहं च योज्यानि गरदोषप्रशान्तये ॥
सुवर्णादिरयं वर्गः षट्संख्यः परिकीर्तितः ॥ Śodhala p.6

Therefore, it can be doubted that except these metalic drugs the remaining portion of the sixth chapter is a later addition. There is also a vast difference of the Miśrakādi chapter of both these Nighaṇṭus. While mentioning the *Guṇasaṃgraha* गुणसंग्रह portion of the Nighaṇṭu, Śodhala has mentioned that-

द्रव्यावली विहीनेषु हीनवर्ग क्रमेषु च ।
अनादिनामनिर्वाण ग्रन्थेष्वर्थकदर्थितम् ॥
शिष्यसंघं समालोक्य हृदि जातदयोदयः । Śodhala p. 90.

This also suggests that the portions of the नामनिर्वाणग्रन्थ Nāmanirvāṇa grantha (i.e. द्रव्यावली Dravyāvalī) are vitiated (कदर्थित) by certain defects. This statement also substantiate the doubt mentioned above.

There are also reasons for the vitiation of the Mṣṣ. There was no printing technology available in those days.Either one has to copy in his own handwriting or to get it copied by the professional copy writers. While copying from one Mss. to another, it is but natural that many mistakes, misreadings, different readings, interpolations, additions etc. might had been entered intentionally or unintentionally. The copy of the Mṣṣ. was meant for the use of the other scholars, students etc. therefore, advancement of knowledge might had been included intentionally. All these things were made on the name of the original compiler. In the case of Nighaṇṭus it is more possible of such additions. Rarely, if the original text is very popular and important, then some scholar might had taken pains to note the different readings and rectify the mistakes. *Jñāneśwarī* ज्ञानेश्वरी in *Marathi* is a very famous example of this. *Jñāneśwarī* which was written at the time of *Yadavas* became so corrupt within a period of two centuries, that the famous *Santa Eknath* had to take lot of efforts to prepare a corrected copy of the same and had to give a strict warning of not making any additions to this *Jñāneśwarī** (ज्ञानेश्वरी).The various different readings mentioned in the commentary of Ḍalhaṇa is an example of such efforts. Under these circumstances the doubts mentioned earlier of additions in this Dhn.Ni. is understandable.However, as mentioned earlier in the preface, Ḳśiraswami had mentioned few readings from *Suvarṇādi Chapter* and *Misrakādi Chapter* from the present Dhn.Ni.therefore it is quite reasonable to infer that he had such Mss for his study while Śoḍhala did not have the Mṣṣ. containing the said portion.

---

* "शके पंधराशे सावोत्तरी । तारणनामसंवत्सरी ।
एकाजनार्दनें अत्यादरी । गीता ज्ञानेश्वरी प्रतिशुद्ध केली ॥
ग्रंथ पूर्वीच अतिशुद्ध । परि पाठांतरे शुद्धाबद्ध ।
ते शोधुनि एवंविध । प्रतिशुद्ध सिद्ध ज्ञानेश्वरी ॥"

** "ज्ञानेश्वरी पाठी । जो ओवी करील मऱ्हाठी ।
तेणें अमृताचे ताटीं । जाण नरोटी ठेवली ॥"

Some modern reserchers believe this verse also an extrapolation
(Prof. Gurava. *Pailatira*- पैलतीर 1997. Diwalispecial number-marathi (मराठी)

Additional Plants

In the published text of the Dhn.Ni. it will be seen that there are some additional plants, mentioned under certain headings. The subject is discussed to some extent in the "Treatise and its constitution" (Page 49). I have shown in the preface that some of these plants are mentioned by क्षीरस्वामी-Kśiraswāmī. Therefore it cannot be conluded that all the additional plants are later additions. But those plants which are not consistant with the heading names either morphologically or pharmacologically or without reference to context can be said to be later additions by other than the complier himself. eg. विजया – Vijayā under the heading मेदा Medā is not consistant with the heading name. It seems that the compiler had added those plants which has some similarity either morphologically or pharmacologically. This is of much importance because it shows the way or the direction how to include the vast number of plants used locally (folk uses) and by the Ayurvedic physicians of the various regions of this country, in our Nighaṇṭu.In the various modern botanical floras, plants are mentioned with their families. As in human families certain hereditary characters are found, similarly, the pharmacological properties may be found in different species of the plants. *eg.* Bhallātaka भल्लातक belonging to the family Anacardiaceae shows उष्ण *Uṣṇa*, तीक्ष्ण *Tīkṣna* and blistering properties. Many of the species of this family show the same properties to a greater or lesser extent. eg.

1) *Anacardium occidentale* Linn.
Sans. Kājutaka, Mar.Kājū. काजू (Gl. Chopra p.17)

2) *Holigarna grahamii* (Wight) Hook f.
Mar. Bipṭā बिपटा (Chopra Gl.p.135)

3) *H. arnottiana* Hook.f. (Chopra Gl. p. 135)
Mumb.Mar. - Bibu बिबु

4) *H.longifolia* Buch. -Ham. ex.Roxb.

Mumbai-Hullugirī- हुलगिरी, Kannad-Kaṭugirī. Juice from the trunk and the rind of the fruit, is poisonous, vesicant (Chopra Gl. 135).

There are some common properties in all of the above plants, therefore these can be mentioned having similar or nearly similar pharmacological and morphological properties under the heading name भल्लातक of Dhn.Ni. Secondly, the plants belonging to the different families but having similar pharmacological properties can also be mentioned under a particular heading. eg.Under the heading दारुहरिद्रा *Dāruharidrā* of Dhn.Ni. following plants of the same family can be mentioned :

1) *Berberis asiatica* Roxb. ex.DC.

2) *B. insignis* Hook. f. & Thoms.

3) *B.lycium* Royle

4) *B. nepalensis* Sprengue.

5) *B. umbellata* Wall.

6) *B. pachyacantha* Koehne. (*B. vulgaris* Linn.)

Along with these the following plants belonging to the Menispermaceae (गुडूची कुल-Guḍūcī family) can also be included. *Coscinium fenestratum* (Gaertn.) Colebr. (Chopra. Gl.p.78) *Fibraurea tinctoria* Lour. (Chopra. Gl. p.78)

This shows the way how the plants used in our country as medicinal or food plants, used by the people and Vaidyas in particular can be documented and mentioned in our Nighaṇṭus .

What is the total number of drugs in Dhn.Ni.:-

As stated earlier the total number of drugs mentioned at the end of the *Miśrakādi Chapter-* मिश्रकादि वर्ग is 373.

शतत्रयं च द्रव्याणां त्रिसप्तत्यधिकोत्तरम् ।

The statement has been made at the end of the chapter. It suggests that the drugs mentioned here are inclusive of all the chapters. If the method of counting of drugs is adopted as by way of heading names eg. under the heading तैलम् - *Tailam*, all the types of तैलानि - *Tailani* are represented by counting them under one heading. Similarly, सर्पिः *Sarpiḥ,* पयः *Payaḥ* etc.are counted as heading names, from the chapter VI and 1) विषाणि *Viṣāṇi* 2)उपविषाणि *Upaviṣāṇi* 3) विषप्रशमनानि *Viṣapraśamanāni* are under 3 heading names from the VII th Chapter, then the total number of 373 drugs can be explained.

There may be a difference of opinion in counting these heading names, and I would like to keep the issue open for discussion. I have prepared the index (serial) of the present book accordingly. It is also to be noted here that the list of headings is prepared according to *Gaṇadravyāvalī* गणद्रव्यावली and not from the remaining part *Paryāyanāmadravyāvalī* - पर्यायनाम द्रव्यावली which includes *Guṇasamgraha* गुणसंग्रह (Properties of the drugs) and additional plants.

Sr. No.	Name of the Chapter	No. of Plants
1	Guḍūcyādi Chapter गुडूच्यादिवर्ग	82 (८२)
2	Śatapuṣpādi Chapter शतपुष्पादि वर्ग	35 (३५)
3	Candanādi Chapter चंदनादि वर्ग	65 (६५)
4	Karavīrādi Chapter करवीरादि वर्ग	48 (४८)
5	Āmrādi Chapter आम्रादि वर्ग	60 (६०)
6	Suvarṇādi Chapter सुवर्णादि वर्ग	80 (८०)
7	Miśrakādi Chapter मिश्रकादि वर्ग	3 (३)
		373 (३७३)

Thus the total number of 373 drugs can be explained on the basis of heading names.

---

* I have found one Mss from the library of the university of Mumbai. In this the *Viṣapraśamanāni* विषप्रशमनानि drugs are mentioned in a separate chapter, and there the total no. of chapters becomes 9 instead of 7.

Two Mss (bearing no. 924 & 1054) of Dhn. ni. from Bhandarkar institute, Pune of which the socalled author is Mahendra also mentions 9 (nine) chapters S.D. Kamat.

अथ गुडूच्यादिः प्रथमो वर्गः

GUDŪCYADIH CHAPTER I

1. गुडूची Guḍūcī

धन्वन्तरिपदद्वंद्वं नत्वा लोकहितार्थिनाम् ।
रसवीर्यविपाकादि द्रव्याणां कथ्यते मया ॥*

This is a salutary stanza in which the compiler after bowing to the feet of the God Dhanvantari begins for the benefit of the people the pharmacological properties of the plants i.e. *Rasa, Vīrya, Vipaka* etc, The word etc. here is meant for the actions on various diseased conditions.

गुडूच्यमृतवल्ली च छिन्ना छिन्नरुहाऽमृता ॥
छिन्नोद्भवाऽमृतलता धारा[१] वत्सादनी स्मृता ॥ १

सैवोक्ता सोमवल्ली च कुण्डली चक्रलक्षणा ।
प्रोक्ता नागकुमारी च छिन्नांगी ज्वरनाशिनी ॥२

जीवनी मधुपर्णी च तन्त्रिका देवनिर्मिता ।
वयस्था मण्डली सौम्या विशल्याऽमृतसंभवा ॥३

रसायनीमृत्तिका च चन्द्रहासा भिषग्जिता ॥
पिण्डामृता बहुच्छिन्ना सा चोक्ता कन्दरोहिणी ॥ ४

अन्या कंदोद्भवा कन्दाऽमृतकन्दागुडूचिका ॥
गुडूची स्वरसे तिक्ता कषायोष्णा गुरुस्तथा ॥ ५
त्रिदोषजन्तुरक्तार्शः कुष्ठज्वरहरा परा ॥

गुडूच्यायुष्प्रदा मेध्या तिक्ता संग्राहिणी बला ॥ ६
ज्वरतृट्पाण्डुवातासृक्छर्दिमेहत्रिदोषजित् ॥

गुडूची कफवातघ्नी पित्तमेदोविशोषणी ॥ ७
रक्तवातप्रशमनी कण्डूवीसर्पनाशिनी ॥

---

* The stanza is important because according to some scholars, herein onwards the compiler may be different one from that of the 1st part i.e. (गणद्रव्यावली) The method of giving various similar terms was the practice of earlier Nighaṇṭukar's. This is perhapas the earliest Nighaṇṭukar who has started the pioneer work of giving similitive terms and pharmacological actions etc. together under one heading. And later on certain plants having either similar pharmacological actions (might be in some respects) or having similar morphological characters were added.

१ 'धरा' इति नि.शे. टीकायाम ।

कन्दोद्‌भवा गुड्‌ची च कटूष्णा संनिपातहा ॥ ८
विषघ्नी ज्वरभूतघ्नी वलीपलितनाशिनी ॥

गुडूची (Guḍūcī), अमृतवल्ली (Amṛtavallī), छिन्ना (Chinnā), छिन्नरुहा (Chinnaruhā) अमृता, (Amṛtā), छिन्नोद्‌भवा (Chinnodbhavā), अमृतलता (Amṛtalatā), धारा (Dhārā), वत्सादनी (Vatsādanī), सोमवल्ली (Somavallī), कुण्डली (Kuṇḍalī), चक्रलक्षणा (Cakralakśaṇā), नागकुमारी (Nāgakumārī), छिन्नाङ्गी (Chinnānigī), ज्वरनाशिनी (Jwaranāśinī), जीवनी (Jīvaṇī), मधुपर्णी (Madhuparṇī), तन्त्रिका (Tantrikā), देवनिर्मिता (Devanirmitā), वयस्था (Vayasthā), मण्डली (Maṇḍalī), सौम्या (Saumyā), विशल्या (Viśalyā), अमृतसंभवा (Amṛtasambhavā), रसायनी (Rasāyani), मृत्तिका (Mṛttikā), चन्द्रहासा (Candrahāsā), भिषग्जिता (Bhiṣagjitā), are the synonyms of Gūḍūcī.

There is an another type, tuberous in origin called as कंदरोहिणी *kandarohiṇī* of which synonyms are पिण्डामृता (Piṇḍāmṛtā), बहुच्छिन्ना (Bahucchinnā), कंदोद्‌भवा (Kandodbhavā), कन्दा (Kandā), अमृतकन्दा गुड्‌चिका (Amṛtakandā Gūḍūcikā).

Guḍucī is bitter and astringent in taste, *uṣṇavīrya* and *guru*. It pacifies all the three *doṣas* and is useful in worms, bleeding piles, skin diseases and fever. It increases longevity, promotes intellect, is bitter in taste, having astringent action, increases strength, and is useful in fevers, thirst, anaemia, gout (*vātarakta*), emesis, diseases characterized by polyuria and pacifies all the three *doṣas*.

Guḍūci pacifies *kaphavāta doṣas,* reduces *pitta* and *meda* and is useful in *Raktavāta* (Gout), pruritus and erysipelas.

कंदगुडूची *Kandaguḍūcī* is pungent in taste, *uṣṇavīrya* and useful in the conditions caused by vitiation of the three *doṣās,* is alexipharmic febrifuge, antiseptic and reduces wrinkles and gray hair at immature age.

(Two plants are included under the heading A-गुडूची (Guḍūci) and B-कन्द गुडूची (Kanda Guḍūcī).

(Fam. Menispermaceae).

I- A-a- ***Tinospora cordifolia*** *(Willd.) Miers
Syn-*Cocculus cordifolia* DC.
b- Roxburgh, c- Throughout India, common,
d- Jain, Apte. For confirmation.

II- A-a- (छिन्नरुहा) (Chinnaruhā), चक्रलक्षणा, (Chkralakśāṇā), जीवन्ती (Jīvantī).

Currently accepted name for. *T. cordifolia* (Wild.) Miers is *T. cordifolia* (Willd.) Hook. f. & Thoms.

(Comp. p. 151)

b- H-Giloe, Gurca, B.-Gulanca; Mar.-Bom.-Guḷwel, Tam-sindalkodi; Cintil; Tel.- Tipp-tige; Somidā; Guḍuci: M.Sittamrytu; Kan.-Amrutballi; Goa-Amrutyel; Eng.-Gulanch.

B-*a*- पिण्डामृता (Piṇḍāmṛtā), कन्दरोहिणी (Kandarohiṇī), कन्दोद्भवा (Kandodbavā), (Piṇḍaguḍūcikā) पिण्डगुडूचिका

b- Eng.- Columba, Radix Columba.

III-b- (1) 27, छद्मकेति, कन्दरोहिणी (Harshe),

(2) गुल्मकः –गुलञ्चकन्दः। (Tripathi- Vātāśmari).

c-(1) अमृतकन्दः (Ras. P.P. 15).

(3) Columba- *Jateorhiza palmata* Miers
Syn. *Cocculus palmata* DC. (Potter's Cyclo.)
Vern-'Kolam Kāp' (कोलम काप).
(Yadavji; Desai; Priyavrata).

(4)*Jateorhiza columba* Miers Syn. *Cocculus palmatus* D.C, (Mat-Med.)-Columba radix. Native of Africa, Ibo, Zambezi. (Waring).

(5) Columba-(B.P.C.)-Columba radix, Roots of *Jateorhiza palmata* (Ghosh).

This plant seems quite allied to and also may be the valid name of *M.columba* Roxb. Both the plants are of the same family and were included in the same genus. The medical names are also the same. But having got no authentic record and therefore it is not confirmad as a valid name of *Menispermum columba* Roxb. *Columba* is used in place of *Pāthā* (पाठा) under the name *'Kolam Kāp'* . (कोलम काप). (Yadavji and Priyavrat) which is suggestive of columba radix.

Following plants are used as (गुडूची) (Guḍūcī) in some parts of India :-

(6) *Tinospora tomentosa* Miers; Syn. *T. malabarica* (Lam.) * Meirs; *Menispermum tomentousm* Roxb.
(Sudarśana), (Bh. Pr.Ni.).

B- (पद्मगुलञ्च) (Padmagulañca)used in Bengal.

(7) *Tinospora crispum* Miers (Chopra).
Menispermum crispum Linn. *Cocculus crispus* DC;
C. verrucosus Wall. *(Vernacular names as those of)*
T. cordifolla (Watt Dic).

(8) *Menispermum verrucosum* Roxb. (Guḍuci, Putra Valli). Used in South India. (Roxb).

---

current names for
Tinospora tomentosa Miers is *T. sinensis* (Lour.) Merr.
T. crispa Miers is *T. crispa* (Linn.) Hook f. & Thomas. (Comp.p.151)

(9) *M. fenestratum* Gaertn.वेणीवेल (Veṇivel); बंगवेल (Bungvel-gatt.) Native of Ceylon (Roxb.) used in Ceylon.

But in Maharashtra and generally all over India, the plant *Tinospora cordifolia* Miers, is used as Guḍuci of Nighaṇṭus.

Note- IV((1) Columba root, Columba rad. (Ainslie).

(2) As, Res. Vol. XI-385.

2. अतिविषा Ativiṣā

अतिविषा शुक्लकन्दा ज्ञेया विश्वा च भंगुरा ॥ ९
श्यामकन्दा प्रतिविषा श्रृंगी चोपविषा विषा ॥

आर्द्रा[१] श्वेता विरूपा च विषदा पित्तवल्लभा ॥ १०
घुणप्रियाऽतिसारघ्नी बालानां रोगनाशिनी ॥

अतिविषा *Ativiṣā* is of two types शुक्लकन्दा *Śuklakandā* and श्यामकन्दा *Śyamakandā*. Śuklakandā is called by the synonyms विश्वा (Viśvā), भङ्गुरा (Bhangurā), *Śyāmakandā* is called as प्रतिविषा (Prativiṣā). श्रृङ्गी (Śṛngi) उपविषा (Upaviṣā), विषा (Viṣā), आर्द्रा (Ārdrā), श्वेता (Śvetā), विरूपा (Virūpā), विषदा (Viṣadā), पित्तवल्लभा (Pittavallabhā), घुणप्रिया (Ghuṇapriyā), अतिसारघ्नी (Atisāraghni) and बालरोगनाशिनी (Bālaroganāśini) are synonyms of अतिविषा *Ativiṣā*.

कटूष्णाऽतिविषा तिक्ता कफपित्तज्वरापहा ॥ ११
आमातिसारकासघ्नी विषच्छर्दिविनाशिनी ॥

Ativiṣā is pungent and bitter in taste and *uṣṇavīrya*. It pacifies *kapha* and *pitta doṣa*. It is useful in fevers, *Āmadoṣa*, diarrhoea, cough, poisons, and emesis.

This heading includes two plants: A-शुक्ल (Śukla and B- श्याम Śyāma.)

(Fam. Ranunculaceae.)

I- A-*a*- ***Aconitum heterophyllum*** Wall.*
b-Dymock, *c*- North-Western Himalayas, *d*-Jain.

B-*a*-***A. palmatum*** Ḍ. Don,**
b-Kamat, *c*-as above.

II- A-*a*-भङ्गुरा (Bhangurā), अतिविषा (Ativiṣā), शुक्लकन्दा (Śuklakandā).

१ 'आद्या' इति साधु पाठः भविष्यति। S.D. K.

* The current name is *Aconitum heterophyllum* Wall. ex Royle

** The current name is *Aconitum bisma* (Buch. Ham.) Rap. (Comp. P.3) *b*-H.-Atis; Mar.-Ativiṣa, atis; B.-Ataich; Tel.- Ati-vasa; Mad.-Ativadyam; Guj.-Ativasa;

B-*a*-प्रतिविषा (Prativiṣa) श्यामकन्दा (Śyāmakandā).

b-H-Bikham.

III-*d;e,g:* -See current names.

3. मूर्वा Mūrvā[2]

मूर्वा मधुरसा देवी पृथक्पर्णी त्रिपर्ण्यपि ॥१२
देवश्रेणी स्वादुरसा स्निग्धपर्णी च मोरटा ॥

मूर्वा स्वादुरसा चोष्णा हृद्रोगकफवातजित् ॥ १३
कुष्ठकण्डूवमीमेहविषमज्वरनाशिनी ॥

मूर्वा (Murvā), मधुरसा (Madhurasā), देवी (Devī), पृथक्पर्णी (Pṛthakparṇī), त्रिपर्णी (Triparṇī), देवश्रेणी (Devaśreṇī), स्वादुरसा (Swādurasā), स्निग्धपर्णी (Singdhaparṇī), and मोरटा (Moratā), are synonyms for *Murvā.*

Murvā is sweet in taste, *usṇavīrya,* and pacifies *kaphavāta doṣa*. It is useful in diseases of heart, skin diseases, pruritus, emesis, diseases characterized by polyuria and intermittant fevers (*visạma jwara.*)

Controversial plant. Several plants are recorded by the commentators and modern writers; but none of them aptly correspond to the texts.

Not confirmed. (Fam. -Capparidaceae).

Note- 'Corasnāyu' may be species of Sanseviera genus. Eng.- Bow string hemp. (Hill.) Murvā (Chopra); (Kokan) Manyar Kānden.

I- *a*- ***Maerua ovalifolia*** Canw.-Syn, *M. arenaria* Hook. f.*

Note- The generic name *'Maerua'* shows striking similarity with the name 'Mūrvā' -But the leaves in *Maerua* are simple and entire. (Mahajan).

II- b- Tel. Moranika; Tam.-Bhumicakkarai; H. Curanahāra, Morahari; Maruā, Dudhi (Balavantaji, Vidyotani and Vaidya)

III- See Moraṭā.

b- (1) 169 मूर्वा मधुरसा क्षीरमोरटा, मूर्वाभेदा (Harshe.)
(2) 172 मूर्वा (Harshe.), (3) मूर्वा-पृथक्पर्णी (Madan Pal).

c- मूर्वा -चोरस्नायु; अन्ये कोविदार सदृश युग्मपत्रा. (Dalhaṇa on sū)

IV Some plants under the name mūrvā are recorded here
(1) *Sansevieria zeylanica* Will. and some other species of this

---

मूर्वा-र्वी-मूर्विका a kind of creeper from the fibers of which bowstring is made. मौर्वी a girdle made of Murva grass to be worn by क्षत्रिय kśatriya (Apte 2-42) D.K.Kamat

* The current name is *Maerua oblongifolia* (Forsk.) A. Rich (Comp. p. 97))

genus. (U.C.Dutta).
(2)*Clematis triloba*- (Vidyotani; U.C.Dutta).
(3)*Maerua arenaria* (Valkum Murahari). (Priyavrata)
(4)*Bauhinia vahlli* (Mālajzan) (Balavantsimhaji, Bihar, Priyavrata).
(5)*Hyacinthoids alestris* -(Sir John Shoar, As, Res. Vol. IV).

मोरटः Moraṭaḥ 1

मोरटः कीर्णपुष्पश्च पीलुपुष्पो मधुस्रवः ॥१४
तेजनी दीर्घमूला च पुरुषः क्षीरमोरटः ॥

ज्वरघ्नो मुखवैरस्य तृष्णादाहविनाशनः ॥ १५
कफपित्तहरश्चासौ विज्ञेयः क्षीरमोरटः ॥

कीर्णपुष्पः (Kīrṇapuṣpaḥ), पीलुपुष्पः (Pīlupuṣpaḥ), मधुस्रवः (Madhusravaḥ), तेजनी (Tejanī), दीर्घमूला (Dīrghamūlā), पुरुषः (Puruṣaḥ), क्षीरमोरटः (Kṣīramoraṭaḥ), are synonyms for मोरटः (Moraṭaḥ).

Moratah is useful in fevers, tastlessness, thirst, and burning sensation. It pacifies *kapha* and *pittadoṣa*.

(Under this heading , it seems that two plants are recorded. One of it may be *Moraṭa* as a reference of Mūrvā (see *Mūrvā*) and the next is A- क्षीरमोरटः (Ksīramoraṭah).

(Fam. Ranunculaceae.)

I- A-*a*- ***Clematis gouriana*** Roxb.*
b- Mahajan. c- Western ghat, Kolhapur District (Mahajan), Mahabaleshwar.

II- A-a- तेजनी (Tejanī).
b- H.-Murahari. Mar.-Morvel; Morvai.

III- b- (1) 531 क्षीरमोरटो मूर्वाभेदः (Harshe).

IV- (1) मोरटा (Moraṭā) *Clematis triloba*. (Dymok; Desai; Chopra, Molswarth).

4. मञ्जिष्ठा Mañjiṣṭhā

मञ्जिष्ठा कालमेषी च समङ्गा विकसाऽरुणा ॥ १६
मञ्जुका रक्तयष्टी च भाण्डी योजनवल्ल्यपि ॥

* *Clematis gouriana* Roxb. is *Clematis gouriana* Roxb. ex. DC. (Comp.p.38)

क्षेत्रिणी विजया रक्ता रक्ताङ्गी वस्त्रभूषणा ॥ १७
जिङ्गी भण्डी तथा काला गण्डाली कालमेषिका ॥

मञ्जिष्ठा मधुरा स्वादे कषायोष्णा गुरुस्तथा ॥ १८
कफोग्रव्रणमेहास्रविषनेत्रामयाञ्जयेत् ॥

मञ्जिष्ठा (Mañjiṣṭhā), कालमेषी (Kālameṣī), समङ्गा (Samaṅgā), विकसा (Vikasā), अरुणा (Aruṇā), मञ्जुका (Mañjukā), रक्तयष्टी (Raktayaṣṭī), भाण्डी (Bhāṇḍī), योजनवल्ली (Yojanavallī), क्षेत्रिणी (K'setriṇī), विजया (Vijayā), रक्ता (Raktā), रक्ताङ्गी(Raktāṅgī), वस्त्रभूषणा (Vastrabhūṣaṇā), जिङ्गी (Jiṅgī),भण्डी (Bhaṇḍī), काला (Kālā), गण्डाली (Gaṇḍālī), कालमेषिका (Kālameṣikā), are synonymous.

Manjisṭhā is sweet and *kaṣāya* (astringent) in taste, *uṣṇavīrya,* and *guru.* It is useful in pacifying *kaphadoṣa,* obstinate sores,diseases charetarized by polyuria, dyscrasia, pacifying posions and diseases of the eye.

I- *a-* ***Rubia cordifolia*** Linn.
b- Dymock, *c*-On higher western ghats, Common throughout India in hilly districts.

II- *a-* कालमेषी (Kālameṣī) विकसा (Vikasā), वस्त्रभूषणा (Vastrabhūṣaṇā)
b- H- Mañjit; B.-Mañjith; Mar.-Mañjit; Tam. Mañjiṣṭh; Savali; Tel.- Manjisṭhige; Kan.- Mañjiṣṭha, Mal.- Mañjiṭhi; Eng.-Turk red; Indian maddar.

III- See मांसरोहिणी (Māmsarohiṇī).
d, e, g - See *Rubia* speices.

5. धन्वयासः Dhanvayāsaḥ

धन्वयासो दुरालम्भा ताम्रमूली च कच्छुरा ॥ १९
दुरालभा च दुःस्पर्शा यासो धन्वयवासकः ॥

दुरालम्भा स्वादुशीता तिक्ता दाहविनाशिनी ॥ २०
विषमज्वरतृट्छर्दिमेहमोहविनाशिनी ॥

धन्वयास (Dhanvayāsa), दुरालम्भा (Durālambhā), ताम्रमूली (Tāmra-mūlī), कच्छुरा (Kacchurā), दुरालभा (Durālabhā) दुःस्पर्शा (Duḥspar'sā), यासः (Yāsaḥ), and धन्वयवासकः (Dhanvayāsakaḥ) are synonymous.

Durālambhā is sweet and bitter in taste, *'sītavīrya* and useful in burning sensation, malarial fevers (prolonged fevers), thirst, vomiting, diseases characterised by polyuria & mental confusion.

(Dh. ni. records A-धन्वयासः but Raj. ni. adds one more B-क्षुद्रदुरालभा which is यासः proper).

(Fam. : Leguminosae), Fabaceae.

I- A-a- ***Alhagi camelorum*** Fisch.*
Syn - *A. maurorum* Baker
Hedysarum alhagi Linn.
b- Roxburgh. c-Gujarath, Rajasthan, Sindh, Syria, ran.
B-a- See (Yāsaḥ) the next plant.

II - A-*a*- दुरालभा (Durālabhā), ताम्रमूली (Tāmramūlī).
b- H.- Mar.-jawāsā; B.-Dulāl labhā; Guj.- Javāso. Tel.- Girikarmik; Eng.- Camel thorn; Persian manna.

III- d, e, f, g-See current names and synonyms.

IV- Manna from twigs containing cane-sugar. (Roxb. & Uphof).

यासः Yāsaḥ 2.

यासो यवासकोऽनन्तो बालपत्रोऽधिकण्टकः ॥ २१
दूरमूलः समुद्रान्तो दीर्घमूलो मरुद्भवः ॥
यवासकः स्वादुतिक्तो ज्वरतृड्रक्तपित्तनुत् ॥ २२

यासः (Yāsaḥ), यवासकः(Yavāsakaḥ), अनन्तः (Ananantaḥ),बालपत्रः (Bālapatraḥ), अधिकण्टकः (Adhikanṭakaḥ), दूरमूलः (Dūramūlaḥ), समुद्रान्तः (Samudrāntaḥ), दीर्घमूलः (Dīrghamūlaḥ), मरुद्भवः (Marudbhavaḥ) are synonymous.

Yavāsakaḥ is sweet and bitter in taste, and useful in fevers, thirst and bleeding disorders.

(Fam.- Zygophyllaceae)

I- a- ***Fagonia cretica*** Linn. syn.-*F.arabica* Linn.
b- Watt. Dict. c-Gujarath, Deccan, Baluchistan, Punjab, W. Rajastan.

II - a- यवासकः (Yawāsakaḥ) बालपत्रः (Bāla patrḥ), मरुद्भवः (Marudbhavaḥ).
b- H.-Ustarkhara, Damahan, Mar.-Dhamāsā; Guj.-Dhamāso; Tel.- Citti-gara.

---

* The current name is *Alhagi psudalhagi* (Bieb.) Desv.

6. वासकः Vāsakāḥ

वासकः सिंहपर्णी च वृषो वासाऽथ[1] सिंहिका ॥
आटरूषः[2] सिंहमुखी भिषङ्माताऽऽटरुषकः ॥ २३

आटरुषो हिमस्तिक्तः पित्तश्लेष्मास्रकासजित् ॥
क्षयहृच्छर्दिकुष्ठघ्नो ज्वरतृष्णाविनाशनः ॥ २४

वासकः (Vāsakaḥ), सिंहपर्णी (Simhaparṇī), वृषः (Vṛṣaḥ), वासा (Vāsā), सिंहिका (Simhikā), आटरूषः (Āṭarūṣaḥ), सिंहमुखी (Simhamukhī) भिषङ्माता (Bhiṣaṅmātā) आटरुषकः(Āṭarūṣakaḥ) are synonymous.

Ātarūṣa is *sītavīrya*, bitter in taste, pacifies, *pitta* and *śleṣmā.* It is useful in bleeding disorders cough, consumption, emesis, skin disorders, fever and thirst.

(Fam. - Acanthaceae).

I- a- ***Adhatoda vasica*** Nees*
b-Dymock; c-Throughout India, d-Apte, Mukerji.

II- a- आटरूषः (Āṭaruṣaḥ); सिंहमुखी (Simhamukhī).
b.-H -Arusā, adolsā; B.-Bakās; Mar.-Adulsā; Tam.-Atātotai; Tel. -Aḍāsaram. Adāpāku; Keral- Atalotakam, Kan, -Adasage, Eng. -Vasaka.

III- b-क्षुद्रमहच्च्येति द्विविधोऽयम् दृश्यते ।(Ayur, O. ni.).
d,e.g- See current name.

Note- *IV*- (1)- *Adhatoda beddomei*, C. B. Clarke. Mal.- Ceriya atotakam, Tam. - Cinnātātotai
This is more powerful and is used in Keral, (Mooss).

7. खदिरः Khadiraḥ

खदिरो रक्तसारश्च गायत्री दन्तधावनः ॥
कण्टकी बालपत्रश्च जिह्मशल्यः क्षतक्षमः ॥ २५

खदिरः स्याद् रसे तिक्तो हिमः पित्तकफास्रनुत् ॥
कुष्ठामकासकण्डूतिकृमिदोषहरः स्मृतः ॥ २६

खदिरः (Khadiraḥ), रक्तसारः (Raktasāraḥ), गायत्री (Gāyatrī), दन्तधावनः

---

१ 'वसोऽथ' क्षीरस्वामी । २ 'अटरूष' क्षीरस्वामी ।

* The current name is *Adhatoda zeylanica* Medik.

(Dantadhāvanaḥ), कण्टकी (Kaṇṭakī), बालपत्रः (Bālapatraḥ), जिह्मशल्यः (Jihmaśalyaḥ), and क्षतक्षमः (Kśatakśamaḥ), are synonymous.

Khadira is bitter in taste, *śitavīrya* pacifies *kapha* and *pittadoṣa.* It is useful in blood disorders, skin diseases, *āmadoṣa,* cough, pruritus and worms.

(Fam.-Leguminosae, Sub. Fam.-Mimosae)

I- *a-* ***Acacia catechu*** * Willd. Syn. - *Mimosa catechu* Linn.
b- Roxburgh. *c*-N.N.W. and C. India.
A. catechu var. sundra Prain.
b- Mahajan, *c*-Throughout Maharashtra, *d*-Apte.

II *a-* रक्तसारः (Raktasāraḥ), गायत्री (Gāyartī), यज्ञाङ्गः (Yajñyāṅgaḥ)
b- H. Mar.- Khair; B.-Khaor; Guj.-Kher, Keral-Ceriya karingāli.

III-*a-* 31 Khadir, RV. iii-53-19; AV. iii-6-1; S. Br. -1-3-5.20 (Harshe).
b- 215 Khadira. *A*. Catechu. Ceria karingāli चेरिय करिंगाली (Krishnan).

सोमवल्कः Somawalkaḥ 3.

खदिरः[1] श्वेतसारोऽन्यः सोमवल्कः पथिद्रुमः ॥
श्यामसारो नेमिवृक्षः कार्मुकः[2] कुब्जकंटकः ॥ २७
श्वेतस्तु खदिरस्तिक्तः शीतः पित्तकफापहः ॥
रक्तदोषहरश्चैव कण्डूकुष्ठविनाशनः ॥ २८

There is another type of *khadira* having heartwood of white colour is having the synonyms श्वेतसारः (Śvetasāraḥ), सोमवल्कः (Somavalkaḥ), पथिद्रुमः (Pathidrumaḥ), (and another type) श्यामसारः (Śyāmsāraḥ), नेमिवृक्षः (Nemivṛkśaḥ), कार्मुकः (Kārmukaḥ), कुब्जकंटकः (Kubjakaṇṭakaḥ).

Śevtakhadira is bitter in taste, *śitavīrya* and pacifies *pitta & kaphadoṣa* and is useful in blood diseases, pruritus and in skin disorders.

This heading includes two plants. A-श्वेतसारः, B-श्यामसारः
For confirmation. (Fam.-as in Khadira 7).

I- A- *a-* ***Acacia ferruginea*** DC.
b- Syn.- *Mimosa ferruginea* Roxb.

---

* The current name is *Acacia catechu* (Linn f.) Willd.

१ "कदर" इति क्षीर. संमत : पाठः

२ ' कामुक' इति नि. शो. टीका संमतः पाठः ।

b- Kamat; *c*-Gujarath, Poona, Kokan (Mahajan), Karnatak, Berar, Deccan.
Acacia leucophloea Willd.*
b- Mahajan. *c*-Deccan, Poona, Gujarath, Khandesh.

B- *a*- *Mimosa suma* Roxb.
Syn.-*Acacia suma* Kurz;**
Syn. - *A. polycantha* Willd.
b- Kamat. d-S.M. Country, Kokan (Cooke), Bengal. Bihar (Chopra), Nasik Dist., on the पारनदी Para river bank from Bahre to Ambegaon. (Kamat and Mahajan).

II- A-*a*- सोमवल्कः श्वेतसारः (Somavalkaḥ Śwetāsaraḥ).
b- Berar - Sonakhair; Mar- Pāndharākhair, Sheṇyākhair; Kan.-Banni; Tel. Anasandra, Mussi.
B-*a*-श्यामसारः (Śyāmasāraḥ).

III- See Śamī (Raj. ni.), Irimeda.
b- (1)216, 217 गोरखदिर वेळ्त्त करिण्णालि ***(Vellutta Kariṇṇali). (Krishnan).
c- (1) सोमवल्क विट्खदिर (Viṭkhadira); (Cakr.-2-77).
(2) सोमवल्क(Aruna and Hemadri. Su.-15-47).

Note-IV-(1) Somavalka- *Acacia polycantha* (Ghanekar-Su.38-82)
(2) Śwetasāra Somavalka,. *Acacia suma*. (Priyavrata, Dwivedi).
(3) *Mimosa suma* Roxb.
Remarkably white bark; wood of black colour (Lisboa).
(4) *A. ferruginea* DC. Somasāra; (Mar.) Pāndharākhair. (Chopra. Watt.).

8. निम्बः Nimbaḥ

निम्बो नियमनो नेता पिचुमन्दः सुतिक्तकः ॥
अरिष्टः सर्वतोभद्रः प्रभद्रः पारिभद्रकः ॥ २९

निम्बस्तिक्तरसः शीतो लघुः श्लेष्मास्रपित्तनुत ॥
कुष्ठकण्डूव्रणान् हंति लेपाहारादि शीलितः ॥ ३०

अपक्वं पाचयेच्छोफं व्रणं पक्वं विशोधयेत् ॥

निम्बः (Nimbaḥ), नियमनः (Niyamanaḥ), नेता (Netā), पिचुमन्दः

* The current name is *Acacia leucophloea* (Roxb.) Willd.
** The current name is *Acacia polycantha* Willd. (Comp. p. 2)
*** 'वेळुत्त करिङ्गालि' read by Miss K. Nalini.

(Picumandaḥ),सुतिक्तकः (Sutiktakaḥ), अरिष्टः (Ariṣṭaḥ), सर्वतोभद्रः (Sarvatobhadraḥ), प्रभद्रः (Prabhadraḥ), पारिभद्रकः (Pāribhadrakaḥ), are synonymous.

Nimba tastes bitter; is *śītavīrya* and *laghu*. It pacifies *kapha pitta doṣas*.It is useful in blood disorders, skin disorders, pruritus, and ulcers by oral ingestion and external application. It ripens the threatened boil & abscess and cleanses the ripen one.

(Fam.-Meliaceae).

I- *a-* ***Azadirachta indica*** A. Juss.
b- Roxburgh; *c-*Throughout India; d-Apte.

II- a- पिचुमन्दः (Picumandaḥ); अरिष्टः (Ariṣṭaḥ); पारिभद्रकः (Pāribhadrakaḥ).
b- H.B., Mar,- Nimba; Bom.- Kaḍulimb; Tel. Tam., Mal.- Vepu; Eng.-Neem; Margos tree.

महानिम्बः Mahānimbaḥ 8.

महानिम्बः स्मृतो द्रेकी कार्मुको[१] विषमुष्टिकः ॥ ३१
केशमुष्टिर्निम्बरको रम्यकोऽक्षीव[२] एव च ॥

महानिम्बो रसे तिक्तः शीतः पित्तकफापहः ॥ ३२
कुष्ठरक्तविनाशी च विसूचीं हन्ति शीलितः॥

महानिम्बः (Mahānimbaḥ), द्रेकी (Drekī), कार्मुकः (Kārmukaḥ), विषमुष्टिकः (Viṣamuṣṭikaḥ), केशमुष्टिः (Keśamuṣṭiḥ), निम्बरकः (Nimbarakaḥ) रम्यकः (Ramyakaḥ), and अक्षीवः (Akśīvaḥ) are synonymous.

Mahānimba is bitter in taste; *śītavīrya* and pacifies *pitta kaphadoṣas*. It is useful in skin disorders, blood disorders and cholera.

(Under the heading two plants are included. A-द्रेकी (Drekī) and निम्बरकः (Nimbarakaḥ).

(Fam. Meliaceae).

I- A-*a-* ***Melia azedarach*** Linn.
b- Kamat; *c-* Naturalized and cultivated throughout india. *d-* Apte.

---

१ 'कामुको' इति नि. शे. टीका संमतः पाठः । २ 'ऽक्षीर' इति आनन्दाश्रम पुस्तके ।

B-a- ***Melia composita*** Willd. *
b- Kamat,
c- Kokan, S.M. Country; W. Ghats, N. Cirkar; E. Himalayas.

II- A-*a*- द्रेकी(Drekī), कार्मुकः (Kārmukaḥ);विषमुष्टिकः (Viṣamuṣṭikaḥ).
b- H.: Pan., B., -Bakāyan, dreki, Ghoranimb; Mar.- Bakāṇanimba; Tam.- Malaiveṃbu; Tel.-Betti vepu, Mal.-Maha veppu., Eng.- Parsian Lilac.

B-*a*- केशमुष्टिः (Keśamuṣṭiḥ),निम्बरकः (Nimbarakaḥ).
b- Bom.-Nimbārā; Guj.- Kaḍu Khajura.

III- *b*- (1) रोमको रम्यको विषमुष्टिकः (Kaiyadeva).
c- (1) रम्यको द्रेका बकाइणिं (Ḍalhan, Si. 39-4).
d, e, f-See current names.

Note -IV-महानिम्ब *Ailanthus excelsa* Roxb, (Deasi, Chopra).
Guj.- Aduraso, S.-Aralu. (Ni. Adarsha).

9. किराततिक्तः Kirātatiktaḥ

किराततिक्तको हैमः काण्डतिक्तः किरातकः ॥ ३३
भूनिम्बोऽनार्यतिक्तश्च किरातो रामसेनकः ॥

नेपालः कथितश्चान्यो जातिभेदो[१] ज्वरान्तकः ॥ ३४
महातिक्तश्च[२] तिक्तश्च निद्रारिः संनिपातहा ॥

किरातको रसे तिक्तोऽनुष्णशीतो लघुस्तथा ॥ ३५
श्लेष्मपित्तास्रशोफार्तिकासतृष्णाज्वरापहा ॥

किराततिक्तकः (Kirātatiktakaḥ), हैमः (Haimaḥ), काण्डतिक्तः (Kāṇḍatiktaḥ), किरातकः (Kirātakaḥ),भूनिम्बः (Bhūnimbaḥ), अनार्यतिक्तः (Anāryatiktaḥ), किरातः

---

* The current name is *Melia dubia* Cav.

१ 'जात्यश्चैष' इति. नि. शे. टीकायाम् ।

२, 'नाडीतिक्तोऽङ्गतिक्तश्च' इति नि.शे. टीकायाम् पाठः ।

Sodhala has mentioned the following varieties of Nimba 1) Nimba 2) Mahānimba of which synonym is Kaiḍarya 3) Kirātatikta & 4) Bakāyini (Soḍhala p.11)

('अनार्यतिक्त' स्थाने 'नाडीतिक्तः ' इति शोढल पाठः ।

कैडर्यनिम्बस्योल्लेखः –

कैडर्यः पिचुमन्दश्च निम्बोऽरिष्टो वरत्वचः ।

छर्दिघ्नो* हिंगुनिर्यासः प्रियशालश्च ** पार्वतः ॥ इ. पाठ. *** आनन्दाश्रम मुद्रित पुस्तके किरात तिक्तांतर्गतः दृश्यते । चौखम्बामुद्रित पुस्तके तु 'महानिम्ब' शीर्षकान्तर्गतः ।राजनिघण्टौ तु महानिम्बः 'अन्य' इति पृथगेव निर्दिष्टः 'कैडर्योऽन्यो महानिम्ब' इति प्रभद्रादिवर्गे।

S.D. Kamat

* छर्दनो' इति नि.शे. टीका संमतः पाठः ।

** 'मालश्च ' इति. नि. शे. टीका संमतः । *** 'पर्वत' इति नि. शे. टीका ।

(Kirātaḥ), रामसेनकः (Rāmasenakaḥ) are synonymous. There is an another type of *Nimba* which is called as नेपालः *Nepālaḥ* of which synonyms are ज्वरान्तकः (Jwarāntakaḥ), महातिक्तः (Mahātikataḥ), तिक्तः (Tiktaḥ), निद्रारिः (Nidrāriḥ), संनिपातहा (Sannıpātahā).

Kirātaka is bitter in taste, neither too *usna* or *sita* in *virya, laghu* and useful in pacifying *slesma, pitta, rakta doṣa,* oedema, pain (body), cough (*Kāsa)*, thirst and fever.

Two plants are recorded under the heading.

A- किराततिक्तकः (Kirātatiktaḥ) and B- नेपालः (Nepālaḥ).

(Fam. Gentianaceae.)

I- A-*a*- ***Swertia chirata*** Buch.-Ham.

b- Dymock, *c*- Temperate Himalayas. *d*- Jain,

(Fam.- Scrophulariaceae).

B-*a*- ***Schweinfurthia sphaerocarpa*** A. Br.*

b- Dymock, *c*-Rajastan, Sindha.

II- A-*a*- भूनिम्बः (Bhūnimbaḥ), अनार्यतिक्तः (Anāryatiktaḥ), हिङ्गुनिर्यासः (Hinguniryāsaḥ)

b- Mar.-Kirāyat; H.B.,-Cireta; Tam., Tel.-Nila vebu; Eng.-Chireta.

B-*a*- सन्निपातहा (Sannipatahä).

b- H., B.-Sannipata; Bom.-Sonpat.

III- *d, e. g*-See Current names.

IV- See current names in Desai; U.C.Dutt.

10. कटुका Kaṭukā

कटुका मत्स्यशकला मत्स्यपित्ता च रोहिणी ॥३६

कृष्णभेदा काण्डरुहा[१] नाम्ना कटुकरोहिणी ॥

अशोकरोहिणी तिक्ता चक्राङ्गी शकुलादनी ॥ ३७

कटुरोहिण्यरिष्टा च प्रोक्ता तिक्तकरोहिणी ॥

आमघ्नी शतपर्वा च विप्राङ्गी जननी जना ॥३८

कटुका पित्तजित्तिक्ता कटुः शीतास्रदाहजित् ॥

बलासारोचकान् हन्ति विषमज्वरनाशिनी ॥ ३९

---

१ 'चन्द्ररुहा' इति. नि. शे. टीका संमतः पाठः । ' चण्डरुहा' इति क्षीरस्वामी ।

* The current name is *Schweinfurthia papilionacea* (Burm. f.) Boiss

कटुका (Kaṭukā), मत्स्यशकला (Matsyaśakalā), मत्स्यपित्ता (Matsyapittā), रोहिणी (Rohiṇī), कृष्णभेदा (Kṛṣṇabhedā), काण्डरुहा (Kāṇḍaruhā), कटुकरोहिणी (Kaṭukarohiṇī), अशोकरोहिणी (Aśokarohiṇī), तिक्ता (Tiktā), चक्राङ्गी (Cakrāṅigi), शकुलादनी (Śakulādanī), कटुरोहिणी (Kaṭurohiṇī), अरिष्टा (Ariṣṭā), तिक्तकरोहिणी (Tiktakarohiṇī), आमघ्नी (Āmaghnī), शतपर्वा (Śataparavā), विप्राङ्गी (Viprāṅgī), जननी (Jananī), जना (Janā), are synonymous.

Kaṭukā pacifies *pitta;* is bitter in taste, *śitavīrya.*, useful in blood disorders, burning sensation, pacify *kaphadoṣa* and in intermittant fevers.

(Fam.-Scrophulariaceae).

I- *a- **Picrorhiza kurroa*** Royle ex Benth.
b- Dymock, *c*-Gujarath, M.P. and Sub-Himalayan tracts. *d*-Jain.

II- *a-* रोहिणी (Rohiṇī),चक्राङ्गी (Cakrāṅgī), शतपर्वा (Śataparvā).
b- H.- Kuṭaki; B.-Kaṭaki; Mar.-Kuṭaki; Tam.-Katurogani; Tel.-Kaṭukaroni; Bom.-Baḷkuṭaki; Keḍarakuṭaki; Eng.-Picrorhiza.

III- *b-* (1) 194 कटुरोहिणी 195 पित्तरोहिणी (Abhi.Manj.):
(2) कटुका(Su.10).Eng.-Black hellebore; *Picrorhiza kurroa* (Vaidya)
d, e-See current name and *Hellebore niger* Linn.

11. मुस्ता Mustā

मुस्ता चाम्बुधरो मेघो घनो राजकसेरुकः ॥
भद्रमुस्तो वराहोऽब्दो गांगेयः कुरुविन्दकः ॥ ४०

जीमूतोऽथ वृषध्वांक्षी जलदोऽथ बलाहकः[१] ॥
नादेयः पिण्डमुस्तोऽन्यो नागरः परिकीर्तितः ॥ ४१

मुस्ता तिक्तकषायाऽतिशिशिरा श्लेष्मरक्तजित् ॥
पित्तज्वरातिसारघ्नी तृष्णाकृमिविनाशिनी ॥ ४२

मुस्ता (Mustā), अम्बुधरः (Ambudharaḥ),मेघः (Meghaḥ), घनः (Ghanaḥ), राजकसेरुकः (Rājakaserukaḥ), भद्रमुस्तः (Bhadramustaḥ), वराहः (Varāhaḥ),अब्दः (Abdaḥ), गांगेयः (Gāngeyaḥ), कुरुविन्दकः (Kuruvindakaḥ), जीमूतः (Jimūtaḥ), वृषध्वाङ्क्षी (Vṛṣadhwāṅkśi), जलदः (Jaladaḥ), बलाहकः (Balāhakaḥ), नादेयः (Nādeyaḥ) are synonymous.

There is an another variety of *mustā* which is is called as पिण्डमुस्तः (Piṇḍamustaḥ) of which synonym is नागरः (Nāgaraḥ)

---

१ जलावहः इति पा

Mustā is bitter and *kaṣāya* (astringent) in taste, very much *śītavīrya* and pacifies *kapha, pitta* and *rakta doṣas.* It is useful in fevers, diarrohea, thirst and worms.

(Several kinds and varieties, which cannot be identified today are included under the heading. Generally two species : A-भद्रमुस्ता and B-नागरमुस्ता are employed in medicine.

(Fam. Cyperaceae).

I- A-*a*- ***Cyperus rotundus*** Linn.
b- Dymock, *c*-Throughout India, *d*-Apte, Mukerji,
B-*a*- ***C.scariosus,*** Linn. Syn.-*C.pertenuis* Roxb.
b- Dymock, *c*-Bengal, U.P. & E.S. parts of India.

II- A-*a*- भद्रमुस्ता (Bhadrmustā).
b- Bom.-Motha; H.B.-Muthā; Tam;.-Korai; Tel.-Tuna Mustā; Bhadra mustā.
B-*a*- नागरमुस्ता (Nāgaramustā).
b- Kokan-Lavālā; Tam.-Muthakach;H., Mar., Guj., B Nāgarmothā; Tel.-Kolalunga-musta; Kan.-Konnari gadde.

III-See Gunḍa and Gunḍakanda (Raj.ni).
c- मुस्ता /ci-7 / नागरमुस्ता *Cyperus pertenuis* गांगेयम्, भद्रमुस्ता and members. (Vaidya).

IV- (1)*Cyperus jeminious* भद्रमुस्तम् (Bhagirath).

जलमुस्तम् Jalamustum 10

जलमुस्तम् दाशपुरं वानेयं परिपेलवम् ॥
कैवर्तमुस्तं शैवालं जलजं च शुकाह्वयम् ॥ ४३

जलजं तिक्तकटुकं कषायं कान्तिदं हिमम् ॥
मेध्यं वातान्ध्यवीसर्पकण्डूकुष्ठविषापहम् ॥ ४४

जलमुस्तम् (Jalamustam), दाशपुरम् (Dāsapuram), वानेयं (Vāneyam),परिपेलवम् (Paripelavam), कैवर्तमुस्तं(Kaivartamustam), शैवालं (Śaivālam), जलजं (Jalajam), शुकाह्वयम् (Śukāhvayam) are synonymous.

Jalamusta is bitter, pungent and *kaṣāya* (astringent) in taste, *śītavīrya* and improves complexion of the body. It is useful in promoting intellect; pacifying *vātadoṣa,* and is useful in blindness,erysipelas, pruritus, skin diseases and as an antipoison.

Not identified

12. पर्पटः Parpataḥ

पर्पटः स्यात्पर्पटको वरतिक्तः सुतिक्तकः ॥४५
रजो रेणुश्च पांशुश्च कवचो वर्मकंटकः ॥

पर्पटः शीतलस्तिक्तः पित्तश्लेष्मज्वरापहः ॥४६
रक्तदाहारुचिग्लानिमदभ्रमविनाशनः ॥

पर्पटः (Parpaṭaḥ), पर्पटकः (Parpaṭakaḥ), वरतिक्तः (Varatiktaḥ), सुतिक्तकः (Sutiktakaḥ), रजः (Rajaḥ), रेणुः (Renuḥ),पांशुः (Pāmsuḥ), कवचः (Kavacaḥ), वर्मकंटकः (Varmakanṭakaḥ) are synonymous.

Parpata is *śītavīrya,* bitter in taste and pacifies *pitta* and *kapha doṣas.* It is useful in blood disorders, burning sensation loss of appetite, languor, intoxicated state and giddiness.

(Several plants are noted as Parparṭa by modern writers. But the traditional 'Parpaṭa' is recorded herebelow).

(Fam.-Fumariaceae.)

I- *a-* ***Fumaria officinalis*** Linn.

b- Dymock, *c*-Deccan plateau (Mahajan) Persia (Chopra).

II- *a-* वरतिक्तः (Varatiktaḥ), वर्मकण्टकः (Varmakanṭakaḥ), रक्तपुष्पः (Raktapuṣpaḥ).

b- S-Yāvana parpata; H.-Pitapapra; B-Banasulpha; Mar.- Pitpapada; Tam.-Tura, Turu; Tel.- Cabarci; Pers.-Sahātarā.

III- *d, e, f, g*-See current name and *F. parviflora* Linn.

IV- (1) *Fumaria officinalis* and *Justicia procumbens*- Pitapāpaḍā (Desai), (2) *Rungia repens* Pitpāpaḍā (Ayur-joti).

13. वालकम् Vālakam

वालकं वारि तोयं च ह्रीवेरं जलमम्बु च ॥
केश्यं वज्रमुदीच्यं च पिङ्गमाचमनं कचम् ॥ ४७

वालकं शीतलं तिक्तं पित्तश्लेष्मविसर्पजित् ॥
ज्वरकुष्ठातिसारघ्नं केश्यं श्वित्रव्रणापनुत ॥ ४८

वालकं (Vālakam), वारि (Wāri) तोयम् (Toyam), ह्रीवेरं (Rhīveram), जलं (Jalam),अम्बु(Ambu), केश्यं (Keśyam), वज्रं (Vajram), उदीच्यं (Udīcyam),पिङ्गम् (Pingam), आचमनं (Ācamanam), and कचम् (Kacam) are synonymous.

Vālakam is *śitavīrya*, bitter in taste and pacifies *pitta* and *kaphadoṣa*. It is useful in erysipelas, fever, skin disorders, and diarrhoea. It is beneficial for hair, and useful in leucoderma and ulcers.

(Vālaka and Uśīra are quite different plants*. Dh. ni. and Raj. ni. have recorded them separately).

(Fam. Gramineae). Poaceae.

I- **a- ***Vetiveria zizanioides*** Nash.**
Syns. -*Andropogon muricatus* Retz.
A. sqarrosus Hook. Fl. (non L., Sp. PL.).
b- Kamat, *c*-All over India, *d*-Blatter and Mc Cann.

II- *a*- ह्रीबेरम् (Rhiberam), उदीच्यम् (Udicyam).
b- Tel.-Vettiver; Tam.-Vettiver; H.-Khas; B.-Khaskhas; Mar.-Vālā, Netra vālā.

III- See उशीरम् (Usiram) (Dh. Ni. p. 86).
b- बालम् हिवेरम्-नेत्रवाला (Netrawälä) (Bhar.uji; Madan-Ni; Vaidya).

14. (१४) पटोलः Paṭolaḥ

पटोलः कुलकः प्रोक्तः पाण्डुकः कर्कशच्छदः[1]॥
राजीफलः पाण्डुफलो राजनामाऽमृताफलः[2] ॥ ४९
वीर्यगर्भप्रतानश्च[3] कुष्ठहा कासमुक्तिदः ॥
पटोलं कटुकं तिक्तमुष्णं पित्तविरोधि च ॥ ५०
कफासृक्कण्डुकुष्ठानि ज्वरदाहौ च नाशयेत् ॥

पटोलः (Paṭolaḥ), कुलकः (Kulakaḥ), पाण्डुकः (Pāṇḍukaḥ), कर्कशच्छदः (Karkaśacchadaḥ), राजीफलः (Rājīphalaḥ), पाण्डुफलः (Pāṇḍuphalaḥ), राजनामा (Rājanāma), अमृताफलः (Amṛtāphalaḥ), वीर्यगर्भप्रतानः (Vīryagarbha pratānaḥ), कुष्ठहा (Kuṣṭhahā), कासमुक्तिदः (Kāsamuktidaḥ) are synonymous.

Paṭola is pungent and bitter in taste, *uṣṇavīrya* and pacifies *pitta, kapha*

---

* Vālaka should be *pavonia odorata* Linn.
** The current name is *Vetiveria zizanioides* (Linn.) Nash.
१ 'कर्कशच्छदी' इति क्षीर. संमतः पाठः ।
२ ' राजिमानमृताफलः' इति. क्षी. संमतः पाठः ।
३ 'वीर्यगर्भप्रतानश्च' इत्यादि पाठः क्षीर. टीकायां, नि. शे. टीकायां न दृश्यते ।
The source of 'Sugandhabālā sold in North India is *Valeriana Wallichii* Dc. In south Coleus vettiveroides K.C. Jacob is accepted.

and *raktadoṣa* . It is useful in pruritus, skin disorders, fevers, and burning sensation of the body.

(Two plants are recorded as 'Paṭola' of old Sanskrit books by modern writers).

(Fam.-Cucurbitaceae).

I- A-*a*- ***Tricosanthes dioica*** Roxb.
b- Roxburgh, *c*-Northern India; wild.
B-*a*- ***T. cucumerina*** Linn.
b- Watt Dict. *c*-Wild throughout India, Kokan.

II- A-and B-*a*- राजीफलः (Rājiphalaḥ), पाण्डुफलः (Pāṇḍuphalaḥ).
b. -H.-Paravara, Parvel; B.-Poṭol; Guj.-Poṭla; Ṭam.-Kombu, ppuḍalai Tel.-Kommu poṭlā; Mal.-Paṭolum; Mar.-Parvar.
B-*b*- H.-Jangli cincoḍā; Mar.-Rānpaḍaval.

III-*d, e, f*- See current names.

स्वादुपत्रफला Swādupatraphalā 11.

पटोली स्याद् द्वितीयाऽन्या स्वादुपत्रफला च सा ॥ ५१
पटोलस्य तु पर्यायैर्योजयेद् भिषगुत्तमः ॥

पटोलपत्रं पित्तघ्नं वल्ली चास्य कफापहा ॥ ५२
फलं त्रिदोषशमनं मूलं चास्य विरेचनम् ॥

There is an other type of पटोलः (Paṭolaḥ) which is called as स्वादुपत्रफला *Swādupatraphalā*. i.e. the leaves and fruits are not bitter. (contrary to the wild one.). The other synonyms are the same as of Paṭola.

The leaves of Paṭola pacify *pittadoṣa*, the stem pacifies *kapha* and the fruits pacify all the three *doṣas* and the root is purgative.

(Fam.- Cucurbitaceae)

I- *a*- ***Trichosanthes anguina*** Linn.*
b- Roxburgh, *c*-Cultivated throughout hotter parts of India.

II- *a*- पटोली (Paṭoli), स्निग्धपर्णी (Snigdhaparṇi).
b- B.-H.-Cincidā; Mar.-Paḍwala; Tel.-Ling poṭlā; Kan.-Paḍwal Kāvi.
This seems Dangari डङ्गरी of pdt. Bhagirath.

15. हरिद्रा Haridrā (१५) निशाद्वयम् Nisādwayam

हरिद्रा पीतिका पिङ्गा रजनी रञ्जिनी निशा ।
गौरी वर्णवती पीता हरिता वरवर्णिनी ॥ ५४

---

* The current name is *Trichosanthes cucumerina* Linn Var. *aunguina* (Linn.) Hains

हलदीका[1] भद्रलता ज्ञेया वर्णविलासिनी ॥ ५४
विषघ्नी च जयन्ती च दीर्घरङ्गा[2] तु रङ्गिणी ।
हरिद्रा स्वरसे तिक्ता रूक्षोष्णा विषमेहनुत् ॥ ५५
कण्डूकुष्ठव्रणान् हन्ति देहवर्णविधायिनी ॥
विशोधनी कृमिहरा पीनसारुचिनाशिनी ॥ ५६

हरिद्रा (Haridrā), पीतिका (Pītikā), पिङ्गा (Piṅgā), रजनी (Rajanī), रञ्जिनी (Rañjinī), निशा (Niśā), गौरी (Gaurī), वर्णवती (Varṇavatī), पीता (Pītā), हरिता (Haritā), वरवर्णिनी (Varavarṇinī), हलदीका (Haladīkā), भद्रलता(Bhadralatā), वर्णविलासिनी (Varṇavilāsinī), विषघ्नी (Viṣaghnī), जयन्ती (Jayantī), दीर्घरङ्गा (Dīrgharaṅgā) and रङ्गिणी (Raṅgiṇī) are synonymous.

Haridrā is bitter in taste, *rūkśa* and *usṇavīrya,* antipoisonous and useful in disorders characterised by polyuria. It is useful in pruritus, skin disorders. It improves the complexion of the body and useful in helminths, is purificatory, in sinusitis and anorexia.

(Two kinds are recorded under the heading. These are noted below).
(Fam.-Zingiberaceae).

I- A-*a*- ***Curcuma longa*** Linn. (proper).
b- Roxburgh, *c*-Cultivated throughout India.
B-*a*- ***C. caesia***, Roxb.
b- Roxburgh. *c*-Wild and cultivated in Bengal.

II- A-*a*- पीतका (Pītakā), हलदिका (Haladikā).
b- H., B.,-Haladi; Guj., Mar.-Haladi; Tam. Manjel, Eng.Turmeric
B-*a*- श्यामा (Śyāmā), जयन्तिका (Jayantikā).
b- H-Narakacūr; Mar.-Kāḷī haḷad.

16. दारुहरिद्रा Dāruharidrā

अन्या दारुहरिद्रा च पीतद्रुः[3] पीतचन्दनम् ॥
निर्दिष्टा काष्ठरजनी[4] सा* च कालेयका स्मृता ॥ ५७
कालीयकं[5] दारुनिशा दार्वी पीताह्व[6]पीतका ॥
कटंकटेरी पर्जन्या पीतदारु पचंपचा ॥ ५८

---

१ 'हलदी हलना श्रेष्ठा' इति. नि. शे. टीकायाम् ।
२ 'दीर्घरक्ता सुरङ्गिणी' इति नि. शे. टीकायाम् ।
३ 'हरिद्रु' नि.शे. क्षीरस्वामी संमतः पाठः ।
४ 'वै कण्टकिनी स च कालेयकः' इति नि.शे. टीका, क्षीरस्वामी संमतः पाठः । ५ 'कालीयको' नि. शे. टीका, क्षीरस्वामी संमतः पाठः । ६ 'पीतद्रुपीतिका' नि.शे. टीका. क्षीरस्वामी संमतः पाठः ।
* स च कालेयकं स्मृतम् । इति आनन्दा. पाठः ।

हैमवर्णवती[१] पीता हेमकान्ता कुसुम्भका ॥
तिक्ता दारुहरिद्रा स्याद् रूक्षोष्णा व्रणमेहजित् ॥५९
कर्णनेत्रमुखोद्भूतां रुजं कण्डूं च नाशयेत् ॥

There is an another plant दारुहरिद्रा (Dāruharidrā) which has the synonyms: पीतद्रुः (Pītadruḥ), पीतचन्दनम् (Pītacandanam), काष्ठरजनी (Kāṣṭharajanī), कालेयका (Kāleyakā), कालीयकं (Kālīyakam), दारुनिशा (Dāruniśā), दार्वी (Dārvī), पीताह्वपीतका (Pītāhvapītakā),[2] कटंकटेरी (Kaṭaṅkaṭerī), पर्जन्या (Parjanyā), पीतदारु (Pitadāru), पचंपचा (Pacampacā), हेमवर्णवती (Hemavarṇavati), पीता (Pītā), हेमकान्ता (Hemakāntā), कुसुम्भका (Kusumbhakā).

Dāruharidrā is bitter in taste, *rūkśa* and *uṣṇavīrya.* It is useful in ulcers, disorders characterized by polyuria, diseases of the ear, eyes, oral cavity and pruritus.

(Fam.-Berberidaceae).

(About four species of *Berberis* are used as Dāruharidrā. Due to difficulty in specific confirmation, only one species has been notea here, as an example).

I- *a-* ***Berberis aristata*** DC.
b- Watt Dict. *c*-Himalayas and Nilagiri. *d*-Jain.

II- *a-* पीतदारु (Pitadārū), काष्ठरजनी (Kāṣṭharajanî).
b- H.-Citrā, Kāśmal; Mar.-Dāruharidrā, Tam. Mal-Kasturi-manjul, Eng.-True turmeric; True berberis.

III- *d, e,g,*-See species of Berberis and *Coscinum fenestratum*[3].

IV- See Dāruharidrā in Nadkarni and Desai.

17 शठी Śaṭhī

शटी शठी पलाशा च ज्ञेया पृथुपलाशिका ॥ ६०
सुगन्धमूलागन्धालीषड्ग्रन्थासुव्रतावधू ॥
चंद्राणी चद्रगन्धा च दुर्विधेयेति संज्ञिता ॥ ६१
शठीस्यात्तिक्ततीक्ष्णोष्णासंनिपातज्वरापहा ॥
कफोग्रव्रणकासघ्नी वक्त्रशुद्धिविधायिनी ॥ ६२

शटी (Śaṭī), शठी (Śaṭhī), पलाशा (Palaśa), पृथुपलाशिका

---

१ 'हेमवर्णवती ' इ. पाठः नि.शे. टीका, क्षीर. टीकायां न दृश्यते.
2 It may be also *Pītāhvā* and *Pītakā*
3 Climber used in south as a substitute of Berberis.

(Pṛthupalāśikā), सुगन्धमूला (Sugandhamūlā), गन्धाली (Gandhālī), षड्ग्रन्था (Ṣaḍgranthā), सुव्रता (Suvratā), वधू (Vadhū), चंद्राणी (Candrāṇī), चंद्रगन्धा (Candragandhā), दुर्विधेया (Durvidheyā) are synonymous.

Śaṭhī is bitter in taste, *tīkṣṇa, uṣṇavīrya* and pacifies *kapha;* it is useful in *Sannipāta Jwara,* septic ulcers, cough and it clears the mouth.

For confirmation.
(Fam. Zingiberaceae).

I- *a- **Kaempferia galanga*** Linn.
b- Kamat and Mahajan, c-Foot of Himalays and Bengal.
II- *a-* सुगन्धमूला (Sugandhamūlā), चन्द्राणी (Candrāṇī).
b- Kāpurkacrī.
III- See Karcura.
d, e, f, g-See current name and *Curcuma zedoaria* Rosc. *Curcuma zerumbet* Roxb. *Hedychium spicatum* Ham.
IV- (1)शठी (Śaṭhī) *Curcuma zedoaria* Rosc. (Dymock; Kirtikar).
(2) शठी (Śaṭhī) *Kaempferia galanga* Linn. (Yadavji, Kirtikar).

गन्धपलाशी Gandhapalāśī 12 *

अन्या गन्धपलाशी च स्थूलका तिक्तकंदका ॥ ६३
तापसी ज्वलनी चैव हरिद्रापत्रकन्दका ॥

कासश्वासहरा हिध्माज्वरशूलानिलापहा ॥ ६४
शटी स्वर्या गन्धमूला कषायकटुका सरा ॥

There is an another plant गन्धपलाशी (Gandhapalaśī) of which synonyms are स्थूलका (Sthūlakā), तिक्तकंदका (Tiktakandakā), तापसी (Tāpasī), ज्वलनी (Jwalanī), and हरिद्रापत्रकन्दका (Haridrā patra kandakā),

Śatī is *kaśāya* (astringent), and pungent in taste and is useful in bronchial asthma, cough,. hiccup, fever, pains (body). It pacifies *vāta doṣa*. *Śatī* having fragrant tubers is beneficial for throat and voice and is sara.

Not identified.

See- Śaṭhī.

---

१ 'शठी ', 'सटी' 'सठी' इ. आनन्दा. मुद्रित पुस्तके पाठः ।
* *Hedychium spicatum* Ham. ex Smith गन्धपलाशी
Kaempferia galanga Linn. चन्द्रमूल के टुकडे भी व्यवहार में लाये जाते हैं जो इसीके समान होते हैं । Chunekar Bha. Pr. P. 247

18 (१७). मूलम् Mūlam

मूलं पुष्करमूलं च पौष्करं पुष्कराह्वयम् ॥
काश्मीरं पुष्करजटा धीरं तत्पद्मपत्रकम् ॥ ६५

तिक्तं पुष्करमूलं तु कटूष्णं कफवातजित् ॥
ज्वरारोचककासघ्नं शोफाध्मानविनाशनम् ॥ ६६

श्वासं हिक्कां जयत्येव सेव्यमानं शनैः शनैः ॥

मूलम् (Mūlam), पुष्करमूलं (Puṣkaramūlam), पौष्करं (Pauṣkaram), पुष्कराह्वयम् (Puṣkarāhvhayam), काश्मीरं (Kāśmīram), पुष्करजटा (Puṣkarajaṭā), धीरं (Dhīram), पद्मपत्रकम् (Padmapatrakam), are synonymous.

Puṣkaramūlam is bitter, pungent, *usṇa vīrya* and pacifies *kapha* and *vāta doṣas*. It is useful in fever, anorexia, cough, oedema and flatulence. It is useful (if used for a long time) to relieve br. asthma and hiccup gradually.

(Fam.-Iridaceae.)

I- *a*- ***Iris germanica*** Linn.

b- Dymock. *c*-Kashmir; N. Himalayas.

II- *a*- पुष्करमूलम् (Puṣkaramūlam), काश्मीरम् (Kāśmīram).

b- H.-Keware kā-mul; Mar.-Pokharmul; Eng.-Oriss root.

III- See Kuṣṭa; Rāsnā, and Peu. (Raj. ni.).

b- (1) पुष्करमूलम् Veḷḷakotam; Puṣkaramūlam. (Krishnan)

(2) Kuṣṭabhed puṣkaramūlam.
Inula racemosa (Vidyotani; Yadavji and Priyarvrata).*

(3) पुष्करमूलम्- *Iris germanica* (Dwivedi).
d, e, g-See current name and other species of Iris.

IV- (1) पुष्कर मूलम् -See Nadakarni.

(2) Puskaramulam -in its absence kuṣtham.Dipikā page 201.

Sodhala has mentioned the following synonyms of Puskaramūlam -पुष्करमूलम् ।
पुष्करमूलके मूलं काश्मीरं पौष्कराह्वयम् ।
पद्मपत्रं च धीरं च श्वासारि ब्रह्मतीर्थकम् ॥
वृक्षारोहं शूलहरं पद्मपुण्यं च सागरम् ॥
पद्माभिधानकं शूरं वैरि वृक्षसहं तथा ।
See Late D. K. Kamats note under श्वासारिः (२३) * Mostly this is accepted.

19 (१८). भाङ्गी Bhārṅgī

भाङ्गी गर्दभशाकं च पद्मा ब्राह्मणयष्टिका ॥ ६७
अंगारवल्ली फञ्जी[१] च सैव ब्रह्मसुवर्चला ॥
शक्रमाता च कासघ्नी भृङ्गजा भार्गवा मता ॥ ६८
भाङ्गी स्यात् स्वरसे तिक्ता चोष्णा श्वासकफापहा ॥
गुल्मज्वरासृक्वातघ्नी यक्ष्माणं हन्ति पीनसम् ॥ ६९

भार्ङ्गी (Bhārṅgī), गर्दभशाकं (Gardabhaśākam), पद्मा (Padmā), ब्राह्मणयष्टिका (Brāhmaṇayaṣṭikā), अंगारवल्ली (Angāravallī), फञ्जी (Phañjī) ब्रह्मसुवर्चला (Brahmasuvarcalā), शक्रमाता (Śakramātā), कासघ्नी (Kāsaghnī), भृङ्गजा (Bhṛngajā), भार्गवा (Bhārgavā), are synonymous of *Bhārgī*.

Bhārṅgī is bitter in taste, *uṣṇavīrya* and pacifies *kapha* and *vātadoṣa*. It is useful in dyspnoea, cough, tumors (or diverticulae,) fever, *vāta rakta rājayakṣmā* (tuberculosis) and sinusitis.

(Under the name Bhārgī the Nighaṇṭus have noted several names which seem to be synonymous, but some modern writers have identified them as different species. This is the difficulty to distinguish them from each other and in consequence those have mistaken one for another all over India. In this situation the authour has selected the following two plants from the authentic record).

For confirmation.

(Fam.-Verbenaceae).

I- A-*a*- ***Clerodendron serratum*** (L.) Moon.
b- Kamat *c*- More or less throughout India.

Note -This seems to be synonymous with *C. serratum.* Spreng as recorded by T. Cooke (Mahajan).

Note- Clerodendron. Syn.clerodendrum (Agharkar; Jain; Chopra)

B-*a*- ***C. indicum*** (L)Kuntze.
Syn.- *C. siphonanthus* (R. Br.) C.B. Clarke.
b- Kamat. *c*-Deccan, Karnatak. W. coast of Madras state, Kumaon cultivated for ornamental purpose.

II- A- and B-फञ्जी (Phañjī), ब्राह्मणयष्टिका (Brāhmaṇayaṣṭikā)
b- H.- Bārangi; Mar.- Bhārangi; H.-Cinārī. B.- Bahmanhaṭṭi.

III- See Kāsaghnī and Angārwallī.

---

१ 'हञ्जी च वर्चो वर्वरकस्तथा ' इति . क्षीर. संमतः पाठः ।

b- भार्ङ्गि -भृगुभवा (Harshe).

d,e, g-Species of the genus Clerodendron

Note- IV-(1) *C.indicum* (L) Ktze. (Mayarm Uniyal, in Ayurveda Vikās 8-1967; Desai; U.C.Dutt.)

(2) *C. serratum* (L) Moon (Not of spreng).(Mayaram see above).

(3) *Premna herbacea;* Roxb. (U.C.Dutt; Mhaskar; Dymock Kirtikar).

(4) *P. integrifolia* Linn. (Dymock).

श्वासारिः Śwāsāriḥ 13.

श्वासारिः* पद्मतीर्थं च पद्मं पुष्परसागरम् ॥
वृक्षरोहं शूलहरं समूलं सुखसंभवम् ॥ ७०

पद्मतीर्थं (Padmatirtham), पद्मं (Padmam), पुष्परसागरम् (Puṣparasāgaram), वृक्षरोहं (Vṛkšaroham), शूलहरं (Śūlaharam), समूलं (Samūlam), सुखसंभवम् (Sukhasambhavam), are synonyms for श्वासारिः (Śvāsāriḥ).

Not identified

Note- This plant seems to be a kind of orchid growing near the surrounding of 'Padmatirtha' (पद्मतीर्थ) in Kashmir. Its name Padmam 'Puṣparasāgaram' (पुष्परसागरम्) is suggestive of its locality similar to 'Puṣkaramūla' (पुष्करमूल) (*Iris germanica Linn.*). It is not recorded by Raj-ni.

20. (१९) पाठा Pāṭhā

पाठाऽम्बष्ठाऽम्बष्ठकी च प्राचीना पापचेलिका ॥
वरतिक्ता[१] बृहत्तिक्ता पाठिका स्थापनी वृकी ॥ ७१

मालती च वरादेवी त्रिवृत्ताऽन्या शुभा मता ॥
पाठा तिक्तरसा वृष्या विषघ्नी कुष्ठकण्डूनुत् ॥ ७२

---

* Raj. Ni. has recorded some of the synonyms of Śwāsāriḥ under the heading 'Mūlam' vide supra pre No. 18. It is perhaps suggestive of some Iris species, or var. of *Iris germanica.* (Var. florentina). S. D. Kamat.

१ 'वृकतिक्ता वनतिक्ता पापिका ' इति नि.शे. टीका संमतः पाठः । 'वृकतिक्ता वने तिक्ता पापिका स्थापिका वृकी इति क्षीर संमतः पाठः ।

छर्दिहृद्रोगज्वरजित् त्रिदोषशमनी परा ॥
पाठाऽतिसारशूलघ्नी कफपित्तज्वरापहा ॥ ७३

पाठा (Pāṭhā), अम्बष्ठा (Ambaṣṭhā), अम्बष्ठकी (Ambaṣṭhakī), प्राचीना (Prācīnā), पापचेलिका (Pāpacelikā), वरतिक्ता (Varatiktā), बृहत्तिक्ता (Bṛhattiktā), पाठिका (Pāṭhikā), स्थापनी (Sthāpanī), वृकी (Vṛkī), मालती (Mālatī), वरा (Varā), देवी (Devī) are synonymous. The other type त्रिवृत्ता (Trivṛttā), has better properties.

Paṭhā is bitter in taste, *vṛṣya,* antipoisonous (alexipharmic) and is useful in skin disorders and pruritus.

Paṭhā pacifies the three *doṣas* and is useful in emesis, diseases of heart, fever, diarrohea and colics.

(Two plants are included. A- प्राचीना Prācīnā) and B- त्रिवृत्ता (Trivṛttā).

(Fam.- Menispermaceae).

I- A-a- ***Cissampelos pareira*** Linn.
Syn. *C.hernandifolia* Wall. (Watt Dic.)
b- Desai c- Throughout tropical and subtropical India, America.

B-a- ***Cyclea peltata*** Hook.

II- A-a- पाठा (Pāṭhā), प्राचीना (Prācīnā), अंबष्ठा (Ambaṣṭhā)
b- H.,B.- Akanādī, Mar.- Pahāḍvel, Eng.- False Pareira Brava

B-a- मालती (Mālatī), त्रिवृत्ता (Trivṛttā), त्रिशिरा (Triśirā), वृत्तपर्णी (Vṛttaparṇi).
b- Sk..-Rājapāthā, Guj.- Kalipathā; Mar.-Kokan - Pādāval, Tānīci vela.

III a - (1) द्वेपाठे (Dwepāṭhe), (Ca CIXVIII Tryūṣaṇādighṛta).
(2) A.V. ii 27 (Harshe) c- (1) प्राचीना Prācīnā (Arun, Sū-15-33)
d,e,f- See current names and synonyms

IV पाठा (Pāṭhās) of other writers-
(1) *Stephania glabra; Stephania hernandifolia*. (Priyavrata).
(2) *Cissampelos hexandra* Roxb.
Syn.-*Stephania hernandifolia* (U.C.Datta).

21(२०). कट्फलः Katphalaḥ

कट्फलः सोमवल्कश्च श्रीपर्णी कुमुदा तथा[१]।
महाकुम्भा च कुम्भीका भद्रा भद्रवतीति च ॥ ७४

---

१ 'महाकषायोग्रगन्धिः क्षिप्रगर्भः प्रचेतनः ।' इत्यधिकः पाठः अस्याग्रे नि.शे. टीकायाम् । क्षीरटीकायाम् न दृश्यते।

कट्फलः कफवातघ्नो गुल्ममेहाग्निमान्द्यजित ॥ ७५
रुचिष्यो ज्वरदुर्नामग्रहणीपाण्डुरोगहा ।

कट्फलः (Kaṭphalaḥ), सोमवल्कः (Somavalkaḥ), श्रीपर्णी (Śrīparṇī), कुमुदा (Kumudā), महाकुम्भा (Mahākumbhā), कुम्भीका (Kumbhīkā), भद्रा (Bhadrā) and भद्रवती (Bhadravatī) are synonymous.

Kaṭphalaḥ pacifies *kapha* and *vāta doṣas* and is useful in tumors (diverticulosis), diseases characterized by polyuria, dyspepsia, is appetite promoting, and useful in fever, haemorrhoides, diseases of *Grahaṇī* and anemia.

(Fam. Myricaceae).

I- *a*- ***Myrica nagi*** Thumb. (Chopra).
b- Dymock, c-Sub-tropical Himalayas.

II- *a*- सोमवल्कः (Somavalkaḥ), महाकुंभा (Mahākumbhā), कुमुदा (Kumudā), रञ्जनकः (Rañjanakaḥ).
b- H.,P.,Bom., Mar., B.-Kāyaphala; Tel.-Kaidaryamu Mal.-Mauta; Tam.-Marudam.

III- *b*- कट्फलः (Su.-15) Laghukāśmarya. *Myrica sapida M. malabarica,* (Jātipatrikāvat) (Vaidya).
d,e,f,g,-See current name and *M. malabarica.*

IV- कट्फल Kaṭphal (Ni.-Adarsha).

22(२१). देवदारुः Devadaruḥ

देवदारु स्मृतं दारु सुराह्वं किलिमं च तत् ॥ ७६
स्नेहविद्धं महादारु भद्रदार्विन्द्रदारु च ॥

देवकाष्ठं भद्रकाष्ठं पूतिकाष्ठं सुदारु च ॥ ७७
सुरदार्विन्द्रवृक्षश्च तथैवामरदारु च ॥

देवदारु रसे तिक्तं स्निग्धोष्णं श्लेष्मवातजित । ७८
आमदोषविबन्धाध्मप्रमेहविनिवर्तकम् ॥

देवदारुः (Devadāruḥ), दारुः (Dāruḥ), सुराह्वं (Surāhvam), किलिमं (Kilimam), स्नेहविद्धं (Snehaviddham), महादारुः (Mahādāruḥ), भद्रदारुः (Bhadradāruḥ), इन्द्रदारुः (Indradāruḥ), देवकाष्ठं (Devakāṣṭham), भद्रकाष्ठं (Bhadrakāṣṭham), पूतिकाष्ठं (Pūtikāṣṭham), सुदारुः (Sudāruḥ), सुरदारुः (Suradāruḥ), इन्द्रवृक्षः (Indravṛkṣaḥ), and अमरदारुः (Amaradāruḥ) are synonymous.

Devadāru is bitter in taste, *uṣṇavīrya, snigdha* (unctuous) and pacifies *Vāta* and *kapha doṣas*. It is useful in *Āmadoṣa*, blockage in the channels, tympanitis, diseases characterized by polyuria including diabetes.

Under the heading two plants are recorded.

A-देवदारुः (Devadāruḥ) and B.-काष्ठदारुः (Kāṣṭhadāruḥ) .

(Fam.-Pinaceae).

I- A-*a*- ***Cedras deodara*** (Roxb.) Loud.*
b- Roxburgh, *c*-North western Himalayas.
B-*a*- Not identified.

II- A-*a*- स्नेहविद्धम् (Snehawiddham), देवकाष्टम् (Dewakāṣṭham).

23(२२). कत्तृणम् Kattṛṇam

कत्तृणं सकलं भूति भूतिदं रोहिषं तृणम् ॥ **
ध्यामकं श्यामकं पौरं पाटलं देवदंशकम्[१] ॥ ७९
कत्तृणं श्वासकासघ्नं हृद्रोगशमनं परम् ॥
विसूच्यजीर्णशूलघ्नं कफपित्तास्रनाशनम् ॥ ८०

कत्तृणं (Kattṛṇam), सकलं (Sakalam), भूतिः (Bhutiḥ), भूतिदं (Bhūtidam), रोहिषं (Rohiṣam), तृणम् (Tṛṇam), ध्यामकं (Dhyāmakam), श्यामकं (Syāmakam), पौरं (Pauram), पाटलं (Pāṭalam), देवदंशकं (Devadam'sakam) are synonymous.

Kattṛṇam pacifies *kapha, pitta* and blood disorders. It is useful in dyspnoea, cough, and heart disease. It is also useful in cholera, indigestion and colics.

Under this heading are included some aromatic grasses; all of them cannot be identified today. Two varieties of them are noted here A-(Laghukāṇḍa) and B-(Dīrghakāṇḍa) .

(Fam.-Gramineae). (Fam.Poaceae)

I- A-*a*- ***Cymbopogon schoenanthus*** (L). Spreng.

---

१ ' देवदण्डकम् इति. पा.

* The current name for *Cedrus deodara* (Roxb.) Loud is *Cedrus deodara* Roxb. ex. D.Don syn *C. libani* Barrel var. *deodara* Hook. *f.*

** "कत्तृणं शकलिर्भूरि भूतिकं रौहिषं ततम् ।
ध्यामकं भूमकं पौरं मुद्गलं देवजग्धकम् । इति
क्षी. संमतः पाठः ।"

Syn.-*Andropogon schoenanthus* Linn.
Andropogon martini Roxb. (Watt p. 249. A)
b- Dymock *c*-Hotter parts of India.

B-*a*- ***Cymbopogon martini*** Stapf. (Roxburgh, Agharkar).
b- Mahajan C- Hotter parts of India, d- Blatter

II-A & B-*a*- **रोहिषम्** (Rohiṣam), **कुतृणम्** (Kutṛṇam), **कत्तृणम्** (Kattṛṇam.)
b- B. Gandha benā; Bom.-Rohisagavat; Mar., H.-Rosāghās, Tel.-rosel; Tam.-Shaknaruppillu, Eng.-Geraninum grass, Rusa oil grass.

III- *d, e, f*- See current names.

IV- (1)**दीर्घकाण्ड** H. -Sophiya; **लघुकाण्ड** H.-Motiya,(Kirtikar).

कपटम् Kaptam 14.

कपटं च सुमङ्गल्यं चिडा* गन्धवधूस्तथा ॥
तरुणं तरुणी तारा वातभूतविनाशनी ॥ ८१

कफवातहरा चोष्णा दीपनी रक्तपित्तजित् ॥

कपटं (Kapaṭam), **सुमङ्गल्यं** (Sumangalyam), **चिडा** (Cidā), **गन्धवधूः** (Gandhavadhūḥ),**तरुणं** (Taruṇam), **तरुणी** (Taruṇī), **तारा** (Tārā) **वातभूतविनाशनी**, (Vātabhūtavināsanī), are synonyms for *kapaṭam.*

Kapaṭam pacifies *kapha* and *vātadoṣas*, it is *uṣṇavīrya,* appetizer and useful in bleeding disorders.

(A kind of grass). Not identified.

गुण्ठः Gunṭhaḥ 15.

गुण्ठो वृत्तगुणः शुण्ठः शृंगभेदीभमूलकः ॥ ८२
शुण्ठं कुण्ठं तृणशुण्ठो वर्तुलः पृथुकन्दकः ॥

कषायानुरसः स्वादुः शीतलो मूत्रकृच्छ्रहा ॥ ८३
रक्तपित्तहरो गुण्ठो रजःशुक्रविशोधनः ॥

गुण्ठः (Gunṭhaḥ), **वृत्तगुणः** (Vṛttaguṇaḥ), **शुण्ठः** (Śuṇṭhaḥ), **शृङ्गभेदी** (Śṛngabhedī), **इभमूलकः** (Ibhamūlakaḥ), **शुण्ठं** (Śuṇṭham), **कुण्ठं** (Kuṇṭham),

---

* The synonym is suggestive of some pine tree, however, as per the context it may be a kind of grass also.

तृणशुण्ठः (Tṛṇaśuṇṭhaḥ), वर्तुलः (Vartulaḥ), पृथुकन्दकः (Pṛthukandakaḥ) are synonyms for *Guṇṭhaḥ*..

Guṇṭhaḥ is sweet in taste and *kaṣāya* (astringent) as secondary taste, *śītavīrya*. It is useful in diseases characterized by oliguria, bleeding disorders and is having purificatory actions on *rajaḥ* (monthly periodic bleeding in female) and *śukram* (male semen.)

(A kind of grass) Not identified.*

24. (२३) शृङ्गी Śṛṅgī

श्रृंगी कर्कटश्रृंगी च कुलीरा कर्कटाह्वया ॥ ८४
कुलीरश्रृंगी वक्रा[1] च महाकोषा[*] नताङ्गिनी[2] ॥
चंद्रास्पदा[3] विषाणी च श्रृंगी वनजमूर्धजा[4] ॥ ८५
तिक्ता कर्कटश्रृंगी च गुरुश्चोर्ध्वसमीरजित् ॥
कासश्वासार्तियक्ष्मघ्नी वान्तितृष्णारुचीर्जयेत् ॥ ८६

श्रृङ्गी (Śṛṅgī), कर्कटश्रृङ्गी (Karkaṭaśṛṅgī), कुलीरा (Kulīrā), कर्कटाह्वया (Karkaṭāhvayā), कुलीरश्रृङ्गी (Kulīraśṛṅgī), वक्रा (Vakrā), महाकोषा (Mahākoṣā), नताङ्गिनी (Natāṅginī), चंद्रास्पदा (Candrāspadā), विषाणी (Viṣāṇī), श्रृंगी (Śṛṅgī), and वनजमूर्द्धजा (Vanajamūrdhajā) are synonyms for *śṛṅgī*.

Karkaṭaśṛṅgī is bitter in taste, *guru* and useful in conditions like eructations, cough, dyspnoea, (Br.asthma), Pulm. t.b., emesis, excessive thirst, and is appetizer.

(Fam. Anacardiaceae).

I- *a*- ***Pistacia integerrima*** Stew. ex. Brandis
Syn.-*Rhus integerrima* Wall.

b- Murray (in Watt. Dict. VI-268).

c- Trans Indus; N.W. Himalayas.

---

* Priyavartaji sharma has identified it with '*Typha elephantina* Roxb.' Rāmabāṇa - रामबाण in marāṭhi Sans. Gundrā - गुन्द्रा (chopra). S.D.Kamat.

१ "चक्रा" इति नि.शे. टीका। २ "नवाङ्गिनी" इति आनन्दाश्रम पुस्तके।

३ "चन्द्रास्वादु" इति नि.शे. टीकायाम्। ४ "प्रोक्ता च निजमूर्द्धजा" इति नि.शे. टीकायाम्।

* 'महाघोषा' इति आनंदा. पाठः।

II- *a-* कर्कटश्रृंगी (Karkaṭaśṛiṅgī),विषाणी (Viṣāṇī).
b- H.-Kākrāsingi. Mar.-Kākaḍśingi; Tam.-Karkaṭaga singi; Tel.-Karkarcingi; Eng.-True Karakatsingi.
(J. Murray. Watt. Dict).
d,e,-See current names and synonyms.

अजशृङ्गी Ajaśṛṅgī 16.

अजश्रृंगी मेषश्रृंगी सर्पदंष्ट्रा च वर्तिका ॥
द्वितीया दक्षिणावर्ता वृश्चिकाली विषाणिका ॥ ८७
अजश्रृंगी हिमा स्वादुः शोफतृष्णावमीर्जयेत् ॥
चक्षुष्याश्वासहृद्रोगविषकासार्तिकुष्ठनुत् ॥ ८८

अजश्रृङ्गी (Ajaśṛṅgī), मेषश्रृङ्गी (Meṣaśṛṅgī), सर्पदंष्ट्रा (Sarpadaṃṣṭrā), वर्तिका (Vartikā); The other type is laevo twiner and called as वृश्चिकाली (Vṛścikālī) and have the synonym विषाणिका (viṣāṇikā).

Ajaśṛṅgī is *śītavīrya*, sweet in taste and useful in odema (inflamations), thirst, emesis, beneficial to eyes, dyspnoea (asthma), cardiac diseases, poisoning, diseases characterized by cough and in skin disorders.

Not identified.

II- A-a- सर्पदंष्ट्रा (Sarpadaṃṣṭrā); वर्तिका (Vartikā).
b- Sk.-Meṣaśṛṅgi; H.-Medāsingi; B.-Mersingi; Bom.-Kāvaḷī; vākhāṇḍi, Medhasingi; Tel.-Podapatra; Tam.-Sirukuranja.
B-a- दक्षिणावर्ता (Dakṣiṇāvartā).

III- a- अजशृङ्गी-त्वयापूर्वमथर्वा (AV.IV-37-6). (Satavlekar), (Karambelkar).
(1) 221, 222 मेषशृङ्गी (Abhi. Manj).
(2) मेषशृङगी –न्योब्युण्णी, मुत्तपनृताठी, वद्दकुरुञ्ची, आदट्ट कोटप्याला (Vaidya)
(3) मेषशृङगी (Gymnema sylvestre. (Vidyotani, Dwivedi).
(4) मेषशृङगीत्वक्क्वाथाभिषुतोगुडप्रतिवापा मैरेयम् (Kautiliya A. Shastra, Surādhyakṣa 43 Chapter).Note-'Maireyam', a kind of Sura.

V- (1) Medhasingi, gudmar.
Medicinal properties similar to (Utarana). (Balawant-Bihar).
*(2) *Gymnema sylvestre* and (Utarna) *Daemia extensa* are written separately but are the same. (Bhagirath p. 77).

---

* The current name for *Daemia extensa* R.Br. is *Pergularia daemia* (Forsk.) Choiv. syn. *Pergularia extensa* N.E.Br. (Comp. P. 115). This may be Ajaśṛṅgī (Utaraṇa) but Guḍamāra (paralyses temporarily sweet taste) is *Gymnema sylvestre* R. Br.

25. शालिपर्णी Śāliparṇī
(24) पर्णिनीद्वयम् Parṇinīdwayam.

शालिपर्णी स्थिरा सौम्या त्रिपर्ण्यतिगुहा ध्रुवा ॥
विदारिगन्धांऽशुमती दीर्घमूलांशुपत्रिका ॥ ८९

शालिपर्णी विशेषः
आलकं पालकं दग्धं सबलं भूमिगन्धकम् ॥
ज्वलनाभं विशुद्धं च गन्धं बोटं कुसुम्भकम् ॥ ९०

शालिपर्णी रसे तिक्ता गुरूष्णा वातदोषजित् ॥
विषमज्वरमेहार्शःशोफसन्तापनाशनी ॥ ९१

शालिपर्णी (Śāliparṇī), स्थिरा (Sthirā), सौम्या (Saumyā), त्रिपर्णी (Triparṇī), अतिगुहा (Atiguhā), ध्रुवा (Dhrurvā), विदारिगन्धा (Vidārigandhā), अंशुमती (Amśumatī), दीर्घमूला (Dīrghamūlā), अंशुपत्रिका (Amśupatrikā), are synonymous. For another type of śāliparṇī the synonyms are आलकं (Ālakam), पालकं (Pālakam), दग्धं (Dagdham), सबलं (Sabalam), भूमिगन्धकम् (Bhūmigandhakam), ज्वलनाभं (Jwalarābham), विशुद्धं (Viśuddham), गन्धं (Gandham), बोटं (Boṭam), and कुसुम्भकम् (Kusumbhakam).

Śāliparṇī is bitter in taste, *guru* and *uṣṇavīrya*. It pacifies *vātadoṣa,* is useful in intermittant fevers, disorders charaterized by polyuria, piles, oedema (inflammation) and burning sensation.

(It seems that more than one plants are recorded under this heading, as well as by the modern writers. Out of them two generally recognised species are recorded here below.

(Fam.-Leguminosae, Sub. fam. Papilionaceae). Fabaceae

I- *A-a-* ***Desmodium gangeticum*** DC.*
Syn.-*Hedysarum gangeticum* Willd.

b- Roxburgh.

For confirmation

B-*a-* ***Desmodium laxiflorum*** DC.

b- Cooke.

---

१ अस्याग्रे " सर्वानुकरिणी तन्वी दीर्घपर्णी च पर्णिका ।" इत्यधिकः पाठः नि.शे. टीकायाम् । 'पृष्णिरिव पर्णान्यस्याः पृष्णिपर्णी सुक्ष्मपर्णा वा । हैमोणादौ 'पृष्णि' शब्दः स्वीकृतोऽस्ति पाणिन्युणादौ अमरादौ च 'पृश्नि' शब्दः स्वीकृतोऽस्ति । ' इति नि.शे. टीकायाम् ।

* Current name for *Desmodium gangeticum* DC. is *D. gangeticum* (Linn.) DC. Syn. *Hedysarum gangeticum* Linn. It is better to call it as Śalaparṇī (resembling leaves of śāla- shorea robusta.)

II- A-*a*- शालिपर्णी (Śāliparṇī), विदारिगन्धा (Vidārigandhā), दीर्घमूला (Dīrghamūlā), अंशुमती (Amśumatī)

b- H.-Sarivan, Sālpan; B,-Sālpani; Mar.-Dāya, Rānbhāl, Sālvaṇ; Guj.-Sālvan, Poona - Rānsewrā.

B-*b*-Mar.-Rānagānjā, Bhuisewrā, Dāya.

III- See Pṛthakparṇī.

a- (1)अंशुमती काण्डिनी, (AV. VIII-7).

(2)अंशुमतीद्वयम् (Amśumatidwayam), शालिपर्णी (Śāliparṇī), पृश्निपर्णी (Pṛṣniparṇī).
(Ashta. San. U.Rasayan. 49).

d,e,f,g-See current names and synonyms.

IV- (1) Many species of Desmodium come across.
(Sachitra Ayur. 10.58).

26. पृष्टिपर्णी Pṛṣṭiparnî* (पृश्निपर्णी Pṛṣniparṇī)

पृष्टिपर्णी पृथक्पर्णी कलशी धावनी गुहा ॥
श्रृगालविन्नाऽङ्घ्रिबला पर्णी क्रोष्टुकपुच्छिका ॥ ९२

(पृश्निपर्णी विशेषः)
सर्वानुकारिणी तन्वी दीर्घपर्णी च पर्णिका ॥
कुमुदाऽतिगुहा चैव विषघ्नी सैव कीर्तिता ॥ ९३

पृश्निपर्णी रसे स्वादुर्लघूष्णाऽस्त्रत्रिदोषजित् ॥
कासश्वासप्रशमनी ज्वरतृड्दाहनाशिनी ॥ ९४

पृष्टिपर्णी (Pṛṣṭiparṇī), पृथक्पर्णी (Pṛthakparṇī), कलशी (Kalaśī), धावनी (Dhāvanī), गुहा (Guhā), श्रृगालविन्ना (Śṛgālavinnā),अंघ्रिबला(Anghribalā),पर्णी (Parṇī), क्रोष्टुकपुच्छिका (Kroṣṭukapucchikā) are synonyms for *Pṛṣniparṇī.*

For other type of *Pṛṣniparṇī* the synonyms are सर्वानुकारिणी (Sarvānukāriṇī), तन्वी (Tanvī), दीर्घपर्णी (Dirghaparṇī), पर्णिका (Parṇikā), कुमुदा (Kumudā), अतिगुहा (Atiguhā) and विषघ्नी (Viṣaghnī).

Pṛṣniparṇī is sweet in taste, *laghu*, *uṣṇa*, pacifier of *rakta* and *tridoṣas*. It is useful in cough and breathlessness (dyspnoea), fever, thirst and burning sensation of the body.

Under this heading two plants are recorded in Dh. ni. It seems that

* "पृश्निपर्णी" इति साधु पाठः ।

Raj. ni has noted only one. A-(Pṛṣṭiparṇī of Dh. ni. and B- (Pṛṣniparṇī) of both Ni. s.

For confirmation. (Fam. Laguminosae) Fabaceae

I- A-*a*- ***Desmodium triquetrum*** DC.*
Syn-*Hedysarum alatum* Roxb.
b- Kamat.

Confirmed.

B-*a*- ***Uraria picta*** Desv.
Syn.-*Doodia picta* Roxb. (Roxb fl.).
b- Dymock.

II- A-*a*- पृथक्पर्णी (Pṛthakparṇī), धावनी (Dhāvanī).
b- Mar.-Rānabhāla, Dāvaḍavalā; Piṭhavaṇ,

B-*a*- पृश्निपर्णी (Pṛṣniparṇī), तन्वी(Tanvī),चित्रपर्णी (Citraparṇī), महागुहा (Mahāguhā).
b- H-Piṭhavan.Dābrā; B.-Sankariaṭā. Mar.- Davalā Tel.-Kālpannā.

III- a- (1) पृश्निपर्णी (Pṛsniprṇī):-
शं नो देवी पृश्निपर्ण्यशं निऋत्या अकः (AV. ii-25-1).
(2) पृश्निपर्णी *Harmonitis cordifolia.* (Shende AV-iii-25)
(3) Pṛ'sniparnī S. B. xiii-8,
(Harshe. intro).
b- द्विधास्यात् पृश्निपर्णिका (Dwidhāsyāt Pṛsniparṇikā).
(Raj. N. Gana. iv. 1).
c- शृगालविन्नाम् (Śṛgālavinnām).
Eke Vidārigandhā paṭhanti, anye Pṛthakparṇī bhedam Dīrghapatrāmāhuḥ. (Dalhaṇ S. Sū.-38).

(4) पृश्निपर्णी (Pṛ'sniparṇī) (Vartulapatrā simhapucchi)
(Cakra, Su. 3-20),
d,e,f,g-See current names and synonyms.

Note - V- Many Vaidyas take शालिपर्णी as पृश्निपर्णी and पृश्निपर्णी as शालिपर्णी Sachitra Ayur. 10-196

27. बृहती Bṛhatī (२५) बृहतीद्वयम् Bṛhatīdwayam

बृहती सिंहिका कान्ता वार्ताकी राष्ट्रिका कुली ॥
विषदा स्थूलकण्टाकी महती तु महोटिका ॥ ९५

---

* Current name for *D. triquetrum* DC is *D. triquetrum* (Linn.) DC., for *Uraria picta* Desv. is *U. picta* (Jacq.)Desv. ex DC.

सिंहिका कफवातघ्नी श्वासशूलज्वरापहा ॥
छर्दिहृद्रोगमन्दाग्निमामदोषांश्च नाशयेत् ॥ ९६

बृहती (Bṛhatī), सिंहिका (Simhikā), कान्ता (Kāntā), वार्ताकी (Vārtākī), राष्ट्रिका (Rāṣṭrikā), कुली (Kulī), विषदा (Viṣadā), स्थूलकण्टाकी (Sthūla kaṇṭākī), महती (Mahatī) and महोटिका (Mahoṭikā) are synonyms for *Bṛhatī.*

Bṛhatī pacifies *kapha* and *vāta doṣa,* breathlessness (Br. Asthma), pains and aches and fever. It is useful in emesis, diseases of the heart,dyspepsia and *āmadoṣa.*

(Fam. -Solanaceae).

I- *a*- ***Solanum indicum*** Linn.
   b- Several writers,

II- *a*- सिंहिका (Simhikā), स्थूलकण्टाकी (Stlūlakaṇṭākī), महोटिका (Mahoṭikā).
   b- Kokan-Dorli: Cicurḍi; B.-Vyakura; Mal.-Nilavatutin H.-Birhaata; Tam.-Papparamulli.

28. कण्टकारी * Kaṇṭakārī

कण्टकारी तु दुःस्पर्शा क्षुद्रा व्याघ्री निदिग्धिका ॥
कण्टालिका कण्टकिनी धावनी दुष्प्रधर्षिणी ॥ ९७

कण्टकारी कटुस्तिक्ता तथोष्णा श्वासकासजित् ॥
अरुचिज्वरवातामदोषहृद्गदनाशिनी ॥ ९८

कण्टकारीद्वयं तिक्तं वातामकफकासजित् ॥
क्षुद्रिकायाः फलं ज्ञेयं कटु तिक्तं ज्वरापहम् ॥ ९९

कण्डुकुष्ठकृमिघ्नञ्च कफवातहरं तथा ।

कण्टकारी (Kaṇṭakārī), दुःस्पर्शा (Duḥsparśā), क्षुद्रा (Kśudrā), व्याघ्री (Vyāghrī), निदिग्धिका (Nidigdhikā), कण्टालिका (Kaṇṭālikā), कण्टकिनी (Kaṇṭakinī), धावनी (Dhāvanī), दुष्प्रधर्षिणी (Duṣpradharṣiṇī), are synonymous .

Kaṇṭākarī is bitter and pungent in taste and *uṣṇavīrya.* It is useful in cough, breathlessness, anorexia, fever, *vāta dosa, āmadosa,* and car-

---

*"भागुरिर्हि द्वयोर्बृहतीत्वं मन्यते, यच्छाश्वतः ।
" क्षुद्रायां क्षुद्रवार्ताक्यां बृहती छन्दसि क्वचित् ।
द्व्यर्थे प्रचोदनी कण्टकारिका च दुरालभा ॥"
इति क्षीरस्वामीटीकायां नि.शे. टीकायां च । S.D.K.

diac disordrs. Both the *kaṇṭakaris* are bitter in taste and pacify *vāta, kapha* and *āmadoṣa.* It is useful in diseases charaecterized by cough. The fruits of *kśudrikā* are bitter and pungent in taste and useful in fevers, *kapha* and *vātadoṣa,* and useful in pruritus, skin disorders and as an anthelmintic.

(Fam.-Solanaceae).

I- *a-* ***Solanum xanthocarpum*** * Schrad & Wendle.
b- Roxburgh.

II- *a-* दुस्पर्शा (Dusparśā), व्याघ्री (Vyāghrī).
b- H.-Kaṭeli; Ben.-Kanṭakāri; Mar.-Kateringṇi; Tel.-Rasagadi; Tam. Kandangattiri; Mal.-Malanjunta

लक्ष्मणा Lakśmaṇā 19.

लक्ष्मणा क्षेत्रदूती च सितसिंही कुवार्तिका ॥ १००
सुश्वेता कण्टकारी दुर्लभा च महौषधी ॥

लक्ष्मणा (Lakśmaṇā), क्षेत्रदूती (Kśetradūtī), सितसिंही (Sitasimhī), कुवार्तिका (Kuvārtikā), सुश्वेता (Suśvetā), कण्टकारी (Kanṭakārī), दुर्लभा (Durlabhā), and महौषधी (Mahauṣadhī) are synonyms for *Lakśmaṇā.*

(This heading includes two kinds A-श्वेतकण्टकारी (Śwetakaṇṭakārī) and B-वार्ताकिनीसिता (Wārtākinīsitā).

(Fam.- Solanaceae).

I- A-*a*-(1) White flowered Kaṇṭākārī.

(2) ***Solanum hirsutam*** Roxb.

b- Kamat.

Note- These plants grow sometimes naturally with white flowers. (Kamat) This seems to be due to hybridization (Mahajan).

II- A-a- श्वेता कण्टकारी(Swetā Kaṇṭakārī).

B-a- "White flowering बृहती (Bṛhati)".

b- Kamat.

b- Vern. names as of those of कण्टकारी but begining with श्वेता (Śwetā)

---

*Current name for *S.xanthocrpurm* Schrad &Wendl. is *Solanum surattense* Burm f. (comp.142)

B-a- श्वेतबृहती (Śwetabṛhatī), चन्द्रपुष्पा (Candrapuṣpā), कट्टुवार्ताकिनी (Kaṭuwārṭākini).

Vern. names as in बृहती but begining with श्वेता (Śwetā)

कासघ्नी Kāsaghnī 20.

कासघ्नी क्षुद्रमाता च क्वचिद् वार्ताकिनी विदुः ॥ १०१
वनजा किंचिदाटव्या कपटा कपटेश्वरी ॥

मलिना मलिनाङ्गी च कट्टुवार्ताकिनीति च ॥ १०२
गर्दभी बहुवाहा च चन्द्रपुष्पी प्रियंकरी ॥

कासघ्नी (Kāsaghnī), क्षुद्रमाता (Kśudramātā), sometimes called as वार्ताकिनी (Vārtākinī), वनजा (Vanajā), आटव्या (Āṭavyā), कपटा (Kapaṭā), कपटेश्वरी (Kapṭeśvarī), मलिना (Malinā), मलिनाङ्गी(Malināngī), कट्टुवार्ताकिनी (Kaṭuvārtākinī), गर्दभी (Gardabhī), बहुवाहा (Bahuvāhā), चन्द्रपुष्पी (Candrapuṣpī), and प्रियंकरी (Priyamkarī) are synonyms of another type of *Kanṭakārī*.

Not identifed. *

21. वृन्ताकी Vṛntākī

वृन्ताकी वार्तिका वृन्ता भण्टाकी भण्टिका मता ॥ १०३
वृन्ताकं स्वादु तीक्ष्णोष्णं कट्टुपाकमपित्तलम् ॥

कफवातहरं हृद्यं दीपनं शुक्रलं लघु ॥ १०४

वृन्ताकी (Vṛntākī), वार्तिका (Vārtikā), वृन्ता (Vṛntā), भण्टाकी (Bhanṭākī), भण्टिका (Bhanṭikā), are synonyms for वृन्ताकी Vṛntākī. (Its fruit) Vṛntākam is sweet *tikśṇa, usṇavīrya* and pungent in *vipāka* but does not aggravate *pitta,* pacifies *kapha* and *vāta,* is cordial, appetizer, increases *śukra* and is *laghu.*

(Fam.-Solanaceae).

I- *a*- ***Solanum melongena*** Linn.
b- Roxburgh, *c*-Cultivated throughout India.

II- *a*- भण्टाकी (Bhanṭāki),महोटिका (Mahoṭikā), चित्रफला (Citraphalā)

---

* It is some wild solanum sp. - S. D. Kamat.

b- Ben.-Bengum; H. Baingan; Tel.-Vagkai; Mar.-Vānge; Vāyangen.

29 (२९). गोक्षुरः Gokśurah

गोक्षुरः[१] स्याद् गोक्षुरको भक्षकः स्वादुकण्टकः ॥१०५
गोकण्टको भक्षटकः षडङ्गः कण्टकत्रिकः ॥

श्वदंष्ट्रो बृंहणो वृष्यस्त्रिदोषशमनोऽग्निकृद् ॥१०६
शूलहृद्रोगकृच्छ्रघ्नः प्रमेहविनिवर्तकः ॥

गोक्षुरः (Gokśurah), गोक्षुरकः (Gokśurakaḥ), भक्षकः (Bhakśakaḥ), स्वादुकण्टकः (Swādukaṇṭakaḥ), गोकण्टकः (Gokaṇṭakaḥ), भक्षटकः (Bhakśaṭakaḥ), षडङ्गः (Ṣaḍaṅgaḥ), and कण्टकत्रिकः (Kaṇṭakatrikaḥ) are synonyms for *Gokśura.*

Gokśura promotes the bulk of the body, is *vṛṣya,* pacifier of the three *doṣas,* increases the digestive (and assimilative) capacity. It is useful in colics, cardiac diseases, strangury and diseases characterized by polyuria.

This heading includes two plants : A-षडङ्गः (Ṣaḍangaḥ) and B- त्रिकण्टक (Trikaṇṭakaḥ).

(Fam. Zygophyllaceae).

I- A-*a-* ***Tribulus terrestris*** Linn.
Syn.-*T.lanuginosus* Willd.
b- Roxburgh.

(Fam. -Pedaliaceae)

B-*a-* ***Pedalium murex*** Linn.
b- Dymock.

II- A-a- स्वादुकण्टकः (Swādukaṇṭakaḥ).
b- H.-Chotāgokharu; Miṭhā-gokharu; Mar.- Saraṭā; Tam.-Nerungi; Eng.-Caltrop; Tribulus fructus.

---

१ गोकण्टो गोक्षुरः कण्टीः षडङ्गः क्षुरकः क्षुरः ।
त्रिकण्टकः कण्टफलः श्वदंष्ट्रो व्यालदंष्ट्रकः ।" इत्यानन्दाश्रम पुस्तके अधिकः पाठः ।
क्षीरस्वामी टीकायाम् उद्धृतः पाठः ।
"गोक्षुरः स्याद् गोक्षुरको भक्षकः स्वादुकण्टकः ।
गोकण्टको भक्षटंकः षडङ्गः क्षुरकः क्षुरः ॥
गोकण्टो गोक्षुरः कण्टी षडङ्गः त्रिकट स्त्रिकः ।
त्रिकण्टकः कण्टफलःश्वदंष्ट्रः व्यालदंष्ट्रकः ॥

B-a- त्रिकण्टकः(Trikanṭakaḥ).

b- H. and B.-Barāgokharu, Mar.- Mothāgokharu; Tam.- Perunerunji, Mal.- Katu nerinjl.

30. (२६) बिल्वः Bilvaḥ

बिल्वः शलाटुः शाण्डिल्यो हृद्यगन्धो महाफलः ॥१०७
शैलूषः श्रीफलः श्याह्वः कर्कटः पूतिमारुतः ॥

लक्ष्मीफलो गन्धगर्भः सत्यकर्मा दुरारुहः ॥१०८
वातसारोऽरिमेदश्च कण्टकाद्योऽसिताननः ।

बिल्वमूलं त्रिदोषघ्नं छर्दिघ्नं मधुरं लघु ॥१०९
बिल्वस्य तु फलं बालं स्निग्धं संग्राहि दीपनम् ॥

कटु तिक्तकषायोष्णं तीक्ष्णं वातकफापहम् ।११०
विद्यात्तदेव संपक्वं मधुरानुरसं गुरु ॥
विदाही विष्टम्भकरं दोषहृत्पूतिमारुतम् ॥१११ S.Su. 46. 174

बिल्वः (Bilvaḥ), शलाटुः (Śalāṭuḥ), शाण्डिल्यः (Śāṇḍilyaḥ), हृद्यगन्धः (Hṛdyagandhaḥ), महाफलः (Mahāphalaḥ), शैलूषः (Śailūṣaḥ), श्रीफलः (Śrīphalaḥ), श्याह्वः (Śryāhvaḥ), कर्कटः (Karkaṭaḥ), पूतिमारुतः (Pūtimārutaḥ) लक्ष्मीफलः (Lakśmīphalaḥ), गन्धगर्भः (Gandhagarbhaḥ), सत्यकर्मा (Satyakarmā), दुरारुहः (Durāruhaḥ), वातसारः (Vātasāraḥ), अरिमेदः (Arimedaḥ), कण्टकाद्यः (Kanṭakādhyaḥ), असिताननः (Asitānanaḥ), are synonyms for *Bilva*.

The roots of *Bilva* are sweet in taste and *laghu,* these pacify three *doṣas* and are useful in vomiting The unripe fruit is *snigdha* (unctuous) astringent (binding), and appetizer, it is pungent, bitter, *kaṣāya* in taste, sharp, *usṇavīrya* and pacifies *vāta* and *kapha doṣas.* But when it is well ripe it's subsidiary test is sweet, and is *guru,* increases epigastric burning, constipating and expels doṣas and foetid flatus.

(Fam.-Rutaceae).

I- *a- **Aeglė marmelos*** Corr.*
b- Roxburgh.

II- *a-* शलाटुः** (Śalāṭuḥ), महाफलः (Mahāphalaḥ); श्रीफलः (Śrīfalaḥ), अरिमेदः (Arimedaḥ).
b- H.-Ben., Bom.-Bel; Tam.-Vilum, Vilva-panzam; Tel.-Maredu,

---

* Current name *Aegle marmelos* (Linn) Corr.
** शलाटुः - Unripe fruit.
१ सदाफल : इति नि.शे. टीकायाम् ।
२ 'हृषीकश्च कण्टकाद्यः सिताननः । 'इति नि. शे. टीकायाम् ।

Palir; Mal- Kuwalap-panzam; Eng.-Baelfruit tree, The Bengal Quince.

III-*d*- See current name.

31. (२८) अग्निमन्थः Agnimanthaḥ

अग्निमन्थोऽग्निमथनस्तर्कारी वैजयन्तिका ।
वह्निमन्थोऽरणी केतुः श्रीपर्णी कर्णिका जया ॥ ११२

नादेयी वह्निमथनो द्वितीयश्चाग्निमन्थनः ।
रक्तांगो मन्थनश्चैव स चैवारणिको मतः ॥ *११३

तर्कारी कटुका तिक्ता तथोष्णाऽनिलपाण्डुजित् ।
शोफश्लेष्माग्निमान्द्यांश्च विबन्धांश्च विनाशयेत् ॥११४

अग्निमंथः (Agnimanthaḥ), अग्निमथनः (Agnimathanaḥ), तर्कारी (Tarkārī), वैजयन्तिका (Vaijayantikā), वह्निमंथः (Vahnimanthaḥ), अरणी (Araṇī), केतुः (Ketuḥ), श्रीपर्णी (Śrīparṇī), कर्णिका (Karṇikā), जया (Jayā), are synonyms of *Tarkārī Agnimantha.* नादेयी (Nādeyī), is the second type of *Agnimantha.* The third type is called as अरणिकः (Araṇikaḥ), of which synonyms are रक्तगङ्गः (Raktāṅgaḥ), and मन्थनः (Manthanaḥ)

Agnimantha is pungent and bitter in taste, *uṣṇavīrya* and pacifies *vātadoṣa.* It is useful in anaemia (Pāṇḍu), oedema, dyspepsia due to *kaphadoṣa* and blocking of channels.

This heading includes three plants. A- तर्कारी (Tarkārī), B- नादेयी (Nādeyī) and C- क्षुद्रांग्निमन्थः (Kśūdragnimanthaḥ)

(Fam - Verbenaceae)

I- A-a ***Clerodendron phlomidis*** Linn**
b- Dymock,
B-*a*- ***Premna integrifolia*** Linn.***
Syn. *Premna spinosa* Roxb.
b- Roxburgh.
C-*a*- ***Clerodendron inerme*** (L) Gaertn.****

---

* अस्याग्रे "क्षुद्राग्निमन्थस्त्वपरः पूर्वनाम नियोजित : ।
क्षुद्राग्निमन्थ इत्यादिनामानि परिचक्षते ॥"
इत्यधिकः पाठः आनन्दाश्रम मुद्रित पुस्तके दृश्यते ।

** Current name *Clerodendrum multiflorum* (Burm. f.) O. Ktze.

*** Current name is *Premna corymbosa* Rottle. Comp.P.125

**** Current name *Clerodendrum inerme* (Linn.f.) Gaertn.

b- Kamat.

Note- Raj. ni. has noted this plant separately.

II- A-*a*- तर्कारी (Tarkārī), अरणी (Araṇī),

b- Bom.-Airaṇa; H.-Arṇi; Mar.- Pāṇḍharī ṭākaḷi; Tam.-Taludalel; Tel. Tekkali.

B-*a*- नादेयी (Nādeyï),रक्तगङ्गः (Raktāngaḥ), अरणी (Araṇī),

b- Sk.-Gaṇikārikā; H.-Ageth; B.-Gaṇiārī; Mar., Bom.-Airaṇa; Guj.-Arni; Tam.- Munnay; Tel. Ghebu-nelli; Mal.-Appal.

C-*a*- Sk, -Kundali; Mar.-Vanajāī, Koyanel

IV- Naravel, Jaya, *Viburnum foetidum* Wall.Confounded with, and used for the same purpose as *Premna coriacea* Clarke and other strong smelling Premnas. (Dymock).

32. (२९) स्योनाकः Syonākaḥ

अरलुः (श्योनाकः) Araluḥ, (śyonakaḥ)

श्योनाकः शुकनासश्च कट्वंगोऽथ कटंभरः ।
मयूरजंघोऽरलुकः प्रियजीवः कुटंनटः ॥ ११५

स प्रोक्तः पृथुशिम्बश्च टिण्टुको दीर्घवृन्तकः ।
भल्लूकः शिल्लको फल्गुवृन्ताको[1] जम्बुको मतः[2] ॥ ११६

टिण्टुकः शिशिरस्तिक्तो बस्तिरोगहरः परः ।
पित्तश्लेष्मामवातातीसारकासारुचीर्जयेत् ॥ ११७

श्योनाकः (Śyonākaḥ), शुकनासः (Śukanāsaḥ), कट्वङ्गः (Kaṭvangaḥ), कटंभरः (Kaṭambharaḥ), मयूरजंघः (Mayūrajanghaḥ), अरलुकः(Aralukaḥ), प्रियजीवः (Priyajīvaḥ), कुटंनटः (Kuṭannaṭaḥ), are the synomyms for *śyonakaḥ*. The other type of *śyonāka* has the synonyms as पृथुशिम्बः Pṛthuśimbaḥ टिण्टुकः (Ṭinṭukaḥ), दीर्घवृन्तकः (Dīrghavṛnatakḥ), भल्लुकः (Bhallūkaḥ), शिल्लकः (Śillakaḥ), फल्गुवृन्ताकः(Phalguvṛntākāḥ) and जम्बुकः (Jambukaḥ).

Tinṭuka is *śītavīrya* and bitter in taste and pacifies *pitta,*and *kapha.* It is useful in the diseases of urinary organs, *āmavātātisāra,* cough and anorexia.

(Under this heading two plants are recorded A-श्योनाक (Śyonāka) and B-टिण्टुक (Ṭinṭuka).

---

१ 'फल्गुवृन्तको' इति. क्षीर. संमतः पाठः।

२ 'नट' इति क्षीर. संमतः पाठः ।

I- *a-* Not identified.

(Fam.-Bignoniaceae).

B-*a-* ***Oroxylum indicum*** Vent.*
Syn. *Bignonia indica* Willd. (Roxb).
b- Mahajan. *c-*Throughout India, W. Ghats.

Note- The plant known as Tetu in Konkan is noted here - Dh.ni.notes medicinal uses of *Tiṇṭuka* only.

II- B-*a-* पृथुशिम्बः(Pṛthuśimbaḥ), टिण्टुकः (Ṭiṇṭukaḥ), दीर्घवृन्तकः (Dīrghavṛntakaḥ), निःसारः (Niḥsāraḥ), पीताङ्गः (Pītāngaḥ), मण्डूकपर्णः (Maṇḍūkaparṇaḥ).
b- Mar.Bom.-Ṭeṭū. Ṭeṭav. Dheḍar; Tam.-Venga marum; Tel.-Pumpen.

III- *b-*(1) कटवङ्गफलम् (Kaṭwāngafalam) Su. 15. (Tuṇṭuka, madana falārthena,Aruna Dattastu Kaṭwāngaphalam Araluka- phalaniṭi (Vaidya).
c- मर्दयेत् टेण्टूजद्रावैः (Mardayetṭeṇṭuja drāvaiḥ). (Wadi Khanḍa, Vanga Vedha).
*d, c, f, g-*See current names and synonyms.

IV- (1)टेण्टू, टिण्टूक, श्योनाक *(Oroxylum indicum)*. (Ni. Adarsha).
(2)अरलुः तदभावे स्योनाकः । P. 142 Aralu puṭapāka
(3)Dhn. Ni. has not separated two plants by noting'अन्यच्च' but has separated them by 'mentioning ' स प्रोक्तः पृथुशिम्बश्च टिण्टुकः but Raj. Ni. has noted by अन्यः । **

33.(३०) काश्मर्यः Kāśmaryaḥ

काश्मर्या काश्मरी हीरा काश्मर्यो मधुपर्ण्यपि ।
श्रीपर्णी सर्वतोभद्रा गम्भारी कृष्णवृन्तका ॥ ११८

श्रीपर्णी स्वरसे तिक्ता गुरूष्णा रक्तपित्तजित् ।
त्रिदोषश्रमदाहार्तिज्वरतृष्णाविषाञ्जयेत् ॥ ११९

काश्मर्या (Kāśmaryā), काश्मरी (Kāśmarī), हीरा (Hīrā), काश्मर्यः (Kāśmaryaḥ),मधुपर्णी (Madhuparṇī), श्रीपर्णी (Śrīparṇī), सर्वतोभद्रा (Sarvatobhadrā), गम्भारी (Gambhārī), and कृष्णवृन्तका (Kṛṣṇavṛntakā), are synonyms for *kāśmarī*.

It is bitter in taste, *guru* and *uṣṇavīrya* and pacifies *Tridoṣa*. It is

---

*Current name *Oroxylum indicum* (Linn.) Vent.
** *Aralu* has been now treated separately as *Ailanthus excelsa* Roxb.

useful in bleeding disorders, fatigue, burning sensation, pains (aches), fevers, thirst and poisons.

(Fam.-Verbenaceae).

I- *a*- ***Gmelina arborea**** Linn.
b- Roxburgh, *c*-Throughout India.

II- *a*- श्रीपर्णी (Śrīparṇī), गम्भारी (Gambhārī); कृष्णवृन्ता (Kṛsṇavṛntā);
b- B.-Gabhāri, Mar.-Kokan-Sivan; Santal-'Kāsmar;' Tel.-Gamadi; Tam.-Gundu-tekku; Kan. Kāsmari, Sivani.

III- *a*- Kāśmarya; TS.V.-2.7.3.4; MS. iii-2-6; S.Br. iii.-4-1-6. (Harshe).

Note- Here serial number (34) is mistaken for (33), in the original book.

34. (३१) पाटला Pāṭalā**

पाटलोत्तमा तु कुम्भीका ताम्रपुष्पाऽम्बुवासिनी ।
स्थाली वसन्तदूती स्यादमोघा कालवृन्तिका ॥ १२०

पाटला तु रसे तिक्ता गुरूष्णा पवनास्रजित् ।
पित्तहिक्कावमीशोफ कफारोचकनाशिनी ॥ १२१

पाटला (Pāṭalā), कुम्भीका (Kumbhīkā), ताम्रपुष्पा (Tāmrapuṣpā), अम्बुवासिनी (Ambuvāsinī), स्थाली (Sthālī), वसन्तदूती (Vasantadūtī), अमोघा (Amoghā), कालवृन्तिका (Kālavṛntikā), are synonyms for *Pāṭalā.*

Pāṭalā is bitter in taste, *guru,* and *uṣṇavīrya.* It pacifies *Vāta, rakta* and *pitta doṣas*. It is useful in hiccup, vomitting, oedema and anorexia due to *kapha doṣa.*

(Fam.-Bignoniaceae).

I- *a*- ***Stereospermum suaveolens*** DC. Proder.
Syn. *Bignonia suaveolens* Roxb.
b- Roxburgh, *c*-Throughout India in drier parts.

II- *a*- पाटला (Pāṭalā), कुम्भीका (Kumbhīkā), ताम्रपुष्पा (Tāmrapuṣpā).
b- H.-Paral; B.-Parul; Mar.-Tāmbaḍi Pāḍaḷ; Tam.-Pādiri; Tel.-Kokes; Kan.-Hude; Mal.-Pupatiri.

III- *b*- पाटला (Pāṭalā), Tāmrapuṣpī, dwitiyā Kāṣṭhapāṭalā. (Bh-Pr-Ni).
d,e,f,g-See current names and synonyms.

---

* The current name is - *Gmelina arborea* Roxb.

** Kṡiraswāmi has mentioned the synonyms of Pāṭalā and Kāṣṭhapāṭalā together.

काष्ठपाटला Kāṣṭhapātalā 23.

द्वितीया पाटला श्वेता निर्दिष्टा काष्ठपाटला ।
सा चैव श्वेतकुम्भीका कुबेराक्षी फलेरुहा ॥ १२२

पाटलायाः गुणैस्तद्वत् किंचिन्मारुतकृत् भवेत् ।

The second type of *Pāṭalā* which is white is called as काष्ठपाटला (Kāṣṭhāpaṭalā) the synonyms for which are श्वेतकुम्भीका (Śveta kumbhī-kā), कुबेराक्षी (Kuberākṣī) and फलेरुहा (Phaleruhā),

It has the properties similar to *Pāṭalā* but slightly aggravates *vāta doṣa*.

(Fam.-Bignoniaceae).

I- *a*- ***Stereospermum chelonoides*** **DC.***
Syn. *Stereospermum tetragonum* DC.
Bignonia chelonoides Wall. (Roxb).
b- Kamat and Mahajan.
c- Throughout India in drier parts.

II- *a*- पाटलाश्वेता (Paṭalāśwetā).
b- A-Pādar; Mar.-Pāṇḍharī Pāḍal; B-Dharamara.

III- *d,c,e, f,g*-See current names and synonyms.

35. (३२) जीवकः Jīvakah

जीवकः श्रृङ्गकः क्ष्वैडो दीर्घायुः कूर्चशीर्षकः ॥१२३
ह्रस्वाङ्गः मधुरः स्वादुः प्राणदश्चिरजीव्यपि ॥

जीवकः मधुरः शीतो रक्तपित्तानिलाञ्जयेत् ।१२४
दाहज्वरक्षयान् हन्ति कफशुक्रविवर्धनः ॥

जीवकः (Jīvakaḥ), श्रृङ्गकः (Śṛṅgakaḥ), क्ष्वैडः (Kṣveḍaḥ), दीर्घायुः (Dīrghāguḥ), कूर्चशीर्षकः (Kurcaśirṣakaḥ), ह्रस्वाङ्गः (Rhasvāṅgaḥ), मधुरः (Madhuraḥ), स्वादुः (Swāduḥ), प्राणदः (Prāṇadaḥ), चिरजीवी (Cirajīvī) are synonyms of *Jīvaka*.

It is sweet in taste, *śītavīrya,* and pacifies *pitta, rakta* and *vātadoṣas* It is useful in burning sensation, fever, and consumption, increases *kaphadoṣa* and *śukra*.

'सर्जो' इति क्षीरस्वामी -निघण्टुशेष टीका संमत : पाठः
* The current name is *S. personatum* (Hassk.) Chatterjee (Comp. p. 145)

Not identified.

The bulbs of *Microstylis wallichi* Lindl and *M. musifera* Ridley are being supplied in their names in U. P market. (Balvantji p. 170)

36. वृषभः Vṛṣabhaḥ (३३) ऋषभकः Ṛṣabhakaḥ

ऋषभो दुर्धरो[1] धीरो मातृको वृषभो वृष : ॥१२५
विषाणी ककुदिन्द्राक्षो बन्धुरो गोपतिस्तथा ॥

ऋषभस्तु रसे स्वादु पित्तरक्तसमीरहा ॥१२६
क्षयदाहज्वरान् हन्ति श्लेष्मशुक्रविवर्धनः ॥

ऋषभः (Ṛsabhaḥ), दुर्धरः (Durdharaḥ), धीरः (Dhīraḥ), मातृकः (Mātṛkaḥ), वृषभः (Vṛṣabhaḥ), वृषः (Vṛṣaḥ), विषाणी (Viṣāṇī), ककुद् (Kakud), इन्द्राक्षः (Indrākṣaḥ), बन्धुरः (Bandhuraḥ), गोपतिः (Gopatiḥ), are synonyms for *vṛṣabha.*

It is sweet in taste and pacifies *pitta, rakta, vāta doṣas.* It is useful in consumption, burning sensation in the body, fever and increases *kapahadoṣa* and *śukra.*

Not identified.

III- जीवकर्षभाविति राज्ञामपि दुर्लभाः । उत्तरापथेत्वसंदिग्ध एव इत्येके ।

Note - These plants may belong to the Orchidaceae family which contain सालंमिश्री (Salam Miśrī), पंजामिश्री (Panjāmisrī) etc.*

37. मेदा Medā (३४) मेदे द्वे Mede dwe

मेदा ज्ञेया मणिच्छिद्रा शल्यपर्णी धराऽपि च ।१२७
महामेदा देवमणिर्वसुच्छिद्रा प्रकीर्तिता ॥

मेदा स्वादुरसा शीता क्षयदाहज्वरापहा ।१२८
सा[2] पित्तं तु जयेच्छुक्रं सकफं च विवर्धयेत् ॥

महामेदा हिमा स्वादुः कफशुक्रविवर्धनी ।१२९
हन्ति दाहास्रपित्तानि क्षयवातज्वरैः सह ॥

---

१ 'धूर्वहो' इति नि.शे. टीका क्षीर संमतः पाठः

* It may be one of the sp. of *Microstylis.*

२ 'सपित्तं तु जयेत्कासं' इति आनन्दाश्रम पुस्तके पाठः ।

मेदा (Medā), मणिच्छिद्रा (Maṇicchidrā), शल्यपर्णी (Śalyaparṇī) धरा (Dharā) are synonyms for *Medā.*

देवमणि (Devamaṇi), वसुच्छिद्रा (Vasucchidrā) are synonyms for महामेदा (Mahāmedā).

Medā is sweet in taste, *śitavirya,* it pacifies *pittadoṣa* and increases *kapha* and *śukra.* It is useful in pthiasis, burning sensation in the body and fever.

Mahāmedā is sweet in taste, *śitavīrya* increases *kapha* and *śukra.* It pacifies *pitta doṣa* and useful in burning sensation of the body, bleeding disorders, consumption and fevers due to *vātadoṣa.*

Not identified.*

विजया Vijayā 24.

विजया रञ्जिका भङ्गा तन्द्राकृद् बहुवादिनी ।१३०
मादिनी मादिका मातुः प्रोक्ता गञ्जाकिनिस्तथा ॥

भङ्गा कफहरी तिक्ता ग्राहिणी पाचनी लघुः ॥ १३१
तीक्ष्णोष्णा पित्तला मोहमदवाग्वह्निवर्धिनी ॥

विजया (Vijayā), रञ्जिका (Rañjikā), भङ्गा (Bhangā), तन्द्राकृद् (Tandrākṛd), बहुवादिनी (Bahuvādinī), मादिनी (Mādinī), मादिका (Mādikā) मातुः (Mātuḥ), and गञ्जाकिनि (Gañjākinī), are synonymous.

Bhangā is bitter in taste, pacifies *kapha,* is *tīkṣna* and *uṣnavīrya.* It is astringent, digestant and *laghu,* and aggravates *pitta,* causes intoxication, giddiness, increases digestive capacity and delirious talk.

(Fam. Cannabinaceae).

I- *a-* ***Cannabis sativa*** Linn.
Syn. *C. indica* Lam. (Roxb).
b- Roxbrgh. *c-*Naturlized in the Himalayan tract, abundant in waste lands in Punjab etc. Cultivated for narcotic drug. Wild in C. Asia.

II- *a-* भङ्गी(Bhangī), रञ्जिका (Rañjikā), बहुवादिनी (Bahuwādinī); तन्द्राकृत् (Tandrākṛt).
b- H.-Ben., Mar.-Bhānga, gānjā; Tel. -Ganjāṭhī; Tam.-Bangi, Mal.-Kanjothu; Eng.-Hemp, Indian hemp.
d,e,f,g- See current name and Syn.

IV- Hill, page 281

---

* *Polygonatum verticillatum* All and *P. cirrhifolium* Royle are used. (Uniyal. Sachi. Ayu. 1966, 1968).

38. काकोली Kākolī
३५ काकोलीद्वयम् Kakolidwayam

काकोली मधुरा शुक्ला क्षीरा ध्वांक्षोलिका स्मृता ॥ १३२
वयःस्था स्वादुमांसी च वायसोली च कर्णिका ॥

काकोली स्वादुशीता च वातपित्तज्वरापहा ॥१३३
दाहघ्नी क्षयहन्त्री च श्लेष्मशुक्रविवर्धिनी ॥

काकोली (Kākolī), मधुरा (Madhurā), शुक्ला (Śuklā), क्षीरा (Kṣīrā), ध्वांक्षोलिका (Dhwānkṣolikā), वयःस्था (Vayaḥsthā), स्वादुमांसी (Swādumāmsī), वायसोली (Wāyasolī), and कर्णिका (Karṇikā), are synonymous.

It is sweet in taste, *śītavīrya,* pacifies the *Vātapitta* (fevers due to *vāta pitta doṣas*). It is useful in burning sensation, consumption and increases *kapha* and *śukra.*

Not identified.*

39. क्षीरकाकोली Kṣīrakākolī

द्वितीया क्षीरकाकोली क्षीरशुक्ला पयस्विनी ॥ १३४
वयःस्था क्षीरमधुरा वीरा क्षीरविषाणिका ॥

रुचिष्या वातपित्तास्रहृद्रोगशमनी मता ॥ १३५
श्वासकासक्षयहरा वृष्या बस्तिविशोधनी ॥

The second one is क्षीरकाकोली (Kṣīrakākolī), the synonyms of which are क्षीरशुक्ला (Kṣīraśuklā), पयस्विनी (Payasvinī), वयःस्था (Vayaḥsthā), क्षीरमधुरा (Kṣīramadhurā), वीरा (Vīrā) and क्षीरविषाणिका (Kṣīraviṣāṇikā).

It promotes appetite and pacifies *vāta, pitta* and *rakta doṣas.* It is useful in bleeding disorders, cardiac diseases, dyspnoea, cough, pthiasis, *vṛṣya* and in diseases of the urinary organs (purificatory action of the bladder.)

Not identified.

---

* *Roscoea procera* Wall. - काकोली *Roscoea alpina* Royle - क्षीरकाकोली
These are being used by many. (Balvantji P. 89)

(३६) पर्णिनीद्वयम् Parṇinidwayam

40. माषपर्णी Maṣaparṇi

माषपर्णी च काम्बोजी कृष्णवृन्ता महासहा ॥१३६
आर्द्रमाषा सिंहविन्ना[१] मांसमाषाऽश्वपुच्छिका[२] ॥

माषपर्णी रसे तिक्ता शीतला रक्तपित्तजित् ॥ १३७
कफशुक्रकरी स्वादुर्हन्ति दाहज्वरानिलान् ॥

माषपर्णी (Māṣaparṇī), काम्बोजी (Kāmbojī), कृष्णवृन्ता (Kṛṣṇavṛntā), महासहा (Mahāsahā), आर्द्रमाषा (Ārdramāṣā), सिंहविन्ना (Simhavinnā), मांसमाषा (Māmsamāṣā), अश्वपुच्छिका (Aśvapucchikā), are synonymous.

Māṣaparṇī is bitter and sweet in taste, *śītavīrya.* It increases *kapha* and *śukra* and useful in haemorrhagic disorders, burning sensation of the body and fever. It pacifies *Vātadosa.*

(Fam. Leguminosae). Fabaceae

I- *a*- ***Teramnus labialis*** Spreng.*
Syn.-*Glycine labialis* Linn.
G. debilis Willd.
b- Roxburgh *c*-Throughout India, willd.

II- *a*- कृष्णवृन्ता (Kṛṣṇavṛntā), मांसमाषा (Māmsamāṣā).
b- H.-Māsoni; Ben.-Māsani; Ma.-Rānauḍīda.

III- *a*- (1)माषओषधि (AV. VI-130-15-13).

Note-IV-(1) *Teramnus labialis* Spreng.
Maṣaprarṇi (Ghanekar; Desai; Yadavji; Priyavrata)

41. मुद्गपर्णी Mudgaparṇī

मुद्गपर्णी क्षुद्रसहा शिम्बी मार्जारगन्धिका ॥ १३८
वनजा रिंगणी[३] ह्रस्वा[४] शूर्पपर्ण्याविभे स्मृते ॥

मुद्गपर्णी हिमा स्वादुर्वातरक्तविनाशिनी ॥ १३९
पित्तदाहज्वरान् हन्ति कृमिघ्नी कफशुक्रकृत् ॥

---

१ 'सिंहवृन्ता' इति नि.शे. टीकायाम् । २ 'मांसमासा' इति आनन्दाश्रममुद्रित पुस्तके पाठः ।
३ 'रङ्गणी इति नि.शे. टीकायाम् । ४ 'ह्रासा' इति नि.शे. टीकायाम् ।

*The current name for *Teramnus labialis* Spreng is *T. labialis* (Linn. f.) Spreng, syn. *Glycine labialis* Linn.f. & *Phaseolus trilobus* Ait. is *Vigna trilobata* (Linn.) Vardcourt (see next page)

मुद्गपर्णी (Mudgaparṇī), क्षुद्रसहा (Kśudrasahā), शिम्बी (Śimbī), मार्जारगन्धिका (Mārjāragandhikā), वनजा (Vanajā), रिंगणी (Ringaṇī) ऱ्हस्वा (Rhasvā) are synonymous. Both Mudgaparni and Māsaparni are called as शूर्पपर्णी (Sūrpaparni). (a common name).

It is sweet in taste, śītavīrya and pacifies *vāta, rakta* and *pitta doṣas.* It is useful in burning sensation of the body, fevers, and worms. It increases *kapha* and *śukra.*

(Fam. Leguminosae, Sub.-Fam. Papilionaceae). Fabaceae

I- a- ***Phaseolus trilobus*** Ait.
   b- Dymock, c-Himalayas and southward to ceylon.Weed in Sindh and Maharashtra.

II- a- मार्जारगन्धिका (Mārjāra gandhikā),वनजा (Vanajā).
   b- H., B.-Mungni; Mar,-Rānamūg; Tel.-Pillippersara; Tam.-Panipayara; Eng.-Three Lobed kidney bean;

III- d,e,f,g-See current name.

IV- (1)*Phasseolus trilbous* Willd. Mudgaparni, (D Candolle p.346; Desai; Ghanekar; U.C.Datt; Priyavrata; Br.Ni. Pade.)

42. (३७) जीवन्ती Jīvantī

जीवन्ती जीवनीया च जीवनी जीववर्धनी ॥ १४०
मांगल्यनामधेया च शाकश्रेष्ठा यशस्करी ॥

चक्षुष्या सर्वदोषघ्नी जीवन्ती मधुरा हिमा ॥ १४१
शाकानां प्रवरा न्यूना द्वितीया किंचिदेव तु ॥ A.sang.7.129

जीवन्ती (Jīvantī), जीवनीया (Jivanīyā), जीवनी (Jīvanī), जीववर्धनी (Jīvavardhanī), माङ्गल्यनामधेया (Māṅgalyanāmadheyā), शाकश्रेष्ठा (Śākaśreṣṭhā), and यशस्करी (Yaśaskarī) are synonymous.

Jīvantī pacifies all the three *doṣas*, is sweet in taste, *śītavīrya* and vision promoting. It is best amongst vegetables.

The second variety of *Jīvantī* is slightly lesser in its propereties and actions.

This heading includes two plants. One A-माङ्गल्यनामा (Māṅgalyanāmā) and B-बृहत्पूर्वा (Bṛhatpūrvā).

(Fam.-Asclepiadaceae).

I- *A-a-* ***Leptadenia reticulata*** W.& A.*
b- Kamat, *c-* Punjab; Western Peninsula, Poona, Baramati.

B-a- ***Marsdenia volubilis*** T. Cooke**
b- Kamat, *c*-Bengal; W.Peninsula; S. Maratha Country; Madras State, Kolhapur, Poona.

II- A-*a-* शाकश्रेष्ठा (Śākaśreṣṭhā), चक्षुष्या (Cakṣuṣyā), शृङ्गाटी (Śṛṅgāṭī)
b- Harandoḍī, Rāyadoḍī, Singuṭ Haraṇael; Tam.-Palakuḍai; Tel.-Palatige.

B-*a-* भूतविद्रावणी (Bhūtavidṛavaṇī), रसनियामका (Rasaniyāmakā).
b- Mar.-Nakachikaṇ Haraṇadoḍī Harikhāndodī Tel.- Dudihlala; Mal.- Waṭṭakka kkakoṭi; Tam.-Kodipalai.

Note- For botanical synonyms of I -A and B see (IV) below.

III- See Vandā (वन्दा).

a- 1) जीवन्ती अरुन्धतीमुन्नयन्ती पुष्प्यां मधुमतीम् । (AV. viii-7);
2) केशवृद्धिकरणकामः काकमाची फलं जीवन्तीफलं भृङ्गराजं वा - (AV-viAnu-13sū-137 ; Kau. sū. 7, referred by Sāyaṇa).
3) जीवन्ती चक्षुष्या शाकानां प्रवरा । (Ashta Sang.in Astā. hṛ. su. 6-86).

b- 1) द्व्यर्थेः - जीवन्ती , गुडूची, वृक्षरुहा (Amara).
2) वन्दा जीवन्तिकेत्यपि । (Maheśhwar);
3) दोडीगुडूची मेदा च काकोली हरिणी तथा ।
जीवन्ती चैव षड्प्रोक्ता जीवन्त्यां च भिषग्वरैः । (Raj.ni.Saḍarthaḥ)
4) जीवन्ती 'शृङगराटी' केयदेवे 'पयस्विनी' 'भावप्रकाशके' शिम्बिराटकी' गणनिघण्टके (Ni. Si. Pade, p.H.);
5) हेमा, तृणग्रन्थि .. स्वर्णपर्णी हेमपुष्पी स्वर्णजीवन्तिका चक्षुष्या । (Raj. nī Parisi 1-16);
6) जीवन्ती (sū6); शाकलता । (Vaidya);
7) १३९ जीवन्ती मङ्गल्या शाकश्रेष्ठा । चेरिय अडकोतिम्बाल Ceriya aḍakothimbāla Aḍapothiyana (Kṛṣṇanan);
8) १४० द्वितीया जीवन्ती पयस्विनी । वलिय अडकोतिम्बाळ Valiya aḍakothimbāl. (Krishnan);
9) १३९ जीवन्ती (Keral) अटवतियम् अटपीतियन् अटकोनियन् ; (Tam.) जीवन्तीलतै (Kan.) हाले, किरिय हाले,(Ayu o. Ni)

---

* The current name is - *L. reticulata* (Retz.) Wt. & Arn.
Syn. *Gymnema aurantiacum* Wall. ex Hook. f. (Comp.p. 91)
**The current name is -*Wattakaka volubilis* (Linn.) Stapf (Comp.p. 160)

10) जीवन्ती - हरण दोडी हरणवेल इति ख्याता (Maheshwara).

11) जीवन्तिका (Mar). लहान हरणवेल, (H.) क्षुपरुकडी . (Dattaram)

12) जीवन्ती शाकश्रेष्ठा.(Madan, ni.).

c- 1) जीवन्ती स्वर्णमूलनालादिका (Cakra-sū. 4.9),

2) जीवन्ती दोडिका इति लोके. लतार्कफला सक्षीरफला ।
अन्ये सुवर्णजीवन्तीमाहुः । (Dalhana; sū. Kākolyādigaṇa);

3) जीवन्तीशुष्कयावनालवर्ण लतौषधि पर्वती । (Dalhana; sū. 43).
जीवन्ती शाकविशेष : । वन्दा वृक्षशाखासु । (Dipika).
जीवन्ती दोडीशाकः । (Gu. Dipika M. 3-17).

d,e,f, -See current names.

IV-Synonyms of plants (1-A and B above) occured in different books.

(1) *Wattakaka volubilis* (L.) Stapf; *Marsdenia volubilis T. Cooke; Dregia viridiflora Benth. ex* Hook. F,. *Hoya viridi flora* R. Br. Sk., Madhumālatī; Mar.- Haranḍoḍī. (Chopra; Watt Dict.; Basu Pl. 819; Cooke Fl., Br. ni. Pade).

(2) *Leptadenia reticulata* W. & A. Mar. -Rāyadodī, Singutī, Jīvantī, (Bhagirath; Ni; Adarsha; Priyavrata; Balavantji, van. Darpan; Yadavji; Ghanekar). The leaves,. tender shoots and follicles arc employed as food (Watt Dict.).

(3) Leptadenia (Bot. महामेदत्ती,) L. spartum सामान्य मेदा (Raghuvir)

(4) See Ayur, Patrika : - 16-11-1962; 1-12-1959; 1-5-1960; 6-6-1960; 16-7 -1960.

Two different kinds of plants are considered under the name Jīvantī namely Jīvantī climber and Jīvantī Vandā. The name ' Jīvantī' (जीवन्ती)is applied to seven plants ; (vide III-b-3- supra), in which includes (1) Latā Jīvantī (लता जीवन्ती) (Vide I II-b-6, 9,10, 11; c-2,3; supra) of the Asclepiadaceae fam. (vide 42 -1-A, B, supra) and (2) Vṛiksharuhā (वृक्षरुहा) or Vandā Jīvantī (वन्दा जीवन्ती) (vide III-b-7;c-4 supra) of the Orchidaceae fam.) Vandā Jīvantī is described by the terms Swarṇa Jīvantī (स्वर्ण जीवन्ती) (vide III-b-5 supra). Vandā Vṛkśaśākhāsu (वन्दावृक्षशाखासु) (vide III -c-4 supra); while Latā Jīvantī (लता जीवन्ती)) by the terms Śṛṅgāraṭī (शृंगारटी)Payaswinī (पयस्विनी) Sākaśhreṣṭhā ,(शाकश्रेष्ठा) Śakalata (शाकलता), Haraṇadoḍī हरण दोडी (vide III-b-4-6, 12; c-3, supra); Doḍī (दोडी). Kśīraphalā (क्षीरफला) (vide III- c-2 supra); Latā Jīvantī (लता जीवन्ती) is supposed to be the traditional Jīvantī (जीवन्ती) from Vedic age (vide III-a-1 supra).

---

१ चेरिय अटकोतिपाळ (अटकोतियन्)

२ वलिय अटकोतिम्बळ Vd. Miss. Nalini K.

3 Raj. ni. has mentioned three types ofजीवन्ती Jīvantī in his Gaṇadravyavāli गणद्रव्यावली Jīvantī trividhā जीवन्ती त्रिविधा and described them under separate headings under *Paryāyanāmadravyāvāli* पर्याय नामद्रव्यावली

4 Amarakośa notesजीवन्ती Jīvantī as a similitive term for Vandaवंदा but Dhn. Ni, does not do so. D.K. Kamat

Śākaśreṣthā - *L. reticulata.* Vandā Jīvantī is *Dendrobium macraei* Lindle

The current name for the this is *Desmotrichum fimbriatam* Blume (U P I. p. 169)

43. (३८) मधुयष्टी Madhuyaṣṭī

मधुयष्टी च यष्टी च यष्टीमधु मधुस्रवा ॥ १४२
यष्टीकं मधुकं चैव यष्ट्याह्वं मधुयष्टिका ॥
स्थलजा जलजाऽन्या तु मधुपर्णी मधूलिका ॥ १४३
मधुयष्टी स्वादुरसा शीता पित्तविनाशिनी ॥
वृष्या शोषक्षयहरा विषच्छर्दिविनाशिनी ॥ १४४

मधुयष्टी (Madhuyaṣṭī), यष्टी (Yaṣṭī), यष्टीमधु (Yaṣṭimadhu), मधुस्रवा (Madhusravā), यष्टीकं (Yaṣṭīkam), मधुकं (Madhukam), यष्ट्याह्वं (Yaṣṭyāhvam), मधुयष्टिका (Madhuyaṣṭikā) are the synonyms for स्थलज (Sthalaja) terrestrial type and for जलज (Jalaja) type the synonyms are मधुपर्णी (Madhūparṇī) and मधूलिका (Madhūlikā).

Yaṣṭīmadhu is sweet in taste, *śītavīrya* and pacifies *pitta*. It is *vṛṣya*, and useful in emaciation and phthisis. It is antipoisonous and antiemetic.

(Fam. -Leguminosae, Sub-Fam.-Papilionaceae.).(Fabaceae)

I- *a*- ***Glycyrrhiza glabra*** Linn.
b- Dymock, *c*-Baluchistan , Sub-Himalayan tract, Andaman, Peshawar (Mukerji).

II- *a*- मधुस्रवा (Madhusaravā), मधुकम् (Madhukam).
b- H.-Jeṭimad, muleṭi Mar.- Jeṣṭamadha; Tam.-Tel.- Atimadhuram, Yaṣṭimadhukam; Kan.- Yaṣṭimadhuka; Mal.- Irraṭṭi madhuram, Eng.- Liquoris root.

III- See Cūdāmani Klītanaka.
a-(1) मधूमन्मूलं ... विरुधां बभूव ...। (AV. VIII-7-12).
(2) Kausika (32-5-7) spell informs us that the herb which is sweet like honey (Madhulā) crushes insects. (Shende).

क्लीतनकम् Klītanakam 25.

तल्लक्षणं क्लीतनकं क्लीतनं क्लीतिका च सा ॥
यष्टिकायुगलं स्वादु तृष्णापित्तास्रजित् हिमम् ॥ १४५

क्लीतनकं (Klītanakam), क्लीतनं (Klītanam), क्लीतिका (Klītikā), is of the same type. Both the types of *madhuyaṣṭi* are sweet in taste and

---

१ 'यष्टीमधूकं मधुकं ' इति क्षीर.संमतः पाठः ।

śītavīrya. It pacifies *pitta* and *raktadoṣa* and is useful in thirst.

This includes two plants: A-जलज (Jalaja) and B-स्थलज (Sthalaja).

I- A-*a*- Not identified.

(Fam. Leguminosae).

B-*a*- ***Taverniera nummularia*** Baker -(Chopra).*

b- Mahājan, *c*-Deccan; Gujarath, Punjab, Baluchistan.

II- B-*a*- क्लीतनकम् (Klītanakam).

b- Mar.-Jeṣṭhīmadha.

III-*d,e,*-See Current name.

44. (३९) ऋद्धिः Ṛddhiḥ

ऋद्धिर्वृद्धिः सुखं सिद्धी रथाङ्गं मंगलं वसु ॥
ऋषिसृष्टा[१] युगं योग्यं लक्ष्मीः सर्वजनप्रिया ॥ १४६
ऋद्धिर्मधुर शीता स्यात् क्षयपित्तानिलाञ्जयेत् ॥
रक्तदोषं ज्वरं हन्ति वर्धनी कफशुक्रयोः ॥ १४७

ऋद्धिः (Ṛddhiḥ), वृद्धिः (Vṛddhiḥ), सुखं (Sukham), सिद्धी (Siddhī), रथाङ्गम् (Rathāṅgam), मंगलं (Mangalam), वसु (Vasu), ऋषिसृष्टा (Ṛṣisṛṣṭā), युगं (Yugam), योग्यं (Yogyam), लक्ष्मीः (Lakṣmīḥ), सर्वजनप्रिया (Sarvajanapriyā) are synonymous.

Ṛddhi is sweet in taste, *śītavīrya* and pacifies *vāta, pitta* and *raktadoṣas*. It is useful in phthisis and fevers. It increases *kaphadoṣa* and *śukradhātu.* **

This includes two plants.

Not identified.**

45. (४०) विदारिका Vidārikā

विदारिका मता शुक्ला स्वादुकन्दा श्रृगालिका ॥
वृष्यकन्दा[२] विदारी च वृष्यवल्ली[३] बिडालिका ॥ १४८

---

१ " ऋद्धि पुष्टा " इति क्षी. संमतः पाठः ।
२ " ऋष्यगन्धा " इति क्षीरस्वामी । ३ " ऋष्यवल्ली " इति क्षीरस्वामी ।

* The current name is *Taverniera nummularia* (Roth.) Arn.

**Dr. Chunekar (in his vān. Anu. Dars.) has suggested Habeneria sp.*Habenuria intermedia* D.Don

विदारी शिशिरा स्वादुर्गुरुः स्निग्धा समीरजित् ॥
पित्तास्रजित् तथा बल्या वृष्या चैव प्रकीर्तिता ॥ १४९

विदारिका (Vidārikā), शुक्ला (Śuklā), स्वादुकन्दा (Swādukandā), शृगालिका (Śṛgālikā) वृष्यकन्दा (Vṛṣyakandā) विदारी (Vidārī), वृष्यवल्ली (Vṛṣyavallī), बिडालिका (Biḍalikā), are synonyms for *vidārikā*.

It is sweet in taste, *sītavīrya*, *guru*, *snigdha* (unctuous) and pacifies *vāta*, *pitta* and *rakta doṣas*. It is strengthgiving (tonic) and *vṛṣya*.

(Fam.-Leguminosae, Sub. Fam. Papilionaceae). Fabaceae

I- A-*a*- ***Pueraria tuberosa*** DC.*
Syn.-*Hedysarum tuberosum* Roxb.
b- Kamat, c-W. Himaḷaya to Sikkim , S. India, Kokan.

II- *a*- शुक्ला (Śuklā), भूकूष्माण्डी (Bhūkūṣmāṇḍī).
b- Kol.- Bhuin kovala; Pattānā; H.-Sihāli; Bilai Kanda; Mar., Kokana Pāndharābhuikohalā, Bendricāwel, Udakyābhuikohalā; Guj.- Bhokolu, Khākarwel, B.-Simiya, Uatraji; Tel.- Dāri, Nelgumuḍu.

III- *b*- (1)विदारी (Sū.6) *Ipomoea paniculata.* सा च द्विधा इति डल्हणः. Bom., Mar.-Dudhibhui-Kohalā B.-Bhumikumra. Tel.- Paḷamodikku, Mullpab tiga. Tam.-Nilpuccani (Vaidya).

क्षीरविदारी Kṣīravidārī 26.

अन्या क्षीरविदारी स्याद् इक्षुगन्धेक्षुवल्ल्यपि ।
क्षीरवल्ली क्षीरकन्दा क्षीरशुक्ला पयस्विनी ॥ १५०
क्षीरविदारिका बल्या वातपित्तहरा च सा ॥
मधुरा बृंहणी वृष्या शीतस्पर्शाऽतिमूत्रला ॥ १५१
स्तन्यदोषस्य हरणी पित्तशूलनिषूदनी ॥

There is other type of *Vidārī* called as क्षीरविदारी (Kṣīravidārī), of which synonyms are इक्षुगन्धा (Ikṣugandhā), इक्षुवल्ली (Ikṣuvallī), क्षीरवल्ली (Kṣīravallī), क्षीरकन्दा (Kṣirakandā), क्षीरशुक्ला (Kṣīraśuklā), and पयस्विनी (Payasvinī).

It is sweet in taste and pacifies *vāta* and *pitta doṣas* and it is strength giving (tonic), body bulk promoting, refrigerating, excessive diuretic, removes defects of breast milk and is useful in pains due to *pittadoṣa*.

---

* The current name is *Pueraria tuberosa* Roxb.ex Willd.

(Fam.-Convolvulaceae).

I- *a-* ***Ipomoea paniculata*** R. Br.* Syn.- *I. digitata* Linn.
b- Watt. Dict. *c*-Throughout India, Kokan, Gujarath, Nasik.

II- *a-* क्षीरकन्दः (Ksīrakandaḥ), इक्षुगन्धा (Iksugandhā), क्षीरवल्ली (Ksīravallī).
b- Mar.-Dudhī bhuikohaḷā; H.-Bilāikanda; B.Bhumi Kumrā.

Note - The tubers of this plant are used in Bengal. In Maharashtra and other parts of India 'Vidārī' (see above 45) is in common usage. Two plants are included under this heading but the other विनाल (vināla) of Rājni. is not idendtified and is not recorded here.

46. (४१) कपिकच्छुः Kapikacchuḥ

कपिकच्छूरात्मगुप्ता स्वयंगुप्ता महर्षभी ॥ १५२
लाङ्गूली कण्डुला चण्डा मर्कटी दुरभिग्रहा ॥

कपिकच्छूः रसे स्वादुस्तित्तग शीताऽनिलापहा ॥ १५३
वृष्या पित्तास्रहन्त्री च दुष्टव्रर्णाविनाशिनी ॥

कपिकच्छुः (Kapikacchuḥ), आत्मगुप्ता (Ātmaguptā), स्वयंगुप्ता (Swayamguptā), महर्षभी (Maharṣabhī), लाङ्गूली (Lāngūlī), कण्डुला (Kaṇḍulā), चण्डा (Caṇḍā), मर्कटी (Markaṭī), दुरभिग्रहा (Durabhigrahā) are synonyms for *kapikacchuḥ*.

Kapikacchuḥ is sweet and bitter in taste, *śītavirya* and pacifes *vātadoṣa*. It is *vrṣya* and useful in haemorragic disorders and bad ulcers. (septic wounds)

(Fam. Leguminosae, Sub.-Fam.-Papilionaceae). Fabaceae.

I- *a-* ***Mucuna prurita*** Hook.**
b- Chopra, c-From Himalaya to ceylon.

II- *a-* आत्मगुप्ता (Ātmaguptā), कपिरोमफला (Kapiromaphalā).
b- H.-Kavanca; B.-Alkusa; Bom., Mar.- Kuhili; Tam.-Soriyanam; Tel. -Dulgondo; Mal.-Punaikkali Eng.- The cow hedge plant.

III- *d,e*-See current name.

दधिपुष्पी Dadhipuṣpī 27.

दधिपुष्पी तु खट्वाङ्गी खट्वा पर्यङ्कपादिका ॥ १५४
ऋषभी सा तु काकाण्डी ज्ञेया शूकरपादिका ॥

---

* The current name is *I. paniculata* (Linn.) R.Br. Syn *I.digitata* auct. (non Linn.)

** The current name is *Mucuna pruriens* (Linn.) DC.

The other climber with latex suggested is *Argyreia strigosa* Roth.) S. & P.

कफपित्तहरा गुर्वी रञ्जनी वातनाशिनी ॥ १५५
उष्णवीर्या स्वादुरसा काकाण्डी माषवद्भवेत् ॥

दधिपुष्पी (Dadhipuṣpī),खट्वाङ्गी (Khaṭvāṅgī),खट्वा (Khaṭvā), पर्यङ्कपादिका (Paryaṅkapādikā), ऋषभी (Ṛṣabhī), काकाण्डी (Kākāṇḍi), and शूकरपादिका (Śūkarapādikā) are synonyms for *Dadhipuṣpī*.

Dadhipuṣpī is sweet in taste, *uṣṇavīrya, guru,* tasteful (Rañjani). It pacifies *kapha, pitta and vātadoṣas*. Its properties are similar to *māṣa* (chapter VI)

(Fam.-Leguminosae, Sub.-Fam.- Papilionaceae). Fabaceae.

I- A-*a*- ***Carpopogon capitatum*** Roxb.
b- Kamat. *c*-Foot of the Western and Eastern Himalayas.

II- *a*- खट्वाङ्गी (Khaṭwāṅgī), वृषभी (Vṛṣabhī), काकाण्डी (Kākāṇḍī), सूकरपादिका (Sūkarapādikā).
b- Tel.-Suruta, B. Khavace, Kokan- Goḍī Kuhiḷī.

III- कोलशिंबिनामाकपिकच्छुविशेषः (Sū.6).
Kolasimbināmā Kapikacchuviśeṣaḥ, c-काकाण्डोला निःशूक कपिकच्छुः (Hemadri Sū.6-21,) 22; Cakra Sū).
d,e,f-See current name.

47 (४२) शितिवारः Śitivāraḥ

शितिवारः सूचिपत्रः सूच्याह्वः सुनिषण्णकः ॥ १५६
श्रीवारकः शितिवरः स्वस्तिकः कुक्कुटः शिखी ॥

शितिवारस्तु संग्राही कषायः सर्वदोषजित् ॥ १५७
हृद्रोगप्लीहगुल्मार्शोबस्तिशुद्धिकरः परः ॥

शितिवारः (Śitivāraḥ), सूचिपत्रः (Sūcipatraḥ), सूच्याह्वः (Sūcyāhvaḥ), सुनिषण्णकः (Suniṣaṇṇakaḥ), श्रीवारकः (Śrīvārakaḥ), शितिवरः (Śitivaraḥ), स्वस्तिकः (Swastikaḥ), कुक्कुटः (Kukkuṭaḥ), and शिखी (Śikhī) are synonymous.

Śitivāra is *kaśāya* in taste and pacifies the three *doṣas* and is astringent (binding). It is useful in cardiac diseases, diseases of spleen, intestinal tumours (diverticulosis), piles and has very much purificatory action on urinary bladder.

Under this name two plants are included. A-शितिवारः (Śitivāraḥ) and B-सुनिषण्णकः (Suniṣaṇṇakaḥ).

(Fam.-Amaranthaceae).

I- A-*a*- ***Celosia argentea*** Linn.
b- Roxburgh, *c*-Common weed, *d*-Mukerji, Apte,

B-*a*- ***Marsilea quadrifoila*** Linn.* (Fam. Marsileaceae.)
b- Roxburgh, *c*- A plant of marshy habitat. Common in W. India Poona, Khandala; Kolhapur.

II- A-*a*- सूचिपत्रः (Sūcipatraḥ),श्रीवारकः (Śriwārakaḥ),कुक्कुटः (Kukkuṭaḥ) शिखी (Śikhī), कुरुटः (Kuruṭaḥ).
b- H.-Saphetmurgā , Guj.- Sāpḍi; B.-Swetamurga, Mar.-Kurḍu, Tel.- Gurugu.

B-*a*- सुनिषण्णकः (Suniṣaṇṇakaḥ), स्वस्तिकः (Swastikaḥ).
b- H.-Siriāri. B.-Susni sāka. Nasik-Pet- Zārezurā; Eng.-Marsilea ; Sk.-Jalakumbhi.

III- *b*- 1) शितिवारः *(Celosia argentea).*
(Br. ni. Pade; Ni. Shi. Pade; Desai; Priyavata).
c- सुनिषण्णकः -सिरिवालीतिलोके। श्रीब्रह्मदेवस्तु-चतुर्दलामाह तल्लक्षणं कथ्यते - 'चांगेरी सदृशैः पत्रैः सुनिषण्णश्चतुर्दलः । शाको जलान्विते देशे चतुःपत्रीति कथ्यते । (Dalhan, Sū- 46-262; Aruna, Su.6.)

IV- सुनिषण्णक *Marsilea quadrifolia* (Ghanekar Su. 46-262. Asi Rs. IV-225; U C.Dutt).

48. (४३) पाषाणभेदकः Pāṣāṇabhedakaḥ

पाषाणभेदकोऽश्मघ्नः शिलाभेदोऽश्मभेदकः ॥ १५८
स चैवोपलभेदश्च नगभिद्[1] दृषदश्मजित् ॥

अश्मभेदो हिमस्तित्तः शर्करा शिस्नशूलजित् ॥ १५९
ह्रोगप्लीहगुल्मार्शोबस्तिशुद्धिकरः परः ॥

पाषाणभेदकः (Pāṣāṇabhedakaḥ), अश्मघ्नः (Aśmaghnaḥ), शिलाभेदः (Śilābhedaḥ) अश्मभेदकः, (Aśmabhedakaḥ), उपलभेदः (Upalabhedaḥ), नगभिद् (Nagabhit), दृषदश्मजित् (Dṛṣadaśmajit), are the synonyms for *Pāṣānabheda.*

Pāṣāṇabheda is *śitavīrya,* bitter in taste, and is useful in urinary calculus, pain in penis, cardiac diseases, spleen diseases, intestinal tumors, piles and has much purificatory action on the bladder (urinary organs).

'शितिवार : सूतपुत्रस्तुल्या च सुनिषण्णकः ।' क्षीरस्वामी ।
१ 'नगविध्वंसकोऽश्मभित' इति नि.शे. टीकायाम् ।
* The current accepted name is - *Marsilea minuta* Linn. (U.P.I. p. 357)

Not identified.

Note- A kind of medicinal stone. Vegetable drugs, noted by some writers do not correspond to the text of Nighaṇṭu.*

II- A-a- उपलभेदः (Upalabhedaḥ), श्वेताचोपलभेदि (Śwetācopalabhedi), शिलगर्भजा (Śilagarbhajā).

49. श्रावणी Śrāwaṇī, (४४) श्रावण्यौ Śrāvaṇyau

श्रावणी स्यान्मुण्डितिका भिक्षुः श्रवणशीर्षिका ॥ १६०
श्रवणाह्वा प्रव्रजिता परिव्राजी तपोधना ॥ **
महाश्रावणिका[१] मुण्डी लोभनीया तथाऽन्यका ॥ १६१
कदम्बपुष्पिका प्रोक्ता छिन्नग्रन्थिनिका च सा ।
मुण्डिका कटुतिक्ता स्यादनिलास्रविनाशिनी ॥ १६२
आमारुचिघ्न्यपस्मारगण्डश्लीपदनाशिनी ॥

श्रावणी (Śrāvaṇī), मुण्डितिका (Muṇḍitikā), भिक्षुः (Bhikśuḥ), श्रवणशीर्षिका (Śravaṇaśīrṣikā), श्रवणाह्वा (Śravanāhvā), प्रव्रजिता (Pravrajitā), परिव्राजी (Parivrājī), and तपोधना (Tapodhanā) are synonyms for *Śrāvaṇī*.

The other type is महाश्रावणी (Mahāśrāvaṇī), of which synonyms are मुण्डी (Muṇḍī), लोभनीया (Lobhanīyā), कदम्बपुष्पिका (Kadambapuṣpikā), and छिन्नग्रन्थिनिका (Chinnagranthinikā),

Muṇḍikā is pungent and bitter in taste and pacifies *vāta, rakta* and *āmadoṣa.* It is useful in anorexia, epilepsy, glands and elephantiasis.

Under this name two plants are recorded. A-श्रावणी (Śrāwaṇi), and B-महाश्रावणी (Mahāśrāwaṇī).

(Fam.-Composite). Asteraceae.

I- A-*a*- ***Sphaeranthus africanus*** Linn.

b- Mahajan, *c*-Swamps, in damp waste grounds; throughout plains of Bengal, Thana Dist; Mulund.

Note- A fragrant plant 8"-24" high, stem compressed with entire wings.

---

१ 'महाश्रावण्यथाऽन्या तु लोचनीया तथाऽपरा ।' इति नि.शे. टीकायाम् ।

**Saxifraga ligulata* Wall. (Chunekar p. 105)

**Nighantuśeṣa निघण्टुशेष has mentioned the authourity of this plant as-
"श्रावणी श्रावितापूर्वं गालवेन महात्मना ।
आत्रेयस्यैषिका प्रोक्ता छिन्नग्रन्थिनिका च सा " इति ।

heads smaller than in *S. indicus* (Mahajan).

B-*a*- ***S. indicus*** Linn.
Syn. *S, mollis* Roxb.
b- Mahajan and Kamat, *c*-Thoughout India and Himalayas.

II- A-*a*- मुण्डिनिका (Muṇḍinikā), श्रवणशीर्षक (Śravaṇaśīrṣaka).
b- Vernacular names as in Mahāśrāwaṇī.

B-a- महाश्रावणिका (Mahāsrāwaṇikā), कदंबपुष्पिका (Kadambap-uṣpikā).
b- H.-Muṇḍi;B.-Murmuriyā Mar.-Gorakhamuṇḍī; Bonḍsarā; Tam.-Kattakarandai; Tel.-Boḍasarum Mal.-Attakkamanni.

III- b- (1) महामुण्डी *Sphaeranthus indicus* (Dwivedi).
(2) श्रावणी (Ci-31) मरा.-बोंडथरा, वरसबोंडी.(Bondatharā, Varasbondi)
S. indicus, S. hirtus (Vaidya).
(3) 163 श्रावणी श्रवणेति -श्रावणी श्राविता पूर्वं गालवेन महात्मना ...... मते ति धन्वतरीयः (Ca.sū. 1-10. Harshe).

50. सारिवा Sāriwā ४५ सारिवे Sarive

सारिवा शारदा[१] गोपा[२] गोपवल्ली प्रतानिका ॥ १६३
गोपकन्या लताऽऽस्फोता[३] श्वेतोक्ता काष्ठसारिवा ॥

सारिवा (Sārivā), शारदा (Śāradā), गोपा (Gopā), गोपवल्ली (Gopavallī), प्रतानिका (Pratānikā), गोपकन्या (Gopakanyā), लता (Latā), आस्फोता (Asphotā), श्वेता (Śvetā) and काष्ठसारिवा (Kāṣṭhasārivā) are synonymous.

(Fam.-Apocynaceae).

I- *a*- ***Ichnocarpus frutescens*** R. Br.*
Syn.-*Echites frutescens* Roxb.
b- Roxburgh, *c*-More or less throughout India , Sawantwadi, Goa. (Mahajan).

II- *a*- शारदा (Śāradā). गोपवल्ली (Gopawallī), श्वेतोक्ता काष्ठसारिवा (Swetoktā Kāṣṭhasārivā).

---

१ 'शारदी ' नि.शे. टीका संमत : पाठः ।
२ 'गोपी' नि.शे. टीकासंमत पाठः।
३ 'लता सीता नि.शे. टीका संमतः. पाठः ।
* The current name is *Ichnocarpas frutescens* (Linn.) R. Br.

b-H.Kālidudhi, B.-Dudho; Tel.-Illukaṭṭi; Tam.-Udaragoḍi; Kan.-Kariumbu.

51. कृष्णमूली Kṛṣṇamūlī

सारिवाऽन्या कृष्णमूली कृष्णा चन्दनसारिवा ॥१६४
भद्रा चन्दनगोपा तु चन्दना कृष्णवल्ल्यपि ॥

सारिवे द्वे तु मधुरे कफवातास्रनाशने ॥ १६५
कुष्ठकण्डूज्वरहरे मेहदुर्गन्धिनाशने ॥

कृष्णमूली तु संग्राहि शिशिरा कफवातजित् ॥ १६६
तृष्णारुचिप्रशमनी रक्तपित्तहरा स्मृता ॥

The other type of sārivā is कृष्णमूली (Kṛṣṇamūlī), the synonyms of which are कृष्णा (Kṛṣṇā), चन्दनसारिवा (Candana sārivā), भद्रा (Bhadrā), चन्दनगोपा (Candanagopā), चन्दना (Candanā) and कृष्णवल्ली (Kṛṣṇavallī).

Two types of *sārivās* are sweet in taste and pacify *kapha, vāta* and *rakta doṣas.* These are useful in skin diseases, pruritus, fever, disorders characterized by polyuria, and foetid smell. Out of these the *kṛṣṇamūlī* is *śītavīrya*, astringent and pacifies *kapha* and *vātadoṣas*. It is useful in thirst, anorexia and haemorrhagic disorders.

(Fam.-Asclepiadaceae).

I- *a*- ***Hemidesmus indicus*** R. Br.*

b- Roxburgh, *c*-Kokan, S. M. country, Bengal, Madhya Pradesh, S. India, *d*-Jain.

II- *a*- अन्या सारिवा (Anyāsārivā), चन्दनसारिवा (Candanasārivā), कृष्णवल्ली (Kṛṣṇawallī).

b- Roxburgh;

b- H.-Jangli chameli; B.-Anantmul;. Mar.-Bom.- Uparsal, Anantmūla;
Tam.-Nannāri; Mal.-Nannari kizhanna; Eng.-Indian Sarsaparilla.

III-*b*- (1) सा द्विधा (Sā dwidhā) श्वेता कृष्णाचेति (Swetākṛṣṇāceti),
इति आदमल्लः *Hemideśmus indicus.* (Vaidya; Dipika Bṛhanmañjiṣṭhādi).

c- (1) शारिवा, कृष्णसारिवा (Dalhana, 38-4).

---

* The current name is *Hemidesmus indicus* (Linn.) R. Br.
stem pieces of *Cryptolepis buchanani* Roem. & Schult. (Jambupartā sarivā) are sold in North Indian markets.

52. (४६) बाकुची Bākucī

बाकुची सोमराजी तु सोमवल्ली सुवल्ल्यपि ॥ १६७
अवल्गुजा[1] कृष्णफला[2] सैव पूतिफला[3] मता ॥

चंद्रलेखेन्दुलेखा च शशिलेखा मता च सा ॥ १६८
पूतिकर्णी[4] कालमेषी दुर्गन्धा कुष्ठनाशिनी ॥

बाकुची शीतला तिक्ता श्लेष्मकुष्ठकृमीञ्जयेत् ॥ १६९
रसायनोपयुक्ता च रुचिमेधाविवर्धनी[5] ॥

बाकुची कटुका पाके ग्राहि कुष्ठव्रणापहा ॥१७०

बाकुची (Bākucī), सोमराजी (Somarājī), सोमवल्ली (Somavāllī), सुवल्ली (Suvallī), अवल्गुजा (Avalgujā), कृष्णफला (Kṛṣṇaphalā), पूतिफला (Pūtiphalā), चंद्रलेखा (Candralekhā), इन्दुलेखा (Indulekhā), शशिलेखा (Śaśilekhā), पूतिकर्णी (Pūtikarṇī), कालमेषी (Kālameṣī), दुर्गन्धा (Durgandhā), and कुष्ठनाशिनी (Kuṣṭhanāśinī) are the synonyms of *Bākuchī*.

Bākucī is bitter in taste, *śīta virya*, pacifies *kapha* and is useful in skin diseases, (esp. leucoderma), is vermicidal, rejuvinating (*Rasāyana*), and increases appetite and is intellect promoting.

Bākucī is pungent in *vipāka,* astringent and useful in ulcers due to skin diseases.

This name includes two plants: A- कृष्णफला (Kṛṣṇaphalā) and B- सिता (Sitā).

(Fam. : Leguminosae). Fabaceae.

I- A-a- ***Psoralea corylifolia*** Linn.
b- Dymock, c-Throughout India.
(For confirmation).

B-a- ***Psoralea plicata*** Del. (Cooke).
b- Mahajan, c-Sindh and Punjab.

Note- The flowers are yellowish, fruits are 'not black', leaves are trifoliate. *P. corylifolia* very rarely bears white flowers, but the fruits are 'black-'(Mahajan).

II- A-a- सोमराजी (Somarājī), अवल्गुजा (Awalgujā), कृष्णफला (Kṛṣṇaphalā), पूतिफला (Pūtiphalā).
b- H.-Bākci, Bābaci; Mar.-Rānbāvacī; B.-Latā Kasturī; Tam.-

---

१ 'अवल्गुजी' २ 'कृष्णफली' ३ 'पूतिफली' ४ 'पूतिपर्णी' इति नि.शे. टीका संमताः पाठाः ।
५ 'मेधाविनाशिनी' इति आनन्दा. पुस्तके पाठः ।

Karpokarisi,Tel.-Bāvanci vittulu, Karu-bogi vittulu.

B-b- Not known.

III- See Bṛhatpālī, Varga II.

c- (1) बाकुची चंद्रिका कृष्णफला (Madaṇ ni).

(2) बाकुची *Psoralea corylifolia* अस्या भाषांतराणि अन्यथा च दृष्यंते (Vaidya).

b- (1) अवल्गुजफलानि । ताऽपिश्वेता गृह्यते (Dalhan Ci. Medhāyuskāmīya).

d- See current names.

53. (४७) मदनः Madanaḥ

मदनः शल्यको राठः पिण्डी पिण्डीतकः फलः ॥
गालवः[1] करहाटश्च च्छर्दनो विषपुष्पकः ॥१७१

मदनः कटुकस्तिक्तस्तथा चोष्णो व्रणापहः ॥
श्लेष्मज्वरप्रतिश्याय गुल्मेषु विद्रधीषु च ॥ १७२· A.H. Kalp.1.9
शोफदोषापहो बस्तौ वमने चेह शस्यते ॥

मदनः (Madanaḥ), शल्यकः (Śalyakaḥ), राठः (Rāṭhaḥ), पिण्डी (Piṇḍī), पिण्डीतकः (Piṇḍītakaḥ), फलः (Phalaḥ), गालवः (Gālavaḥ), करहाटः (Karahāṭaḥ), छर्दनः (Chardanaḥ), विषपुष्पकः (Viṣapuṣpakaḥ), are synonyms for *Madanaḥ*.

Madanaḥ is pungent and bitter in taste, *uṣṇavīrya* and useful in ulcer, fevers caused by *kaphadoṣa*, coryza, tumours, abscesses and oedema, for the therapy of *Bastī* and *vamana* (emesis) therapy.

Fam. (Rubiaceae)

I- a- ***Randia dumetorum*** (Linn.) Lam .-Chopra.*
Syn.-*Gardenia floribunda* Roxb. (Watt Dict.).
Randia brandisi Gamble.

b- Dymock, c-Sub:Himalayan tract; Western India.

II- a- शल्यकः (Śalyakaḥ).पिण्डीतकः (Piṇḍītakaḥ); करहाटकः (Karahāṭakaḥ),

54. (४८) कटुकालाम्बुनी Kaṭukālāmbunī

कटुकालाम्बुनी तुम्बी लम्बा पिण्डफला च सा ॥ १७३
इक्ष्वाकुः क्षत्रियवरा[2] तिक्तबीजा महाफला ॥

---

१ 'तस्करः' इति नि.शे. टीका, क्षीर. संमतः पाठः।
२ 'क्षत्रियधनः' इति क्षीर. संमतः पाठः
* The current names *Xeromphis spinosa* (Thunb.) Keay Syn. *Gardenia floribunda* Roxb.

कासश्वासच्छर्दिहरो विषार्ते कफकर्षिते ॥ १७४
इक्ष्वाकुर्वमने शस्तः प्रताम्यति च मानवे ॥ A. H. Kalp.1.27 C. Kalpa 3. 4

कटुतुम्बी कटुस्तिक्ता वातकृत् श्वासकासजित् ॥ १७५
कफघ्नी[१] शोधनी शोफव्रणशूलविषापहा ॥

कटुकालम्बुनी (Kaṭukālāmbunī), तुम्बी (Tumbī), लम्बा (Lambā), पिण्डफला (Piṇḍaphalā), इक्ष्वाकुः (Iks'vākuḥ), क्षत्रियवरा (K'satriyavarā), तिक्तबीजा (Tiktabījā), महाफला (Mahāphalā), are synonyms for *Kaṭukālāmbunī*.

It is useful as an emetic especially when the patient is languored by cough, dyspnoea, vomiting, poisoning and *kaphadoṣa*.

Katutumbī is pungent and bitter in taste, aggravates *vātadoṣa* and is purificatory by action on *kaphadoṣa*. It is useful in oedema, obstinate ulcers, colics and poisons.

The fruit of this plant occurs in many forms such as तुम्बी (Tumbi), लम्बा (Lambā), पिण्डफला (Piṇḍaphalā), महाफला (Mahāphalā) etc. etc.

(Fam.-Cucurbitaceae).

I- *a*- ***Lagenaria siceraria*** Standle* = *L.vulagaris* Seringe
b- Dymock, *c*-Indigenous to India. *d*-Apte.

II- *a*- तुम्बी (Tumbī), कटुतुम्बी (Kaṭutumbī).
b- H.-Kās'īphal, Kaddū; B.-Kaḍalau; Mar.-Kaḍu Bhopḷā; Dudhī; Tel.-Sarakaya; Tam.-Sorakkai, Soriai-kari; Mal.-Bella-Scora; Eng.-Bottle shaped gourd, Indian club shaped gourd, Pilgrims gourd, Kalambash, Trumpet gourd.

Note- By the result of cultivation over hundreds of years the bitter taste of the fruit is resulted into sweet taste.

III- *a*- Alābu. AV. vii; 10-29, 30; Maitr . Sam. iv 2.13. (Harshe).
b- इक्ष्वाकुः कटुतुम्बीस्यात् । तुम्ब्यलाबु उभे समे । (Bhanuji).

55. (४९) जीमूतकः Jīmūtakaḥ

जीमूतको देवताडो वृत्तकोशो गरागरी ॥ १७६
प्रोक्तःऽऽखुविषहा वेणी देवदाली च ताडका ॥

जीमूतको ज्वरश्वास कासहिध्मारुचिक्षये ॥ १७७ A.H. Kalp.1.19
शोफपाण्डुविषध्वंसी गरेषु वमने हित : ॥

---

१ 'कासघ्नी' इति पाठः ।

* *Lagenaria siceraria* (Molina) Standle.

जीमूतकः (Jīmūtakaḥ), देवताडः (Devatāḍaḥ), वृत्तकोशः (Vṛttakośaḥ), गरागरी (Garāgarī), आखुविषहा (Ākhuviṣahā), वेणी (Veṇī), देवदाली (Devadālī), ताडका (Tāḍakā), are synonyms of *Jīmūtaka.*

Jimūtaka is useful in the therapy of emesis . It is beneficial in the treatment of fevers, dyspnoea, cough, hiccup, anorexia, consumption, oedema, anaemia, poisons, and artificial poisons.

(Fam.: Cucurbitaceae)

I- a- ***Luffa echinata*** Roxb.
b- Roxburgh c-Sindh, Gujarath, Bengal.

II- a- देवदाली (Devadālī), लोमशपत्रिका (Lomaśa patrikā).
b- B.-Devatāḍa; H.-Kukurvel, Binḍāla; Mar., Kan.- Devadangara; Guj.- Kukurvela.

II- c- जीमूतकम् (Aruna. Kalp. I-20, 22).

56. (५०) त्रपुसम् Trapusam

त्रपुसं कटुकं तिक्तं विपाण्डुर्हस्तिपर्णिनी ॥ १७८
दीर्घपर्णी मूत्रफला लताकर्कटिकाऽपि च ॥

त्रपुसं छर्दिहृत् प्रोक्तं मूत्रबस्तिविशोधनम् ॥ १७९

त्रपुसम् (Trapusam), कटुकं (Kaṭukam), तिक्त (Tiktam), विपाण्डुः (Vipāṇḍuḥ) हस्तिपर्णिनी (Hastiparṇinī), दीर्घपर्णी (Dīrghaparṇī), मूत्रफला (Mutraphalā), लताकर्कटिका (Latākarkaṭikā), are synonyms.

It is useful in emesis and has purificatory action on urine and urinary organs.

Includes two kinds : A-कटुकम् (Kaṭukam. Dhn. ni.)and B- रुच्यम् (Rucyam, Raj. ni.);

(Fam.-Cucurbitaceae)

I- A-*a-* ***Cucumis trigonus*** Roxb.*
b- Roxburgh.

B-*a-* ***Cucumis trigonous*** Roxb,* *var. ***pubescens,***

---

* The current name is *Cucumis callosus* (Rottle) Cogn; Syns. *C. psudocolocynthis* Royle, *Brayonia callosa* Rottle.

** According to Av. & Rv. उर्वारुः Urvāruḥ may be *Cucumis melo* proper. But according to De candole all present varieties of cucumis genus are developed from *C.melo.* (Vide Watt. Dict.) D.K.Kamat *b*- 1-B.-Gomuka; H.-Bisalambī; Tam.- Kaṭṭumaṭṭi; Kokan- Kārīṭ.

B-*a*- तुन्दिलफला (Tundilaphalā), मधुरम् (Madhuram).

b- Mar.-Takamaken; Kokan-Āmble.

III- *a*- 43 Trapu-AV.X-3-8; ksii-11-5; T.S. iv.-7-5-1 (Harshe)

d; e,g: -See current names.

Note- IV- (1) 23 इन्द्रायणभेद (Indrāyaṇabheda). *Cucumss trigonus* Roxb. In Pahādi area of U. P., the fruit of this plant is sometimes called 'Indrāyan' or 'Viṣalambhi'. This is substituted for Indrāyaṇa. (Balavant. Bihar).

Note- Dhn. ni's and Raj. ni's plants are different.

उर्वारुः Urvāruḥ 34.

उर्वारुः कर्कटी प्रोक्ता व्यालपत्रा च लोमशा ॥
स्थूला तोयफला चैव हस्तिदन्तफला मुनिः ॥१८०*

उर्वारुकं पित्तहरं सुशीतलं मूत्रामयघ्नं मधुरं रुचिप्रदम् ।
संतापमूर्च्छापहरं सुतृप्तिदं वातप्रकोपाय घनं तु सेवितम् ॥ १८१

उर्वारुः (Urvāruḥ), कर्कटी (Karkaṭī), व्यालपत्रा (Vyālaptrā), लोमशा (Lomaśā), स्थूला (Sthūlā), तोयफला (Toyaphalā), and हस्तिदन्तफला (Hastidantaphalā), are synonyms for *Urvāruḥ*.

It is sweet in taste, pacifies *pittadoṣa,* is *śītavīrya* and appetizer. It is useful in urinary diseases, burning sensation, giddiness and is satiating but if used in excess it aggravates *vātadoṣa.*

(Fam.-Cucurbitaceae).

I- *a*- ***Cucumis melo***** var. ***momordica*** Duthie and Fuller

Syn.-*C.momordica* Roxb.

b- Roxburgh, c-Cultivated.

II- *a*- कर्कटी (Karkaṭī),व्यालपत्रा (Vyāḷapatrā),तोयफला (Toyaphalā), हस्तिदन्तफला (Hastidantaphalā).

b- Mar.-Kākaḍi, Tovasen.

III- *a*- छिन्नंह्यस्य बन्धनं मूलं उर्वार्वा इव । (AV-vi-14).

d,e,f-See current names.

Note- See Melon (D. Candolle pp. 25-61).

---

* Synonyms restricted ? Probably taken from Raj. ni.

** The current name is *Cucumis melo* Linn. var. *culta*

वालुकम् Vālukam 35.

वालुकं काण्डकं वालु तच्छीतं मधुरं गुरु ।
रक्तपित्तहरं भेदि लघूष्णं पक्वमग्निकृत् ॥१८२

वालुकं (Vālukam), काण्डकं (Kāṇḍakam), and वालु (Vālu), are the synonyms for *Vālukam*.

It is sweet in taste, *śītavīrya* and *guru*. It pacifies *rakta* and *pitta doṣa* (haemorrhagic disorders), when fully ripe it is purgative, *laghu; usṇavirya* and stimulates digestive capacity.

(Fam.-Cucurbitaceae).

I- A-*a*- form of *Cucumis melo* var. *momordica*.
b- Kamat, *c*-Self-grown.

II- *a*- क्षेत्रकर्कटी (Kśetra karkaṭī- kind of Karkaṭī), मधुरफला (Maḍhuraphalā).

शीर्णवृन्तम् Sīrṇavṛntam 38.

शीर्णवृन्तं चित्रफलं विचित्रं पीतवर्णकम् ।
शीर्णवृन्तं लघु स्वादु भेद्युष्णं वह्निपित्तकृत् ॥१८३

शीर्णवृन्तम् (Sīrnavṛntam), चित्रफलं (Citraphalam), विचित्रं (Vicitram) पीतवर्णकम्, (Pītavrṇakam), are synonymous.

It is *laghu*, aggravates *pittadoṣa,* is sweet in taste, purgative, *uṣṇavīrya* and useful for stimulating digestive capacity.

(Fam.-Cucurbitaceae).

I- *a*- ***Cucumis melo*** Linn. (proper).
b- Kamat, *c*-Cultivated.

II- *a*- चित्रफलम् (Citraphalam), *c*-पीतवर्णकम् (Pītawarṇakam).
b- H.-Kharbuja; B.-Kharmuj; (Santāl-Tarbuj), Tam. -Vellarivarai; Mulampazam; Tel. -Kharbuja-dosā; Eng.-Melon; Guj.-Tarbucha; Mar.-Chibūḍa.

III- See Urvāru. *d*-See current name.

चिर्भटम् Cirbhaṭam 41.

चिर्भटं धेनुदुग्धं च ज्ञेयं गोरक्षकर्कटी ।
चिर्भटं मधुरं रूक्षं गुरु पित्तकफापहम् ॥ १८४

चिर्भटं (Cirbhaṭam), धेनुदुग्धं (Dhenudugdham), and गोरक्षकर्कटी (Goraksakarkaṭī) are synonymous. It is sweet in taste, pacifies *pitta* and *kaphadoṣas, guru* and *rūksa.*

(Fam.Cucurbitaceae).

I- *a-* A form of ***Cucumis trigonus*** Roxb. var ***pubescens.***
b- Dwivedi.

II- *a-* धेनुदुग्धम् (Dhenudugdham), गोरक्षकर्कटी (Goraksakarkaṭī).
b- H.-Phūṭ; Mar.-Sendāḍa.

IV- 1) Pubescent cucumber चिर्भटम् H. -Phut;** Sindhi- cebhira (Jaitly). *Cucumis pubescensse* (Dwivedi).

डङ्गरी Ḍangrī 43.*

डंगरी डांगरी चैव दीर्घोर्वारुश्च डङगरिः।
डांगारी नागशुण्डी च गजदन्तफला मुनिः ॥१८५
डंगरी शीतला रुच्या दाहपित्तास्रदोषजित्
शोषहृत्तर्पणी गौल्या जाड्यहा मूत्ररोधनुत् ॥१८६ Raj. ni. ch. 7.

डङगरी (Ḍangarī), डाङ्गरी (Ḍān lgarī), दीर्घोर्वारुः (Dīrghorvāruḥ), डङ्गरिः (Dangariḥ), डाङ्गारी (Dāngārī), नागशुण्डी (Nāgasuṇḍī) and गजदन्तफला (Gajadantaphalā), these seven are synonymous.

Ḍangarī is sweet in taste, *sitavirya* and pacifies *pitta* and *raktadoṣas*. It promotes appetite and is useful in burning sensation of the body, alleviates thirst (?emaciation), is nutrient, removes dullness and is useful in obstruction to the flow of urine.

Not confirmed.

(Fam.-Cucurbitaceae).

I- *a-* May be a kind of ***Cucumis trigonus*** Roxb.
b- Bhagirath.

II- *a-* दीर्घोर्वारुः (Dīrghorvāruḥ), नागशुण्डी (Nāgasuṇḍī), गजदन्तफला (Gajadantaphalā).
b- H.Dungarī, Dāngarī.

Note- IV-1)डङ्गरी-कर्कटिका-डङ्गरी, डांगरी, दीर्घ उर्वारुक, उर्वारु *Cucumis momordica;* त्रपुसारणी. *C. sativa* (C.ci-26-71). (Bhagirath).

---

* This plant name seems to be copied from Raj. ni. chap.7.

१ 'बल्या इति चौखम्बामुद्रित पुस्तके पाठः।

** The current name is *C. melo* Linn. var. *momordica* Duthi & Full.

कूष्माण्डिका Kūṣmāṇḍikā 44.

कूष्माण्डिका कुम्भफला तथा स्थिरफला मता ।
कूष्माण्डी सोमसृष्टा च पीतिका च बृहत्फला ॥१८७

वल्लीफलानां प्रवरं कूष्माण्डं वातपित्तजित् ।
बस्तिशुद्धिकरं वृष्यं हृद्यं चेतोविकारजित् ॥ १८८

A.H. Su.6.88 (also A. sang.)

कूष्माण्डिका (Kūṣmāṇḍikā), कुम्भफला (Kumbhaphalā), स्थिरफला (Sthiraphalā), कूष्माण्डी (Kūṣmāṇḍī), सोमसृष्टा (Somasṛṣṭā), पीतिका (Pītikā) and बृहत्फला (Bṛhatphalā), are synonymous.

Kūṣmāṇḍa is the best fruit vegetable amongst creepers. It pacifies *vāta* and *pitta doṣas.* It is purificatory of urinary organs, *vṛṣya,* cordial and useful in psychological disorders.

(Fam.-Cucurbitaceae).

I- *a*-***Benincasa hispida*** Cogn*. = ***B. cerifera*** Savi.
Syn.-*Cucurbita pepo* Willd. (non Linn.)
b-Kamat; *c*-Cultivated all over India.

II- *a*-कुम्भफला (Kumbhaphalā).
b-H.-Peṭhā; B.-Calkumarā; Mar.-Kohālā; Tam.-Buḍiḍ gamṭe; Tel.-Burḍa-gumḍu; Mal.-Kampalaṇṇa Eng.-Ash gourd, White gourd.

वंध्यकर्कोटकी Vandhyakarkoṭakī 46.

वंध्यकर्कोटकी देवी मनोज्ञा च कुमारिका ।
नागारिः सर्पदमनी विषकण्टकिनी तथा ॥ १८९

विज्ञेया नागदमनी सर्व भूतप्रमर्दिनी ।
वन्ध्यापुत्रप्रदा चैव ज्ञेया योगेश्वरी तथा ॥१९०

वंध्यकर्कोटकी (Vandhyakarkoṭakī), देवी (Devī), मनोज्ञा (Manojñyā), कुमारिका (Kumārikā), नागारिः (Nāgāriḥ), सर्पदमनी (Sarpadamanī), विषकण्टकिनी (Viṣakaṇṭakinī),नागदमनी(Nāgadamanī),सर्वभूतप्रमर्दिनी (Sarvabhūtapramardinī) वन्ध्यापुत्रप्रदा (Vandhyāputrapradā) and योगेश्वरी (Yogeśvarī) are synonymous.

---

* *Benicasa hispida* (Thunb.) Cogn. is the current accepted name (comp.21)

Fam.-Cucurbitaceae).

I- a- The male plant of ***Momordica dioica*** Roxb.*

b- Kamat. c-Wild throughout India; Cuiltivated in Deccan, Himalaya.

II- a- नागारिः (Nāgariḥ),कुमारिका (Kumārikā).

b- Vernacular names as in कर्कोटकी (Karkoṭakī) but beginning with Vandhyā.

कर्कोटकी Karkoṭakī 47.

कर्कोटकी स्वादुफला मनोज्ञा च कुमारिका ।
अवन्ध्या चैव देवी च विषप्रशमनी तथा ॥१९१

कर्कोटकी युगं तिक्तं हन्ति श्लेष्मविषद्वयम् ।
मधुना च शिरोरोगे कन्दस्तस्याः प्रशस्यते ॥१९२

कर्कोटकी (Karkoṭakī), स्वादुफला (Swāduphalā), मनोज्ञा (Manojñyā), कुमारिका (Kumārikā), अवन्ध्या (Avandhyā), देवी (Devī), विषप्रशमनी (Viṣapraśamanī) are synonyms for *karkoṭakī*.

Both of these are bitter in taste, pacify *kaphadoṣa* and both types of poisons. Its tuber with honey is used in certain diseases of the head.

(Fam.-Curcurbitaceae).

I- a- Female plant of ***Momordica dioica*** Roxb.

b- Kamat; *c*-Wild throughout India as in 46 above.

II- *a*- स्वादुफला (Swāduphalā), अवन्ध्या (Awandhyā).

b- Mar.-Karṭolī; Santal-Karlā (fruit); Bom.-Kāṭlen; Tam.-Palu-pagel-kalunga; Tel.-Puāgākār; Kan.-Giḍā hāgelu.

57 (५२) धामार्गवः Dhāmārgawaḥ

धामार्गवः कोशफला राजकोशातकी तथा ।
कर्कोटकी पीतपुष्पा महाजालिनिरुच्यते ॥**१९३

---

* The current name is *Momordica dioica* Roxb. ex. Willd. H. kheksā

** According to śodhala Ni. this seems to be included in (vide suprapost No. 47) There is a scope to rearrange the reading see note under (Post No. 50) कोशातकी S.D.Kamat

कोशफला (Kośaphalā), is the synonym for धामार्गव (Dhāmārgava), and for राजकोशातकी (Rājakośātakī), the synonyms are कर्कोटकी (Karkoṭakī), पीतपुष्पा (Pītapuṣpā), and महाजालिनि (Mahājālini)

Two plants are included under this headisng. A-धामार्गव (Dhāmārgawa); and B-राजकोशातकी (Rājakosātakī).

I- A-*a*- Bitter kind of ***Luffa cylindrica*** (L). M.Roem
Syn.-*L.pentandra* Roxb.
b- Kamat; c-Wild.

B-*a*- Sweet kind of *Luffa cylindrica* (L) M. Roem.
b- Kamat, c-Cultivated.

II- A-*a*- कोशफला (Kośaphalā), धामार्गवः (Dhāmārgavaḥ), शोधनी (Śodhanī).
b- Sk.-Kaṭu Kośātakī; Eng.-Bitter sponge, smooth gourd.

B-*a*- राजकोशातकी (Rājakosātakī), हस्तिघोषा (Hastighoṣā).
b- H.Ghiyā turai; B.-Danḍal; Bom.-Mar.- Ghosālen; Kolhapur, Mar.-Gilake.

(५१) कृतवेधनम् Kṛtavedhanam *
कोशातकी Kośātakī 50.

महाकोशातकी त्वन्या हस्तिघोषा महाफला ।
धामार्गवो गदेष्विष्टः स्थिरेषु च महत्सु च । १९४

In the *Gaṇadravyāvalī* गणद्रव्यावली *Kṛtavedhanam* कृतवेधनम् is mentioned first followed by *Dhāmārgava,* both of these are the types *of Kośātakī* only. Therefore the types are 1) राजकोशातकी Rajkośātakī 2) महाकोशातकी Mahākośataki together called as *Dhāmārgava* धामार्गव and 3) कोशातकी Kośātakī called as *Kṛtavedhanam* कृतवेधनम्. These are further divided as bitter तिक्त and स्वादु sweet; धारा कोशातकी (acutely angled) and वृत्तकोशातकी (round body) see Raj. ni. chapter 7. In the present context of emesis (वमनाधिकार) bitter variety is indicated. S. D. Kamat.

अष्टांगहृदयकल्पस्थानपाठमनुसृत्य अत्र पाठशुद्धिः इत्थं भवितुमर्हतीति चिन्तनीयं विद्वद्भिः ।
धामार्गवः कोशफला राजकोशातकी तथा ।
कर्कोटकी पीतपुष्पा महाजालिनिरुच्यते । १ ॥
महाकोशातकी त्वन्या हस्तिघोषा महाफला ।
कोशातकी सुतिक्तोष्णा पक्वामाशयशोधनी ॥ २ ॥
कासगुल्मोदरगरे वाते श्लेष्माशयस्थिते।
कफे च कण्ठवक्त्रस्थे कफसंचयनेषु च ॥ ३ ॥
धामार्गवः गदेष्विष्टः स्थिरेषु च महत्सु च ।
अन्या स्वादुस्त्रिदोषघ्नी ज्वरस्यान्ते हिता स्मृता ॥ ४॥
इति । स.दि. कामत.

कोशातकी सुतिक्तोष्णा पक्वामाशयशोधिनी ।
कासगुल्मोदरगरे वाते श्लेष्माशयस्थिते ॥ १९५

कफे च कण्ठवक्त्रस्थे कफसंचयनेषु च ।
अन्या स्वादुस्त्रिदोषघ्नी ज्वरस्यान्ते हिता स्मृता ॥ १९६

कोशातकी कृतच्छिद्रा जालिनी कृतवेधनी ।
क्ष्वेडा सुतिक्ता घण्टाली मृदङ्गफलिका मता ॥ १९७ C. Kalp. 3.4

क्ष्वेडस्तिक्तः कटुस्तीक्ष्णोऽप्रगाढश्च[१] प्रशस्यते ।
कुष्ठपाण्ड्वामयप्लीहशोफगुल्मगरादिषु ॥ १९८ A.H. Kal.1.41

महाकोशातकी (Mahākośātakī), is another type of which synonyms are हस्तिघोषा (Hastighoṣā), and महाफला (Mahāphalā).

Dhāmārgava is useful in diseases which are deeply rooted (in tissues) and are very extensive. *Kośātakī* is bitter in taste *uṣṇavīrya* and has purificatory action on stomach and intestines. It is useful in cough, tumors, ascites, artificial posioning and when *vātadoṣa* has invaded the natural locations of *kapha doṣa,* and when *kapha* is accumulated in bronchi and throat.

The sweet variety of *koaśātakī* pacifies all the three *doṣas* and is beneficial after fever.

कृतवेधनी (Kṛtavedhanī) has the synonyms as कोशातकी (Kośātakī), कृतच्छिद्रा (Kṛtacchidrā), जालिनी(Jālinī), क्ष्वेडा (Kśveḍā), सुतिक्ता (Sutiktā), घण्टाली (Ghanṭālī) and मृदङ्गफलिका (Mṛdaṅgaphalikā).

Kśveḍa is bitter and pungent in taste, *tīkśṇa* and is used in diseases which are deeply situated (in tissues) as skin diseases including leprosy, anaemias, spleen diseases, oedema, tumors and artificial posoning.

This heading includes three varieties: A-सुतिक्ता (Sutiktā) and B-धाराफला ((Dhārāphalā), C-स्वादुफला ((Swāduphalā)

(Fam.-Curcurbitaceae).

I- A-*a*- ***Luffa acutangula*** Roxb. var. ***amara*** clarke.*
b- Kamat. *c*-Willd.

B-*a*- ***Luffa acutangula*** Roxb.
b- Kamat, c-Cultivated.

II- A-*a*- क्ष्वेडा (Kśweḍā), सुतिक्ता (Sutiktā), घण्टाली (Ghanṭālī), मृदङ्गफलिका

---

* The current name is *Luffa acutangula* (Linn) Roxb. Var. amara Clarke.

१ 'प्रगाढेषु च शस्यते' प्रगाढेषु प्रशस्यते' इति वा साधु पाठः अ. हृ. कल्प. २.४१ इत्यनुसारेण । अत्यर्थ कटुतीक्ष्णोष्णं गाढेष्विष्टं गदेषु च' इति चरक पाठः । अत्यर्थ गाढेषु कुष्ठादिषु इति चक्रः । कटुतिक्तोष्णं प्रगाढेषु च शस्यते । इति वा साधु पाठः । S. D. Kamat.

(Mṛdaṅgaphalikā).

b- Kokan-Vātoḷen Kadu Ghosāḷen, Sātaputen.

B-*a*- स्वादुफला (Swāduphalā), धाराफला (Dhārāphalā).

b- H.-Jingā, Torai; B.-Ghosā; Mar.-Sirāḷen, Doḍakā.

III-C-(1) कोशातकी Kosātakī; Kaḍu Doḍaki (Rasa P. 1-74).

(2) क्ष्वेड Kśwed Tikta Kosātakī (Aruna Kalpa.1-41).

(3) क्ष्वेड : कोशातकी चोक्तं मृदङ्गफलमेवच । अत्यर्थ कटुः । (Ca. Kalp. 6-

58.(५३) अश्मन्तकः Aśmantakaḥ

अश्मन्तकश्चन्द्रकस्तु[1] कुद्दाली चाम्लपत्रकः ।
श्लक्ष्णत्वक् मालुकापर्णः[2] स्मृतो यमलपत्रकः ॥१९९

अश्मन्तकः कषायस्तु हिमः पित्तकफापहः ।
मधुरः शीतसंग्राही दाहतृष्णाप्रमेहजित् ॥२००

अश्मन्तकः (Aśmantakaḥ), चन्द्रकः (Candrakaḥ), कुद्दाली (Kuddālī), अम्लपत्रकः (Amlapatrakaḥ), श्लक्ष्णत्वक् (Ślakśṇatwak), मालुकापर्णः (Mālukāparṇaḥ), यमलपत्रकः (Yamalapatrakaḥ), are synonymous.

Aśmantaka is *kaṣāya* (astringent) and sweet in taste, *śītavīrya* and pacifies *pitta* and *kapha doṣas,* astringent in action. It is useful in burning sensation, thirst (*tṛṣṇā*) and diseases characterized by polyuria.

There may be included more than two plants but two are identified here. A-अश्मन्तक : (Asmantakaḥ proper) and B-अम्लपत्रकः (Amlapatrakaḥ).

(Fam.-Leguminosae; Sub.fam.-Caesalpinae). Caesalpinaceae.

I- A-*a*- ***Bauhinia racemosa*** Lam.

b- Dymock, *c*-Throughout India, *d*-Apte.

B-*a*- ***Bauhinia malabarica*** Roxb.

b- Priyavrata, *c*-Sub-Himalayan tracts, S. India.

II- A-a- अश्मन्तकः (Aśmantakaḥ), चन्द्रकः (Candrakaḥ).

b- H.Zinjorā; Mar.-Apṭā; Guj.-Asondaro; Tam.-Arikka; Tel.-Pacnāre, Ari.

B-a- अम्लपत्रकः (Amlapatrakaḥ).

b- H.-Khaṭṭā patrowālā zinjorā; Mar.-Koraḷā; Tel.-Pulla dendur; kan.-Ceppuru; B.-Karamai.

---

१ 'श्चेन्द्रकस्तु' इति पा. २ 'वालुकापर्णः' इति पा.

III- b- अश्मन्तकस्तु शफरी चाम्लपत्रक इति भावमिश्रः । युग्मपत्रः । (Harshe).

c- (1)अश्मन्तक Khaṭṭā patrowālā Kacanāra. (Tripathi; Cakradutta, Aṣmari ci.)

(2)अश्मन्तकःअम्ललोटः (Aśmantakaḥ Amlaloṭaḥ)(Cakra Su. i-15-33)

59. (५४) कोविदारः Kowidāraḥ*

कोविदारेऽथं कुद्दालः कुम्भारः कुण्डली कुली ।
ताम्रपुष्पश्चमरिको महायमलपत्रकः ॥ २०१

कोविदारः कषायस्तु संग्राही व्रणरोपणः ।
गण्डमालागुदभ्रंशशमनः कुष्ठकेशहा ॥ २०२

कोविदारः (Kovidāraḥ), कुद्दालः (Kuddālaḥ), कुम्भारः (Kumbhāraḥ), कुण्डली (Kuṇḍalī), कुली (Kulī), ताम्रपुष्पः (Tāmrapuṣpaḥ), चमरिकः (Camarikaḥ), महायमलपत्रकः (Mahāyamalapatrakaḥ) are synonymous.

Kovidāra is *kaṣāya* in taste and astringent in action. It is useful in wound healing, scrofula, anal prolapse, diseases of the skin and hair.

Under this heading it seems four plants are included. A- कोविदारः (Kowidāraḥ), B-काञ्चनारः (Kāñcanāraḥ), C-चमरिकः (Chamarikaḥ) D-सुवर्णारः (Suwarṇāraḥ).

(Fam.-Leguminosae, Sub-fam. Caesalpinae).

I- A-*a*- ***Bauhinia candida*** Willd.

b- Roxburgh, (Mahajan).

B-*a*- Not identified.

C-*a*- ***B.purpurea*** Willd.

D-*a*- ***B.tomentosa*** Willd.

b- C-*a* & D-*a*-Kamat,

II- A-*a*- कोविदारः(Kovidāraḥ).

---

१ कोविदारः काञ्चनारः इति आनन्दा. मुद्रित पुस्तके पाठः ।

*कोविदारादि द्रव्याणि वमनोपयोगित्वादत्र निर्दिष्टानि । तत्तु हृदये (अ.हृ.क.१,६.८)
अथादाय ततो मात्रां जर्जरीकृत्य वासयेत् ।
शर्वरीं मधुयष्ट्या वा कोविदारस्य वा जले ॥
कर्बुदारस्य बिम्ब्या वा नीपस्य विदुलस्य वा ।
शणपुष्प्याः सदापुष्प्याः प्रत्यक्पुष्प्युऽदकेऽथवा ॥
ततः पिबेत्कषायं तं प्रातर्मृदित गालितम् ॥८ ॥
इत्यत्र द्रष्टव्यम् ।
वमनद्रव्योपयोगी द्रव्याणि अधिकारानुसारेण अवस्थान्तराणि च वीक्ष्य प्रयोज्यानि । S.D.K.

b- H.-Kacanāra; B.-Kancāna; Tel.-Kāncana; Mar. Bom.-Pāṇdharā Kāncana.

C-*a*- ताम्रपुष्पः (Tāmrapuṣpaḥ), चमरिकः (Camarikaḥ), महायमलपत्रकः (Mahāyamalapatrakaḥ).

b- H.Sona, Koliār; Kaniār; B.-Devakāncan, Rakta Kāncana Korial; Mar.-Deva Kancan, Rakta Kāncan, Tel.-Pedda-āre; Tam Peuyāre, Mandarca; Kan.-Sarul, Surūl Kancivala.

D-*a*- पीतपुष्पः (Pītapuṣpaḥ).

b- H.-Kacanār; Guj.-Asundro; Kokan - Cāmel; Mar.-Piwaḷā Kāncana; Tam.-Kancani.

d,e,f,g,-See current names.

F-(1) *B.tomentosa* Willd.

Flowers large, of a pale sulphur colour (Roxb).

(2) *B. purpurea* Willd.

Leaves from five to six inch long. (Roxb.)

60. (५५) आवर्तकी Āwartakī *

विषाणिकः Viṣāṇikaḥ (?) (विषाणिका) Viṣāṇikā (Raj. Ni.)

आवर्तकी बिन्दुकिनी[1] विभाण्डी पीतकीलका[2] ।
चर्मरंगा पीतपुष्पा महाजालिनिरुच्यते ॥ २०३

आवर्तकी च कुष्ठघ्नी सोर्ध्वाधोदोषनाशिनी ।
कषाया शीतला वृष्या त्रिदोषघ्न्यतिसारजित् ॥२०४

शोफगुल्मोदरानाह कृमिजालविनाशिनी ।

आवर्तकी (Āvartakī), बिन्दुकिनी (Bindukinī), विभाण्डी (Vibhāṇḍī), पीतकीलिका (Pītakīlakā), चर्मरङ्गा (Carmaraṅgā), पीतपुष्पा (Pītapuṣpā), महाजालिनी (Mahājālinī) are synonymous.

Āvartakī is *kaṣāya* (astringent) in taste, *śītavīrya;* is useful in skin disorders and removes the *doṣas* from both the routes (oral and anal). It is *vṛṣya,* pacifies three *doṣas* and useful in diarrohea. It is used in oedema, tumors, ascites, tympanitis and (intestinal) helminths.

(Fam.-Sterculiaceae).

---

* गणद्रव्यावल्ल्यां 'विषाणिकः' इति पदं दृश्यते । तत्स्थाने पर्यायनामद्रव्यावल्ल्यां गुणसंग्रहे च 'आवर्तकी' ति-पदं दृश्यते । तत्र तु 'विषाणिकः' इति पदं पर्यायनामेषूचितम् । 'सोर्ध्वाधोदोषनाशिनी' इति गुणसंग्रहोऽपि अवधेयः'। 'विषाणिका' इति पर्यायः गुणभिन्नत्वं च । राजनिघण्टौ तु 'विषाणिका' इति पर्यायः। स.दि. कामत.

१ " तिन्दुकिनी " इति आनन्दाश्रम मुद्रित पुस्तके पाठः ।

२ " पीठिका लता " इति नि.शे. टीकायां पाठः ।

I- *a*- ***Helicteres isora*** Linn. Willd.
b- Kamat, *c*-Throughout India. Abundant in W. Ghasts.
d- Apte.

II- *a*- तिन्दुकिनी(Tindukinī),विषाणी(Visāsṇī),पीतकीलकः (Pītakīlakaḥ), महाजाली (Mahājālī), वामावर्ता (Wāmāvartā).
b- B.-Atamor; H.-Marorphali; Kokan-Kewaṇ, Muruḍāseng; Eng.-The East Indian Screw Tree.

III- See Āhulyam (Raj.ni.).
b- (1)आवर्तकी महाजालिनिका स्याद् नीलपुष्पिका। 1230 'रक्तपुष्पिका रेचनी (Bh. Pr. Ni).
(2)' रक्तः आहुलीं, तमरवल्ली, रक्तपुष्पी वामविषाणिका 'द्रव्य रत्नाकरे' (Ni. Shi. Pade).
d,c,f,g,-See current names.

IV- (1) मरोरफली आवर्तकी (Abhi. Butti Darpa.; Desai; Priyavrata; Bhagirath).

61.(५६) शणपुष्पी Śaṇapuṣpī

शणपुष्पी बृहत्पुष्पी सा चोक्ता शणघण्टिका ॥२०५
महाशणो[१] माल्यपुष्पी वमनी कटुतिक्तका ॥
शणपुष्पी रसे तिक्ता वमनी कफपित्तजित् ॥ २०६
वातघ्नी कण्ठहृद्रोगमुखरोगविनाशिनी ॥

शणपुष्पी (Śaṇapuṣpī), बृहत्पुष्पी (Bṛhatpuṣpī), शणघण्टिका (Śaṇaghaṇṭikā), महाशणः (Mahāśaṇaḥ), माल्यपुष्पी (Mālyapuṣpī), वमनी (Vamanī), and कटुतिक्तका (Kaṭutiktakā) are synonymous.

Śaṇapuṣpī is bitter in taste and emetic, It pacifies three *doṣas* and is useful in diseases of throat, heart and mouth.

(Fam.-Leguminosae, Sub-fam.-Papilionaceae). Fabaceae.

I- A-*a*- ***Crotalaria retusa*** Linn.
b- Mahajan, *c*-tropical regions of India from Himalaya to Ceylon.

II- *a*- शणघण्टिका (Śaṇaghaṇṭikā), महाशणः (Mahāsaṇāḥ).
b- H.-Zuṇazuniā, Ban sun; Mar.-Ghagarī, B.-Pipuli zuṇjhun.

१ 'महाशणा' इति चन्द्रनन्दन टीकायामुल्लिखितः ध.नि. पाठः ।

62. (५७) बिम्बी Bimbī

बिम्बी रक्तफला तुण्डी तुण्डिकेरफला च सा ।२०७
ओष्ठोपमफला गोल्हा पीलुपर्णी च तुण्डिका ॥
तुण्डिका कफपित्तासृक्शोफपाण्डुज्वरापहा ॥२०८
श्वासकासापहा तज्जं फलं वातकफावहम् ॥

बिम्बी (Bimbī), रक्तफला (Raktaphalā), तुण्डी (Tuṇḍī), तुण्डिकेरफला (Tuṇḍikeraphalā), ओष्ठोपमफला (Oṣṭhopamaphalā), गोल्हा (Golhā), पीलुपर्णी (Pīluparṇī), and तुण्डिका (Tuṇḍikā), are synonymous.

Bimbī pacifies *kapha -pitta* and *rakta doṣas* It is useful in odema anaemia. fever and dyspnoea and cough. It's fruit aggravates *vātakapha doṣa.*

This includes two kinds : A-कटुबिम्बी (Kaṭubimbī) and B-स्वादुबिम्बी (Swādu bimbī).

(Fam.-Cucurbitaceae).

I- B-*a-* ***Coccinia indica*** W. & A.*
=*Cephalandra indica* Naud.
Syn.-*Momordica monadelpha* Roxb.
b- Roxburgh, (Mahajan), *c-*Throughout India.

II- *a-* रक्तफला (Raktaphalā), तुण्डी (Tuṇḍī); तुन्डिका (Tuṇḍikā).
b- H.-Kundri, Mar.-Toṇḍali; B.-Tetākaci, Tel.-Dondodaya.

63. हरीतकी Harītakī (५८) त्रिफला Trifalā

हरीतक्यभया पथ्या प्रपथ्या पूतनाऽमृता ॥२०९
जयाऽव्यथा हैमवती वयःस्था चेतकी शिवा ॥
प्राणदा नन्दिनी चैव रोहिणी विजया च सा ॥२१०
कषायाऽम्ला च कटुका तिक्ता मधुरसान्विता ।
इति पञ्चरसा पथ्या लवणेन विवर्जिता ॥ २११
अम्लभावात् जयेद्वातं पित्तं मधुरतिक्तकात् ।
कफं रूक्षकषायत्वात् त्रिदोषघ्नी ततोऽभया ॥२१२
प्रपथ्या लेखनी लघ्वी मेध्या चक्षुर्हिता सदा ।
मेहकुष्ठव्रणच्छर्दिशोफवातास्रकृच्छ्रजित् ॥२१३

---

* Current accepted name -*Coccinia grandis* (Linn.) Voigt.

वातानुलोमनी हृद्या सेन्द्रियाणां प्रसादनी ।
संतर्पणकृतान् रोगान् प्रायो हन्ति हरीतकी ॥२१४

तृष्णायां मुखशोषे च हनुस्तम्भे गलग्रहे ।
नवज्वरे तथा क्षीणे गर्भिण्यां न प्रशस्यते ॥२१५

हरस्य भवने जाता हरिता च स्वभावतः ।
सर्वरोगांश्च हरते तेन ख्याता हरीतकी ॥ २१६

हरीतकी (Harītakī), अभया (Abhayā), पथ्या (Pathyā), प्रपथ्या (Prapathyā), पूतना (Pūtanā), अमृता (Amṛtā), जया (Jayā), अव्यथा(Avyathā), हैमवती (Haimavatī) वयःस्था (Vayaḥsthā), चेतकी (Cetakī), शिवा (Śivā), प्राणदा (Prāṇadā), नन्दिनी (Nandinī), रोहिणी (Rohiṇī), विजया (Vijayā), are synonymous.

Harītakī is *kaṣāya* (astringent), sour, pungent, bitter and sweet in taste. Except salty taste all the tastes are present in *Harītakī.*

Because of its sour taste it pacifies *vāta doṣa,* due to the presence of sweet and bitter taste it pacifies *pitta doṣa* and due to *rūkṣa* guṇa and *kaṣāya* taste it pacifies *kapha doṣa.* Hence *Harītakī* is said to pacify all the three *doṣas.*

It is *lekhana* (emaciating), *laghu,* intellect promoting and always beneficial to vision. It is useful in diseases characterized by polyuria, skin diseases,ulcers, emesis, oedema, gout and diseases characterized by difficulty in micturition. It is carminative, beneficial to heart and clears the organs of perception. It is usually useful in diseases caused by excessive bulk promoting substances and habits.

Harītakī is not usually indicated in conditions like thirst, dryness of mouth, lockjaw, dysphagia, early stage of fever, emaciation and in pregnancy.

As it originates in the homeland of the God Hara (i.e. the Himalaya), and greenish in appearance, and useful in all types of diseases, it is called as *Harītakī.*

The forms noted by Nighaṇṭus are not yet identified and confirmed. The following plants are named *Harītakī* by the natives and the fruits of them are used as *Harītakī* proper.

(Fam.-Combretaceae).

I- A-*a*- ***Terminalia chebula*** Retz. & Willd.*

For confirmation.

B-*a*-***T.citrina*** Roxb. Var. Malayana Kurz

* The current names *Terminalia chebula* (Gaertn.) Retz.

C-*a*-***T.angustifolia*** Willd.
D-*a*-***T. gangetica*** Roxb.
b-Roxburgh.

Note- The plants B and D are noted as varieties of *T. chebula* Watt. Dict. These varieties are confirmable with the kinds recorded by the Nighaṇṭus

II- A-*a*- हरीतकी (Harītakī), अभया (Abhayā).
b- H.-Harara; B.-Haritaki; Kol-Rola, Hardā; Santal-Rol; Bom., Mar.-Hirdā, Hardā; Guj.-Hardi; Tam.-Kaḍakāi; Tel.-Keraka; Kan.-Hirḍā, Eng.- Black or Indian Myrobalan. The Chebulic myrobalaṇ.
B,C,D-Vernacular names go by the same names as in A-b supra.

III- *d,c,f,g*-See current names and varieties.

64. बिभीतकः Bibhītakaḥ

बिभीतकः कर्षफलो वासन्तोऽक्षः कलिद्रुमः ।
संवर्तको भूतवासः कल्किहार्यो बहेडकः ॥२१७

बिभीतकः कटुः पाके लघुर्वैस्वर्यजित् सरः ।
कासाक्षिवक्त्ररोगघ्नः केशवृद्धिकरः परः ॥२१८

बिभीतकः (Bibhītakaḥ), कर्षफलः (Karṣaphalaḥ), वासन्तः (Vāsantaḥ), अक्षः(Akśaḥ), कलिद्रुमः (Kalidrumaḥ), संवर्तकः (Samvartakaḥ), भूतवासः (Bhūtavāsaḥ), कल्किहार्यः (Kalkihāryaḥ), बहेडकः (Baheḍakaḥ), are synonymous.

Bibhītakaḥ is pungent in *vipāka* and *laghu*. It is laxative and useful in hoarseness of voice. It is used in cough, diseases of the eyes and mouth. It promotes the profuse growth of the hair.

Roxburgh has recorded two plants under the same vernacular name and fruits of both the plants are used for the same purpose.

(Fam.-Combretaceae).

I- A-*a*- ***Terminalia bellirica*** Roxb. (Cooke).*
b- Roxburgh (Cooke), *c*-Throughout the forests of India, *d*-Apte.
B-*a*- ***T.moluccana*** Willd. (Roxb). *b*-Roxburgh.

II- A-*a*- कर्षफलः (Karṣaphalaḥ), वासन्तः (Vāsantaḥ), अक्षः (Akśaḥ),बहेडकः (Beheḍakaḥ), कल्किधर्मघ्नः (Kalkidharmaghnaḥ),

* *Terminalia bellirica* (Gaertn.) Roxb. current accepted name.

b- Kokan-Bhelā; H. Behedā, Sagonā, Ben.-Baherā; Guj.-Behadā; Tam.-Kattuelacpay; Tel. Bahadraha; Kan.-Berdā, Yehale; Eng.-Belleric Myrobalan.

B-*a*- As in II-As-a above.

b- Goes by the same names as in (II-A-b-supra).

Note- In Watt Dict. B-a is recorded as a variety of A-a.

65. वयस्था Vayasthā

वयःस्थाऽऽमलकं वृष्यं जातीफलरसं शिवम् ।
धात्रीफलं श्रीफलं च तथाऽमृतफलं स्मृतम् ॥ २१९

कषायं कटुतिक्ताम्लं स्वादु चामलकं हिमम् ।
सरं त्रिदोषहृद् वृष्यं ज्वरघ्नं च रसायनम् ॥ २२०
हन्ति वातं तदम्लत्वात् पित्तं माधुर्यशैत्यतः ।
कफं रूक्षकषायत्वात् फलं धात्र्यास्त्रिदोषजित् ॥ २२१

वयःस्था (Vayaḥsthā), आमलकं(Āmalakam), वृष्य (Vṛṣyam), जातीफलरसं (Jātīphalarasam), शिवम् (Śivam), धात्रीफलं (Dhātrīphalam), श्रीफलं (Śrīphalam), and अमृतफलं (Amṛtaphalam), are synonyms of *Āmalakī*.

It is *kaṣāya* (astringent), pungent, bitter, sour and sweet in taste, *śitavīrya,* laxative, pacifies the three *doṣas,* is *vṛṣya,* and useful in fever and is *rasāyana.*

The fruit of *Āmalaka* because of its sourness pacify *vāta*, *pitta doṣa* is pacified because of its sweet taste and *śitavīrya* and *kaphadoṣa* due to *rūkṣa guṇa* and *kaṣāya* taste and thus it is a pacifier of all the *doṣas.*

(Fam.-Euphorbiaceae).

I- *a*- ***Emblica officinalis*** Gaertn.

b- Roxburgh, *c*-Common in forests of India.

II- *a*- आमलकम् (Āmalakam), धात्रीफलम् (Dhātrīphalam.)

b- H., B.-Āmlā; Kol.-Aurā; Santal-Meral; Bom., Mar.-Āwali; Guj.-Āmlī; Tam.-Nelli-kai, Tel.-Usereki; Kan.-Nelli, Nilika; Eng.-The embellic myrobalan.

III-*a*-12 Ämalak-Ch. Up.-vii-3-1 (Harshe).

प्राचीनामलकम् Pracīnāmalakam 52.

प्राचीनामलकं प्राचीनारंगंरक्तकं मतम् ।
तत्पक्वं पित्तकफकृद् दुर्जरं गुरु वातजित् ॥ २२२

प्राचीनामलकं (Prācīnāmalakam), प्राचीनारंगं (Prācīnārangam), and रक्तकम् (Raktakam), are synonymous.

The ripe fruit of it aggravates *pitta* and *kapha doṣas,* is difficult to digest and is *guru* and pacifies *vātadoṣa.*

(Fam.-Flacourtiaceae).

I- *a*- ***Flacourtia jangomas*** (Lour.) Raeusch.
Syn.-*F.cataphracta* Willd.(Roxb).
b- Dymock. *c*-Kumaon, Lower Bengal, Assam, Orissa.

II- *a*- प्राचीनारङ्गम् (Prācīnārangam)
b- H.-Pāniāl; Mar.-Pāṇāwalā. Tāmbat; Eng.-Many spined Flacourtia, Guj., Pers.-Talispatra.

III- *Cf.Talisam.*
b- (1)45 प्राचीनामलकम् - जलामलकम् । 'पानीयामलकम् मतम्' इति भावमिश्रः । (Harshe).
d- Cf. current name.

66. (५९) आरग्वधः Āragvadhah*

आरग्वधो दीर्घफलो व्याधिहा चतुरङ्गुलः।
आरेवतस्तथा कर्णी कर्णिकारोऽथ रेचनः ॥ २२३

आरग्वधो रसे तिक्तो गुरूष्णः कृमिशूलनुत् ।
कफोदरप्रमेहघ्नः कृच्छ्रगुल्मत्रिदोषजित् ॥ २२४

आरग्वधः (Āragvadhaḥ), दीर्घफलः (Dīrghaphalaḥ), व्याधिहा (Vyādhihā), चतुरङ्गुलः (Caturangulaḥ), आरेवतः (Ārevataḥ), कर्णी (Karṇī), कर्णिकारः (Karṇikāraḥ) and रेचनः (Recanaḥ) are synonymous.

Āragavadha is bitter in taste, *gurū*, *usṇavirya* and useful in helminthic infestation and colics. It is used in ascites caused by *kaphadoṣa,* and diseases of urinary organs characterized by polyuria, and difficulty in passing urine, and tumors. It pacifies all the *three doṣas.*

---

* ज्वरहृद्रोगवातासृगुदावर्तादिरोगिषु ।
राजवृक्षोऽधिकं पथ्यो मृदुर्मधुरशीतलः ॥A.H. Kalpa 2.30
This verse from A.H. perhaps suggests two varieties of आरग्वध Āragvadha.
(S. D. Kamat)

This heading includes two plants : A-आरग्वधः (Āragwadhaḥ) ,तिक्तः (tiktaḥ, of Dh. Ni.), and B-आरग्वधः मधुरः (Āragwadhaḥ madhuraḥ of Raj. ni.)

For confirmation.

(Fam.-Leguminosae). Caesalpinaceae.

I- A-*a*- ***Cassia rhombifolia*** Roxb.

b- Kamat, *c*-Throughout India.

Confirmed.

B-*a*- ***C. fistula*** Linn. & Willd.

b- Roxburgh, *c*-Throughout India.

II- A-*a*- दीर्घफलः (Dīrghaphalaḥ) ,चतुरङ्गुलः (Caturaṅgulaḥ), कर्णिकारः (Karṇikāraḥ), रेचनः (Recanaḥ), रसेतिक्तः (Rasetiktaḥ).

b- Mar.-Bhāwā, Kadu bhāvā; H.-Choṭā amalatās; Tel.-Kiragakke, Rālā, Gaud-Kotta sonālu, Choṭṭā sonalu-gaccha; B.-Sondalai; Mal.-Valiya Konnā: Keral-Kshudra āragwadha.

B-*a*- अन्य आरग्वधः (Anya āragwadhaḥ), मन्थानः (Manthānaḥ), कर्णाभरणकः (Karṇābharaṇakaḥ), कर्णिकारो महादिः (Karṇikāromahādiḥ, 1st Edn,), (आनन्दाश्रम) महाद्रि (Mahādri, 2nd Edn.),अतिमधुरः (Atimadhuraḥ).

b- H.-Amalatās; Guj.-Garmāḷo; Gaud-Vadsonḍāl, Badā sonālu, Tam,- Konnarai; Mar.-Bahāvā, Bhāvā, Mal.- Konnā, Khani-Khonnā, ceria konrā; Kan.-Kaku; Eng.-Indian laburnam; Purging cassia.

Note-' Valiya ' small ' Ceriya' large (Krishnan).

कर्णिकारः Karṇikāraḥ 55.

कर्णिकारो राजवृक्षः प्रग्रहः कृतमालकः ।
आरोग्यशिम्बी शम्पाको व्याधिघातो व्यथान्तकः ॥ २२५

कृतमालो लघुः शीतः पित्तघ्नो मधुरः सरः ।
तत्फलं मधुरं बल्यं वातपित्तामजित्सरम् ॥ २२६

कर्णिकारः (Karṇikāraḥ), राजवृक्षः (Rājavṛkṣaḥ), प्रग्रहः (Pragrahaḥ), कृतमालकः (Kṛtamālakaḥ), आरोग्यशिम्बी (Ārogyaśimbī), शम्पाकः (Śampākaḥ), व्याधिघातः (Vyādhighātaḥ), and व्यथान्तकः (Vyathāntakaḥ), are synonymous.

Kṛtamāla is *laghu, śitavīrya,* pacifies *pittadoṣa,* sweet in taste and laxative. Its fruit is sweet in taste, pacifies *vāta* and *pitta,* and is useful in *āma* and is laxative.

This heading includes two plants : A-कर्णिकारः Karṇikāra Madhuraḥ (of Dhn.ni.)., This is B-plant under the heading आरग्वधः (Aragvadaḥ) (Vide No. 66-IB-a supra), and the next is B-कर्णिकारो रसेतिक्तः (Karṇikaro rase tiktaḥ). (of Raj.ni.). This is A-plant under the same heading आरग्वधः (*Āragvadaḥ)* (Vide No. 66-I-A-a supra). Alteration of heading names is occured here, such as the name of Raj., ni.'s कर्णिकार (Karṇikāra)is standing here for Dhn. ni.'s आरग्वध (Āragavadha),and vice versa. (Vide No. 66 supra). This arrangement aptly corresponds to the plants included under the headings A and B of Karṇikāra and Äragvadha of both the Ni. s. Traditionally the two plants are termed A-बडा अमलतास (*Baḍā-Amalatās a*nd B-छोटा अमलतास (*Choṭā Amalatās)* respectively to A-कर्णिकारो मधुरः and B- कर्णिकारो रसेतिक्तः).

(Fam.-Leguminosae). Caesalpinaceae.

I- A-*a*- ***Cassia fistula*** Linn. & Willd.

b- Roxburgh, *c*-As in Aragwadha of Raj. Ni. (66-1-B-a supra).

For confirmation.

II- A-*a*- ***C.rhombifolia*** Roxb.,

b- Kamat.

c- as in Āragwadha of Dh. Ni. (66-1-A-a supra).

A-*a*- राजद्रुः (Rājadruḥ), कृतमालः (Kṛtamālaḥ), आरोग्यशिम्बी (Ārogyaśimbī), मधुरः (Madhuraḥ), शम्याकः (Śamyākaḥ), सरः (Saraḥ), फलं मधुरम् (Phalam madhuram).

b- Vernacular names as in आरग्वधः (Āragwadhaḥ 66-11-B-b supra).

B-*a*- सुफलः (Suphalaḥ), परिब्याधः (Parivyādhaḥ), पङ्क्तिबीजकः (Paṅktibījakaḥ), रसेतिक्तः (Rase tiktaḥ), ब्याधिरिपुः (Vyādhi ripuḥ).

b- Vernacular names as in आरग्वध (66-11-A-b supra).

III- *a*- (1)कर्णिकारद्वयम् (Raj. ni. Varga 9th).

(2) 56आरग्वध-शंप्याक (Ceriya konrā) (Krishnan).

(3) 57 कर्णिकार-आरग्वधो द्वितीयो राजाह्वः कोशफलः । abhi. Manj. valiya konna - (Krishnan).

(4) कर्णिकारः कटुः तिक्तः शोधनो लघुः (Bh. Pr. ni.);

(5) अथ द्रुमोत्पल कर्णिकारः द्रुमेउत्पलम् कर्णिकामियर्ति । 'ऋ गतौ'। कट-चंपक इति ख्यातस्य । (Bhanuji).

(6) 422 कर्णिकारः काण्ठचम्पक इति रामः । + दीर्घफलः कनकपुष्पिका । (Harshe).

(7)आरग्वधः; केरळ - वंकोन्ना . हेमक ता. कोंन्ना. महा.. बहावा; हि,-अमलतास; वंग-सोनालु (Ayur. 0. Ni.)

(8)कर्णिकारः; के.-चेरुकोन्ना; माहा.-लघु बहावा. मदनपाल निघण्टौ गणनिघंटौ कर्णिकार आरग्वध पर्यायौ दृश्येते. (Ayur.O.Ni.).

IV- (1) *Cf.* कर्णिकार (Ni. Adarsha).

(2) गणेरुका कर्णिकारश्च (Dh. ni. Āmrādi Varga V; Vargetara).

(3) A-कनियार वा कनकचंपा *Pterospermum acerifolium;* B-अमलतासभेद, छोटा अमलतास , क्षुद्रसोनालु. लघुबहावा ; तेलगु - किरुबक्के. (Ayur. Vishwa Kosh).

(4) आरग्वध-वृक्षविशेषः । कर्णिकार-आरग्वध विशेषः "पिण्ड बीजकः लघ्वावारग्धः' कोटद् सोनालु इति भाषा; (Shabda Kalpa, Part II).

(5) A-कर्णिकार-थोरबहावा, वृक्ष कमल. B-व्याधिघात-थोरबहावा,लघुबहावा (Joshi).

Note- (The author Bhagirath, in his book has scored all points raised on these plants and lastly apporaches to the conclusion that "by following Shastra we must take notice that the name, कर्णिकार (Karnik̄ara) we must include अमलतास and गणिकारिका (Gaṇikārikā) only. No any other plant is कर्णिकार(Bhagirath).

(6) 17 *Cassia fistula* Linn, Āragwadha. H. Amalatās; Mal.-Konna, Khani Konnā. two varieties of Aragwadha, viz, Kṛtamāla (Ceriya Konna) and Caturaṅgula (ValiyaKonnā) are described in Abhi. Manj. (Moos).

(7) According to Raj. Ni. Chotā Amalatās is identified as कर्णिकार, (Dwivedi).

(8) कर्णेषु योग्यं नवकर्णिकारम् (Rtu. Sam. VI-5 Kalidas).

(9)आकृष्ट हेमद्युति कर्णिकारम (Ku. Sam., iii-53 Kalidas). सुवर्णादपि कान्तिमन्नइति यावत्कर्णिकारस्तदारव्य कुसुमानि यस्मिन्तत (Gajendragadakar).

(10) हुतहुताशनदीप्ति वनश्रियः (Raghu. VI-90- Borwankar).Tika आज्यादि प्रज्वलित अग्निप्रभं यत्कुसुमम् । कर्णिकारमित्यर्थः। (Mallinath).

(11) वर्णप्रकर्षे सति कर्णिकारं दुनोति निर्गन्धतया स्मचेतः ।

(Ku. Sam. vi. 6-20).

Following plants are recorded as कर्णिकार (Karnikāra) by some modern writers.

(12) *Pterospermum acerifolium* Linn.(Chopra, Desai, Dymock, Watt. Dict.)

Note- This is a kind of Mucakunda tree.

(13) *Erythrina species.* Indian Coral tree Pānderavo; Pāngrā.

Note- Flowers of the above plants are shining red.

(14) *Pavetta indica* Linn. Indian Pavet (W.Jones IV-248).

Note- Nasik Tryamback adivasi- Papat; flowers, white. This may be

गणिकारिका (Gaṇikārikā) गणेरुका (Gaṇerukā) of Nighaṇṭus and Bhagirath. (Vide Note under IV- 5 supra).

(15) *Bauhinia species (*Ni. Adarsh).

Note- In this genus includes युग्मपत्र (Yugmapartra) species of कांचनार (Kāñcanār) अश्मन्तक (A'smantaka) etc.

(15) *Cassia auriculata* and *marginata* (Moos). Note- Tarawada, āhulī etc.

(16) *Abroma augusta* Linn. Fl. Ulaṭakambal. (Pdt. Bhagirath).

67. (६०) दन्ती Dantī

दन्ती शीघ्रा निकुम्भा स्यात् उपचित्रा मुकूलकः ॥ २२७
तथोदुम्बरपर्णी च विशल्या च घुणप्रिया ॥

दन्ती तीक्ष्णोष्णकटुका कफवातोदरान् जयेत् ॥ २२८
अर्शोव्रणाश्मरीशूलान् हन्ति दीपनशोधनी ॥

दन्ती (Dantī), शीघ्रा (S'ighrā), निकुम्भा (Nikumbhā), उपचित्रा (Upacitrā), मुकूलकः (Mūkūlakaḥ), उदुम्बरपर्णी (Udumbaraparṇī), विशल्या (Vis'alyā), घुणप्रिया (Ghuṇapriyā) are synonymous.

Dantī is *tīkshṇa, uṣṇavīrya,* pungent in taste and pacifies *kapha* and *vātadoṣa.* It is used in ascites, piles, ulcers, calculus affections and colics. It has purificatory action and stimulates digestive capacity.

This heading includes two plants : A-उदुम्बरपर्णी(Udumbara parṇi), B-एरण्डपत्रिका (Eraṇḍa patrikā, (Raj. ni.)

(Fam.-Euphorbiaceae).

I- A-*a*- ***Baliospermum montanum*** Muel.- Arg.*
Syn.-*Croton polyandrus* Roxb.

b- Desai, *c*-From Kasmir to Bhutan, W. India.

B-*a*- See द्रवन्ती (Dravantī, infra).

II- A-*a*- विशल्या (Vis'alyā), निकुम्भा (Nikumbhā), दन्ती (Dantī).

b- H.-B.-Dāti; Mar.-Dātī; Tel.- Adavi, Amudam, Konda-amumdam.

B-*b*- See द्रवन्ती (Dravantī).

---

*The current name is - *Baliospermum montanum* (Willd.) Muel. - Arg.

III- *Cf.* Nāgadantī and Putraśreṇī of Raj. ni.

b- (1) 40 दन्ती Nākkānanti (Abhi. Manji.).

(2) 23 दन्ती (Sū. 9) Maḷ.- Nirwalamar., Tel.- Konda amadum *Baliospermum montanum, Jatropha montana.* (Vaidya).

(3) लघुदन्ती, वृषदन्ती- (Vidyotani).

d- See current names.

IV- (1) See दन्ती (Dantī). Vaidya Jangale.-Kirtikar, Priyavrata.

Note- *Croton polyandrum* Wight, *C. axilare* Bl. are synonyms of *Baliospermum* montanum.

अरणी Araṇī 56.(वरणी Varaṇī)*

अरणी च वराङ्गी च तथैव च जयावहा ॥ २२९
आवर्तकी केशरुहा तथैव विषभद्रिका ॥
वरणी तु रसे तिक्ता शूलत्वग्दोषनाशिनी ॥ २३०
कफवातोदरार्शांसि हन्ति दीपनशोधनी ॥

अरणी (Araṇī), वराङ्गी (Varāṅgī), जयावहा (Jayāvahā), आवर्तकी (Āvartakī), केशरुहा (Keśaruhā) and विषभद्रिका (Viṣabhadrikā) are synonymous.

Varaṇī is bitter in taste and pacifies *kaphavāta doṣas.* It is useful in colics, diseases of skin, ascites, piles and stimulates the digestive capacity and has a purificatory action.

Not confirmed.
(Fam. -Euphorbiaceae).

I- a- ***Jatropha multifida*** Linn.

b- Chopra, c-Cultivated in gardens.

Note- Introduced from New World, but When? Is it not a naturlized plant ?

रेचकः Recakaḥ 57.

रेचको जयपालश्च सारकस्तिन्तिडीफलम् ॥ २३१
दन्तीबीजं मलद्रावी निकुम्भो बीजरेचकः ॥

---

* 'वरणी'इति चौखम्बामुद्रितपुस्तके पाठः । 'अरणी' इति आनन्दा. पुस्तके पाठः । बरणी रित्यपि पाठभेदः क्वचित् पुस्तकेषु । S.D.K.

कुम्भीबीजं निकुम्भाह्वबीजं तत्कुम्भिनीफलम् ॥ २३२
जेपालः कटुरुष्णश्च कृमिहारी विरेचनः ।
दीपनः कफवातघ्नो जठरामयनाशनः ॥२३३

रेचकः (Recakaḥ), जयपालः (Jayapālaḥ), सारकः (Sārakaḥ), तिन्तिडीफलम् (Tintiḍiphalam), दन्तीबीजं (Dantībījam), मलद्रावी (Maladrāvī), निकुम्भः (Nikumbhaḥ), बीजरेचकः (Bījarecakaḥ), कुम्भीबीजं (Kumbhībījam) निकुम्भाह्वबीजं (Nikumbhāhvabījam), and कुम्भिनीफलम् (Kumbhinīphalam), are synonymous.

Jepāla is pungent in taste, and pacifies *kapha-vāta doṣas*, It is useful as anthelmintic and purgative. It stimulates appetite and is used in ascites.

(Fam. Euphorbiaceae).

I- *a-* ***Croton tiglium*** Linn.
b- Roxburgh, *c*-Naturlīsed and cultivated throughout India. (Chopra).

II- *a-* जयपालः (Jayapālaḥ), दन्तीबीजम् (Dantībījam).
b- H.Bom.-Jamālgota; Mar-Jepāḷ;Tel.-Nepal; Tam.-Mal.-Nerawalam.

III- *Cf.* Dantī. *c*-दन्ती (Jayapāla mūlam). (Gu. Dip. Bindughṛta).

IV- (1) See Vaidya Phadake.

68. (६९) द्रवन्ती Drawantī

द्रवन्ती शम्बरी चित्रा न्यग्रोधा मूषकाह्वया ॥
प्रत्यक्श्रेणी वृषा चण्डा[१] पुत्रश्रेण्यारवुपर्णिका ॥ २३४

द्रवन्ती ग्रहणीतृष्णा त्रिदोषशमनी हिता ॥
अभिष्यण्णतनौ ग्रथ्यां प्रमेहे जठरे गरे ॥ २३५

कफपित्तामये पाण्डौ कृमिकोष्ठभगंदरे ॥
द्रवन्ती ह्द्रोगहरा कफकृमिविनाशिनी ॥ २३६

द्रवन्ती (Dravantī), शम्बरी (Śambarī), चित्रा (Citrā), न्यग्रोधा (Nyagrodhā), मूषकाह्वया (Mūṣakāhvayā), प्रत्यक्श्रेणी (Pratyakśreṇī), वृषा

---

१ 'रण्डा ' इति नि.शे. टीका संमतः पाठः ।
It is to be noted that Raj.ni. has mentioned 'द्रवन्ती' in his पर्पटादि parpaṭādi chapter V while he had mentioned पुत्रश्रेणी (Putraśreṇī) in his Guḍūcyādi 3rd chapter . It is mentioned under the heading आखुकर्णी and is not purgative . S.D. Kamat

(Vṛṣā), चण्डा (Caṇḍā), पुत्रश्रेणी (Putraśreṇī), आखुपर्णिका (Ākhuparṇikā), are synonymous.

Dravantī is useful in diseases of *Grahaṇī,* thirst and pacifies the three doṣas, when the body has become dull, in glandular swellings on the body, diseases charecterized by polyuria, ascites and artificial posionoing.

It is used in anaemias due to *kapha* and *pitta dosas,* helminthic infestations, fistula in ano, in the diseases of heart, and in the parasitic infestations due to *kapha doṣa.*

Not Confirmed.
(Fam. Euphorbiaceae).

I- A-*a*- ***Jatropha glandulifera*** Roxb.

II- *a*- शम्बरी (Śambarī); चित्रा (Citrā), न्यग्रोधी (Nyagrodhī), आंखुकर्णिका (Ākhukarṇikā) पुत्रश्रेणी (Putraśreṇī).

b- B.-Śāmbarī; Guj.-Moto nepālo. Ratanjota; H.-Mugalāī eraṇḍa; Mal.-Veluta nakananti.

III- *Cf.* Danti Sutaśreṇī (Raj. ni.).

b- (1)41 द्रवन्ती Veluta nākananti (Abhi. Manj.)

(2) द्रवन्ती (Su. 15श्यामागण)+ ताम्रवर्ण विशिष्टमूलो एरण्डतुल्यबीजो सक्षीर स्वनामख्यात विशेषः + Jatropha curcusपुत्रश्रेणीतिपाठः । एरण्डसदृशफलपत्राल्पविटपा संबरीति लोके इति डल्हणः । समुद्रैरण्ड इति केचित्. (Vaidya).

IV- (1)द्रवन्ती *Jatropha curcas*. (Ni. Adarsha).

Note- *Jatropa glandulifera* may be identified with putraśreṇī of (parishiṣṭa) Raj.ni. (see Roxb. *J. glandulifera*).

69. (६२) नीलिनी Nīlinī

नीलिनी नीलिका काला ग्राम्या दोला[१] विशोधनी ।
तुत्था श्रीफलिका मोचा भारवाही[२] च रञ्जनी ॥ २३७

नीली तिक्ता रसे चोष्णा कटिवातकफापहा ॥
केश्या विषोदरं हन्ति वातासृक् कृमिनाशिनी ॥ २३८

नीलिनी (Nīlinī), नीलिका (Nīlikā), काला (Kālā), ग्राम्या (Grāmyā), दोला (Dolā), विशोधनी (Viśodhanī), तुत्था (Tutthā), श्रीफलिका (Śriphalikā), मोचा (Mocā),भारवाही (Bhāravāhī), and रञ्जनी (Rañjanī) are synonymous.

---

१ 'मेला' इति क्षी. संमतः पाठः ।
२ 'सारवाही' इति. क्षीर. संमतः पाठः ।

Nīlī is bitter in taste and *uṣṇavīrya* . It is useful in backaech, promotes growth of hair, ascites due to poison, gout and worms.

(Fam.-Leguminosae). Fabaceae.

I- A-*a*- ***Indigofera oblongifolia*** Forsk.
Syn.- *I. paucifolia* Delib., and other speices of *Indigofera.*
b- Kamat; *c*-Throughout India.

II- A-*a*- काला (Kālā), विशोधनी (Viśodhanī), भारवाही (Bhārawāhī), रञ्जनी (Rañjanī), क्लीतनी (Klītanī).

70. (६३) स्नुक् Snuk

स्नुक् स्नुही[1] च महावृक्षो गुडा निस्त्रिंशपत्रिका ॥
समन्तदुग्धा गण्डीरः[2] सेहुण्डो वज्रकण्टकः ॥ २३९

सेहुण्डस्तु रसे तिक्तो गुरूष्णः कफवातजित् ॥
दुष्टव्रणाश्मरीं हन्ति तथा वातविशोधनः ॥ २४०

स्नुहीक्षीरं विषाध्मानगुल्मोदरहरं परम् ॥

स्नुक् (Sunk), स्नुही (Snuhī), महावृक्षः (Mahāvṛkśaḥ), गुडा(Guḍā), निस्त्रिंशपत्रिका (Nistriṃśapatrikā), समन्तदुग्धा (Samantadugdhā), गण्डीरः (Gaṇḍīraḥ), सेहुण्डः (Sehuṇḍaḥ), and वज्रकण्टकः (Vijrakaṇṭakaḥ) are synonymous.

Snuk is bitter in taste, *guru, usnavirya* and pacifies *kapha* and *vāta.* It is useful in nonhealing (septic) wounds, calculus and has purificatory action on *vāta doṣa.*

The milky juice of *Snuhī* is very useful in poisons, tympanitis, tumors and ascites.

(Several forms or speices are recorded under this heading. Some of them are noted herebelow : A-शाखाकाण्डा (Śākhākāṇḍā), B-निस्त्रिंशपत्रिका (Nistrimsapatrika), C-वज्रवृक्षः (Vajravṛkśaḥ), and D-त्रिधारा (Tridhārā).

(Fam. Euphorbiaceae).

I- A-*a*- ***Euphorbia neriifolia*** Linn. (Watt).
Syn.-*E. ligularia*. Roxb.
B-*a*- ***E. nivulia*** Buch.-ham. (Watt).

---

१ 'सुधा' नि.शे. टीकायाम् ।

२ 'गण्डीरा' इति. नि.शे. संमतः पाठः ।

C-*a*- ***E. tirucalli*** Linn. (Watt).

D-*a*- ***E. antiquorum*** Linn.

b- All are identified by Kamat.

II- A-*b*- Mar.-Minguṭa, Nivaḍunga.

B-*a*- Mar.-Newarunga, Niwaḍunga.

C-*b*- Mar.-Sera, Thoṛa, H.-Sehunḍa, B.-Lankāsija.

D-*b*- Mar.-Tinadhārī niwaḍunga.

Note- Medicinal virtues of एरण्डपत्रिका are not recorded here by the Nighaṇṭus.

71. (६४) सातला Sātalā

सातला सप्तला सारी[1] विदुला विमलाऽमला ॥ २४१
बहुफेना चर्मकषा फेना दीप्ता मरालिका[2] ॥

सातला शोधनी तिक्ता कफपित्तास्रदोषनुत् ॥ २४२
शोफोदराध्मानहरा किञ्चित् मारुतकृत् भवेत् ॥

सातला (Sātalā), सप्तला (Saptalā), सारी (Sārī), विदुला (Vidulā), विमला (Vimalā), अमला (Amalā), बहुफेना (Bahuphenā), चर्मकषा (Carmakaṣā), फेना (Phenā), दीप्ता (Dīptā), and मरालिका (Marālikā), are synonymous.

Sātalā is bitter in taste and has purificatory action on *kapha, pitta* and *rakta doṣas.* It is useful in oedema, ascites, tympanitis and aggravates *vātadoṣa* slightly.

For confirmation.
(Fam.-Legumionosae). Mimosaceae.

I- a- ***Acacia concinna*** DC. var. ***rugata***

b- Dymock; c-Himalayas.

a- *A. concinna* DC.*

b- Dymock, c-Tropical jungles of India.

II- a- सारी (Sārī), विमला (Vimalā), अमला (Amalā), बहुफेना (Bahuphenā), चर्मकषा (Carmakaṣā), शोधनी (Sodhanī), विषाणिका (Viṣāṇikā), स्वर्णपुष्पी (Swarṇa puṣpī), चित्रघना (Citraghanā).

b- H.-B.-Bana riṭhā; Guj. Cikākāī; Tel.-Sikaya; Tam.- Sikai; Mar.- Sikekāī; Eng.-Soap-nut acacia.

---

१ 'सारा' इति क्षी. पाठः । २ 'सनालिका' इति. क्षीर. पाठः ।

* The current accepted name is *Acacia rugata* (Lamk.) Merr.

Note- Vernacular names of both the plants are the same.

III- a- 5-Amalā-J.Up. Br.- 1-38-6; Ch. UP. VIII-3-1 (Harshe).

b- (1) सातला (Sū. 6) सातला नामाख्या रिठाकरंजः *Acacia-concinna* Soap-nut acacia; Mar., Sikekāi; Tel. Cikāy; Tam.-Ciyākkā, Cinikkā; Mal.-Cikkākāī, (Vaidya)

c- 1-सप्तला यवतिक्ताभेदा, स्नुहिभेदः । (Dalhan Ci. 31-5)

(2) सातला-पीत सेहूंड, चोक (Coka). (Dipika, Hapushadi and Maha-Khandava churna).

(3) सातला -सप्तला सेहुण्डभेदः (Dalhan Kalp. A.5; Su. A-44).

(4) 473 विमलेति सातला सेहुण्ड भेदः (Harshe).

Note-IV- (1) सातला -स्नुहिभेद. (Priyavrata, Vidyotani, Dwivedi).

(2) सप्तला - सिकेकाई (Sikekāī), (Ghanekar Sū.38-28; Athawale, Nadkarni, Dymock).

72. क्षीरिणी Kśīriṇī (६५) कांचनक्षीर्यौ Kāñcanakśīryau

क्षीरिणी कांचनक्षीरी कटुपर्णी च कर्षणी ॥ २४३
तिक्तदुग्धा हैमवती हेमदुग्धा हिमावती ॥

तिक्ता तु काञ्चनक्षीरी पित्तकृमिविषापहा ॥ २४४
शोधनी दोषसंघातशमनी रक्तपित्तजित् ॥

क्षीरिणी (Kśīriṇī), कांचनक्षीरि (Kāñcanakśīrī), कटुपर्णी (Kaṭuparṇī), कर्षणी (Karṣaṇi), तिक्तदुग्धा (Tiktadugdhā), हैमवती (Haimavatī), हेमदुग्धा (Hemadugdhā), and हिमावती (Himāvatī) are synonymous.

Kāñcanakśīrī is bitter in taste and has purificatory action on *doṣas*. It is useful in *pittadoṣa,* helminthic infestation and is antipoisonous. It is used in haemorrhagic disorders.

For confirmation.
(Fam.-Euphorbiaaeae).

I- A-a- ***Euphorbia thomsoniana*** Boiss.

b- Kirtikar, c-Kashmir above 1000ft.

II- a- कांचनक्षीरी(Kāñcanakśīrī),

b- Hiravi, Hirṭiza, Hiyāwalī.

III- *Cf.* Sarwakśirī; infra.

IV- See Ghanekar Sū. 39-3.

सर्वक्षीरी Sarvaksīrī 59. स्वर्णक्षीरी Swarṇaksīrī

स्वर्णक्षीरी स्वर्णदुग्धा सुवर्णक्षीरिकाऽपि च ॥ २४५
हेमाह्वा कनकक्षीरी हेमक्षीरी च कांचनी ॥
क्षीरिणीयुगुलं तिक्तं कृमिपित्तकफापहम् ॥ २४६

स्वर्णक्षीरी (Swarṇakśīrī), स्वर्णदुग्धा (Swarṇadugdhā), सुवर्णक्षीरिका (Suwarnakśīrikā), हेमाह्वा (Hemāhvā), कनकक्षीरी (Kanakakśīrī), हेमक्षीरी (Hemakśīrī), and कांचनी (Kāñcanī) are synonymous.

Both the types of *kśiriṇī* are bitter in taste and useful in helminthic infestations and pacifiy *kapha* and *pitta doṣas.*

(Fam.-Papaveraceae).

I- *a*- ***Argemone mexicana*** Linn.

b- Kamat, *c*-Throughout India.

II- *a*- स्वर्णदुग्धा (Swarṇa dugdhā), कांचनक्षीरी (Kāñcanakśīrī),कांचनी (Kāñcanī).

b- Eng.-The Mexican poppy, Prickly poppy; Santāl- Gokhul -junum; (Awari) Bilāya; N. W.P. -Bhārbhurvā, Kawah; Mar.-Piwaḷādhotrā, Coka, Kaḍasarā, Pisoḷā, H. -Satyānāsī, Ujarkanṭ, Siyālkanṭa; Guj.-Daruḍi.
For Tamil and Maliyal names see Krishnan, Vaidya and Ayur. O. Ni. (III 3, 4 and 5 infra).

III- *a*- कांचनक्षीर्यौ (Su. ci-8-3.9).

b- (1) हेमाह्वा तस्य मूलम् चोकमुच्यते; 'नेत्रे क्षिप्तं घृताप्लुतं' । शुक्रं च अधिमांसं च + नाशयेत् (Ni. Shiromani; Ramateja).

(2) चोषनाम गुणाः हेमाह्वा, सत्यानासी चौषमूलम् (Ramprasad.);

(3) 59, 60 कांचनक्षीरी, पीतपुष्पः कंकुष्टम् . Malayaruma, Swarṇa kśiri. (Krishnan).

(4) H.-कटुपर्णी (Kaṭuparṇī) Keral; मलयेरुम्, एरुमक्कल्ली; Tam.-कुकुनीर द्विविधैषास्ति इति नृसिंहः । (Ayur. O-Ni).

(5) कांचनक्षीरी (Kāñcanakśīrī). (ci.15).कंटकी कंटपत्रा च + iti Siva-ni. Argemone mexicana.
Tel. Brhamadanḍi; Kan.-Arisin ummatta, Gola golike; Datturi gida, Cikkanike; Tam.-Kuttiyotti; Piramataṇṭu Mal.-Ponumattam Kaṭuparṇī चोकमूल Bh. Pr. (Vaidya) .

(6) कटुपर्णी(चोक Coka). हेमाह्वा + तस्यामूलं चोक *Argemone mexicana,* Satyānāsi (Coka). (Vidyotani).

c- (1) स्वर्णक्षीरी. कनकपुष्पी. (Cakra Ci. 7-3, Su. 4-9-4; Ci-8-67; Dalhan Su. 44-49; 39.3).

(2) हेमाह्वा ह्वात्री -चोक (Rasa. Pp. 1.165; 5-161.)

(3) हेमाह्वा ह्वात्री -चोक (Coka).चोष.
(Dipika; Gud.-Dipika; Hapushādi Churṇa; Narāyāṇa Churṇa Icchābhedi; Swarṇa kshiri rasa).

d- The name *Argemone* is derived from small ulcer in the eye' (Watt, p. 325).

Note- (Vide supra III-B-1).

Note- The plant सत्यानासी (Satyānāśī) पिवळा धोत्रा (Pivaḷa dhotrā) the vulgar name of which is recorded as चोष, चोक and also is recorded a synonym for सुवर्णक्षीरी (Suvarnakśirī) by the commentators of the 11th century, is now identified by the botanists of to-day as *Argemone mexicana,* Linn. This identifcation of commentators proves that the plant *A. maxciana* was present in India before the arrival of Portuguese.

IV- (1) दारुडी (गु) पिवळा धोत्रा (Mar.)-*Argemone mexicana,* but ancient Swarṇakśirī is not this. "What evidence have we do say it native? " (Ni. Adarsha).

(2) Hiravi- is not Choka. Ayurvedic "Choka" is the root of 'Satyānāsī Swarṇakshirī (Ayurved Vijnyān year viii-10).

(3) It is not possible to say whether *Argemone mexicana* and similar American plants were introduced either before or after the discovery of America. (Chief Botanist, Botanical Survey of India, Havra, Calcutta).

Note- A reply to the author.

(4) स्वर्णक्षीरी - *Cleome felina*-Syn-*Polanisia felina* (U.C.Dutt).

(5) काटे धोत्रा Kāte Dhotrā, Pivḷā Dhotrā, Pisorā 'Chok', (Ni. Ratnakar; Dra. Ratnakar).

(6) Two kinds of Swarṇakśirī, one is Satyānāsī and the next is Hirvī (Yadavji).

(7) Ayur. Patrika-15-2-1971, P. 241.

73. (६६) श्यामा Śyāmā

श्यामा त्रिवृन्[१] मालविका मसूरविदला च सा ॥
कालाऽर्धचन्द्रा पालिन्दी[२] सुषेणी कालमेष्यपि ॥ २४७

१ अरुणा त्रिवृत् Aruṇā trivṛt is not noted by Dhn. Ni. & Raj. Ni. D. K. Kamat
२ "कालिन्दी " इति आनन्दाश्रम मुदित पुस्तके पाठः ।

त्रिवृता कटुरूष्णा तु कृमिश्लेष्मोदरज्वरान् ॥
शोफपाण्ड्वामयप्लीहान् हन्ति श्रेष्ठा विरेचने ॥ २४८

श्यामा (Śyāmā), त्रिवृत् (Trivṛt), मालविका (Mālavikā), मसूरविदला (Masūravidalā), काला (Kālā), अर्धचन्द्रा (Ardhacandrā), पालिन्दी (Pālindī), सुषेणी (Suṣeṇī), and कालमेषी (Kālameṣī), are synonymous.

Trivṛt is pungent, and *usṇavīrya.* It is useful in worms, ascites caused by *kapha,* fevers, oedema, anaemia, diseases of spleen and is the best amongst purgatives.

(For confirmation).
(Fam.Convolvulaceae).

I- A-*a*- ***Ipomea pes-caprea*** Sweet.*
Syn.-*I.biloba* Forsk; *Convolvulus pes-caprea*, Linn. Sp. Pl.; *C. bilobatus* Roxb.
b- Kamat. *c*-Throughout peninsular India -abundant along sea shores.
B-*a*- ***Lettsomia atropurpuria***. (Nadkarni).
b- Nadkarni, *c*-Nepaḷ and Sikkim.

II- A & B-*a*- त्रिवृन्मालविका(Triwṛnmālavikā), श्यामाऽर्धचन्द्रा (Śyāmārdhacandrā),कालिन्दी (Kālindī),कालमेषी (Kālameṣī) त्रिवेलावनिऽचन्द्रा (Trivelā-awanicandrā), श्रेष्ठाविरेचने (Śreṣṭhāvirecane).
A-*b*- Sk.; Sāgaramekhalā, Vṛddhadāraka, Maryādavallī , H.-Tam.- Dopātillatā, B.-Chagalkhuri; Guj.- Ārvel; Mar.- Maryādvel; Adambu; Kan.-Adumb, Mal.- Cukanna atampu; Tel. - Civulpillitige
B-*b*- Eng.-Black turpethum. Vern. names not known.

III- *Cf.* Vṛddha dāraka; Śukrabhāṇḍī.
b- (1) 44 श्यामा(Śyāmā), Mālavikā; Kālameṣī, Karuthā trikop Konnā. (Krishnan).
(2) 45 महाश्यामा (Mahāśyāmā)- Nāikkolpa Konnā (Kṛṣṇan).
c- (1) श्यामा (Śyāmā); Mālavikā.trivṛt (Aruna). Kṛṣṇamūlātrivṛt (Hemadri. Sū. 15-45)
श्यामा, महाश्यामा (Syāmā) (Mahāsyāmā) (Dalhan, Sū. 38-29).
d, c- See current names.

IV- (1) Black turpethum. *Lettsomia atropurpuria.* Nepal, *Ipomoea pescaprea.*
(Mhaskar, Jangale, Nadakarni; Desai).

---

* The current name *Ipomea pes-caprea* (Linn.) Sweet.

शुक्लभण्डी Śuklabhaṇḍī 60.

शु[1]क्लभण्डी त्रिभण्डी स्यात् काकाक्षी सरला त्रिवृत् ।
सर्वानुभूतिस्त्रिपुटा त्र्यस्रा कुमुदगन्धिनी ॥ २४९
कषाया मधुरा चोष्णा विपाके कटुका त्रिवृत् ।
कफपित्तप्रशमनी रुक्षा चानिलकोपनी ॥२५० A.H.Kal. 2.1& ca. Kal.7.5

शुक्लभण्डी (Śuklabhaṇḍī), त्रिभण्डी (Tribhaṇḍī), काकाक्षी (Kākākṣī), सरला (Saralā), त्रिवृत् (Trivṛt), सर्वानुभूतिः (Sarvānubhūtiḥ), त्रिपुटा(Triputā), त्र्यस्रा (Tryasrā) and कुमुदगन्धिनी (Kumudagandhinī) are synonymous.

It is *kaṣāya* (astringent) and sweet in taste, pungent in *vipāka*. It pacifies *kapha* and *pitta* doṣas, is *rūkśa* and therefore aggravates *vātadoṣa*.

This heading includes two plants. A-अरुणत्रिवृत् (Aruṇatrivṛt), and B-रक्तमूलत्रिवृत् (Raktamūlātrivṛt). (Raj.ni).

For confirmation.
(Fam.-Convolvulaceae).

I- A-*a*- ***Operculina turpethum*** Silva Manso*
b- Kamat, *c*-Throughout India, cultivated in gardens .

II- A-*a*- शुक्रभाण्डी(Śukrabhāṇḍī), त्रिवृत् (Trivṛt), बहुरेचनी (Bahurecanī).
b- H.-Nisoth; B.-Dudhia Kalmi; Santāl-Bana etka; Bom.-Nisottar, Phutkarī; Tam.-Sivadai; Tel.-Tella tigeda; Eng.-Turpeth root; Indian jalapa, False jalapa.
कुटरणी -शुक्लात्रिवृत् Dalhan Su. Sū. 15.30
कुटरणी -त्रिवृत् - पदा.चन्द्रि. कुटरणी - अरुणमूला त्रिवृत् Hemadri

III- *d,e,g*-See current names.

74. (६७) ऐन्द्री Aindrī

ऐन्द्रीन्द्रवारुणीन्द्राह्वाऽथेन्द्रवारु[2]र्मृगादनी ॥
गवादनी क्षुद्रफला वृ[3]षभाक्षी गवाक्ष्यपि ॥ २५१

---

१ 'शुक्ला चापि त्रिभण्डी स्यात् काकाक्षी सरला त्रिवृत् ।
सर्वानुभूति स्त्रिपुटा त्र्यस्त्रा कूटरबृंहिणी ॥
आम्भसी रेचनी चैव कण्ठविक्षोभणी तथा ।" इति क्षीर. संमतः पाठः ।
२ 'इन्द्रैर्वारुर्विषादनी ' नि.शे. टीकायाम् ।
३ 'विशालाक्षी इति नि.शे. टीकायाम्
* The current name is *Merremia turpethum* (Linn.) Shah & Bhatt

इन्द्रवारुणिकाऽत्युष्णा रेचनी कटुका तथा ॥
कृमिश्लेष्मव्रणान् हन्ति हन्ति सर्वोदराण्यपि ॥ २५२

ऐन्द्री (Aindrī), इन्द्रवारुणी (Indravāruṇī), इन्द्राह्वा (Indrāhva), इन्द्रवारुः (Indravāruḥ), मृगादनी (Mṛgādanī), गवादनी (Gavādanī), क्षुद्रफला (Kśudraphalā), वृषभाक्षी (Vṛṣabhākṣī), and गवाक्षी (Gavākṣī) are synonymous.

Indravāruṇī is exessively *uṣṇavīrya,* purgative, and pungent in taste. It is useful in worms, *kaphadoṣa* and wounds (ulcers) and in all types of ascites.

This heading includes two plants. A-ऐन्द्री (Aindrī proper) and the next B-रक्तेर्वारु (Rakterwāru).

(Fam.-Cucurbitaceae).

I- A-*a*- ***Citrullus colocynthis*** Schrad.*
b- Dymock, c-Self sown in cultivated fields.
B-*a*- See विशाला next plant.

II- A-*a*- इन्द्रवारुणी (Indrawāruṇī), गवादनी (Gawādanī).
b- H.-Indrāyaṇa; B.-Indrāyana, mākhāl; Mar.-Indrāwaṇa, Kaḍu indrāwaṇa; Tam.-Peykonmati, Pedikāri; Tel.-Paparbudam; Kan.-Havumekee

III-*Cf.* Trapusa.

75(६८). विशाला Viśālā

अन्येन्द्रवारुणी प्रोक्ता विशाला च महाफला ।
आत्मरक्षा चित्रफला त्रपुसी[१] त्रपुसा च सा ॥ २५३

इन्द्रवारुद्वयं तिक्तं कटुपाके रसे लघु ॥
वीर्योष्णं कामलापित्तकफश्लीपदनाशनम् ॥ २५४

The other kind of इन्द्रवारुणी *Indravāruṇī* is called as विशाला Viśālā of which synonyms are महाफला (Mahāphalā), आत्मरक्षा (Ātmarakśā), चित्रफला (Citraphalā), त्रपुसी (Trapusī), and त्रपुसा (Trapusā).

Both types of *Indravāruṇī* are bitter and pungent in taste, and

---

* current name *Citrullus colocynthis* (Linn.) schrad.

१ 'तुवसी' इति क्षीर. संमतः पाठः ।
'तुम्बसी त्रपुसी इति नि.शे. टीकायाम् ।

vipāka, laghu and *uṣṇavīrya.* They are useful in jaundice, *pitta, kapha doṣas* and filariasis.

(Fam.-Cucurbitaceae).

I- *a*- ***Trichosanthes bracteata*** (Lam.) Voigt.
Syn.-*T. palmata* Roxb.

b- Dymock, *c*-Throughout India.

II- *a*- अन्येन्द्रवारुणी (Anyendrawāruṇī), महाफला (Mahāphalā), चित्रफला (Citraphalā), महेन्द्रवारुणी (Mahendrawāruṇī), रम्या (Ramyā), दीर्घवल्ली (Dīrghavallī).

b- Sk.-Mahākāla; H.-Lal indrāyana; B.-Mākāl-Kokan-Kawaṇḍala; Peth-Nasik -Dholambā; Guj.- Rātā indrawaṇa; Kan.- Kaka mandali; Tel.-Abbaguda; Tam.-Kurattai.

d,e,f-See current name and synonym.

IV- See Desai, Vidyotani, Dwivedi.

श्वेतपुष्पी Śwetapuṣpī 61.

श्वेतपुष्पी मृगाक्षी च मृगैर्वारुर्मृगादनी ॥
हस्तिदन्ती नागदन्ती वारुणी गजचिर्भटा ॥ २५५

कण्ठरोगापचीश्वासकासप्लीहकफोदरान् ॥
मूढगर्भं च हरति कुष्टदुष्टव्रणान् जयेत् ॥ २५६

There is an another type of *Viśāla* called as श्वेतपुष्पी *Śvetapuṣpī* of which synonyms are मृगाक्षी (Mṛgākśī), मृगैर्वारु (Mṛgairvāru), मृगादनी (Mṛgādanī), हस्तिदन्ती (Hastidantī), नागदन्ती (Nāgadantī), वारुणी (Vāruṇī) and गजचिर्भटा (Gajacirbhaṭā).

It is useful in diseases of throat, scrofula, dyspnoea, cough, diseases of spleen and ascites due to *kpahadoṣa.* It removes foetal obstruction, diseases of skin and in chronic ? (septic) wounds (ulcers).

Not identified.

76. (६९) त्रायमाणा Trāyamāṇā

त्रायमाणा कृतत्राणा त्रायन्ती त्रायमाणका ॥
बलदेवा बलभद्रा वार्षिकी गिरिसानुजा ॥ २५७

---

१ गिरिजानुजा' इति पाठा.। 'गिरिसानुजम् इति क्षीर.

त्रायन्ती कफपित्तास्रगुल्मज्वरहरा मता ॥
उष्णा कटुकषाया च सूतिकाशूलनाशिनी ॥२५८

त्रायमाणा (Trāyamāṇā), कृतत्राणा (Kṛtatrāṇā), त्रायन्ती (Trāyantī), त्रायमाणका (Trāyamāṇakā), बलदेवा (Baladevā), बलभद्रा (Balabhadrā), वार्षिकी (Vārṣikī), गिरिसानुजा (Girisānujā) are synonymous.

Trāyantī is pungent and *kaṣāya* (astringent), *uṣṇavīrya* and useful in pacifying *kapha, pitta* and *rakta doṣas*. It is also useful in tumors, fevers and purpureal colics.

There is a difference of opinion regarding the identification of this drug. Majority of writers, among whom are B.L. Gupte, C. Chakravarti, Nadkarni, Dhurye, and Dr. Waring have identifed A- *Thalictrum foliolosum* DC., but by some other writers B-*Delphinium zalil* Aitch. is identified as Trāyamāṇā (त्रायमाणा).

For confirmation.
(Fam.-Ranunculaceae).

I- A-*a*- ***Thalilctrum foliolosum*** DC.
b- Nadakarni, *c*-Inner vallies of Himalayās W. Tibet.
B-*a*- ***Delphinium zalil*** Aitch. & Hemsl.*
b- Yadavji, c-Afaganistan and Persia.

II- A & B-*a*-वार्षिकम् (Vārṣikam), गिरिसानुजा (Girisānujā),त्रायन्ती (Trāyantī), बलदेवा (Baladewā), तिक्तवल्कला (Tiktawalkalā).
A-*b*- Sk.-Trāyamāṇā; H.-Mamirā, Pinjarī, (P.B.), Gur-biyani, Pili pinjar;
Khasi-Caitrā.
B-*b*- Sk.-Trāyamāṇā, H.-Asabar; Bom.-Gulzala;Yunanī Gule gāphis; Arab-Gāfis, Zarria, Pers.-Asaphrak, Zalila; Panj.-Asabarg, Gāphis.

III- *a*- त्रायमाण त्रैकुदाञ्जनम् (AV.iv.-9-1.).

IV- (1) त्रायमाण (Trayamāṇā).**
In 'Muhite Ajam' Gule.-gaphis is noted as Trāyamāṇā (Yadavji; Abhi. butti. Darp; C.A.D.).
(2) *Delphinium zalil* DC. Aitch and Hemsl.
H. -Asburgh (the dye), Gāphis (Medicine); Khorasan -Zalil, Arab-Zarir, Bom.-Trāyamāṇā, Gul Zarir, Pers,-Asfrak; Asperag, Trāyamāṇa (Watt Dict).

Note - The plant (I-B-a supra) may be the 'Trayaman' of Vedic age when according to the Theory of Historians, these Vedic people were in Central, Asia.

---

* Current name - *Delphinium semibarbatum* Blenert ex Boiss.

** Ach. Yadavji introduced *Gentiana kurroo* Royle as its source plant which is now accepted.

77. (७०) यवतिक्ता Yawatiktā (शंखिनी Śaṅkhinī)

यवतिक्ता शंखिनी तु दृढपादा विसर्पिणी ॥
नाकुली चाक्षपीडा च नेत्रमीला यशस्करी ॥ २५९
शंखिनी कटुतिक्ताम्ला गुरुः स्निग्धा विशोधनी ॥
त्रिदोषशमनी कुष्ठश्वयथूदरनाशनी ॥ २६०

यवतिक्ता (Yavatiktā), **शंखिनी** (Śaṅkhinī), **दृढपादा** (Dṛḍhpādā), **विसर्पिणी** (Visarpiṇī), **नाकुली** (Nākulī), **अक्षपीडा** (Akṣapiḍā), **नेत्रमीला** (Netramīlā), **यशस्करी** (Yaśaskarī), are synonymous.

Śaṅkhinī is pungent, bitter and sour in taste, *guru*, unctuous, and purificatory. It pacifies three *doṣas*, and useful in skin diseases, anasarca and ascites.

This heading includes two plants : A-**शंखिनी**(Śaṅkhinī) and B-**यवतिक्ता** (Yawatikatā).

For confirmation.
(Fam. Convolvulaceae).

I- A-*a*- ***Ipomoea grandiflora*** Roxb.
Syn.-*I. bona-nox Jack* (Roxb.Fl).
Syn.-*I -bona-nox* Linn. (Watt Dict.)
Calonyction bona-nox Boj-var. *grandiflora*.
Syn.-*I.bona-nox* Linn. (Balwant Simha, Bihar). *C.aculeatum* House.
Syn.-*I.-bona-nox* Linn. (Chopra).
b- Kamat.

Confirmed.

B-*a*- ***Ipomoea caerulea*** Roxb.*
Syn.-*Ipomoea hedracea* Jacq. =*I. caerulea* Koen.
Convolvulus nil Linn. (Roxb). *Pharbitis choisy*. (Kirtikar).
b- Kamat, *c*-Throughout India. cultivated and wild, in Himalaya above 6000 ft.

II- A-*a*- **विसर्पिणी** (Visarpiṇī), **तण्डुली** (Taṇḍulī), **नेत्रमीला** (Netramīlā), **तिक्ताम्ला** (Tiktāmlā), **पत्रतण्डुली**(Patrataṇḍuli).
b- B.-Dudhiya-Kalami; H.-kouḍenā, Cāndani; Mar.-Moṭhī bhovari;Guj.-Kumpānā velā; Eng.-Moon flower (Watt Dict); Sk. Kṛṣṇa bijā; Yavatiktā-bheda, Kālānjañī sadṛsāswetapuṣpā.

B-*a*- **महातिक्ता** (Mahātiktā),**सूक्ष्मपुष्पी** (Sūkṣmapuṣpī).
b- Sk.-Kālāñjanī. Kṛṣṇa bijā, B.-Nil kamal; H.-Kālā dānā, Kouḍenā,

---

* Current name - *Ipomea nil* (Linn.) Roth. (Comp. p. 83)

III- b-(1) शंखिनी (Śankhinī), (Su.15) शंखिनी Śankhinī śweta budhnyām iti Medini.

(2) H.- Yavocī; Kokan-Mhaisikārt; Mar.-Yavoci, Tiṭavi, Sākhavel,
Tel.- Poṭṭi budamu, Kudarubudā; Kan.-Maniṭopanṭe kanda. pavatte walli; Mal-Mukka pirum, Kiriwalli. *Mukia scabrella; Bryonia scabrella* Yawatiktā 'Kalamegha' iti Bhāsyākaraḥ (Vaidya)

c- (1) शंखिनी (Śankhinī) Yawatiktā bheda, bṛhatpatrā-Yawatiktā bheda,
Swetabudhnā (Dalhan Su. 39-4, 38-29),

(2) शङ्खिनी-कालाञ्जनी सदृशश्वेतपुष्पा । (Hemadri Su. 15-2).

(3) अक्षिपीडकः -पीडयित्वा यद्रसोऽक्षिण दीयते सो अवपीडोऽक्षिपीडकः इति गंगाधरः । (Foot note Ca-Viṣa 22-215).

d,f-See current names and synonyms.

Note- बुघ्नः A bottom of a vessel; The + lowest part. (Apte). कोटर :-रं - Hollow of a tree (Apte) *Cf.* -अंतः कोटरपुष्पी शंखिनी -श्वेतबुघ्ना (Cakara. Ca,. Su. 1-81-82)

IV- (1) Kālādānā यवतिक्ता (Yawatikā). Let us accept also for the time being as the कालमेघ (Kālamegha).
Andrographis paniculata Nees, Sachitra Ayur. 10-1961)

(2) There is another kind of this climber which is '*Calonyction bononox* Boj var, *grandiflora.* Syn. *Ipomoea bona-nox* Linn. 'Candrakāntī' Cāndaṅi (Moon flower). Flowers very odorous, white and open only at night. (Balwantji, Bihar).

(3) *Ipomoea grandiflora* Roxb. Flowers remarkably large pure-white. (Roxb).

78. (७८) अङ्कोटः Ankotah

अङ्कोटोऽङ्कोलको रेची निर्दिष्टो दीर्घकीलक ॥
पीतसारस्ताम्रफलो गन्धपुष्पो निकोचक : ॥ २६१

अंकोलः स्निग्धतीक्ष्णोष्णः कटुको वातनाशनः ॥
कुक्कुराखुविषं हन्ति ग्रहजन्तुविषापहः ॥ २६२
भूतहृद् विषहृच्चैव कण्ठ्यः सूतस्य शोधनः ।

अंकोटः (Ankoṭaḥ), अंकोलकः (Ankolakaḥ), रेची (Recī), दीर्घकीलकः (Dīrghakīlakaḥ), पीतसारः (Pītasāraḥ), ताम्रफलः (Tāmraphalaḥ), गन्धपुष्पः

(Gandhapuṣpaḥ), and निकोचकः (Nikocakaḥ), are synonymous.

Aṅkola is pungent in taste, *tikṣṇa*, unctuous (*snigdha*), *uṣṇavīrya* and pacifies *vātadoṣa.* It is useful in dog and rat's poisons, disorders caused by *grahas* (seizures) (or psycological disorders) (or micro organisms), poisons, is beneficial to throat and in purificatory process of mercury.

(Fam.-Alangiaceae).

I- *a*- ***Alangium salvifolium*** Wang.*
Syn.-*A. lamarckii* Thwait.
b- Dymock, *c*-Northern India, Common from Punjab to Bengal, rare in Poona Dist.

II- *a*- अंकोलकः (Aṅkolakaḥ), रेची (Recī), दीर्घकीलकः (Dīrghakīlakaḥ), ताम्रफलः(Tāmraphalaḥ),गूढमल्लिका (Gūḍhamallikā).
b- H.-Akola; Mar.-Akoli, Akali; Tel.-Akolum; Tam.-Alangi.

III- c- श्वेतअखोल (Rasa P. Cintamani tail).

79. (७२) अपामार्गः Apāmārgah

अपामार्गस्तु शिखरी प्रत्यक्पुष्पी मयूरकः ॥ २६३
अधःशल्योऽथ किणिही दुर्ग्रहा खरमञ्जरी ॥
स चैवोक्तः शैखरिको मर्कटी दुरभिग्रहः ॥ २६४
पराक्पुष्पी वशिरश्च कण्टी मर्कटपिप्पली ॥

अपामार्गस्तु तिक्तोष्णः कटुश्च कफनाशनः ॥ २६५
अर्शः कण्डूदरामघ्नो रक्तहृद् ग्राहिवान्तिकृत् ॥

अपामार्गः (Apāmārgaḥ), शिखरी (Śikharī), प्रत्यक्पुष्पी (Pratyakpūṣpī), मयूरकः (Mayūrakaḥ), अधःशल्यः (Adhaḥśalyaḥ), किणिही (Kiṇihī), दुर्ग्रहा (Durgrahā), खरमञ्जरी (Kharamañjarī), शैखरिकः (Śaikharikaḥ), मर्कटी (Markaṭī), दुरभिग्रहः (Durabhigrahaḥ), पराक्पुष्पी (Parākpuṣpī), वशिरः (Vaśiraḥ), कण्टी (Kaṇṭī) and मर्कटपिप्पली (Markaṭpippalī) are synonymous for *Apāmārga.*

Apāmārga is bitter, pungent and *uṣṇavīrya* and pacifies *kapha*. It is useful in piles, prutitus, ascites, *Āmadoṣa,* haemorrhgic disorders, and is astringent and emetic.

---

*Current name *Alangium salvifolium* (Linn. f.) Wang

(Fam.-Amaranthaceae).

I- *a- **Achyranthes aspera*** Linn.
b- Roxburgh, *c-*Throughout India. Weed.

II- *a-* मयूरकः (Mayūrakaḥ), खरमञ्जरी (Kharamañjarī).
b- H.-Lātajirā, ciracirā; Mar.- Aghāḍā; Guj.-Aghāḍo; Kan.-Uttaraṇi, Tel. -Uttareni; Tam.-Nyaruwi Nayakkuruwi; Kocarink, Mal.-Katalāti, Vankatalati.

III- a- (1) प्रतीचीन फलोहित्वपामार्गरुरोहिय- (AV-Kanda-vii-65, vi-18).

रक्तपुष्पः Raktapuṣpaḥ 62.

अन्यो रक्तो रक्तपुष्पो वशिरः कपिपिप्पली ॥ २६६
क्षुद्रापामार्गको रक्तः ख्यातको रक्तपूर्वकः ॥

अपामार्गोऽरुणो वातविष्टम्भी कफनाशनः ॥२६७
व्रणकण्डूविषघ्नश्च संग्राही वान्तिकृत्परः ॥

There is an another red kind of *Apāmārga* of which synonyms are रक्तपुष्पः (Raktapuṣpaḥ), वशिरः (Vaśiraḥ), कपिपिप्पली (Kapipippalī), क्षुद्रापामार्गकः (Kśudrāpāmārgakaḥ), रक्तः (Raktaḥ), रक्तपूर्वकः (Raktapūrvakaḥ).

Raktāpāmārgaḥ pacifies *kaphadoṣa* causes flatulance and is useful in wounds (septic), pruritus, and poisons. It is astringent in action and powerful emetic.

I- a- Red flowering kind of *Achyranthes aspera* Linn.
b- Kamat, c-As in (79 supra).

II- a- अघट्टकः(Aghaṭṭakaḥ); रक्तोऽपामार्गः (Rakto pāmārgaḥ).
b- Vernacular names as in (79-II-A-b supra).

80. (७३) तेजस्विनी Tejaswinî

तेजस्विनी तेजवती तेजोह्वा तेजनीति च ॥ २६८
अश्वघ्नी वल्कला शीता पारिजाता महौजसी ॥

तेजोह्वा श्लेष्मवातघ्नी रुच्या दीपनपाचनी ॥ २६९

---

१ 'तेजनी तिजा' इति नि.शे. टीकायाम ।
(तेजस्विनी) This may be a form of *Celastrus paniculatus* S.D. Kamat,.

तेजस्विनी (Tajasvinī), तेजवती (Tejavatī), तेजोह्वा (Tejohvā), तेजनी (Tejanī), अश्वघ्नी (Aśvaghnī), वल्कला (Valkalā), शीता (Śītā), पारिजाता (Pārijātā), and महौजसी (Mahaujasī) are synonymous.

Tejasvinī pacifies *kapha* and *vāta doṣas*, improves desire for food, is appetiser and digestant.

The heading includes two plants, A-तेजोवती (Tejowatī) and B-तेजस्विनी (Tejaswinī).

For confirmation.
(Fam.-Rutaceae).

I- A-*a*- Bark of ***Zanthoxylum alatum*** Roxb.
b- Kamat, *c*-Sub-tropical valleyes of the Himalayas.

Confirmed.
(Fam.-Celastraceae).

B-*a*- ***Celastrus paniculatus*** Willd.
b- Dymock. *c*-Sub-Himalayan tracts, M. Pradesh, Hilly parts of Bombay and Madras State.

II- A-*a*- तेजवती (Tejawatī),वल्कला (Valkalā),कनकप्रभा (Kanakaprabhā), बहुरसा (Bahurasā).
b- Mar.-Tiraphal, Ciraphala; Sk. -Tumbaru; B.-Nepālidhaniā Tāmbula H.P.-Tejabalā, Urdu-Kabābe; Kan.-Tumaruḍu.

B-*a*- सुवर्णनाकुली (Suwarṇanākulī), अग्निदीप्ता (Agnidīptā), कङ्गुणी (Kanguṇī), सुतैला (Sutailā), पीततैला (Pītatailā), मेघ्या (Medhyā).
b- Sk.-Jyotiṣmatī, Kaṅguṇī; Bom.-Kangaṇicīvel; Mar.-H., B.-Mālkangoṇī.

III- *Cf* jyotiṣmatī, Karnasphoṭā and Tejaphala in Raj. ni. Parishiṣṭa.
a- ज्योतिष्मती (Jyotiṣmatī)-Mūlani, तेजस्विनी (Tejaswinī)-Twacā (Aṣtānga, San. Si. Virechan, A. 14).
b- (1) पीततैला (Pīta tailā) Valli Tejowati samā/ Jotismatya. (Harshe).
(2) 254तेजोव्हा–Tejaswinī तेजबल इति प्रसिद्धा (Harshe).
(3) 180 -तेजोवती (Tejowatī)- Jyotiṣmatī (Harhse)
(4) 202 कङगुणिका (Kanguṇikā Pitatailā ज्योतिष्मती Jyotiṣmatī) Kanguṇikā तेजवती(Tejawatī) (Tejohvā/Harshe).
(5) तेजोवती ((Tejovati) (Ci.4)-महाज्योतिष्मती.
Mar.-Tejabala; Eng.-Tooth ache tree.
Zanthoxylum hostil. Cavike ti Cakraduttah (Vaidya).
(6) ज्योतिष्मती (Jyotiṣmatī (Sū. 21)मालकांगणी, कानपुटी, शिवजाला; *Cardiospumum halicacabum* (Vāidya). (used in Bengal).

(7) तेजोवती (Tejowatī), Jyoṣtismatī; (Malkangaṇī), (Tripathi, Visarp. A-14).

(8) 298 तेजवती (Tejawatī), Pīta tailā Kangūnikā ceti. (Abhi. Man).

(9) 299 तेजस्विन्नापरा (Tejaswinnāparā), Kaṭabhī lawaṇāgnibhāsā (Abhi. Man.).

IV- (1) अश्वघ्नी तेजस्विनी (Tejaswinī Tejavatī).
H.Guj.-Tejabala; Mar.-Tirphal; *Zanthoxylum budranga, Z.alatum; Z, rhetsa (*Bhagirath).

Note - *Z.budranga* Wall. syn. *Z.rhetsa* DC. (Chopra).

(2) Synonyms to-
Celastrus paniculata Willd. Syn. -*C. alnifolia* Don.
C. depandens Wall. *C. nutans* Roxb.
C.multiflora Roxb. (Watt Dict.).

Note- The names तेजोवती (Tejovati) and तेजस्विनी (Tejaswini) are indiscriminately used for the plants तेजोवतीवल्कला and तेजवती. But the synonmys कङ्गुणी,पीततैला अग्निदीप्ता are particulariy applied to तेजस्विनी (1-B-a supra), These synonyms correspond to and are identified as *Celastrus paniculata.*

Note - Dhn. ni. notes *Tejovati* only but Raj. ni. adds *Tejaswini* plant more.

81. (७४) ज्योतिष्मती Jyotismatī

ज्योतिष्मती तु कटभी सुवर्णलतिकेति च[1] ॥
ज्योतिष्कायाऽग्निभासा[2] च लवणोक्ता च दुर्जरा ॥२७०

ज्योतिष्मती कटुस्तिक्ता सरा कफसमीरजित् ॥
अत्युष्णा वमनी तीक्ष्णा वह्निबुद्धिस्मृतिप्रदा ॥२७१

ज्योतिष्मती (Jyotiṣmatī), कटभी (Kaṭabhī), सुवर्णलतिका (Suvarṇalatikā), ज्योतिष्काया (Jyotiṣkāyā), अग्निभासा (Agnibhāsā), लवणोक्ता (Lavaṇoktā), and दुर्जरा (Durjarā) are synonymous.

Jyotiṣmatī is pungent and bitter in taste and laxative. It pacifies *kapha* and *vāta doṣas,* is excessively *uṣṇavīrya tīkṣṇa,* emetic. It promotes digestive (assimilative) capacity, intellect and memory.

Not identified.*

१ 'स्यात् सुवर्णलतेति च' नि.शे. टीकायाम् ।
२ 'चाग्निभा सा च लवणोदा च दुर्दिनी ' इति नि.शे. टीकायाम् ।
३ 'लवणोत्का च दुर्दिना' इति क्षीरस्वामी संमतः पाठः
* It is better to identify this as *celastrus painculatus*

82. (७९) रास्ना Rāsnā

रास्ना युक्तरसा रस्या श्रेयसी रसना रसा ॥
सुगन्धमूलाऽतिरसा सैव पूतिरसा¹ स्मृता ॥ २७२

रास्ना गुरुश्च² तिक्तोष्णा विषवातास्रकासजित् ॥
शोफकम्पोदरश्लेष्मशमन्यामस्य पाचनी ॥२७३

रास्ना (Rāsnā), युक्तरसा (Yuktarasā), रस्या (Rasyā), श्रेयसी (Śreyasī), रसना (Rasanā), रसा (Rasā), सुगन्धमूला (Suandhamūlā), अतिरसा (Atirasā), and पूतिरसा (Pūtirasā) are synonyms.

Rasnā is *guru*, bitter in taste, *uṣṇavīrya*, and alleviates effects of poisons, *vātarakta,* cough, oedema, shaking of body (? parkinsonism), ascites. It pacifies *kapha* and digests *āmadoṣa.*

For confirmation.
(Fam.-Compositae).

I- *a-* ***Inula helenium*** Linn.
b- Bhagirath *c-*See Potters cyclo. (IV-2infra).

II- *a-* रसना (Rasanā),सुगन्धमूला (Sugandhamūlā),अतिरसा (Atirasā),
b- Sk.-Rāsnā; Arab.-Janjabil-i-šāmi; Eng.-Elecampana, scab wort.

III- *Cf.* Nākulī, Mahasugandhā, Vandakā.
a- अगुरु(1) रास्ना(2) रुहा (3) रोहा (4) नाकुली (5) गन्धनाकुली (6).
(Ca.Ci. 3-2 67).

Note- Agaru (1), Rāsnā (2), Ruhā (3), Rohā (4), Nākulī (5), Gandhanākulī (6)
These six plants are noted together in one stanza. This arrangement shows that everyone of these members are considered separately as a different plant from each other, "Vandāka should be substituted if Rāsnā is not available" says Bhavamishra,

b-(1) त्र्यर्थेश्रेयसी –Rāsnā , Harītakī, Hastipippalī, (Kṣīraswāmi 2-4- 60).
(2) व्यर्थेसुवहा- Rāsnā, Sephālikā, Gandha nākulī. (Amar 2-4-71).
(3)त्र्यर्थेरसा – Rāsnā , Sallakī, Pāthā. (Kṣīraswāmī 2-4-85).
(4) रास्ना (Rāsnā) एलापर्णी (Bh. Pr. Ni. Harītakyādi).
(5) रास्ना (Rāsnā), (Sā.15).

Rāsnābhāve ca Vandākaḥ iti Bhavamisraḥ.

H.-Rāyasan; B.-Rāsnā; Mar.-Nāwalichyā mulyā Tel.-Sannarastramu; Tam.- Araitti; Mal.-Aratta, Arab.- Janjabil-i-

---

१ 'पुत्तिरसा' इति आनन्दाश्रम मुद्रित पुस्तके ।
२ 'गुर्वी' –इति साधु पाठः । S.D. Kamat
'युत्तफ्ला' इति क्षी. 'युत्तरसा' इति. नि.शे. टीकायाम् ।

shami; Lat.-*Vanda roxburghi* (Vaidya) .

(6) 245 रास्नेति (Rāsneti) (Bhujangākšī laghu Rāsnā 'Sarpākšiti/ Rāsnā +rasanā rase ti' *Kaiyadevaḥ*/Rāsnā bhujangapatrā + laghurāsnāsyā' diti', Rāsnā smṛtā bhujangākhyāmelā parṇyām ca kathyate iti Viswaḥ / Elāparṇī tu suwahā tyamaraḥ. (Harshe).

(7) (Cakradutta Abhāva, Chapter). *Inula helenium* Linn. Eng.-Elecampana; Greeks-Elenion; Roman -The Inula.

The old Persian name Rasna lead us to suppose that it was possibly the original Rasna of the Hindoos. The properties attributed to these roots in the same books (Ni.s) are those of Elecampana. All the Indian Mohomedan writers mention this drug under the name 'Rasna' Kusta-i-shami' or Zanjibil-i-shami i.e. Syrian ginger.

(Dymock P. 168 and App. II).

IV- (1) *Asli Rāsnā*, (a) *Inula racemosa;* (b) *I.helenium.* In France and in Germany it is called *'Ayurvedaki asali Rāsnā mool"* (Bhagirath).

(2) Elecampana-*Inula helenium.* Eng. -Scab wort, Habitat-Temperate Europe and Asia Cultivated for medicinal use in Europe. (Potters cyclo).

(3) *I.helenium*-Diaphoretic, tonic, diuretic, expectorant, chronic bronchitis, cough, chronic diarrhoea. (Uphof).

(4) (Vāyasuraīrāsnā) *Pluchiea lanceolata* Oliver (Jaipur Akhil Bharatiya Vaidyak Sammelan referred in Abhi. Butt. Darp., Ni. Adarsha; Priyavrata).*

83. (७६) अश्वगंधा Aśwagandhā

अश्वगंधा वाजिगन्धा कञ्चुकाऽश्वावरोहकः ॥
वराहकर्णी तुरगी बल्या वाजीकरी स्मृता ॥२७४

अश्वगन्धा कषायोष्णा तिक्ता वातकफापहा ॥
विषव्रणक्षयान् हन्ति कान्तिवीर्यबलप्रदा ॥ २७५

अश्वगंधा (Aśvagandhā), वाजिगन्धा (Vājigandhā), कञ्चुका (Kañcukā), अश्वावरोहकः (Aśvāvarohakaḥ), वराहकर्णी (Varāhakarṇī), तुरगी (Turagī), बल्या (Balyā), and वाजीकरी (Vājīkarī) are synonyms.

---

१ 'कुम्भको' इति नि.शे. टीकायाम ।

* Accepted in North whereas in South *Kuliñjana* is accepted as *rāsnā*

Aśvagandhā is *uṣṇavīrya, kaṣāya* (astringent), and bitter, pacifies *vāta* and *kaphadoṣas*. It is useful in poisons, wounds, consumption; improves complexion, and gives strength and energy.

(Fam. -Solanaceae).

I- *a*- ***Withania somnifera*** Dunal.*
Syn.-*Physalis flexuosa* Linn.

b- Roxburgh, *c*-In the drier parts of India.

II- *a*- **वाजिगन्धा** (Vājigandhā), **कञ्चुका** (Kañcukā), **वराहकर्णी** (Vāraha karṇi), **मदगन्धिका** (Madagandhikā).

b- H.-Asagandha; Bom.-Jagam; Mar.-Askand, Dhoragunja; Guj.-Asandh, Ghoḍā, ahan; Tam.-Amukiram, Aswagandhi; Mal. Amukiram, Pivande; Kan.-Amerakeru; Tel.-Piliandra penneru , Aswagandhi.

III-*a*-(1) **सर्वथा होमा** (Homā) **सम्भवे अश्वगन्धारसं (इति मन्त्रेण)दक्षिण नासाया - मासिच्योपगमनं कार्यम् ।**
(Dharmasindhu, Garbhādhāna Samskāraḥ).
(2) 9 Asmagandha-Sr. -Kosh-p-791.
d,e,f-See current name.

IV- (1) The following writers have identified *Withania somnifera* with **अश्वगन्धा** (Aśvagandhā) of Nighaṇṭus.
Ni. Adarsha. Yadavaji, Jangle, Kirtikar.
(2) *Cf.* Desai and Com. Prod. India p. 1120.

84. (७७) पुनर्नवा Punarnavā

पुनर्नवा विशारवश्च कठिल्लश्च शिवाटिका[१] ॥
वृश्चीरः क्षुद्रवर्षाभूर्दीर्घपत्रः कठिल्लकः ॥२७६

पुनर्नवा भवेदुष्णा तिक्ता रूक्षा कफापहा ॥
सशोफपाण्डुहृद्रोगकासोरःक्षतशूलनुत् ॥२७७

---

* The current name is - *Withania somnifera* (Linn.) Dunal. (Comp. p. 160)
W. ashwagandha Kaul
"Cultivated plants of *W.somnifera* differ from the wild ones not only morphologically but also in theraputical activity, though the same alkaloids are present. In view of these differences, some botanists consider the cultivated plants distinct from the wild ones and have assigned a new specific name mentioned above " U.P.I. ed. 1986 p. 689
S.D. Kamat

१ 'शशिलाटकः' इति नि.शे. टीका 'स शिलाटकः इति क्षी. ।
चरिय तमिळाम, -क्षुद्रवर्षाभू ; श्वेतमूलपुनर्नवा- वलिय तमिळाम (कैरली) Miss K. Nalini
Mrs. Chitra K.

पुनर्नवा (Punarnavā), विशाखः (Viśākhaḥ), कठिल्लः (Kaṭhillaḥ), शिवाटिका (Śivāṭikā), वृश्चीरः (Vṛścīraḥ), क्षुद्रवर्षाभूः (Kśudravarṣābhuḥ), दीर्घपत्रः (Dīrghapatraḥ), कठिल्लकः (Kaṭhillakaḥ), are synonyms for *Punarnavā*.

Punarnavā is bitter, *uṣṇavīrya, rūkśa* and pacifies *kaphadoṣa*. It is useful in oedema, anaemia (*Pāṇḍu*), heart disease, cough, cavities in the lungs (*uraḥkśata*), and for relief of pain.

This heading includes perhaps more than two plants, but two are indentified. Those are: A-कठिल्लकः (Kaṭhillakaḥ) and B-वृश्चीरः (Vṛsciraḥ).

(Fam.-Nyctaginaceae).

I- A-*a*- ***Boerhaavia diffusa*** Linn. (Cooke Fl.).
Syn.-*B. procumbense* Roxb. Fl.).
b- Roxburgh, *c*-A weed throughout India.
B-*a*- ****Boerhaavia repanda*** Willd. (Cooke Fl.).
b- Kamat, *c*-As in (I-A-a-supra, Poona in the hedges of gardens).

II- A-*a*- विशाखा (Viśākhā), कठिल्लकः (Kaṭhillakaḥ).
b- H.-Sant; B.-Gadaha purnā, Punarnavā; Bom.-Khāpra, Punarnawā; Mar.-Gheṭoḷi, Mālagheṭoli; Guj.-Vakha-khāpro; Tel.-Alika māmiḍi; Kan.-Kariya-beḷladakilu; Tam.-Makkarate-kire,Mukukarattai; Eng. The spreading Hog weed.
B-*a*- वृश्चीरः (Vṛścīraḥ),दीर्घपत्रः (Dīrghapatraḥ), सितवर्षाभू (Sita varṣ-ābhu).
b- Mar.-Gheṭoḷī, Malegheṭoḷi; Kan.-Biliyaḍu beleḍa kilu; (Vernacular names of (I-A-b-) are also applied to this plant).

III- *Cf.*Krūraḥ.
a- (1) अग्निर्घासो अपाङ्गभोयारोहन्ति पूनर्णवा (AV.viii-7).
b- (1) पुनर्नवात्रयंप्रोत्तम् (Raj. ni. Gana. 5-5).
(2) 154 वृश्चीवः (Wṛscīvaḥ)-
Boerhaavia diffusa Ceriya tamizāmā, (Tazhutma,Tavizhamā). (Note-"Here ZH" is to be pronounced as 'L' in Nagari). (Krishnan).
c- (1) वर्षाभूः (Dalhan, Sū).
(2) वृश्चीरः स्थिरः कठिल्लकः (Cakra; Sū. 4-6;Sū.27).
(3) वर्षाभ्वौ-हस्व महत्यौ रक्तःश्वेत पुननंवा. (Hemadri Sū. 6-97).

III- *d,e,f,g*-See current names and synonyms.

IV- (1) *B. diffusa* Linn.
It is a protean plant changing appearance according to soil and situation, (Cooke Fl.).

Currently accepted spelling of ' Boerhaavia * is -Boerhavia

(2) *Trianthema monogyna* Linn.
Therefore it should be called Raktapunarnavā and Śwetpunarnava to the species of *Boerhaavia* and Raktavarṣhābhū and Śwetawarṣābhū to the species of *Trianthema.* (Balwantji Bihar). Classifacation of Punarnawas and Varshābhū (including Vasuka).

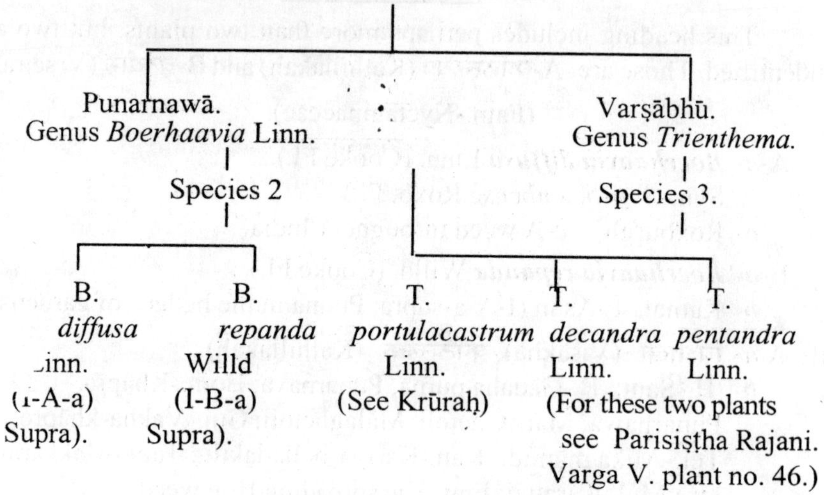

Krūraḥ क्रूरः 63.

पुनर्नवोऽपरः क्रूरः सद्योमण्डलपत्रकः ॥
श्वेतमूलो वर्षकेतुर्महावर्षाभूरुच्यते ॥ २७८

रक्ता पुनर्नवा तिक्ता सारिणी शोफनाशिनी ॥
रक्तप्रदरदोषघ्नी पाण्डुपित्तप्रमर्दिनी ॥ २७९

The other type of पुनर्नवा (Punarnavā) is having the following synonyms. क्रूरः (Krūraḥ), सद्योमण्डलपत्रकः (Sadyomaṇḍalapatrakaḥ), श्वेतमूलः (Śvetamūlaḥ), वर्षकेतुः (Varṣaketuḥ) and महावर्षाभूः (Mahāvarṣābhuḥ).

Rakta punarnavā is bitter in taste, and mild laxative. It is useful in oedema, conditions characterised by bleeding per vagina, anaemia (*Pāṇḍu*), and *pittadoṣa.*

(Fam.-Ficoideae).

I- *a*- ***Trianthema portulacastrum*** Linn.
Syn.- *T. monogyna* Linn.
b- Kamat, *c*-Thoughout India.

II- *a*- मण्डलपत्रिका (Maṇḍalapatrikā), रक्तकाण्डा (Raktakāṇḍā); रक्तपत्रिका (Raktapatrikā).

b- H.-Lāla sābuni; Mar.-Pāṇḍharīgheṭoḷī; Tel. -Galijeru Bom.- Visakhāparā; Tam.-Sarānaha.

III-a-(1) 155महावर्षाभू (Mahāwarṣābhū) + Śwetamūlaḥ sadyomaṇḍala-partrakaḥ + virecanī / Kaṭhillakāḥ VALIYA TAMIZHĀMĀ (Krishnan).

(2) 55-अत्र वर्षाभूः क्षुद्रवर्षाभूः । क्रूरको रक्तवृन्तकः इति केयदेवः ।
(Harshe).

85. (७८) सैरेयकः Saireyakaḥ

सैरेयकः सहचरः सैरेयश्च सहाचरः ॥
पीतो रक्तोऽथ नीलश्च कुसुमैस्तं विभावयेत् ॥ २८०

पीतः कुरण्टको ज्ञेयो रक्तः कुरबकः स्मृतः ॥
कुरण्टको हिमस्तिक्तः शोफतृष्णाविदाहनुत् ॥२८१
केश्यो वृष्योऽथ बल्यश्च त्रिदोषशमनो मतः ॥

सैरेयकः (Saireyakaḥ), सहचरः (Sahacaraḥ), सैरेयः (Saireyaḥ), सहाचरः (Sahācaraḥ), are synonymous. These can be attributed by पीत (Pīta) (Yellow), रक्त (Rakta), (Red), नील (Nīla), (Blue-Bluish black), varieties of flowers. That one with yellow flowers is कुरण्टकः (Kuraṇṭakaḥ), with red flowers is कुरबकः (Kurabakaḥ).

Kuranṭaka is bitter in taste, *śītavīrya* and useful in oedema (inflammation), thirst and burning.

It is beneficial for hairs, is *vṛṣya* and strength giving. It pacifies all the three *doṣas*.

The heading includes three plants: A-पीतः (Pītaḥ), B-रक्तः (Raktaḥ), and C- नीलपुष्पा (Nīlapuṣpā).

(Fam.-Acanthaceae).

I- A-*a*- ***Barleria prionitis*** Linn.

b- Roxburgh, *c*-Throughout the hotter parts of India.

B-*a*- ***B.involucrata*** Nees.

b- Dymock, *c*-Throughout India.

C-*a*- ***B. cristata*** Linn.

b- Roxburgh, *c*-W. India, Kolhapur.

Ī I- A-a- पीतः (Pītaḥ),पीतः कुरण्टकः (Pitaḥ Kuranṭakaḥ).

b- H.-Kata saraiyā; Mar.-Piwaḷī Korānṭi; B.-Kanṭajati; Tam.& Mal.-Semmuli; Tel.-Mullugoranṭa.

B-*a*- रक्ताम्लानः (Raktāmlānaḥ).कुरबकः (Kurabakaḥ),

C-*a*- आर्तगला (Ārtagalā), दासी (Dāsī), नीलाम्लानः (Nilāmlanaḥ).

b- Sk.-Zintī; Mar.-Niḷī Korānṭi; Tam.- Udamulli.

86 (७९) बला Balā

बला भद्रौदनी वाटी समङ्गा खरयष्टिका ॥ २८२
महासमङ्गौदनिका शीतपाक्योदनाह्वया ॥

बला स्निग्धा हिमा स्वादु वृष्या बल्या त्रिदोषनुत् ॥ २८३
रक्तपित्तं क्षयं हन्ति बलौजो वर्धयत्यपि ॥

बला (Balā), भद्रौदनी (Bhadraudanī), वाटी (Vāṭī), समङ्गा (Samaṅgā), खरयष्टिका (Kharayaṣṭikā), महासमङ्गा (Mahāsamaṅgā), ओदनिका (Odanikā), शीतपाकी (Śitapākī), and ओदनाह्वया(Odanāhvayā) are synonymous.

Balā is sweet in taste, *śitavīrya* and unctuous (*snigdha*). It pacifies all the three *doṣas,* promotes strength, and is *vṛṣya*. It is useful in haemorrhagic disorders (*Raktapitta*), consumption and promotes strength and *ojas*.

Not confirmed.

(Fam.-Malvaceae).

IV- (1) बला (Balā) *Sida cordifolia*.(Yadavaji and several other writers).

(2) बला (Balā), अतिबला (Atibalā) and नागबला (Nāgabaḷā), expepting these three, *Sahadevā, Viśwadevā, Bhadraudanī, Sitapākī* and *Odanapākī*, which have occured in (Samhitās) are diffcult to confirm. The commentators and the writers of the Nighaṇṭus have not definitely interpreted their meanings. The medicinal qualities of these different kinds (included in Balā Varga) are similar. Therefore one can be substituted for the other. (Yadavji).

महाबला Mahābalā 65.

महाबला वाट्यपुष्पी तथा वाट्यायनी स्मृता ॥ २८४
सहदेवा देवसह्रा पीतपुष्पा बृहत्फला ॥

महाबला तु ह्द्रोगवातार्शःशोफनाशिनी ॥ २८५
शुक्रवृद्धिकरी हन्याद् विषमं च ज्वरं नृणाम् ॥

महाबला (Mahābalā), वाट्यपुष्पी (Vāṭyapuṣpī), वाट्यायनी (Vāṭyāyanī) सहदेवा (Sahadevā), देवसहा (Devasahā), पीतपुष्पा (Pītapuṣpā), and बृहत्फला (Bṛhatphalā) are synonymous.

Mahābalā is useful in heart diseases, piles due to *vātadoṣa* and oedema. It promotes semen (*Śukra*) and useful in intermittant fevers (*viṣama jwara*).

Confirmed.

(Fam.-Malvaceae).

I- *a-* ***Abutilon indicum*** G. Don.*

b- Kamat, *c-*Throughout the hotter parts of India.

II- *a-* देवसहा (Devasahā), बृहत्फला (Bṛhatphalā), देवार्हा (Devārhā), पीतपुष्पा (Pītapuṣpā), सहदेवा (Sahadevā).

b- Eng.-Country Mallow; H.-Kāngli, Kānguni - Peṭari; B- Petārī Goa-Tupakaḍi; Bom.- Kanguṇi, Tutturu benḍa; Tam.-Tutti (Kaccha) Balabija; Guj.-Khāpāt, Mar.- Petārī; Kanguṇī. Mudrā.

III-a (1) शर्मयच्छत्वोषधिः सहदेवी । करतपयरचन्तं गोष्टमय क्ष्माँ उत पुरुषान् ।
(AV.vi-59).

c- (1) पेटारीबीजम् (Petārī bījam), (Vadikhanda Vajrāmaraṇa).

(2) देवाद्वयेति पाठः (Devādwayeti pāṭhaḥ). Ekā Sahadevā dwitīya Viswadewā. (Aruna Su. 15-10).

(3) देवसहा (Devasahā) -Sahadevi Balābhedaḥ pītpuṣpā 'Kāṅkasī iti loke, Anyā Balā nīlapuṣpāmāhuḥ. (Dalhan, Su. 38:4).

IV- 1 *Argeratun conyzoides* Linn.
This plant is sometimes confounded with *Vernonia cineria*** Less, 'Sahadevi' of purple flowers (Watt. Dict.).

Note- These two plants noted by Watt should not be confounded with Mahābalā -Devasahā of Nighaṇṭus.

2. Synonym-
Abutilon indicum G. Don Syns. *Abutilon asiaticum* W. & A. (Non-*Sida asiatica* Linn). *Sida indica* Linn., *S. populifolia* Lam. H.-Kāngani; B.-Poṭārī; Bom.-Chakrabhenḍ. (Watt Dict).

3.- *Sida asiatica* Willd. Tel. Tutte bendo.

---

* Current accepted name-*Abutilon indicum* (Linn.) Sw.

** The current accepted name is *vernonia cineria* (Linn.) Less. (Comp. P. 157). This *sahadevei* should not be included in *Balābheda*. *Sahadevi* may be a variety of Balā. (sida sp. or Abutilon sp.)

7- *Abutilon indicum* (L) SW. Syn. -*A. indicum* G. Don
4.- *A. asiaticum* G. Don Syn. -*Sida asiatica* Linn.
H.-Kaṅgni; B.-Poṭāri;

A. asiaticum G. Don, *A. indicum* G. Don these two species are so nearly allied botaniclly that from the economic point of view they may be regarded as one and the same. (Watt. Dict.).

गाङ्गेरुकी Gāṅgerukī 66.

गांगेरुकी नागबला खरगन्धिनिका झषा ॥ २८६
विश्वदेवा तथारिष्टा खण्डा ऱ्हस्वगवेधुका ॥

गांगेरुकी मधुराम्ला कषायोष्णा गुरुस्तथा ॥ २८७
कटुस्तिक्ता च वातघ्नी व्रणपित्तविकारजित् ॥

गांगेरुकी (Gāṅgerukī), नागबला (Nāgabalā), खरगन्धिनिका (Kharagandhinikā), झषा (Jhaṣā), विश्वदेवा (Visvadevā), अरिष्टा(Ariṣṭā), खण्डा (Khaṇḍā), and ऱ्हस्वगवेधुका (Rhasvagavedhukā) are synonymous.

Gāṅgerukī is sweet, sour, *kaṣāya* (astringent), pungent and bitter in taste, *uṣṇavīrya* and *guru.* It pacifies *vātadoṣa* and useful in wounds and diseases caused by *pittadoṣa.*

This heading includes two plants. A-गाङ्गेरुकी (Gāṅgerukī) and B-uncertain kind of बला (Balā).

(Fam.-Tiliaceae).

I- A-*a*- ***Grewia populifolia*** Vahl.
b- Kamat, *c*-Panjab, Sindh, Western India, down to Nilgiris.
B-*a*- Uncertain kind of बला (Balā).

II- A-*a*- गाङ्गेरुकी (Gāṅgerukī), चतुष्फला (Catuṣphalā), महोदया (Mahodayā),महाशाखा (Mahāśākhā), महापत्रा (Mahāpatrā), महाफला (Mahāphalā), मधुराम्ला (Madhurāmlā), कटुस्तिक्ता (Kaṭustiktā).
b- H.-Gangeran, Gāngo; Gangera, Gulaśakri.
B-a- झषा (Zaṣā), ह्रस्वगवेधुका (Rhaswagawedhukā), नागबला (Nāgabalā), खरगन्धिनिका (Kharagandhinikā).
b- Sk.-Nāgabalā and such other names of Balā kinds.

III- a- (2) गाङ्गेरुकं + मधुरं सकषायम् (Ca-Su. 27).
(3) पिबेन्नागबला मूलम् (Ca. Ci. 11).

b- गाङ्गेरुकम् (Gāṅgerukam) Tasya phalam himam swādū
(Madan ni, I-180)

(2) विश्वदेवा (Viśwadewā), गाङ्गेरुकी (Gāṅgerukī);
(Dalhan Su. 38-41; 15-163),

d- See current names.

IV- (1) गाङ्गेरुकी *Grewia populifolia.* Small tree, 5' to 10' high. The fruit of this tree is said बोजोडियुं (Bojoḍiyun) on Girnar mountain. The root is very tonic (Ni. Adarsh).

(2) नागबला -गांगेरुकी *Cf.* Bhagirath.

(3) गांगेरुकी *Sida spinosa.** (Br. ni. -Pade; Abhi. Butti Darpan, Chopra).

बलिका Balikā 67.(& बलात्रयम् Balātrayam)

बलिकाऽतिबला प्रोक्ता वाट्यपुष्पी च कंकता ॥ २८८
ऋष्यप्रोक्ता[१] ऋष्यगन्धा सैव भूरिबला मता ॥
वातपित्तापहं ग्राहि बल्यं वृष्यं बलात्रयम् ॥ २८९

बलिका (Balikā), अतिबला (Atibalā), वाट्यपुष्पी (Vāṭyapuṣpī), कंकता (Kamkatā), ऋष्यप्रोक्ता (Ṛsyaproktā), ऋष्यगन्धा (Ṛsyagandhā) and भूरिबला (Bhūribalā) are synonymous.

Three types of *Balā* pacify *vāta* and *pitta doṣa.* Together these are called as Balātrayam. It is astringent, promote strength and is *vṛsya.*

The text is too ambigous and incomplete to confirm the plant. It may be included in ATIBALA and BHŪRIBALĀ).

Not identified.

बला Balā 68.(बलापञ्चकम्)

बला चातिबला चैव महाबलबला बला ।
अन्या राजबला चैव बलायाः पञ्चकं मतम् ॥२९०

---

१ 'वृष्या प्रोक्ता वृष्यगन्धा' इति आनन्दाश्रममुद्रित पुस्तके ।
* The current name for *Sida spinosa* Linn. is *Sida alba* Linn.
Raj. Ni.'s Mahābalā महाबला is not coroborating with Dhn.Ni.'s as it is वृक्षरुहा Vṛkṣaruhā (epiphytic) D.K.Kamat.

तत्पित्तवातजिद्ग्राही बल्यं वृष्यं च कृच्छ्रजित् ।
स्निग्धं मधुरमायुष्यं वातासृग्दरनाशनम् ॥ २९१

बला (Balā), अतिबला (Atibalā), महाबला (Mahābalā), नागबला (Nāgabalā), and राजबला (Rājabalā), these five constitute बलापञ्चक (Balā pañcaka).

Balāpañcaka is sweet in taste, and is astringent, strength promoting, *vṛṣya,* unctuous, promotes longevity. It is useful in conditions where there is difficulty in urination, and excessive vaginal bleeding due to *vātadoṣa* (*vātāsṛgdara*).

This seems to be a later addition and should have been mentioned after प्रसारिणी (Prasāriṇī) the next plant. The reading appears in Anandāśram edition which was used by Late vd. D. K. Kamat.

Not confirmed.

Under the heading it is included five kinds of BALĀ which are as follows:- बला (Balā), अतिबला (Atibalā), महाबलबला (Mahābalabalā), बला (Balā). This may be बलिका supra and राजबला (Rājabalā).

Note- The first BALĀ and the third MAHĀBALĀ may be *Sida cordifolia* and *Abutilon indicum* G. Don (Vide supra 86 and 65 respectively). ATIBALĀ may be *Abutilon asiaticum* G. Don. and RAJĀBALĀ may be PRASĀRAṆĪ (*Paederia foetida Linn.*)

87. (८०) प्रसारणी Prasāraṇī

प्रसारणी सुप्रसरा सरणी सारणी च सा ॥
चारुपर्णी राजबला भद्रपर्णी प्रतानिका ॥ २९२

प्रसारणी गुरुस्तिक्ता सरा सन्धानकृन्मता ॥
त्रिदोषशमनी वृष्या तेजः कान्तिबलप्रदा ॥ २९३

प्रसारणी (Prasāraṇī), सुप्रसरा (Suprasarā), सरणी (Saraṇī), सारणी (Sāraṇi), चारुपर्णी (Cāruparṇī), राजबला (Rājabalā), भद्रपर्णी (Bhadraparṇī) and प्रतानिका (Pratānikā), are synonyms for *Prasāraṇī*

Prasāraṇī is of bitter taste and pacifies all the three *dosas,* it is *guru,* mild laxative, union promoting, *vṛṣya* and promotes glow, complexion and strength.

---

१ 'प्रसारिका' इति क्षीरसंमतः पाठः ।

(Fam.-Rubiaceae).

I- *a*- ***Paederia foetida*** Linn. *
b- Dymock, *c*-Throughout India.

II- *a*- सुप्रसरा (Suprȧsarā), सारणी (Sāranī), चारुपर्णी (Cāruparnī), राजबला (Rājabalā), प्रतानिका (Pratānikā), चन्द्रवल्ली (Candrawallī).
b- H.-Gandhāli; Tel.-Savirelā; Mal.-Talanili; B.-Gandhabandhuli; Mar.-Cāndawela.

III- *d,e,f,*-See current name.

IV- (1) *P. foetida* Willd. Somarāji (AS Res. Vol. IV-261).
(2) 274 प्रसारणी *Convolvulus arvensis*. Haranapaga. (Ni. Adarsha).

88. शतावरी Śatāwarī (८९) शतावर्यौ Śatāvaryau

शतावरी शतपदी पीवरीन्दीवरी वरी ॥
ऋष्यप्रोक्ता द्वीपिशत्रुर्द्वीपिका चोर्ध्वकंटका ॥ २९४

शतावरी हिमा तिक्ता रसे स्वादुः क्षयास्रजित् ॥
वातपित्तहरा वृष्या रसायनवरा स्मृता ॥ २९५

शतावरी (Śatāvarī), शतपदी (Śatapadī), पीवरी (Pīvarī), इन्दीवरी (Indīvarī), वरी (Varī), ऋष्यप्रोक्ता (Ṛṣyaproktā), द्वीपिशत्रुः (Dwipiśatruḥ), द्वीपिका (Dwīpikā), and उर्ध्वकंटका (Ūrdhvakaṇṭakā) are synonymous.

Śatāvarī is sweet and bitter in taste, *sitavīrya*, pacifies *vāta* and *pitta doṣas,* is *vṛsya, rasāyana*. It is useful in consumption and haemorragic disorders (*raktapitta*).

This heading includes two plants.:A-इन्दीवरी (Indiwarī) and B-द्वीपि (Dwīpi).

(Fam.-Liliaceae).

I- A-*a*- ***Asparagus racemosus*** Willd.
b- Roxburgh, *c*-Tropical and sub-tropical India, Himalayas.
B-*a*- ***A.officinalis*** Linn.
b- Kamat, *c*-vide iii-g. Dymock -infra.

II- A-*a*- शतपदी(Śatapadī), पीवरी (Pīvarī), सुक्ष्मपत्रा (Sūkśmapatrā), नारायणी (Nārāyaṇī), शतवीर्या (Śatavīryā), दुर्मरा (Durmarā), आत्मशल्या (Ātmaśalyā), ऋष्यप्रोक्ता (Ṛṣyaproktā).

---

* The current name for *Paederia foetida* Linn. is *Paederia scandens* (Lour.) Merr

b- H.-Satawar, Sada-bori; B.-Sat-mooli, Kokan-Aswali, Sitācawarī; Tam.-Simai-Sadawari, Pāniyanaku; Tel.-Cala gadda; Poona-Diwas-mawali; Nasik-Peth-Kolyāci-ghongadi; Kan.-Asadiyu.

B-a- द्वीपि (Dwipi), शत्रुर्द्वीपिका (Śatrurdwipikā), अमरकंटका (Amarkaṇṭakā), ऊर्ध्वकंटका (Ūrdhwakaṇṭakā).

b- Per., H.-Nāk-doun, Haliyoon; B.-Hilyoon; Arab- Hulyoon, Isperaj; Eng.-Asparagus.

III- g- *A.officinalis* L. Habitat-Europe, Southern Russia, Turkey, Cultivted in Persia and Northern India. Fruit-Halian (in Ind. baz.) (Dymock).

सहस्रवीर्या Sahasravīryā 69.

सहस्रवीर्याऽभीरुश्च तुङ्गिनी बहुपुत्रिका ॥
महापुरुषदन्ता च शतावर्यूर्ध्वकंटिका ॥ २९६

सहस्रवीर्या मेध्या तु हृद्या वृष्या रसायनी ॥
शीतवीर्या निहन्त्यर्शोग्रहणीनयनामयान् ॥ २९७

तदंकुरस्त्रिदोषघ्नो लघुरर्शःक्षयापहः ॥

सहस्रवीर्या (Sahasravīryā), अभीरुः (Abhīruḥ), तुङ्गिनी (Tunginī), बहुपुत्रिका (Bahuputrikā), महापुरुषदन्ता (Mahāpuruṣadantā), शतावरी (Śatāvarī), उर्ध्वकंटिका (Ūrdhvakaṇṭikā), are synonymous.

Sahasravīryā (Śatāvarī), is intellect promoting, cordial, *vṛṣya, rasāyan,* and *sītavīrya*. It is useful in piles, *grahaṇī* and diseases of the eye.

Its off shoots pacify all the three *doṣas,* are *laghu* and useful in piles and cousumption.

(Fam.-Liliaceae).

I- *a*- ***Asparagus sarmentosus*** Linn.
b- Dymock, *c*-Throughout India.

II- *a*- Vernacular Names as in शतावरी (Śatāwarī supra).
b- Arab, Pers. H.Śakākul; Tam.-Kitavari, Tannir-vittankicangu; Tel. Pilli-picara, calla-gaddulu; Mal.-Satāvrrîkiz-hanna, Satāvli; Kan.-Majjge-gadde.

III- *d,e,g*-See current name.

IV- Vide Sachitra Ayurved Patrika 10-1961 शतावरी (Śatāwarī).

89. (८२) एरण्डः Erandah

एरण्डः तरुणः शुक्लश्चित्रो गन्धर्वहस्तकः ॥ २९८
पञ्चाङ्गुलो वर्धमान आमण्डो दीर्घदण्डकः ॥
रक्तोऽपरो हस्तपर्णो[1] व्याघ्रो व्याघ्रदलो रुबुः ॥ २९९
रुबुको हस्तिकर्णी च चञ्चुरुत्तानपत्रकः[2] ॥
एरण्डस्तु रसे तिक्तः स्वादूष्णोऽनिलनाशनः ॥३००
उदावर्तप्लीहगुल्मबस्तिशूलान्त्रवृद्धिनुत् ॥
गुरुर्वातप्रशमनो विकाराञ्शोणिताञ्जयेत् ॥ ३०१
फलं स्वादु च सक्षारं लघूष्णं भेदि वातजित् ॥
एरण्डयुगलं वृष्यं स्वादु पित्तसमीरजित् ॥३०२

एरण्डः (Eraṇḍaḥ), तरुणः (Taruṇaḥ), शुक्लः (Śuklaḥ), चित्रः (Citraḥ), गन्धर्वहस्तकः (Gandharvahastakaḥ), पञ्चाङ्गुलः (Pañcāṅgulaḥ), वर्धमानः (Vardhamānaḥ), आमण्डः (Āmanḍaḥ), दीर्घदण्डकः (Dīrghadanḍakaḥ). The other type is called as रक्तएरण्डः (Raktaeranḍaḥ) has the synonyms as हस्तपर्णः (Hastaparṇaḥ), व्याघ्रः (Vyāghraḥ), व्याघ्रदलः (Vyāghradalaḥ), रुबुः (Rubuḥ), रुबुकः (Rubkaḥ), हस्तिकर्णी (Hastikarṇī), चञ्चुः (Cañcuḥ) and उत्तानपत्रकः (Uttānapatrakaḥ).

Eraṇḍa is bitter and sweet in *taste;* guru, *uṣṇavīrya* and pacifies *vāta* and *raktadoṣa.*

It alleviates *udāvarta,* diseases of spleen, tumors, relieves vesicular colics and useful in inguinal hernia.

Its fruits are sweet, salty, *laghu, uṣṇavīrya, vātahara* and breaks faecal mass.

Both the kinds are sweet in taste, *vṛṣya* and pacify *vāta* and *pitta doṣa.*

This heading includes two plants : A- शुक्ल (Śukla) and B-रक्त (Rakta).

(Fam.-Euphorbiceae).

I- A-*a*- ***Ricinus communis*** Linn.
b- Roxburgh, *c*-Cultivated and self sown.
B-*a*- Red shading form of *R. communis* Linn.
b- Kamat, *c*-As in Eranḍa, supra.

II- A-a- शुक्लः (Śuklaḥ), गन्धर्वहस्तकः (Gandharvahastakaḥ), पञ्चांगुलः (Pañcāṅgulaḥ).
b- H.-Aranḍu; B.-Bheranḍa; Mar.-Eranda, Eranḍī; Kan.-Mandan;

---

१ 'कर्णो' नि.शे. टीकायाम् ।
२ 'पर्णश्चञ्चुरुत्तानपत्रकः ' इति नि.शे. टीकायाम् ।

Tam.-Amanakku, Tel.-Eranḍamu, Mal.- Earanḍam, Eng.-Crotonplant, castor oil plant.

B-a- हस्तिकर्णः (Hastikarṇaḥ), रुबुः (Rubuḥ), उरुबूकः (Urubūkaḥ).

b- Vernacular names as in (II-A-*b*)Sweta-eranda.

III- *a*- (1) 17 Eranḍa-Sānkh. A. xii-8. (Harshe).

d- See current names and Harshe, intro.p.xiii.

There are two chief forms met with, but that under each of these there are numerous modifications. The one form is a tall bush The second race is an annual plant, some times grown as a pure crop. (Watt. Dict. p. 523)

गुडूच्यादिरयं वर्गः प्रथमः परिकीर्तितः ।
ऊर्ध्वाधोदोषहरणः सर्वामयविनाशनः ॥

Thus has been told the first Guḍūchyādi chapter, in which the drugs are mentioned for removal of *doṣas* from both the routes, upper and lower and generally for all the types of diseases.

वृषमेधा Vṛsamedhā

वृषमेधा च मेषान्त्रिर्बस्तान्त्रिच्छगलान्त्रिका ।
वृषगंधा रसे तिक्ता कषाया मधुरा कटुः ॥ १ ॥
विपाकशमनी शीता लघ्वी मारुतकोपनी ॥ १/२ ॥

वृषमेधा (Vṛṣamedhā), मेषान्त्रि (Meṣāntri), बस्तान्त्रि (Bastāntrī), च्छगलान्त्रिका (Chagalantrikā) are synonymous.

Vṛṣagandhā is bitter, *kaṣāya* (astringent), sweet and pungent in taste.After *vipāka* it pacifies the *doṣas*, is *laghu* and aggravates *vātadoṣa*.

This plant is not included in पर्यायनाम द्रव्यावलि (Paryāyanāmadravyāvali); but is recorded after the end of the same Varga).

(Fam.-Convolvulaceae).

I- *a*- ***Ipomoea obscura*** Ker.-Gaul.

b- Kamat, *c*-Throughout India.

II- *a*- मेषान्त्रि (Meṣāntri), बस्तान्त्रि (Bastāntrī), वृत्तपत्रिका (Vṛttapatrikā), बोकडी (Bokaḍī).

Mar. Bokaḍī Pungaḷī, Pinguḷi, Painguli; Tam.-Seruttali; Mal.-Cherutali; Tel.-Nalla-kokkita.

III- *Cf.*Vrddhadaraka.

b- (1) बस्तांत्री -बोकडी, पुंगळी -वृषगन्धा, बीजदा, गर्भदा, छगलांत्री, केयटेवे (Ni.Si.Pade).

(2) बस्तांत्री (Su. 15); H., Mar.--बोकडी, Guj.- पुंगळी
Argyreia speciosa - बस्तांत्री -वृषगन्धाख्या 'वृद्धदारक' हेमाद्रि ।
H.-विधारा; Mar. वरधारा. (Vaidya).

IV- (1) वृषमेधा (Bhagirath and Jangale 11-21, Wṛddhadaraka).

Note- The leaves of this plant with leaves of other edible plants are used as pot-herb in Konkan. The leaves are supposed to have cooling and tonic effect. The leaves have curious smell which flavours the boiled pot herb.

इति गुडूच्यादिः प्रथमो वर्गः समाप्तः ।

Thus ends the Guḍūcyādi Chapter First.

शतपुष्पादिर्द्वितीयो वर्गः ।

ŚATAPUṢPĀDIḤ CHAPTER II

1 शतपुष्पा Śatapuṣpā

शतपुष्पा मिशिर्घोषा पीतिका माधवी शिफा ।
अतिच्छत्रा त्ववाक्पुष्पी शताह्वा कारवी स्मृता ॥ १

शताह्वा कटुका तिक्ता स्निग्धोष्णा श्लेष्मवातजित् ।
ज्वरनेत्रव्रणान् हन्ति बस्तिकर्मणि शस्यते ॥ २

शतपुष्पादलं चोक्तं वृष्यं रुधिरगुल्मजित् ।
वातघ्नं दीपनं स्तन्यपित्तकृत् रुचिदायकम् ॥३

शतपुष्पा (Śatapuṣpā), मिशिः (Miśiḥ), घोषा (Ghoṣā), पीतिका (Pītikā), माधवी (Mādhavī), शिफा (Śiphā), अतिच्छत्रा (Aticchatrā), अवाक्पुष्पी (Avākpuṣpī), शताह्वा (Śatāhvā) and कारवी (Kāravī) are synonymous.

Śatāhvā is pungent and bitter in taste, *snigdha* (unctuous), *uṣṇavīrya* and pacifies *kapha* and *vāta doṣas.* It is useful in fevers, diseases of eyes and in wounds. It is recomended in the procedure of *Basti* (enema).

The leaves of *śatapuṣpā* aggravate *pitta doṣa* and pacify *vātadosa.* It is *vṛṣya,* stimulates lactation and digestive capacity, is appetising and useful in haematoma (or uterine fibroid).

Fam. Umbelliferae. Apiaceae

I- a ***Anethum sova*** Kurz
Syns. -*Peucedanum graveolens* Benth. & Hook. f.**
b- Roxburgh (Fl. Indica). C-Tropical and subtropical India. Cultivated in some parts.

II- a माधवी (Mādhavī), अतिच्छत्रा (Atichatrā), शिफा (Śiphā), कारवी (Kāravī), शताह्वा (Śatāhvā).
b Mar.-Bom.-बाळंतशेप (Bāḷantaśepa), शापू (Śāpū); H.B. सुल्फा - (Sulphā), सोवा (Sovā); Guj-सुवा (Suwā); Tam; -शतकुप्पा - Satakuppā, Eng.: *the Dill, Sovā*. Mal.- चटकुप्पा (Chatakuppā).

III- Cf. मिश्रेया - *Miśreyā.*

---

१ शिफका नि. शे. टीकायाम् । षाडका इति क्षीरस्वामी ।

** Syn. *Peucedanum graveolens* (Linn.) in part (U.P. I. p. 41.), *P. graveolens* (Linn.) Hiern (Comp. P. 12) a शतपुष्पा Ca. Su. 4.25.-26; Su. Su. 10.4; Ast. hr. Sa. 1,88.

b- 1) 69 मिसिरुद्दिष्टा घोषाशतपुष्पा सेतिका षष्पचेति ।
कारव्यूत्कटपुष्पी मागधी मधुपुष्पिकातिछत्राः । (Abhi. Man.)

2) 407 मागधी -वनशतपुष्पा 'सेतिका योनिशूलघ्नी । मधुरा मागधीषडे' ति केयदेवः ।
शालेयं स्याच्छीतशिवश्छत्रामधुरिकामिसीत्यमरः ॥ (Harshe)

3) शतपुष्पाद्वयमिति लघु स्थूल भेदेन । एका 'सौफ' अपरा 'सोवा' ....(Dipika p. 190).

IV- 1. शतपुष्पा ŚATAPUṢPĀ.
Peucedanum graveolens Linn.
SATĀHVĀ, Foeniculum vulgare Mill. (Balawantji p. 388).

The Plant *Pimpinella anisum* Linn. introduced into India, is native of Europe but not known to the ancient Hindus ."
Modern Names: Mar. Bom. -*Soumpha* Eng.-Ervādosa;

B.- *Mithājira*, Guj.-*Sova, Anis*,.
The bazar names in Bombay are the same as those for *The Dill*. (Dymock-II 182. Watt Dic.).

2 मिश्रेया Miśreyā

मिश्रेया तालपर्णी[1] तु तालपत्री[2] मिशिस्तथा ।
शालेयः स च शालीनो नाम्ना शीतशिवो मतः ॥४

तिक्तग स्वादु हिमा वृष्या दुर्नामक्षयजिन्मिशिः ।
क्षतक्षीणहिता बल्या वातपित्तास्रदोषजित् ॥ ५

मिश्रेया (Miśreyā), तालपर्णी (Tālaparṇī), तालपत्री (Tālapatrī), मिशिः (Miśiḥ), शालेयः (Śāleyaḥ), शालीनः (Śālinaḥ) and शीतशिवः (Śītaśivaḥ), are synonymous.

Miśreya is sweet and bitter in taste, *śītavīrya*. It pacifies *vāta, pitta* and *rakta doṣas*. It is strength promoting, *vṛṣya* and useful for those who are weakened by wounds (or cavities in lungs). It is used in piles and consumption.

Fam-Umbelliferae. Apiaceae.

I- a - ***Foeniculum vulgare*** Mill,

---

१ तालकर्णी इति नि.शे. टीकायाम् । २ तालपर्णी इति. नि. शे. टीकायाम् ।

Anethum foeniculum Linn. *A. panmorium* DC. (Roxb.). *Foeniculum capillaceum* Gilib.

b- Dymock & Watt. Dic.

c- Commonly cultivated in India but sometimes is found wild.

II- a- मिशि(Miśī), तालपर्णी (Tālaparṇī), मधुरिका (Madhurikā) शालेया (Śāleyā), शीतशिवः (Śitaśivaḥ), छत्रा (Chatrā).

b- H-बरीसोंफ (Barisoumph); B.-पानमुरी (Pānmurī); Bom.- बरिआरि (Bariārī); Mar.-बडिशेप (Baḍiśepa); Kan.-Badisopa, Tam.-Sahikires; Tel : Pedda-jillakuru; Eng.*Fennel, Anis, Arva dosa.*

III- See शतपुष्पा Śatapuṣpā (III-b-1,2,3)

a- 1) शताव्हाAst. hr. śa-1.88; Su. Ci-8-39.

b- 1) मिश्रेया-शतपुष्पा (See शतपुष्पा, III)

2) शतपुष्पामिशिवचाणाम्
(Gaṇadravyāvali Dhn. ni. p. 3; Śatapuṣpā-Chapter II-1)

Note: Śatapuṣpā and Misi. are denoted as separate two plants.

3) अतिछत्रा-मधुरिका (Cakra Ci. 1-6.).

4) छत्रा-मधुरिका अतिछत्रा- शतपुष्पा (Cakra-Ci.6-46).

5) छत्रातिछत्रे-छत्रा-शतपुष्पा । (Aruṇa).
छत्रातिछत्रे-शतपुष्पाद्वयम् । (Hemadri Sū29-26).

IV- 1) शताव्हा Śatāhvā. *Foeniculum vulgare* Mill. सोंफ *Soumpha.* syn. शतपुष्पा Śatapuṣpā and Satāhvā have been used for both Sovā and Soumpha. (Balwantji P. 388).

2) Foeniculum-A genus of glabrous herb-having 3 to 4 species which are widely distributed from Canaris to Western Asia. Several cultivated species seem to grow in India.... but are not recognised botanically. (Watt Dic. III-405).

3) See Desai p. 365.

4) Atichatrā.

*Chatrā*छत्रा and अतिछत्रा *Atichatrā* invariably occur together in the texts. in C. S. they, together with *Śatapuṣpā*-have been placed in Madhuraskandha. In S. S, besides their highly antiseptic (Rakśoghna रक्षोघ्न) use, in Ci.30-14, 15 they have been included among the Soma like powerful drugs where they have been described in the following words :-

"Chatrā " and 'Atichatrā' are antiseptic and obtained from tubers. They resemble Śwetakāpotī and prevent old age and death." (Balwantaji p. 10 11)

Pimpinella anisum Linn.
San. Śatapuṣpā; H. Soumpha, B.Movāri; Tam. Perunskirangnm sombu.

...Originally in Egypt... It is not the true native of Indian soil but ...introduced by Mohamedan invaders of Persia, however it is naturlised into India (Chopra-Handa 1958, p. 219).

Discussion - Miśreyā : मिश्रेया.
The equivalents which now find under the heading Śatapuṣpā and Miśreyā in Dhn. ni . are included under the heading Śatapuṣpā alone in Bṛhattrayī (Caraka, Suśrut and Vāgbhat) the classical books of Ayurveda. This means that the compilers of Bṛahattrayī have not recorded these two plants separately. But the name (*Miśī*) might have been used for मिश्रेया (*Miśreyā*). In *Gaṇa-drawyāvali,* the first part included in the present edition of Dhn. ni. (See *Śatapuṣpā* Chap. II p. 3) which is a compilation prior to the present compilation of Dhn. ni. (See) has also recorded two names as " *Śatapuspā* and *Miśreyā* separately.

In Amarkosh, the *Śatapuṣpā* of the classical books is recorded as two plants namely *Śatapuṣpā* and *Miśreyā* (Tivari Pp. 110; 122). In Dipika commentary of Adhamalla, *Śatapuspā* and *Miśreyā* are recorded as two separate plants noting their modern names *Sowā* and *Soumpha* (See *Śatapuspā* III-b-3).

Arunadatta notes on *Chatrā* (छत्रा) as (शतपुष्पा) Śatapuṣpā while Hemadri notes *Chatrātichatre* as *Śatapuspādwayam* (two). (छत्रातिछत्रे शतपुष्पाद्वयम्) (Aṣṭa. Hr. Su. 29-26).

Cakra commenting on *Chatrātichatrā* (छत्रातिछत्रा) notes as *Chatrā* (छत्रा)- *Madhurikā* (मधुरिका) and *Atichatrā* (अतिछत्रा) *Śatapuspā* (शतपुष्पा) (C.Ci.9.46). From these references it is clear that our present *Śatapuṣpā* (शतपुष्पा) and *Miśreyā* (मिश्रेया) now known as *Sowa* (सोवा) and *Soumph* (सौंफ) have traditional background of these names prior to 10th century i.e. prior to Dīpikā commentary, also prior to the compilation of present edition of Dhn. ni. (See above).

Our Nighaṇṭus have given *Chatrā Atichatrā* as equivalents to *Miśreyā* (मिश्रेया) and *Śatapuṣpā* (शतपुष्पा).

In Carak Samhitā *Chatrā* (छत्रा) and *Atichatrā* (अतिछत्रा) are occuring together with *Śatapuspā* in *Madhuraskandha* (मधुरस्कंध) (IV-4 above). In S. S. Ci. 30-14,15 *Chatrātichatrā* (छत्रातिछत्रा) are occuring together which have tubers and antiseptic in quality. Our Nighaṇṭus do not note tubers to *Śatapuṣpa* and *Miśreyā*. From this it is clear that the nighaṇṭus *Miśreyā* and *Śatapuṣpa* are different plants from *Chatrātichatrā* of Samhita plants.

3. वचा Vacā

वचोग्रगन्धा गोलोमी जटिलोग्रा च लोमशा ।
अन्या श्वेतवचा मेध्या षड्ग्रन्था हैमवत्यपि ॥ ६

वामनी कटुतिक्तोष्णा वातश्लेष्मरुजापहा ।
कण्ठ्या मेध्या च कृमिहृत् विबन्धाध्मानशूलहृत् ॥ ७

वचाद्वयं तु कटुकं रूक्षोष्णं मलमूत्रलम् ।
दीपनं कफवातघ्नं मेध्याऽयुष्यं च पाचनम् ॥ ८
जन्तुघ्नं चोग्रगन्धं स्याल्लघु कण्ठास्यरोगजित् ।

वचा (Vacā), उग्रगन्धा (Ūgragandhā), गोलोमी (Golomī), जटिला (Jaṭilā),उग्रा (Ugrā), and लोमशा (Lomaśā) are synonymous. There is an an another type of *vacā* called as श्वेतवचा (Śvetavacā) of which synonyms are मेध्या (Medhyā), षड्ग्रन्था (Ṣaḍgranthā) and हैमवती (Haimavatī).

Vacā is emetic, pungent and bitter in taste, *uṣṇavīrya* and alleviates the diseases due to *vāta* and *kapha doṣas*. It is beneficial to throat, intellect, is insecticidal, relieves constipation and flatulence.

Two types of *vacās* are pungent in taste, *rukśa* (roughning), *uṣṇavīrya*, pacifies *kapha* and *vāta doṣas*, expels faeces and urine (after normalization) stimulates digestive capacity, are intellect promoting, provide longevity, and digestant, insecticidal, have sharp smell, are *laghu*, and useful in the diseases of the mouth and the throat.

(Generic name-compiler records two plants under this heading, of which one is A-उग्रगन्धा (*Ugragandhā*) and the next is B.- श्वेतवचा मेध्या (*Śwetavvacā medhyā*). Raj. ni. records the first under this heading but the next श्वेतवचा (*Śwetavacā*) records separately under the heading मेध्या (*Medhyā*) which are Post No. (1) infra.

Fam. Araceae.

I- A-a-***Acorus calamus*** Linn.

---

¹"वचोग्रगन्धा गोलोमी षड्ग्रन्था जटिला तथा ।
जटिला शतपर्वाऽन्या लोमशा हैमवत्यपि ॥ इति. नि. शे. टीका संमतः पाठः

b- Dymock. c-Originally native of Asia. Probably spread and made its home in Europe and N. America. (Watt. Dic.'A' p.99).

II- a- A-उग्रगन्धा(Ugragandhā) गोलोमी (Golomī),जटिलोग्रा (Jaṭilogrā), लोमशा(Lomaśā).

b- H.-घोडवच (Ghoḍvaca); B.-वच (Vaca): Mar.-Maha. St.Gaz (III-84). वेखंड (Vekhaṇḍa); घोडवच (Ghoḍwaca); Guj.-गोधिलोबज; (Godhilobaja), घोडो बेज (Ghodabeje). Tel.: - Vadaja Vasa; Kan;- Basegid; Tam.:-चटिन चटक्कोत्तन. Vashambu; Mal.: -Vayambam (वयबँ). Wayaman; Vashampā,Wasampu; Eng.:-Calamus root. The sweet Flag

III *Cf.*कुष्ठ Kuṣṭha, मेध्या Medhyā

a- 1) वी ते मदं मदावती ॥४॥ परिग्राममिवाचित...:.वचसा स्थापयामसि ॥ (Satavalekar AV-IV-7).

2) वचा (Vacā), उग्रगन्धा (Ūgragandhā). C.S. Ci. 26-2 ; S. S. U. 50-54; A. H. U. 39-46t (Balawantji, p. 48).

3) श्वेतवचा (Vayambum) (वयम्बँ) (वयमनँ) (Shri Krishnan). *

Note- In some books it finds a name as (*Mahābharīvacā*) -Plant of this name is not included in Dhn. ni. or in Raj. ni. but under the genus *Zinjiber* Dr. Roxburgh records a species *Zingiber zerumbet* Rosc. ex. Smith giving its modern name as *Mahābharī vacā*) and Chopra records its names *Sthūla granthī*.

मेध्या Medhyā (I) (Raj ni.)

मेध्या श्वेतवचा त्वन्या षड्ग्रन्था दीर्घपत्रिका ।
तीक्ष्णगन्धा हैमवती मंगल्या विजया च सा ॥

श्वेतवचाऽतिगुणाद्या मतिमेधायुः समृद्धिदा कफनुत् ।
वृष्या च वातभूतक्रिमिदोषघ्नी च दीपनी च वचा ॥ (Raj. ni.)

श्वेतवचा (Śvetavacā), is another type of *vacā* having the synonyms मेध्या (Medhyā), षड्ग्रन्था (Ṣaḍgranthā), दीर्घपत्रिका (Dīrghapatrikā), तीक्ष्णगन्धा (Tīkṣṇagandhā), हैमवती (Haimavatī), मङ्गल्या (Maṅgalyā) and विजया (Vijayā).

Śvetavacā is more potent in action; it pacifies *kapha* and *vātadoṣa*, is intellect promoting, promotes prosperity. It is *vṛṣya*, insecticidal, useful in *vāta*, *bhūta* (?psychological disorders), worms and stimulates digestive capacity.

---

* श्वेतवचा – वेल्वयम्बु (Abhi. Mañj. p. 13)
(Vd. Miss Nalini K., Vd. Mrs. Chitra K.

(This plant of Raj. ni. is श्वेतवचा (Śwetavacā)of Dhn. ni. Pre. No. 3 Supra. Under this name modern writers recognise the following plants.

(Fam. Iridaceae). For Confirmation.

I- a- 1) ***Iris versicolor.*** Linn

b- Yadavaji; Priyavrat. c-As in 2 below.

2) *Iris kumaonensis* Wall.*

I- ***I . nepalensis.*** D. Don.

b- Balawantji C-Western Himalaya, Punjab, Kashmir, Komaon, Tibet.

3) *Iris soongariea*, Schrenk.

b- Priyavrataji, C-Baluchistan.

II- a) श्वेतवचा (Swetawacā), दीर्घपत्रिका (Dīrghapatrikā*)* हैमवतीवचा (Haimavati-vacā*)*.

b) Mar.पांढरे वेखंड (Pāṇḍhare Wekhaṇda),बाळ वेखंड (Baḷa Wekhaṇḍa); Mal : वेळ वयंपु (Velavayampu). Tam : वेळ्ळे वयंपु(Velevayampu). Bazarname वेखसोन (Vekhson*)*; Arab-*Irsā, Susan.* Eng. Sweet flag root, Orris root.

III *Cf* . Vacā Kusta, *Moolam (puskara).*

III- a- 1) C-Sū-1-78; Si. Sū-38-58; 44-36. Asta. H.S*ū*. 40-88

b- 1) प्रोक्ता वचोग्रगन्धा जटिलोग्रा रोमशा गोलोमी च रक्ता ॥ ३२ ॥
अन्या श्वेतवचा मेध्या षड्ग्रंथिका च हैमवती ॥ ३३ ॥
(33 Abhi-Man).

2) 395,वचा-हैमवती 395, 530, 507, 496 (Harshe).

3) 33 अन्या श्वेतवचा : Vel vambu. (Krishṇan). वयम्पु (Asta H. Kosh).

IV- 1) There is also a second variety of *Vacā* called *'Swetavacā* or *'Haimavati vacā '* whose identity is doubtful.Some species of *Iris* as *I. germanica* Linn. (Orris Root) may be its source ...For the determination of this white variety of *Vacā* the Himalayan species (See above I-a) should be examined. (Balwantji p. 355).

2) वचा *Acorus calamus* Linn. (Ayur. Patrika. IV.-3-289).

4. हपुषा Hapuṣā

हपुषा विपुषा विस्रा विस्रगन्धाऽतिगन्धिका । ९

* currently accepted name for *Iris kumaonensis* Wall. is *Iris kumaonensis* Wall. ex Don. The current valid name for *Iris nepalensis* G. Don is *Iris decora* Wall.

अपरा चाश्वत्थफला कच्छूघ्नी ध्वांक्षनाशिनी ॥
हपुषा कटुतिक्तोष्णा गुरुर्वातबलासजित् ।१०
अर्शांसि गुल्मशूलानि हन्ति जन्तूदरैः सह ॥
प्लीहोदरविबन्धघ्नी शूलगुल्मार्शसां हिता ॥ ११

हपुषा (Hapuṣā), विपुषा (Vipuṣā), विस्रा (Visrā), विस्रगन्धा (Visragandhā), अतिगन्धिका (Atigandhikā), are synonymous.

The synonyms for another kind which is called as अश्वत्थफला (Aśvatthaphalā), are कच्छूघ्नी (Kacchūghnī), and ध्वांक्षनाशिनी (Dhwankṣanāśinī)

Hapuṣā is pungent and bitter in taste, *uṣṇavīrya,* pacifies *vāta* and *kaphadoṣās*. It is beneficial in piles, tumors (diverticulae.), colics, helminthic infestations, ascites due to spleen disorders, relieves constipation and painful conditions due to tumors and piles.

(Under this heading two kinds of plants are included. One of it is A-अतिगन्धिका (Atigandhikā) and the next B- अश्वत्थफलाAswatthaphalā)

Fam. Euphorbiaceae. Cupressaceae.

I-A a- ***Juniperus communis*** Linn.

b- Desai and Yadavji.

c- A large shrub of North-west Himalaya from Komaon West-ward. Distribution throughout Asia, Europe and North-America.

For confirmation. Fam : Euphorbiaceae.

B a- ***Homonoia riparia*** Lour.

b- Kamat. c-(See IV-1 below).

II- a- A अतिगन्धिका (Atigandhikā), विपुषा (Vipuṣā), विस्रगन्धा (Visragandhā).

b- A हाऊबेर (Hāuber); असर (Asara); हावुशा (Hāvuśa); Tel. Ceppunegringal: Tam.-Cirakarantai, Varantāi. Kan: Thathur; Arab; अबहाल (Abhal); अबलअरहर (Abala arahar). Mal; अट्यक्कामणियन् (Atyakāmaṇiyan): कोटैकरलै इति द्राविडश्चैके। Eng-Juniper. (Asta. Hr. Kosh).

a- B अश्वत्थफला(Aśwatthaphalā), अपराजिता(Aparājitā); . मत्स्यगन्धा(Matsyagandhā).

b- B Mar: -मोठी शेरणी (Mothi śeraṇī). Guj: Hosa. Tel : Capunje; Rinjale; San; -पाषाणभेद (Pasāṇabheda)

.Current name for. *Juniperus communis* Linn. is *Juniperus communis* Var. *saxatilis* Pallas Comp. to Gloss P. 86.

III- a- 1) C. S. Sū. 23-19; S.S. Ci. 5-28, 38-43; A. H. Sū. 14-26.

b- 1) हपुषा 40 (Hapusā) ; Mar; थोर शेरणी(Thoraśeraṇī);

2) 41 विश्रगन्धा राजनिघण्टे । कुष्ठघ्नी विषदूषणी ॥
लघुशेरणी, खडशेरणी (मराठी).
तथा स्वल्प फलाचैव...अपराजिता-रा. नि., के.।
अश्वत्थफलाचैव प्रोक्ता धन्वन्तरौ । यक्षघ्ना विश्रगन्धा
"मत्स्यगन्धा" केयदेवके विश्रगन्धा च दुर्गन्धा
गणनिघन्टके । (Nighanṭa Śiromaṇi p. 35)

3) जम्बुवत् विटपविशेषः । (Dipikā p. 192-189)

4) हपुषाः-शेरणीति लोके (Rasapadhati) p. 82).

5) द्वितीयामश्वत्थफलासदृशं मत्स्यगन्धान् (Dipikā p. 2).

6) हपुषा के. अट (क्का-यक्का) वाणियन् अटचक्कामणियन्
ता. चिरकारत्तै, मा. शेरणीहोष, क. हम्बे.
Eng: - Sphaeranthus, (Aynr. O. Ni).

IV- 1) *Homonoia riparia* Lour - A rigid evergreen shrub; leaves linear oblong, 3.6 x 3/8-3/4 in. linear lanceolate, entire,capsules globus 1/8 in. in diameter-found in rocky and stony river lands Assam, Khasia Hills, Andaman, Bundel-khand and in the Deccan peninsula from Kokan Southwards,
" *Sherani* " (Cooke fl .). also occurs in the Muthā river bed near Pune (Mahajan)

2) हपुषा (Hapuṣā), शेरणी (Śeraṇi), (Vaidya, Navare Shārn. Samhitā. Narayan Cūrṇa).

V- *Hapuṣā* : हपुषा

1) There is no mention of the existance of two varieties in the text. It has also been named ' *Viśra gandhâ* '(विश्रगन्धा) and *Palāṣī* (पलाशी) which are interpreted as to mean that the drug resembles flesh in colour and smell. This attracts notice towards a plant '*Casearia tomentosa* Roxb.' known as *Cillā* (चिल्ला) Another species ' *C. esculanta Roxb*..... useful in etc.
It is therefore, suggested that '*Casearsia*' fruits may be examined. (Balwantji p. 464).

Note: We think, commentaries on Sanskrit books and modern writers literature confirm śeraṇī as हपुषा Hapuṣā. Balwantji would have also accepted शेरणी Śeraṇī as second हपुषा of Sanskrit books and he would have not suggested the plant-names recorded by him for Hapuṣā.

2) *Thevetia nerifolia Juss,* हपुषा of some modern writers. Lately intoduced into Inidia from New World and it is deadly poisonous as *Nerium species (Karawira)*.(abbreviated from Watt. Dic.'T' p. 6-7,3).

3) *Sphaeranthus*. (See III-b above Ayur. O. Ni.)
This plant is श्रावणी *Srāvaṇi* of Dhn. ni.(Chap. I Plant pre. No. 49).

Note: *For these reasons* शेरणी *Seraṇi (I-B-a) Homonoia for the present, should be accepted as Hapuṣa, the second plant of Nighaṇṭu and accepted by modern writers and commentators.*
The plant suggested by Balwantaji (See V-i-above) is not supported by modern writers and according to Dr. Roxburgh the fruits of this plant are used for fish poison. Balwantaji and also Dr. Roxburgh do not note the smell of the fruits of these trees. The fruits of the both हपुषा *Hapuṣa have a particular smell. This is an important point to recognise the compilers' plant.*

5. विडङ्गम् Vidangam

विडंगा जन्तुहन्त्री च कृमिघ्नी चित्रतण्डुला ।
तण्डुली कृमिहाऽमोघा कैरला[1] मृगगामिनी ॥ १२
रूक्षोष्णं कटुकं पाके लघु वातकफापहम् ।
ईषत्तिक्तं विषान् हन्ति विडंगं कृमिनाशनम् ॥ १३

विडङ्गा (Viḍangā), जन्तुहन्त्री (Jantuhantrī),. कृमिघ्नी (Kṛmighnī), चित्रतण्डुला (Citratanḍulā), तण्डुली (Tanḍulī), कृमिहा (Kṛmihā), अमोघा (Amoghā), कैरला (Kairalā), and मृगगामिनी (Mṛgagāminī) are synonymous.

Viḍaṅga is pungent and bitter in taste, *uṣṇavīrya, pungent* in *vipāka, laghu,* roughning, pacifies *kapha* and *vāta doṣas* and is useful in poisons and *helminths.*

Fam.-Myrsinaceae.

I- a- ***Embelia ribes*** Burm, b-Dymock
c Hilly parts from Central Himalaya to Ceylon.

II- a- चित्रतण्डुला (Citrataṇḍulā), कैरला (Kairalā), किमिघ्नी (Krimighnī) तण्डुली (Tanḍulī).
b- II बबेरंग (Baberanga).बाबरंग (Bābarang);Mar: वावडिंग (Wāvaḍing);

---

१ 'केशला' इति क्षीरस्वामी। 'करला' इति नि. शे. टीका।

Bom; वायविरंग (Wāyaviranga): कर्कनी (Karkani);Kan:-वायुविरंग (Wāyuvirang); Tam; वायु विलंगम (Wāyuvilangam). Eng:-*Embelia,* Mal;- विषालरि वियालरि (Ast. Hr. Kosha).

III- a- 1) C. S. Sū-1-80; 2-23; S. S. Sū.-14.35; A. H. Su 14.24.

IV- 1) Chunekar, p. 69; 2) Mukarji; 3) Desai;

Note : in Kokan and also in bazar the fruits of *Embelia robusta* *C. B. Clarke (Mar- Āmṭī) are used and sold as (Viḍaṅga).

6. कुटजः (Kuṭajaḥ)

कुटजः कौटजः कौटो वत्सको गिरिमल्लिका ।
कलिंगो मल्लिकापुष्प इन्द्रवृक्षोऽथ वृक्षकः ॥ १४
कुटजः कटुकस्तिक्तः कषायो रूक्षशीतलः ।
कुष्ठातीसारपित्तास्रगुदजानि विनाशयेत ॥ १५

फलानि तस्येन्द्रयवाः शक्राह्वाः स्युः कलिंगकाः ।
तथा वत्सकबीजानि प्रोक्ता भद्रयवास्तथा ॥ १६

शक्राह्वाः कटुतिक्तोष्णास्त्रिदोषघ्नाश्च दीपनाः ।
रक्तार्शांस्यतिसारं च घ्नन्ति शूलवमीस्तथा ॥ १७

कुटजः (Kuṭajaḥ), कौटजः (Kauṭajaḥ), कौटः (Kauṭaḥ), वत्सकः (Vatsakaḥ), गिरिमल्लिका (Girimallikā), कलिङ्गः (Kaliṅgaḥ), मल्लिकापुष्पः (Mallikāpuṣpaḥ), इन्द्रवृक्षः (Indravṛksaḥ), and वृक्षकः (Vṛksakaḥ) are synonymous.

Kuṭaja is pungent, bitter and *kaṣāya* in taste, *śītavīrya* and is roughning. It is useful in skin disorders, diarrhoea, bleeding disorders and piles.

The fruits of *kuṭaja* have the following synonyms इन्द्रयवाः (Indrayavāḥ), शक्राह्वाः (Śakrāhavāḥ), कलिंगकाः (Kalingakāḥ), वृक्षकबीजानि (Vṛksakabijāni) and भद्रयवाः (Bhadrayavāḥ).

Indrayava is pungent and bitter in taste, *usṇavīrya,* pacify all the three *dosas,* stimulate digestive capacity. These are useful in hemorrhoides (with bleeding), diarrhoea, colics and emesis.

---

* The current name for
Embelia robusta C̦BC̦ is *Embelia tsjeriam - cottom* A.DC. (Comp. to Gloss Page 59.)

Fam. Apocynaceae.

(Under this heading the compiler of Dhn. ni. has recorded only one plant which is A-कुटज (Kuṭaja) but Raj-ni adds one more B असित कुटज (Asita Kuṭaja) in describing गुणाः (Medicinal properties of the plant).

I- A-a-***Holarrhena antidysenterica*** Wall.
Syn.-*Wrightia antidysenterica* (J. Graham)*
b- Dymock. c-Tropical Himalaya extending the dry forest of India.

I- B-a- ***Wrightia tinctoria*** R. Br.
b- Kamat. c-As in I-a-A above.

I- a- Aवत्सक (Vatsaka), कलिङ्ग (Kalinga),पांडुरद्रुमः (Pāṇḍuradrumaḥ), इंद्रवृक्षः (Indravṛksaḥ), गिरिमल्लिका (Girimallikā)

B-b- H.कुर्चि (Kurci), कुरा (Kurā): Kokan कुडा (Kuḍā), कुडय (Kuḍaya),पांढरा कुडा(Pāndharā Kuḍā) Nasik-Peth Adivāsi काळी कुडय (KāḷīKuḍaya): Tam: Kudasappali. Tal: Kodisepal Palakods

B:-तित्तइंद्रजव (Tiktaindrajava). Mal;- कुटकप्पाला (Ast H.Kosa). Eng-Tellecheri bark

B-a- असित कुटज (Asita Kuṭja):

B-b- मिठ्ठा इंद्रजव (Miṭṭha indrajava): South Kokan काळाकुडा (Kālā Kuḍā), Naisk peth धवली कुडय (Dhavali Kuḍaya).
Tam :-Nepali: Mal:-Kola Kappal;Tel :- Jalpadal :Kan:- Kirikodesijam.

III- a- 1) C.S. Su. 1-82, 2-23, S. S. Sū. 46-32.
A.H. Sū. 15-1, 3, 35.
2) कुटज Kutaja (Agrawal 4-3-136).

IV- 1) Mukerji: 2) Chopra-Handa; 3) Desai: 4) Chunekar.

Note- In South Kokan the plant कुटज (I-A-a) is called पांढरा कुडा (*Pāṇḍharā Kuḍā*) and the next असित कुटज (I-B-a) is called काळा (Black) कुडा Kāḷā Kudā but in the hilly tribes of Naisk District, these plants are recognised reversely such as काळी कुडई (*Kāli kudaī*) to l (I-A-a) and ढवळी कुडई (Dhavalī = white to (I-A-a above.)

/. इंद्रयवः Indrayavḥ

I- A-a- ***Seeds of Holarrhena antidysenterica*** Wall.
b- Kamat c- See *Kutaja* कुटज Supra.

*The current name for. *H. antidysenterica* is *H. antidysenterica* (Roth.) DC. (comp. to Gloss P. 77)

II- a & b वत्सक बीजानि Vatsaka bījāni, भद्रयवः (Bhadrayavaḥ), कृष्ण तण्डुलः (Kṛṣṇa taṇḍulāḥ), कलिङ्गः (Kaliṅgaḥ), Mar. इंद्रजव (Indrajava) H. इन्दरजव (Indarjava), Eng. Kurchi seeds. Mal. कुटकप्पालरी (Kutakappālari).

V- i See Desai and Mukerji.

Note : The seeds of *Holarrhena antidysenterica* Wall. are bitter in taste, these are *Indrajava* proper of Books which are used in medicine but the seeds of *W. tinctoria* R. Br. are not bitter in taste and are not used as medicine. These are known as (Mīthā indrajav).

8. यवक्षारः Yavakśāraḥ

(८) त्रिक्षारा Trikśārā

यवक्षारः स्मृतः पाक्यो यवजो यवशूकजः।
यवाह्वः शूकजो यव्यो यावशूको यवाग्रजः ॥ १८

यवक्षारः कटूष्णश्च कफवातोदरार्तिजित् ।
आमशूलाश्मरीकृच्छ्रविषदोषहरः सरः ॥ १९

ऊष्णो विरूक्षणस्तीक्ष्णो दीपनः कफवातजित् ।
पित्तास्रदूषणो हृद्यो यवजः क्षार उच्यते ॥ २०

Kśāras being non vegetable (plants) these are not commented upon by Late vd. D. K. Kamat.

पाक्य (Pākya), यवजः (Yavajaḥ), यवशूकजः (Yava,sūkajaḥ), यवाह्वः (Yavāhavaḥ), शूकजः (Śūkajaḥ), यव्यः (Yavyaḥ), यावशूकः (Yāvaśūkaḥ), यवाग्रजः (Yavāgrajaḥ) are synonyms of यवक्षार (Yavakśāra)

Yavaksara is pungent in taste, *uṣṇavīrya* and pacifies gastrointestinal disorders due to *kapha -vāta doṣas*. It is useful in colics and pains due to *āmadoṣa*, urinary calculus, dysuria and as antipoisonous.

It is *uṣṇavīrya* tīkśṇa, appetizer pacifies *kapha vāta doṣas*, causing dryness or roughning,cordial and vitiates *pitta* and *rakta doṣas*.

9. स्वर्जिकाक्षारः Swarjikākśāraḥ

क्षारोऽन्यः स्वर्जिकाक्षारः स्वर्जिकाऽथ सुवर्चिका ।
सुवर्चिकः सुवर्चोऽथ सुखवर्चः स एव च ॥ २१

स्वर्जिकोष्णा कटुः क्षाररसा वातकफौ जयेत् ।
गुल्माध्मानकृमीन् हंति मेदोजठरनाशिनी ॥ २२

स्वर्जिकाक्षारः (Swarjikāk's arah), स्वर्जिका (Swarjikā), सुवर्चिका (Suvarcikā), सुवर्चिकः (Suvarcikaḥ), सुवर्चः (Suvarcaḥ), सुखवर्चः (Sukhavarcaḥ) are synonymous.

Swarjikā is pungent and salty in taste, *uṣṇavīrya,* pacifies *vāta kaphadoṣas.* It is useful in int. tumors (diverticulosis), flatulence and worms, It is used in disorders of fatty tissues and those of gartrointestinal tract.

10 टंकणक्षारः Taṅkaṇak's ārah

टंकणष्टंकणक्षारो मालतीरससम्भवः ।
द्रावी द्रावणकश्चैव लोहानां शुद्धिकारकः ॥ २३

कथितष्टंकणक्षारः कटूष्णः कफनाशनः ।
स्थावरादिविषघ्नश्च कासश्वासापहारकः ॥२४ S.S. Su. 46. 325

विरूक्षणोऽनिलहरः श्लेष्महा पित्तदूषणः ।
अग्निदीप्तिकरस्तीक्ष्णः टंकणक्षार उच्यते ॥ २५

टंकणः (Taṅkaṇaḥ), टंकणक्षारः (Taṅkaṇak's ārah), मालतीरससम्भवः (Mālatirasasambhavaḥ), द्रावी (Drāvī), द्रावणकः (Drāvaṇakaḥ), लोहशुद्धिकारकः (Loha's uddhikārakaḥ) are synonymous.

Taṅkaṇaks'āra is pungent in taste, *uṣṇavīrya* and pacifies *kaphadoṣa.* It is useful in poisons of immovable and movable in origin, dyspnoea and cough. It is roughning (drying), pacifies *vāta* and *kapha doṣās* and vitiates *pittadoṣa.* It sharpens the digestive capacity and is *tīk'saṇa.*

(९) लवणानि Lavaṇāni

10 सैंधवम् Saindhavam

सैन्धवं सिन्धु सिन्धूत्थं नादेयं सिंधुजं शिवम् ।
शुद्धं शीतशिवं चान्यत् मणिमन्थं शिलात्मकम् ॥ २६

सैंधवं शिशिरं स्निग्धं लघु स्वादु त्रिदोषजित् ।
हृद्यं हृन्नेत्ररोगघ्नं व्रणारोचकनाशनम् ॥ २७

अन्यच्च
सैंधवं स्वादु चक्षुष्यं वृष्यं रोचनदीपनम् ।
अविदाहि विबन्धघ्नं सुखदं स्यात् त्रिदोषजित ॥ २८

सैंधवम् Saindhavam etc. लवणानि *Lavaṇāni* not being vegetables (plants) these are not commented upon by Late vd. D.K. Kamat.

सिन्धु (Sindhu), सिन्धूत्थं (Sindhūttham), नादेयं (Nādeyam), सिंधुजम् (Sindhujam), शिवम् (Śivam), शुद्ध (Śuddham), शीतशिवम् (Sitaśivam), मणिमन्थं (Maṇimantham) शिलात्मकम् (Śilātmakam) are the synonyms.

Saindhava is sweet in taste, *śītavīrya, snigdham* (unctuous), *laghu* and pacifies three *doṣas*. It is cordial, useful in diseases of heart, diseases of the eyes, and alleviates anorexia and is useful in wounds.

According to another text

Saindhava is sweet in taste, pacifies the three *doṣas, vṛṣya* beneficial for the eyes, promotes desire for food, stimulates digestive capacity, does not cause burning sensation in the epigastrium (*Avidāhī*), removes constipation and is useful for health.

12 बिडम् Bidam

बिडं कृत्रिमकं धूर्तं क्षारं द्रविडमासुरम् ।
सुपाक्यं खण्डलवणं कृतकं चेति नामतः ॥ २९
सक्षारं दीपनं शूलहृद्रोगकफनाशनम् ।
रोचनं तीक्ष्णमुष्णं च बिडं वातानुलोमनम् ॥ ३० S.Su. 46.316

कृत्रिमकम् (Kṛtṛimakam), धूर्तं (Dhūrtam), क्षारं (K'sāram) द्रविडम् (Draviḍam), आसुरं (Āsuram), सुपाक्यम् (Supākyam), खण्डलवणं (Khaṇḍalavaṇam), कृतकं (Kṛtakam), are synonyms of बिडलवणं (Biḍalavaṇam).

Bidalavaṇa is salty, stimulates appetite, pacifies *kapha doṣa,* is *uṣṇavīrya, tīkṣṇa* (sharp), promotes desire for food and carminative. It is used in intestinal colics and heart disease.

13 सौवर्चलम् Sauvarcalam

अक्षं सौवर्चलं प्रोक्तं रुचकं हृद्यगन्धकम् ।
तिलकं कृष्णलवणं तत्काललवणं स्मृतम् ॥ ३१

लघु सौवर्चलं पाके वीर्योष्णं विशदं कटु ।
गुल्मशूलविबन्धघ्नं हृद्यं सुरभि रोचनम् ॥ ३२ S.Su. 46.317

सौवर्चलं (Sauvarcalam), अक्षम् (Akśam), रुचकं (Rucakam), हृद्यगन्धकम् (Hṛdyagandhakam), तिलकं(Tilakam), कृष्णलवणं (Kṛṣṇalavaṇam), काललवणं (Kālalavaṇam) are synonymous.

Sauvarcala is pungent in taste, *laghu* after *vipāka* (final transformation after digestion), *uṣṇavirya*, nonslimy, cordial, sweet smelling, promotes desire for food. It is useful in (intestinal) tumors (diverticulosis) and to remove constipation.

14 औद्भिदम् Audbhidam

औद्भिदं पांशुलवणं रोमकं वसुकं वसु ।
ऊषरं पांसवक्षारमौर्वं सार्वगुणं तथा ॥ ३३

लघु तीक्ष्णोष्णमुत्क्लेदि सूक्ष्मं वातानुलोमनम् ।
सतिक्तं कटुकं क्षारं विद्यात् लवणमौद्भिदम् ॥ ३४ S.Su. 6.319

औद्भिद (Audbhida), पांशुलवण (Paṁśulavaṇa) रोमकं (Romakam), वसुकं (Vasukam), वसु (Vasu), ऊषरं (Ūṣaram), पांसवक्षारं (Pāmsavakśāram), और्वम् (Aurvam), सार्वगुणं (Sārvaguṇam) are synonymous.

Audbhida Lavaṇa is slightly bitter, pungent and salty in taste, *uṣṇavīrya, ṭikśna* (sharp) causing excessive moistening, penetrating (entering minute channels) and carminative.

15 सामुद्रम् Samudram

सामुद्रलवणं प्राहुः क्षारं च शिशिरं तथा ।
समुद्रजं सागरजं लवणोदधिसंभवम् ॥ ३५

सामुद्रलवणं पाके नात्युष्णमविदाहि च ।
भेदनं स्निग्धमीषच्च शूलघ्नं नातिपित्तलम् ॥ ३६ S.Su. 46.315

सामुद्रलवणं (Sāmudralavaṇam), क्षारं (Ksāram), शिशिरं (Śiśiram), समुद्रजं (Samudrajam), सागरजं (Sāgarajam), लवणोदधिसंभवम् (Lavaṇodadhisambhavam) are synonymous.

Sāmudralavaṇa after *pāka* is not excessive *uṣṇa vīrya* and does not cause burning with hyperacidity and poor digestion (*avidāhī*), is *bhedana* (breaking of a mass), slightly unctuous, relieves colics and does not aggravate *pitta doṣa* too much.

16. (१०) हिंगु Hingu

हिंगु रामठमत्युग्रं जन्तुघ्नं भूतनाशनम् ।
अगूढगन्धं बाल्हीकं जरणं सूपधूपनम् ॥ ३७

हिङ्गूष्णं कटुकं हृद्यं सरं वातकफौ कृमीन् ।
हन्ति गुल्मोदराध्मानबन्धशूलहृदामयान् ॥ ३८

हिङ्गु (Hiṅgu), रामठम् (Rāmaṭham), अत्युग्रं (Attyugram), जन्तुघ्नं (Jantughnam), भूतनाशनम् (Bhūtanāśanam), अगूढगन्धं (Agūḍhagandham), बाल्हीकं (Bālhīkam), जरणं (Jaraṇam) and सूपधूपनम् (Sūpadhūpanam) are synonymous.

Hingū is pungent in taste, *uṣṇavīrya*, cordial, *sara* (laxative), pacifies *vātakaphadoṣas* and helminths. It is useful in tumors (dirverticulosis), abdominal swelling (ascites), tympanitis, constipation, colic and heart disease.

(Gum-resin obtained from the following plants)
Fam: Umbelliferae. Apiaceae.

I- a- ***Ferula foetida*** Regel.
Syn; *F.assafoetida* Boiss. and other allied species.

b- Dymock.C: Southern, Persia; Khorasan and Afaganistan near Herat.

II- a- रामठम् (Rāmaṭham); जन्तुघ्नम् (Jantughnam); बाल्हीकम् (Bāhlīkam); जरणम् (Jaraṇam); भूतनाशनम् (Bhūtanāśanam); सहस्रवेधी (Saharavedhī).

b- H. Mar. Bom. Bazar-name: हिंग्रा (Hingrā): Mal; Kayam; परुकायम (Parukāyam).

III- *Cf.* हिंगुपत्री (Hiṅguparti Plant pre No. 17 infra).
a- 1) हिंगु C.Sū. 2-29. Su. Sū. 38-22; 3-37.
1) *Ferula narthex Boiss.* (Chopra Handa p. 174-1958).

---

*The current name for *F. foetida* Regel is *Ferula assafoetida* Linn.

IV- Kannaya Lall Day, Desai, Chunekar p. 76.

Note: Several kinds and forms are now obtained from the plants included in the genus Ferula and are given different names according to the original gumresin. eg. Hiṅgrā, Abushāhi Hiṅga etc. (See Watt. Dic. Vol. III 328-336).

Hira hing: The term is applied to a liquid of treacly consistance found in the centre of the bales which is squeezed out and sold at a high price (Watt Dic. Vol. III P. 332 para 75).

17. हिंगुपत्री Hiṅgupatrī

हिंगुपत्री तु कबरी पृथ्वीका पृथुला पृथुः ।
बाष्पिका दीर्घिका तन्वी बिल्विका दारुपत्रिका ॥ ३९
बाष्पिका कटु तीक्ष्णोष्णा हृद्या वातकफापहा ।
कृमि प्लीहविबन्धार्शोगुल्महृत् बस्तिशूलनुत् ॥ ४०

हिंगुपत्री (Hiṅgupatrī), कबरी (Kabarī), पृथ्वीका (Pṛthvīkā), पृथुला (Pṛthulā), पृथुः (Pṛthuḥ), बाष्पिका (Bāṣpikā), दीर्घिका (Dīrghikā), तन्वी (Tanvī), बिल्विका (Bilvikā) and दारुपत्रिका (Dārupatrikā), are synonymous.

Bāṣpikā is pungent in taste, *uṣṇavīrya, tīkṣṇa* (sharp), pacifies *vāta, kaphadoṣas* and wholesome for heart. It is useful in worms, disorders of spleen, constipation, piles, tumors and renal colic.

Controversial plant

I- a- पृथ्वीका (Pṛthwīkā), बाष्पिका (Bāṣpikā) दारुपत्रिका (Dārupatrtikā), पृथुला (Pṛthulā), बिल्विका (Bilvikā).

III-a- 1) हिङगुपर्णी C. S. Ci. 9.63 हिङगुपत्रिका C. S. Ci. 9-66 (72). हिङगुशिवाटिका C.S. Ci. 10-35 (37).पृथ्वीका C.S. Sū. 2-3 5-20 बाष्पिका A. hr. Sû. 7-25; 15-4. (Balwantji p. 73.)

b- 1) 95 पृथ्विका पृथुलास्याच्छिकरिका हिङगुपत्रिका तंत्रि । बिल्वी खदिरपर्णी पृथुदीर्घा वार्षिका चेति ॥ (Abhi. Manj.)

2) 380 हिङगुपत्री (Hiṅgupatrī),बाष्पिका (Bāṣpikā), पृथ्वीका (Pṛthwīkā). (Harshe).

3) हिङगुपत्री-विटप विशेषः तस्याः पत्राणि हिङगुगन्धसदृशाणि भवन्ति । सा-द्विविधा एकाचारुणपत्रिका तन्त्री अपरा वेणुपत्रिका हिङगुफला ॥ (Dipika p. 190)

4) हिङगुपर्णी (Hinguparṇī), हिङगुशिवाटिका (Hinguśiwāṭikā); Lastly regarding the botanical source of *Hingupatrikā* हिङगुपत्रिका two varieties of Gum-resins i.e. those obtained from 1) *Gardenia gummifera* Linn. or (2) an allied species of Ferula such as *F.narthex Boiss* etc. may be examined. (Balwantji. Pp. 472-73)

Note: But the compiler of Dhn-ni. has recorded Hingupartikā, Nāḍī Hingu. (Dikāmāli *Gardenia gummifera* Linn Fl.) and Hingu (Ferula species) separately. Therefore Hingupatri is neither Dikāmāli nor Hingu of Dhan. ni.

The smell of *Hinguptrī* is similar to that of *Hingu*, so that the name *Hingupatrī* is applied to this plant. (Dipika III- 3 above).

18. (११) नाडीहिङ्गु Nāḍīhingu (Hinguśivāṭikā) (हिङ्गुशिवाटिक)

नाडीहिङ्गु पलाशाख्या जन्तुका रामठी च सा ।
वंशपत्री वेणुपत्री पिण्डा हिङ्गुशिवाटिका ॥ ४१

नाडीहिंगु कटूष्णं च कफवातार्तिशान्तिकृत् ।
विष्टम्भनविबन्धामदोषघ्नं दीपनं परम् ॥ ४२

नाडीहिङ्गु(Nāḍīhingu), पलाशाख्या (Palāśākhyā), जन्तुका (Jantukā), रामठी (Rāmaṭhī), वंशपत्री (Vamśapatrī), वेणुपत्री (Veṇupatrī), पिण्डा (Piṇḍā) and हिङ्गुशिवाटिका (Hinguśivāṭikā), are synonymous.

Nāḍihingu is pungent in taste, *uṣṇavīrya*, and pacifies the disorders caused by *kapha* and *vātadoṣa.* It is a strong appetiser and useful in constipation, flatulance and *āmadoṣa.*

Fam. Rubiaceac.

I- a- ***Gardenia gummifera*** Linn fl.
b- Dymock, c-Central and South India from Satapura range south ward.

II- a- पलाशा (Palāśā), जन्तुका (Jantukā), शिवाटिका (Śivātikā),
b- डिकामाली-Dikamālī; Tam; टिक्कामल्ली (कमले) (Tikkāmalli);कंबई (kambai); tel. करिंगुव (Karinguva), गोरिबिक्की (Goribikki); Mar:डिकामाली (Dikāmālī).

Note : There is another plant of the same genus *Gardenia lucida* *

*The current name for *Gardenia lucida* Roxb. is *Gardenia resinifera* Roth. (comp. p.68)

Roxb. from which the gum is obtained similar to above species and is used medicinally as Ḍikāmāli, Mar. H. Dikamali, Tam-Kumbi, Tel-Kuringuya, Kurungi, Tellamanga.

Modern names for the gum obtained from this plant are the same as those of *G. gummiferra* Linn.

19 (१२). तुम्बरुः Tumbaruḥ

तुम्बरुः सौरंभः सौरो वनजः सानुजोऽग्निकः ।
तीक्ष्णवल्कस्तीक्ष्णफलस्तीक्ष्णपत्रो महामुनिः ॥ ४३

तुम्बरुः कटुतीक्ष्णोष्णः कफमारुतशूलजित् ।
अपतन्त्रोदराध्मानकृमिघ्नो वह्निदीपनः ॥ ४४

तुम्बरुः (Tumbaruḥ), सौरभः (Saurabhaḥ), सौरः (Sauraḥ), वनजः (Vanajaḥ), सानुजः (Sānujaḥ), अग्निकः (Agnikaḥ), तीक्ष्णवल्कः (Tīkṣṇavalkaḥ), तीक्ष्णफलः (Tīkṣṇaphalaḥ), तीक्ष्णपत्रः (Tīkṣṇapatraḥ), and महामुनिः (Mahāmuniḥ) are synonymous.

Tumbaruḥ is pungent in taste, *tīkṣṇa* (sharp) and *ūṣṇavīrya*. It pacifies colics due to *kapha* and *vāta doṣas*. It is useful in *Apatantra* (a disease caused by *vātadoṣa*), ascites, tympanitis, anthelmintic and as a stimulant for digestive capacity.

Fam : Rutaceae.

I- a- ***Zanthoxylum alatum*** Roxb., b- Desai, c-Hot vallies of Sub-tropical Himalayas, Punjab, Komaon, Bhutan, Khasia Hills. (Watt. Dic.)

II- a- सौरभः (Saurabhaḥ), द्विजः (Dwijaḥ), तीक्ष्ण वल्कलः (Tīkṣṇavalkalaḥ), स्फुटफलः (Sphuṭaphalaḥ), सुगन्धिश्च (Sugandhiśca) तीक्ष्णपत्रः (Tīkṣṇaspatraḥ)

b- H.:तेजबल(Tejabala); B.- नेपाली धनिया Nepālidhaniā;Kan तुंबरुड्ड (Tumbarudu); Mar.; चिरफल(Chirphaḷa); तिरफळ (Tiraphaḷa); Mal- तुम्प्युनल, तुम्प्युणी

III- *Cf.* तेजफल(Tejaphlaḷa) of Raj. ni. P. 374 Plant No. 65 and तेजस्विनी (Tejaswinī) of Dhn. ni. Chap. 1 plant No. 80.

The tree *Z. rhetsa* DC. of S. India is used as *Tumbaru*. It is

---

१ 'सारसः' इति नि.शे. टीकायाम ।
२ 'सानुजो द्विजः' इति आनन्दाश्रम मुद्रित पुस्तके पाठः ।
For. *Z. alatum* Roxb. the current name is *Z. armatum* DC. (Comp. p. 161)
According to U.P.I. the current name for *Zanthoxylum rhesta* DC is *Z. limonella* (Dennst.) Alston Syn. - *Z.budrunga* Wall. ex DC. (p. 698).

तिरफळ (Tirphal), चिरफल (Chirphal) of Konkan, Tel.Rhetsāmaram. Kan-Gumi maran.

Z. rhetsa DC and *Z. budranga* Wall. are recorded two separate species in Watt. Dic.

20 (१३) सूक्ष्मैला Sūkṡmailā

सूक्ष्मैला द्राविडी तुत्था कोरङ्गी बहुला त्रुटिः ।
एला कपोतवर्णा च चन्द्रबाला च निष्कुटिः ॥ ४५
सूक्ष्मैला मूत्रकृच्छ्रघ्नी श्वासकासक्षये हिता ।
सूक्ष्मैला शीतला स्वादु हृद्या रोचनदीपनी ॥ ४६

सूक्ष्मैला (Sūkṡmailā), द्राविडी (Drāviḍī), तुत्था (Tutthā), कोरङ्गी (Koraṅgī), बहुला (Bahulā), त्रुटिः (Truṭiḥ), एला (Elā), कपोतवर्णा (Kapotvarṇā), चन्द्रबाला (Candrabālā), and निष्कुटिः (Niṣkuṭiḥ) are synonymous.

Sūkṡmailā is sweet in taste, *ṡītavīrya,* cordial, palatable and stimulates appetite. It is useful in dysuria, dyspnoea, cough and consumption.

Fam. Zingiberaceae.

I- A-a- ***Elettaria cardamomum***. Maton*
Syn. *Alpinia cardamomum* Roxb.

b- Roxburgh (Clarke ed. p. 24)
(Watt. Dic. p. 'E' 229).

c- Indigenous in West and South india growing abundantly in South Kanara, Mysore, Coorg. Travankor and Malabar and is said to be native of Cochinchina (Watt. Dic.)

II- a- द्राविडी (Drāviḍī), कोरंगी (Koraṅgī),कायस्था (Kāyasthā). Raj. ni.त्रुटि (Truṭi), उपकुञ्ची (Upakañcī). Raj.ni.
गर्भारिः (Garbhāriḥ).

b- Bom. Marathi; वेलची(Welacī), H.B.; छोटी एलची(Choṭī-elacī), Tam; Elakai : Tel : Elakkayalu, Eng : *Cardamoum, Lesser cardamoum.*

III Cf.भद्रैला (Bhadrailā).

---

* *Current accepted name is
Elettaria cardamomum (Linn). Maton (Comp. P. 58)

भद्रैला Bhadrailā (10)

भद्रैला बृहदेला तु त्रिपुटा त्रिदिवोद्भवा ।[१]
स्थूलैला त्वक्सुगन्धा च पृथ्वीका कन्यका पुटा ॥ ४७

एला तिक्तग च लघ्वी स्यात् कफवातविषव्रणान् ।
बस्तिकण्ठरुजो हन्ति मुखमस्तकशोधिनी ॥ ४८

भद्रैला (Bhadrailā), बृहदेला (Bṛhadelā), त्रिपुटा (Tripuṭā), त्रिदिवोद्भवा (Tridivodbhavā), स्थूलैला (Sthūlailā), त्वक्सुगन्धा (Twaksugandhā), पृथ्वीका (Pṛthvīkā), कन्यका (Kanyakā), and पुटा (Puṭā) are synonymous.

Bhadrailā is bitter in taste, *laghu* and pacifies *kapha-vāta doṣas*. It is useful in poisons and wounds, pains in urinary bladder, throat- pain and has purificatory action on mouth and head.

Fam. : Zingiberaceae.

I- a- 1) ***Amomum aromaticum*** Roxb.
b- Roxburgh . c-Native of villages on eastern frontier of Bengal and Nepal (Watt. Dic.)
a- 2) ***A. subulatum*** Roxb.
b- Roxburgh (Clarke ed. p. 13). c-Native of Nepal (Watt Dic.)

II- a- त्रिपुटोद्भवा (Tripuṭodbhavā),बृहदेला (Bṛhadelā), त्रिपुटा (Tripuṭā), त्वक्सुगन्धा (Twak sugandhā), पृथ्वीका (Pṛthvīkā), कन्यका (Kanyakā).
.b- San; त्रिदिवोद्भवा । सुरभि । - Tridivodbhava, Surabhī.
H.: बराएलची Barā elci, Tam : Peria elukkaya,
Tel. : Pedda yelukkayalu; Kan.: Bedda elakki;
Eng.: Greater cardamom, Grains of Paradise (Watt), *
H.B. मोरंग एलची(Moranga elachi); Mar.वेलदोडा (Veladoḍā).

Note : A fruit of a size of nutmeg containing smelling seeds. Raj. ni. and Watt. notes its native place asत्रिदिवोद्भवा (*Tridivodbhavā*) This name seems exactly alike Tibet. But Dhn. ni. notes त्रिपुटोद्भवा (*Tripuṭodbhavā*) which means as seeds covered in three caupsules (Puta = capsule).Raj. ni's त्रिदिवोद्भवा may be corruption of Dhn. ni.s त्रिपुटोद्भवा or a mistake may have been occured in copying or otherwise.

III- a- 1) A. H. U. 6 -26-See एला Ela.
2) C.S. Sū. 2-3, S. S. U. 28-21,22.

---

१ 'धान्यका ' इति नि. शे. टीकायाम् ।

* The grains of paradise is the name given to *Aframomum melegueta* Rosc.K. Schum; syn. *Amomum melegueta* Rosc. (U.P. I. p. 18)

21 (२४) नागपुष्पम् Nāgapuṣpam (Kesaram) केसरम्

नागपुष्पं मतं नागं केसरं नागकेसरम् ।
चाम्पेयं नागकिञ्जल्कं कनकं हेमकाञ्चनम् ॥ ४९

नागकेशरमल्पोष्णं लघु तिक्तं कफापहम् ।
बस्तिरुग्विषवातास्रकण्डूघ्नं शोफनाशनम् ॥ ५०

नागपुष्पं (Nāgapuṣpam), नागं (Nāgam), केसरम् (Kesaram), नागकेसरम् (Nāgakesaram), चाम्पेयं (Cāmpeyam), नागकिञ्जल्कं (Nāgakiñjalkam), कनकं (Kanakam), and हेमकाञ्चनम् (Hemakāñcanam), are synonymous.

Nāgakeśara is bitter in taste, *laghu* (easily digestible), slightly *uṣṇavīrya* and pacifies *kaphadosa.* It is useful in pain in the urinary bladder, poison, *vātarakta* (gout), pruritus and oedema.

Fam. Guttiferae. Clusiaceae.

I- a- ***Mesua ferrea*** Linn.
Syn. *M. coromondaliana* Roxb.

b- Roxburgh. c-Mountains East Himalayas and East Bengal, Asam and green rain forests of N. Kanara and S. Kokan -from S. Karwar to Travankor.

II- a- नागकेसरम् (Nāgakesaram), नाग किञ्जल्कम् (Nāgakiñjalkam), चाम्पेयम् (Cāmpeyam), हेम किञ्जल्कम् (Hema Kiñjalkam), नागीयकाञ्चनम् (Nāgīyakāñcanam).,

b- H. B. नागकेसर(Nāgakesara); Bom: - Mar-नाग चाफा Nāgacāpha), Tam-Shirk nāgappu, Nāngal; Mal: Nāngal, Tel: Kesaramu Guj: Puṣpam Mal: Nagacampakam. Behett- Champagum, Velutta campagam.

III- *Cf* चम्पक (Campaka), सुरपुन्नाग (Surapunnāga); किंकिरात (Kinkirāta) and क्षुद्रचम्पक (Kśudracampaka), described by Raj. ni. in.चम्पक

a- 1) Su. Su. 45-12; Ast. Hr. Ci. 5-54; C. ci. 28-154.

a- 1) नागप्रियाणि केसरवन्ती पुष्पाण्यस्य नागकेसरः । आह च- "नागपुष्पे मतो नागः केसरो नागकेसरः । चाम्पेयो नागकिञ्जल्कः कनकं हैमकाञ्चनम् ॥" (Ksiraswami, Amara 2-4-45; Tiwari P. 101)

2) 'चाम्पेयश्चम्पके स्वर्णवर्ण किञ्जल्के नागकेसर नागाख्य केसरः । इति मेदिनी' । स्वर्णभ्यः सर्पाख्य नागकेसरः षट्पदप्रियः इति रभसः । चम्पेयः केसरो नागकेसरः काञ्चनाह्वयः । (Bhanuji).

3) पुन्नागपुष्पम् (Punnāgapuṣpam), पुन्नागस्तुङ्गः अन्ये सुरपर्णिका

सुगन्धिपुष्पा दक्षिणापथे सुरपति (सुरङ्गी) इति ख्यातः ।
(Dalhan Su. 38-45).

4) नागपुष्पं-नागकेसरम् । अन्ये नागकेसरपुष्पो महातरुरितिख्यातः ।
(Dalhan Su-38-24)

Note: Dalhans's महातरु Mahātaru seems the tree *Ochrocarpus longifolius* Benth and Hook F. सुरपर्णी (Suraparṇi), सुरङ्गी Surangī

IV- 1) *Mesua ferrea* Linn with large globe of bright-gold coloured anthers in the centre of the flower. (Robura).

2) नागचम्पक (Nāgacampaka) See Ayur. Patrika 16-12-62.

3) *Mesua ferrea* Linn. नाग चाफा (Nāgacāpha). (See Desai & Cooke.)

4) नागकेसर (Nāgakesara). *Mesua ferrea* Linn.
भुजङगपुष्पम्, नागचम्पक, वारण केसर, अहिकेसर, कनक, नागाह्व.
C. S. Ci. 28-153, S.S. Su. 38-26, A. H. 21-79; u; 5-32, 6-27.
The anthers are used as genuine Nāgakesara, for which other substances such as the flower buds of *Ochrocarpus longifolius* Benth. and Hook. f. *

Calophyllum inophyllum Linn.-and fruits of some *Cinnamomum species* are used at present as substitutes (Balawantji Gloss, p. 220).

Note : The true नागकेसर (*Nāgakesar*) is the yellow किञ्जल्क (*Kinjalka*-Stamens and परागकोश (Parāgakosa-Anthers) of the flowers of नागचम्पक (Nāgacampaka).
These substituted substances are sold under the names लाल नागकेसर Lāla nāgakesara, कालेकेसर Kālekesara. The substituted trees are also recorded as Nāgakesara.

5) नागकेसरम् *Nāgakesaram* (J.R.I. M. II No. I.1967 p. 58).

6) क्षुद्रादिचम्पक *Kśudrādicampaka Nāgāhvacampaka* of South India (J.R. I. M. II. No. 1 of 1967 p. 58).

V- 1) नागचम्पक *Plumeria acutifolia Poir.* (Dr. Mhaskar).

Note: Mar. खडचाफा (*Khaḍacāphā*), खुरचाफा (*Khurcāphā*).

2) किंकिरात (*Kinkirāta*) of Dhn. ni. Bom: सुरंगी (*Surangi*); H.B.: Nāgakesara; Kan. Surungi; Tam : Surapuannai; Tel : Surapunnāgamu, *Ochrocarpus longifolius* Benth. Hook.f .* (Chopra).

3) नागकिंञ्जल्क नागपुन्नाम पुन्नाग केसर (Dr. Mhaskar p. 46).

---

* The current accpted name for *O. longifolius* Benth. & Hook. f. is *Mammea suriga* (Ham. ex Roxb.) Kosterm

Discussions :

Dr. Mhaskar has recorded पुन्नागकेसर (*Punnāga kesara*) for नागकेसर (*Nāgakesara*) i.e. the stamens of (V.3 above) and gives its botanical name as *Plumeria acutifolia* Poir.* (V-I above), पुन्नाग *Punnāga* is a South Indian tree and its botanical name is *Calophyllum inophyllum* Linn. and its South Indian names are *Punn, Punnāgam, Punnai;*- Mar.उण्डी *Uṇḍī* while the names of *P. acutifolia* Poir. are Mar. *Khaḍa cāphā, Khur-chāphā* Mal. *Vellachampakam;* Tam. *Porungallii* introduced into India from New World (See Chopra) - Milky juice; purgative, stamens few inserted in the base of petals. In short Dr. Mhaskar's *P. acutifolia* Poir. is not *Punnāga* and *Punnāga* is not नागकेसर *(Nāgakesara)* of Ayurvedic Books, True *Nāgakesara* of the Books is *Mesua ferrea* Linn. which is known as *Nāgacampaka, Nāgakesara* (See III-1,2,3, 4 and IV-1 to above). But the buds of सुरंगी, सुरपर्णी *Ochrocarpus longifolius* Benth. and Hook. f. *Calophyllum inophyllum* Linn. and Cinnamomum buds are substituted (See III-1 to 4 an IV-4 above) for true नागकेसर *Nāgakesara.*

22 (२५). त्वक् Twak

त्वचं वराङ्गं भृङ्गं त्वक्चोचं शकलमुत्कटम् ।
सैहलं लाटपर्णं च मुखशोध्यं वनप्रियम ॥ ५१

वराङ्गं लघु तीक्ष्णोष्णं कफवातविषापहम् ।
कण्ठवक्त्ररुजो हन्ति शिरोरुग्बस्तिशोधनम् ॥ ५२

त्वचं (Twacam), वराङ्गं(Varāngam), भृङ्गं (Bhṛngam), त्वक् (Twak), चोचं (Cocam), शकलम् (Śakalam), उत्कटम् (Utkaṭam), सैहलम् (Saihalam), लाटपर्णं (Lāṭaparṇam), मुखशोध्यं (Mukhaśodhyam), वनप्रियम् (Vanapriyam) are synonymous.

Twacam is *laghu, tīkṣṇa* (sharp) and pacifies *kapha vāta doṣas*. It is antipoisonous, useful in diseases of throat, mouth and head and purifies urinary organs.

Fam : Lauraceae

I- a- ***Cinnamomum zeylanicum*** Blume **

b- Watt. Dic. c-Native of Ceylon forest. Wild in the Southern coastal

---

* For *Plumeria acutifolia* Poir is *Plumeria rubra* Linn. forma *acuminata* Sant, Irani ex Shah. (comp. p. 121) (current name)

* * For *C. zeylanicum* Blume the current name is *C. verum* J.S.Presl. (comp p.37)

regions of Western India

II- वराङ्गम् (Warāṅgam), त्वक्चोचम् (Twak cocam); सैहलम् (Saihalam); गन्धवल्कम् (Gandhawalkam); शकलमुत्कटम् (Śakalamutkaṭam). H. B. Bom. Mar. दालचिनी(Dālchinī); Tel. Lavangamu, Lavangap-paṭṭa; Sanjling Kan. Dālcini, Lavangapatti.
Tam: Lavangap-paṭṭi Karruwa, Karuvap-paṭṭi; Eng,-True Cinnamon. Bark of *C. Zeylanicum* (Watt) Mal: Lavangap-patta.

III- *Cf. C.tamala,* Nees & Eburm.*

a- A.hr. Sū 6-158, 20-18; Su. Sū. 44-17.

IV- 1) The roots of this tree yeild camphor. The bark of *Cassia cinnamon* is adulterated in *true cinnamomum,* (Watt. Dic.)

23. (१६) तमालपत्रम् Tamālapatram

तमालपत्रं पत्रं स्यात्पलाशं च्छदनं दलम् ।
रामं तापसजं वासो गोपनं वस्त्रमंशुकम् ॥ ५३
पत्रकं कफवातार्शो हृल्लासारोचकापहम् ।

तमालपत्रं (Tamālapatram), पत्रं (Patram), पलाशं (Palāśam), च्छदनं (Chadanam), दलम् (Dalam), रामं (Rāmam), तापसजं (Tāpasajam), वासः (Vāsaḥ), गोपनं (Gopanam), वस्त्रं (Vastram), and अंशुकम् (Amśukam) are synonymous.

Tamālapatra pacifies *kapha* and *vāta doṣas* and is used in piles. It is useful in nausea and anorexia.

Fam. Lauraceae

I- a- ***Cinnamomum tamala*** Nees & Eburm.
Syn. *Laurus cassia* Roxb. (Watt. Dic).

b- Dymock. c-A moderate sized tree on the Himalaya from Indus to Satalaz.

II- a- पलाशम् (Palāśam), छदनम् (Chadanam), दलम् (Dalam), वासस्तापसम् (Wāsastāpasam).

B-b- तेजपत्र (Tejapatra); Bom-Mar; तमालपत्र (Tamālplatra), Tam, Tel:- तालिशपत्तरि (Tāliśa-pattari). Mal.:करुवयिला इलवङ्गतिज्जिला; Lavangada paṭṭa. (Ast. H. Kos.)
Eng - Cassia Lignae. China Cinnamon.

---

* For *C. tamala* Nees & Eburm. the current name is *C. tamala* (Ham.) Nees & Eburm.

IV- 1- *Cassia buds* of China is kept distinct from *C. tamal* by some writers, (Watt. Dic.).

2- *Cassia buds:*

These are the immatured fruits yielding Cassia Lignus. They are something as *cloves*...... They possess properties similar to those of *Cassia bark*.......... two kinds are found in Bombay makret Chinese and Malabar. (Watt. Dic. p. 32).

Bazar name of these buds is नागकेसर(*Nāgakesara)* and is used in spices by Mohamedens and are also substituted for *true Nāgakesara* (नागकेसर) (See नागकेसर Balwantaji).

24. (१७) तालीसकम् Tālisakam

तालीसकं तु तालीसं पत्रं तालीसपत्रकम् ॥५४
नीलमामलकीपत्रं पत्राढ्यं च शुकोदरम् ॥
तालीसं श्वासकासघ्नं दीपनं श्लेष्मपित्तजित् ॥५५
मुखरोगहरं हृद्यं सुपत्रं पत्रसंवृतम् ॥

तालीसकं (Tālisakam), तालीसं (Tālisam), पत्रं (Patram), तालीसपत्रकं (Tālisapatrakam), नीलं (Nilam), आमलकीपत्र (Amalakipatram), पत्राढ्यं (Patrāḍhyam), and शुकोदरं (Śukodaram) are synonymous.

Tālisa is useful in dysponea and cough, stimulates digestive capacity and pacifies *kapha pitta doṣas*. It is also useful in diseases of the mouth, सुपत्रं (Supatram) and पत्रसंवृतम् (Patra saṃvṛtam) are also its synonyms.

(Two species are used as Tālisam for compiler's plant, which are recorded here below.)

For Confirmation

A Fam : Pinaceae; Coniferaceae.

I- A-a- ***Abies webbiana*** Lindle.= *A-spectabills* (D. Don) Spach.

b- Kirtikar. c-Khassia, Sikkim and Bhutan, Fam: Taxaceae.

I- B-a- ***Taxus baccata*** Linn.

b- Th.Balawantji (p.10-179).

For *Abies webbiana* Lindl. the current name is *A. spectabilis* (D. Don) Spach. syn. *Pinus webbiana* Wall. (Comp. Gloss. p. 1)

For *Taxus baccata* Linn. the current name is *T. wallichiana* Zucc. syn *T. baccata auct.* (non Linn.) (comp. Gloss. p. 149.)

c- Temp. Himalayas, Kassia Hills.

II-A&B-a तालीस पत्रकम् (Tālis-patrakam), नीलामलकी पत्रम् (Nîlāmalakī-patram), नीलम् (Nīlam), तालम् (Tālam), नीलांबरम्(Nilāmbaram), तलाह्वयम् (Talāhvayam), पत्राढ्यम् (Patrāḍhyam), शुकोदरम् (Śukodaram),धात्रीपत्रम् (Dhātrīpatram), अर्कवेधम् (Arkawedham), घनच्छदम् (Ghanacchadam),

Note: Theses names are applicable to both the plants.

A-b H.चिलिराघ (Cilirāgha); Nepal; गोब्रासल (Gobrāsal); Eng. Himalayan Silver fer.

B-b- H.P. and Kashm: Birmi. B. Bhirmi; Bom: Barmi; Khasia-Dingsablih (Chopra).

III- *Cf.* प्राचीनामलकम् *Flacourtia jangomas* Raeusch (Watt Vol. I. P. A) तमालपत्रम् (*Cinnamomum tamal* Nees & Eburm).

a- 1) C.S. Sū. 1-80; 2-2; S.S. Su. 14-35; A.H. Sus. 14-24. (Balawantji p.368)

IV- 1) The dried leaves used by the Kaviraj as under the name of *Tālilsapatra*, were idedntified at the herbarium of the Royal Botanic Garden to be the leaves of *Pinus webbiana*. (U.C.Dutt).

2) In Ainslie and earlier writers on Indian Eco. Botany, तालीसपत्र *Tālisapatra* are the vernacular names for the dried leaves of *Flacourtia catafracta* Roxb* theपानीयाल *Pāniyāla* of Bengal. Mr.Gamble gives तालीसपत्र as the Hindi name for *Flacourtia catafracta* Roxb;

It seems difficult, however, for a man of Dr. Ainslie's ability mistaking the ovate leaf of *flacourtia* for the needle shaped leaves of *Fir (or Fer),* he must have personally identified the plants of which he wrote and acertained locally that the *Flacourtia* was the *Talīsapatra* of the shops of South India. It seems however that in different parts of the country different plants are prescribed as and it is quite probable that one of them are *true Talīsapatra* of Sanskrit writers. (Watt. Dict.)

3) It seems likely however that the leaves of *Abies webbianus* Lindl. are the original or true *Tālīspatra* . (Kirtikar II 1239).

4) *Abies webbianus* Lindl.
No cases of poisoning by this plant have been recorded in India but considering the common use as drug through-out the country such accident must have happened especially as the native doctors do not have appear to be aware of its poisonous properties.

* For *Flacoritia cataphracta* Roxb. the current name is *F. jangomas* (Lour.) Raeusch

Several cases of poisoning by Yew have recorded in England most of which have ended fatally..... (Dym III 377).

5) *Tālīspatra of Bombay Bazar..*

It is rather surprising that the plant *T. baccata* has no vernacular name, bears the *Talis,* but as modern application.

It is remarkable that in Bengal the *Tālispatra* as sold in Bazar, should be an *Abbies,* a plant possessed of carminative, expectorant and stomachic properties while in Bombay it should be the posionous leaves of the *Yew* which possessed emmenagogue, sedative and anti-spasmodic properties.

(Dr. Kirtikar).

(See Th. Balavantaji P. 177).

Note: The leaves of following trees are used as Tālispatra in the following parts of India.

1) Tamālapatra in South India.
2) Taxus baccata in Bombay.
3) Abies webbiana in Bengal.
4) Flacourtia jangomas Raeusch in Western India.
6) Ayur. A. P. IV-3-76 p. 294.
7) *Yew -Taxus baccata,* Linn.
Habitat-It grows in England and America and other parts of the world.
Description -Excepting the pulp of the fruit all parts are poisonous to man and animals. (Potter's cyclo).
8) *Taxus baccata* L. Plant poisonous, alk. taxine is vigourously active heart poison. (Chopra).

Discussion :

The confusion about the plant तालीसकम् *Tālīsakam* seems to have arisen due to similarity of the names occured in the text, such as: धात्रीपत्रम् आमलकीपत्रम्, तालम् etc. These similative terms of Sanskṛt books may have caused the confusion in the search of the तालीसकम् (*Tālīsakam*). When Ayurvedic Society was sperading East-ward and Southward may have selected a plant of somewhat similarity in morphological and having pharmacological properties. In this way different plants in different parts and in different regions may have utilised by different societies and the true drug-plant remained in confusion.

It is said that some parts of *Taxus baccata* are poisonous and if it would be proved by examination or analysis then *Abies webbianus* Lindl. should be examined and accepted as तालीसकम् (*Tālīsakam*) of the Sanskṛt books.

The other plants used in different parts are not acceptable as *Tālisakam* to our compiler's.

25 (१८) (तुगा) वंशरोचना (Tugā)Vaṁśarocanā

स्याद वंशरोचना वांशी तुगाक्षीरी तुगा शुभा ।५६
त्वक्क्षीरी वंशजा शुभ्रा वंशक्षीरी च वैणवी ॥

वंशक्षीरी स्मृता वंश्या यवजा यवसंभवा ।।५७
गोधूमसंभवा चान्या षष्टितण्डुलजोद्‌भवा ॥

कषाया मधुरा तिक्ता कासघ्नी वंशरोचना ।।५८
मूत्रकृच्छ्रक्षयश्वासहिता बल्या च बृंहणी ॥

पलाशगंधा (ध.नि.) Palāśagandhā (11)
अन्या पलाशगंधा च तवक्षीरी प्रकीर्तिता ।।५९
त्वक्क्षीरी मधुरा रूक्षा कषायाऽस्रारुचिव्रणान् ॥ Ast. San.Sū.12
पित्तश्वासक्षयान्हन्ति कासदाहनिषूदनी ।।६०

वंशरोचना (Vaṁśarocanā), वांशी (Vāṁśī), तुगाक्षीरी (Tugākśīrī), तुगा (Tugā), शुभा (Śubhā), त्वक्क्षीरी (Twakkśīrī), वंशजा (Vaṁśajā), शुभ्रा (Śubhrā), वंशक्षीरी (Vaṁśakśīrī), and वैणवी (Vaiṇavī) are synonymous.

Vaṁśakśīrī is derived from vaṁśa (Bamboo). There are other types like यवजा (Yavajā), which is derived from *Yava*; गोधूमसंभवा (Godhūmasambhavā) and षष्टितण्डुलजोद्‌भवा (Ṣaṣṭitaṇḍulajodbhavā) are other types.

Vaṁśarocanā is sweet, *kaṣāya* (astringent) and bitter in taste. It is useful in cough, dysuria, consumption, dyspnoea, is strength promoting and body weight promoting.

पलाशगन्धा (Palāśagandhā)

There is an another type of त्वक्क्षीरी (Twakkśīrī); पलाशगन्धा (Palāśagandhā) and तवक्षीरी (Tavakśīrī) are its synonyms.

Twakkśīrī is sweet, *kaṣāya* (astringent) in taste, *rūkśa* (roughning) and pacifies *pitta doṣa*. It is useful in *raktapitta* (haemorrhagic disorders), in anorexia, wounds, dyspnoea, consumption, cough and burning sensation.

(Under this heading name both the compilers have recorded two kinds of वंशरोचना (Vaṁśarocanā). The one of it is *'A'* तुङ्गा (Tuṅgā) तुगाक्षीरी (Tugākśīrī), a group of seven materials and the next is *'B'* वंशरोचना (Vaṁśarocanā); *Tugākaśīrī* is a generic name of the substance derived from the materials and plants noted herebelow while 'B' *Vam'sarocanā* group is a substance obtained from *Bamboo* varieties.

I-a-A तुङ्गा Tungā Group

Under this following materials and plants are included by the compilers.

I- a- i- यवजा (*Yavajā*) viz. starch derived from *Hordeum species* (Barley).

a- ii- गोधूम (*Godhūm*) viz. starch derived from wheat.

a- iii- षष्टितण्डुलोदभवा-मासद्वयोदभवा i.e. starch derived from the rice which ripes within two months.

a-iv- अन्या पलाशगंधा(*AnyāPalā'sagandhā*) i.e. Starch derived from the root-stock of the following plants.

Fam : Zingiberaceae.

(a) *Hedychium spicatum* Ham. ex Smith.

(b) *H. coronarium* Linn.

Note: The plant पलाशगंधा (*Pala'sagandhā*) is, in this edition recorded under a separate heading but it is actually a part of तुगाक्षीरी (*Tugāk'sīri* 1-A-a above), being so we have not given a separate heading name to this plant. Besides the above noted group of तुगाक्षीरी *(Tugāk'sīri)* Raj.ni. includes the following materials in तुगाक्षीरी (*Tugāk'siri)* under the heading name पलाशगन्धा (*Palā'sgandhā*).

a-iv- गवयोद्भवम् *Gavayodbhavam* i.e. obtained from cow' milk.

a-vi-वनगोक्षीरम् *Vanagok'sīram* obtained from wild cow's milk.

a-vii- ताल संभूतं तालक्षीरादि नामकम् (*Tāla sambhutam Tālak'sirādi nāmakam*) obtained from various species of Tāla (Palms).

II- A-a- तुङ्गा (तुगा) क्षीरी (*Tugāk'sīri), तुगा* (*Tugā*), शुभ्रा.(*'Subhrā*),श्वेता (*'Swetā*).

A-b- H:-तिक्कुर तवक्षीर, सागु (*Tikkūra*), (*Tavak'sīra*), (Sāgu), Eng.: *Sago Starch, Manna.*

These are the seven kinds of starch included under the heading तुगा Tugā(A group).

I-a-B-वंशजा Vamsajā Group.

I- B-a-***Bambusa arundinacea*** Willd. and allied species of Bambusa.

b- Watt Dic. IV-10. c- Wild and cultivated.

II- B-a- वंशजा (Vam'sajā), पिङ्गा (Pingā), वंशक्षीरी (Vam'sak'sīri), वंशरोचना (Vam'sarocanā).

B-b- वंश (Vams̓a):H.B-Bās, Mar: Kaḷaka; Bom; Māṇagā, Tam; & Mal-Māngal; Tel-Bangu, (Bambu?) venduru, Eng: Bamboo(Tree). *Bamboo-Manna*-(The substance).

III- b- 173 तुकाशुभा तुकाक्षीरीत्वक्क्षीरी धवला शुभा ।
शुभापुष्पा कुग्गीनीति प्रोक्ता प्रदरनाशिनी ।
(Abhi. manji. Moos).

Foot Note: Maranta arundinacea,
केषुचित् प्रदेशेषु तुकाभावात् वंशरोचनोपज्युते ॥
तेन गणेऽपठिताया वंशरोचनाया पर्यायाणामत्र
वक्तुमुचितत्वात् तेऽपि निगद्यते । (Abi. Man. 173 Moose).

IV- 1) ....and indeed considerable confusion existed in the species of *Curcuma, Amomum, Alpinia* and *Hedychium.*
(Watt. Dic. 'H' P. 207).

2) पलाशा *PALĀSA;*
C.S.Si. 3-37.
In both these places the version is disputed to be either *Palās̓a* पलाश or *Palās̓ā* पलाशा. If the latter is correct, कर्चूर (*Karcūra*) or शठी (S̓aṭhī) should be taken. (Balvantaji P. 241).

3) *Hedychium spicatum* Ham. ex Smith.(see I-A-a, iv -ai-above).

Note: There are two varieties. The Indian and Chinese. The latter is larger and less pungent. The powder of roots is the chief ingredient in Abir. (Watt. Vol. ;N' p. 207), but according to Dr. Desai the Indian variety is preferred for practice. Indian variety has more pleasant flavour than that of China variety.

4) *Hedychium coronarium* Linn. (See I-a-A-iv-b-above).

5) पृथु पलाशिका (Pṛthu Palās̓ikā) broad leaved, सुगन्धमूला (Sugandhamūlā), चंद्राणी (Candrāṇī), हिमोद्भवा (Himodbhavā) (flowers appear in Winter season), सठी (Saṭhi), सठिका (Saṭhikā).(Dhn. Ni.Pp.18,19).

Note: Cooke notes its Marathi name as *(Sonatakka).* This is actually called सोनटक्का (Sonaṭakkā) in Marathi in Poona, Satara and Kolhapur Districts. (Mahabaleshwar also). Roots are not horizontal, it is underground *stem rhizome.* (Mahajan).

Note : We have accepted this plant as शढी *S̓adhi* of Dhn. ni.
(See Vol. I-p. 15).

6) तवक्षीरी (*Tavasksīrī*) A. H. Sū. 30-51; Ci. 3-66.
This is the starch separated from rhizomes of *Curcuma angustifolia,* Roxb, and called *Tikkura* and used as arrowroot as a substitute of true *arrow root* (*Maranta arundinacea* Linn). This appears to have been used by Vagbhat as substitute of *True Vams̓alocana* वंशलोचन as well . (Balavantji p. 176).

Note: Balvantji appears to recognise *Curcuma angustifolia* Roxb, as तवक्षीर Tavaksira occured in Vagbhat, but our compiler has not included *Curcuma* species under this heading. It is true that several species of *Curcuma* genus are now used as Tavaksira. *Maranta arundinacea* Linn is introduced in the Old World after 1831. (see IV-7-below).

7) *Maranta arundinacea* Linn.
West Indies Arrowroot.
The first introduction of Maranta into India........... First plantation in Good Hope in 1831.

8) सुगा* (Sago) तालसंभूता (Tālasambhutā of Raj. ni. (I-a-A-VII above).

9) The proper *Sago Palm (Metroxylon sagu)* is not indigenous to Indian peninsula but large quantities of sago of commerce are obtained in India from other sources. (Watt Dic. 'M' 180-182)

10) *Bambusa arundinacea* Retz.
History uses (P. 586-87)
Young shoots are eaten, action on the uterus: used by females to cause free flow of the lochial discharge.......(abide p. 180-82)

Description :

Bamboo manna is the Vamsha lochan of the Hindoos, *Tabakshira* consists of irregularly shaped fragments opque white or bluish opalescent colour.; The larger pieces are about an inch in diameter *'concave-convex* and have evidently derived from the joints (nodes) of the bamboo in which the deposit has collected. The raw article is blackened and dirty having apparently been obtained by burning the bamboos or on account of the presence of insects; to make it fit for use it is calcined when it becomes perfectly clean. Chemical composition.... (Dymock Vol. III P. 590.)

26 (१९) उपकुञ्ची (पृथ्वीका) Upakuñcī (Pṛthvikā)

उपकुञ्चा चोपकुञ्ची[१] कालिका चोपकालिका ।
सुषवी कुञ्चिका कुञ्ची पृथ्वीका स्थूलजीरकः ॥ ६१

पृथ्वीका कटुका पाके रुच्या पित्ताऽग्निदीपनी ।
श्लेष्माध्मानहराऽजीर्णजन्तुघ्नी च प्रकीर्तिता ॥ ६२

१ 'कुञ्चिका चोपकुञ्ची च कालिका चोपकालिका ।
सुषवी कुञ्चिका कुञ्ची पृथ्वी कृष्णे च जीरके ॥' इति नि.शे. टीकायाम् ।

* (? तुगा - तवक्षीरं - तालसम्भूतम् ।)S. D. K.

उपकुञ्चा (Upakuñcā), उपकुञ्ची (Upakuñcī), कालिका (Kālikā), उपकालिका (Upakālikā), सुषवी (Suṣavī), कुञ्चिका (Kuñcikā), कुञ्ची (Kuñcī), पृथ्वीका (Pṛthvīkā), and स्थूलजीरकः (Sthūlajīrakaḥ) are synonymous.

Pṛthvīkā is pungent in *vipāka* (final transformation after digestion), appetite promoting, aggravates *pitta* and pacifies *kapha*. It stimulates digestive capacity, is carminative, digestant and anthelmintic.

(This plant is a kind of जीरक (Jīraka), Cumin but of black colour).

Fam. Ranunculaceae.

I- a- ***Nigella sativa*** Linn.
Syn. *N. indica* Roxb.

b- Roxburgh. c-Punjab, Bihar and parts of India, cultivated and occasionally weed of cultivation, (Chopra).

II- a पृथ्वीका (Pṛthwīkā), सुषवी (Suṣavī), स्थूलजीरक (Sthūlajīraka), कालिका (Kālikā), कुञ्चिका(Kūñcikā).

b- San.कृष्ण जीरक (Kṛṣṇa jīraka);
H.: मंगरेला (Mangarailā); कलौञ्जी (Kalauñji);
B : कालीजिरा (Kālijīrā); Bom: काळे जिरे(Kaḷenjire);
Tel : Nulda jilakara; Tam: Karun jiragam, Eng.: Small fennel, Blackcumin.

III- *cf. Carum nigrum* Royle (Watt.) *C. carvi* Linn.

Note : जीरक (Jīraka), जरण (Jaraṇa), is a generic name. There are several forms and species in this genus of Indian and foreign nativity with slight difference in their colour. उपकुञ्ची and कृष्णा infra are a slight black purple colour.

a- उपकुञ्ची (Upakuñcī).C.S.Su.-8-70; 73. S.S.Su.-46-230. A. hr. ci. 8-45.

b- 1) 103 'उपकुञ्ची' ति कृष्णजीरः कृष्णाजाजी (Harshe)

IV जीरक (Jīraka)

(a) *Cuminum cyminum Linn.*
श्वेत (Śwet) or Saphet जिरा (Jirā);

(b) *Carum carvi* Linn. and *C. bulbocastaum* Koch,कालाजीरा (Kālājirā);(Syāhaīira)

(c) *Nigella sativa* Linn.
By Jīrakadwaya जीरकद्वय the first two varities ie. *śveta* and *Kṛṣṇa* are understood, *Upakūñcikā* and *kāravi* कारवी are exclusively used for the third and second varieties respectively. *Ajājī* अजाजी, it seems, has been used for either of the first two

and *Pṛthvīkā* पृथ्वीका if used for any varieties of *Jīraka,* should indicate the third variety." (Balavantji P. 169)

27. (२०) दाडिमः Dāḍimaḥ

दाडिमो दाडिमीसारः कुदिटमः फलषाडवः ।
स्वाद्वम्लो रक्तबीजश्च करकः शुकवल्लभः ॥ ६३

स्निग्धोष्णं दाडिमं हृद्यं कफपित्ताविरोधि च ।
द्विविधं तच्च विज्ञेयं मधुरं चाम्लमेव च ॥ ६४

दाडिमः (Dāḍimaḥ), दाडिमीसारः (Dāḍimīsāraḥ), कुट्टिमः (Kuṭṭimaḥ), फलषाडवः (Phalaṣāḍavaḥ), स्वाद्वम्लः (Swādvamlaḥ), रक्तबीजः (Raktabījaḥ), करकः (Karakaḥ), and शुकवल्लभः (Śukavallabhaḥ) are synonymous.

Dāḍima is *snigdha* (unctuous), *uṣṇavīrya,* palatable and is not contraindicated in the conditions due to *kapha-pitta doṣas*. It is of two kinds sweet and sour.

I- a- ***Punica granatum*** Linn.

b- Roxburgh c-Asiatic plant-Wild in the Salt ranges and in the Himalayas. Cultivated in many parts of India (See Decandole) wild in Persia, Kurdistan, Afaganistan, Balucistan, (Watt. P. 369).

II- a- रक्तबीजः(Raktabījaḥ), कुचफलः (Kucaphalaḥ), शुकवल्लभः (Śukavallabhaḥ).

b- H : दारिम (Dārim), अनार (Anāra).
B : दालिम (Dālim), Mar: डाळिंब (Ḍāḷimba). Tam : Madulai; Magilam;
Tel : Dālimba. Eng : The Pomegranate
Kan : Dallimbe-gid, Mal; Maṭalam, pazham, जालिमालक, उसमाम्यकम्

III- 1) A decoction of the bark of the root has been found to be a sovereign remedy for the *Tenia* or Tape-worm. (C.B.C.P.402).

28 (२१) धान्यकम् Dhānyakam

धान्यकं धान्यका धान्या धानी धानेयकं तथा ।
कुस्तुम्बरुश्चाल्लका च च्छत्रधान्यं वितुन्नकम ॥ ६५

आर्द्रा कुस्तुम्बुरुः कुर्यात् स्वादुसौगन्ध्यहृद्यताम् ।
सा शुष्का मधुरा पाके स्निग्धा तृड्दाहनाशिनी ॥ ६६

S.S.Su.46. 230

धान्यकं कासतृट्छर्दि ज्वरहृच्चक्षुषो हितम् ।
कषायतिक्तम्मधुरं हृद्यं दीपनपाचनम् ॥ ६७

धान्यकं (Dhānyakam), धान्यका (Dhānyakā), धान्या (Dhānyā), धानी (Dhānī), धानेयकं (Dhāneyakam), कुस्तुम्बरुः (Kustumbaruḥ), अल्लका (Allakā) च्छत्रधान्यं (Cchatradhānyam) and वितुन्नकम् (Vitunnakam) are synonymous.

Ārdra kustumburuḥ (the green plant of Dhānyakam), is sweet, fragrant and palatable. when dried it is sweet in *vipāka* (final transformation after digestion) and useful in thirst and burning sensation.

Dhānyaka is *kaṣāya*, bitter and sweet in taste, appetizer and digestant and useful in cough, thirst, emesis, fever and beneficial to heart and eyes.

Fam : Umbelliferae. Apiaceae

I- a- ***Coriandrum sativam*** Linn.
b- Roxburgh c-cultivated all over India.

II- a- धानेयकम् (Dhāneyakum), कुस्तुंबुरु (Kustumburu), चावलिका (Cāwalikā).

II- a- धानेयकम् (Dhāneyakam), कुस्तुंबुरु (Kustumburu), चावलिका (Cāwlikā).
b- H.धनिया, (Dhāniyā), धान (Dhāna):
B-Mar. Bom; धने (Dhane) कोथिंबीर (Kothimbira) (Green plant);
Tam : Koth-malli, Kotamalli, Kan : Dhanialu, Kothamilu;
Kothimir, Tel : Dhanialu, Kothamilu; Kothimir,
Mal :Kothumpalari Eng.: Coriander,
Assyrian ; *Kuetimbari,* (Harshe into .P. XLVIII).

29 (२२) जीरकम् Jīrakam

जीरकं दीर्घकं हृद्यमजाजी दीप्यमागधम् ।
मनोज्ञं वरुणं रुच्यं पीताभं पूज्यमानकम् ॥ ६८

जीरकं कटुकं रूक्षं वातहृद्दीपनं परम् ।
गुल्माध्मानातिसारघ्नं ग्रहणीकृमिहृत्परम् ॥ ६९

जीरकं (Jīrakam), दीर्घकम् (Dīrghakam), हृद्यम् (Hṛdyam), अजाजी

(Ajājī), दीप्यम् (Dīpyam), मागधम् (Māgadham), मनोज्ञम् (Manojñyam), वरुणम् (Varuṇam), रुच्यम् (Rucyam), पीताभं (Pītābham), and पूज्यमानकं (Pūjyamānakam) are synonymous.

Jīraka is pungent in taste, *rūkśa* (roughning), pacifies *vātadoṣa,* stimulates appetite. It is useful in tumors (diverticulosis), tympanitis, diarrhoea, *grahaṇī* (disorders of *Grahaṇī*) and worms.

Fam. : Umbellifere. Apiaceae

I- a- ***Cuminum cyminum*** Linn.

b Roxburgh c-cultivated throughout India except Bengal and Assam (Chopra).

II- a अजाजी (Ajājī), दीप्यम् (Dīpyam),मागधम् (Māgadham), H-जीरा (Jirā); Mar.Jiren; Tam : Siragam, Tel : Jiraka; Kan : Kirag, Mal : Jorakam, Eng. : Cumin.

III- *cf.*कृष्णा Kṛṣṇā उपकुञ्ची (Upakuñcī).

IV- 1) "But we are justified in accepting the opinions....... that it is a native of Meditarranean region...... The uniformity in which through all the languages of India, the Sanskrit name Jiraka and the Persian name Zira re-appear, points atleast to a common centre from which the plant spread over the East.

(Watt. Dict. P. 'C' 643)

2) Native of Persia and some parts of Western Asia.

(Fl. indi. C.B.C. Edit. P.271)

शुक्लः Suklaḥ (12)

शुक्लाजाजी कणा ख्याता दीर्घकः कणजीरकः ।
स्तन्यो दीर्घकणा गौरजीरको दीर्घजीरकः ॥ ७०

गौराजाजी हिमा रुच्या कटुर्मधुरदीपनी ।
कृमिघ्ना विषहन्त्री च चक्षुष्याऽध्माननाशनी ॥ ७१

शुक्लाजाजी (Śuklājājī), कणा (Kaṇā), दीर्घकः (Dīrghakaḥ), कणजीरकः (Kaṇajīrakaḥ), स्तन्यः (Stanyaḥ), दीर्घकणा (Dīrghakaṇā), गौरजीरकः (Gaurajīrakaḥ) and दीर्घजीरकः (Dīrghajīrakaḥ), are synonymous.

Śuklajīraka is pungent and sweet in taste, *śitavīrya*, palatable, promotes appetite, is anthelmintic, antipoison, beneficial to eyes and carminative.

I- a- A kind of *C. cyminum* Linn. but may be a rather whitish colour and little longer

b- Kamat. C. Cultivated.

II- a शुक्लाजाजी (Śuklājājī), कणजीरकः (Kaṇajīrakaḥ), दीर्घकणकः (Dīraghakaṇakaḥ).

Modern names as in जीरकम् (Pre No. 29 supra).

III- *cf.* जीरकम् च शुक्लम् (Gud. Dip. p. 124).

IV 1) There are many forms of Zīrā (Watt. Dic.)

2) Vol. II part Pp. 113-114 (Dymock).

कृष्णजीरकम् Kṛṣṇajīrakam (13)

कृष्णाजाजी तु जरणा सुगन्धः कणजीरकः ।
कश्मीरजीरका वर्षा कालिः स्यात् कालपेशिका ॥ ७२
जरणा कटुरुष्णा च कफशोफनिकृन्तनी ।
रुच्याऽजीर्णज्वरघ्नी च चक्षुष्या ग्राहिणी परा ॥ ७३

कृष्णाजाजी (Kṛṣṇājājī), जरणा (Jaraṇā), सुगन्धः (Sugandhaḥ), कणजीरकः (Kaṇajīrakaḥ), कश्मीरजीरका (Kaśmīrajīrakā), वर्षा (Varṣā), कालिः (Kāliḥ) and कालपेशिका (Kālapeśikā) are synonymous.

Kṛṣṇajīraka is pungent in taste, *uṣṇavīrya,* pacifies *kaphadoṣa* and relieves oedema. It is useful as appetizer, in indigestion, beneficial to eyes and as astringent.

Fam : Umbelliferae. Apiaceae.

I- a- ***Carum caravi*** Linn.

Syn ; C. *bullbocastanum* koch.

b Dymock

c- Cultivated in the plains of India, Baltistan and Kashmir.

II- a- कृष्णजीरक (Kṛṣṇajīraka); कश्मीरजीरका (Kaśmīrajīrakā), नीलकणा (Nīlakaṇā).

b- H.कालाजिरा (Kālājirā), शिआजिरा(Śiājirā); Bom : विलायती जिरे Vilāyatijire),शहाजिरे (Sahājire), Tam.: Shimai-shembu; Kekuviral, Pilappu Shiragam; Tel. : Simai-sappu, Sima-jilakara.Mal : Simajilakara, Mal: Shima-jirakam, कारीजिरकं Eng;Indian Caraway.

III- *cf.*उपकुञ्ची (Upakuñcī),

b- 1) कृष्णजीरक (Kṛṣṇajīraka),
438-उपकुञ्ची (Upkuñcī),
135-कालाजीरा (Kālājīrā) (Harshe).

2) कृष्णजीरकं पाश्चात्यम् । (Kṛṣṇajīrakam Pāścātyam).
तच्च खुरासन (Khurāsana) वाच्यम् (Gu. Dip. P. 194).

IV- The existence of the name of Vilāyatī zirā. The name might simply mean that part of the country it was first brought to the attention of Natives by the Europeans. (Watt. Dic. P. C.197)

बृहत्पाली Bṛhatpālī (14) (Vanya Jīrakam वन्यजीरकम्)

बृहत्पाली सूक्ष्मपत्रा वन्यजीरः कणा तथा ।
वन्यजीरः कटुः शीतो व्रणहा जन्तुनाशनः ॥ ७४

बृहत्पाली (Bṛhatpālī), सूक्ष्मपत्रा (Sūkṣmapatrā), वन्यजीरः (Vanyajīraḥ), and कणा (Kaṇā) are synonymous.

Vanyajīraḥ is pungent in taste, *śitavīrya.* It is useful in wounds and as an anthelmintic.

Fam: Compositae. Asteraceae.

I- a- ***Centratherum anthelminticum*** (Willd) Kuntze*
Syn: *Vernonia anthelmintica* Willd.

b- Desai, Roxburgh c-Throughout India, Himalaya and Khasia Hills, Troublesome weed in winter- crops.

II- a- वन्यजीरः (Vanyajīraḥ), अरण्यजीरः (Araṇyajīraḥ)

b- H.B. Somarāji; Bom; Kadūjiren; Mal : Kaṭu-jirkam Tam : Kattu-Shiragam; Tel. : Adavi jilakamu, Eng : The Purple Flea Bane.

III- cf बाकुची (Bākucī) Dhn. ni. Chapter I.)

a- 1) S.S. ci. 9-2, 25-18; A.H. ci. 9-12, 19-45; 53. (Balawantji).

IV- 1) Araṇyajīraka (Yadavji).
2) *Vernonia anthelmintica* Willd.
Somarāji, Bākucī.
Dymock; Kirtikar, Ghanekar, Su. Su. 42-29, 46-269).
(Balavantsimhaji Bihar; Watt. Dic).

---

* The current name for *Centratherum anthelminticum* (Willd.) Kuntze is: *Centratherum anthelminticum* (Linn.) Kuntze; syns. *Serratula anthelmintica* Roxb., *Vernonia anthelmintica* Willd.(comp. to Gloss. p. 33)

Note - अरण्यजीरक (Araṇya jīraka) is not (Bākucī) of Dhn. ni.; Dhn.ni's Bākucī is *Psoralia corylifolia* Linn.

30 (२३) पिप्पली Pippalī

पिप्पली मागधी कृष्णा चपला तीक्ष्णतण्डुला ।
उपकुल्या कणा श्यामा कोला शौण्डी तथोषणा ॥ ७५

पिप्पली कटुका स्वादुर्हिमा स्निग्धा त्रिदोषजित् ।
तृड्ज्वरोदरजन्त्वामनाशिनी च रसायनी ॥ ७६

पिप्पली (Pippalī), मागधी (Māgadhī), कृष्णा (Kṛṣṇā), चपला (Capalā), तीक्ष्णतण्डुला (Tikṣṇataṇḍulā), उपकुल्या (Upakulyā), कणा (Kaṇā), श्यामा (Śyāmā), कोला (Kolā), शौण्डी (Śauṇḍī), and ऊषणा (Ūṣaṇā) are synonymous.

Pippalī is pungent and sweet in taste, *śītavīrya,* unctuous (*snigdha*) and pacifies all the three *doṣas*. It is useful in thirst, fever, ascites, worms, *āmadoṣa* and as *rasāyana* (rejuvinating).

(Pippalī is a generic name and under this *generic group* three to four species are included which see infra).

Fam. Piperaceae.

I- a- ***Piper longum*** Linn. Sp. Pl.

b- Roxburgh c-Hotter states of India; particularly in Bengal.

II- a- मागधी (Māgadhī), वैदेही (Vaidehī), उपकुल्या (Upakulyā),कणा (Kaṇā), कोरंगी (Korangī), तिक्ततण्डुला (Tiktataṇḍulā).

b- Kan : Vippali, Yippali;
H.: पिप्पलमूल (Pippalamula); Mar: Lenḍi-Pimpḷi;
Tel : Pippuli, piplalachetu; Mal; Pippali, pippalu,
Tam : (Tippali; Eng : Long pepper.)

III- *cf;* चव्य (Cavya),श्रेयसी (Śreyasī),

a- 1) तां देवा समकल्पनीयं जीवितं वा अलम् ॥.. ॥
(Av. VI-109)
हे पिप्पली त्वा त्वाम् असुरः पूर्वदेवाः न्यखनत ॥ (Sayana).

b- 1) चतुर्धा पिप्पली प्रोक्ता (Raj. ni. Dhn ni. p. 345)

2) सं. पिप्पलीः के. तिप्पली. त. -तिप्पिली, क.-हिप्पली; ते. पिप्पलु; म-लेंडी पिंपली.(Ayur. 0. Ni.).

IV- 1) *Piper longum* Willd.
S.-Kṛṣṇā (etc.) Tel: Pippal-chetu (Plan), Pippaloo (root); (Roxb. j.)
2) Long Pepper is obtained from *Piper retrofractum* of Java and *Piper longum* of India. The former is a climbing woody plant, native to Malaya, is culitivated in Java, Bali and adjacent islands. (Hill).

31 (२४) मूलम् Mūlam (Pippalīmūlam) (पिप्पलीमूलम्)

मूलं च पिप्पलीमूलं ग्रन्थिकं चविकाशिरः[1] ।
कोलमूलं कटुग्रन्थि सर्वग्रन्थिकमूषणम् ॥ ७७

कटूष्णं पिप्पलीमूलं श्लेष्मसंघातनाशनम् ।
वातोच्छित्तिकरं हन्ति कृमीन् वह्निप्रदीप्तिकृत् ॥ ७८

मूलम् (Mūlam), पिप्पलीमूलं (Pippalimūlam), ग्रन्थिकं (Granthikam), चविकाशिरः (Cavikāśiraḥ), कोलमूलं (Kolamūlam), कटुग्रन्थि (Kaṭugranthi), सर्वग्रन्थिकम् (Sarvagranthikam) and ऊषणम् (Ūṣaṇam) are synonymous.

Pippalīmūlam is pungent in taste, *uṣṇavīrya,* removes accumulation of *kaphadoṣa,* pacifies *vātadoṣa,* useful in worms and stimulates digestive capacity.

I- a- 1) Roots of *Pippalī* and *Chavya.*
b- Kamat. c-See Pippalī and Chavya.

II- a- पिप्पली मूलम् (Pippalī mūlam), चविका शिरः (Cavikāśiraḥ)
b- Mar : Pimpaḷamuḷa, H. Cāba; Guj; Cavaka;
Tel: Seciasu; Bom: Pimpaḷ muḷa.

32 (२५) चविका Cawikā

चविका कोलवल्ली च चव्यं चविकमेव[2] च ।
चव्यं च कटुकोष्णं स्याज्जन्तुहृद्दीपनं परम् ॥ ७९

कफोद्रेकहरं वातप्रकोपशमनं भवेत् ।

---

१ 'चटकाशिरः' इति नि. शे. संमतः पाठः । 'चविकाशिरः' इति रा. नि. संमतः पाठः ।
२ 'चवनमेव' इति नि. शे. टीकायाम् ।

चविका (Cavikā), **कोलवल्ली** (Kolavallī), **चव्यम्** (Cavyam), and **चविकम्** (Cavikam), **करिकणा** (Karikaṇā) are synonymous.

Cavya is pungent in taste, *uṣṇavīrya,* pacifies *vāta* and *kapha doṣas.* It is useful against worms and strongly stimulates digestive capacity.

Fam. Piperaceae.

I- a- ***Piper chaba*** W. Hunter,*
Syn; *Piper longum* Rumph. and *P. glabrum* Roxb

b- Roxburgh. c-Native of Molluca, cultivated in India. (Watt).

II- a- **कोलवल्ली** (Kolawalli), **करिकणा** (Karikaṇā), **चव्यम्** (Cawyam).

b- H.**चाब** (Cāba); B : **चोइ** (Coī), Mar : Guj : **चवक** (Cavaka).; Tel : Sevasu. Eng : Long Pepper (root). Mal : **अतिपालके.**

III- *cf. Pippali, Śreyasī,*

a- 1) **चविका** (Cawikā).
C.S. ci.-18-158, S. S. Su-39-247 A. Hr. Su 6-165.

b- 1) **चवन मूलम् चव्यम्** (Madan, Ni).
2) **चव्यम्** (Dipikā Citrakadi Churṇa).

IV- 1) *Piper chaba* W. Hunter.

Sans : *Chawyam, Chawak* ; B-Choi; Kaṭu tipal, Rheed (As res. Soc. IX 301).

The aromatic fruit is also used all over India as long pepper ......much cultivated for its roots which the native call Pippal mul. (Watt. Dic.).

श्रेयसी Śreyasī (15)

तस्याः फलं विनिर्दिष्टं श्रेयसी गजपिप्पली ।८०

(अन्यच्च)
तत्फलं श्रेयसी हस्तिमगधा गजपिप्पली ।
गजकृष्णा करिकणा इभकणा द्विपपिप्पली ॥ ८१

---

* The current name for *Piper chaba* Hunter is *Piper retrofractum* Vahl (Comp. to Gloss.p. 119)

गजपिप्पलिका स्वादुः कटुरुष्णा च कीर्तिता ।
बलासं हन्ति वातेन सार्धं जन्तुजयप्रदा ॥ ८२

The fruit of it (*Cavikā*) is called as श्रेयसी (Śreyasī) and गजपिप्पली (Gajapippalī) are its synonyms.

(From other sources)

It's (Cavikā) fruit is श्रेयसी (Śreyasī), the synonyms of which are हस्तिमगधा (Hastimagadhā), गजपिप्पली (Gajapippalī), गजकृष्णा (Gajakṛṣṇā), करिकणा (Karikaṇā), इभकणा (Ibhakaṇā) and द्विपपिप्पली (Dwipapippalī).

Gajapippalī is sweet and pungent in taste and *usṇavīrya* It pacifies *vāta* and *kapha doṣas* and is useful in worms.

Dhn. ni. has recorded two plants under this heading, one of it is 'A' -श्रेयसी गजपिप्पली (Śreyasī gajapippalī) and the next is 'B' `द्विप पिप्पली, (Dwipa pippalī, करिकणा Karikaṇā), Rāj. ni. has recorded only the first under this heading and the next द्विप पिप्पली of Dhn. ni. has noted under a separate heading सैंहली (Saimhalī) This different arrangement of Raja. ni. clearly means that the first 'A' plant is of Indian nativity while the द्वीपी (Dwīpī) 'B' plant, the nativity of which is सिंहलद्वीप (Simhal dwīpa) as foreign nature.

I- A-a- ***Fruits of Piper chaba*** Hunter
  b- Desai, c-as in चविका (Cavikā supra).

I- B-a- ***Fruits of P. officinarum*** DC
  Syn : *P. retrofractum* Vahl
  b- Kamat. c.-The nativity of this species may be Ceylon, Singapor, Java, Sumatra etc., cultivated in India.

II- A-a- चव्यफला (Cavyaphalā), चव्यजा (Cavyajā), हरित मगधा (Haritamagadhā), गजपिप्पली (Gajapippalī).
  A-b- H : -Gajapippali; Mar : थोर पिंपळी (Thor pimpaḷī).
  Eng : Long pepper.
  B-a- सर्पदण्डा (Sarpadaṇḍā), सैंहली (Saimhalī), सिंहलस्था (Simhalasthā), ब्रह्मभूमिजा (Brahmabhūmijā), लम्बबीजा (Lambabījā), उत्कटा (Utkaṭā), शैलजा मूलम् (Śailajāmūlam).

Note : Raj. ni's सैंहली is (Dwipapippalī) of Dhn. ni., Raj. ni's terms of सैंहली (Saimhalī) correspond to द्विप पिप्पली (Dwpapippalī) of Dhn. ni. so that Raj. ni's terms of सैंहली are noted here for the द्विप पिप्पली (see under श्रेयसी of Dhn. ni.).

  B-b- Mar :स्वाहेली पिंपळी (Swāhelī pimpaḷī: Bazarname सिंगापुरी पिंपळी Singāpurī pimpḷī);

Eng : Long pepper.

III- *cf.-Pipppalī; Cavyam.*

b चव्यम्-विटप विशेषः तस्य फलम् गजपिप्पली (Dīpikā Citrakādi chūrṇa).

Gajapippali

Gajapippalī has long been a drug of controversial origin. According to Bhāvamiśra, *cavikā* (चविका) or *Chawya* (चव्य) is also the part of this. *Piper chaba* Hunter and *Scindapsus offcinalis* Schott have usually been considered as probable source plants. It appears difficut to decide between the two. Piper chaba may have the properties claimed, for '*Gajapippal*i' and '*Cavya'* and it may be safe to accept it for use under the above names but due to rare occurrence it is not easily available on a large scale, This apart, *Scindapsus* fruit being used since long and it is interesting to note that in Garhawal it is called 'Hatkola' no doubt means *Gajapippalī.* (Balwantji p. 132 abide p. 155 Cavya).

IV- 2) Desai (*Cavikā*); 3) Ghanekar, Su. Su. 38-21; 4) Asia. Res, Soc-IX- 301, Piper chaba.

Discussions :

Some modern writers, under the name *Gajapippalī* have recorded the plant '*Scindapsus officinalis* Schott* Fam. -Araceae. H.B. -Gajapipal; Mar.-Thora pimpḷi; Mal. Attitippali. Tam.-Anaittippali. Tel.-Enugatippali (Chopra). But Nighaṇṭus note clearly चविकायाः फलं गजपिप्पली etc. and चविकाया फलम् is *Piper chaba* adopted even by some modern writers. Therefore it is clear and without doubt that plant *Scindapsus officinalis* Schott गजपिप्पली (*Gajapippalī*)of some modern writers is not that of our Nighaṇṭus. *Gajapappli* is the fruit of *Piper chaba.*

(See Pre. No. 32 Cavicā II-a A. syns. Śreyasī श्रेयसी Post No.(15) Syns.II-a-A *Cavya phalā*; चव्यफला *Gajapippalī* गजपिप्पली etc.,and III-b- 1) चव्यम् *Cavyam* तस्या फलम् *tasya phalam* गजपिप्पली *(Gajapippalī).*

33 (२६). चित्रकः Citrakaḥ

चित्रको दहनो व्यालः पाठीनो दारुणोऽग्निकः ।
ज्योतिष्को वल्लरी वह्निः पाली पाठी कटुः शिखी ॥ ८३

* The present accepted name is *Scindapsus officnalis* (Roxb.) Schott. (Comp. p. 137)

कृष्णारुणोऽनलो द्वीपी चित्रभानुश्च पावकः ।
चित्रकोऽग्निसमः पाके कटुकः कफशोफजित ॥ ८४
वातोदरार्शो ग्रहणीक्षयपाण्डुविनाशनः ।

चित्रकः (Citrakaḥ), दहनः (Dahanaḥ), व्यालः (Vyālaḥ), पाठीनः (Paṭhīnaḥ), दारुणः (Dāruṇaḥ), अग्निकः (Agnikaḥ), ज्योतिष्कः (Jyotiṣkaḥ), वल्लरी (Vallarī), वह्निः (Vahniḥ), पाली (Pālī), पाठी (Pāṭhī), कटुः (Kaṭuḥ), शिखी (Śikhī), कृष्णः (Kṛṣṇaḥ), अरुणः (Aruṇaḥ), (See comments) अनलः (Analaḥ), द्वीपी (Dwīpī), चित्रभानुः (Citrabhānuḥ) and पावकः (Pāvakaḥ) are synonymous.

Citraka is excessively *uṣṇavīrya*, pungent in *vipāka* (final transformation after digestion) and pacifies *kaphadoṣa*. It is useful in oedema, ascites due to *vātadoṣa, grahaṇī,* consumption and anaemia.

(Generic name. Under this heading compiler has recorded four varieties-These are :)

A- कृष्णः (Kṛṣṇaḥ). B-अरुणः (Aruṇaḥ),

C- अनलः (Analaḥ), and the fourth. D-द्वीपी (Dwīpī), All of the same genus).

Fam : Plumbaginaceae.

I- A-a- ***Plumbago indica*** Linn.
Syn. *P. rosea* Linn.
P. coccinia Boiss.

b- Roxburgh, C. Perhaps a native of Khassia and Sikkim; cultivated in gardens throughout India.

B-a- ***Vogelia indica*** Gibs.
Syn : *V. arabica* Boiss.

b- Bapalalji (Sachitra Ayurveda 10-1961). Wild in Girnar hills, Native of the N. W. frontiers, Baluchistan, Afaganistan.

I- C-a- ***Plumbago zeylanica*** Linn.

b- Roxburgh . C-Throughout India. Much cultivated in gardens; wild in Western Peninsula, Bengal.

I- D-a- ***Plumbago capensis*** Thunb.*

b- Th. Balwantji (P. 127).

c- Native of Cape of Good Hope. Introduced to India, cultivated in gardens as an ornamental plant.

---

* For *Plumbago capensis* Thunb. the current valid name is *Plumbago auriculata* Lam. (U.P. I. Page 470)

II- A-a- दारुणोग्निः (Dārṇognih), रक्त चित्रः (Rakta citraḥ),
A-b- Mar. तांबडा चित्रक (Tāmbaḍā citraka).
H. लाल चित्रक (Lāla citraka), Tam: Akkinisivapp-chitra;
Mal : Cettikottuveti ; Tel : Erra chitra.

II- B-a- अरुणः (Arunaḥ);
b- Guj. रातोचित्रो (Rato chitro).

II- C-a- अनलः (Analaḥ).
b- Mar : पांढरा चित्रक (Pāndharā citraka), H.:-चित्ता (Cittā);
Tam : Chitragam. Chitra mulam, Tel.: Chitramulam;
Keral : Koṭṭuve, Vena cittira; Kan : Velli chitraka,

II- D-a- द्वीपी (Dwīpī).
b- Mar: काळा चित्रक(Kāḷā citraka).

III- a- 1) Ca. su. 2-17, 28; Su 11-11; Ast. Hr, su 6-16; 9-26.
2) द्वीपी (Dwīpī), कृष्ण चित्रक (Kṛṣṇa-citrak), (Kāsyap Sam. Kukuṇaka cikitsā.13-56).
b- 1) 9 चित्रको गुल्मकः साग्रवृत्तपत्रस्त्रिधासुमैः । सित पीतारुणैः कृष्ण पुष्पैरेष गुणोत्तर इति । (Harshe)
2) कृष्णपुष्पः (Ast. hr. Kosha su. 15).
3) चित्रकः कृष्णपुष्प ग्राह्यः (Dalhan, ci-Medhyāuṣkāmīya).
4) द्वीपी चित्रक (Shivadas, Ast. hr. u. 22-57; 30-38).

IV- 1) *Vogelia indica* Gibs. a rare plant in Bombay Presidency. Native of Arabia. Abundant below Mount Abu. Naturalized in India (Cooke fl.)

Note : (Kṛsṇa citraka of commentators may be रक्तचित्रक (Raktacitraka) (1-a-A) of Nighaṇṭu. The term कृष्ण (Krṣṇa) may have been used to differentiate it from अरुण (Aruṇa).

Discussion :

Dhan. ni. has recorded द्वीपी चित्रक *Dwīpī citraka* which directs to mean a foreign plant. The plant (1-a-D) noted above is an African i.e. a foreign plant. The flowers of this plant are blue black and is found in cultivated state. The above noted two comments (III-a-1 and b2) have identified द्वीपी as चित्रक. Dhn. ni. notes only one plant as under the चित्रक (citraka) heading and among the *Citrakas* noted by Raj. Nighaṇṭu is only one plant in genus *Plumbago* and it is the *P. indica* Gilas. रुद्राह्व चित्रक (*Rudrāhva citraka*) of Raj. ni. is not identified. The plant *Vogelia indica* Gibs. not originally an Indian plant but it might have naturalized in India at the period of the compiler. पीत चित्रक Pīta citraka is notknown or has not been recorded in modern writers books.

34 (२७) शुण्ठी Śuṇṭhī & आर्द्रकम् (Ārdrakam)

शुण्ठी महौषधं विश्वं नागरं विश्वभेषजम ॥ ८५
विश्वौषधं शृङ्गवेरं कटुभद्रं तथाऽऽर्द्रकम ॥

स्निग्धोष्णा कटुका शुण्ठी वृष्या शोफकफारुचीन् ॥८६
हन्ति वातोदरश्वासपाण्डुश्लीपदनाशिनी ॥

कफानिलहरं स्वर्यं विबन्धानाहशूलजित् ॥ ८७
कटूष्णं रोचनं वृष्यं हृद्यं चैवार्द्रकं स्मृतम ॥

शुण्ठी (Śuṇṭhī), महौषधं (Mahauṣadham), विश्वं (Viśvam), नागरम् (Nāgaram), विश्वभेषजम् (Viśvabheṣajam), विश्वौषधं (Viśvauṣadham), शृङ्गवेरं (Śṛṅgaveram), कटुभद्रं (Kaṭubhadram), and आर्द्रकम् (Ārdrakam) are synonymous.

Śuṇṭhī is pungent in taste, unctuous, *uṣṇavīrya,* pacifies *kapha (Vāta) doṣas.* It is useful in oedema, anorexia, ascites due to *vātadoṣa,* dyspnoea, anaemia and filariasis.

Ārdrakam is pungent in taste, *uṣṇavirya.* It removes constipation, tympanitis and intestinal colics. It is appetizer, *vṛṣya* and beneficial to heart.

I- a- Dried rhizomes of आर्द्रकम् (Ārdrakam).
b- Kamat. c-See आर्द्रकम् (Ārdrkam),

II- a- महौषधम् (Mahauṣadham), नागरम् (Nāgaram),
Mar : सुंठ(Suṇṭha).
b- Tam : Shukku, Tel.-Sonthi.
आर्द्रकम् (Ārdrakam) (19),

Fam : Zingiberaceae.

I- a- ***Zingiber officinale*** Rosc.
b- Roxburgh. c-Widely cultivated throughout India,
A native of Tropical Asia.

II- a- शृंगबेरम् (Śṛṅgaberam), आपाकशाकं चार्द्रकम् (Āpākaśākam cārdradkam).
Eng : Ginger,
b- H. : Adraka; Mar.-Ālen; Kan ; Husi-sunthi;
Tam : Enje. Inji, Mal-Inchi Andrakam;
Tel : Ardrakamu, allum, Arebic-Zanzabic.

35 (२८) मरिचम् Maricam

मरिचं पलितं[1] श्यामं वल्लीजं[2] कृष्णमूषणम् ॥ ८८
यवनेष्टं शिरोवृत्तं कोलकं धर्मपत्तनम्[3] ॥

मरिचं कटुतीक्ष्णोष्णं पित्तकृत् श्लेष्मनाशनम् ॥ ८९
वायुं निवारयत्येव जन्तुसन्तानननाशनम् ॥

श्वेतमरिचम् (ध.नि.)_
मरीचं शुभ्रमरिचं बीजं शिग्रोस्तु शिग्रुजम् ॥ ९०
नात्युष्णं नातिरूक्षं च वीर्यतो मरिचं सितम् ॥ S.S. Su. 46. 225

मरिचम् (Maricam), पलितं (Palitam), श्यामं (Śyāmam), वल्लीजं (Vallījam), कृष्णं (Kṛṣṇam), ऊषणम् (Ūṣṇam), यवनेष्टं (Yavaneṣṭam), शिरोवृत्तम् (Śirovṛttam), कोलकम् (Kolakam) and धर्मपत्तनम् (Dharmapattanam) are synonymous.

Marica is pungent in taste, *tīksṇa* (sharp), *ūṣṇavīrya*, aggravates *pitta* and pacifies *kapha* and *vātadoṣas*. It is useful in worms.

श्वेतमरिचम् (*Śvetamaricam*)

मरिचम् (Maricam), शुभ्रमरिचम् (Śubhramaricam), शिग्रुबीजं (Śigrubījam) and शिग्रुजम् (Śigrujam) are synonymous.

Sitamaricam is not excessively *uṣṇavīrya* and not excessively *rukṣa* (roughning) in its action.

Fam : Piperaceae

I- a- ***Piper nigrum*** Linn, b-Roxburgh.

c- Wild in the forests of Circars and cultivated in the hot damp parts of India for its fruits.

II- a- श्यामम् (Śyāmam), मलिनम् (Malinam), वल्लीजम् (Vallījam), शाकाङ्गम् (Śākāṅgam), यवनेष्टम् (Yavaneṣṭam),

b- 1 Mar. Mirī, Kaḷemirī; H.-Gola mircha:
Kan-Shime-jirage; Tam Mitagu, Shimai.
Kan : Mirialu, Kare mensasu, shiragam, Moluvakhdi,
Tel. Maricamu, Miryahtig Mal-Karu mulanka,
Eng : Black pepper.

III- a- A. hr. su.-6-16 , 164-, 165, S.Su. 38-21.

---

१ 'मलिनं' इति नि. शे. टीकायाम् ।
२ 'वेल्लजम्' इति नि. शे. टीकायाम् ।
३ 'धार्मं' इति नि. शे. टीकायाम् ।

Note : B.C.Arrian the author of Periplus of the Erythrean sea, written about A. D. 618 states that pepper was then imported from Barake the shipping place of Nelkunda, localities which have been identified with points on the Malabar Coasts.

(Watt. vol. VI I.P.264)

मरिचम् Maricam (20).(श्वेतमरिचम्)

(Under this heading occur two drugs, the first 'A' is of Dhn. ni. and the second 'B' is of Raj. ni).

I- A-a- शिग्रु बीजम् Seeds of *Moringa species* (Dhn.ni).

b- Kamat and Mahajan. c-See *Moringa species.*

I- B-a- Husked berries of Black Pepper (Raj.ni).

b- Hill (iv-2 below).

II- A-a- शिग्रु बीजम् (Śigru bījam), शुभ्र मरिचम् (Śubhra Maricam),

B- सितवल्लिजम् (Sitawallijam),

III *cf.* मरिचम् Maricam-

b- 1) शिग्रु बीजं शोभाञ्जनम् -श्वेत मरिचमिति प्रसिद्धम् ॥

(Dipika-P.182).

IV- 1) मरिच *Marica* सित *Sita,* what is called सित मरिच(Sitamarica) is either the (seeds) of Śigru शिग्रु or the decorticated and dried Marica fruit (Balwantaji P. 299).

2) White pepper is prepared from berries that are nearly ripe. They are picked and piled in heaps to ferment or are soaked in water. The pulp and outer coating of the seeds are then removed. Frequently white pepper is prepared from black pepper by grinding outer parts by machinery. (Hill).

36 (२९) यवानी Yawānī (दीप्यकम् Dīpyakam)

यवानी दीप्यको दीप्यो यवसाह्वो यवाग्रजः ॥ ९१
यवानिकोग्रगन्धा च दीपनीया च दीपनी ॥

यवानी कटुतिक्तोष्णा वातार्शःश्लेष्मनाशिनी ॥ ९२
हन्ति गुल्मोदरं शूलं दीपयत्याशुचानलम् ॥

यवानी (Yavānī), दीप्यकः (Dīpyakaḥ), दीप्यः (Dīpyaḥ), यवसाह्वः (Yavasāhvaḥ), यवाग्रजः (Yavāgrajaḥ), यवानिका (Yavānikā), उग्रगन्धा (Ugragandhā), दीपनीया (Dīpanīyā), and दीपनी (Dīpanī), are synonymous.

Yavanī is pungent and bitter in taste, *uṣṇavīrya,* pacifies (*vāta*) and *kapha doṣas.* It stimulates digestive capacity immediately and is useful in piles due to *vatadosa*, tumor (diverticulosis), ascites and colic.

Fam : Umbelliferae. Apiaceae

I- a- ***Trachyspermum ammi*** Sprague.
Syn. *Carum copticum* Benth. & Hook. f.
(Watt. & Chopra).
Lisgunticum ajovan Roxb; *Ptychotis ajowan* DC.

b- Roxburgh. C. cultivated throughout in India for its seeds.

II a- दीप्यकः (Dīpyakaḥ), भूकदम्बकः (Bhūkadambakaḥ), तीव्रगन्धः (Tīvragandhaḥ).

b- H : अजोवान (Ajowān), Bom.; - अजवान (Ajawāna), Tam : Ommum; Tel.: Omamu; Kan : -Omu; B:- Jowan, Mar : ओवा (Owā); Eng : Bishop's weed, Ajova seeds, Lovage.

III cf Yawānīkā (Post No. 21), Yawānī (Post No. 22) and Pre-No 39 infra.

IV- 1) See Chunekar P. 152.

2) Omum Water ; Ajawan Ka phul. Thymol obtained from *Carum copticum* Benth. and Hook. fl. (Watt. Dic).

3) यवानी *Trachyspermum ammi* Sprague.
Syns : अजवायन, खराह्वा, यमानी , and यवानिका.
C. Sū-23-19; 27-167, 302; S. S. Ci. b-13, i 38-27.
A. H. Su. 14-25-Ci-3-20 (Balawantji p. 328).

Discussion :

Under the names अजमोदा (*Ajamodā*), ओवा (*Owā*) and यवानी (*Yawānī*) four plants occur in this chapter (See pre No. 36) post Nos (21), (22) and Pre No. 39 of Dhn. ni.). Yadavji has recorded these four plant names. Balwantji does not record Post No. (21) चौहार यवानी *Cauhāra yavānī* and Kudtarkar Shastri does not record Pre No. 36 यवानी *yawānī.* Balawantji quotes reference of Caraka under the name खराह्वा (*Kharāhvā*) confirming plant name (Post No. 21-See V-2). He has recorded different names together under the heading name yavānī of Dhn. ni. (See Pre No. 36-IV supra).

(*Ajamodā*) Post Nos. (21) and (22) are included in this Book after the compilation of गणद्रव्यावलि, the first part of this Nighaṇṭu. Before that, it seems the Indian plant *Artemisia vulgaris* Linn. might have been in practice.

यवानिका Yawānikā (Chauhāraḥ) चौहारः (21)

यवानिका यवानी स्याच्चौहारो जन्तुनाशनः ॥ ९३
चौहारस्तद्‌गुणः प्रोक्तो विशेषात् कृमिनाशनः ॥

यवानिका (Yavānikā), यवानी (Yavānī), चौहार (Chauhāra), and जन्तुनाशनः (Jantunāsanaḥ), are synonymous.

Chauhāra has similar properties to those of *Yavānī* but is more useful in worms.

Fam : Compositae. Asteraceae.

I- a- ***Artemisia maritima*** Linn.*
Syn : *A. officinale* Lam, . *A. absinthium* Linn . *Absinthium vulgare* Gaertn.

b- Dymock and Watt. Dic. c-Western Himalaya from Kashmir to Komaon and W. Tibet, commercially obtained from Russia.

II a- चौहार (Cauhāra), जन्तुनाशनः (Jantunāśanāḥ), यवानी (Yawānī).

II b- San-गदाधर (Gadādhara); H.Kiramāl, Vilayati ovā; Mar. Bom. किरमाणी ओवा (Kiramāṇī owā). Eng : Worm seed, Old woman, Ajeno, Lavant, The Absinth, Santonica. (Watt. Dic. I. 354).
III-b-1) 252 जन्तुघ्न मिति......... चौहारो जन्तुनाशनः । पारसीय यमानी (Harshe).

IV- 1) *Artemisia vulgaris* Linn. Syn; *A. indica* Willd.
Indian Wormwood.
H. Nāgadaunā; Mar.Nāgadauṇā; Tam. Surabanda, Baz. name-Afsuntin. Sans.-Nāgadamanī. Granthiparnî. Throughout the mountain parts of india, N. Burma..... The Western Ghats of Konkan, southwards to Ceylon-Distributed to temparate Europe and Asia. Following plants referred to by Indian authors *A. indica; A. dubia; A. myriantha; A.paniculata;* etc. etc.One or two of the forms of these species along with *A. absinthium* constitute the official *worm wood......* It is used as tonic, anthelmintic....... especially in diseases of children. (Watt. Dic. Vil I-P.32).

Artemisia maritima Linn.
Late vd. D.K. Kamat had mentioned the synonyms following Dr. Watt. *A. absinthium* Linn. and *A. vulgaris* Linn. are different species. However, चौहार (Chauhara), चोर ओवा (Cora owā), किरमाणी (Kirmāṇī owā) is identified correctly by Late vd. D.K. Kamat. Dr. chopra in his Glossary had also mentioned *A. indica* Willd. for *A. vulgaris* Linn. but these are again diffent species (See IV-1)

S.D. Kamat

2) Kharāhvā C.S. Sū. 23-14; 27-169.
It has been identified with *Ajamoda, Yavānī* or *Pārasīkya Yawānī* पारसिक्य यवानी *(Hyoscyamus niger* Linn. (Balwantji p. 130).

Note : The name खराह्वा occurs in Dhn, ni. only under the name 39 अजमोदा Ajamodā .Dhn, ni's (Kharāhvā) is Ajamodā (Pre No. 39 infra.) *Trachyspermum roxburghianum* (DC.) Sprague.

यवानी Yawānī (22) (Turuṣkayavānī) (तुरुष्कं यवानी)

यवानी यावनी तीव्रा तुरुष्को मदकारिणी ॥ ९४
यवानी यावनी रूक्षा ग्राहिणी मादिनी कटुः ॥

यावनी यवानी (Yāvanī Yavānī), तीव्रा (Tīvrā), तुरुष्क (Turuṣka) and मदकारिणी (Madakāriṇī) are synonymous.

Yāvanī Yavānī is *rūkṣa* (roughning), astringent, naroctic and pungent in taste.

Fam : Solanaceae.

I- a- ***Hyoscyamus niger*** Linn.

b- Dymock. c-Native of Temperate Western Himalaya from Kashmir to Gaharwal. Distributed over Western and Northern Aisa, Europe and Southern Africa. (Watt.Dict).

II- a- यावनी (Yāwanī), तुरुष्कः (Turuṣkaḥ), मदकारिणी (Madakāriṇī), यवानी (Yawānī).

b- Sans : पारसिक्य (Pārasikya); Bom. खोरासनी (Khorāsanī); Keral - पाशिदेशतिङल (Pasidesattinkal), उण्टाकुग्न करामशानि (Unṭākugna Karām'sānī); Tel : Kurashanī-vamum, Kirinji vamum, Tam : Khurāsani yomum. Eng. : *Black henbane,* (Hill).

III *cf* यवानी, यवानिका, अजमोदा.

b- 1) पारसिक यवानी (Shārngadhara Sam. p. 177),

2) पारसिक यमानी, (Ayur. O.Ni).

3) म्लेंच्छदीप्याः (Ras. Yog Sagar P. 646).

IV- 2) Black henbane -Hill.

1) 233 पारसिक यवानी, तुरुष्क, मदकारिणी (हि.) खुरासनिक (म.) खुरासनी ओवा. (ले.) *Hyoscyamus reticulatus* Linn. (Jadavaji p. 286)...

Note : There is difference of opinion about the native place of this plant. Many writers note its foreign nativity. Even Dhn. ni.notes its foreign nativity. Local equivalents are also prevalent with foreign names. But only Watt states its nativity.

37 (३०) वृक्षाम्लम् Vṛkśāmlam

वृक्षाम्लं तित्तिडीकं च शाकाम्लं रक्तपूरकम् ॥ ९५
अम्लवृक्षोऽम्लशाखः[१] स्यादपरोऽम्लमहीरुहः[२] ॥
तित्तिडीकं च वातघ्नं ग्राह्युष्णं रुचिकृल्लघु ॥ ९६

वृक्षाम्लं (Vṛkśāmlam), तित्तिडीकं (Tittiḍīkam), शाकाम्लं (Śākāmlam), रक्तपूरकम् (Raktapūrakam), अम्लवृक्षः (Amlavṛkśaḥ) and अम्लशाखः (Amlaśākhaḥ) are synonymous. There is an another *Vṛkśāmla* called as अम्लमहीरुहः (Amlamahīruhaḥ)

Tittiḍīka pacifies *vātadoṣa,* is *laghu,* astringent, *uṣṇavīrya* and appetiser.

Fam. Guttiferae. Clusiaceae.

I- A-a- ***Garcinia indica*** Chois.*
Syn : *G. purpurea* Roxb.
b- Kamat. C-Kokan and North Canara, Western Ghat, Coorg, yanad. Also cultivated in garden for its frutis.

Fam. Anacardiaceae.

I- B-a- ***Rhus parviflora*** Roxb.**
b- Yadavji. C. Persia Asia, Minor, Afaganistan, Komaon, Nepal, Panchamahal.

II- A-a-वृक्षाम्लम् (Vṛkśāmlam), शाकाम्लम् (Śākāmlam), रक्तपूरकम् (Raktapūrakam), अम्लशाखा (Amlasākhā), चूडाम्लबीजम् (Cūḍāmlabījam), फलं च चुक्रादि (Phalam ca cukrādi), तित्तिडीकम् (Tittiḍīkam).

b- Modern names :
H.B. Bom : Kokam, Amsol; Tam : Murgal mara; Mal. Punamppuli;

---

१ 'अम्लशाकम्' इति नि. शे. टीकायाम् ।
२ 'तदम्लपूरो महीरुहः इति नि. शे. टीकायाम् ।
* *Garcinia indica* Chois; The current accepted name is *Garcinia indica* (Dupetit Thouars) Chois.
** *Rhus parviflora* Roxb, the current name is *Rhus parviflora* Roxb. ex DC.
(Comp. to Gloss p. 68 & 131)

Keral -Maram-ppuli; Kan; Tittiḍika, Eng : *Kokam Butter; Mangostan Oil.*

II-B- a- महीरुहम् (Mahīruham).

b- Modern names :

Sans.: Tittiḍīka, Tintiḍīka, H.B. Tatrak, Tunga, Raitunga, Sumāka.
(Fruit) : Punjab-bazar name : - Tantarika, Marawad-Dāsariyā
Eng.: Sumach. Kashmir : Sumaka.

III- *cf Amlaḥ* (अम्लः)

a- i) Vṛksāmlam वृक्षाम्लम्

Ca. Su 4-10, Su U. 42-29. A. Su. Su. 6-129.
(Balvantji P.376).

2) *Tintiḍika* तिन्तिडीक

Ca. Su. 26-112; V. 8-147, Su-Su-42-139, A.H.Ci. 5.55, 7-40
(Balavantji P. 182).

b- 1) वृक्षः के. मारमुपुली (Maramppuli); मा-आमसोल (Amsol) तित्तिडीक (Tittiḍīka) (G.) कोकम (Kokam). (Ayur 0. Ni.)

2) वृक्षाम्लः (Vṛksāmlaḥ):

६२ 'वृक्षाम्लं तिन्तिडीकं च साम्लकं रक्तपूरक' मिति धर्मदासः ।
(Harshe).

3) 14 तिन्तिडी वृक्षाम्लं । 'अथ पादपः तिन्तिडीकः (फलं तस्य) चिञ्चार्धं दाडिमीदलः । दलं कषायमम्लं च फलं तद्रसशोषकं । फलानि चास्य शुष्काणि तिन्तिडीकमुदाहृतम् ।उदीच्यां नात्सिद्धतरं शुष्कं मङ्गल्यका कृति' ति । 'डासरया' इति लोके । (Harshe).

4) 378 तिन्तिडीकं वृक्षाम्लम् ।

"चुक्री' चाङ्गेरिकायां स्यात् 'चुक्र' वृक्षाम्लके । (Harshe).

5) अम्लं वृक्षाम्लं वृक्षभेदः सच फलाम्लः (Dipika P. 192)

6) तिन्तिडीक स्थाने वृक्षाम्लम् (Dipika P. 185).

IV- 1) *Vrksāmlam :*

Garcinia indica Chois. (Balwantaji 376)

2) *Tintiḍīka* (तिन्तिडीक) *Rhus parviflora* Roxb. The seeds are sold in market under the name *Samākadānā* (समाकदाना) or *Dāyasariyā.* (डायसरिया)

Rhus parviflora Roxb.

It is substituted by foreign seeds obtained from *Rhus coriaria* Linn.

It should not be confused with Amilkā (अम्लिका) or वृक्षाम्ल Vrksāmla (Balwantaji P. 182).

3) The Sumāch or Sumāk.

The berries of the following plants are known by the name SUMAK.

The following plants 'a to c' are recorded by Watt.

a- *Rhus coriaria* Linn.
The Sumach tree of Europe (Watt.)
Sicilian Sumach (Hill).
(H) Tatrak, (B), Sumak, (Bom) Sumak.
The berries are not used by the Hindus but by Mohamedans.

b- *R. parviflora* Roxb :*
(H) Tuṅga. Raituṅga (Mārwāḍ) Dāyasariā, (Bazar name in Punjab), seeds 'Tantirika', (Kashmir) Sumak. The Tantirika of the the Bazar appears to be the fruits of this plant. Its fruits are used by Hindoos and mixed with salt is said to act as 'Tamarind' (Stewart). An uncertain shrub of Western Himalaya from Komaon to Nepal.
The leaves are reported to be used in Garhaval instead of Tobacco. (Watt. Dic. P. -495. 98 and Chopra).

c- *R. semeialata* Murray : **
Syn : *R. chinensis* Mill., *China sumach* (Chopra). The beries have sharp acid taste and are sometimes eaten by the Nepalis and Lepachas. (Watt. Dic. P. R-498).
Rhus parviflora Roxb :
A small shrub arborious bushy tree; fruit when mixed with salt acts like Tamarind. (Roxburgh fl.).

Discussion

The Compiler (Dhn. ni) has recorded two plants "A" Vṛkṡāmla and 'B' Mahīruham (महीरुहम्) but without giving similitive terms of *Mahīruham.* He has given synonym 'Tintiḍīka' to Vṛkṡāmla. But there is also a different plant by name '*Tittidika*' which is mentioned by commentators on Ayurvedic books and identified by modern writers with the botanical name *Rhus parviflora* Roxb. with its modern names *'Sumāk'*, *'Dāyasariā'* (डायसरिया) *'Tantarika'* etc. (See iv-2, 3 above).The Punjab bazaar name *'Tantarika'*(तंतरिक)seems to be corruption of *'Tinttiḍīk'* (तिन्तिडीक) or *Tittiḍ ika.*(तित्तिडीक).

The fruits of *Tittiḍīka* and *Vṛkṡāmla* are used medicinaly for the same purpose and are substituted for one another. (See III b 6, above).

current valid names:
* For *Rhus. parviflara* Roxb. is *R. parviflora* Roxb. ex DC.
** For *R. semialata* Murr. is *R.javanica* Linn.
Syn. *R. chinensis* Mill. (Comp. to Gloss p. 131)

The leaves and young stocks of Vṛkṣāmla are used for curry. The fruits of both the plants are used as acid taste in domestic preparations.

The compiler has not recorded the medicinal properties of *'Mahīruham'* but as both the plants are included under the same heading it can be presumed that both the plants have the same medicinal properties and as such he might have neglected to record those of Mahīruham. Several examples of such kind would be available in this book. The difference between these two plants is shown by naming *Mahīruham* i.e. shrublike plant.While the other is a large tree. This is the difference between these two plants recorded by the compilers.

The next point for consideration is the identification of the name *Mahīruham* and the equivalent *Tittiḍīka* applied to *Vṛkṣāmla* (See II-A-a-and B above)

Tittiḍīka is a traditional name of a plant which is also recorded in classical books (See III-a-2 above) and is always accompanied (See III-b above) and substituted by *vṛkṣāmla* (See III-b-6 above).

The compilers of the classical-books were inhabitants of the region from Nepal to Kashmir. (See pp. LIVII of our 1st Vol.) and as they have included this plant in their books, then it follows that the plant *Tittidika* was also before them. Hence the nativity of the plant in question was at that time also the same. But as followers of the classical books spread out in other parts of the country the book described traditional plant became unavailable, and to overcome this difficulty they might have selected from the region where they were settled the plant *Vṛkṣāmla* (वृक्षाम्ल) as a substitute for the original traditional *'Tittidīka* (तित्तिडीक) and the same name was also applied as an equivalent to *Vṛkṣāmla* (See III-b e 6, above).

The compiler has recorded *'Mahīruham'* as a separate plant from *Vṛkṣāmla*.commentators record *'Tittiḍīka'* with *Vṛkṣāmla*. Medicinal qualities of both the plants as discussed above are the same and both the plants are substituted for one another.
(*Vṛkṣāmla-Mahīruham* -compilers: *Tintiḍīka* commentators)

Hence compiler's Mahīruham and commentators', *Tittiḍīka* or *Tintiḍika* are the same plants and as modern writers have identified *Tintiḍika* to be *R. parviflora* Roxb. it follows that compiler's Mahiruham also must be identified as *R. parviflora* Roxb.

This is our conclusion about the name (Mahīruham).

38 (३१) अम्लः Amlah (Amlavetasaḥ)

अम्लोऽम्लवेतसो भीमः रसाम्लो वीरवेतसः ।[1]
रक्तस्रावी वेतसाम्लः शतवेधी च भेदकः[2] ॥ १७

कषायं कटु रूक्षोष्णमम्लवेतसकं विदुः ॥
तृट् कफानिलजन्त्वर्शोहृद्बाधाश्मरिगुल्मजित् ॥ १८

अम्लः (Amlaḥ), अम्लवेतसः (Amlavetasaḥ), भीमः (Bhīmaḥ), रसाम्लः (Rasāmlaḥ), वीरवेतसः (Vīravetasaḥ), रक्तस्रावी (Raktasrāvī), वेतसाम्लः (Vetasāmlaḥ), शतवेधी (Śatavedhī) and भेदकः (Bhedakaḥ) are synonymous.

Amlavetasa is sour, pungent, and *kaṣāya* in taste *rūkṣa* (roughning) and *uṣṇavīrya*. It pacifies *kapha* and *vātadoṣas* and is useful in worms, thirst, piles, heart disease, calculous affections and tumors (diverticulosis).

(Under this heading the compiler has recorded only one plant but Raj. ni. has added one more plant.)

A- अम्लवेतसः *Amlavetasaḥ.*
B- फलाम्ल, अम्लनायकः *Phalāmla, amlanāyakḥ.*

Fam. Salicaceae.

I- A-a- ***Salix tetrasperma*** Willd. (Roxb.)
b- Yadavji (See below IV-5).
c- Throughout tropical and sub-tropical India (Chopra).

Not identified

B-a- Confirmed *Citrus species.* b- Desai.
c- See *IV*-below.

II- A-a- रसाम्लः Rasāmlah,रक्तस्रावी (Raktasrāvī), वेतसाम्लः (Vetasāmlaḥ), वीरवेतसः(Vīravetasaḥ).
B-a- फलाम्लः (Phalāmlaḥ), अम्लनायकः (Amlanāyakaḥ), वीराम्लः (Vīrāmlaḥ), सहस्रवेधी (Sahasravedhī), शंखमांसादि द्रावी (Śaṅkha māmsādi drāvī).
B-b- H Amlabed, Bijora Nimbu, Amlabed; Nimbu, Bhutan - Amlabed; Varhad-Suḷe limbu; Nepal-Cukutri,Śankatry-Desai (See IV- 1 below).

III- a- 1) अम्लवेतसो भेदनीयदीपनीयानुलोमिकवातश्लेष्महराणाम् ।
(Ca.Su. 2.)

---

१ 'बिल्व वेतसः' इति नि. शे. टीकायाम ।
२ 'वेधकः' इति नि. शे. टीकायाम ।

2) अम्लवेतस *Amlavetasa* दीपनीय (C.Sū-4-9-6).

3) द्राक्षाकाश्मर्य......पीलूनीतिविरेचनोपगानि (Ca-Sū- 4-13,26).

Note : *In this Gaṇa* अम्लवेतस *is not included.*

4) अम्लस्कन्ध (Amlaskandha),
अम्लोधात्रीफलाम्लिका........अम्लवेतसम् (Ast. hr, Su. 10-17).

5) मदन विदुल दहन...। छर्दनानि । विदुल जलवेतस (Aruna 15-1)

6) वञ्जुलवानीरोपशोभित तीराभिः । सद्‌भूभिःकूपगतभूमिभागः (Ca. Kal-1-8)

7) नल वञ्जुल वानीर शतपत्राणि शैवलम् ॥ (Ca.Si. 10-21)

b- 8) द्विपी शत्रोश्च द्विपी चित्रकः शत्रु (*Śatru*) अम्लवेतस(*Amlavetasa*) (Tripaṭhi Kukuṇakā ci. 1-3-59).

9) अम्लवेतस् (Su.10).
अम्लवेतसो वेतसश्च नम्रत्वात् । (Rumex vesicarius; R. crispus.)
मल्या-कटप्पुळी (अरि जा म्युली इति बहवः) (Vaidya).

10) 14- अम्लकमिति- अम्लवेतसो रसाम्लः ।
'रसाम्लो वेतसाम्लश्चाप्यम्लकश्चाम्लवेतस'-इत्यजयः ।
'रसाम्लश्चाम्लविदुलो वेतसाम्लोऽम्लवेतस'-इतिहृदयदीपकः।
(Harshe)

11) 377 वेतसाख्यम्
'जम्बीर फलसम्भूतरसः संशोषितो रवौ ।
मृदमत्रे वेतसाख्यं लोके तच्चूक संज्ञक' मिति ।
अम्लवेतसः सहस्रवेधी ।"(Harshe)

Note : This reference directs to mention फलाम्लवेतस Phalāmlawetasa.

12) 473 वेतसो नम्रकः प्रोक्तो 'वानीर वंजुलस्तथेति ।
(Harshe).

13) 474 'विदुलस्तुभवेद् अम्लवेतसे वेतसेऽपि च' इति शाश्वतः ।
विदुल इति अम्लवेतसः वेतसाम्लः (Harshe).

14)165- 'लसनो मञ्जरी नम्रः सुषेणो गंधपुष्पक' इति धर्मिष्टः ।
(Harshe).

15) अम्लवेतस थैकलम् (Shivadas).

16) अम्लवेतसः (Keral)
ओरियाञ्जपुळी, पिपारनपुळी, कुटंपुळी, कोट्टक्का पुळी Tam.पुळीवच्चि (Ayur. O.Ni).

IV- 1- अम्लवेतस (Amlavetas), *Citrus* बिज़ोरा निंबू (*'Bijora Nimbu'*), अम्लबेद(*Amlabed*),चकुत्री *Cakutrī,* Nepal: शखुत्री; Varaḍ- सुळे लिंबु *Sule Limbū*. This kind of Bijaurānimbū is found in Bhutan, Nepal, Silhet Bihar, Komaon, Khasi Hills. The fruit is like महाळुंग (*Mahāḷung*) (*Citrus medica* Linn.) but very sour.If a pin is rushed in the fruit, it melts but being unavailable the following substances are substituted:- In Bengal थैकल (*Thaikal*), *Garcinia pedunculata* Roxb. In Punjab the stalks of रेवाचिनी (Revācinī)- *Rheum species*. But these fruits (Cakotri *Citrus-species* are used as अम्लवेतस (*Amlavetas*) where they are available. (Desai p. 176).

2) वेतस Vetas may be *Salix caprea* Linn., known as वेदमुष्क (*Vedamuṣka*) while वंजुल (vañjula) may be *S. tetrasperma* Roxb. also known as *Jalavetas*. (जलवेतस) (Balwantji p. 364).

3) Either *Thaikal* (थैकल) of Bengal or चकुत्री *(Cakutrī)* of Nepal as described by A. Yadavaji, this acid fruit should be used as अम्लवेतस (*Amlavetas*), (Sachitra Ayurved 5-1972).

4) 246 अम्लवेतस (*Amlavetas*) Varāḍ-Sulenimbu Lat. (Acido Zypholi (Pade Br. Ni.).

5) 294 वेतस वेदमुष्क (*Vetas; Vedamuṣka*) name : *Vetasa, Vānīra; Bedamuṣka*; Punjab-*Bedamuṣka*; Arab: *Khilaphul balki*; Lat. *Salix caprea*, Iran and N.W. Provinces : 295 जलवेतस (Jalavetasa) San. *Vañjula;* Parsi; Bed, *Bedamuṣka*: Kan-*Vira;* Mar : *Vāluṇja.* Lat. *Salix tetrasperma* Roxb. Habit.-On the banks of rivers (A. Yadavji PP. 343-44).

6) *Amlavetas* is an acid fruit according to Caraka. (Balvantji p. 21).

7) History and uses of *'Willow'* (See Dymock Vol. III, 365-66).

8) *Salix tetrasperma* Roxb. Bom. *Vañjul;* B.H.: *Beda*; Tam. : *Aruppalai;* Kan.: *Niranjal;* Tel.: *Beti-pā*. A moderate sized deciduous tree, found throughout India on river banks and in moist places-Himalaya, Java, Burma. (Watt. Dic. 'Sa' P. 394).

9) *Salix tetrasperma* Willd.
B-*Pani-Jama*-This is the only species of *Salix* I have yet found in India. This is a middle sized tree which is a native of rivuletes and moist places (C.B.C. Edi.p.712).

10) *Salix* (N.O. Salicaceae).
Salix tetrasperma Roxb. Cor Pl.
A much branched tree 20-40 feet high. Bark rough with deep vertical furrows......... Flowers appearing after the leaves, catkins, hairy 2-5 inches long. Peduncles; silky-villous. Flower October-November. Vern. Wālunj.
Deccan, Poona, Mahabaleswar, Belgaum; (Kolhapur, Karad-Mahajan)

11) 1203-*Salix tetrasperma* Roxb.

........Male catkins 2-4 in. on leafy branchlets sweet scented... Female catkins 2-5 in. long.

uses=Bark is said to be of some account as *frebrifuge*

1205 *S. caprea* Linn. (Kirtikar).

Habitat=Cultivated in Rohikhand and N.W. India.

Uses=.....The distilled water from the flowers is useful in *palpitation* of the heart (Dr. Perry in Watt. Dic.)

Chemical composition=*Willow bark*........ salicin, wax, fat, gums and a tannin which gives with ferric salt...... a kind of sugar...... glucoside, banzoholicin etc........ *Willow honey* etc. (Watt Dic.)

1206 *S. alba* Linn.

Cultivated in N.W. Himalaya and Tibet.

Uses=The bark yields *salicin,* a drug, used in acute rheumatism. It is recognised as antiseptic, antipyretic, and antiperiodic (Kirtikar Basu Pp. 216-221) *Amlavetas.*

38 *Amlavetas* is kind of a citrus fruit similar to *Mahāḷunga*(महाळुंग) =*Cirus medica* Linn. These plants are grown at Khāsi.(खासी) The fruits are very sour चणकाम्ल (*Caṇakāmla guṇam jñeyam Loha-sūcī-dravatwakṛt.*(Bha.Ni.) (Kudatarkar).

Note : The description given above is simlar to that of Dr.Desai (IV-1 above) and it is फलाम्लवेतस(Phalamlavetas) of Raj. ni. (1-a-B - above).

IV- 1) The traditional use of *Rheum stalks,* however, may be allowed to continue as a substitute for it. (i.e.for *Amlavetas*). (Balavantaji p. 21).

2) *Amlavetas: Rumex vesicarius* Linn. (Dr. Pendse).

3) *Amlavetas : Rumex crispus*L;. *R. acitosa* Linn. Eng : 'Dick Sorrel (Chopra, Watt Dic.)

Note : These two plants are speices of.चुक्र

4) Does it indicate that name *Vetas* now given to *Salix species* was given also to *Garcinia pedunculata fruit?* (Balvantji p. 21).

Note : Very surprising suggestion: species different.

5) *Hindi Revandachīnī; Himalayan rhubarb* (para 217) *Rheum emodi* Wall.* H. :-Hindi revand chīnī. Bom : *revandachīnī.* Tam : Nattu.-ereval chini, Nattumanjal chini ; chinal-Kishangu.

Tel. : Nattu pusapu. Chinagadda.

Himalayan rhubarb is used as purgative and astringent, tonic, less active and is pronounced worthless' (Watt Dic. Salix-para 227).

* The current name for *Rheum emodi* Wall. is *R. emodi* Wall. ex Meissn

Discussion-Amlavetas

The compiler of Dhn.ni. has noted *Amlavetas* under the heading *Amlaḥ*. But the term Amlaḥ used by the compiler as heading is confusive.It can direct to mean either *Rumex* species or *Salix* species or even *Garcinia* species, for the term *Amlaḥ* is a generic term (See III 9, 12, 14 above; 37 Vṛksāmla IV-7)

But the similative terms those followed in the text are clearly applicable to *Salix species*.

In Śatapuspā class, the II chapter of *Gaṇadrawyāvali* (गणद्रव्यावली) occurs the term *Sāmlavetas* साम्लवेतस (Ānandāśram edition) which directs to the terms रसाम्ल, अम्लवेतस followed in the text under the heading. From this it is clear that the compiler's *Amla* term under the heading is used for *Vetas* species.

Some modern writers on this subject have accepted *Rumex species* which are Cukra class (See V above).

But *Cukra* proper or Cukraka species are different from those of *Salix (Vetas)* species. *Cukra* is also a common term or generic name in A) which includes वृक्षाम्ल, (Vṛkśāmla) अम्लवेतस (Amlavetas) and चुक्रक (Cukraka) (See III. B above) *Cukraka* is substituted in the absence of Amlavetasa. Amlavetas is a tree of medium height having catkinous flowers (See iv-8. 9.10; III b-9,10,12 ,14) while Cukraka is a herbacious plant and it has no catkins.

Foot Note-1) Cukrakam : Vṛkśāmlam (378 Harshe)

2) Cukram: Kśudramla; Amlavetasaḥ; Cukram (Dhn. ni.P. 439-41).

3) Amlaḥ : Cincā; Jambira, Mātuluṅga (Dhn. ni. P. 418)

The term Amlavetas (अम्लवेतस) is prevalent atleast from the compilation of Caraka Samhita (III 1-7). The compiler of Sivakośa describes it as *Namrakaḥ* (III-11) which is indicative of the catkinous plant. *Salix species* is also catkinous plant (III-9,12, 14, IV-8) and *Amlavetasa* of the Books is now recognised and identified to be *Salix* species (IV.2,8 above).

Note : *Catkin. The pendulous uni-sexual flowers of the Willow Burch etc.* (Assell's concise Eng. Dic.)

There are various kinds and species included in *Salix family* but two to three are recognised and accepted (वृक्षाम्ल iv-3.) In Kāśyapa

Samhitā it is remarked *Satrośca* (शत्रोश्च)(III-8 above) to *Amlavetas*, meaning in the territory of 'enemy' (III-8 above) or foreign nativity of IV-3 and IV-5 IV-10 above plants. Others have suggested some species of this genus as Amlavetasa (IV-5 7,8.) But Ayurvedic *Amlavetas*(अम्लवेतस) is(जलाम्लवेतस) *Jalāmlavetas* (वञ्जुल) *Vañjula* (III-a -5, b-9, 10.) Which are synonyms for *Jalavetas* and now it is identified as *Salix tetrasperma* Roxb. (1-a-A IV-5, 12, 13).

Raj. ni has recorded a kind Phalāmla Vetas(I-B-a) which is not recognised botanically yet. Shivadas and some modern writers suggest to accept *Thaikal* (थयकल)for it (III-b-15 V-4, 5-6). *Thaikal* is identified tobe *Garcinia pedunculata* Roxb. (V-6). Some modern writers suggest a *Citrus species* which is generally known as *Suḷelimbu*(सुळेलिंबु), *Amlabeda* (अम्लबेद) the shape of which is like *Citrus medica* Linn. (जम्बीरफल) (Jambīraphala) C (III-11) above but very acidous or sour. It is said if a pin is rushed in the fruit it melts (IV-1 above). If it is unavailable the fruit of *Thaikal* is substituted for it (IV-11, 3).

The compiler of Śivakośa records a kind of Vetasāmla (III-11) Jambīra-phala (जम्बीरफल). This seems *Citrus species* to which he records the *name Amlavetas, Sahasravedhi* (III-b11).

The references of Śhivakośa seems to be based on traditional information. This species and Dr. Desai's species seem to be similar and identical with Raj. ni's *Phalāmla vetas* and the fruit of *Thaikal* should be used as substituted for Raj. ni's accepted *Phalāmlavetasa*. The substance of both fruits seems to be similar. Hence the fruit of citrus species should be recognised as *Phalāmla -vetas* of Raj. ni. and the fruit of *Thaikal* should be used as substitute for Raj. ni.'s *Phalāmlavetas*.

Besides this plant of (अम्लवेतस)*Amlavetas* other two plants, different from this under the heading (वेतस) Vetasa (See Chap V)are mentioned . According to compiler of this Nighaṇṭu the plants recorded there are quite different from the plant recorded here but the species are the same.

But it is strange to say that such an important medicinal plant is not recognised and identified botanically. Vaidya Pade has recorded botanical name as *Acido zeypholia* but this name is not found in modern books on this subject.

In short it is suggested that Ayurvedic *Amlavetas* should be accepted as *Salix tetraspema* Roxb. and Raj. ni's *Phalāmlavetas* should be accepted as *Citrus species* which is discussed above.

39 (३२) अजमोदा Ajamodā

अजमोदा बस्तमोदा दीप्यको लोचमर्कटः ।
खराह्वा कारवी वल्ली[१] मोदा हस्तिमयूरकः[२] ॥९९

अजमोदा च शूलघ्नी तिक्तोष्णा कफवातजित् ।
हिक्काध्मानारुचीर्हन्ति कृमिजिद् वह्निदीपनी ॥१००

अजमोदा (Ajamodā), बस्तमोदा (Bastamodā), दीप्यकः (Dīpyakaḥ), लोचमर्कटः (Locamarkaṭaḥ), खराह्वा (Kharāhvā), कारवी (Kāravī), वल्ली (Vallī), मोदा (Modā) and हस्तिमयूरकः (Hastimayūrakaḥ) are synonymous.

Ajamodā is bitter in taste, *uṣṇavīrya,* pacifies *kapha vātadoṣas* and stimulates digestive capacity. It is useful in hiccup, tympanitis, anorexia and worms.

For Confirmation

Fam. -Umbelliferae. Apiaceae.

I- a- ***Trachyspermum roxburghianum*** (DC.) Sprague.*
Syn.- *Carum robxburghianum* Benth. & Hook. f.
Apium involucratum Roxb., *Pimpinella involucratum* W.& A.
Ptychotis roxburghiana DC.

b- Watt Dic. & Chopra.

c- Extensively cultivated throughout India from Himalyas, Bengal to Singapore and Ceylon.

II- b- दीप्यकः (Dīpyakaḥ),अजमोदा (Ajmodā),खराह्वा (Kharahvā), उग्रगन्धा (Ugragandhā), कारवी (Kāravī), गन्धदला (Gandhadalā), शिखिमोदा (Śikhimodā), फलमुख्या (Phalamukhyā)

b- H- Ajamoda; Guj-Bodiajmoda, C.P.-Rānadhanī; Bom. Ajawān; Mar.-Korānjhā, Ajamodā-owā, Kan.-Ajamud voman; Tel.-Ajamuda-Vomun, Asumanṭaga vomum. Tam.-Ashamtawam; Ashmotman. Keral. Ayamodakam, Kaccarakku-Arab.Bazarul Karaphs Per-Tukme Karaphas.

III- *cf.* (Pre No. 36 and Post No. 22 Supra).

b- 1) (Ayur O. Ni.)

2) ३० अजमोदा 'अलंकारे यवान्यां च दीप्यको लोचमस्तकम्' इति रभसः । 'अजमोदाद्वयं प्रोक्तं द्वयं तनुदलं तनु । क्षेत्रे विचीर्णपत्रे च

---

* The current name for *Trachyspermum roxburghianum* DC. is *T. roxburghianum* (DC.) Wolff. Syn. *Carum roxburghianum* Benth. & Hook. f.

The Synonyms mentioned I-a by D. K. Kamat are according to Watt Dictionary Vol !'. P. 201, Vol. I-P. 272. etc.

१ 'वह्निर्मोदा' इति आनन्दा. पुस्तके पाठः ।

२ 'हस्तिमयूरिका' इति आनन्दा. पुस्तके पाठः ।

तत्रतीक्ष्णेऽजमोदकः । सूक्ष्मः सरो सबीजस्तु सदा पथ्यो भृशं कटुरिति
(Harshe)

Note : Some modern writers on this plant have recognised and identified Ajamodā (अजमोदा) to be *Apium graveolens* Linn. But it is a kind of Celery used by Europeans and its native place is also England and the Persia, Arabia.Hindi names given to this plant are more generally applied to *Carum roxburghinum* Benth. (Watt. Dic.Vol. III, p.271; Desai p. 370-371).

We have identified and accepted Ajamodā (अजमोदा) of Dhn.ni. to be *Carum roxburghiamum* Linn.Ajamodā of Dhn. ni. is a medicinal plant and is used for the same purpose (Watt. Dic. II, 201, Desai P. 366). but it is not used in India as Celery seeds.Being such difference between these two plants *A. graveolens* cannot be accepted to be Ajamodā of Dhn. ni.

40. (३३) अजगन्धा Ajagandhā

अजगन्धा खरपुष्पा बस्तगन्धा विगन्धिका ।
कारवी[१] बर्बरा गन्धा तुङ्गी पूतिमयूरिका[२] ॥ १०१

अजगन्धा वातहरा वीर्योष्णा तु ज्वरापहा ।
गुल्माष्ठीलाकफानाहशूलजित् वह्निकृत्परा ॥ १०२

अजगन्धा (Ajagandhā), खरपुष्पा (Kharapuṣpā), बस्तगन्धा (Bastagandhā), विगन्धिका (Vigandhikā), कारवी (Kāravī), बर्बरा (Barbarā), गन्धा (Gandhā), तुङ्गी (Tuṅgī), and पूतिमयूरिका (Pūtimayūrikā), are synonymous.

Ajagandhā is *uṣṇavīrya* and pacifies *vāta* and *kapha doṣa*. It strongly stimulates the digestive capacity and is useful in fevers, tumors, (diverticulosis), *aṣṭhīlā* (prostatic hypertrophy ?) and colic due to typanitis.

(Under this heading the compiler Dhn.Ni. has recorded a plant अजगन्धा without giving its morphological identity but Rāj. ni. records it as पीताचेदंजने हिता (*Pīatācedañjane hitā*). At present two varieties are found under the name अजगन्धा (*Ajagandhā*) one of it is 'A' पीता (*Pītā -yellow*) and the next is 'B' श्वेता (*Sweta -white)* both of the same family.

---

१ " कवरी " इति क्षीर. संमतः पाठः ।

२ " पीतमयूरकः " इति क्षी. संमतः पाठः ।

Fam : Capparidaceae.

I- A-a- ***Polanisia icosandra*** (Linn)* W & A., Syn-*Cleome viscosa* Linn.
b- Kamat. C-A common weed throughout the warmer parts of India.

I- B-a- ***Gynandropsis gynandra*** (Linn.) Briquet, Syn, *G.pentaphylla DC.*, *Cleome pentayhalla* Linn.
b- Kamat C-A common weed abundant throughout the warmer parts of India.

II- a A & B
खरपुष्पा (Kharapuṣpā), बस्तगन्धा (Bastagandhā), बर्बरगन्धा (Barbaragandhā), पूतिमयूरिका (Pūtimayūrikā), अजगन्धा (Ajagandhā), सुरपुष्पी (Surapuṣpī), ब्राह्मी (Brāhmī).
1) *Kharpuṣpā*-severe, hurtful.
2) *Bastgandhā*-a Basta- a goat.
3) *Barbarā*-not an Aryan, barbarian,
4) *Pūti mayūrikā*-Putrid, stinking inflorescene (Putrid, bad).

A-b- Sanṣ-तिलपर्णी (Tilaparṇī), आदित्यभक्ता (Ādityabhaktā), H : Kānapuṭī, Hurahura ; Hurahuriā (Watt. Dic.) Mar : पिवळा तिळवण (Pivalātiḷavaṇa); Dec-चेरिय अजवान (Ceriya ajawāna); Bom : जंगली अजवान (Jangalīajawana), तिळवण (Tiḷavaṇa). Eng.: *Wild mustard.*
b- H-Karāliya; Mar : पांढरा तिळवण (Pāndharā tilavaṇa -white). Mal. : Taivel, Tam: Kaduga : Tel : Vamit. Mal. वेला कारवेला-अटट्ट नारिवेला.

III- *cf.* बर्बरः (Barbaraḥ), Dhn. ni. p. 373-20. ब्राह्मी (Brāhmi) Dhn. ni. p. 154 . सुवर्चला (Suvarcalā) Dhn. ni. p. 153; चोरकः (Corakaḥ). Dhn. ni. p. 110

a- 1) अजगन्धा बस्तगन्धा (Ca. Su. 1-77); Su-Sū. 36-16. Ast. hr. Ci.-1-160 (Balawantji p. 6).

b- 1) अजगन्धा तिलपर्णिका (Raj. ni. Tryarthe).
2) 375-बर्बरी कबरीतुङगी खरपुष्पा अजगन्धिका-इत्यमरः (Harshe)
3) 168 तिलपर्णीति-तिलपर्णी खरच्छदा । सुदित्या पूतिगन्धा च

---

* I-a-A The current name for *Polanisia icosandra* (Linn.) W.&A. is *Cleome viscosa* (Linn.) Syn.*C. icosandra* Linn. (Comp. to Gloss. p.39)
I-a-B For *Gynandropsis gynandra* (Linn.) Briq, The current name is *Cleome gynandra* Linn.
Syn. *C. pentaphylla* Linn. ; *Gyandropsis pentaphylla* DC. (Comp. to Gloss. p.39)

हुलहुल...इति डल्हणः (Harshe)
बर्बरः तिलपर्णी बदरको -कैय्यदेवः
4) तिलपर्णी सूर्यावर्तेषु । रस रत्नाकरे । (Rasa. p. 15)
b- 5) अजगन्धा वीर्योष्णा - गुल्माष्ठिला कफानाह शूल' इति ॥
ब्राह्मी .Dhn. ni. p. 90.
कर्णव्रणार्ति शूलघ्नी पीताचेदंजने हिता । Raj. ni
6) सुर्वचला (भा.नि.) Suvarcalā, सूर्यभक्ता वरदा वरदापि च ... सूर्यावर्ता. पराब्रह्मसुवर्चला... गुणा हिमारूक्षा स्वादुपाका ... अपित्तला कटु... विष्टंभकफवातजित ॥ २८९ ॥
अन्या सुवर्चला तिक्ता कषायोष्णा लघुः कटुः ॥ २८० ॥
(Bh. ni. P. 141 b)
ब्राह्मी ....सोमवल्ली सरस्वती तिलपर्णी-सूर्यावर्ता
(Cleome viscosa) U.C. Dutta, Desai.

III-*cf* 7) Hulahula. (Rasayogasagar, Bhasmāmṛt).
8) Ajagandhā, Hulahulā (Ni.Adarsha).
9) Tilaparṇi. Hulahulā. (Ni. Adarsh).

IV- 1) *Cleome icosandra* Linn., *C. viscosa* Linn. Bom-Hurahura, kānaphuṭi, pivaḷā Tiḷavaṇa; San. Ādityabhaktā, Suvarcalā (Chopra-Handa. p. 32 b).

2) *Cleome viscosa* Linn.The juice of the leaves is poured into the ear to relieve *earache*. According to Rheed the juice mixed with oil is a popular remedy in Bombay for purulent discharge from the ear. As a drug *C.viscosa* Linn. is more superior to *C.pentaphyla* DC. *C. viscosa* posseses a distinct *foetid smell* and *vesicant* property. (Watt Dic. p. 'C' 371).

3) In C. S. and A. H. This variety of *Suvarcalā* appears to have been mentioned under the name of *Tilaparṇī* (C,S. 27-94 and A.H. Su. 6.76) (Balavntaji p. 440)

4) ...*Tilaparṇī*...is usually indentified with *Gynandropsis gynandra Briquet* called तिलपर्णी which can be called *sūryāvartā* or *sūryabhaktā*...moreover there is a section of Vaidyas in Bengal which also believe *Hulhula* to be the source of *Brahmasuvarcalā.* Thus *Gynandropsis* may be tentatively accepted as the second variety of *Suvarcalā* and named as *Tilaparṇikā* and *Brahmasuvarcalā,* the so-called *divine drug of the same name*. It is not uncommon for a divine drug name to be also used for common drugs such as छत्रा *Chatrā* etc.
(Balawantji p. 441)

V- 1) *Ocimum basillicum* Linn :
Mañjarikā H .B. Bābuī Tulas; Bom & Marathi - Subjā

Tam : Tirunt patchi; Tel. : Bhutulsi; Mal :Tirunitru, P. Bābri. (Chopra).

2) बर्बरः सुमुखश्चैव गरघ्नः गन्धपत्रः सुराहवयः ॥
सुगन्धिर्वान्तिनाशनः ।
त्वक्दोषशमनस्तथा ॥ (Raj. ni. Dhn. ni. p. 372)

3) a- *Helianthus annuus* Linn. Eng. : Sunflower

4) *Sunflower* native of N.W. America, a recent intorduction into India. (Cook fl.).

5) *H. annuus* Willd-of this several varieties are introduced from China and Persia and although originally from Peru."
(Roxb. III-444).

6) आदित्यपर्णी(Ādityaparṇī).In औषधीशब्दसिंधु (Oṣadhī Śabdasindhu))describing आदित्यपर्णी *Āditya parṇī* is recorded as : या सूर्यकान्तेति भाष्यते क्षीरं यस्या सुवर्णाभं पुष्पाणि यस्या च सूर्यमण्डलाकाराणि । (Balvantji)

7) आदित्यपर्णी *Āditya parṇi* C.S. Ci.1-A; Su.S.Ci.Ci.15 43,90.5 S 20-91...Caraka described it as having golden latex and flowers like the orb of The sun (See Balvantji Gloss. p. 35).

8) *Helianthus annuus* Linn., Eng-Sunflower. Sushrut has discribed this drug for promoting the healthy granulation in wounded area.... etc. (Udupa A.S.R.M. p.273).

41 (३४) कपित्थः Kapitthaḥ

कपित्थोऽथ दधित्थस्तु ग्राही गन्धफलश्च सः[1] ।
अक्षसस्यो[2] दधिफलश्चिरपाकी कपिप्रियः ॥ १०३

कपित्थमामस्वर्यं कफघ्नं ग्राहि वातलम् ॥
कफानिलहरं पक्वं मधुराम्लरसं गुरु ॥ १०४
श्वासकासारुचिहरं तृष्णाघ्नं कण्ठशोधनम् ॥

कपित्थः (Kapitthaḥ), दधित्थः (Dadhithaḥ), ग्राही (Grāhī), गन्धफलः (Gandhaphalaḥ), अक्षसस्यः (Akśasasyaḥ), दधिफलः (Dadhiphalaḥ), चिरपाकी (Cirapākī), and कपिप्रियः (Kapipriyaḥ), are synonymous.

Unripe fruit of *kapittha* is harmful to voice, pacifies *kaphadoṣa* and aggravates *vātadoṣa* and is astringent.

---

१ 'फलसुगन्धकः' इति नि. शे. टीकायाम ।
२ 'अक्षिस्पन्दो' इति. नि. शे. टीकायाम ।

The same when ripe (fruit) is sweet and sour in taste, pacifies *kapha vata doṣas* and is *guru.* It is useful in dyspnoea, cough, loss of appetite, thirst, and purifies throat.

Fam : Rutaceae.

I- a- ***Feronia limonia*** (Linn.) Swingle
Syn : *F. elephantum* Correa.

b- Roxburgh c-Sub Himalayan forest, throughout the greater parts of the plane of India, Bengal, Bombay and Madras, indigenous to S. India.

II- a- गन्धफलः (Gandhaphalaḥ), दीर्घफलः (Dīrghaphalaḥ) कपिप्रियः (Kapipriyaḥ), अक्षसस्यः (Akśasasyah).

b- Marathi - Kavith, Kaith; B: Katabel; Tel : Velaga, Kapittha; Tam Nerivil, Kavit, Vela, Velium; Kan : Bela, Belada, Bilwa Haṇṇu. Mal. विळारमरं Eng : Elephant apple, Wood apple.

III- a वीर्यश्रदानवेऽन्न उन्नमयित्रीम् ओषधीम् कपित्थकाख्यं वयं खनामसि खनामः ॥ भाष्य पुरुषस्य वीर्यकर कर्मणी कपित्थक मूलं ओषाधिवत् खात्वा... वीर्यकामाय पुरुषः पिबेत् । (Av. III-106)

2) Ca. Su. 3-13; Su-Su. 46 139, 147 Asht. Hr. Sū. 6-126; 10-26.

42 (३५) शर्करा Śarkarā (Sugar)

शर्करोत्तग तु मीनाण्डी श्वेता मत्स्यण्डिका सिता ॥ १०५
अहिच्छत्रा तु सिकता शुद्धा शुभ्रा सितोपला ॥
शर्करा शीतवीर्या तु सर्वदाहविनाशिनी ॥ १०६
रक्तपित्तप्रशमनी छर्दिमूर्च्छातृषापहा ॥

शर्करा (Śarkarā), मीनाण्डी (Mīnāṇḍī), श्वेता (Śvetā), मत्स्यण्डिका (Matsyaṇḍikā), सिता (Sitā), अहिच्छत्रा (Ahicchatrā), सिकता (Sikatā), शुद्धा (Śuddhā), शुभ्रा (Śubhrā) and सितोपला (Sitopalā) are synonymous.

Śarkarā is *śītavīrya* and useful in all types of burning sensations, alleviates bleeding disorders, emesis, syncope and thirst.

मधुशर्करा (ध.नि.) Madhuśarkarā (23)
शर्कराऽन्या मधुभवा माधवी मधुशर्करा ॥ १०७
माक्षीकशर्करा प्रोक्ता शर्करा मदनोद्भवा ॥
शर्करा मधुसंभूता छर्द्यतिसारनाशिनी ॥१०८

There is an another type of *Śarkarā* (sugar) of which synonyms are मधुभवा (Madhubhavā), माधवी (Mādhavī), मधुशर्करा (Madhuśarkarā), माक्षीकशर्करा (Mākṣīka śarkarā) and मदनोद्भवा शर्करा (Madanodbhavā śarkarā).

Madhuśarkarā is useful in emesis and diarrhoea.

यवासशर्करा (ध. नि.) Yawāsaśarkarā.

यवासशर्करा चान्या निर्दिष्टा यासशर्करा ।
स्वेदनी ह्लादनी रूक्षा कषाया स्वादुपाकिका ॥ १०९
(यवासशर्करा शीता रसे स्वादुज्वरास्रजित् ॥)

There is an another type of *Śarkarā* called as यवासशर्करा (Yavāsaśarkarā) of which synonym is यासशर्करा (Yāsaśarkarā).

Yāsaśarkarā is diphoretic, pleasing, *rūkṣa* (drying), *kaṣāya* in taste and sweet in *vipāka* (final transformation after digestion.).

Yavāsaśarkarā is *śītavīrya,* sweet in taste and useful in fevers and bleeding disorders.

(Generic name of various kinds of sugar produced from sugarcane. But under this heading the kinds A- मीनाण्डी (Mīnāṇḍī) and B-अहिच्छत्र सितोपला (Ahichatrā sitopalā) are recorded which are produced from (Guḍa) i.e.Jageri.

I- A-a- Mīnāṇḍī i.e. of small particles like the size of eggs of fishes.

b- Kamat.

B-a- अहिच्छत्रा (Ahichatrā) Name of a kind of sugar which was manufactured at अहिच्छत्र (Ahichatra) a name of the seat of Pāñchāls kingdom. Now it may be known as रामपुर (Rampur) in U.P.

II- B-a- श्वेता (Śwetā), (Matsyāṇḍkiā). B-a-(Ahichatrā), (Sikatā), (Śuddhā), (Sitopalā).

A-b- (Not known).

B-b- (Not known).

Cf. (Madhu Śārkarā), (Yāwanāli) and (Ṭavarāja śarkarā) of Raj. ni. (Post Nos. 23, 24 & 25). (Madhuśarkarā). Post No. is 23.25).

(Under this heading two kinds of (Śarkarā-Sugar) are included which are A मधुभवा (Madhubhawā), and Bयवासशर्करा (Yāwāsa Śarkarā). Raj. ni. has recorded this separately under the heading,तवराजशर्करा (Tawarāja Śarkarā) (Post No. 25). (Yawasa) and(Tawarāja) are the names of the same plant, hence description of (Tawarāja) is added hereunder.

II- A-a- Crystalised settled particles of honey.

b- Kamat.

II- B-a- Sugarlike sweetish particles obtained from the following plants.

Fam. Leguminosae. Fabaceae.

Alhagi pseudalhagi

b- Watt. Dic.

c- This is chiefly collected in Khorasan, Kurdistan and Humdan. Turanjbin of Bazar is imported into Bombay from Persia and Baluchistan. (Watt Dict).

I- A-a- (Madhubhawā) (Mādhavī). (Mākśikā Śarkarā), (Madanodbhawā)(Sitākhaṇḍā), (Khaṇḍajā), (Atimadhurā).

A-b- Honey collected by bees.

B-a- यवासशर्करा (Yāvasa Śarkarā) तवराजः (Tawarājaḥ).

B-b- जवासा साखर (Javāsā sākhara), Pers-Turanjabin.तुरंजबिन् Eng. : Manna is known as Turanjabin.

III-a (Yāsa sugar) Su. Su-Su.45-167.

IV- The Sanskrit writers do not appear to refer to the '*Manna*' (a-1) or sweet sugary extraction obtained naturally from the plant by shaking its twigs over a cloth . (Watt.) (Dymock) 1-418). Watt Dic 'M' -p-165).

शतपुष्पादिको वर्गः द्वितीयः परिकीर्तितः ।
कायाग्निदीपनो बल्यो वक्त्रसौगन्ध्य तीक्ष्णकृत ॥

Thus has been told the शतपुष्पादि (Śatapuṣpādi) 2nd chapter. The drugs mentioned in it, stimulate and strengthen the digestive (Metabolic) capacity of the body. These improve taste, and odour of the mouth'

इति शतपुष्पादिर्द्वितीयो वर्गः समाप्तः ।

Thus ends the Śatapuṣpādi Chapter Second.

चंदनादिस्तृतीयो वर्गः
CANDANADIḤ CHAPTER III

1 चन्दनम् Candanam

चंदनं गंधसारं च महार्हं श्वेतचन्दनम् ।
भद्रश्रीस्तु मलयजं गोशीर्षं तिलपर्णकम् ॥ १

श्रीखण्डं शीतलं स्वादु तिक्तं पित्तविनाशनम् ।
रक्तप्रसादनं वृष्यं अंतर्दाहापहारकम् ॥ २

पित्तास्रविषतृड्दाहकृमिघ्नं गुरु रूक्षणम् ।
सर्वं सतिक्तमधुरं चन्दनं शिशिरं परम् ॥ ३

चंदनं (Candanam), गंधसारं (Gandhasāram), महार्हं (Mahārham), श्वेतचन्दनम् (Śvetacandanam), भद्रश्रीः (Bhadraśrīḥ), मलयजं (Malayajam), गोशीर्षं (Gośīrṣam), and तिलपर्णकम् (Tilaparṇakam) are synonymous.

Śrīkhaṇḍa (Candana) is sweet and bitter in taste, *śītavīrya,* pacifiy *pittadosa*, is blood purifying, *vṛṣya* and useful in internal burning sensation.

All kinds of candana are sweet and bitter in taste, *śītavīrya,* pacify *pitta* and *raktadoṣa,* bad effects of poisons. thirst, burning sensation and worms. These are *guru, rūkṣa* (roughing). and causes much refrigerant action.

Generic name, under this heading the compiler's have recorded five kinds.

I- A-a- गंधसारम् (Gandhasāram). B- श्वेतचन्दनम् (Śwetacandanam), C- भद्रश्री (Bhadraśrī), D - गोशीर्षम् (Gośīrṣam), E-तिलपर्णकम् (Tilaparṇakam),

Besides these kinds some other sorts are noted by the compilers (See post numbers (3), (4), (5) infra)

(Fam. Santalaceae)

I- A-a- ***Santalum album*** Linn. sp. Pl. and Willd.
Syn. *S.verum* Linn.
b- Roxburgh (Fl. Indi).
c- See below IV-2

Note : The above recorded kinds of Candanas are not botanically recognised so the accepted name given above should be treated, for the present, for all kinds noted above.

II- a- चंदनम् (Candanam), महार्हम् (Mahārham), मलयजम् (Malayajam),

b- Kan - Śrigandhadamar, Mar. - Bom.- Candana ; Hind - Candan, Sandal; B. Candan, Srikaṇḍa; Tam. Sandal, Sandanak - Katti (The Wood)
Tel - Gandhapu - Cekka, Haricandan, Teḷtacandanam; Kan. Gandhan Gandad (- tree) Malay, - Candanamatti, (-tree), Tsjandan-marum (-wood)
Guj. Serkets, Sukad; Sind - Sukhand; Eng. The White Sandal Wood Tree.

III- See - Kalīyakam (3) Barbarkakam (4) Hari candanam (5) infra

a-1) चंदन (Candana) (Patañjali -see 4-3-141 Agarval Pp-209-212)

b-1) 136 चन्दनं गन्धसारम् । खादने कटुकं शीतमिषत् पीतं च घर्षणे ।
छेदनेरक्तवर्णं यश्चन्दनं तद्वरं परमिति धर्मिष्ट : ॥ (Harshe)

2) 162 चन्दनं श्रीखण्डः । ' रोहणश्चन्दनद्रुममिति ' हारावलिः । (Harshe)
" मलयस्तुस्याच्छ्रीखण्डो रोहणश्च स' इति पुरुषोत्तमः । (Harshe)

IV-a-1) श्रीखण्डः or white variety, पीत चन्दनं or yellow variety. These varieties are found on the difference in the depth of colour in the heart wood, and not on any specific difference in the plants."
(Dr. U.C. Dutt)

2) The Genus *Santalum* is ... composed of eight species, all closely allied to one another. They are indigenous to East India. The Malaya Archipelago, Australia and the islands of the Pacific ocean - *Santalum album* is described in Flora British India only Indian representative of the genus. Santalum L. The white Sandal wood. English
Syn : *S. myrtifolium* Roxb.
S. verum Linn.
Sirium myrtifolium Roxb.
Habitat - Drier parts of Mysore, Coimbatore, south to Madras and North to Kolhapur, Watt. VI- II P. 461-62

3) *Santalum album* Linn. Sp. pl. ed. Willd.
Syn : *S. verum,* Linn. Mat. Med.
S. myrtifolium R.
Syn. : *Sirium myrtifolium* (Roxb. Carom pl.)
I think it nearer the truth to consider them to be distinct species of the same genus or varieties of the same species. For my own part I think them distinct species. Therefore, I call the narrow leaved one *Santalum myrtifolium* Roxb. C.B.C. p. 148.

4) See चंदन Candan, पीत चंदन Pīta Candan (Chunekar Bh.Pr.p.187-190)

Note : चंदन सामान्य गुणाः (candan sāmānya gunāḥ) noted under कालीयकम् kālīyakam see: चंदन under कालीयक

रक्तचन्दनम् Raktacandanam (1)

रक्तचन्दनमप्यन्यल्लोहितं हरिचन्दनम् ।
रक्तसारं ताम्रसारं निर्दिष्टं क्षुद्रचन्दनम् ॥४

रक्तचन्दनमप्याहु रक्षोघ्नं तिक्तशीतलम् ।
रक्तोद्रेकहरं हन्ति पित्तकोपं सुदारुणम् ॥५

There is an another type of candanam called as रक्तचन्दनम् (Raktacandanam) of which synonyms are लोहितं (Lohitam), हरिचन्दनम् (Haricandanam), रक्तसारं (Raktasāram), ताम्रसारं (Tāmrasāram) and क्षुद्रचन्दनम् (Kśudracandanam).

Rakta candana is bitter in taste, *śītavirya,* antiseptic (or destroys evil spirits), pacifies severe *rakta* and *pittadoṣas.*

I- a) ***Pterocarpus santalinus*** Linn.f.
b) Roxburgh
c) Burma and Andaman Islands.

II- a) लोहितम् (Lohitam), ताम्रसारम् (Tāmrasāram), अर्कचन्दनम् (Arkacndanam)
b) (Sk. B) Raktacandana; (H. Mar.) Lālacandana; (Tel.) Raktacandanamu; (Tam.) Sena śadana; (Mal.) Rakta śandanam; (Eng.) Red sandal wood; The Andaman red wood. The Andaman red wood.

III- 1) *Adenanthera pavonia* Willd. (Linn).

IV Sk. Kucandana, Raktacandana which means Red Sandal whereas we consider *P. santalinus* to be the true which yields that wood ... (Roxb. Fl. Ind.)

कुचन्दनम् Kucandanam (2) (पतङ्गम् - Patangam)

कुचन्दनं पतङ्गं च रक्तकाष्ठं सुरङ्गकम् ।
पत्राङ्गं पट्टरागं च पट्टरञ्जनमेव च ॥ ६

स्वादुपाकरसे शीतं पतंगं नातिशीतलम् ।
कुचन्दनं तु तिक्तं स्यात्सुगन्धि व्रणरोपणम् ॥ ७

कुचन्दनं (Kucandanam), पतङ्गं (Patangam), रक्तकाष्ठं (Raktakāṣṭham), सुरङ्गकम् (Surangakam), पत्राङ्गं (Patrāngam), पट्टरागं (Paṭṭarāgam), and पट्टरञ्जनम् (Paṭṭarañjanam) are synonymous.

Patanga is sweet in taste and in *vipāka,* not excessivley *śītavīrya. kucandana* is bitter in taste, fragrant and useful in wound healing.

(Fam. Leguminosae) Caesalpiniaceae

I- a ***Caesalpinia sappan*** Linn.

b -Roxburgh

c-Eastern & Western peninsula, Pegu & Tenaserim, Cultivated in C. India. (Watt. Dict. II-10)

II- a) पतङ्गम् (Patangam), रक्तकाष्ठम् (Rakta Kāṣṭham), पत्राङ्गम् (Patrāngam)

b) (SK) Paṭṭarañjanam; (Santal) Teri; (Mar.) Patanga; (H.B.) Bakkam, Patanga; (Guj.) Patangno lākḍo; (Tam.)patanga kaṭṭa, Bakapu; (Kan) patanga ceke, sapanga. (Eng.) The sappan wood.

III-b-1) 195 कुचन्दनम् - पत्राङ्गम् (Harshe)

2) 166 "पट्टरञ्जनं चतुर्थं कुचन्दनं पत्तरं पतंगम् ।
रक्तकाष्टं सुगन्धं पाण्डुरागमिति ॥" (Abhi. Man.)

कालीयकम् Kālīyakam (3)

कालीयकं[1] तु पीतं स्यात्तथा नारायणप्रियम् ।
मलयोत्थं पीतकाष्ठं चतुर्थं[2] हरिचन्दनम् ॥ ८

कालीयकं पवित्राद्यं शीतलं रक्तपित्तजित् ।

कालीयकं(Kālīyakam), पीतं (Pītam), नारायणप्रियं (Nārāyaṇapriyam), मलयोत्थं (Malayottham), पीतकाष्ठं (Pītakāṣṭham), हरिचन्दनम् (Haricandanam) are synonymous.

Kālīyakam is *śītavīrya,* useful in bleeding disorders (rakta pitta) and is too much auspicious.

---

१) 'कं पतंगं स्यात।' २) 'चतुर्थं पीत चन्दनम् इति पा. आनंदा.

(Under this heading the compiler has recorded four kinds* of Candanam. These are as follows :)

II- a) कालीयकं पतङ्गाख्यम् (Kālīyakam patangākhyam),
b) नारायणप्रियं (Nārāyaṇapriyam),
c) मलयोत्थं (Malayottham), पीतकाष्ठम् (Pītakāṣṭham),
d) हरिचन्दनम् (Haricandanam).

बर्बरिकं (ध.नि.) Barbarikam (4)

अथ बर्बरिकं श्वेतं निर्गन्धं बर्बरोद्भवम् ॥९
पित्तासृक् कफदाहघ्नं कृमिघ्नं गुरु रूक्षणम् ॥

सर्वाण्येतानि तुल्यानि रसतो वीर्यतस्तथा ॥१०
गन्धेन तु विशेषः स्यात् पूर्वं श्रेष्ठतमं गुणैः ॥

बर्बरिकं (Barbarikam), श्वेतं (Śvetam), निर्गन्धं (Nirgandham), बर्बरोद्भवम् (Barbarodbhavam) are synonymous. It pacifies *pitta, rakta* and *kapha doṣas,* alleviates burning sensation, is *guru* and *rūkṣa*. (roughning).

All these kinds are similar in taste and *vīrya,* but there is a differance in the fragrance.These are serially better in qualities in the reverse order.

II- a) अथ बर्बरिकं श्वेतं निर्गन्धं बर्बरोद्भवम् ।
Barbarikam swetam nirgandham
Barbarodbhavam (i.e. growing in Barbara country or in a region having such name.)

III-b-1) 272 निर्गंधं चन्दनम् गन्धरहितं श्वेतचन्दन जाति (Harshe)
(This is a kind of a white and odourless candanam).

हरिचन्दनम् Haricandanam (5)(Raj. ni.)

हरिचन्दनं सुरार्हं हरिगन्धं चन्द्रचन्दनं दिव्यम् ॥
दिविजं च महागन्धं नन्दनजं लोहितं च नवसंज्ञम् ॥(रा. नि.)

---

* It may be perhapes that three kinds i.e. 1) श्रीखण्डम् Śrīkhaṇḍam 2) रक्तचंदनम्, Rakta candanam., 3) कुचंदनम् Kucandanam are already discribed and the fourth is 4) कालीयकम् Kālīyakam the synonyms of which are mentioned here. - S.D.Kamat

There is a kind of (Candana) having nine synonyms which are हरिचन्दनम् (Haricandanam) सुरार्हं (Surārham), हरिगन्धं (Harigandham), चन्द्रचन्दनं (Candracandanam), दिव्यम् (Divyam), दिविजं (Divijam), महागन्धं (Mahāgandham), नन्दनजं (Nandanajam) and लोहितम् (Lohitam).

II- a- हरिचन्दनं सुरार्हम् (Haricandanam Surārham); दिव्यं, दिविजम् (Divyam, divijam), महागन्धम् (Mahāgandham), (Raj. ni.)

III-b-1) 164 नारायणप्रियमपरममलं मालेयकं हिमं शीतम् ।
हरिचन्दनं च पीतं पीततरुः स्याध्दरिश्यामः ॥ (Abhi. manj.),

2) 283 पीतचन्दनमिति । कालीयको "दारुनिशे" ति रुद्र : । (Harshe)

3) 287 हरिचन्दनं त्रिदिशानां महीरूहो देववृक्षः "हरिद्व पीतचन्दन " मिति निघण्टुः । (Harshe)

4) 56 हरिचन्दनं । पीतसारं "कालीयकं च पीतं स्यात् तथा नारायणप्रियम् । कालीयकं पीतसारं पीताभं हरिचन्दन " मिति धन्वतरि : । Harshe

५) चन्दन सामान्य गुणा : -
सर्वाण्येतानि तुल्यानि रसतो वीर्यतस्तथा ।
गन्धेन तु विशेषः स्यात्पूर्वं श्रेष्ठतमं गुणैः ॥
अन्यच्च :
चन्दनानि समानानि रसतो वीर्यतस्तथा । भिद्यन्ते किन्तु गन्धेन तत्राद्यं गुणवत्तरम् ॥

IV- 1) कालीय (Kālīya), कालीयक (Kālīyaka) ,कालेयक (Kāleyaka) *Coscinium fenestratum* (Gaertn.) Colebr. Maramañjalu मरमञ्जलू (South), *Kālīyam* and other allied names refer to this south Indian plant. (Baivantaji p. 95)

2) चन्दन Candana

1) *Santalum album* Linn
श्वेत चन्दन Śweta candana

2) *Pterocarpus santalinus* Linn f.
Rakta candana रक्तचन्दन

3) *Coscinium fenestratum* (Gaertn.) Colebr.
Kaleyaka कालेयक
The references for candana only have been noted here for which Śweta or Rakta kinds are used according to the nature etc. of the preparations and their uses. (Balavantaji p. 152)

Foot note : ४ दारुनिशा *Berberis aristata* DC. (Kamat) ५ हरिद्व *Adina cordifolia* (Roxb.) Benth. & Hook. f. or *Wrightia tomentosa* Roem. & Schult. S.S. Ci. II- 9 (Va कुटज or हरिद्रा वृक्ष (Balvantaji P. 466) D.K Kamat.

2 कुंकुमम् Kumkumam

कुंकुमं रुधिरं रक्तमसृगस्रं च पीतकम् ॥११
काश्मीरं चारु बाह्लीकं संकोचं पिशुनं वरम् ॥

कुंकुमं कटुकं तिक्तमुष्णं श्लेष्मसमीरजित् ॥१२
व्रणदृष्टिशिरोरोग विषहृत्कायकान्तिकृत् ॥

कुंकुमं (Kumkumam), रुधिरं (Rudhiram), रक्तम् (Raktam), असृग् (Asṛg), अस्रं (Asram), पीतकम् (Pītakam), काश्मीरं (Kā śmīram), चारु (Cāru), बाल्हीकं (Bālhīkam), संकोचम् (Samkocam), पिशुनं (Pi śunam) & वरम् (Varam) are synonymous.

Kumkumam is pungent and bitter in taste, *usṇavīrya,* and pacifies *vāta & kapha doṣas.* It is useful in wounds (ulcers), diseases of the eyes and head, in poisons and to improve the complexion (lustre) of the body.

Fam. Iridaceae.

I- a- ***Crocus sativus*** Linn.
b- Dymock
c- See below IV- i; IV ii

II- a- रुधिरम् (Rudhiram); काश्मीरम् (Kāsmīram); बाह्लीकम् (Bāhlīkam);
b- (H.) Kesar; (Ben.) Safrana; (Guj. Bom. Mar.) Kesara; (Tam.) Kungumapu; (Tel.) Kunkumapu; (B) Safran; (Eng.) Crocos; Saffron

a-1) ... C.S.Ci. 23-53
S.S. Sa 28.13s
Asta. H. Su. 3.11 (Balvantji)

b-1) 34 'कुसुंभसदृशैर्गुच्छैस्तृणकैः कुंकुमं समम् ।
भोटकाश्मीर विषये तनुवाटतया द्विधा ।
उत्तरं शुभमद्रौ चे' ति । '' (Harshe 34)

IV- 1) *Crocus sativus* Linn.
Asia minor, persia and Kashmir have been a long time the countries which export the most. India gets it from Kaṣhmir at the present day ...
Now ... genus crocus, based on a long observations .... connects with C. sativus.Six forms which are found wild.. from Itali to Kurdistan. None of these are identical with the cultivated variety, but certain forms described under other names (C. orisii ....) hardly differ from it. Those are from Italy and Greece (D Candolle)

2) *Crocus sativus* Linn. Saffron ... ... Beng. - Jafran; Tam. Kungumapu; Tel. Kunkumapuva.
Habitat ... It is cultivated in Kashmir at pampur ... The Indian supply is obtained from France, China, Kashmir and small quantity from Persia in form of cakes known as Kesar-Ki-rote...
" Indian saffron adlterated with Saffowers (*Carthamus tinctorius*)" -speaks Ainslie ... .. (abbreviated from Watt Dict.)

3 उशीरम् Uśīram

उशीरं च मृणालं स्यादभयं समगन्धिकम् ॥१३
व्रणप्रियं वीरतरं वीरं वीरणमूलकम् ॥

अन्यच्च- उशीरं वीरणीमूलं वालकं तृणवालुकम् ॥१४
उशीरं शीतलं दाहक्लान्तिहरं च तत् ॥

वातघ्नं ज्वरतृष्णमेहनुद् रक्तं हन्ति योगतः ॥१५
उशीरं स्वेददौर्गन्ध्य पित्तघ्नं स्निग्धतित्तकम् ॥

उशीरं (Uśīram), मृणालं (Mṛṇālam), अभयं (Abhayam), समगन्धिकम् (Samagandhikam), व्रणप्रियं (Vraṇapriyam), वीरतरं (Vīrataram), वीरं (Vīram), वीरणमूलकम् (Vīraṇamūlakam) are synonymous.

[From other sources उशीरं (Uśīram), वीरणीमूल्म् (Vīraṇīmūlam), वालकं (Vālakam), तृणवालुकम् (Tṛṇavālukam) are synonymous.

Uśīram is *śitavīrya* and useful in burning sensation. and removes fatigue.]

Uśīra is bitter in taste, *snigdha* (unctuous), pacifies *pitta* and *vāta doṣas*. It useful in fever, thirst, *meha* (disorders characterised by polyuria), bleeding disorders, and bad odour of perspitation.

Controversial, Confirmed
(Fam. Graminae) Poaceae

I- a- ***Andropogon squarrosus*** Linn. Sp. pl. (non Hook. f.)**
Syn. *Panicum paludosum,* Roxb.
b- Kamat (Following Roxb.)

---

१ 'अमृणालम्' इति रा. नि. संमतः पाठः । २ 'रणप्रियम्' इति आनन्दाः मुद्रित पुस्तके अन्यः पाठः राः निः संमतश्च

** The current accepted name is *vetiveria zizanioides* (Linn.) Nash.

c- See below IV-I Roxburgh.

II- a- अमृणालम् (Amṛṇālam), अभयम् (Abhayam), समगन्धिकम् (Samagandhikam), वणप्रियम् (Vraṇapriyam), वारितरम् (Vāritaram), वीरणमूलकम् (Vīraṇamūlakam), जलवासम् (Jalavāsam), अभयम् (Abhayam), जलामोदम् (Jalāmodam), शुभ्रम् (Śubhram), वालकम् (Vālakam)

b- (SK) Sugandhika, Uśīra; (H.) Khasa, Gāndara Jaḍa. (Maly.) velutta Ramaccam (Shri Krishnan)

III-a- उशीर वालक

1) (Patanjali) Su. IV-5-53 iv-2.80 (Agrawal P. 212)
2) वीरण IV- 5.53; IV- 2.80 (Agrawal P. 212)
3) सेव्यद्वयम् - उशीरं लामज्जकद्वयम् (Asta.) Sang. A. 47. P. 389)
4) Virana Sh . Br. Xii- 8. 1. 15 Sad.Br. V. 2 (Harshe p. X.)
5) नलद, उशीर, -ह्रीबेर (Ast. Sang. A. 14)
6) वालकोशीर (C.S. Vi. 8.143)

b- 1) उशीरम्- हिं. खस; बं. वेणरमूल; तं. आपुकराइ, नेलदम् , करुवेरु, चिडवली. क.वालदगेरु, गंडगंजल, गरिके, उशीर; मल्या. -रामचं; त. वेटीवेर, इजामच्चै,. (Ast. Hr. Kosh)

2) उशीरम् (Uśīram); Keral- Ramaccam; Tam . Itamaccai ; Virana mulam usiram. Tel. Awaru gatti Vang: Venara mula; (H) Gandar -Khasa. (Ayu. O. Ni.)

3) 159 प्राहुरुशिर वीरणम् अभयम् ... बहुमूलम् (Harshe)

4) 160 वालकमुक्तमुदीच्यं -ह्रीबेरम् .... (Harshe)

5) 97 लामज्जमुशिरम् (Harshe)

6) 479 उशीरः - वीरणम् - दीर्घमूलम् (Harshe)

7) उशीरसवालकम् (Uśīra Sa Wālakam).
Usira -khas (Kāśyp. S. Bhāṣā ṭīkā p. 170)

8) वालक (Wālaka) : Netrawalā.
(Kasyp. S. Katutail Kalp.) P. 182

9) अमृणालम् (Amṛṇālam) : Uśiram.
(Cakra. Ca. Vi. 8.135)

10) उशीरम् (Uśīram) : Sugandhakam (Sharn. S. Khand 2.2)

11) ह्रीबेरम् (Rhiberam) "Vālakam, Udīcyam (Sharn. S. Kuaṭjāriṣṭa)

IV- 1) .. Dr. Coning was too accurate a botanist to describe this conspicuous plant under the two names :

a- *Andropogon squarrosus* Linn. Sp. pl. (Willd IV. 908) and

b- *Andropogon muricatus*

The former is eveidently a different species and found by him in Ceylon, floating on pools of water; whereas *A. muricatus* (which was formerly called aromaticus) is always rigidly erect whether growing in water or on dry land. Its root is delightfully aromatic as mentioned by Coning himself and by Sir William Jones particularly when moistened in water.
I am inclined to think Koning's *A. squarossus* is my *Panicum paludosa* a species with thick spongy culms which is generally found swimming of pools of sweet water (C.B.C. 89)

2) उशीरम्, सेव्यम् , वालकम्, नलद, अमृणाल–हीबेरम्
उशीरम् त्रिविधम् – कृष्णम् , पीतम्, श्वेतं च
Kinds of Usira are three - Kṛṣṇam, Pītam and Śvetam- Vaidya Phadke.

Note - No authority is cited for Kṛṣṇa Uśīra by writer of the above book.

V. 1) काळो वाळो, उशीर, वीरणमूलम्
Kāḷo waḷo- Usisra - Vıraṇamulam Guj. Virana na vala; Kāḷo vaḷo *Pavonia odorata* kāḷa waḷā (Narua Sahib)· *P. odorata* - wala, Rhiber (Dr. Kirtikar)
Syn. *Andropogon squarrosus* (U.C. Datta)
These are the names given for Kāḷā wāḷā. Therefore kālā wālā is ambiguous, Katobhatta calls 'Kālo walā to Usira. (Ni. Adarsha.)

2) सुगन्ध वाला, काला वाला
Pavonia odorata Linn, (Chunekar p. 237.)
उशीर (Uśira) This is a kind of Uśīra which is known in Hindi as गांडरजड (Gāṇḍār Jaḍa) H. Khas. (Acha. Yadavji).

3) अथोशीरम्.– वीरण, खस,
Andropogon muricatus Retz.
Vetiveria zizanioides (Linn)· Nash
H.वीरणमूल. गांडर, बेना,
B. वेणरमूल. खसखस
Tel. वेट्टिवेलु ता.वेंट्टिचेर Eng. Cuscus
(Chunekar Bh. Pr. Ni. p. 239-240)

4) Serpentary roots. *Asristolochia serpentaria* Linn.
The verginian snake root. Native of America. Used by native practitioners under the name of Kala wala (Watt Dict.)

4. प्रियङ्गुः Priyanguh

प्रियङ्गुः प्रियवल्ली च फलिनी कङ्गुनी प्रिया ॥१६
वृत्ता गोवन्दनी श्यामा करम्भा वर्णभेदिनी ॥

प्रियंगुः शीतला तिक्ता मोहदाहविनाशिनी ॥१७
ज्वरवान्तिहरा रक्तमुद्रित्तं च प्रसादयेत् ॥

प्रियङ्गुः (Priyanguḥ), प्रियवल्ली (Priyavallī), फलिनी (Phalinī), कङ्गुनी (Kangunī), प्रिया (Priyā), वृत्ता (Vṛttā), गोवन्दनी (Govandanī), श्यामा (Śyāmā), करम्भा (Karambhā) and वर्णभेदिनी (Varṇabhedinī) are synonymous.

Priyangu is *śitavīrya,* bitter in taste and pacifies *rakta doṣa* (purificatory action on *rakta*). It is useful in syncope, burning sensation, fever and emesis.

Fam. Rosaceae

I- a- ***Prunus mahaleb*** Linn.
b- Kamat (see below III)
c- See below IV

II- a- फलिनी (Phalinī), गोवन्दनी (Govandanī), श्यामा (Śyāmā), फलप्रिया(Phalapriyā), भङ्गुरा (Bhangurā), प्रियवल्ली (Priyavallī), कङ्गुनी (Kangunī)

b- Mar. Gahulā. B. Gandha priyangu;
Tel. -Prengana Cettu. Kan.- Nerpilangu. Tam. Yanlal H. Gavala. (Asta. Hr. Kosha)

III-a-1) प्रियङ्गुः Ca. S. a- पुरीषसंग्रहणीय (Su. 4. 15) b- मूत्रविरजनीय (Sy. 4. 15) c- शोणितास्थापनीय (Su. 18. 46) d- संधानीय (Su. 4.6) e-प्रजास्थापनीय (Su. 4.18)

2) चरके वमनोपगानिः- मधु, मधुक, कोविदार. विदुल, बिम्बी, शणपुष्पी ।

3) प्रियङ्गु गन्धप्रियङ्गु (Asta. Sang. Agrya अग्र्य Adhyāya 13)

4) प्रियङ्गु । (Shrauta Kosha Eng. p. 5. 77)

b-1) 116 प्रियङ्गु, कङ्गु., कान्ता, श्यामलता, गोवन्दनी (Abhidhan Man.)

2) 285 प्रियङ्गु., फलिनी
284 लता -प्रियङ्गु 332 श्यामा-प्रियङ्गु लताविशेषः । तस्या फलानि । (Harshe)

3) Priyangulata Viśeṣaḥ : Tasyā phalāni न तु वृक्षप्रियङ्गु
Natu Vṛkśapriyanguh: + + + वृक्षप्रियङ्गुरन्या Vṛkśapriyanguranyā, सा ज्ञेया - वमनकल्पिका (sā jñeyā wamana kalpikā) i + i
(Dipika Shar. Churna M. Khand) 2.14

4) लता गोवन्दनी फलिनीत्यमरः । लता प्रियङ्गु श्यामा तु महिलाह्वया । अथाऽद्रौ "प्रियङ्गुर्बकुलाभासदलस्तन्मंजरी तनु" रिति । (Harshe)

IV- 1) *Prunus mahaleb* Linn.- Habitat : A small tree a native of Central Asia and Europe; cultivated in Baluchistan.
(Watt. Dict. 'P'. 348.)

2) प्रियङ्गु *Prunus mahaleb*
(H.) Priyaṅgu, Phulpriyaṅgu, (Mar.) Gahulā, san. Gandha priyaṅgu,
Habitat: Baluchistan, Kashmir. (Kurtadkar p. 402)

3) 144 गन्धप्रियङ्गु Gandha priyaṅgu,
Prunus mahaleb - *Majja* of Priyaṅgu known as 'Gahulā' is sold in Bombay market, shape and size as *Ciraunjī* चिरौंजी and odorous. (Yadvaji p. 197)

V- *Aglaia roxburghiana* Miq.*
(Fam. Meliaceae)
Habitat : A large tree of the Westersn peninsula from the Konkan and Midnapur Southward, Ceylon, Malaya. (Watt.)

Note - In Watt. Dict. the medicinal properties of this tree are accepted from Dr. U.C. Dutt, who has applied wrongly medicinal properties of Priyaṅgulatā (Prunus mahaleb.) See- Deepika III b. 2. Vṛk'sa priyaṅgu of Deepika. This tree is accepted as Priyaṅgu of Ayurvedic books by some modern writers.
Priyaṅgu प्रियङ्गु.
Callicarpa macrophylla. **
(AMOAP II. 1976 p. 523 Uniyal)
Priyaṅgu प्रियङ्गु.

1) *Prunus mahaleb* Linn.
2) *Aglalia roxburghiana* Miq.
3) *Callicarpa macrophylla* Vahl **
(Chunekar Bh. Pr. pp. 249-50)

5 तूणिः Tūṇiḥ

तूणिस्तूणीकमापीतस्तूणिकः कनकस्तथा ॥१८
कुठेरकः कान्तलको नन्दिवृक्षोऽथ नन्दिकः ॥
तूणी त्रिदोषहृद्वृष्यः कण्डूकुष्ठव्रणापहः ॥१९
गण्डमालापहरणः सन्निपातनिकृन्तनः ॥

तूणिः (Tūṇiḥ), तूणीकः (Tūṇīkaḥ), आपीतः (Āpītaḥ), तूणिकः (Tūṇikaḥ), कनकः (Kanakaḥ), कुठेरकः (Kuṭherakaḥ) ,कान्तलकः (Kāntalakaḥ), नन्दिवृक्षः

* The current accepted name is *Aglaia elaeognoidea* (Juss.) Benth. (Comp. p. 6) (U.P. I. p. 21). The dry fruits are sold in North Indian market.

१ "तुणिस्तुन्नक आपीतस्तुणिकः कच्छकस्तथा।
कुबेरकः कान्तलको नन्दिवृक्षोऽथ नन्दकः ॥" इति क्षी. संमतः पाठः ।

** Very small fruits of this are mostly accepted as its source.

(Nandivṛkśaḥ), and नन्दिकः (Nandikaḥ) are synonymous.

Tūṇīḥ pacifies all the three *doṣas* and is *vṛṣya*. It is useful in pruritus, disorders of skin, wounds, scrofula and *sannipāta*

I- a- ***Cedrela toona*** Roxb * (Fam. Meliaceae)

b- Roxburgh

c- tropical Himalaya from Indus towards and through the hilly districts of Central and South India

II- a कनकः (Kanakh:), पीतकः (Pītakah:), नन्दिवृक्षः (Nandivṛkśaḥ).

b- Sk. Nandivṛkśa, Tūni; H.B. Tūna, Tuna; Mar. Tuna, Kurava, Kudak; Tel. Nandicethu; Tam. Tunu maram; Kan. Biligandhagiri; Mal. Madagiri Vemba, Malaraveppu.
Eng. Molmein Cedar, The Toona or Indian Mahagani.

6 रोचना Rocanā

रोचना पिङ्गला पिङ्गा मेध्या गौरी च गोमती ।।२०
माङ्गल्या वन्दनीयाऽग्र्या पावनी रुचिरा रुचिः ।।
रोचना पाचनी शीता विषनेत्ररुजो हरेत् ।।२१
सौभाग्यकरणी भूतग्रहदोषं च नाशयेत् ।।

रोचना (Rocanā), पिङ्गला (Piṅgalā), पिङ्गा (Piṅgā), मेध्या (Medhyā), गौरी (Gaurī), गोमती (Gomatī), माङ्गल्या (Māṅgalyā), वन्दनीया (Vandanīyā), अग्र्या (Agryā), पावनी (Pāvanī), रुचिरा (Rucirā) and रुचिः (Rucih) are synonymous.

Rocanā is digestant, *śītavīrya,* and brings fortune. It is useful in poisons, diseases of the eyes and destroys *bhūtagraha* (seizures).

This is being an animal in origin is not commented upon by Late Vd. D.K. Kamat

Eng. Gall stone, serpent stone; Latin- Bezoar.

The stone or concretion obtained from the gall bladder of a cow of a size about a betelnut to a small lemon, either rounded or triangular.

The properties are supposed to be different from the purified ox gall (Extractum fellis bovini) and should not be used for one another.

---

* The Current accepted name is *Toona ciliata* Roem.

7 तुरुष्कः Turuṣkaḥ

तुरुष्को यावनः कल्कः पिण्याकः पिण्डितः कपिः ॥२२
कपिजः कृत्रिमो धूम्रो धूम्रवर्णश्च सिल्हकः ॥

सुगन्धिः कृतकश्चैव युक्तियुक्तश्च पिण्डकः ॥२३
कपितैलमिति ख्यातं तथा पिङ्गलनामकम् ॥

तुरुष्कः कटुतिक्तोष्णः स्निग्धो वातबलासजित् ॥२४
स्वादुश्च कटुकः पाके सुरभिर्देवताप्रियः ॥

तुरुष्कः (Turuṣkaḥ), यावनः (Yāvanaḥ), कल्कः (Kalkaḥ), पिण्याकः (Piṇyākaḥ), पिण्डितः (Piṇḍitaḥ), कपिः (Kapiḥ), कपिजः (Kapijaḥ), कृत्रिमः (Kṛtrimaḥ), धूम्रः (Dhūmraḥ), धूम्रवर्णः (Dhūmravarṇaḥ), सिल्हकः (Silhakaḥ), सुगन्धिः (Sugandhiḥ), कृतकः (Kṛtakaḥ), युक्तियुक्तः (Yuktiyuktaḥ), पिण्डकः (Piṇḍakaḥ), कपितैलम् (Kapitailam) and पिङ्गल (Pingala) are synonymous.

Turuṣka is sweet, pungent and bitter in taste, *uṣṇavīrya*, pungent in *vipāka* (final transformation after digestion), pacifies *vāta* and *kapha doṣās*. It is fragrant and is agreeable to deities.

(Generic, name. includes two species. A. कल्कः (Kalkaḥ) and the next is B - पिण्डकः (Piṇḍakaḥ) A- gumlike substance obtained from the tree known as सिलारस (Silārasa).

(Fam. Hamamelidaceae).

I- A-a- ***Liquidamber orientalis*** Miller
b- Dymock c- See below IV-I
(Fam. - Styracaceae)
B-a- ***Styrax officinalis*** Linn.
b- Dymock, c- See below IV-I

II-A&B-a- यावनः (Yāvanaḥ), कृत्रिमः (Kṛtrimaḥ), सिल्हकः (Silhakaḥ), युक्तियुक्तश्च पिण्डकः (Yukti Yuktasca Piṇḍakaḥ), कल्कः (Kalkaḥ).
A-b-Turuṣka (H.B.Bom.) Silāras; Tel. Silarasamu; Tam. Neruju Sippala.
Eng. Liquid styrax; Tam- Citārasam; Mal.निर्यासु नारिवातं Niaryāsu nārivatam अरबी -कुन्तुरकं kunturakam (Ast. H. Kosa)
B-b- Silajit (Bom. Baz.) Usturaka
Eng. Solid Styrax.
The true styrax tree, sumatra bnezoin

III-a-i) C.S.Ci. 28. 151 S.S.Su. 38. 24.
A.H. Su. 1 5. 43 (Balvantji)

6-1-77- मुखमण्डनक .... इति , । धूम्रवर्ण तुरुष्कः इति कैयदेव :
(Harshe)

IV- 1) *L. orientalis* Miller. A handsome tree forming forest in the extreme South -Western part of Asia minor (Watt. Dict .)
Styrax officinalis Linn. a native of the Levant, Asia minor and Syria. (Watt. Dict.)

2) A similar but of inferior quality of balsam found from an Indian species *Altingia excelsa* Norohna. (Balvantji p. 188).

3) Styrax or storax. The most important type which the styrax of antiquity is known as levant styrax. This is obtained from Liquidambar orientalia, common along the coasts of South Western Asia minor. (Hill)

4) Hanbury's investigations have proved that the solid styrax of the ancients, which was derived from *Styrax officinalis* Linn. of the ancients, which was valuable, has in modern times entirely disappeared and has been replaced by Liquidambar orientalis ....
(Watt. Dict.) (Vol. I. pp. 504 to 96)

5) *Liquidambar orientalis*, Miller
Eng. Liquid storax; Verna.-silaras (Ind.); Neri-arishippal (Tam.); Silarasam (Tel.)

We learn from the Periplus of the Ery-threan sea that as long ago as the first century storax was exported via the sea to India.

About this time Silhak (Silaras)is mentioned as one of the ports at the port of Thane on the Western Coast....................
In India it is called silaras and described as product of Turkey..... Three kinds are generally mentioned, viz.- 1st that which exudes naturally; and that which is obtained by pressing the bark; and the third that which is obtained by boiling it. These three kinds, however, are not at the present time distinguished in commerce in Bombay. ... .

In one sample that had been kept more than 20 years, the resin at the bottom formed a transparent pale golden brown.... ...
It has a pleasesnt balsamic smell, especially after it has been long kept; when recend ..... far from agreeable.... ...

Under the name of Usturak, a bark is sometimes found in the Indian drug shops, it is said to be imported from Turkey .... it is probably the bark of *Storax officinalis* Linn. The tree which produced the storax of the ancients. (*Cf.* Pliny. XII. SS)
(Dymock I - 596)

8 अगरु Agaru

अगरु प्रवरं लोहं कृमिजग्धमनार्यकम् ॥२५
कृष्णागरु स्वाद्वगरु योगजं विश्वरूपकम् ॥
कटुतिक्तोष्णमगरु स्निग्धं वातकफापहम् ॥२६
श्रुतिनेत्ररुजं हन्ति माङ्गल्यं कुष्ठनुत्परम् ॥

अगरु (Agaru), प्रवरं (Pravaram), लोहं (Loham), कृमिजग्धं (Kṛmijagdham), अनार्यकम् (Anāryakam), कृष्णागरु (Kṛṣṇāgaru), स्वाद्वगरु (Swādvagaru), योगजं (Yogajam), and विश्वरूपकं (Viśvarūpakam) are synonymous.

Agaru is bitter and pungent in taste, *uṣṇavīrya, snigdha* (unctuous), pacifies *vāta* and *kapha doṣas*. It is useful in diseases of ears and eyes is auspicious and very good for disorders of of skin.

(Generic name; includes A अगरु (Agaru) and कृष्णागरु (Kṛṣaṇāgaru). The second is योगजम् (Yogajam) - obtainable by chance only.)

I-

A-a- ***Aquilaria agallocha*** Roxb. (Thymeleaceae); *Aquilaria ovata* Willd.

b- Roxburgh. (Fl. indica)

c- See IV- I below

B-

a- Gharki kind

b- Kamat c- See IV-1 below

II- a- लोहम् (Loham), अनार्यकम् (Anāryakam), कृमिजग्धं (Kṛmijagdham)

b- H.B.); Agara, Agaru; (Mar.) - Agara; (Tam.) Agali candan; (Tel.) Agru, Agallochan; (Eng.) Aloe wood; Eagle wood; Calambae.

B-a- कृष्णागरु (Kṛṣṇāgaru), योगजम (Yogajam), विश्वधूपनम (Viśwadhūpanam).

B-b- Gharki ūda

III- See

a-1 C.S. Su. 4-37, 3-27
S.S.Su. 5.18
A.H. Su. 3-11-20 (Balvantji)

---

१ 'अनार्यजम्' इति. नि.शे. टीका संमतः पाठः ।
२ 'जोङ्गकम्' इति.नि. शे. टीका संमतः पाठः ।
३ 'विश्वधूपकम्' इति आनन्दाश्रम मुद्रितपुस्तके पाठः ।

b-1) 33 जोऽगकम् - लोहम् ... लोहं कृमिजोऽगकम् (Harshe)

2) 97 अगरु प्रवरं लोहं .... अनार्यकम् ... मलिनं कालेयम् (Harshe)
अगरुद्रुस्तु द्व्यंगुलिच्छदनः सुमं अल्पं न च फलम् काष्ठं जन्तु
जग्ध्वावशिष्टकं सारः सोऽगुरुरस्मात्तु प्राग्जः कृष्णो विशिष्यते ।
(Harshe)

IV- *Aquilaria agallocha* Roxb.
History - since the time Dr. Roxburgh described this plant .. the conclusion he arrived it seems correct namely that the much prized wood is obtained from Eastern India, and from the forests to the East and South East of sylhet extending through Mainpur, Chitgong, Arakan, to Murgui Sumatra..... ....

It is found in fragments of various shapes and sizes in the centre of the tree, and usually, if not always, where some former injury has been received. ... ...

The best kind for medicinal use is Gharki from sylhet; it should be bitter, odoriferous, oily and a little astringent ... it is after buried in wet ground. Parts which have unodorus, the change above mentioned become oily heavy and black. They are cut out and tested by being thrown into water, then which sink are called 'Gharki'
(Watt. Dict. I. 280.)

2) *Carissa spinarum* A. DC.
Kangra authority remarks that the very old wood gets into very black and fragrant and is sold at a high price as aggar or ud-hindi.
(Watt. Dict. III - 167)

कालेयकम् Kaleyakam (7)

कालेयकं ससारं च पीतवर्णं च शब्दतः ॥२७
वर्णप्रसादनं चैव लघुचन्दनमेव च ॥

कालेयकं (Kāleyakam), ससारं (Sasāram), पीतवर्णं (Pītavarṇam), वर्णप्रसादनं (Varṇaprasādanam) and लघुचन्दनं (Laghucandanam) are synonymous.

I- Not confirmed.

a- ***Vepris bilocularis***, Engler*
(Rutaceae)

b- Chopra.

---

* The current accepted name is - *V. bilocularis* (W.& A.) Engler

II- a- पीतवर्णं च शब्दतः (Pītawarnamca Śabdataḥ), कृष्ण काष्ठकम् (Kṛṣna Kāṣṭhakam.)
b- (Sk) Kṛṣṇāgaru (Chopra)

III-a-1) कृष्णवर्ण चन्दन विशेषः । मलयाद्रिचन्दनं इति लोके । (Dalhan Su. Su.)

IV- *Aquilaria agallocha* Roxb.
Syns.कालागुरु, कृष्णागुरु, जोङ्गक
C. Su. 3.27, 4.37, 42; etc.
S. Su. 5.18 etc.
A.H. Su. 3.11-20, 10 38 etc.
(Balvantji p.3)

9 कस्तूरी Kastūrī (Musk)

कस्तूरिका मृगमदो मृगनाभिर्मृगाण्डजा ॥२८
मार्जारि वेधमुख्या च मदनी गन्धचेलिका ॥
कस्तूरिका रसे तिक्ता कटुः श्लेष्मानिलापहा ॥२९
विषघ्नी दोषशमनी मुखशोषहरा परा ॥

कस्तूरिका (Kastūrikā), मृगमदः (Mṛgamadaḥ), मृगनाभि (Mṛganābhi), मृगाण्डजा (Mṛgāṇḍajā),मार्जारी (Mārjārī), वेधमुख्या (Vedhamukhyā), मदनी (Madanī), गंधचलिका(Gandhacelikā) are synonymous.

Kastūrī is bitter and pungent in taste. It pacifies *vāta* and *kapha doṣas*, poisons, other *doṣas* and is very much useful in dryness of mouth.

Musk is supposed to be a very important stimulant medicine.

Being animal in origin this is not commented upon by late Vd. D.K. kamat.

There is one synonym mentioned here is मार्जारी (Mārjārī) which brings our attention to the musk like substance obtained from the civet cat (Latin-*Viverra zibetha* Linn.). It is described in Bh. Pr. Ni. under the heading 'गन्धमार्जार वीर्यम्'.

(S.D.K)

10 कर्पूरः Karpūraḥ

कर्पूरः शीतलरजः शीताभ्रः स्फटिको हिमः ॥३०
चन्द्रस्तुषारस्तुहिनः शशीन्दुर्हिमवालुकः ॥

कर्पूरं कटुतिक्तं च मधुरं शिशिरं विदुः ॥ ३१
तृण्मेदोविषदोषघ्नं चक्षुष्यं मदकारकम् ॥

कर्पूरः (Karpūraḥ), शीतलरजः (Śītalarajaḥ), शीताभ्रः (Śītābhraḥ), स्फटिकः (Sphaṭikaḥ), हिमः (Himaḥ), चन्द्रः (Candraḥ), तुषारः (Tuṣāraḥ), तुहिनः (Tuhinaḥ), शशी (Śaśī), इन्दुः (Induḥ), and हिमवालुकः (Himavālukaḥ) are synonymous.

Karpūra is sweet, pungent and bitter in taste, and *śītavīrya* . It is useful in thrist, *medodoṣa*, poison is beneficial for eyes and intoxicant (mild).

(Generic name includes four kinds. A.शीतलरजः (Śitalrajaḥ) and B- चन्द्रस्तुषारः (Candrastuṣārahaḥ) of Dhn. Ni. and C- पोतासो भीमसेनः (Potāso Bhīmsenaḥ), D- पक्विका (Pakwikā) of Raj. ni. These four kinds of camphor are obtained from camphor giving plants which are as follows :

I- A & B a- Ambiguous
(See IV- 1 & 2 below)

C-a- ***Dryobalanops aromatica*** Gaertn.

D-a- ***Cinnamomum camphora*** F. Nees*

b- Watt Dict C- See IV 2 below

b- Watt Dict. C; See IV -1 below

II- a-c- भीमसेनः (Bhīmsenḥ), पोतासः (Potāsaḥ).

b-c- (Bazar name) Bhimasenī Kāpura
Eng. Borneo camphor, Kapur Baras, The Barass Camphor.

a-d- चीन कर्पूरः (Cīna Karpuraḥ), कृत्रिमः (Kṛtrimaḥ), धवलः (Dhavalaḥ)

b- (Bazar name) Cini Kapur, Jāpāni Kapur
(Eng) Formosa Camphor, Cina Camphor, Japan Camphor.

III- See स्थौणेयकम् (Sthauṇeyakam)

a- 1) C.S. Su. 5.77
S.S. Su.s 46 .202;
A.H. Ka. 1.7

b-1) कर्पूरः; तै.कर्पूरमु; क. कर्पूर; त. कर्पूरं; मल. कर्पूरं, पच्च कर्पूरं
(Ast. H. Kosha)

IV- 1) Forms of Camphor :
1st-*Cinnamomum camphora*. Nees, Formosa in Japan and through out Central China.

---

* The current accepted name is-
Cinnamomum camphora (Linn.) Sieb. (Comp. p. 36)
syn : *Cinnamomum camphora* (Linn.) Nees & Eburm.

2nd-The Borus Camphor (From Borus a town in Sumatra) is also known as Bornio camphor and Malaya camphor and in Indian trade returns as Bhīmsenī Kapur.

It is obtained as coarse crystls formed naturally in the stems of *Dryobalanops camphora* Colebr. (*D. aromatica* Gaertn.) This is a large tree. The formation of cyrstaline substances within the tissues .. ... Similar to that Khersal in the interior of the stems of *Acacia catechu* or *Aquilaria agallocha*.

3rd-The blumea or Nagi Camphor. This is scarcely known out of China but consignment ... was sent to Europe from Tenasserim ... in China. It is preferred from ... member of ... genus 'Blumea' most probably from *B. balsmifea*.* It occurs also in Khasia hills, Chitgong, Pegu and Burma.

The boiled camphor referred to (by the Sanskrit writers) may also be Blumea or Nagi Camphor. The substance which at the period of Sanskrit writers may have been manufactured in India or imported from China.

As a matter of fact this camphor (Nagi) is more nearly related to the Malayan than to the China camphor, and is extensively consumed in China partly as medicine and partly in the finer qualities of China ink. Watt. Dict. II. P. 86-87.

2) २) कर्पूरः (१) भद्रश्रियं पारलोहित्यं जातिवर्णम्
(२) आन्तर्वत्यमुशीरवर्णम् उभयं कुष्ठगन्धिश्चेति 11 70-71.72.

** The camphor which is produced beyond the river "लोहित्य" (Lohitya) in Assam is like मालतीपुष्प (Malatī flower) and it is called भद्रश्रिय (Bhadraśriya) and that which is produced on the banks of "अन्तर्वती" (Āntarvatī) (in or near about to) is like उशीर (Uśira) and it is called 'आन्तर्वत्य' (Āntsarvatya). The both have the smell like कुष्ठ (Kuṣṭha). (Kaut. Arth. A. 11.A.2 Pr.19) (Translated summararily from Hindi Bhāṣā Ṭīkā)

Note- These two kinds may be the camphor of Dhan. nighantu's A. & B

4) If the patient is suffering from retention of urine and constipation the practising priest ties on his body a substance like "Haritakī" (gall nut) or Karpura (Camphor) which promotes mictutrittion while reciting. (Atharvavedic Civilization by Dr. Karambelkar)

---

* *Blumea balsamiferra* (Linn.) DC. (U.P.I. p. 125) (U.P.I. p. 75)

(** It seems that Late vd. D.K. Kamat has relied on Hindi translation of कौटिलीय अर्थशास्त्र (Kauṭilīya Artha Śāstra) but this seems to be incorrect. The Sutras भद्रश्रियं पार लौहित्यं etc. should be attributed to (चन्दन) Candana and not to कर्पूर (Karpūra), Ref. Dr.Kangale's translation of कौटिलीय अर्थशास्त्र S. D. Kamat)

11 जातिपत्री Jātipatrī

जातिपत्री जातिकोशा सुमनःपत्रिकाऽपि च ॥३२
मालतीपत्रिका चैव प्रोक्ता सा मलनाशिनी ॥

जातिपत्री कटूष्णा स्यात् सुरभिः कफनाशिनी ॥३३
वक्त्रदौर्गन्ध्यहृत् वर्ण्या विषहृत् कायशान्तिदा ॥

जातिपत्री (Jātipatrī), जातिकोशा (Jātikośā), सुमनःपत्रिका (Sumanaḥ patrikā), मालतीपत्रिका (Mālatīpatrikā)and मलनाशिनी (Malanāśinī) are synonymous.

Jātipatrī is pungent in taste, *uṣṇavīrya*, fragrant and pacifies *kaphadoṣa*. It removes foetid smell from the mouth, improves complexion of the body, is antipoisonous and useful in burning sensation of the body. (? useful for calmness).

---

a- Mace (The aril of Nutmeg)
b- Dr. W. Dymock (In Pharm. Indi)
II- a- जातिपत्री (Jātipatrī), जातिकोशः (Jātikośaḥ), मलनाशिनी (Malanāśinī)
b- (Mar.) Jaypatri; (Tel.) Jajipatri; (Kan) Jayapatri; (Tam.) Jatipattiri.

12 जातीफलम् Jātīphalam

जातीफलं जातिसस्यं[१] शालूकं मालतीफलम् ॥३४
मदशौण्डं जातिशृङ्गं पुटं सौमनसं फलम् ॥

जातीफलं कषायोष्णं कटुकण्ठमयार्तिजित् ॥३५
वातातिसारमेहघ्नं लघु वृष्यं च दीपनम् ॥

जातीफलं (Jātīphalam), जातिसस्यं (Jātisasyam), शालूकं (Śālūkam), मालतीफलं (Mālatīphalam), मदशौण्डं (Madaśauṇḍam), जातिशृङ्गं (Jātiśṛṅgam), पुटं (Puṭam), and सौमनसं फलम् (Saumanasam phalam) are synonymous.

Jātīphalam is *kaṣāya* (astringent) and pungent in taste *uṣṇavīryā, laghu, vṛṣya* and stimulates digestive capacity. It is useful in pain due to diseases of throat, diarrhoea due to *vāta* and *meha* (disirders characterized by polyuria).

(Fam. Myristicaceae)

a- ***Myristica fragrans*** Houtt.

---

१ 'जातिसूतं' इति पा.

Syn. *M. maschata* Willd. (Roxb.)
M. officinalis Linn.

b- Roxburgh (in. Fl. Ind.)

c- Wild in Molucca.

II- a- शाल्कम् (Śālūkam), मदशौण्डम् (Madaśauṇḍam)

b- (Sk) Jātiphalam; (Tam.) Jadikkaya (Tel.) Jajikaya, Advikaya; (Mal) Katulatika; (Mar. H.B.) Jāyphala; (Keral) Jattika; (Eng.) Nutmeg.

III-

IV- 1) Nutmeg - *Myristica fragrans,* Native of Mollucca or Spica island; It is doubtful whether these species were known to the ancients. (Hill)

2) Nutmeg. The seeds of *Myristica fragrans* and allied species contain about a yellow fat with flavour and consistancy of tallow. Several varieties of nutmeg butter are on the market (Hill).

3) Nutmeg -*Myristica fragrans* Houtt. Syn. *Myristica officinalis* Linn.

Nux moschata.

Description - average size nuts 60-100 to the lb..... long nutmeg about 1 ½ inch long of the genuine kind ... and these can be distinguished from the Papua .... which otherwise resembles true 'nutmeg'. In Bombay long nutmegs also occur in commerce, but these lack fragrance ... 2 inches long.

V- False jātīphala
Myristica malabarica Lam.; Bom. Rāmpatrī; San.Kamuka; Tam. Kattuchadi; Tel. Advijajikaya; Māl. Kattujatika. Evergreen forest of Konkan, Ghats, Kanara and Malabar (Chopra).

Note - महाराष्ट्रात याचे फळाला कायफळ म्हणूनहि म्हणतात. याचेवर जायफळ प्रमाणेच पत्री असते. तिला रामपत्री म्हणतात. व बाजारांत जायपत्री ऐवजी विकतात. पण फळाला व या रामपत्रीला सुगंध मात्र नसतो.

D.K. Kamat.

The fruit of this tree in Maharashtra is also called as कायफळ *Kāyaphala* and the aril of the fruit is called as रामपत्री *Rāmpatrī.* It is somtimes sold as *Jāypatrī* but both the fruit and aril are inodorus.

(free translation - S. D. Kamat)

13 कङ्कोलम् Kamkolam

कंकोलकं कृतफलं कोलकं कटुकं फलम् ॥३६
चूर्ण कन्दफलं द्वीपमरिचं माधवोचितम ॥

कंकोलं कटुतित्तगोष्णं वक्त्रवैरस्यनाशनम ॥३७
मुखजाड्यहरं रुच्यं वातश्लेष्महरं परम् ॥

कंकोलकं (Kamkolakam), कृतफलं (Kṛtaphalam), कोलकं (Kolakam), कटुकं फलं (Kaṭukam phalam), चूर्ण (Cūrṇam), कन्दफलं (Kandaphalam), द्वीपमरिचं (Dwīpamaricam) and माधवोचितं (Mādhavocitam) are synonymous.

Kamkola is pungent and bitter in taste, *ūṣṇavīrya,* pacifies *vāta* and *kaphadoṣas.* It is useful in tastelessness and stiffness of mouth and promotes desire for food.

(Fam. Piperaceae)

a- ***Piper cubeba*** Linn.

b- W. Dymock (Pharm. Indi.)

c- Native of Java and Molucca, cultivated in India.

II- a- द्वीपम् (Dwīpam), मरिचम् (Maricam), कोलकम् (Kolakam)

b- (Sk) Sugandh Marica, (Bom. Mara.) Kankola; (H.B.)Kabābcīnī, Śītalamirca; (Eng.) Cubebs.

Note - At the time of compiler, it seems, the fruits of this plant were imported from out of India hence the equivalent द्वीपी (Dwīpī) is occured.

14 पूगफलम् Pūgaphalam

स्यात्पूगफलमुद्वेगं स्रंसि घोण्टाफलं स्मृतम ॥३८
चिक्कणं चिक्कणा चिक्का गुवाकः खपुरं च तत ॥

भेदिसंमोहकृत्पूगं कषायं स्वादुरोचनम ॥३९
कफपित्तहरं रुक्षं वक्त्रक्लेदमलापहम ॥

पूगफलं (Pūgaphalam), उद्वेगं (Udvegam), स्रंसि (Sramsi), घोण्टाफलं (Ghonṭāphalam), चिक्कणं (Cikkaṇam), चिक्कणा (Cikkaṇā), चिक्का (Cikkā), गुवाकः (Guvākaḥ), and खपुरं (Khapuram) are synonymous.

Pūgaphala is *kaṣāya* and sweet in taste, pacifies *kapha* and *pitta doṣas, rukśa* (roughning), *bhedi* (purgative), intoxicating, delightful, removes moistning of mouth and cleanses mouth.

I-Generic name, includes two kinds A -घोण्टाफलम् (Ghoṇṭāphalam= Common) and B- चिक्कणम् (Cikkanam= boiled) Both of the same species.

Fam. Palmae.. Arecaceae.

A-a- ***Areca catechu*** Linn.

b- Dr. Roxburgh (in.fl. ind.)

c- Cultivated in South India, coastal region of Eastern & Western India, Bengal.

B-a- Boiled young fruits of *Areca catechu.*

II- A-a- गुवाकः (Guwākaḥ),*क्रमुकः (Kramukaḥ), दीर्घपादपः (Dīrghapādapaḥ), दृढवल्कः (Dṛḍhawalkaḥ), वल्कतरुः (Valkataruḥ),

b- (Sk) Pūgīphalam, Guwāk; (Guj.) Sopari; (H.Pers.) Supārī; (Tel.) Poka chetu, Vekhā; (B) Gūa (Tam) Kamugu, Pakhū; (Mal.) Adhaka; (Mar.) Pophal (whole fruit), supārī (husked nut); (Kan.) Adike

Eng. The Areca, Betelnut palm.

B-a- चिक्कणम् (Cikkaṇam)

b- (Mar.) (Cikaṇī Supārī).

15 लवङ्गम् Lavaṅgam

लवङ्गं देवकुसुमं भृङ्गारं शिखरं लवम् ॥४०
दिव्यं चन्दनपुष्पं च श्रीपुष्पं वारिसंभवम् ॥

लवङ्गकुसुमं हृद्यं शीतलं पित्तनाशनम् ॥४१
चक्षुष्यं विषहृद् वृष्यं माङ्गल्यं मूर्धरोगहृत् ॥

लवङ्गम् (Lavaṅgam), देवकुसुमं (Devakusumam), भृङ्गारं (Bhṛṅgāram), शिखरं (Śikharam), लवम् (Lavam), दिव्यं (Divyam), चन्दनपुष्पं (Candanapuṣpam), श्रीपुष्पं (Śrīpuṣpam), and वारिसंभवम् (Vārisambhavam) are synonymous.

Lavaṅgakusma is *śitavīrya* and pacifies *pitta doṣa*. It is cordial, beneficial to eyes, is *vṛṣya,* antipoison, auspicious and useful in diseases of head.

Fam. Myrtaceae

*Dh.Ni. has mentioned only the fruit while क्रमुकः (Kramukaḥ) tree is mentioned by Raj. Ni. (S.D.K.)

I- a-1- ***Syzygium aromaticum*** Merr. Perry.*
Syn. *Eugenia aromatica* Kuntz, Thunb.
Caryophyllus aromaticus Linn.

b- देवकुसुमं (Devaksumam), श्रीपुष्पम् (Śrīpuṣpam), वारिसंभवम् (Wārisambhavam), शृङ्गारम् (Śṛṅgāram)

b- (B. Bom.) Lavriaga; (Mal.) Canki; (Tam.) Kirāmbu, Ilavangu; (Mal). Canki.Eng. Caryophylum.
(त). किरांपु (ते.) लवंगलु, लवंगमु (मल्या) करयांपूवु, करांपू (क.) लवङ्ग कलिका (Ast. Hr. Kosha).

IV- 1) Clove - *Caryophyllus aromaticus* Linn.
Clove must have originally from *Malaccas. Rumphius* considers that ... *Caryophyllus sylvestre* belong to the same species, and this plant is wild throughout the Moluccas. A native told him that the cultivated clove trees degenerate into this form ... ...As a rule, the aromatic properties are more developed in the wild plant of a species than in the cultivated plants.
If it is true, as Roxburgh says, that the Sanskrit language had a name *Lavunga* for the clove, the trade in this space must date from very early epoch, even supposing the name to be modern than the true sanskrit. But I doubt its genuine character, for the Romans would have known of a substance to easily transportable into Europe before the discovery of the Malaccas by the Portugues. (De candolle)

2) *Caryophyllus aromaticus* Linn.
Syn. *Eugenia caryophyllata* Thumb.
(Pers.) Mekhaka; (Tel.) Lavangalu; (Tam.) Kiramber, Kirambu, ilvangappu, Karu vappui crambu; (Mal.) Chanki.... ... ... The cloves met with in Indian bazars are generally old and worthless.
(Watt. Dict.) (abbreviated)

3) *Caryophyllus aromaticus* Linn.
Habitat - Moluccas. cultivated everywhere.
Vern. Lavanga (Mar. Can.); Lavangalu, Lavangap-pu (Tel.); Kirambu, lavangap-pu, karavappu (Tam.); The fruit Narlavang. (Ind. Bazar)
History - The clove tree is said to be indigenous only in the five small islands, which constitute the Moluccas proper ... and it was afterwards introduced into neighbouring islands ... and at latter period into Zanjibar and Pemba ....
It is difficult to say when they were first introduced into India.They are mentioned in Charak. (Abreviated from Dymock)

* The current accepted name is *S. aromaticum* (Linn.) Merr. & L.M. Perry.

16 नलिका Nalikā

नलिका विद्रुमलता कपोतचरणा नली ॥४२
सुषिरा धमनी शून्या निर्मध्या[१] नर्तकी नटी ॥
नलिका रक्तपित्तघ्नी चक्षुष्या विषनाशिनी ॥४३
नलिका वातला तिक्ता गुर्वी च मधुरा हिमा ॥

नलिका (Nalikā), विद्रुमलता (Vidrumalatā), कपोतचरणा (Kapotacaraṇā), नली (Nalī), सुषिरा (Suṣirā), धमनी (Dhamanī), शून्या (Śūnyā), निर्मध्या (Nirmadhyā), नर्तकी (Nartakī), and नटी (Naṭī)

Nalikā is bitter and sweet in taste, *śītavīrya* and *guru.* It aggravates *vātadoṣa*, is useful in bleeding disorders, beneficial to eyes and antipoison.

Fam. Boraginaceae

I- For confirmation
- a- ***Onosma echioides*** Linn.*
- b- Dr. Chopra (Gloss Indi. Medi. Plants).
- c- Hispid erect herb found in Western Himalaya from kashmir to kumaon.

II- a- कपोतचरणा (Kapotacārаṇā), धमनी (Dhamanī), शून्या (Śūnyā), नटी (Naṭī), नर्तकी (Nartakī), रक्तदला (Raktadalā), विद्रुमलतिका (Vidrumalatikā)
- b- (H.) Ratanjot; (P.) Maharangi, Gaozaban., (Tam.) Gaozbaban; (Sk.) Dhamanī

III-b- 225 नटी -नली । Naṭī -Nalī ...Nalikā Uttarāpathe 'पवारी' (Pawārī) prasiddha 'सुगन्धा प्रवाला कृति' iti Bhāvamiśraḥ. (S.kosha)

IV- 1) ...Red dye for wool. It is empolyed ... to stain their images... imparts a rich red colour. In Nepal these roots are boiled with oil and used as a dye for the hair ...
Habitat- Kashmir to kumaon, widely distributed from siberia and Cabul to France. (Watt. Dict. 486)

2) धमनी - नलिका *Onosma echioides* Linn.
Levaes - purgative to childern and alterative
Flowers - cordial and stimulant in rheumatism and palpitation of heart .
Roots impart a rich red colour to medicinal oils, oils as a dye for the hairs. Roots employed to stain images . Impart a rich red colour.

---

१ 'निर्मथ्या' इति नि.शे.टीका संमतः पाठः ।

* The current accepted name is *Onosma hispidum* wall. ex G. Don
Dr. Chunekar (Bh. Pr. p. 267) has mentioned *Cinnamomum* sp. available in North Indian market. *Onosma* sp. mentioned here is accepted as a type of Ratanjot.

17 (नलदम्) Naladam मांसी Māmsī

मांसी कृष्णजटा हिंस्रा नलदा जटिला[1] मिशी[2] ॥ ४४
जटा च पिशिता पेशी क्रव्यादी च तपस्विनी ॥

मांसी स्वादु कषाया स्यात् कफपित्तास्रनाशिनी ॥ ४५
विषमारुतहत् बल्या त्वच्या कान्तिप्रसादनी ॥

मांसी (Māmsī), कृष्णजटा (Kṛṣṇajaṭā), हिंस्रा (Himsrā), नलदा (Naladā), जटिला (Jaṭilā), मिशी (Miśī), जटा (Jaṭā), पिशिता (Piśitā), पेशी (Peśī), क्रव्यादी (Kravyādī) and तपस्विनी (Tapasvinī) are synonymous.

Māmsi is sweet and *kaṣāya* (astringent) in taste, pacifies *vāta, pitta, kapha* and *rakta doṣas*. It is antipoison, strength promoting, beneficial for skin and improves lustre.

I- a- ***Nardostachys jatamansi*** DC.*
b- Watt. Dict. (Syns. See below)
c- a perenial herb of the Alpine Himalaya, Garhwal, Sikkim.

II- a- कृष्णजटा (Kṛṣṇasjaṭā), हिंस्रा (Himsrā), नलदा (Naladā), चक्रवर्तिनी (Cakravartinī), भूतजटा (Bhūtajaṭā)
b- (H.B.Mar.) Jatāmānsī; (Bom.) Sambhul; (Tam.) Jatāmānsī; (Tel.) Jatamānsī; Mal.) Jatamancī; (Kan.) Jatamāvasī; (Eng.)Spikenard.
Syn. *N. grandiflora* DC.
Patrinia jatamansi Don.
Valeriana jatamansi Wall. (Watt. Dict.)

गन्धमांसी Gandhamāmsī (12)

द्वितीया गन्धमांसी स्यात्केशी भूतजटा स्मृता ॥४६
पिशाची पूतना केशी भूतकेशी च लोमशा ॥

मांसीद्वयं कषायं च वर्ण्यं पित्तकफापहम् ॥४७
रक्षोघ्नं च सुगन्धि स्याद् वातघ्नं केश्यमुत्तमम् ॥

There is an another type of *māmsī* called as गन्धमांसी (Gandhamāmsī) of which synonyms are केशी (Keśī), भूतजटा (Bhūtajaṭā), पिशाची (Piśācī), पूतना (Pūtanā), केशी (Keśī), भूतकेशी (Bhūtakeśī) and लोमशा (Lomaśā).

---

१ 'जटिलाऽऽ मिषी' इति नि. शे. टीका. संमतः पाठः ।
२ 'मेषी' इति नि. शे. टीका. संमतः पाठः ।
* The current accepted name is *N. grandiflora* DC.

Both types of *māmsī* are *kaṣāya* (astringent) in taste, pacify *pitta, kapha* and *vāta doṣas,* are beneficial for complexion, antiseptic, fragrant and beneficial for hairs.

For Confirmation
(Fam. Cyperaceae)

I- a- ***Cyperus stoloniferus*** Retz.
Syn. *C. juncifolius* Klein,
b- D. K. Kamat (Following Watt. II. 638)
c- The term is applied in South India to several species of Cyperus.

II- भूतजटा (Bhūtajaṭā), भूतकेशी (Bhūtakeśī), लघुमांसी (Laghumāmsī), मांसीद्वयम् The former no. 17 plant and this plant.

IV- 1) *Cyperus stoloniferus*, Retz.
As with other scented species the tubers of this plant are used for varioius purposes of perfumery. Referring to the name 'Jaṭāmāmsī' Sir Walter Elliot says "In applying this botanical name, we have followed Heyne." (Watt. Dict. II. 688).

2) *Jaṭamāmsī*
Cyperus stoloniferus Retz.
Tubers stomachic, stimulant for heart. (Chopra)

3) जटा-Jaṭā
S.S. Ka. 6.15 (Both Jatā and Māmsī), U. 60.47s (both Jatā and Bhūtkeśī)
A.H. U. 5.2 (both Jaṭā & Bhutakeśī)
6.38 (Jaṭā & Murā)
Jaṭā has been mentioned side by side with *Māmsī, Bhūtakeśī* and Murā. According to Ḍalhaṇa it is another variety of *Māmsi* known as Gandhamāmsī गन्धमांसी. It appears that *Jatā* and *Jatāmāmsi* identified as *Nardostachys jatamansi* DC. and known as Bāḷachaḍa बाल्छड are synonyms and the inferior variety of *Māmsi,Bhūtkeśī* * and *Murā* are different plants.
(Balavantji p. 163)

V- 1) गन्धमांसी
Nardus indicus (Dr. Desai)

१८ कुष्ठम् Kuṣṭham

कुष्ठं रोगोऽगदो व्याधिरुत्पलं पाकलं रुजा ॥४८
वाप्यं वानीरजं रामं कौबेरं[1] पारिभद्रकम्[2] ॥

---

१ 'कौवीरं ' क्षी. संमतः पाठः ।
२ 'पारिभव्यकम् 'इति क्षी .संमतः पाठः ।
* *Corydalis govaniana* Wall. is accepted as *Bhūtakeśī*

कुष्ठं कटूष्णं तिक्तं स्यात् कफमारुतरक्तजित् ॥४९
त्रिदोषविषकण्डूंश्च कुष्ठरोगांश्च नाशयेत् ॥

कुष्ठं (Kuṣṭham), रोगः (Rogaḥ), अगदः (Agadaḥ), व्याधिः (Vyādhiḥ), उत्पलं (Utpalam), पाकलं (Pākalam), रुजा (Rujā), वाप्यं (Vāpyam), वानीरजं (Vānīrajam), रामं (Rāmam), कौबेरं (Kauberam), पारिभद्रकम्,(Pāribhadrakam), are synonymous.

Kuṣṭha is pungent and bitter in taste, *uṣṇavīrya.* It pacifies all the three *doṣās and raktadoṣa.* It is useful in poisons, pruritus and disorders of skin.

(Fam. Compositae) Asteraceae

I- a- ***Saussurea lappa*** C.B. Clarke*
Syn. *Auclandia lappa* Falkoner
Aplotaxis auriculata DC.

b- Dymock (Pharm. indi II. 296)

c- A tall very stout herb with annual stem and a thick perenial herb indigenous to the moist open slopes surrounding the valley kashmir to the bassins of Chenab and Jhelam at 1000-15000ft. (Watt. p. 481).

II- a- वाप्यम् (Vāpyam),वानीरजम् (Vānīrajam), कौबेरं (Kauberam), त्वग्दोषमुत्पलम् (Twagdoṣamutpalam), पद्मकम् (Padmakam).

b- (H.) Kuṭ, Kuṣṭa, talk , Pācak; (B) Pācaka, Kut; (Bom) uplet, Kuṣṭa; (Guj) Kuṣṭa; (Tam.) Kuṣṭam, Goṣtam, Pācakam; (Arab, Pers.) Kuṣta; (Eng.) Sassuria costus; Arabian costus. (Pers.) 'Kusta-i- talkah' to pungent kut (Tîkta Kuṣṭa) and 'Kusṭa-i-Sirin' to sweet kuṣṭa (Madhura Kuṣṭa)

III-a-1) यो गिरिश्च जायथा (AV-V-4; IXX-33) (Kamat).
2) कुष्ठ (Kuṣṭa) (AV-V-4, Vi-102) (Harshe)

b-1) कुष्ठम् (केरळ) कोट्टम् (त.) कोट्टम् (क.) कोष्ट (गु.) उपलेट. (Ayu. O.Ni.)

2) तै. चइगल कोष्ठं त. कोष्ठं, मल्या. कौट्ट (Ast. Hr. Kosha)

3) 122- कुष्ठं वाप्यम् ।'कुष्ठं गदाह्वयं मूलं त्वस्य पुष्करमूलकं' मिति त्रिकाण्डशेषः । 'रुक् पुष्करावभिन्नौ तु विटपौ तुरगीदलौ । सितासित समित्कौ च गिरौ मूलककन्दिना' विति । (Harshe)

4) 141 कुष्ठं - पारिभाव्यम् । 'कौबेरं भास्वरं कुष्ठं पारिभाव्यं गदाह्वय' मिति रभसः (Harshe)

5) 419 कुष्ठं - पारिभाव्यम् । पुष्करं पुष्करमूलम् । (Harshe)

---

* The current accepted name is *S.lappa* (Decne.) Sch.-Bip. (Comp. p. 137)

6) पुष्करमूलाभावे कुष्ठम् ग्राह्यमिति व्यवहारः । शारंग. म १०.७८; २.८१.

IV- 1) For a long time *kut* was referred most probably to that of 'orris root' or ' *costus speciosus* Sm. But Now it is proved beyond doubt that the *kut* of upper India was the root of 'Auclandia Costus' (Now reduced to Saussurea lappa) ... (Watt.Dict)

2) कुष्ठ-कूट –*Saussurea lappa*

... Doctors of the present day have identified 'Madhur kut' as orris root' which according to their opinion is 'Puṣkaramūla' पुष्करमूल

... "*Puṣkarmūla* is different from Kuṣṭa" (Bh. Pr. Ni.) Modern researches have identified पुष्करमूल (Puṣkarmūla) with *orris root* (Ni. Adarsha)

१९ रेणुका Reṇukā (हरेणुः)(Hareṇuḥ)

रेणुका राजपुत्री च नन्दिनी कपिला द्विजा ॥ ५०
कपिलोला पाण्डुपत्नी स्मृता कौन्ती हरेणुका ॥
रेणुका शिशिरात्यन्ता तृष्णां कण्डूं च नाशयेत ॥ ५१
विषघ्नी दाहदौर्बल्यमुन्मूलयति योजिता ॥

रेणुका (Reṇukā), राजपुत्री (Rājaputrī), नन्दिनी (Nandinī), कपिला (Kapilā), द्विजा (Dwijā), कपिलोला (Kapilolā), पाण्डुपत्नी (Pāṇḍupatnī), कौन्ती (Kauntī) and हरेणुका (Hareṇukā) are synonymous.

Reṇukā is excessively *śītavīrya* and useful in thirst, pruritus, poisons, burning sensation and debility.

For Confirmation
(Fam. Rutaceae)

I- a- ***Murraya paniculata*** (L.) Jack.
Syn. *M. exotica* Linn.
Communium sinense Rump.
Chalacas paniculata Linn.
M. sumatrana Roxb.

b- Kamat

c- See IV-1 below

II- a- द्विजा (Dwijā), राजपुत्री (Rājaputrī), कपिला (Kapilā), कौन्ती (Kaunti), हरेणुका (Hareṇukā), सुपर्णी (Suparṇī), शान्ता (Śāntā), शिशिरा

१ 'पाण्डुफला' इति क्षी .संमतः पाठः ।
२ 'भस्मगन्धा' इति क्षीर. संमतः पाठः ।

(Śiśirā), हैमवती (Haimawatī),

b- (B.) Kāminī; (H) Marchula juti, Bisbar; (Bom). Marchula juti; (Mar.) Kunti; (Tel.) Naga golunga.

III-a

b-1) रेणुका ... । जयेत् त्रिदोषजां छर्दिं पर्पटः पित्तजां तथा । रेणुका कौन्तीति पर्यायनामा प्रसिद्धा । निर्गुण्डी बीजानि रेणुकाशब्दवाच्यानि इत्येके ।
Dipika M. Kh. 2.83.

2) 47 कौन्ती - हरेणु 'हरेणु रेणुका कौन्ती' ति हृदयदीपकः कौन्त्यास्तु पादपो वृत्तपत्रो पुष्पफलस्य च । बीजं तु कौन्तिका संज्ञा तिक्त' मिति ।
(Harshe)

IV- 1) *Murraya exotica* Linn.
Kuntī, Kāminī. A shrub or small tree in the outer Himalaya ... ascending to 4000 ft. in Bihar .. often planted for ornament ..... In Burma the fragrant bark is more universally used as a cosmetic than sandal wood. (Watt. Dict. V. 288)

2) *Murraya paniculata* (L) Jack.
Syn. *M. exotica* Linn.
(H.) Marchul; (B) Kamini; (Bom) chuljuti; (Kan.) Panduy; (Tam.) Simrikkonji; (Tel.) Nagagolunga.Ground bark of root eaten and rubbed on in body ache. *Powdered leaf* - application to the fresh cuts. *Decoction of leaves* in dropsy, *Leaves* Stimulant, astringent, administered in diarr. and dysentery ......
Outer Himalayas, Satpura range and ranges of the peninsula.
(Chopra)

20 तगरम् Tagaram

तगरं कुटिलं वक्रं दीनं जिह्मं नतं शठम् ॥ ५२
कालानुसार्यमनृजु कुञ्चितं नहुषं नृपम् ॥
तगरं स्यात् कषायोष्णं स्निग्धं दोषत्रयप्रणुत् ॥ ५३
दृक्शीर्षविषदोषघ्नं भूतापस्मारनाशनम् ॥

तगरं (Tagaram), कुटिलं (Kuṭilam), वक्रं (Vakram), दीनं (Dīnam), जिह्मं (Jimham), नतं (Natam), शठं (Saṭham), कालानुसार्यं (Kālānusāryam), अनृजु (Anṛju), कुञ्चितं (Kuñcitam), नहुषं (Nahuṣam) and नृपम् (Nṛpam) are synonymous.

Tagara is *kaṣāya* (astringent) in taste, *uṣṇavīrya, snigdha* (unctuous) and pacifies all the three *doṣas.* It is beneficial to eyes, and useful in diseases of head, poisons, bhūtabādhā (antiseptic ? antimicrobial) and in epilepsy.

Fam. Valerianaceae

I- a- ***Valeriana wallichii*** DC.*
Syn. *V. officinalis* Linn.
b- Dymock (Pharm.indi.), Chopra (Gloss.Ind. Med. Pl.)
c- Temparate Himalaya from Kashmir to Bhutan.

II- a- नतम् (Natam), कालानुसार्यम् (Kālānusāryam),
b- (Market) Sugandhabālā; (H.B.) Muṣkabālā; agar; (Guj.) Tagargathona; (Eng.) Indian valerian.

III-a- C.S. Su. 4.42, S.S. Sū. 14. 36. A.H. Su. 10. 28. (Balavantji 173)
b- ते. गन्धतगरचेट्टु; क. तगर; मल्या. तकरं , अशारुन् (Ast. Hr. kosh)
There is a plant of similar name as (Tagara) but it is quite different from that of Dhn. ni. Now it is identified as *Ervatamia coronaria* Stapf. (See watt. Dict.).

21 परिपेल्लवम् Paripellawam

परिपेल्लं प्लवं वन्यं गोपुटं स्यात्कुटन्नटम् ॥ ५४
सितपुष्पं दासपुरं गोनर्दं जीर्णपुष्पकम् ॥

परिप्लवं सुगन्धि स्यात् प्रस्वेदमलकण्डुजित् ॥ ५५
जयेद् वातकफौ चापि मेध्यं कान्तिप्रदं भवेत् ॥

(अन्यच्च - परिप्लवं वातकफौ जयेन्मेध्यं च कान्तिदम् ।
कफतृष्णाहरं प्रोक्तमस्रपित्तविनाशनम् ॥)

परिपेल्लं (Paripellam), प्लवं (Plavam), वन्यं (Vanyam), गोपुटं (Gopuṭam), कुटन्नटं (Kuṭannaṭam), सितपुष्पं (Sitapuṣpam), दासपुरं (Dāsapuram), गोनर्दं (Gonardam), and जीर्णपुष्पकम् (Jīrṇapuṣpakam) are synonymous.

Pariplavam pacifies *vāta* and *kapha doṣas,* is fragrant, is useful in excessive sweating, pruritus, intellect promoting and improves complexion. (***From other sources*** - *Pariplavam* pacifies *vāta* and *kapha doṣas,* is intellect promoting, improves complexion, removes thirst due to *kaphadoṣa* and useful in bleeding disorders.)

I- Not identified

II- a- वन्यम् (Vanyam), सितपुष्पम् (Sitapuṣpam), जीर्णपुष्पकम्

---

* The current accepted name far *V. wallichii* DC. is *V. jatamansi* Jones. *V. officinalis* Linn. is a distinct species having current accepted name as *V. dubia* Bunge (Comp. p. 156)

(Jirṇapuṣpakam), प्लवम् (Plavam), वन्यम् (Vannyam), गोनर्दम् (Gonardam), कुटन्नटम् (Kuṭannaṭam), दासपुरम् (Dāsapuram),

III-b-1) परिपेल्लवम् (Paripellavm), Su. 15. Jālamusta -Śaiwāla madhye Jāyamāno mustākāra Padarthaḥ ityeke ...Jāyante maṇḍukākāram Sajñyeyam. (Ast. Hr. Kosa)

2) 346 (Kśudramustā) ... Paripellavam .. (Dr. Harshe)

3) परिपेलवम् C.S. Vi. 8.15 ka. 1.26.
S.S. K. 2.51 U.47.31
A.H. Su. 15.26 U. 22. 84

See synonyms प्लव & शैवाल See further reading
Balavantji Page 264-265.

22 नखम् Nakham

नरवः कररुहः शिल्पी करजोऽथ खुरः शफः ॥ ५६
शुक्तिः शङ्खः चलः कोशी हनुर्नागहनुः सहः ॥

नखं कटुकमुष्णं च विषं हन्ति प्रयोजितम् ॥ ५७
कुष्ठानि सादयत्येव कफं खण्डयति क्षणात् ॥

नरव (Nakha) and व्याघ्रनख (Vyāghranakha) being animal in origin are not commented upon by Late Vd. D.K. Kamat. In English it is called as Landsnail and its scientific name is *Helix aspera; Achatina fulica.*

नरव (Nakha), कररुह (Kararuha), शिल्पी (Śilpī), करज (Karaja), खुर (Khura) ,शफ (Śapha), शुक्तिः (Śuktiḥ), चलः (Calaḥ), कोशी (Kośi), हनुः (Hanuḥ),नागहनुः (Nāgahanuḥ) and सहः (Sahaḥ) are synonymous.

Nakha is pungent in taste, *uṣṇa,* and if used correctly it is antipoisonous. It is useful in disorders of skin and removes quickly *kaphadoṣa.*

23 व्याघ्रनखम् Vyāghranakham

नरवमन्यद् व्याघ्रतलं पुटं व्याघ्रायुधं मतम ॥ ५८
अस्त्रं व्याघ्रतलं पादं कूटस्थं वज्रकारकम् ॥

ग्रहभूतोपशमनं पवित्रं द्वीपिजं नखम् ॥ ५९
व्याघ्रनखस्तु तिक्तोष्णः कषायः कफवातजित् ॥

कण्डुकुष्ठव्रणघ्नश्च वर्ण्यः सौगंध्यदः परः॥ ६०

See Pre no. 22 नरवम् । The second type of *nakham* is called as व्याघ्रनखम् (Vyāghranakham), व्याघ्रतलं (Vyāghratalam), पुटं (Puṭam), व्याघ्रायुध (Vyāghrāyudham), अस्त्रं (Astram), व्याघ्रतलं (Vyāghratalam), पादं

(Pādam), कूटस्थं (Kuṭastham), वज्रकारकं (Vijrakārakam), ग्रहभूतोपशमनं (Grahabhūtopaśamanam), पवित्रं (Pavitram), and द्वीपिजं नखं (Dwīpijam nakham) are synonymous.

Vyāghranakha is bitter and *kaṣāya* (astringent) in taste, *uṣṇavīrya* and pacifies *kapha* and *vāta doṣas*. It is useful in pruritus, disorders of skin, helaing of ulcers, and improves complexion and gives fragrance.

24 स्पृक्का Spṛkkā

स्पृक्काऽसृग्[1] ब्राह्मणी देवी मालाली कोटिका मता ॥
प[2]ञ्चमुष्टिर्देवपुत्री निर्माल्या पिशुना वधूः ॥ ६१

[3]स्पृक्का शीता सुगन्धा स्यात् तृष्णां मुष्णाति योजिता ॥
विषं हन्ति हिनस्त्येव दाहं देहसमुद्भवम् ॥ ६२

स्पृक्का सुगन्धा कुष्ठघ्नी दौर्गन्ध्यस्वेदनाशिनी ॥

स्पृक्का(Spṛkkā), असृग् (Asṛg), ब्राह्मणी (Brāhmanī), देवी (Devī), मालाली (Mālālī), कोटिका (Koṭikā), पञ्चमुष्टिः (Pañcamuṣtiḥ), देवपुत्री (Devaputrī), निर्माल्या (Nirmālyā), पिशुना (Piśunā) and वधूः (Vadhuḥ) are synonymous.

Spṛkkā is *śītavīrya,* and fragrant. It is useful in thirst, poisons and burning sensation of the body.

Spṛkkā is fragrant, useful in skin disorders, removes foul smell and perspiration.

I- A controversial plant.

Fam. Leguminosae. Fabaceae.

a- ***Melilotus officinalis*** Lam.*
Syn. *M. altisima* Thuill not of Wall. and other species of the same genus.

b- Pt. Bhagirath

c- Nubra and Ladakah. Cultivated here and there in India.
(Watt. V. 224)

II-a- असृग् (Asṛg), ब्राह्मणी (Brāhmaṇī), देवपुत्री (Devaputrī), सुगन्धा (Sugandhā), समुद्रकान्ता (Samudrakāntā),सुकुमारा (Sukumārā), भूतलिका (Bhutalikā), लघ्वी (Laghvī), नखपुष्पी (Nakhapuṣpī)

b- (H) Asparak (B) Banpiranga (Watt. Dict.)

स्रक = माला इत्यपि साधु पाठः भविष्यति । जाद्वतः राजनिघण्टुकारेण । स .दि. कामत

* The current accepted name is *M. officinalis* (Linn.) Medik.

II- See Ārāmśitalā of Raj. Ni; Methikā.

a- C.S. Ci. 12. 64
A.H. Su. 15.43 (Balvantji p. 459)

b- 1- स्पृक्का (Spṛkkā) Su. 15 Sugandhā Śāka Viśeṣaḥ Kuṭila puṣpā Sugandhi dravyamiti uttarāpathike iti suśruta ṭīkāyam. Lankodarpura iti Loke prasidha iti Bhāvaprakāśe
(H) Asaburgh Laṅkādhikā; (Mar.) Karpura walli, Kappuri madhuri; (Guj.) Kapuri Madhuri ; (Kan.) Hikke, Peymarutti. (Mal.) Conakapullu , Parnikkarkka.
(Lat.) *Trifolium officinalis*, *Trigonella corniculata* iti kecit, *Anisomelis malabarica* ityapare. (Ast. Hr. Kośa)

2- 13-स्पृक्का - स्पृक्केति माल्यवती मोहने ।
स्पृक्का वल्ली स्थिरा तिक्ता सुगंधी 'कोल' संफला । अरिपत्रा दाक्षिणात्या सिद्धा लोके तु 'पानरी' ॥ 'मुनिर्माल्यवती माला मोहना कुटिला लते' ति वाचस्पतिः। (Harshe)

IV- 1) *Melilotus alba* Lam. and *M. parviflora* Desf. grow in India. The first species has delicate odour of European Melilot ... In Makhzan an Indian variety of Melilot ... is called 'Pirang' (Dymock I- 405)

2) *Melilotus officinalis* Willd, *M. hamosa* Link; *M. parviflora* Desf.contain coumarin. (Watt. Dict. V. 224-25)

3) *Melilotus officinalis* Willd.
Syn. *M. macrorhiza* Pers.
M. altissisma Thuill, not of Wall. *Trifolium officinale*, Willd.
(H.) Asparak; (B.) Ban pirang; (Pers.) zirir; wild in Nubra and Ladak ... ... It is described in all mohammadan works as Jhilil-el-malic (Dymock)

4- *Melilotus parviflora* Desf.*
Syn. *M. indica* All.; *M. minima* Roth; *Trifolium indicum* Linn.
(H.B.) Banmethī; (Sans.) Vanamethī (Roxb.Fl. Indi.)
A slender herb met with in the Bombay Presidency, Bengal, NWP. & The Punjab.Cultivated or found as cold season cultivation.
Medicine .. like those of M. officinale .... like most of the other species of this genus it contains coumarin.
M. officinalis Willd.
(H.) Aspurk, Banpirang
M. parviflora Desf.
(H.) Banmethi (sans.) Vanmethikā. (Watt. 'M' 224-225)

---

* The current accepted name is *M. indica* (Linn.) All. (comp. p. 100)

5) स्पृक्का (Spṛkkā) The description of *sprkkā* occured in Dhn. Ni. & Raj. Ni. aptly corresponds to *Melilotus officinalis* Billad. (H.) Asara.
Trigonella corniculata (Mālyā, Asbarag), *Anisomelis malabarica; Marcilecia budrifolia* are wrong and unscientific. (Pt. Bhagirath)

V- *Trigonella uncata* Boiss imported from Persian gulf to Bombay to be the meliliotus of Dioscorides ... the author of Makhjan -el-Adwia gives Meliotus as the Greek name for Eklil -el-malik. (Arab) (Dymock Vol. I- 405)

2) *Trigonella corniculata* Linn.
It is called 'Tirup' in Belgam, It is the 'Mālyā' of Sanskrit writers. (Dymock Vol. I. 405)

25 बोलम् Bolam

बोलं गन्धरसं पिण्डं निर्लोहं बर्बरं रसम् ॥ ६३
गोपकं नालिकं पौररसं गन्धरसं विदुः ॥

बोलं तिक्तं हिमं रक्तमुद्रित्तं हन्ति योगतः ॥ ६४
कफपित्तामयान् हन्ति प्रदरादिरुजापहम् ॥

बोलं (Bolam), गन्धरसं (Gandharasam), पिण्डं (Piṇḍam), निर्लोहं (Nirloham), बर्बरं (Barbaram), गोपकं (Gopakam) नालिकं (Nālikam), पौररसम् (Paurarasam) and गन्धरसं (Gandharasam) are synonymous.

Bola is bitter in taste, *śītavīrya,* pacifies disorders caused by *kapha* and *pitta doṣas*, bleeding disorders and bleeding per vagina (*Raktapradara*) etc.

(Fam. Burseraceae)

I- a- ***Commiphora myrrha*** (Nees) Engl. & speices
Syn. *Balsamodendron myrrha* Nees

b- Dymock and Hill

c- See IV- 1,2, below

II- a- गन्धरसम् (Gandharasam), पिण्डम् (Piṇḍam), निर्लोहम् (Nirloham), बर्बरम् (Barbaram), रक्तगन्धम् (Raktagandham), व्रणारिः (Vraṇāriḥ), शुभगन्धम् (Śubhagandham).

b- (Sk) Rasagandhī, Bola; (H) Bola; (B) Gandharasa, Bola; (Mar.) Hirābola; (Kan). Bola; (Madras) vellaippalam; (Singapore) Bolam, Gandharasam; (Eng.) Harbol myrrha.

III- See Guggul, Kundaru, Śriwāsa.

b- 34 बोलो गन्धरसः । (Bolo gandharasaḥ)

श्रीवासः सरलो बोलः कुन्दरुश्चेति पादपाः ।
पृथक्प (य) वनदेशस्थाः क्रमात्तेषामथाकृतिः॥
करवीरोपमः पूर्वः सरलः शाल्मली समः ।
कुमारीच्छदनो बोलः कुन्दरुः शल्लकीसमः ।
एषां द्रवाः स्रुता वृक्षादाच्छियन्ते च ते शकै रिति । (Harshe)

2) जातिरसः । Su. 15. Jātirasaḥ Raktabolaḥ Elādigaṇe gandharasaḥ bola iti Dalhaṇaḥ. (Guj.) Hirābola; (Tam.) Iratta poḷam, Veḷai poḷam; (Mal.) Narumpaśa, Pancamppaluka. (Ast. Hr. Kosa)

IV- 1) *Myrrha* one of the oldest and most valuable gum resin ... ... Two forms (A) Harbol Myrrha is dervied from *Commiphora myrrha* a large shrub or small tree of Abyssinia, Somali land and Arabia.

The pale yellow liquid gradually solidifies and becomes brown even black in colour. (B) Bisbol Myrrha or sweet Myrrha is derived from Commiphora erythreca an Arabian species of similar appearance.

This is the *Myrrha* of Antiquity. (Hill)

3) *History* There are several substances which in English, go by the name of Myrrha .....

Commercial forms of the myrrha ... ...of commerce there are two or three distinct varieties, and each on assortment of stuffs is of differeent commercial value, There is the east coast African myrrha known in Bombay as *'Karam'* and the south Arabian and the Sayam Myrrha the 'Meetiya'.

The myrrha a good quality is also sent from Persia. The latter two forms are really only substitutes,.however, for Myrrha, the 'Karam' obtained from Africa may be said to be the true commercial myrrha, but it is by no means proved that this is entirely obtained from *B. myrrha* Nees. The principal market for myrrha is in Bombay, the chief firms having three agents at Aden and Mukulla. .... The bags of these on arrival at Bombay are said to contain *1st* a large proportion of roundish masses of fine myrrha, *2nd* a considerable proportion of small semi transperant pieces of myrrha, *3rd* numerous pieces of dark coloured myrrha mixed with refuge, *4th* a small proportion of gum resin. The packages coarse assorted the best quality shipped for Europe as also the darker pieces declared as second quality while the refuge is exported to china .

Vern. Bol (Pers, Hind); Gandharasa. bol (Bengal); Morr (Hebrew); (Tel.) Balimtra polam; (Kan.) Bola; (Tam.) Vellaip-polam; (Singapor)Bolam, Gandharasam. (Watt. Dict.)

26 दमनः Damanaḥ

दमनः पाण्डुरागः स्यात् दान्तः गन्धोत्कटो मुनिः ॥ ६५
पुण्डरीको ब्रह्मजटस्तपस्वी ऋषिपुत्रकः ॥

दमनः स्याद् रसे तिक्तो विषघ्नो भूतदोषनुत् ॥ ६६
त्रिदोषशमनो हृद्यः कण्डूकुष्ठापहः स्मृतः ॥

दमनः (Damanaḥ), पाण्डुरागः (Pāṇḍurāgaḥ), दान्तः (Dāntaḥ), गन्धोत्कटः (Gandhotkaṭaḥ), मुनिः (Muniḥ), पुण्डरीकः (Puṇḍarīkaḥ), ब्रह्मजटः (Brahmajaṭaḥ), तपस्वी (Tapasvī), and ऋषिपुत्रकः (Ṛṣiputrakaḥ) are synonymous.

Damana is bitter in taste, pacifies the three *doṣas,* is antipoison, antiseptic, cordial, and useful in pruritus and disorders of the skin.

Fam. Compositae. Asteraceae

I- a- ***Artemisia pallens*** Wall. cat.*
Syn. *A. paniculata,* Roxb.

b- kamat c-Jejuri, Āḷandī in Pune dist, and Alibag, Revdandā in Coloba Dist, **

II- a- पाण्डुरागः (Pāṇḍurāgaḥ), गन्धोत्कटः (Gandhotkaṭaḥ), पुण्डरीकः (Puṇḍarīkaḥ), तपस्वी (Tapaswī), तापसपत्रः (Tāpasapatraḥ) पवित्रः (Pavitraḥ), देवशेखरः (Devasekahraḥ)

b- (Mar.) Davaṇā; (Sk) Damanaka.

III- 1) 64 दमनः पुष्पचामरः। 'दोना मरुआ' इति लोके। 'सर्वाङ्ग सुरभिः पुष्पादि वर्जितश्च। साहजिक रूपवत्या वपुषि भवत्याविभूषणं भारः 'सर्वाङ्गे सौरभिण्या दमनकवन्याः किमालिकुसुमैः' ति कश्चित्। (Harshe)

IV-a-1) *Artemisia pallens* Wall. cat.
Syn. *A. paniculata* Roxb
Vern. Davṇā. Herbaceous ½ ft. high erect, branched wooly canescent, very aromatic, stem rather thick ...... cultivated at Āḷandi and Jejurī in the Deccan for use as offerings at the Ramnavami festival ... ...Roxburgh ... States that he has not been able to ascertain its native country. (Cooke fl.)

(Note : This kind of (Davṇā) is brought for sale to Poona on the Ramnavami the nineth day of first fortnight of Caitra)

---

* The current name : *A. pallens* Wall. ex DC. (U.P.I.p. 55)

** Now Raigad Dist.

दमः Damaḥ (14)

दमनोऽन्यो दमः शान्तः ऋषिर्दमवशान्वितः ॥६७
क्षमाशान्तिपरः साधुः साधुकः साधुगन्धिकः ॥

There is another type of *Damanaḥ* called as दमः (Damaḥ) of which synonyms are शान्तः (Śāntaḥ), ऋषिः (Ṛṣīḥ), दमवशान्वितः (Damavaśānvitaḥ), क्षमा शान्तिपरः (Kśamāśāntiparaḥ), साधुः (Sādhuḥ), साधुकः (Sādhukaḥ), and साधुगन्धिकः (Sādhugandhikaḥ).

I- Controversial.
Fam. Compositae. Asteraceae.

II- a- शान्तिपरः (Śāntiparaḥ), साधुगन्धिकः (Sādhugandhikaḥ), वन्यदमनः (Vanyadamanaḥ)

27 मुरा Murā

मुरा गन्धवती दैत्या गन्धाढ्या गन्धमालिनी[१] ॥ ६८
सुरभिर्भूरिगन्धा च कुटी गन्धकुटी स्मृता ॥

मुराऽत्यन्तं भवेच्छीता तिक्ता सुरभिगन्धिनी ॥ ६९
क्षिणोति क्षतपुञ्जांश्च पित्तशान्तिं नियच्छति ॥

मुरा (Murā), गन्धवती (Gandhavatī), दैत्या (Daityā), गन्धाढ्या (Gandhāḍhyā), गन्धमालिनी (Gandhamālinī), सुरभिः (Surabhiḥ), भूरिगन्धा (Bhūrigandhā), कुटी (Kuṭī), and गन्धकुटी (Gandhakuṭī)are synonymous.

Murā is bitter in taste, very *śita,* fragrant, pacifies *pittadoṣa* and useful in ulcers on the skin.

I- Controversial

II- a- गन्धवती (Glandhavatī), दैत्या (Daityā), गन्धमालिनी (Gandhamālinī), भूरिगन्धा (Bhūrigandhā)

IV- 1) It has been used as a constituent of a preparation in insanity (उन्माद-*Unmāda*). It, therefore to be what has been called *Muramāmsī* मुरामांसी by others. It may be *selinum tenuifolium* Wall.* called

---

१ गन्धमादनी ' इति नि. शे. टीका .संमतः पाठः ।

*It is interesting to note that useful plants of India has noted another species of selinum (Fam.Umbelliferae.) *S. vaginatum* C.B. Clarke which in kumaun area is called as मुर (Moor) and in Kahsmir area as Pushwari, Bhoot-keshi. Its roots are used as a nervine sedative, also employed as incense, yield essential oil with hypotensive, sedative and analgesic properties (S.D. Kamat)

Mūra मूर in the Garhavala region and also being collected and supplied in place of *Murā.* At present curcuma or Hedychium species are being used in its place by many. (Balvantji p. 311)*

28 स्थौणेयकम् Sthauṇeyakam

स्थौणेयकं बर्हिचूडं शुकपुष्पं शुकच्छदम् ॥ ७०
विकर्णं शुकबर्हं च हरितं शीर्णरोमकम् ॥

स्थौणेयं कफवातघ्नं सुगन्धि कटुतिक्तकम् ॥ ७१
पित्तप्रकोपशमनं बलपुष्टिविवर्धनम ॥

स्थौणेयकं (Sthauṇeyakm), बर्हिचूडं (Barhicūḍam), शुकपुष्पं (Śukapuṣpam), शुकच्छदं (Śukacchadam), विकर्णं (Vikarṇam), शुकबर्हं (Śukabarham), हरितं (Haritam), and शीर्णरोमकम् (Śīrṇaromakam) are synonymous.

Sthauṇeya is pungent and bitter in taste, pacifies *vāta, pitta* and *kapha doṣas,* is fragrant and promotes strength and nourishment.

Fam. Compositae. Asteraceae.

I- a- ***Blumea lacera*** DC.**
B. aromatica DC.

b- Kamat c-throughout the plains of India, Himalaya, Travancore to ceylon.

II- a- बर्हिचूडम् (Barhicūdam), शुकपुष्पम् (Śukapuṣpam), हरितम् (Haritam), शीर्णरोमकम् (Śīrṇaromakam), विकीर्णम् (Vikīṇam)

b- Kukurudru; (Mar) Nirmuṇḍi, Nirmuḍi; (H) Kukarondhā Kakarondha; (B.) Kukukarsunga; (Tel.) Karupogaku; (Tam) Narakkandai, Kalumulangi.

III-b-1) (स्थौणेयक श्रीवेष्टक। (Sthauṇeyaka Śrīveṣṭaka) (Su .Su. 38.23)

2) ग्रन्थिपर्णम् (Granthi parṇam) Śukam Barhi Puṣpam sthauṇeyam

---

१ 'वह्निचूडम्' इति नि.शे. टीका संमत पाठः ।
२ 'शुकपुच्छम्' इति आनन्दाश्रम मुद्रित पुस्तके पाठः ।
'शुकगुच्छम्' इति नि.शे. टीका संमतः पाठः ।
३ 'विकचम्' इति नि.शे. टीका संमतः पाठः ।

** The current accepted name is *Blumea lacera* (Burm. f.) DC.

" ग्रन्थौ पर्णान्यस्य Granthau parṇānyasya ... कुक्कुरोऽस्यास्ति (Kukkurosyāsti), कुक्कुरशब्दस्तद्गन्धि (Kukkuraśabdastadgandhi) कुकुरवद्रा (Kukurawadra)
कुक्कुरशब्दस्तद्गन्धि लाक्षणिकः Kukkuraśabdastatagandhi lākśaṇikaḥ iti khyātā.(Bhanuji; Amar 2.4)

3) स्थौणेयम् (Sthauṇeyam) Su 15... ग्रन्थिपर्णस्येव भेदः इषत् सुगन्धः (H) Thuner - *Clerodendron infortunatum* ityeke.(Ast. Hr. Kosā)

4) स्थौणेयकम् Keral- Tuṇiyānka Asya Kandaḥ Chede haritaḥ Tukākśiriviśeṣam; (Tam.)Tantileṇṇai (Ayu. O. Nigh).

5) 383 स्थौणेयकं विकर्ण शुकवर्ण शीर्णरोमकं हरितम् । अविकर्णं शुकपुच्छं शुकच्छंदं शाड्वलं विशिष्टं च ।... तैलबीजकम् । (Abhi. manj.)

6) 12 स्थौणेयः शुकच्छदः । स्थौणेयकं बर्हिचूडं शुकवर्णं शुकच्छदमिति निघण्टुः । (Harshe)

7) 171 शुकपर्णमिति
स्थौणेयकं शुकच्छदं 'स्थौणेयकं बर्हिचूडं शुकवर्णमिति' गुणरत्नमाला. (Harshe)

IV- 1) कुक्कुरद्रु (Kukkuradru) - *Blumea lacera* (Priyavratji)

2) *Blumea balsamifera* DC.
B. densiflora DC.
Sanskrit writers call kakurudru, Kukkundra, 'dogbush'
Camphorous Blumeas - Because their pungent odour is attractive to those animals in addition to the two plants placed at head of this article *B. lacera DC,* and *B. aromatica DC* are considered by the Hindus. (Dymock)

3) *Blumea lacera* DC.
(H.) Kukaronda, kukurvanda and kakaronda and other vernacular names are applied to more than one allied species of *Blumea* and *Laggera* without much regard to the colour and their flavour. It smells strongly of turpentine. Kakaronda is used as febrifuge and also to stop bleeding. (Watt.)

4) स्थौणेयक - C.S.Ci. 3.266; 12.63; 28.122 ka. 1.26.
S.S.Su. 38. 23; ka.5.66; 6.19.
A.H. S. 15.43; 21.13 Ci 1.137; 17.22; 21.79

on the basis of its popular name '*Thuṇeraka* थुणेरक' mentioned by Dalhana and Bhavamisra, *Taxus baccata* Linn. *Thuṇera* थुणेर in Garhaval, was first suggested to be *sthauṇeyaka* in *Vanauśadhi Darshikā*. Its leaves when dried emit fragrance and are being used as Tālisapatra तालीसपत्र. *Granthi parṇikā* ग्रन्थिपर्णिका is mentioned by Ḍalhaṇa as a synonym of *sthauṇeyaka* while, according to Bhavamisra it is a variety of *sthauṇeyaka*. It is felt that *Granthiparṇikā* may better be identified with any species of *Valerian* or *Angelica* rather than considering it to be the same as *sthauṇeyaka*. (Balvantaji p. 459.)

29 चोरकः Corakāḥ

चोरकः शङ्कितश्चण्डा दुष्पत्रः[१] क्षेमको रिपुः ॥ ७२
गणहासः कोपनकः[२] कितवः फलचोरकः ॥

चोरकः शिशिरोऽत्यन्तं विषरक्तगन्तकारकः ॥ ७३
कुष्ठकण्डूव्रणान् हन्ति क्षणात् दोषान् प्रयोगतः ॥

चोरकश्चोग्रगन्धश्च तिक्तकृमिसमीरजित् ॥ ७४

चोरकः (Corakaḥ), शङ्कितः (Śankitaḥ), चण्डा (Caṇḍā), दुष्पत्रः (Duṣpatraḥ), क्षेमकः (Kśemakaḥ), रिपुः (Ripuḥ), गणहासः (Gaṇahāsaḥ), कोपनकः (Kopanakaḥ), कितवः (Kitavaḥ) and फलचोरकः (Phalacorakaḥ) are synonymous.

Coraka is excessively *śītavirya*. It is useful in poisons, bleeding disorders, *doṣas* of skin disorders, pruritus and wounds immediately by proper use.

Coraka is strong smelling, bitter in taste, and pacifies *vātadoṣa* and is useful in worms.

For confirmation

(Fam. Labiatae). Lamiaceae.

I- A-a- ***Coleus amboinicus*** Lour.
Syn. *C.aromaticus* Benth.
Plectranthus aromaticus Roxb.

b- Kamat C- Native of Molucca, cultivated in gardens in India. or

(Fam. Umbelliferae). Apiaceae

B-a- ***Angelica glauca*** Edg.

b- Priyavratji C- From kashmir to simla above kangra valley (Watt. Dict.)

II- a-A & B ग्रन्थिलः (Granthilaḥ), पर्णचोरकः (Parṇa corakaḥ), चण्डा (caṇḍā) ग्रन्थिपर्णः (Granthi parṇaḥ) ,ग्रन्थिदलः (Granthidalaḥ), फलचोरकः

---

१ 'दुष्पुत्रः' इति क्षी. संमतः पाठः ।
२ 'कोहनकः' इति क्षी. संमतः पाठः।

(Phalacorakaḥ), तीव्रगन्धः (Tīvragandaḥ)

A-b- (Mar.) Pānācāowā; (Bom.) owā; (H.) Pātharchūra

B-b- (B.) Patharchur; (Sans.) Paṣāṇabheda;
(Eng.) Country Borage; (P.) Cora, Curā.

III-a-1) C.C.Sū. 3.23 4.28 etc.
S.S.Sū. 98.23 etc.
A.H. Su. 15.43 etc. (Balvantji)

2) स्पृक्का चोरक .... स्थौणेय जातीरस ः। (A.H.Su. 15.31)
Teekā चोरको ग्रन्थिपर्णी (Aruṇa-Hemadri)

3) नखशुक्तिः चण्डा स्थौणेयक - चोरक। (S.S.Su. 38. 24)

b- 1) 328 चोरक चण्ड; चण्डः चोरकभेदः। ' ईषत् कृष्णः अजमोदाकारः इति एलादि गणे डल्हणः। 'चोरकः ग्रन्थिपर्णभेदस्तदाकार एवेति एलादि गणे डल्हणः। (Harshe)

2) 544 चोरको गणहासकः ग्रन्थिपर्णभेदः। (Harshe)

3) 144 क्रोधमूर्च्छिता - चण्डा धनहरी क्षेमद्धः पुत्रगणहासकः। अमरः (Harshe)

4) चोरकः। चि. १ स्वनामख्यात गन्धद्रव्यविशेषः। एलादिगणे व्याख्यायां ग्रन्थिपर्ण एवेति हेमाद्रिः अरुणदत्तश्च। हिं भटेऊर, बं. चौरा, म. भटोरा, क. भटोरा. ' चोरकस्तीव्र गन्धश्च ऊष्ण तिक्तः ... कृमिदोष विनाशन ः। (A.Hr. Kosha)

5) *चोरक* विषमो विषगन्धः .... गन्धाली।
षड्गन्धा दुष्पत्रो धूर्तश्च ... ॥
ग्रन्थिपर्णो ... गन्धिनी वधू ः
सुगन्ध मूलौषधी च निशाचरा ॥
आर्द्रगन्धा पलाशश्च ... पृथुपलाशिका ॥
चोराभिधाना ॥ ३७९ ॥
अन्या कृष्णशटी .... शीतशिवा।
शीताश्च ... ... सितगन्धा
अजाप्रियो ग्रहावासः ... कृष्णचोरकः ॥ ३८०
स्थौणेयकं विकीर्ण शुकवर्णं शीर्णरोमकं हरितम्।
... शुकपुच्छं ... ॥ धूमाहवयं ... तैलबीजकम् ॥ ३८३ ॥
चण्डा तु कोपिका गणहास चोरकः।
दुष्पत्रः ... कितवः फलचोरकः ॥
आर्द्रकन्दा ग्रन्थिकेशी केशिनी च निशाचरी ॥ ३९५ ॥ (Abhi. Manj).

---

३७९ चोरक - अटविक्कच्चोल चण्ण, मञ्जक्कूव। ग्रन्थिपर्ण - करिञ्चण्ण, नरुञ्चण्ण.
पृथुपलाशिका -Curcuma zedoaria कच्चूर किलंगु शटी - कच्चोलम्

३८० कृष्ण चोरकः करुन्तकच्चूरं।

३८३ स्थौणेयक - तुणीयाड्गम। Abhi. Manji

(Miss - Nalini- Mrs. Chitra.)

३९५ चण्डा- चण्ण।

There seems some confusion while giving the serial prenumbers of plants 377-78-79 in Abhi Manji. S.D. Kamat.

IV- 1) *Cleome viscosa* Linn.
Eng. Wild mustard.
The seed are known in bazar as 'churiajwan' (Kannyalal)
(SeeAjagandhā -अजगन्धा)

2) *Angelica glauca* Edgew.
It is also used in obstinate constipation, Roots added to food to give flavour. (Watt. Dict. I- 224)

3) *Coleus aromaticus* Benth.
Country Borage
Powerful aromatic, carminative, pungent, given in cases of colic in children. According to some it is intoxicting but only in large doses. Applied in cases of conjunctivitis ....useful in urinary diseases, ch. dyspepsia etc. Watt.II. 504 505

4) चोरक Coraka
Suśṛuta has used this drug only once under the name of *Taskara* (तस्कर) and has mentioned it twice under the group of drugs i.e.'Elādi Gaṇā' (Su. 38.23) and 'Ekasara Gaṇa' (Ka.5.84) Dalhaṇa in these two places has described it as a variety of Granthiparṇa ग्रन्थिपर्ण and similar to it and he again identifies it with *sthauṇeyaka* स्थौणेयक. The identity of *Coraka* with *A. glauca* having been decided, those of *caṇḍā* चण्डा *granthiparṇa* ग्रन्थिपर्ण and *sthauṇeyaka* स्थौणेयक remain still undecided.
(Balvantji 161)

Note- 1-चोरको वरुणः कुष्ठं ....। Ekasara group (S.Su. 5.84)
2- नखशुक्तिः चण्डा स्थौणेयक चोरक । Elādi group. S.S. kạ. 38. 24.

5) *Plectranthus aromaticus* Roxb.
(See above I-a-A Syn.)
Perennial, villous, leaves short petioled, round cordate, crenated, fleshy rugose, crenulate spikes solitary, bracts caducous.
This most agreeable fragrant plant, every garden in India.
Stems creeping round,... Branches erect ... hairy from one or two ft. high, leaves short petioled, fragile, broad cordate, crenulate, a little hairy, spikes terminal erect, with four rows of ... bracts. The leaves and generally all parts delightfully fragrant ... eaten with bread and butter. ... flowers numerous blue.
(Roxb. Fl. Ind. CBC. 466)

30 शैलेयम् Śaileyam

शैलेयं पलितं वृद्धं जीर्णं कालानुसार्यकम् ॥
स्थविरं च शिलादद्रु शिलापुष्पं शिलोद्भवम ॥ ७९

शैलेयकं हिमं प्रोक्तं दाहजिद् विषनाशनम् ॥
रक्तदोषहरं चैव कण्डूनिर्मूलनं स्मृतम् ॥ ७८

(शैलेयं तिक्तकं शीतं सुगन्धिकफपित्तजित् ॥
दाहतृष्णा वमिश्वासव्रणदोषविनाशनम् ॥)

शैलेयं (Śaileyam), पलितं (Palitam), वृद्धं (Vṛddham), जीर्णं (Jīrṇam), कालानुसार्यकं (Kālānusāryakam), स्थविरं (Sthaviram), शिलाद्रु (Śilādadru), शिलापुष्पं (Śilāpuṣpam). and शिलोद्भवम् (Śilodbhavam) are synonymous.

Śaileya is *śītavīrya*, and useful in burning sensations, poisons, blood disorders and pruritus.

[*Śaileya* is bitter in taste, *śītavīrya,* fragrant and pacifies *kapha* and *pitta doṣas*. It is useful in thirst, burning sensation, emesis, dyspnoea and in the *doṣa* of wounds (septic wounds).]

(Fam. Lichens)

I- a- ***Cetraria islandica*** (Linn.) Ach. (Watt. Dict.)
b- Watt. Dict.

II- a- शैलेयम् (Śaileyam), शिलाद्रुः (Śilādadruḥ), शिलापुष्पम् (Śilāpuṣpam), शिलोद्भवम् (Śilodbhavam), वृद्धम् (Vṛddham), जीर्णम् (Jīrṇam)
b- (H) Patharkā phūl, Carhelā; (Tam.) Kaḷapāsi; (Tel.) Ratipacchi, Ratha-pu; (Mar.) Dagaḍphul; (Eng.) The Iceland moss, Rock flower.

III- 1) 447-448 .शैलेयं शिलापुष्पम् । शैलेयनद्धेषु शिलातलेषु' इति कुमारः ॥ (Harshe)
2) 360 शैलजं शिलापुष्पम् । 'छडीले' इति ख्याता । (Harshe)

IV- 1) *Oak moss* Valuable addition to the raw materials of the perfume industry. It comprises various *Lichens* that grow on the bark of the trees......
These lichens contain oleoresinous substance which are extracted by means of solvent .... It is an essential element in lavender perfume. (Hill)

2) *Lichens* - At present day only one species is regarded as really of remedial valule, namely *Cetraria islandica* or the *island moss. This is above mentioned, contains a very large proportion of lichenine, and undoubtedly a valuable demulcent in various dyes-peptic and pulmonary complaints. several species of the same genus occur in India..... ....
The only lichens which are described as in general use as

The iceland moss (U.P.I.-118)

medicine in India are

Parmelia parlata and *P. perforata*.......

The lichen being employed as food in India is called in Telguratha-pu or rock, flower is used as a food. (Watt. Dict. Vol. IV. p. 638)

31 एलवालुकम् Elavālukam

[१]ऐलावालुकमालूकं वालुकं हरिवालुकम् ।
एल्वालुकं कपित्थं स्याद्दुर्वर्णं प्रसरं दृढम् ॥ ७७

एलावालुः सुगंधिः स्याच्छीतोऽत्यन्तं प्रकीर्तितः ।
विषविध्वंसनोऽत्युग्रः कण्डूकुष्ठव्रणान्तकृत ॥७८

एलावालुकं (Elāvālukam), आलूकं(Ālukam), वालुकं (Vālukam), हरिवालुकं (Harivālukam), एल्वालुकं (Elvālukam), कपित्थं (Kapittham), दुर्वर्णं (Durvarṇam), प्रसरं (Prasaràm), and दृढम् (Dṛḍham) are synonymous.

Elāvāluḥ is exteremely *'sītavīrya* and fragrant. It is antipoisonous and useful in pruritus, skin disorders and wounds.

Ambiguous

II- a- आलुकम् (Ālukam), वालुकम् (Vālukam), हरिवालुकम् (Harivālukam), एलागंधिकं (Elāgandhikam), सुगंधिकम् (Sugandhikam).

III-a-1) एरवारु (Ervāru); (के). वलिय वेळ्ळरि, आट्ट वेळ्ळरी; (ते.)डोसा काया (त.) वेळ्ळरी (Ayu. O. Ni.)

b-2) एलवालु सु. ३९ । कइकोल सदृशं कुष्ठगन्धि । (हिं) एलवा; (म) एलवालुक, कलंगडले; (ते). कुतुमवुडम चेट्टु, कुतुखुडमः, (क.) कलंगडे;, (सिं.) पेत्तिकपुरु (मल).एलवा । अस्य बीजं ग्राह्यम् ।एलवालुक कृष्णगन्धिक सदृशफलमिति डल्हणः । तेजपत्र वृक्षस्य फलमिति केचित् ।
(Ast. Hr. Kosha)

3) 238 हरिवालुक एलावालुकम् । सुगन्धिमरिचाकारि मुखशीतलताकारि द्रव्यम् ।'शीतलचिनी 'इति ख्यातम् । (Harshe)

4) 39 'एलावालुकमैलेयं सुगन्धि हरिवालुकम्' इत्यमरः । 'शीतलचिनी ' लोके प्रसिद्धम् । ' काष्ठसदृशं ' सुगन्धि द्रव्यम् इति भाव-मिश्रः । (Harshe)

IV- 1) Elāvāluka
Prunus cerasus (H.) Gilās.Sour cherry. (Watt VI. I. 346)

2) Ālubālu, *Prunus gilab,* Bark bitter, astringent, kernel nerve tonic, used for same purpose as hydrocynic acid. (Hill)

3) *Gisekia pharanceoides* Linn.

---

१ 'एलवालुक ' इति. पा.

(H.) Bālu-kā-sāg; (Mar.) Vaḷūchī bhājī (Tam.) Manlikkirai; (M) Panekirai (Dymock II Desai p. 357, chopra; watt. III 502)

4) Elavāluka had long remained unidentified but its possible botanical source was first pointed out in Vanaushadhi Darshika to be *Prunus cerasus* Linn. which is known as Āluālu आलुवालु in Punjab. (Balvantji p. 58)

32 सरलः Saralaḥ

सरलः पूतिकाष्ठं च चिडा पूतिद्रुमो मतः ॥
दीपवृक्षः स्निग्धदारुः प्रोक्तो मारीचपत्रकः ॥ ७९

सरलः स्निग्ध तिक्तगोष्णः कफमारुतनाशनः ।
वक्त्रस्रावस्वरभ्रंशनेत्ररोगव्रणान्तकृत् ॥ ८०

सरलः (Saralaḥ), पूतिकाष्ठं (Pūtikāṣṭham), चिडा (Cidā), पूतिद्रुमः (Pūtidrumaḥ), दीपवृक्षः (Dīpavṛk'saḥ), स्निग्धदारुः (Snigdhadāruḥ), and मारीचपत्रकः (Māricapatrakaḥ) are synonymous.

Sarala is bitter in taste, *uṣṇavīrya, snigdha,* pacifies *vāta kapha doṣas.* It is useful in excessive salivation, hoarseness of voice, diseases of eyes and wounds.

(Fam. Coniferae). Pinaceae

I- a- ***Pinus roxburghii*** Sargent
Syn. *P. longifolia* Roxb.

b- Roxburgh (Fl. indi.)

c- Outer and drier of Himlalayan slopes from Indus to Bhutan.

II- a- पूतिकाष्ठम् (Pūtikāṣṭham), दीपवृक्षः (Dīpavṛk'saḥ), स्निग्धदारुः (Snigdhadāruḥ), तुम्बी(Tumbī), उत्थितोपतरुः (Utthitopataruḥ), पीतद्रुः (Pītadruḥ)

b- (Sk.) Sarala; (H.) Cira, Cīḍa, ciḍā; (Mar.) Sarala devadāra; (Maly.) saralam; (Tel.) Saral; (Bom.) oleo resin = Gandha biroaza; (Eng.) The long leaved or three leaved pine.

III- 1) सरलः देवदारु विशेषः । सरलः पूतिकाष्ठे नाऽधोदारावक्रयोस्त्रिषु । इति मेदिनी । 'सरलं स्निग्धमत्यर्थं ...' इति भावमिश्रः । हिं चीर का पेड; तै. गरिके देवदारी चेट्टु; मल. चरळ.। (Ast. Hr. Kosha)

---

१ 'उत्थितो दीपतरु' इति चौखम्बा मुद्रिते पुस्तके साधु पाठः । तच्च पुस्तकं नोपलब्धं स्व.दि.का. कामत महोदयानां समये ।
'बीजपूतिद्रुरुच्छ्रितः' इति नि, शे. टीकासंमतः पाठः ।

IV- 1) *Pinus longifolia* Roxb.
(H.) Shāla, chir, oleoresin - Gandha birozā; (Bom.) Saral, oleoresin sarala drava, *śrīvāsa,* oil of terpentene is extracted from the crude product. The residue (Pale resin colophony) is called sundras in Bijanur.
Medicine - Oil long standing gonorrhoea .. diseases of urinary organs...bronchitis and haemorrhages. (Watt.Dict .VI-I. 244-45)

33 सप्तपर्णः Saptaparṇaḥ

सप्तपर्णः शुक्तिपर्णश्छत्रपर्णः सुपर्णकः ॥
सप्तच्छदो गूढपुष्पस्तथा शाल्मलिपत्रकः ॥ ८१

त्रिदोषशमनो हृद्यः सुरभिर्दीपनः सरः ॥
शूलगुल्मकृमीन् कुष्ठं हन्ति शाल्मलिपत्रकः ॥ ८२

सप्तपर्णः (Saptaparṇaḥ), शुक्तिपर्णः (Śuktiparṇaḥ), छत्रपर्णः (Chatraparṇaḥ), सुपर्णकः (Suparṇakaḥ), सप्तच्छदः (Saptacchadaḥ), गूढपुष्पः (Gūḍhapuṣpaḥ), and शाल्मलिपत्रकः (Śālmalipatrakaḥ) are synonymous.

Saptaparṇa pacifies three *doṣas,* is cordial, fragrant, stimulates digestive capacity, and is laxative. It is useful in colics, tumours (diverticulosis), worms and skin disorders.

Fam. Apocynacceae.

I- a- ***Alstonia scholaris*** R.Br.*

b- Dymock (in Pharm. indica)

c- Sub Himalayan tract from Jamna eastwards in Bengal, Burma and South India.

II- a- छत्रपर्णः (Chatraparṇaḥ), सुपर्णकः (Suparṇakaḥ), सप्तच्छदः (Saptacchadaḥ), शाल्मलिपत्रकः (Salmalipatrakaḥ),

b- (Sk.) Saptaparṇa; (H.) Satauṇā, Chatibana; (B) Chātim, Catwan; (Kol) Catin; (Santal) Chatina; (Tam.) Ezhilaipplai, wodrase; (Tel.)Edakula pāla palagaruda, edākula ariti, Edakula-ponna; (Mal.) Mukampala -pala; (Kan.) Janthala; (commercial name) Dita bark; (Med.) Alstonia (Alston) Chatim; (Cortex) Dala bark.

---

१ 'शक्तिपर्ण' इति क्षी. संमतः पाठः ।
* The current accepted name is - *A. scholaris* (Linn.) R. Br.

34 लाक्षा Lāk'sā

लाक्षा पलंकषा रक्ता दीप्तिश्च कृमिजा जतु ॥
क्षतघ्नी[२] रङ्गमाता च द्रुमव्याधिरलक्तकः ॥ ८३

लाक्षा तिक्तकषाया स्यात् स्निग्धा शोणितपित्तनुत् ॥
कृमिश्लेष्मव्रणान् हन्ति भूतज्वरार्तिनाशिनी ॥ ८४

('पित्तश्लेष्महरा रुच्या विशदा सुरभिर्लघुः ।
नेत्ररोगप्रशमनी व्रणशूलविनाशिनी॥')इति क्वचित् पुस्तके पाठः।

लाक्षा (Lāk'sā), पलंकषा (Palankaṣā), रक्ता (Raktā), दीप्तिः (Dīptiḥ), कृमिजा (Kṛmijā), जतु (Jatu), क्षतघ्नी (K'sataghnī), रङ्गमाता (Rangamātā), द्रुमव्याधिः (Drumavyādhiḥ) and अलक्तकः (Alaktakaḥ) are synonymous.

Lak'sā is bitter and *kaṣāya* (astringent) in taste and *snigdha* (unctuous). It is useful in bleeding disorders, worms, wounds, *bhūtabādhā* (antiseptic) and in fever.

According to some books - It pacifies *pitta - kapha doṣas,* is appetising, cleansing, fragrant and *laghu.* It is useful in diseases of the eye, and pains in wounds.

I- a- Lac.

II- a- पलंकषा (Palankaṣā), कृमिजा जतु (Kṛmijā Jatu), क्षतघ्नी (K'sataghnī), रङ्गमाता (Rangamātā), द्रुमव्याधिः (Drumavyādhiḥ), अलक्तकः (Alaktakaḥ).

b- (H) Lākh; (B), Gālā; (Mar.Guj.) Lāk, Lākha; (Tam.) Komburruki; (Tel.) Kommolaka.

III- 1) लाक्षा (Lāk'sā)वृक्षं वृक्षमारोहसी ... । ३॥
यद्दण्डेन यदिश्वा यद्वारुहसा कृतम् ॥३ ॥
तस्य त्वमसि निष्कृतिः ... ॥ ४॥ (AV.V. 7-5.)
लाक्षा लिङ्गाभिदुग्धे फाण्टान् पाययति । (Kauśika Su. 4. 4)

IV- 1) The name "Lac" is applied to the resinous incrustation formed on the bark or twigs of certain trees by the action of the lac-insect *Coccus lacca.* (Watt. IV- 570)
See कोशाम्रम of Raj. Ni.

2) *Lac* resinous substance secreted on the twigs of many trees by an insect *Trachardis lacca.* (Hill)

---

२ शतघ्नी इति चौ. मुद्रित पुस्तके पाठः ।

35 तामलकी Tāmalakī

तामलक्यजटा ताली तमालं तु तमालिनी[1] ॥
वितुन्नभूता[2] तमकं भूधात्री भ्वामलक्यपि[3] ॥ ८५

भूधात्री मधुरा तिक्ता वीर्यतः शिशिरा स्मृता ॥
पित्तं हन्ति कफास्रघ्नी दृष्टिदाहविनाशिनी ॥ ८६

तामलकी (Tāmalakī), अजटा(Ajaṭā), ताली (Tālī), तमालं (Tamālam), तमालिनी (Tamālinī), वितुन्नभूता (Vitunnabhūtā), तमकं (Tamakam), भूधात्री (Bhūdhātrī) and भ्वामलकी (Bhvāmalakī) are synonymous.

Bhūdhātrī is sweet amd bitter in taste, *śitavīrya*, pacifies *pitta, kapha,* and *rakta doṣas.* and is useful in the burning of the eyes.

Fam. Euphorbiaceae

I- a- ***Phyllanthus niruri*** Linn*

b- Roxburgh (Fl. Indi.)

II- a- अजटा (Ajatā), तमालिनी (Tamālinī), भूधात्री (Bhūdhārtī), भ्वामलकी (Bhwāmalakī), वितुन्ना (Vitunnā), उच्चटा (Uccatā) (H)Jarāmlā; (Sindhi) Niruri; (B) Bhuiāmla; (Mar.) Bhuiāwaḷi; (Tel.) Nelanelli; (Tam.) Kiḷakāya nelli; (Kan.) Kerunnelli; (Mal.) Kiḷanelli.

b- Jarāmlā. (Sindhi) Niruri; (B.) Bhuiāmla; (Mar.) Bhuiāwali; Tel. Nelanelli; (Tam.) Kilakāyanelli; (Kan.) Kerunnelli; (Mal.) Kiḷanelli See Watt Dict. *Phyllanthus urinaria* Linn.
(H) Lāla bhui āwalī, Hajārdanā; (Tel.) eravirica; (Tam.) Śivapuneḷḷi

IV- 1) भूम्यामलकी .... *Phyllanthus urinaria* (Ach. Priyavratji)

2) See Pandt. Bhagirath अजटा Ajaṭā

Note - There are two species 1) *P. niruri* Linn. and 2) *P. urinaria* Linn., Both the species are known and used as भूम्यामलकी of the basic books. The difference in appearance is only the stems and branches of the latter seem reddish tinted and the fruits are many more than the former, hence it is called 'Hājārdāna' and is generally found in cultivated area in winter season. It has much more stronger stem and many spreading branches than the former.

---

१ 'पुलाकिनी' इति क्षी. संमतः पाठः
२ '(वितुन्नकस्त्वज्झटा च झाटा साऽमलकीति च ।)' इति क्षी. संमतः पाठः
३ 'तामलक्युत्तमा ताली तमालं तु तमालिनी वितुन्नकस्त्वज्झटा च झाटासाऽमलकीति च ॥'
इति नि.शे. टीका संमतः पाठः।

* The current accepted name is *P. fraternus* Webster . Syn. *P. niruri auct.* (non. Linn).

36 लामज्जकम् Lāmajjakam

लामज्जकं सुनालं स्यादमृणालं लवं लघु ॥
इष्टकापथकं शीघ्रं दीर्घमूलं जलाश्रयम् ॥ ८७

लामज्जकं भवेत्तिक्तं हिमं चात्यन्तमिष्यते ।
पित्तप्रशान्तिजननं विषरक्तविनाशनम् ॥ ८८

लामज्जकं (Lāmajjakam), सुनालं (Sunālam), अमृणालं (Amrṇālam), लवं (Lavam), लघु (Laghu), इष्टकापथकं (Iṣṭakāpathakam), शीघ्रं (Śighram), दीर्घमूलं (Dirghamūlam), जलाश्रयम् (Jalāśrayam), are synonymous.

Lāmajjaka is bitter in taste, excessively *śitavirya,* pacifies *pittadoṣa.* It is useful in poison and blood disorders.

Not-identified

I

II- a- सुनालम् (Sunālam), अमृणालम् (Amrṇālam), दीर्घमूलम् (Dirghamūlam), जलाश्रयम् (Jalāśrayam), हिमम् (Himam), लघु (Laghu), तृड्दाह .... रक्तपित्तज्वरापहम् (Tṛḍdāha..raktapitta-Jwarāpaham).

III- See Uśira, Vālaka
97 लामज्जमुशीरम् । 'वीरणमूलं' लामज्जकमुशीरवत् पीतच्छवितृणविशेष' इति केचित् । (Harshe)

IV - 1) *Cymbopogon jwarankusa* Schult.*
(H) Lamajjak- used in cough and ch. rhumatism and cholera. (Chopra).

2) See acha. Yadavji लामज्जक (Lāmajjaka)
According to one veiw *Cymbopogon jwarankusa* Schult. a highly aromatic grass with aromatic roots should be accepted as *Lāmajjaka*. Ach. yadavji on the other hand, holds the view that if it is the *Ijakhir* of Unani Hakims as generally supposed, it can not be *Lāmajjak,* because ijakhira is 'hot ' (*Uṣṇavirya* ऊष्णवीर्य and *Lāmajjaka* is cold (*Śitavirya* शीतवीर्य).It is felt that this arrangement cannot hold unless the *Virya* of Ijakhir and its identity with *C. jwarancusa* is finally established...**(Balvantji p. 350)

---

१ 'लयम्' नि. शे. टीका । २ 'जलाशयम्' नि.शे. टीका संमतः पाठः ।

* The current accepted name is- *C. jwarancusa* (Jones) Schult.

** Acording to Ach. yadavji, *C. Jwarancusa* is *Ijakhira* (इजखिर) and is identified with भूतृण (भूस्तृण). It is observed that the roots of gramineac family (तृणकुल e.g. तृणपञ्चमूल are cold *'Sitavirya'* शीतवीर्य in action) Ach. Priyavratji considers भूतृण (भूस्तृण) belonging to the family *Labiate* (तुलसीकुल) and may be *Hyptis suaveolens* Poit. and लामज्जक to be a variety of *vetiveria . zizanioides* (Linn.) Nash. S. D. Kamat.

37 पद्मकः Padmakaḥ

पद्मको मलयश्चारुः पीतरक्तो मरुद्भवः[१] ॥
सुप्रभः शीतवीर्यश्च पाटलापुष्पवर्णकः ॥ ८९

पद्मकं शिशिरं स्निग्धं कषायं रक्तपित्तनुत् ॥
गर्भस्थैर्यकरं प्रोक्तं ज्वरच्छर्दिविषापहम् ॥ ९०
मोहदाहज्वरभ्रान्तिकुष्ठविस्फोटशान्तिकृत् ॥

पद्मकः (Padmakaḥ), मलयः (Malayaḥ), चारुः (Cāruḥ), पीतरक्तः (Pītaraktaḥ), मरुद्भवः(Marudbhavaḥ), सुप्रभः (Suprabhaḥ), शीतवीर्यः (Śītavīryaḥ), and पाटलापुष्पवर्णकः (Pāṭalāpuṣpavarṇakaḥ) are synonymous.

Padmaka is *kaṣāya* (astringent) in taste, *snigdha* (unctuous) and *śītavīrya.* It is useful in bleeding disorders, stabilising foetus, in fever, emesis, poisons, mental confusion, burning sensation of the body, delirium in fevers, skin disorders and eruptions on the skin.

Fam. Rosaceae

I- a- ***Prunus cerasoides*** D. Don
Syn. *P. puddum* Roxb. ex. Wall.[1]

b- Watt. Dict. (Vol. VI. I. 350)

II- a- पीतरक्त (Pītarakta), मरुद्भव (Marudbhawa), पाटलापुष्पवर्णकः (Pātalāpuṣpa varṇakaḥ), पद्मकाष्ठम् (Padamkāṣṭham),

b- (Sk.) Padmaka;(Mar. Bom.) Padmakāṣta; (H) Padam; (Eng.) The wild cherry of the Himalayas.

III- पद्मकम् सू.७ पद्मकम् । (के.) पद्मकुचेट्ट, एणुगुसहदेवी (मल). पतिमुकं पस्तुमुकं (Ast. Hr. Kosha)

38 धातुकी Dhātukī (धातकी – Dhātakī)

धातकी ताम्रपुष्पी च कुञ्जरा मद्यवासिनी[२] ॥९१
पार्वतीया सुभिक्षा च वह्निपुष्पा च शब्दिता ॥

धातकी कटुकोष्णा च मदकृत् विषनाशिनी ॥ ९२
अतिसारहरा गर्भस्थापनी कृमिरक्तनुत् ॥

धातकी (Dhātakī), ताम्रपुष्पी (Tāmrapuṣpī), कुञ्जरा (Kuñjarā), मद्यवासिनी

---

१ ' पीतरक्तश्च सुप्रभः ' इति नि.शे. टीका संमतः पाठः
२ 'मद्यपावनी ' इति. क्षी. संमतः पाठः
1 *P. Puddnm* Roxb. ex Brandis, non Miq.
Himalayan wild cherry. (U.P.I. p.494)

(Madyavāsinī), पार्वतीया (Pārvatīyā), सुभिक्षा (Subhikśā) and वह्निपुष्पा (Vahnipuṣpā) are synonymous.

Dhātakī is pungent in taste, *uṣnavīrya* and intoxicating. It is useful in poisons, diarrhoea, worms and bleeding disorders. It stabilises foetus.

(Fam. Lythraceae)

I- a- ***Woodfordia fruiticosa*** Kurz.
Syn. *W. floribunda* Salisb.

b- Dymock (Pharm.Ind.)

II- a- धातकी (Dhātakī), ताम्रपुष्पी (Tāmrapuṣpī), मद्यवासिनी (Madyawāsinī), लोध्रपुष्पिणी (Lodhrapuṣpiṇī), मद्यपुष्पा (Madyapuṣpā)

b- (H.B.) Dhāī; (Mar.) Dhāyatī, Dhāwasī, Dhāwaḍi; (Kan) Belā; (Tam.) Welakkai; (Tel.) Dhātaki.

III- b-1) धातकी सु. १०
ते सौरिंगि, जार्गी, पर्वापूर्वु. धातुकी पुड. त. काट्टात्तिपु, तातरिप्पुकु मल. तात रिप्पुवु. (Ast. Hr. Kosha)

39 प्रपौण्डीरकम् Prapauṇḍarīkam

प्रपौण्डरीकं चक्षुष्यं पुण्डर्यं पुण्डरीयकम् ॥९३
सितपुष्पं सुपुष्पं स्यात् श्रीपुष्पं सानुजानुजम् ॥

प्रपौण्डरीकं मधुरं कषायं तिक्तःशीतलम् ॥ ९४
पित्तरक्तव्रणान् हन्ति ज्वरदाहतृषापहम् ॥

प्रपौण्डरीकं (Prapauṇḍarīkam), चक्षुष्यं (Cakśuṣyam), पुण्डर्यं (Puṇḍaryam), पुण्डरीयकं (Puṇḍarīyakam), सितपुष्पं (Sitapuṣpam), सुपुष्पं (Supuṣpam) and सानुजानुजं (Sānujānujam) are synonymous.

Prapauṇḍarīka is sweet, *kaśāya* (astringent) and bitter in taste. It is *sītavīrya* and pacifies *pitta* and *rakta doṣas*. It is useful in wounds and alleviates burning sensation and thirst in fevers.

I Controversial

III- See चक्षुष्या (Cakśuṣyā), पद्मचारिणी (Padmacāriṇī),

1) 182 पुण्ड्रमिति प्रपौण्डरीकम् स्थलकमलम् । 'गुलाब' इति ख्यातम् । (Harshe)

---

* The current accepted name is - *W. fruiticosa* (Linn.) Kurz.

2) स्थलपद्मं – प्रपौण्डरीकम् । (Kṡīraswāmī) 2.4.28.

3) 382 'साधुपुष्प' स्थलपद्मम् द्वृष्टिकृत् पुण्डरीयकम्' इति रभसः । (Harshe)

4) 353 चक्षुष्यमिति कतको अम्बुप्रसादनः । (Harshe)

5) 171 पुण्ड्रः प्रपौण्डरीकं चक्षुष्यं मूलसाधकं मधुकम् । (Harshe)

6) प्रपौण्डरीकम् नेत्राश्चोतनार्हम् द्रव्यम् । अन्ये श्रीपुष्पमाहुः । (डल्हण)
*Vangueria spinosa. (Dr. Ghanekar)

10) पुण्डरीकः चि. ८ । शालपर्णी तुल्यपत्रको ऱ्हस्व वृक्षभेदः । स्वनामख्यातं यष्टीमधुद्रव्यात् स्थूलं मधुररसं नेत्राश्चोतनार्हं द्रव्यमिति डल्हणः ।अन्ये श्रीपुष्पमाहुः । (मरा.) पुण्डरीकवृक्ष, (त.) वरळ् त्तामरै (मल.) वीरपुणरै ।
(Ast. Hr. Kosha)

IV- It has till today evaded the identification of its botanical source and Puṇḍarīka पुण्डरीक has been recommended to be used in its place ... ... etc. (Balvantji p. 261)

40 कर्चूरः Karcūraḥ

कर्चूरो गन्धमूलश्च द्राविडः कार्शं[1] एव च ॥ ९५
वेधमुख्यो दुर्लभश्च कस्यचित् संमतः[2] शठी ॥

कर्चूरः कटुतिक्तोष्णो रुच्यो वातबलासजित् ॥ ९६
दीपनः प्लीहगुल्मार्शः शमनः कुष्ठकासहा ॥

कर्चूरः (Karcūraḥ), गन्धमूलः (Gandhaumūlaḥ), द्राविडः (Drāviḍaḥ), कार्श (Kārśa), वेधमुख्यः (Vedhamukhyaḥ), and दुर्लभः (Durlabhaḥ) are synonymous. Some have confounded it with शठी (Śaṭhī),

Karcūra is pungent and bitter in taste, *uṣṇavīrya*, appetiser and pacifies *vāta* and *kapha doṣas*. It simulates digestive capacity and is useful in disorders of spleen, tumours (diverticulosis), piles, disorders of skin and cough.

I- Several fragrant rhizomes of family *Zingiberaceae* are used as कर्चूर (Karcūra) by the practitioners.

Controversial

II- a- गन्धमूलः (Gandhamūlaḥ), द्राविडः (Drāvidaḥ), दुर्लभः (Durlabhaḥ), and शठी (Śaṭhi).

---

* *Vangueria spinosa* Roxb. (Sk.) Piṇḍītaka; (H.) Muyuna; (Bom) Alu ...etc. (Chopra Glossary) (p.252)
Syn. *Meyna laxiflora* Robyns. (U.P. I. p. 369, & 668)

१ 'काल्य' इति. क्षी. संमतः पाठः ।
२ 'कस्यचित् संमता शठी' । इति. क्षी. संमतः पाठः ।

b- (Mar.) Kacora, Kāpurkācarī

IV- See Palāśagandhā, Gandhapalāśā
Tavakśira & Śaṭhi

1) *Curcuma zedoaria* Rosc.*
Syn. *C. zerumbat* Roxb.
(Dr. Dymock, Dr. Kirtikar, Ach. yadavaji)

2) कर्चूर (Karcura)
Hedychium spicatum Ham. ex Smith.
(Chopra; Br. Ni. Pade; Dr. Mantri, Dymock)

3) कापुर काचली (Kāpur Kācalī)
Curcuma zedoaria Roxb.
Syn. *C. aromatica* (Salisb.) Roxb.
(Dr. Kirtikar) wild turmeric (Watt.)

4) C.S. Su. 27.159; 8.Su. 39.6 (Vā.) What is known at present *Karchura* (*C. zedoaria* Rosc.) is rhizome and not a fruit. Its inclusion in the group of fruits (फलवर्ग) is not understandable. (Balavantji p. 82.)

5) शठी चन्द्रमूल, गन्धपलाश
Kaempheria galangal Linn.
चंद्रमूल, कापुर कचरी, शठी, कचुल, गलंगुल.
Chopra, Kirtikar, Dymock.

6) *Hedychium spicatum* Ham. कापुर कचरी, सठी, the Sanskṛt name for *C. zedoaria* is sometimes erroneously applied to this plant, which is not mentioned in राजनिघण्टु.

Two kinds of कापुर काचरी Kāpura Kācari are found in Bombay market Viz.Chinese and Indian. The latter was supposed by Royle to be '*Sittarittee, lessor galangal* of Ainslie but Moidin sherif states that the *Sitarittee* of the Tamils is true *Lessor Galangal* which statement appears to be correct. (Dymock)

41 मनः शिला Manaḥśilā

मनःशिला मनोगुप्ता मनोह्वा कुनटी शिला ॥९७
मनोज्ञा नागजिह्वा च गोला नेपालिका कला ॥

मनःशिला कटुस्तिक्ता तथोष्णा विषनाशनी ॥९८
भूतावेशभयं हन्ति प्रलेपतिलकादिभिः ॥

D. K. Kamat has not commented on this durg as this is a mineral in origin. It is Arsenicum rubrum; *Realgar*. (Eng.)

* The current accepted name is - *C. zedoaria* (Berg.) Rosc.

मनः शिला (Manaḥśilā), मनोगुप्ता (Manoguptā), मनोह्वा (Manohvā), कुनटी (Kunaṭī), शिला (Śilā) मनोज्ञा(Manojñyā), नागजिह्वा (Nāgajihvā), गोला (Golā), नेपालिका (Nepālikā) and कला (Kalā) are synonymous.

Manaḥśilā is pungent, bitter in taste, *uṣṇavīrya*.It is antiposionous and by external application eg. *Tilaka* etc. is antiseptic. *(Bhūtaghna.)*

42 सिन्दूरः Sindūraḥ

सिन्दूरं रक्तरेणुश्च नागगर्भं च नागजम् ॥ ९९
शृङ्गारभूषणं श्रीमद् वसन्तोत्सव मण्डनम् ॥

सिन्दूरमुष्णकटुकं विषदुष्टव्रणापहम् ॥ १००
त्वग्दोषकुष्ठवीसर्प जीर्णज्वरहरं परम् ॥

This is not commented upon by late vd. D. K. Kamat. being mineral in origin.

Red lead. *Plumbi oxidum rubrum*.सिन्दूरः

सिन्दूरं (Sindūram), रक्तरेणुः (Raktareṇuḥ), नागगर्भम् (Nāgagarbham), नागजं (Nāgajam), शृंगारभूषणं (Sṛṅgārabhūṣaṇam), श्रीमद् (Śrīmad), वसन्तोत्सव मण्डनम् (Vasantotsavamaṇḍanam) are synonymous.

Sindūra is pungent in taste, *uṣṇavīrya*. It is useful in poisons, septic wounds, skin disorders, erysipelas and chronic fevers.

गिरिसिन्दूरम् Girisindūram *(15)

महागिरिषु चाल्पीयान् पाषाणान्तःस्थितो रसः ॥१०१
शुष्कः शोणः स निर्दिष्टः गिरिसिन्दूर संज्ञकः ॥

त्रिदोषशमनं भेदि रसबन्धनमग्निदम् ॥१०२
देहलोहकरं नेत्र्यं गिरिसिन्दूरमीरितम् ॥

* In the mountainous parts of some regions, there appears a red coloured substance within the stones. This red coloured dried substance is called as गिरिसिन्दूर *Girisindūra*. The stanza appears in Rasendra cūḍāmanī (Chapter II). According to some scholars it is red oxide of mercury. To differantiate it from सिन्दूर vide supra the adjective गिरि (*Giri*) is used here.

It pacifies all the three *doṣas* and is *Bhedi*, useful in the *bandhanakarma* of mercury (रसबन्धनं), improves digestive (meatabolic) capacity of the body, makes the body strong and is beneficial for eyes (*cakśuṣya*.)

43 सौराष्ट्री Saurāṣtrī (Alum)

सौराष्ट्री चामृतासङ्गा काङ्क्षी काक्षी सुराष्ट्रजा ॥ १०३
अजिता तुवरी स्तुत्या मृत्सा मृत्स्ना मृतालकम् ॥

(अन्यच्च-सौराष्ट्री चामृता काङ्क्षी फटिका मृत्तिका मता ।
आढकी तुवरी त्वन्या मृत्स्ना मृत् सुरमृत्तिका ॥")

कांक्षी कटुकषायास्यात्केश्या चैव विषापहा ॥१०४
कण्डूविसर्पश्वित्राणां नाशनी व्रणरोपणी ॥

(This is not being a plant has not been commented upon by late vd. D.K. Kamat).

सौराष्ट्री (Saurāṣṭrī), अमृतासङ्गा (Amṛtāsangā), काङ्क्षी (Kāṅkśī), काक्षी (Kākśī), सुराष्ट्रजा (Surāṣṭrajā), अजिता (Ajitā), तुवरी (Tuwarī), स्तुत्या (Stutyā), मृत्सा (Mṛtsā), मृत्स्ना (Mṛstnā), मृतालक (Mṛtalaka) are synonyms.

There is another reading (अन्यच्च) written here which has mentioned another drug that is सौराष्टी (मृत) (a kind of Earth or clay or alum in powder form) the synonyms of which are सौराष्ट्री (Saurāṣṭrī), अमृता (Amṛtā), काङ्क्षी (Kāṅkśī), फटिका (Phaṭikā), मृत्तिका (Mṛttikā), आढकी (Āḍhakī), तुवरी (Tuwarī), अन्या मृत्स्ना (Anyā Mṛtsnā)and सुरमृत्तिका (Suramṛttikā).

Kāṅkśī is pungent, and *kaśāya* (astringent) in taste. It is beneficial to hairs and useful in poison, pruritus erysipelas, leucoderma and healing of wounds.

४४ *गन्धकद्वयम् Gandhakadwayam

गन्धको गन्धपाषाणो लेलीतो गन्धमादनः ॥१०५
पूतिगन्धो बलिवसा गन्धाश्मा धातुहा बली ॥

गन्धकः कटु तीक्ष्णोष्णस्तीव्रगन्धोऽतिगन्धकृत् ॥१०६
विषघ्नः कुष्ठकण्डूतिकच्छ्रत्वग्दोषनाशनः ॥

---

* Here the different types of readings in गणद्रव्यावली should be noted. शोढल (Soḍhala) in गणद्रव्यावली of Dhn. Ni. has accepted the reading as मनःशिला ससिन्दूरं सौराष्ट्री गन्धकोमची । (p.4)
Anandāśram reading is मनःशिला ससिन्दूरं सौराष्ट्री गन्धकद्वयम् ।
Insted of गन्धकद्वयम् Gandhakadwayam it has also mentioned another reading as 'गन्धमारिका' but if it is accepted as 'गन्धमाचिका' then the drugs will be as गन्धक & माचिका.
Taking into cousideration the next plant 'माचिका' and according to the पर्याय- गुणसंग्रह नामावली of Dhn. Ni., the reading माचिका seems to be correct. It is also to be noted that the MSS containing माचिका was defintely before Śoḍhala as he had mentioned the synonyms of माचिका.-अम्बष्ठा after गन्धक also in his गणद्रव्यावली ,पर्याय नामावली & गुणसंग्रह see Pages 4. (stanza 42), (Stanza 444);. Page 92 (Stanza 32); Page 122 (Stanza 360) of शोढल नि. Soḍhala Ni.

S.D. Kamat.

Late vd. D.K. Kamat has not commented upon this drug as this is mineral in origin . गन्धक (Gandhaka) = Sulphur. Two types of गन्धकः (Gandhakaḥ),has the synonyms as गन्धपाषाणः (Gandhapāṣāṇaḥ), लेलीतः (Lelītaḥ), गन्धमादनः (Gandhamādanaḥ), पूतिगन्धः (Pūtigandhaḥ),बलिवसा (Balivasā),गन्धाश्मा (Gandhaśamā), धातुहा (Dhātuhā), and बली (Balī).

Gandhaka is pungent in taste, *uṣṇavīrya* , having sharp smell, and causes excessive smell, is antipoisonous. It is useful in disorders of skin, pruritus, scabies and improves complexion of skin.

वटसौगंधिकः Vaṭasaugandhikaḥ

वटसौगंधिको गन्धो गन्धको गन्धमादनः ॥१०७
लेलीनो गन्धपाषाणो लेलीतश्च निकृन्तनः ॥

त्वग्दोष कुष्ठवीसर्प लोहसंहारि सूतहा ॥१०८
रसायनवरो ह्येष कटूष्णो गन्धको मतः ॥

Though the reading वटसौगंधिक is accepted here according to Ānanda'srama, the 'Soḍhala Nighaṇṭu has acccepted the reading as पट्टसौगंधिक (Paṭṭasaugandhīka) which seems a better one.

गन्धः (Gandhaḥ),गन्धकः (Gandhakaḥ), गन्धमादनः (Gandhamādanaḥ), लेलीनः (Lelīnaḥ), गन्धपाषाणः (Gandhapāsānaḥ), लेलीतः (Lelītaḥ), and निकृन्तनः (Nikṛntanaḥ), are synonyms for वटसौगंधिकः (Vaṭasaugandhikaḥ).

It is useful in skin disorders like कुष्ठ *Kuṣṭha*, वीसर्प *Vīsarpa* (erysipelas). It is used as लोहसंहारी Lohasamhārī and सूतहा (Sūtāhā). i.e .māraṇa process of metals and mercury It is pungent (*kaṭu)* in taste, *uṣṇavīrya* and useful as *rasāyana.*(rejuvinating).

45 माचिका Mācikā (अम्बष्ठा - Ambaṣṭhā)

माचिका प्रथिताऽम्बष्ठा तथाऽम्बाऽम्बालिकाऽम्बिका ॥१०९
अम्बष्ठका कषाया च सा प्रोक्ता मुखवाचिका ॥

अम्बिका तु रसे तिक्ता तथोष्णा कफनाशिनी ॥ ११०
अर्शोघ्नी श्वयथूत्थान परिपंथितया स्मृता ॥

(अन्यच्च -
माचिका तु कषाया च कण्ठ्या वातबलासजित ॥
पित्तप्रकोपशमनी व्रणशोधनरोपणी ॥)

---

१ 'अम्बष्ठा माचिकायां च चांगेरी पाठयोरपि ॥' 'Sodhala p. 84

माचिका (Mācikā), अम्बष्ठा (Ambaṣṭhā),अम्बा (Ambā), अम्बालिका (Ambālikā), अम्बिका (Ambikā), अम्बष्ठका (Ambaṣṭhakā), कषाया (Kaṣāyā), and मुखवाचिका (Mukhavācikā) are synonymous.

Ambikā is bitter in taste, *uṣṇavirya*, pacifies *kaphadoṣa* and useful in piles and oedema.

According to other source.

Mācikā is *kaṣāya* (astringent) in taste, beneficial for throat, pacifies *vāta, kapha* and *pitta doṣas* and useful as wound cleansing and healing.

Fam. Malvaceae

I- a- ***Hibiscus cannabinus*** Linn.

b- Watt. Dict. (IV-230). C- Cultivated in India for its fibres. Wild in the East of the Northern Ghat.

II- a- माचिका (Mācikā), अम्बष्ठा (Ambaṣṭhā), दृढवल्का (Dṛḍhavalkā), चित्रपुष्पी (Citrapuṣpī), छिन्नपत्रा (Chinnapatrā),

b- (Sk), Ambaṣṭha, Mācikā; (H.) Āmbārī; (B) Patasana, Sana; (Bom). Āmbārī (B); Mest Pāt; (Mar.) Āmbāḍī; (Tam.) Pulicāyi, Patungi; (Tel.) Gongura; (Konkan) Āmbaḍā; (Mal.) Kattu bellurana; (Kan.)Pudon; (Eng.) Brown hemp. Deccan hemp.

III- See Śwetāmli, Kśudrāmlikā

b- 1) द्विधाऽम्बिका (Dwidhāmbikā) (Raj. Ni. Śatā. Gaṇa.)

2) अम्बष्ठा (Ambaṣṭhā) -Āmbāḍī (Ni.Sir. Pade)

3) अम्बिका *Hibiscus cannabinus* ityeke. (Ast. Hr. Kosha).

46 सिक्थकम् Sikthakam. (Bee's wax).

सिक्थकं मधुकं सिक्थं मधूच्छिष्टं मधूत्थितम् ॥ १११
मधुशेषं मदनकं मधुजं माक्षिकाश्रयम् ॥

सिक्थकं स्निग्धमधुरं भूतघ्नं भग्नसंधिकृत्त ॥ ११२
हन्ति वीसर्पकण्डवादीन् व्रणरोपणमुत्तमम् ॥
भेदनं पिच्छिलं स्वादु कुष्ठवातास्रजिन्मृदु ॥११३

This has not been commented upon by Late vd. D.K. Kamat as it is not a plant in origin.

सिक्थकं (Sikthakam), मधुकं (Madhukam), सिक्थं (Siktham), मधूच्छिष्टं (Madhucchiṣṭam), मधूत्थितम् (Madhūtthitam), मधुशेषं (Madhūśeṣam),

मदनकं (Madanakam), मधुजं (Madhujam) माक्षिकाश्रयम् (Mākśikāśrayam) are synonyms.

Sikthaka is sweet in taste, *snigdha* (unctuous), antiseptic, union promoting in fracture. It is useful in erysipelas, pruritus, wound healing, and is *bhedana, picchila* (slimiy), and useful in disorders of skin, *vātarakta* (gout) and is *mṛdu* (soft).

47 (सर्जरसः) रालः Rālaḥ

रालः सर्जरसः शालः क्षणः कलकलोद्भवः ।।
ललनः शालनिर्यासो यक्षधूपोऽग्निवल्लभः ।। ११४

रालः स्वादुः कषायोष्णः स्तम्भनो व्रणरोपणः ।।
विषादिभूतहन्ता च भग्नसन्धानकृत् मत : ।।११५

रालः (Rālaḥ), सर्जरसः (Sarjarasaḥ), शालः (Śālaḥ), क्षणः (Kśaṇaḥ), कलकलोद्भवः (Kalakalodbhavaḥ), ललनः (Lalanaḥ), शालनिर्यासः (Śālaniryāsaḥ), यक्षधूपः (Yakśadhūpaḥ) and अग्निवल्लभः (Agnivallabhaḥ) are synonymous.

Rāla is sweet and *kaṣāya* (asgtringent) in taste, *uṣṇavīrya, stambhana* (astringent in action), wound healer, antipoison, antiseptic and union promoter in fractures.

(Fam. Dipterocarpaceae)

I- a- Resin exudated from the tree
Shorea robusta Gaertn.*

b- Watt. Dict. Vol. VI-2. 674

c- See below IV-2

II- a- सर्जरसः (Sarjarasaḥ), शालनिर्यासः (Śālaniryāsaḥ), अग्निवल्लभः (Agnivallabhaḥ), बहुरूपः (Bahurūpaḥ),व्रणरोपणः (Vraṇaropaṇaḥ)

b- (H.) Śāla (tree), Ral; Dhūpa (resin); (B) Sāla, (resin) ral; (santal) Sarjam; (Mar.)Rāla, guggulu; (Tam.) Kungilium=resin; (Tel.) Gugultree, Gugilamu-resin; (Kan.) Kabbu-tree, guggala=resin (Eng.) Thesal tree.

Note - The gum resin exuded from this tree is known as रालः (राला) (Rālā). It is not श्रीवेष्ट (Śrīveṣṭa) of Dhn. Ni. It is recorded यक्षधूप (Yakśadūpa) by Dhn. Ni; Raj. Ni. notes देवेष्टा (Deveṣṭā) which

---

* The current accepted name is - *S. robusta* Gaertn. f.

is contrary to देवेष्ट (Deveṣṭā) of Dhn. ni. See श्रीवेष्ट (Śrīveṣṭa) infra.

III-b-1) सर्जक इति । 'असनो बीजकः शालः सर्जः प्राहुः शालं सर्ज च सुरय' इति हलायुधः । 'शालः सर्जः सर्जरसः कान्तो मरिचपत्रक' इति केयदेवः ।

2) अजकर्ण शालप्रभेदः । 'सर्जकोऽन्योऽजकर्णः स्याच्छालो मरिचपत्रक' इति भावमिश्रः । (Harshe)

3) 447 'साले तु सर्ज काश्र्याश्वकर्णकाः सस्यसंवर' इत्यमर : ॥
See श्रीवेष्टकः, सर्जकः, सरलः

4) सर्जरसः 'राल' इति प्रसिद्धः । Dalhana S.Su. 38. 24.

5) शालः ।सू.३ । Engl. white damar tree; Indian copal tree; *Vateria indica, Shorea robusta; Vateria malabarica; Pinus damar.* सर्जकोन्योऽजकर्णः भा.प्र । This large evergreen tree is indigenous to south western India. See. सर्ज
(Ast. Hr. Kosha)

IV- 1) Greeks and Romans were familiar with many of resinous materials that are in use today. As for example Ambar, Mastic, sundrus. (Hill)

2) *Habitat* - It occurs along the base of tropical Himalaya from sutelja to Assam, Eastern districts of central India.
(Watt. Dict. VI.IIs. 673)

48 कासीसम् Kāsīam. Ferrous sulphate.

कासीसं धातुकासीसं केसरं तप्तलोमशम् ॥
कासीसं तु कषायोष्णमम्लं वातबलासजित् ॥ ११६
विषनेत्ररुजः श्वित्रं हन्ति कुष्ठव्रणानपि ।

(This is being mineral in origin not commented upon by Late Vd D.K. Kamat)

कासीसम् (Kāsīsam), धातुकासीसं (Dhātukāsīsam), केसरं (Kesaram), तप्तलोमशम् (Taptalomaśam) are synonyms.

Kāsīsa is *kaṣāya* (astringent) and sour in taste, *uṣṇavīrya* and pacifies *vāta* and *kapha doṣas.*

It is useful in poisons, diseases of the eye, leucoderema and ulcers due to skin disorders (or leprosy).

49 (पुरः Puraḥ) गुग्गुलुः Gugguluḥ.

गुग्गुलुः कालनिर्यासो जटायुः कौशिकः पुरः ॥ ११७
नक्तंचरः शिवो दुर्गो महिषाक्षः पलंकषः ॥
गुग्गुलुः पिच्छिलः प्रोक्तः कटुस्तिक्तः कषायवान् ॥ ११८
वर्ण्यः स्वर्यो लघुः सूक्ष्मो रूक्षो वातबलासजित् ॥

गुग्गुलुः (Gugguluḥ), कालनिर्यासः (Kālaniryāsaḥ), जटायुः (Jaṭāyuḥ), कौशिकः(Kauśikaḥ), पुरः (Puraḥ), नक्तंचरः (Naktancaraḥ), शिवः (Śivaḥ), दुर्गः (Durgaḥ), महिषाक्षः (Mahiṣākśaḥ) and पलंकषः (Palamkaṣaḥ) are synonymous.

Guggulu is pungent, bitter and *kaṣāya* (astringent) in taste and slimy (*Picchila*). It improves complexion, beneficial to voice, is *laghu, sukśma* (penetrating), *rukśa* (roughning) and pacifies *vāta* and *kapha doṣas*.

I- Generic name, includes more than one species but without clear description. Some species of Indian trees from which गुग्गुलुः *Gugguluḥ* is obtained are noted herebelow. Besides these Indian species several Arabian and African varieties of Guggula are imported into India for which the readers may see the books referred below.

(Fam. Burseraceae)

I A-a- ***Commiphora mukul*** Engl.*
Syn. *Balsamodendron mukul* Hook. ex Stocks

b- Dr. Waring (Pharma. Ind.)

c- Sind, Kathiawar, Rajputana.

B-a- ***Commiphora roxburghii*** Engl.
Syn. B. *roxburghii* Arn.

b- Dymock (Pharm. Indi.)

c- Bengal and Assam.

II-A & B -a-कालनिर्यासः (Kālaniryāsāḥ), कौशिकः (Kauśikaḥ), पुरः (Puraḥ), महिषाक्षः (Mahiṣākśaḥ), पलंकषः (Palaṅkaṣaḥ), मरुद्देशः (Maruddeśaḥ)

A &B b- (H.B.) Gugal, Mukul; (Kan.) Guggal; (Mar.) Guggu!a; (Tam.) Gukkal, Gukkulu; (Tel.)Maisaci gugul; (Eng.) Gum Gugul, Guggula of Indian Mat. Medi.

III-a- Guggul AV-XIV-38.2
S.Br.iii-5.2-16; A.Br. 1-28
T.S. VI -2-8.6; Ys. iii-8-5 (Harshe)

---

*The current accepted name is *Commiphora wightii* (Arnott) Bhandari

IV- 1) *Balsamodendron roxburghii* Arn.
Covered with dirt and hair, paper of greenish yellow colour with tinge of red, waxy, soft, brittle ... with water it forms greenish white emulsion, when inflamed it swells and sputters instead of burning with clear flame like of गुग्गुल of *B. serrata.* (Dymock)

2) *Opopanax bdellium* -Bdellium is a bitter aromartic gum resin obtained from *Comiphora mukul* of India and *C.africana* of Africa. Macca balsam is obtained from *C. opobalsumum* an african species (Hill)

3) The medicinal properties of Bdellium aproximate closely to those of Myrrha and as it is much cheaper, it may be substituted for it in Dispensary practice. (Dr. Waring)

4) *Balsamodendron berryi* Arnott
Habitat - A tree of forests on the East side of the Nilgiris.
Gum.- It is very fragrant and yields a gum resin.

5) *Balsamodendron kataf* Kunth.
African Bedillium
Syn. *Balsamea erythrea* Angler.
Amyris kataf Forsk.
Hemprichia erythrea Erhenbung
Vern. (Bom) Bysabol; (Cutch) Mahisasbol; (Sans) Mahisabol.
Gum. This gum resin reaches Bombay from Berbera. The purer kinds very much resembling Myrrha, with which it has been confused by many authors.... Bysabol darker and more reddish than the myrrha.

6) *B. pubecense* Stocks.
opaque Bdellium.
Vern. (Mar.) Bayisa gugal.
Habitat - Baluchistan, Sindh, Karachi. Gum Resin - Small quantity tasteless inodorus gum, almost entirely soluble in water (Watt. Volu. I- 365 . 368)

7) Guggul exported to India from Arabia and Africa is obtained from the following trees.

a- *Balsamodendron opobalsamum* Kunth.
Gum. The famous Balsam of Gelad or Balsum of Mucca is imported into Bombay from Arabia.

b- *B. kataf* Kth.
African Bdellium .This gum resin reaches Bombay from Barbar Sank and cutch -Mahisha bol.

c- *B. myrrha*
Myrrha M. bol - a small tree of Arabia and of african coast at the Red sea. often cultivated in western India. (Watt. Dict.)

50 कुन्दुरुः Kunduruḥ

कुन्दुरुः स्यात् कुन्दुरुकः शिखरी कुन्द्रगोपुरः ॥ ११९
सुकुन्द्रस्तीक्ष्णगन्धश्च पालिंदो भीषणो बली ॥
कुन्दुरुः कटुकस्तित्तगे वातश्लेष्मामयापहः ॥ १२०
पाने लेपे च शिशिरः प्रदरामयशान्तिकृत् ॥

कुन्दुरुः (Kunduruḥ), कुन्दुरुकः (Kundurukaḥ), शिखरी (Śikharī), कुन्द्रः (Kundraḥ), गोपुरः (Gopuraḥ), सुकुन्द्रः (Sukundraḥ), तीक्ष्णगन्धः (Tīkṣṇagandhaḥ), पालिंदः (Pālindaḥ), भीषणः (Bhīṣaṇaḥ) and बली (Balī) are synonymous.

Kunduru is pungent and bitter in taste and pacifies the diseases due to *vāta* and *kapha*. It causes coolness or refregertion after external application and oral use. It is useful in vaginal discharge.

I- a- Exuded substance like gum from the tree सल्लकी (Sallakī) (infra No.52)

b- Roxburgh (Fl. indi)

II- a- तीक्ष्णगन्धश्च (Tīkṣṇagandhaśca), पालिन्दः (Pālindaḥ), सौराष्ट्री (Saurāṣṭrī), गोपुरकः (Gopurakaḥ), बहुगन्धः (Bahugandhaḥ)

b- (H.) Kundur, salai, Salgā; (B) Luban, kundar, Salai; (Bom.) 'sale dup; (Tel.) Palangi Sāmraṇi; (Tam.) Kundurukam, Mādimar; (Mal.)Citinni; (Kan.) Mādimar; (Gond) Salla; (Santal) Sālga; (Guj) Sāledo, Dhupdo; (Mar.) Sāler, Salay.

Note - These vernacular names are applied also to the kundaru giving trees.
(Eng.) Piney , white damar, Indian Copal, White damar of India.

51 श्रीवेष्टकः (सरल निर्यासः) Śrīweṣṭakaḥ

श्रीवेष्टको धूपवृक्षः क्षीरशीर्षः[1] खरद्रुमः ॥ १२१
श्रीवासः पायसः[2] श्याह्वः क्षीरस्रावस्तथा दधि ॥

---

१ 'क्षीरः शीर्षः' फलद्रुमः' । इति आनन्दा. पाठान्तरम् : ।
२ पायसश्चाह्वः इति आनन्दाश्रममुद्रिते पुस्तके पाठः।

श्रीवेष्टः स्वादुतिक्तःस्तु कषायो व्रणरोपणः ॥ १२२
कफपित्तास्रजान् हन्ति ग्रहघ्नः शीर्षरोगनुत् ॥

श्रीवेष्टकः (Śrīveṣṭakaḥ), धूपवृक्षः (Dhūpavṛkśaḥ), क्षीरशीर्षः (Kśīraśīrṣaḥ), खरद्रुमः (Kharadrumaḥ), श्रीवासः (Śrīvāsaḥ), पायसः (Pāyasaḥ), श्याह्वः (Śryāhvaḥ), क्षीरस्रावः (Kśīrasrāvaḥ), and दधि (Dadhi) are synonymous.

Śrīveṣta is sweet, bitter and *kaṣāya* (astringent) in taste and useful in diseases due to *kapha -pitta - rakta* and in wounds. It is destroyer of *grahās* (Seizures) and diseases of head.

I (A resinous substance of white or straw colour exuded from certain Indian trees some of which are noted herebelow. Besides these Indian trees there are also African trees of which the resinous white substance is imported into India under the name candrus).

Fam. Dipterocarpaceae.

I A-a- ***Vateria indica*** Linn.
Syn *V. malabarica* Blume.

b- Watt. Dict. Vol. VI. -IV 223 -225

c- See below IV.

II- A-a- धूपवृक्षः (Dhūpavṛk'saḥ), क्षीरः (K'sīraḥ), शीर्षफलद्रुमः (Sirṣaphaladṛumaḥ), श्रीवासः (Srīvāsaḥ).पायसश्चाह्वः (Pāyasa'scāhvaḥ), क्षीरस्रावः (K'sīrasrāvaḥ), दधि (Dadhi)

IV- 1) *Vateria indica* Linn.
A large evergreen tree of Western peninsula from Kanara to Travankore.
(H.) safed damar, sundras; (Bom.) Rāl; (Tam.) vellui damar; (Tel.) Dipa damaru, Tella damaru; (Kan). Dupa marum.
The tree yields a true resin ... known as white damar or piney resin It occurrs in three forms
1st Compact Piney resin
2nd Cellular Piney resin
3rd dark coloured Piney resin.
Resin ... In south canara it is used for chalking boats (P. 224)
Oil - from fruits *Medicine*- Diarrhoea. It closely resembles the solid fats of Garcina Indica-kokum butter. (Watt. IV-223-25)

2) *Hopea odorata* Roxb.
The rock Dammar of commerce.
Syn. *H. eglandulosa* Roxb.
Burma Thengan.
... This seems such a nice, pure white resin ....

Habitat . A large evergreen tree common in the forests all over Burma from chittagong and Martaban down to tenasserium .. Copal like resin pure white. (Watt. Dict. IV. 271)

52 शल्लकी Śallakī

शल्लकी वल्लकी ह्लादा सुरभिः सुस्रवा च सा ॥ १२३
अश्वमूत्री कुन्दुरुकी गजभक्षा महेरणा ॥

शल्लकी स्यात् कषायाऽतिशीता वीर्ये प्रकीर्तिता ॥ १२४
बलासं हन्ति पित्तस्य प्रकोपशमनी मता ॥

शल्लकी (Śallakī), वल्लकी (Vallaki), ह्लादा (Lhādā), सुरभिः (Surabhiḥ), सुस्रवा (Susravā), अश्वमूत्री (Aśvamūtrī), कुन्दुरुकी (Kundurukī), गजभक्षा (Gajabhakśā) and महेरणा (Maheraṇā) are synonymous.

Śallakī is *kaṣāya* (astringent) in taste and excessively *śītavīrya.* It pacifies *kapha* and *pitta doṣas.*

(Fam. Burseraceae)

I- a- ***Boswellia serrata***, Roxb.*
Syn. *B. thurifera* Roxb. ex Flem.
B. glabra Roxb.

b- Roxburgh (Fl. Indi.)

c- Sub. Himalayan tract from sutlej to Nepal, Berar to Rajputana, Deccan, Konkan. common over hills around Pune (Mahajan)

II- a- सुरभिः (Surabhiḥ), सुस्रवा (Susrawā), कुन्दुरुकी (Kundurukī) गजभक्षा (Gajabhaksā),

b- for vernacular names see कुन्दरुः (Kundaruḥ)
(Eng.) Indian frankincense tree. Indian olibanum.

III- See कुन्दरुः Kundaruḥ

a-1) C.Su. 4.32; 5.19.
S.Su. 25. 28. A.H. Su. 21. 15. (Balvantji)

2) कुन्दरुक Kunduruka
C.Ci. 26. 64
S.Su, 26.64.
A.H. Su. 21. 15 (Balvantji)

b-1) 33 शल्लकी गजभक्ष्या । 'सुगान्धिद्रवका नित्या पङ्क्तिपत्रा तु शल्लकी ।
(Harshe)

IV- 1) कुन्दरुकं

* The current accepted name is - *B. serrata* Roxb. ex Coleb.

The gum of Boswellia serrata Roxb. (शल्लकी चोपः Dalhan)

2) शल्लकी Śallakī

Kunduruka has been defined by Dalhan as Śallakicopa शल्लकी चोपः or the gum obtained from the trunk of the tree.

(Balvantji p. 392).

53 कम्पिल्लकः Kampillakaḥ

कम्पिल्लकोऽथरक्तगङ्गो रेची रेचनकस्तथा ॥ १२५
रञ्जनो लोहिताङ्गश्च कम्पिल्लो रक्तचूर्णकः ॥
कम्पिल्लको विरेची स्यात् कटूष्णो व्रणनाशनः ॥ १२६
गुल्मोदरविबन्धाध्मश्लेष्मक्रिमिविनाशनः ॥

कम्पिल्लकः (Kampillakaḥ), रक्तगङ्गः(Raktāngaḥ), रेची (Recī), रेचनकः (Recanakah),रञ्जनः (Rañjanaḥ), लोहिताङ्गः (Lohitāngaḥ), कम्पिल्लः (Kampillaḥ) and रक्तचूर्णकः (Raktacūrṇakaḥ) are synonymous.

Kampillaka is pungent in taste, *uṣṇavīrya* and purgative. It is useful in healing wounds, tumors (diverticulosis), ascites, constipation, tympanitis and worms due to *kaphadoṣa.*

I- General understanding of modern writers on this drug which is identified as *Mallotus philippinensis* Muel* - Arg.; Eng. Monkey face tree and commentators on Caraka, Suśruta and Vāgbhat express the same view. But the followers of रसवैद्यक (Rasavaidyaka)** suggest it as mineral substance obtainable at Saurastra and the same description is laid down by the compilers of Dhn. Ni. & Raj.Ni.

a- A sandy substance of 'Red hue '

b- Watt Dict. (Vol. V. 116- Mallotus)

नि.शे. टीकायां कम्पिल्लकस्य वृक्षकाण्डे निर्देशः । तत्र च ध.नि. पाठ. इन्दोश्च पाठः उद्धृतः ।
'काम्पिल्यकोऽथ रक्ताङ्गो रेची रेचनकस्तथा ।
रजनो लोहिताङ्गश्व कर्कशो रक्तचूर्णकः ॥ ध.नि. पाठः ।
'कर्कशाख्यः करम्भः स्यात् स काम्पिल्यः पटोदकः । इन्दुः ।

* The current accepted name is *Mallotus phlippinensis* (Lam.) Muel.- Arg.

** This is suggestive more of tree i.e. *Mallotus philippinensis* (Lam.) Muel - Arg.

It is dificult to confirm with the help of similitive terms or synonyms of Dhn. ni. & Raj. ni. whether the source of the drug material is plant in origin or mineral in origin . But along with the reference of Ni. Shesh if we read the Śodhala Niighanṭu the confusion gets cleared.

कंपिल्लकेऽथ रक्तगङ्गो रेची रेचनकस्तथा ।
रंजनो रक्तचूर्णश्च कर्कशः चंद्रसाह्वयः ॥ ४५७
नदीवासो रक्तफलो बहुपत्रो बहूफलः ॥ Śodhal

As the said Śodhal Ni. was published in 1978 it was not available to the author Late Vd. D. K. Kamat (S.D. Kamat)

II- a- रक्ताङ्गः (Raktāṅgaḥ), रेची (Recī), रक्तचूर्णकः (Raktacūrṇakaḥ), रञ्जनः (Rañjnaḥ), लोहिताङ्गः (Lohitāṅgaḥ)

b- A kind of mineral drug.
(Mar. Tam.) Kapilā.

III-b- साधारण रसः (Sādhāraṇa Rasaḥ), 'कम्पिल्ल' गौरीपाषाण (Kampilla-Gaurīpāṣaṇā) (Dhn. Ni. Misra. Varga 7)

2) सामान्यरसाः (Samānya rasāḥ) कम्पिल्लः । Raj. Ni. XII. 7

3) उपरसः गन्धो ...कंकुष्ठकम् सौराष्ट्रम् । (Dhn.Ni. Misrak. varga)

4) कम्पिल्लः । ... रक्तचूर्णविशेषः । इष्टिकाचूर्ण संकाश ... सौराष्ट्रदेशखनिजः सहि कम्पिल्लको मतः इति ग्रन्थान्तरे । (Ast. Hr. Kosa)

5) सौराष्ट्र देशोत्पन्न इष्टिका चूर्णवत् ... 'कमले' इति लोके ।(Rasapaddhati Stanza 58)

IV- 1) See (Kampilla, Kamlā)(Thakurdatta sharma vaidya)

2) In the 10th century Masundi wrote at ' Kambil ' as a sandy substance of 'red hue' which is useful as an anthelmintic and in the treatment of cutaneous diseases. (Watt. V. 116)

54 कंकुष्ठम् Kankuṣṭham

कंकुष्ठं कालकुष्ठं च विरङ्गं रङ्गदायकम्[१] ॥ १२७
रेचकं पुलकं ऱ्हासं शोधनं कालपालकम् ॥

---

१ रंगनायकम् इति पा. ।

कंकुष्ठ has remained a controversial material for a long time just like कंपिल्ल (Kampilla); it may be having all the three original sources mineral as well as plant and animal.

"हिमवत्पाद शिखरे कंकुष्ठमुपजायते ।
तत्रैकं रक्तकालं स्यात्तदन्यदण्डकं स्मृतम् ।
पीतप्रभं गुरु स्निग्धं श्रेष्ठं कङ्कुष्ठमादिशेत् ।
श्यामं पीतं लघु त्यक्तसत्त्वं नेष्टं तथाण्डकम् ॥ "
अन्यच्च .
हिमवत्पाद शिखरे कङ्कुष्ठमुपजायते ।
तत्रैकं नालिकाख्यं च तच्चान्यद्रेणुकं मतम् ।
पीतप्रभं गुरु स्निग्धं तत्र श्रेष्ठमादिमम् ।
श्यावं श्वेतं पीतलघु त्यक्तसत्त्वं हि रेणुकम् ।
केचिद्वदन्ति कङ्कुष्ठं सद्योजातस्य दन्तिनः ।
वर्चश्च श्यावपीताभं रेचनं परिकथ्यते ॥
कतिचित्तेजिवाहानां नालं कङ्कुष्ठ संज्ञितम् ॥
वदन्ति श्वेतपीताभं तदतीव विरेचनम् ।
आनन्दा पुस्तके तलस्थटीकायां पाठः ।

अनेक विद्वानोंने 'गॅम्बोज्' को कंकुष्ठ माना है जो उचित मालूम पडता है । ... ... गॅम्बोज् को बाजारमें उसारें रेवन्द(रेवंदचिनी का सत) कहते हैं किन्तु यह रेंवदचीनीका उसारा नहीं है । गॅम्बोज् (उसारे रेवंद) यह एक वृक्ष (गार्सिनिआ) का निर्यास है और रेवंद चिनी यह एक गुल्मकी (हीउम्) जड है । रेवंद चिनी के जड के सत्त्व की तरह गॅम्बोज में गुण होने के कारण संभवतः गॅम्बोज को भी उसारे रेवंद कहा जाता होगा । (डॉ. चुनेकर पृ. ६२४ भा. प्र.)

कंकुष्ठं तिक्तकटुकं वीर्ये चोष्णं प्रकीर्तितम् ॥ १२८
गुल्मोदावर्तशूलघ्नं रसरञ्जं व्रणापहम् ॥

कंकुष्ठं (Kaṅkuṣṭham), कालकुष्ठं (Kālakuṣṭham), विरङ्ग (Viraṅgam), रङ्गदायकं (Raṅgadāyakam), रेचकं (Recakam), पुलकं (Pulakam), ह्रासं (Rhāsam), शोधनं (Śodhanam), and कालपालकं (Kālapālakam) are synonymous.

Kaṃkuṣṭha is bitter and pungent in taste, and *uṣṇavīrya*. It is useful in tumours (diverticulosis), *uadāvarta* (upward movement of *vāyu*), colic, giving colour to mercury (*Rasarañjam*) and in wound healing.

I- Not identified

II- a- कालकुष्ठम् (Kāla kuṣṭham), रंगदायकम् (Raṅgadāyakam),

III- See सर्वक्षीरी । गुडूच्यादिवर्ग १

b- कंकुष्ठम् (Kaṅkuṣṭham), (Keral) Kakuttam, Sakuporijāra; (Mar.) Muddārsing, (Kan) Kaṅkuṣṭa; (Ben.) Parvatiya mṛttikā viśeṣaḥ (Ayu.O.Ni.)

2) उपरसः गन्धो .. 'कंकुष्टकं' सौराष्ट्री । (Dhn. Ni.)

3) उपरसः - खेचराञ्जन 'कङ्कुष्ठ' (Raj. Ni. Varga 12-16)

55 भल्लातकः Bhallātakaḥ

भल्लातकः स्मृतोऽरुष्को दहनस्तपनोऽग्निकः ॥ १२९
अरुष्करो वीरतरुर्भल्लातोऽग्निमुखो धनुः ॥

भल्लातः कटुतिक्तोष्णो मधुरः कृमिनाशननः ॥ १३०
गुल्मार्शोग्रहणीकुष्ठान् हन्ति वातकफामयान् ॥

भल्लातकः (Bhallātakaḥ), अरुष्कः (Aruṣkaḥ), दहनः (Dahanaḥ), तपनः (Tapanaḥ), अग्निकः (Agnikaḥ), अरुष्करः (Aruṣkaraḥ), वीरतरुः (Vīrataruḥ), भल्लातः(Bhallātaḥ), अग्निमुखः (Agnimukhaḥ) and धनुः (Dhanuḥ) are synonymous.

Bhallātaka is pungent, bitter, and sweet in taste, and *uṣṇavīrya*. It is useful in worms, tumours (diverticulosis), piles *grahaṇī* (disordrs characterized by ch. diarrhoea), skin disorders and diseases caused by *vāta* and *kapha doṣās.*

(Fam. Anacardiaceae)

I- a- ***Semecarpus anacardium*** Linn.*

b- Roxburgh (Fl. indi.)

c- Sub Himalayan tract from Satlej eastwards ascending to altitude of 3000 ft. and throughout the hotter parts of India.

II- a- अरुष्कर (Aruṣkara), बीजपादपः (Bījapādapah), स्फोटकः (Sphoṭakaḥ)

b- (B) Bhela, Bholatuki; (Tel.) Nella jeddi; (H.) Bhilāwā; (Tam.) Sankotei, serngottai; (Mal.) Then kotta, Tempraku; (Eng.) Marking nut tree; (Med.) Anacardium.

56 तुत्थम् Tuttham (Copper sulphate)

तुत्थं कर्परिकातुत्थममृतासङ्गमेव च ॥ १३१
मयूरग्रीवकं चान्यच्छितिकण्ठं च तुत्थकम् ॥

द्वितीयं कर्परीतुत्थं कर्परीतुत्थकं तथा ॥१३२
नेत्रनैर्मल्यकारि स्यात् तत्तुत्थममृतोपमम् ॥

तुत्थकं दृष्टिरोगघ्नं शीतं श्वित्रविनाशनम् ॥ १३३
विषवेगप्रशमनं प्रशस्तं कथ्यते बुधैः ॥

This is being mineral in origin, not commented upon by Late vd. D.K.Kamat. It is Copper Sulphate.

तुत्थं (Tuttham), कर्परिकातुत्थं (Karparikātuttham), अमृतासङ्गम (Amṛtāsangam), मयूरग्रीवकं (Mayūragrīvakam), शितिकण्ठ (Sitikaṇṭham) and तुत्थकं (Tutthakam) are synonymous. The other kind of Tuttha is called by the synonyms कर्परीतुत्थं (Karparikatuttham), and कर्परीतुत्थकम (Karporitutthakam)

That *tuttha* which cleanses the eyes is supposed to be of the best variety.

Tutthaka is useful in the diseases of the eyes, *śitavirya* and vitiligo. It is used in poisons.

---

* *Semicarpus anacardium* Linn. f. - is the current accepted name.

57 ताप्यं (हेममाक्षिकम्) Tāpyam (Hemamākśikam)
(copper pyrite)

हेममाक्षिकमावर्तं तापीजं धातुमाक्षिकम् ॥ १३४
ताप्यं च माक्षिकंधातु मधुधातु विनिर्दिशेत् ॥

माक्षिकं कटु तिक्तोष्णं रसायनमनुत्तमम् ॥ १३५
बस्तिरोगहरं हन्यादर्शःशोफोदरक्षयान् ॥

त्रिदोषशमनं वृष्यं चक्षुष्यं च विषापहम् ॥ १३६
मन्दानलत्वं बलाहानिमुग्रां विष्टम्भतां नेत्ररुजं च कुष्ठम् ॥
करोति मालां व्रणपूर्विकां च माक्षिकधातुर्गुरुप्यपक्वः ॥१३७

This being mineral in origin is not commented upon by Late Vd. D.K. Kamat.

Copperpyrite; (H.) Sonāmākhi; (Mar.) Suvarṇa Mākśhika.

हेममाक्षिकं (Hemamākśīkam), आवर्त (Āvartam), तापीजं (Tāpījam), धातुमाक्षिकं (Dhātumākśikam), ताप्यं (Tāpyam), माक्षिकधातुः (Mākśīkadhātuḥ), and मधुधातुः (Madhudhātuḥ) are synonymous.

Mākśika is pungent and bitter in taste, *uṣṇavīrya, rasāyana* (rejuvinating), and pacifies all the three *doṣas.* It is useful in diseases of urinary organs, piles,oedema, ascites and consumption. It is *vṛṣya,* beneficial to eyes and antipoisonous.

If not purified and not converted to *bhasma,* produces weakness of digestive capacity, great loss of strength, constipation, diseases of the eyes, and skin disorders and ulceration in glands around the neck (scrofula).

58 अञ्जनम् Añjananm (Eng. Galena)

अञ्जनं मेचकं कृष्णं सौवीरं च सुवीरजम् ।
कपोतं यामुनेयं च स्रोतोजं सारितं तथा ॥१३८

सौवीरमञ्जनं प्रोक्तमत्यन्तं शिशिरं बुधैः ।
विषहिध्माविकारघ्नमक्षिरोगविषापहम् ॥ १३९

This being mineral in origin is not commented upon by Late vd. D.K. Kamat

(Eng.) Galena; (H. Mar. etc.) सुरमा (Suramā).

II अञ्जनम् (Añjanam), मेचकं (Mecakam), कृष्णं (Kṛṣṇam),सौवीरं (Sauvīram),सुवीरजम् (Suvīrajam), कपोतं (Kapotam), यामुनेयं (Yāmuneyam), स्रोतोजं (Srotojam), and सारितं (Sāritam) are synonymous.
Sauvīra añjana is excessively *śītavīrya*. It is useful in poisons, hiccup and diseases of the eyes.

59 (गैरिक) धातुः (Gairika) Dhātuḥ (Eng. Ochre)

गैरिकं रक्तधातुः स्यात्ताम्रधातुः गवेधुकम् ।
पाषाणगैरिकं चैव द्वितीयं स्वर्णगैरिकम् ॥ १४०

पाषाण गैरिकं प्रोक्तं कठिनं ताम्रवर्णकम् ।
विशदो गैरिकः स्निग्धः कषायो मधुरो हिमः ॥१४१
चक्षुष्यो रक्तपित्तघ्नः छर्दिहिध्माविषापहः ।

This being mineral in origin is not commented upon by Late Vd.D.K. Kamat.

According to गणद्रव्यावली by the word 'धातु' (Dhātū), गैरिक (Gairika) Ochre has been accepted. It is mentioned serially after अञ्जन (Pre No. 57) but the present published works on Dhn. Ni. (Ānandāśram, Chauwkhamba, (Sharma) (zarkhande) have mentioned it afterअञ्जन (Añjana) समुद्रफेनं, चक्षुष्या, रसाञ्जनं, पुष्पाञ्जनं, शिलाजतु and then गैरिक.However here the serial No. of (Gaṇadravyāvalī) गणद्रव्यावली is accepted.
(Eng.) *Ochre;* (H. & Local languages) *Geru* .
गैरिकं. (Gairikam), रक्तधातुः (Raktadhātuḥ), ताम्रधातुः (Tāmradhātuḥ), गवेधुकम् (Gavedhukam), are synonymous.
It is of two types A) पाषाण गैरिकं (Pāṣāṇa Gairikam) & (B) स्वर्णगैरिकं (Swarṇa Gairikam),
Pāṣāṇagairika is hard and coppery red coloured.
Gairika is *kaṣāya* (astringent) sweet, *śītavīrya;* unctuous, and cleansing.
It is beneficial to eyes, and useful in bleeding disorders, emesis, hiccup and poison.

सुवर्णगैरिकम् Suvarṇa Gairikam (24) (Eng. Ochre)

सुवर्णगैरिकं चान्यत्ततो रक्तरजो विदुः ॥ १४२
अत्यन्तशोणितं स्निग्धं मसृणं स्वर्णगैरिकम् ॥

स्वादुस्निग्धं हिमं नेत्र्यं कषायं रक्तपित्तजित् ॥ १४३
हिध्मावमिविषघ्नं च रक्तघ्नं स्वर्णगैरिकम् ॥

This is being mineral in origin has not been commented upon by Late Vd. D. K. Kamat .

It is mentioned previously as (B) type

The second type of *Gairika* is called as सुवर्णगैरिक (Suvarṇagairika) which has the synonym रक्तरजः (Raktarajaḥ). It is very red in colour, unctuous, and smooth.

Suvarṇagairika is *kaṣāya* (astringent) and sweet in taste, *śītavīrya,* beneficial to eyes. It is useful in hiccup, emesis, poisons and bleeding disorders.

60 समुद्रफेनम् Samudraphenam (Os Sepiae)

समुद्रफेनं फेनं च शुष्काशुष्कं पयोधिजम् ॥१४४
विद्यादुदधिफेनं च प्रोक्तं सागरजं मलम् ॥

समुद्रफेनं शिशिरं कर्णपाकनिवारणम् ॥१४५
लेखनं नेत्ररोगाणां हिमं विषविनाशनम् ॥
चक्षुष्यं रक्तपित्तघ्नं गुल्मप्लीहहरं स्मृतम् ॥१४६

This is not being plant in origin has not been commented upon by Late Vd. D. K. Kamat.

Os sepiae

(H. & Mar.) Samudraphena

समुद्रफेनं (Samudraphenam),फेनम् (Phenam), शुष्काशुष्कं (Śuṣkāśuṣkam), पयोधिजम् (Payodhijam), उदधिफेनं (Udadhiphenam), सागरजं मलम् (Sāgarajam malam) are synonymous.

Samudraphena is *śītavīrya* and useful in otorrhoea. It is *lekhana* (Scarificient) for diseases of the eye and poison. It is beneficial to eyes, bleeding disorders, tumors (diverticulosis), and disorders of spleen.

61 चक्षुष्या Cakṣuṣyā

चक्षुष्या दृक्प्रसादा च सैव प्रोक्ता कुलत्थिका ।
कुलाली लोचनहिता कुम्भकारी मलापहा ।१४७

हिमा प्रोक्ता कषाया च विषं स्थावरजंगमम् ।
निहन्ति योजिता सम्यक् नेत्रस्रावाननेकशः ॥१४८
सा च विस्फोटकण्ड्वर्तिव्रणदोषनिबर्हणी ।

चक्षुष्या (Cakśuṣyā), दृक्प्रसादा (Dṛkprasādā), कुलत्थिका (Kulatthikā), कुलाली (Kulālī), लोचनहिता (Locanahitā), कुम्भकारी (Kumbhakārī) and मलापहा (Malāpahā) are synonymous.

It is *kaṣāya* (astringent) in taste and *Śītavīrya.* It is useful in both, movable and immovable types of poisons. It is useful in conjunctivitis, (and discharge from the eyes), in eruptions, pruritus and wounds.

Fam. Leguminosae. Caesalpiniaceae.

I- a- ***Cassia absus*** Linn.

b- Kamat. C- The seeds are exported from Sindh and Kacha (See below IV -1)

II- a- दृक्प्रसादा (Dṛkprasādā), कुलत्थिका (Kulatthikā), कुलत्था (Kuḷatthā), कुम्भकारी (Kumbhakārī),

b- (Mar.) रानकुळीथ (Rānkuḷītha), (H) चाकसू (Cāksu)

III- S.Ci. 16.26

IV- 1) An erect annual herb 2-3 ft. high growing into the foot of western Himalaya and from there distributed to ceylon.
History The seeds of the plant were used by the Egyptians in the treatment of opthalmia and through them Romans and Greeks and from the latter Mohamedan writers became aware of their properties.*
Arabic name ' Hub-us-Soudām' and 'Tashmizai' are corruptions of Persians 'Chashmīzak',.... The Soudian seeds are the best. (Watt.II. 211)

Note - Shri Kailashpati Pandeya has written an article in Ayurveda Maha sammelan Patrikā (- -) in which he has recorded 76 plants under the heading 'चक्षुष्या' (Cakśuṣyā).

रसाञ्जनम् Rasāñjanam (20)

रसाञ्जनं तार्क्ष्यशैलं रसजातं रसोदभवम् ॥१४९
रसगर्भं रसाङ्ग्रं च दार्वीक्वाथसमुद्भवम् ॥

* काश्यप संहिता (Kāśyapa saṃhitā) has a separate chapter on चक्षुष्या (Cakśusyā)

रसाञ्जनं हिमं तिक्तं रक्तपित्तकफापहम् ।१५०
हिध्माश्वासहरं वर्ण्यं मुखरोगविषापहम् ।

It is prepared from the decoction of दारुहरिद्रा (Dāruharidrā) eg. *
Berberis asiatica, B. lycium etc.

Extractum Berberis

(Eng.) Extract of Indian berberis

(H.) Rasaut, Rasot; (Mar.) Rasavat; (Tel.) Rasāñjanamu. etc.

रसाञ्जनं (Rasāñjanam), तार्क्ष्यशैलं (Tārkśya śailam), रसजातं (Rasajātam), रसोद्भवम् (Rasodbhavam), रसगर्भं (Rasagarbham), रसाग्र्यं (Rasāgryam), दार्वीक्वाथ समुद्भवम् (Darvī kwātha samudbhavam) are synonymous.

Rasāñjana is bitter in taste, *śītavīrya* and pacifies *rakta, pitta* and *kapha doṣas* and bleeding disorders.

It is useful in hiccup, dyspnoea, is beneficial for the complexion, diseases of mouth and poison.

This is not commented upon by Late vd. D.K. Kamat .

दारुहरिद्रा (Dāruharidrā has been already commented in the 1st chapter. .The previous plant चक्षुष्या is useful for eye conditions, similarly रसाञ्जन (Rasāñjana) is also useful for opthalmic conditions. It's regular application in the eyes once in a week is prescribed in Aṣṭāṅga Hṛdaya. It is not mentioned in गणद्रव्यावली. (Gaṇadravyāvalī)

*(दार्वीक्वाथमजाक्षीरं पादं पक्त्वा यदा घनम् ।
तदा रसाञ्जनाख्यं तन्नेत्रयोः परमं हितम् ॥) (S.D. Kamat)

61 रीतिः, पुष्पाञ्जनम् Rītiḥ, Puṣpāñjanam

Eng. Zinc oxide

पुष्पाञ्जनं पुष्पकेतुः कौसुमं कुसुमाञ्जनम् ॥ १५१
रीतिजं रीतिकुसुमं रीतिपुष्पं च पौष्पिकम् ॥

पुष्पाञ्जनं हिमं हन्ति हिक्कामत्यन्तदुस्तराम् ॥ १५२
अक्षिरोगचयं हन्याद् विषं निर्विषतां नयेत् ॥

This is not commented upon by Late D.K. Kamat being mineral in origin.

अत्र तु 'रीति' पदेन 'रीतिजं ' गृह्यते । 'पित्तल' धातोः रीत्यर्थे सुवर्णादिवर्गे पृथक ग्रहणाद । 'सुवर्णरौप्यताम्राणि त्रपुरीतिश्च सीसकम् ।' इति सुवर्णादि

वर्गे पठितत्वात् शोढल संमतत्वाच्च । एकदेशविकृतमनन्यवत् । Here the word *Rīti* is meant for *Rītijam* or *Puspāñjanam* i.e. zinc oxide. *Rītiḥ dhātuḥ* (Brass) has been separately mentioned in Suvarṇādi chapter (Chapter VI). शोढल *(Śoḍhala)* has also accepted this reading. पुष्पाञ्जनं (Puṣpāñjanam), पुष्पकेतुः (Puṣpaketuḥ) , कौसुमं (Kausumam), कुसुमाञ्जनम् (Kusumāñjanam), रीतिजं (Rītijam), रीतिकुसुमम् (Rītikuṣumam), रीतिपुष्पं (Rītipuṣpam), पौष्पिकम् (Pauṣpikam), are synonymous.* S.D. Kamat.

Puspāñjana is *śītavīrya* and is useful in obstinate hiccup, diseases of the eye and poison.

शिलाजतु Śilājatu. (22)

शिलाजतु स्यादतिथिः शैलेयं गिरिजाश्मजम् ॥१५३
जत्वश्मजं चाश्मजतु प्रोक्तं धातुजमद्रिजम् ॥
शिलाजतु भवेत्तिक्तं कटूष्णं च रसायनम् ॥ १५४
मेहोन्मादाश्मरीशोफकुष्ठापस्मारनाशनम् ॥
क्षयशोफोदरार्शांसि हन्ति बस्तिरुजो जयेत् ॥१५५

Does not belong to the plant kingdom and hence not commented upon by Late Vd. D.K. Kamat.

शिलाजतु (Śilājatu), अतिथिः (Atithiḥ), शैलेयं (Śaileyam), गिरिजाश्मजम् (Girijāśmajam), जत्वश्मजम् (Jatwaśmajam), अश्मजतु (Aśmajatu), धातुजमद्रिजम् (Dhātujamadrijam) are synonymous.

Śilājatu is bitter and pungent in taste, *uṣṇavīrya* and *rasāyana* (rejuvinating). It is useful in disorders characterized by polyuyria, insanity, calculi, oedema, disorders of skin, epilepsy, consumption, anasarca, piles, and urinary colics.

63 कतकम् Katakam

कतकं छेदनीयञ्च कतं[1] कतफलं मतम् ।
अम्बुप्रसादनफलं श्लक्ष्णं नेत्रविकारजित् ॥१५६

---

* पुष्पाञ्जनपरिचयः रसस्तरंगिण्यामित्थं प्रदर्शितः ।
'रीतिका द्रावणविधौ रीतिस्थं यशदं द्रुतम् ।
समेत्यम्बरपीयूषयोगेन सितचूर्णताम् ॥ ४९
तदेव सितचूर्णन्तु पुष्पाञ्जनमुदीरितम् ।
भस्त्राध्मातं पुष्पितं तु यशदं वा तदाह्वयम् ॥ ५० रसतरंगिणी पृ. ५७९

१ 'शीर्ष शोढल. पाठः ।
काच्छ चान्द्रायणफलं चक्षुष्यं शोधनं परम् । इति शो. अधिकः पाठः ।

कतकं शीतलं प्राहुस्तृष्णाविषविनाशनम् ।
नेत्रोत्थरोगविध्वंसि विधिनाऽञ्जनयोगतः ॥१५७
कतकस्य फलं तित्तं चक्षुष्यं शीतलं मृदु ।
वारिप्रसादनं कृच्छ्रशर्करामश्मरीं जयेत् ॥ १५८

कतकं (Katakam), छेदनीयं (Chedanīyam), कतं(Katam), कतफलं (Kataphalam), अम्बुप्रसादनफलं (Ambuprasādanaphalam), श्लक्ष्णं (Ślaksṇam) and नेत्रविकारजित् (Netravikārajit) are synonymous.

Kataka is *śītavīrya* and useful in thirst, poiosn, diseases of the eye by the procedure of appliction (of collyrium).

The seeds of *kataka* are bitter in taste, beneficial for eyes *sītavīrya* and soft. It is useful for purification of water, dysuria, urinary calculus and gravels.

(Loganiaceae)

I- a- ***Strychnos potatorum*** Linn.f.
b- Dymock c- A small tree in Deccan, central and south India.
II- a- अम्बुप्रसादनम् (Ambuprasādanam), नेत्र विकारजित् (Netra vikārajit)
b- (H.P.B. Bom.) Nirmalī.
III-b- कतकः (Katakaḥ); (Keral) Tettamaram, Tetta paralam; (Tel.) Tettāmaram, katakam; (Tam.) Teṭṭāñ koṭaṭai; (Kan) cilli kāyi; (Vang) Nirmal Phal. (Ayu . O. Nighaṇṭu)

64 लोध्रः Lodhraḥ

लोध्रोरोध्रः शाबरकस्तिल्वकः[1] तिलकस्तरुः ॥१५९
तिरीटकः[2] काण्डहीनो[3] भिल्ली[4] शबरपादपः[5] ॥
लोध्रः शीतः कषायश्च हन्ति तृष्णामरोचकम् ॥१६०
विषविध्वंसनः प्रोक्तो रूक्षो ग्राही कफापहः ।

लोध्रः (Lodhraḥ), रोध्रः (Rodhraḥ), शाबरकः (Śābarakaḥ), तिल्वकः (Tilvakaḥ), तिलकः (Tilakaḥ), तरुः (Taruḥ),तिरीटकः (Tirīṭakaḥ), काण्डहीनः

---

१ चिल्लकः २ तिरीटः ३ कालहीनश्च ४ चिल्ली इति नि.शे. संमताः पाठाः ।
५ 'शम्बर पादप. इति पा. ।
१ तिल्वकश्च तथा तरुः । शो. ३ काककीलश्च । शो. ४ चिल्ली । शो.
"तिल्वको हस्तिलोध्रः स्यादतिसाराक्षिभेषजम् ।
उत्सादनो हेमपुष्पः शीतत्वक् चाक्षिरोगहृत ॥" इति शोढलपाठः ।

(Kāṇḍahīnaḥ), भिल्ली (Bhillī), and शबरपादपः (Śabarapādapaḥ) are synonymous.

Lodhra is *kaṣāya* (astringent) in taste, *śītavīrya,* pacifies *kaphadoṣa* and is *rūkṣa* (dry). It is useful in thirst, anorexia and as an antipoisonous.

I- Generic name. Two plants are included by both the compilers under this heading. One of it is 'A' शाबरकः तिल्वकः (Śābarakaḥ, Tilvakaḥ), and the next 'B' is तिरीटकः काण्डहीन (Tirīṭakaḥ kāṇḍahinaḥ). But medicianl properties are not given of these plants separately. Kṣīraswāmī also records two kinds under this heading (See III-I below). From this it seems that either the medicinal properties of these two plants may have been the same or the plant 'B' may have been neglected. Modern writers also record two kinds of लोध्रः, one of it 'A' as above and the next क्रमुक (Kramuka) which is recorded also by our compiler under the same heading which see post No. 25 infra.

Fam. Symplocaceae

I- A-a- ***Symplocos racemosa*** Roxb.
Syn. *S. hamiltonia* Wall.
S. nervosa A.D.C.

b- Roxburgh (C.BC. p. 415)

B-a-Not identified. It may be *S. beddomi* or *S. stocksii* (See Birdwood)

II- A-a- शाबरकः (Śābarakaḥ), तिल्वकः (Tilwakaḥ), तिलकः (Tilakaḥ), (Dhn. Ni.) काण्डकीलकः (Kāṇḍakīlakaḥ), भिल्लतरुः (Bhillataruḥ), शाबरकः (Śābarakaḥ), हेमपुष्पकः (Hemapuṣpakaḥ), Raj. Ni.

b- (SK) Lodhra, Śābara rodhra; (H.B.) Lodha; (Tel.) Lodhag; (Mar.) Lodhra; (Eng.) Lodh.

B-a- तिरीटकः (Tirīṭakaḥ), काण्डहीनः (Kāṇḍahīnaḥ),भिल्ली (Bhillī), शबरपादपः (Śabarapādapaḥ),

B-b- Modern names as b-above

III-b-1) 54 तिल्वकः अक्षिपीडः सितलोध्र महत्पत्रश्वेतत्वचस्तिरीटश्च ।
शिखरी त्रिकण्टक इति प्रोक्ताः पयार्यवाचकाः शब्दाः ॥ ५४

(Mal.) Karutta kanvetti, Velutha kanjetti; (Kanpoti), Kammattippala.

Execaria comettia.According to Mr. Krishnan *

"केचिदत्र लोध्रपत्राकारतया तिल्वकस्य लोघ्र इत्यर्थ वदन्ति । तन्न युक्तम् ।
तिल्वकस्तु विरेचन गणान्तःपातितत्वाद् विरेचनकरः । 'अक्षिपाककृ'-

---

*वेळुत्त कण्वेट्टि, कण्पाट्टि, कमबदटि, कम्बट्टिटण्पाल According to Vd. Miss Nalini K. & Mrs. Chitra Krishnan.(Personal correspondence) S. D. Kamat.

दित्यनेन नेत्रपाककारी च । लोधस्तु 'अतिसारभेषज' मित्यनेन ग्राही ।
नेत्रभेषजं च । तस्माल्लोध्रपत्राकारः कश्चिदौषधिविशेषःएव तिल्वकः ।
Editor Abhi. Mañjari (Page 19)

b-1) 'गालवः शाबरो लोध्रस्तिरिटः तिल्वमार्जने । 'आद्यौ श्वेतरोध्रे
तिरीटाद्य रक्तरोध्रे ॥ Amarkosh
गालयति (Srāvayati Ak'si गालवः (Gālavaḥ)
तिरिटः Tirayati rogam
तिल्वः Tilati Snihyatyangam anena 'Tilvaḥ'
मार्जने .... Udvartane Marjane
आहच –
लोधः शाबरकः चिल्लकः तिल्वकः तिरीटः काण्डहीनश्च ...
द्वितीयः पटिटकारोध्रो गालवः ... पट्टी लाक्षाप्रसादनः ।
(K'siraswāmī - Amara)
रोध्रः शाबरकः श्वेतत्वक् अतीसारभेषजम् ।
द्वितीयः पट्टिकारोध्रो ..... पट्टी लाक्षाप्रसादनः ।
बृहत्वक्कः जीर्णबुध्नो .....

2) 17 रोध्रभित् शबरदेशजः श्वेतरोध्रः । 'तिरीटस्तिल्वको रोध्रश्चान्यः
शबरदेशजः ।श्वेतरोध्रः शाबरोक्षिभैषज्यं शबरोद्भव' मिति हृदयदीपक : ।
(Harshe)

3) रोध्रः तिल्वकः शाबरको द्वितीय रोध्रः । रोध्रः अक्षिभेषजापरासंज्ञा ।
शाबरकोरोध्रः श्वेतरोध्रः । (Arun, Hemādri Su. 15.26)

4) लोध्र साबररोध्र स्तम्भी । लोध्रःलाक्षाप्रसादनो रक्तः । साबर रोध्रः
श्वेतमूलम् । (Dalhana S.Sū 38.14. 15)

IV- 1) *Sympolcos racemosa* Roxb.- The Loda or Lodh.
An abundant small tree of the plains and lower hills of Bengal Assam and Burma ... Bowels, eye diseases and ulcers. considered cooling, astringent. Decoction of the wood in spongy and bleeding gums etc.

2) *S. racemosa* Roxb.
Symplocos cortex, S. bark, Lodh.
Flowers - white fading yellow. (Watt. VI- iii- p. 398)

3) *Symplocos racemosa* Roxb.
Syn. *S. hamiltonia* Wall.
S. nervosa A.Dc.
(Sk) Sābar rodhra; (B.) Lodha.
A small tree, 12-20 ft. high, Trunk, 20 in circum.
Bark somewhat rough with a spongy friable exterior gray coat, when fresh of a very pale yellowish colour . *Taste* milky astgringent.*Flowers* colour lively yellow.
The bark of the tree is in request among the dyers of red abira, the red powder used by the natives during the Holi Holidays.
(Roxb. C.B.C. p. 415)

क्रमुकः Kramukaḥ (25)

क्रमुकः पट्टिकारोध्रो वल्कलः[1] स्थूलवल्कलः ॥ १६१
जीर्णपर्णो[2] बृहत्पर्णः[3] पट्टी लाक्षाप्रसादनः[4] ॥

लोध्रयुग्मं कषायं तु शीतं वातकफास्रजित् ॥ १६२
चक्षुष्यं विषहृत्तत्र विशिष्टो वल्कलोध्रकः ॥

क्रमुकः (Kramukaḥ), पट्टिकारोध्रः (Paṭṭikārodhraḥ), वल्कलः (Valkalaḥ), स्थूलवल्कलः (Sthūlavalkalaḥ), जीर्णपर्णः (Jīrṇaparṇaḥ), बृहत्पर्णः (Bṛhatparṇaḥ), पट्टी (Paṭṭī), लाक्षाप्रसादनः (Lākṣāprasādanaḥ) are synonymous.

Both the *Lodhras* are *kaṣāya* in taste, *śitavīrya* and pacify *vāta, kapha* and *raktadoṣas.* Especially, *valkarodhra* is specific as beneficial to eyes and antipoisonous.

(Fam. Symplocaceae)

I- a- ***Symplocos paniculata*** Wall.*
Syn. *S. cratagoides* Buch.- Ham.

b- Watt. Dict. (VI-iii-327)

c- See IV bellow

II- a- क्रमुकः (Kramukaḥ), पट्टिकारोध्रः (Paṭṭikārodhraḥ), वल्करोध्रः (Valkarodhraḥ), अक्षिभेषजः (Akṡibheṣajaḥ), लाक्षाप्रसादनः (Lākṡāprasādanaḥ), बृहत्पर्णः (Bṛhatparṇaḥ), स्थूलवल्कलः (Sthūlavalkalaḥ)

b- (H.) (Guj.) (Mar.) Paṭhānī Lodhra, Tāmbaḍā lodhra; (Tel.) Tella Lottuga chettu; (Tam.) Cebbalotti; (Mal.) Pāchyoṭṭi; (Kan) Bāla ledduginamara; (Eng.) see Lodhra II-B

III-b- रोध्र सू. १५ । लाक्षा प्रसादन रक्तः । ...रोध्रस्य विरेचनकत्वात् आचार्य डल्हणस्य तन्नाभिमतः । हिं पठाणी लोध्र, म. पाच्योटि, ते. लुड्डुगुचेट्टु, (के.) बाललंडुगी नमर, पाचेट्ट;(त.) चेब्रालोट्टी ... स द्विविधः ... तत्र विशिष्टो वल्क लोध्रः । (Asta. Hr. Kosha)

2) पट्टिका लोध्रः क्रमुक स्थूलवल्कल ... लाक्षा प्रसादनः । (Ramteja Bh. Pr. Ni.)

3) अक्षिपीडः (Akṡipīḍaḥ)
अक्षिपीलोऽपरः प्रोक्तः तिल्वकः प्रतितिल्वकः । कृष्णत्वगक्षिपाकी च
Akṡipilo paraḥ proktaḥ Tilwakaḥ pratitilvakaḥ kṛṣṇa twagakṡi-pākica (Karutta Kanvetti - Shrikrishnan) (Abhi. Man. 55)

---

१ कल्करोध्रः । इति पा.
२ 'जीर्णपुष्पो' इति शोढलः ।
३ 'मार्जनो जीर्णबुध्नश्च रोमशः शुष्कवल्कलः । 'इति शोढल पाठः ।
* The current accepted name is *S. chinensis* (Lour.) Druce.

4) धातुकी ताम्रपुष्पी ... लोध्रपुष्पी च । (See Pre No. 38 of this chapter)

5) तिल्वक कम्पिल्लके च लोध्रे ऽपि तिल्वकः संप्रयोज्यते ।
(Tilwaka kampillake ca Lodhrepi Tilwakaḥ samprayojyate)
(Abhi. Manj. p. 256)

65 शंखः Sańkhaḥ Eng. Conch

शंखो वारिभवः कम्बुर्जलदो दीर्घनिस्वनः ॥१६३
सुस्वरो दीर्घनादश्च धवलः श्रीविभूषणः ॥

शङ्खः स्वादुः कटुः पाके वीर्ये चोष्णः प्रकीर्तितः।१६४
परिणामं जयेच्छूलं चक्षुष्यो रक्तपित्तजित् ॥½

This does not belong to the plant kingdom and is not commented upon by Late Vd. D.K.Kamat.

शङ्खः (Śańkhaḥ), वारिभवः (Vāribhavaḥ), कम्बुः (Kambūḥ), जलदः (Jaladaḥ), दीर्घनिस्वनः (Dīrghaniṣwanaḥ) सुस्वरः (Suswaraḥ), दीर्घनादः (Dīrghanādaḥ), धवलः (Dhavalaḥ), श्रीविभूषणः (Śrīvibhūṣaṇaḥ) are synonymous. (Śankha = conch)

Śańkha is sweet in taste, pungent in *vipāka,* and *uṣṇavīrya,* it is useful in colic, when the food is in digestive stage (duodenal ulcer), is beneficial to eyes and bleeding disorders.

चन्दनादिरयं वर्गस्तृतीयः परिकीर्तितः ।
श्रीमतां भोगिनामर्हः प्रायो गन्धगुणाश्रयः ॥

Thus has been told the Candanādi 3rd chapter in which the drugs are mentioned having aromatic perfumary properties which are mainly useful to the kings and wealthy people.

वर्गेतराणि

१ ताम्बूली २ चूर्णम् ३ जिंगिणी ४ कपर्दिका ५ मृत्तिका ६ पर्वतः

These drugs are mentioned in certain MṢṢ as well as in Ānandāśram published edition. These are additional drugs mentioned by some other vaidyas for their own study, These seem to be mostly copied down from Śoḍhala Nighaṇṭu.However (१) ताम्बूली & (३) जिंगिणी belonging to the plant kingodm are commented upon by Late Vd. D.K. Kamat.

जिंगिणी Jingiṇī

जिङ्गिणी झिञ्झिणी ज्ञेया मोदकी गुडमञ्जरी ।
पार्वतेया सुनिर्घोषा तथा मदनमञ्जरी ॥

वातघ्नी मधुरोष्णा च व्रणघ्नी योनिशोधनी ।
जिङ्गिणी कटुका पाके तथाऽतीसारनाशनी ॥

जिङ्गिणी (Jingiṇī), झिञ्झिणी (Ziñziṇī), मोदकी (Modakī), गुडमञ्जरी (Guḍamañjarī), पार्वतेया (Pārvateyā), सुनिर्घोषा (Sunirghoṣā) and मदनमञ्जरी (Madanamañjarī) are synonymous.

Jingiṇī is sweet in taste, pungent in *vipāka, uṣṇavīrya* and pacifies *vātadoṣa.* It is useful in wounds, alleviates disorders in female genital tract and useful in diarrhoea.

Fam. Anacardiaceae.

I- a- ***Lannea grandis*** (Dennst) Engle.*
Syn*. *Odina wodier* Roxb.

b- Dymock (Pharm. indi.) c-IV-1 below.

II- a- गुडमञ्जरी (Guḍamañjarī), पार्वतेया (Pārvateyā), मदनमञ्जरी (Madanamañjarī)

b- (Bom) Mojā, Simtī, Moi, Moya; (Mar.) Same as (Bom.); (Tam.) Wodier maram, Oilyam; (Tel.) Gumpti, Gumpana, Duprl; (Kan.) Shimpti, Gojal, Panil , Simlī; (Mal.) Oti.

III-a- जिङ्गिणी C.S.VI.- 8.151; S.Su. 38. 14

IV- 1) *Odina wodier* Roxb.
Met with throughout hotter parts of India from the Indus eastwards Himalayan tract, is found also in Assam, Madras, Burma, Andaman, Islands and ceylon. (Watt.- V. 445).

2) Balvantji P. 168
जिङ्गिणी *Lannea grandis* (Dennest) Engl.

ताम्बूली Tāmbūli

बहुला च बलाऽनन्ता भद्रा पातालवासिनी ।
मुखरागकरी सौम्या अमृता त्वमृतोद्भवा ॥
कामदा कामजननी जीवन्ती यावनीप्रिया ।
आमोदजननी हृद्या देवानां दानवप्रिया ॥

---

*The presently accepted name is *Lannea coromandelica* (Houtt). Merr. (U.P.I.p.315)

ताम्बूलवल्ली ताम्बूली दाहदा श्रमभञ्जनी ।
नागवल्ली च नागाह्वा रञ्जनी तीक्ष्णमञ्जरी ॥

बहुला (Bahulā), बला (Balā), अनन्ता (Anantā), भद्रा (Bhadrā), पातालवासिनी (Pātālavāsinī), मुखरागकरी (Mukharāgakarī), सौम्या (Saumyā), अमृता (Amṛtā), अमृतोद्भवा (Amṛtodbhavā), कामदा (Kāmadā), कामजननी (Kāmajananī), जीवन्ती (Jīvantī), यावनीप्रिया (Yāvanīpriyā), आमोदजननी (Amodajananī), हृद्या (Hṛdyā), देवानां प्रिया (Devānām priyā), दानवप्रिया (Dānavapriyā), ताम्बूलवल्ली (Tāmbūlavalli), ताम्बूली (Tāmbūlī), दाहदा (Dāhadā), श्रमभञ्जनी (Śramabhañjanī), नागवल्ली (Nāgavallī), नागाह्वा (Nāgāhvā), रञ्जनी (Rañjanī), and तीक्ष्णमञ्जरी (Tīkṣṇamañjarī) are synonynous.

Fam. Piperaceae

I- a- ***Piper betle*** Linn.

b- Roxb. (Fl. indica) c- Probably native of Java. Cultivated in hotter and damp parts of India and ceylon.

II- a- पातालवासिनी (Pātālavāsinī), ताम्बूलवल्ली (Tāmbūlavallī), नागवल्ली (Nāgavallī), यावनीप्रिया (Yāvanīpriyā)

b- (H.B.) Vidāpān (Leaf); (Mar.) Nāgvel, Pānvel. (Tam.) Vettilai, vettale; (Tel.) Vitika; (Mal.) Tambulam.

Note- Raj. Ni. has noted fourteen kinds according to the taste and nativity.

इति चन्दनादिस्तृतीयो वर्गः ।

Thus ends the Candanādi Chapter Third.

करवीरादिश्चतुर्थो वर्ग :।

KARAVĪRĀDIḤ CHAPTER IV

(१) करवीरः Karavīraḥ

करवीरोऽश्वहाऽश्वघ्नो हयमारोऽश्वमारकः ।
श्वेतकुन्दः[१] श्वेतपुष्पः प्रतिहासोऽश्वमोहकः ॥ १

द्वितीयो रक्तपुष्पश्च चण्डको लगुडस्तथा ।
चण्डातको गुल्मकश्च प्रचण्डः करवीरकः ॥ २

करवीरः कटुस्तिक्तो वीर्ये चोष्णो ज्वरापहः
चक्षुष्यः कुष्ठकण्डूघ्नः प्रलेपाद् विषमन्यथा ॥ ३

करवीरद्वयं तिक्तं सविषं कुष्ठजित्कटु ॥

करवीर (Karavīraḥ), अश्वहा (Aśvahā), अश्वघ्नः (Aśvaghnaḥ), हयमारः (Hayamāraḥ), अश्वमारकः (Aśvamārakaḥ), श्वेतकुन्दः (Śvetakundaḥ), श्वेतपुष्पः (Śvetapuṣpaḥ), प्रतिहासः (Pratihāsaḥ), and अश्वमोहकः (Aśvamohakaḥ) are synonymous.

The synonyms for the other type of *karvīrakaḥ* are रक्तपुष्पः (Rakatapuṣpaḥ), चण्डकः (Caṇdakaḥ), लगुडः (Lagudaḥ), चण्डातकः (Caṇḍātakaḥ), गुल्मकः (Gulmakaḥ), and प्रचण्डः (Pracaṇḍaḥ).

Karavīra is pungent and bitter in taste, *usṇavīrya* .It is useful in fever, beneficial to eyes, disorders of skin, pruritus by external application, otherwise it is a poison.

Both the types of *karavīra* are bitter and pungent in taste, poisonous and useful in disorders of skin.

Generic name, includes three plant names A-श्वेतपुष्पः (Śwetapuṣpaḥ), B-रक्तपुष्पः (Raktapuṣpaḥ), and C- पीतपुष्पः (Pītapuṣpaḥ). Raj. ni. has included a kind of कृष्णकुसुम (Kṛṣṇakusma). This may be included in double petalled kind of red coloured *Karavīra* and single petalled wild variety, the flowers of which fade into purple shed).

(Fam. Apocyanaceae)

I- A-a- ***Nerium indicum*** Mill.
Syn. *N. odorum,* Soland.
b- Roxburgh (Flora indica)
B-a- Red Flowered variety of *Nerium indicum*, Mill.

---

१ शतकुन्दः इति पा.

b- Roxburgh (C.B.C.p. 242)

For Confirmation :

C-a- *Nerium pisidium* Roxb.
Nadkarni & Fl. inid. C.B.C.p. 245.

II-A,B-a अश्वहा (Aśwahā), श्वेतपुष्पः (Śwetapuṣpaḥ), प्रतिहासः (Pratihāsaḥ), अश्वमोहकः (Aśwamohakaḥ)

A-b (B) Śweta Kurubi; (H) Śweta Karput; (Marathi) Pāṇḍahrī Kaṇhera; (Tam.Tel.Mal.)Karaviram; (Tam.)Alari; (Tel.) Kasturipattaander; (Eng.) Indian Oleander,

B-a. गणेशकुसुमः (Gaṇeśakusumaḥ), चण्डीकुसुमः (Caṇḍīkusumaḥ), रविप्रियः (Rawipriyaḥ), रक्तकरवीरः (Raktakaravīraḥ)

b- (H) Lalakarpud; (B) Rakta Kurubi, Padma Kuruba (=double pet alled)

C-a पीतप्रसवः (Pītaprasavaḥ), सुगन्धिकुसुमः (Sugandhi Kusumaḥ)

b. (H.) Pīlī Kanera; (Mar.) Pīvaḷī Kaṇhera.

III

IV *Nerium odorum* Willd.
(Ben.) Kurubaka., Raktakurubak (the red variety); Śweta Kurubak (the white vaiety); Padma kurubak (the double petalled vaiety); (H.) Lal Karpud (The single petalled rose coloured); *safed* or *śwet karpud* (Single petalled white), Padma Karpud (The double petalled variety).

2. *N. coccineum* Roxb. (?)
Stem (old plants or even seven years old) short but straight and to the base decorated with numerous branches. Flowers terminal, solitary, ... large of a deep but rather dull red ... . In its native soil it grows to a large timber tree.

3. *N. pisidium* Roxb.
Stem and large branches ligneous and ramble to a vast extent. Flowers many large pale yellow (C.B.C.p. 242-45)

4. करवीर Karvaīra
Nerium indicum Mill.
C.S.Su. 3.2,9,14;
S.S.Su.36.11; 39.5
A.H.Ci. 15.78.
The two colour forms (white and red flowers have difference in respect or their pharmacology, chemical coustituents an1 clinical effects which are indicated by the fact that in some yogas only śweta (White) form has been used. Balvantji (77).

V. 1 *Nerium oleander* Linn.
Pīta karavīra (Eng.) Oleander.

2. *Thevetia peruviana* Schum.
Syn. *T. nerifolia,* Juss. ex Steud.
Cerebra thevetia, Linn.
(Eng.) Yellow Oleander; (Mar.) Piwaḷī Kanher, Biṭṭī.

2 (२) चक्रमर्दः Cakramardaḥ

चक्रमर्दस्त्वेडगजो मेषाक्षिकुसुमस्तथा ॥ ४ ॥
प्रपुन्नाटस्तरवटश्चक्राह्वः चक्रिकस्तथा ॥

([1]अन्यच्च –
चक्रमर्दस्त्वेडगजो मेषाक्षोऽण्डगजस्तथा ॥
प्रपुन्नाटः प्रपुन्नाडश्[2]चक्री व्या[3]वर्तकस्तथा ॥)

चक्रमर्दः कटूष्णः स्यात् प्रोक्तो वातकफापहः ॥ ५ ॥
दद्रुकण्डूहरः कान्तिसौकुमार्यकरो मतः ।

चक्रमर्दः (Cakramardaḥ), एडगजः (Eḍagajaḥ), मेषाक्षिकुसुमः (Meṣāk'sikusumaḥ), प्रपुन्नाटः (Prapunnāṭaḥ), तरवटः (Taravaṭaḥ), चक्राह्वः (Cakrāhvaḥ), and चक्रिकः (Cakrikaḥ), are synonymous.

(From the other text :- चक्रमर्दः (Cakramardaḥ), एडगजः (Eḍagajaḥ), मेषाक्षः (Meṣāk'saḥ), अण्डगजः (Aṇḍagajaḥ), प्रपुन्नाटः (Prapunnāṭaḥ), प्रपुन्नाडः (Prapunnāḍaḥ), चक्री (Cakrī), and व्यावर्तकः (Vyāvartakaḥ) are synonymous.)

Cakramarda is pungent, *uṣṇavīrya,* and pacifies *vāta kapha doṣas*. It is useful in *dadru* (ring worm), pruritus, and is beneficial for complexion and softness (of skin).

I (a) ***Casia tora*** Linn. & Willd.
Syn. *C.obtusifolia* Linn.
Senna tora Roxb.
(b) W. Dymock (Pharm. ind.)

II (a) एडगजः (Eḍgajaḥ), प्रपुन्नाटः (Prapunnāṭaḥ), तरवटः (Taravaṭaḥ), दद्रुघ्नः (Dadrughnaḥ).
(b) (SK) Cakramarda; (Mar.) Ṭākḷā; (H.B.) Cakundā; (Tel.) Tantemu; (Tam.) Tagarai.

---

१ नि.शे.टीका संमतः पाठः ।
२ 'प्रपुन्नाटश्चक्री' नि.शे. टीका संमतः पाठः ।
३ त्वावर्तकः स च नि. शे. टीका संमतः पाठः ।

3 (३) धत्तूरः Dhattūraḥ

धत्तूरः कनको धूर्तो देवता कितवः शठः ॥ ६
उन्मत्तको मदनकः कालिश्च हरवल्लभः ॥

धत्तूरः कटुरुष्णश्च कान्तिकारी व्रणार्तिनुत् ॥ ७
कुष्ठानि हन्ति लेपेन प्रभावेण ज्वरं जयेत् ॥

त्वग्दोषकृच्छ्रकण्डूतिज्वरहारी भ्रमावहः ॥ ८ ॥

धत्तूरः (Dhattūraḥ), कनकः (Kanakaḥ), धूर्तः (Dhūrtaḥ), देवता (Devatā) कितवः (Kitavaḥ), शठः (Śaṭhaḥ), उन्मत्तकः (Unmattakaḥ), मदनकः (Madanakaḥ), कालिः (Kāliḥ), and हरवल्लभः (Haravallabhaḥ) are synonymous.

Dhattūra is pungent, *uṣṇavirya*, improves complexion, relieves pains from the wounds, and is useful in external applications, in skin disorders, by *prabhāva* it is febrifuge. It is useful in skin disorders, obstinate pruritus, in fevers and is intoxicant.

(Generic name, includes the following plants - A-श्यामःलोहितः (Śyāmaḥlohitaḥ), B-कृष्ण (Kṛṣṇa), C- सित (Sita), D –नील(Nīla), E –पीत (Pīta), F राजधत्तूरः (Rājadhattūraḥ). All of the same genus.

I- A-a- ***Datura fastuosa*** (Cooke)*
 b- Cooke Fl. (See IV-1 below).
 B-a- ***D.fastuosa*** Willd.
 Syn. *Stramonia indica Tertia;* (Roxb. p. 188)
 Datura rubra Rumph.
 Black datura (Watt. Dict.)
 b-C.B.C. p. 188 below . Beng. Kala dhootura,
 C-a- ***D. fastuosa*** Linn.,var ***alba*** C.B. Clarke. white datura (See IV-2) below.
 c- Cooke flora, Watt. dict.
 D - Not identified.
 E- a- ***D. metal*** Mukerji
 b Mukerji (See -IV-3 below.)
 F -a- ***D. stramonium*** Linn.
 b Desai (See IV. 4 bellow)
II- A – कनकः (Kanakaḥ), कितवः (Kitavaḥ), उन्मत्तः (Unmattaḥ), हरवल्लभः (Haravallabhaḥ), कालिः (Kāliḥ), श्यामः (Śyāmaḥ), कालपुष्पः (Kālapuṣpaḥ), कण्टकफलः (Kaṇṭaka-phalaḥ).
 (b) (Mara.) Kāḷā dhotrā

---

*The current valid name is -
D. metal Linn. (Comp. p. 50)

B-a कृष्णधत्तूरकः (Kṛṣṇadhattūrakaḥ), कनकः (Kanakaḥ), सचिवः (Sacivaḥ), क्रूरधूर्तः (Krūradhūrtaḥ) + b - (Mar.) Kaḷādhotrā

C-a सित (Sita)

b (Mara.) Pāṇḍhrādhotrā 22.

D-a Not identified

E- a पीत (Pīta)

b- (Mar.) Dhotra, Duttura.

F-a राजधत्तूरः (Rājadhuttūraḥ), महाशठः (Māhāsaṭhaḥ), भ्रान्तः (Bhrāntaḥ), राजस्वर्णः (Rajaswarṇaḥ); Mara. Dhotrā.

III

IV 1) *Datura fastuosa* Linn. काला धतूरा

.... Flowers purple outside, usually white inside, often double. Capsule nodding, covered all over with numerous straight sharp prickels, seeds yellowish brown (Cooke fl.)

2) *Datura fastuosa* Linn. var. *alba*. C.B. Clarke.

Flowers rather smaller than those of *D. fastuosa,* proper, single, not double. Flowers white or cream coloured (cooke-fl.)

3) *D. metal* Linn.

is indigenous to India, flowers erect, calyx purple, tubuler, angular, 5, toothed; Corolla white often violet outside to yellowish. The limb in cultivation often double, capusle nodding, subglobus, short spiny. Dr. Mukherji.

4) *D. stramonium* Linn. (Chopra)

Sans. Rājadhattūra, H. Dhattur, Himalayas, Kashmir, Sikkim, Afganistan, Iran. Seeds-Blackish, Kidney shaped, flat, rough (Desai).

5) धुत्तुर

D. metal Linn.

Syn. उन्मत्त, कनक, धत्तूर

Su. Ci. 17.37; Ka. 7.52,53

Another species i.e. *D. stramonium* Linn. may also be a variety of it, called on the basis of seed colour.

There are other species and varieties of Dhattūra, usually differing in colour of flowers, stem and leaves as mentioned in Raj. ni. which, however, are not differentieted by characters other than morphological ones. (Balvantji p. 214.)

6) It has to be admimtted that at the utmost we can say of the Indian daturs is a confusion of defective knowledge. (Watt. Dict. 'D' page 31)

Note : The interested readers should go through the pages 29-32 of this dictionary where the subject is discussed vastly under the 'History of Datura.'

4 (४) कलिकारी Kalikārī (लाङ्गली-Lāṅgalī)

कलिकारी तु हलिनी विशल्या गर्भपातिनी ॥
लाङ्गल्यग्निमुखी सीरी[1] दीप्ता नक्तेन्दुपुष्पिका[2] ॥ ९

लाङ्गली कटुरुष्णा च कफवातविनाशनी ॥
तिक्ता सरा च श्वयथुगर्भशल्यव्रणापहा ॥ १०

कलिकारी (Kalikārī), हलिनी (Halinī), विशल्या (Viśalyā), गर्भपातिनी (Garbhapātinī), लाङ्गली (Lāṅgalī), अग्निमुखी(Agnimukhī), सीरी (Śīrī), दीप्ता (Dīptā), and नक्तेन्दुपुष्पिका (Naktendupuṣpikā) are synonymous.

Lāṅgalī is pungent, bitter *uṣṇavīrya*, pacifies *kaphavātadoṣas*. It is laxative, and useful in oedema, difficult labour and wounds.

I (a) ***Gloriosa superba*** Linn.
(b) Dr. Dymock (Pharma-indi.)

II (a) हलिनी (Halinī), गर्भपातिनी (Garbhapātinī), लाङ्गली (Lāṅgalī),नक्तेन्दुपुष्पिका (Naktendupuṣpikā), स्वर्णपुष्पा (Swarṇapuṣpā), अग्निजिह्वाAganijihvā).
(b) (Sk) Kalihārī, Śakrapuṣpī; (B) Viṣalānguli; (Bom.) Kaḷalāwī; (Mar.) Khaḍyānāg, Vagnaktā;(Guj.) Dudhiyo bacanāga; (Tam.) Akkinī, Chilam, Kāndala; (Tel.) Aganīśkhā, Masonī; (Kan.) Kolikuttum; (Santal) Sirif Samano.

5 (५) भृङ्गराजः Bhṛṅgarājaḥ

भृङ्गराजो भृङ्गरजो मार्कवो भृङ्ग एव च ॥
भृङ्गारको भृङ्गरेणुर्भृङ्गारः केशरञ्जनः ॥ ११

भृङ्गराजः समाख्यातस्तिक्तोष्णो रुक्ष एव च ॥
कफशोफामपाण्डुत्वग्घ्रद्रोगविषनाशनः ॥ १२

---

१ 'सौरी' इति क्षी. संमतः पाठः ।
२ 'इन्द्रपुष्प्यपि' इति.क्षी. संमतः पाठः ।

भृङ्गराजः (Bhṛṅgarājaḥ), भृङ्गरजः (Bhṛṅgarajaḥ), मार्कवः (Mārkavaḥ), भृङ्गः (Bhṛṅgaḥ), भृङ्गारकः (Bhṛṅgārakaḥ), भृङ्गरेणुः (Bhṛṅgareṇuḥ) भृङ्गारः (Bhṛṅgāraḥ), and केशरञ्जनः (Kes'arañjanaḥ) are synonymous.

Bhṛṅgarāja is bitter in taste, *uṣṇavrīya*, roughning and pacifies *kaphadoṣa*. It is useful in oedema, *āmadoṣa*, anaemia, disorders of skin, heart and poisons.

Generic name includes three plants A. मार्कवः पितृप्रियः (Mārkawaḥ pitṛpriyaḥ), B. पीतो हरिप्रियः (Pīto Haripriyaḥ) and third C. महानीलः * (Mahānīlaḥ).

Fam. Compositae. Asteeraceae.

a-A- ***Eclipta alba*** Hassk.**
Syn. *E. prostrata* Linn.
E. erecta L.

b- Dymock (Phar. indi.)

a-B ***Wedelia calendulacea*** Less J. Murray (Watt. Dict.)***

For confirmtion.

C-a ***Caesulia axiillaris*** Willd.

b Roxburgh iv.

II a-A केश्यः (Kes'yaḥ), मार्कवः(Mārkavaḥ), केशरञ्जनः (Kes'arañjanaḥ), कुन्तलवर्धनः (Kuntalavardhanaḥ), पितृप्रियः (Pitṛpriyaḥ)

(b) (SK) Bhṛṅgarāja; (H.) Bhāṅgrā; (Mara.) Mākā

(B) Kesuti, Kesutijā (Tam.) Gāruga, (Tel) Galgara.

a-B स्वर्णभृङ्गारः (Swarṇa bhṛṅgāraḥ), देवप्रियः (Devapriyaḥ)

(b) (H.) Bhāngrā;(B) Kesuria, Bāngrā; Kesraj; (Mara.) Pivaḷa mākā; (Tam.) Postaley Kaiantgerai.

a-C Mākā (Roxburgh)

IV- 1 *Caesulia axillaris,* Roxb. (Mākā) A succulent prostrate herb, 6-18 inches high, stem stout, more or less branched, striate, Leaves sessile, 1½.6 by .3/1.6-in. lanceolate, acute, distally serrulate. Heads axillary, sessile, flowers pale blue or white, ... Anthers black, Distribution throughout the greater part of India in rice field. Caesulia (Cooke flora p. 35)

2 *Eclipta erecta* Linn.
Syn. *E. prostrata* Linn.
E. alba Hassk, माका, भांग्रा (Cooke Fl.), मार्कवः Mārkavaḥ and

---

* These three types of plants are mentioned according to Raj. Ni. (S.D.K.)

** The current valid name is - *E. alba* (Linn.) Hassk.

*** *W. chinensis* Merrill
Syn. *W. calandulacea* Less. non Rich. (U.P.I.p.687) (Present accepted name)

Pīta Bhṛṅgarāja पीतभृंगराज. The first variety is suggested to be used for medicinal purpose while the second is indicated to be used in the worship of Deities. The third variety महानील *Mahānīla* and मार्कवः *Mārkavaḥ* are not differentiated by the practitioners.

---

6 (६) अर्कः Arkah

अर्कः सूर्याह्वयः पुष्पी विक्षीरोऽथ विकीरणः ॥
जम्भलः क्षीरपर्णी स्यादास्फोटो भास्करो रविः ॥ १३

अर्कस्तु कटुरुष्णश्च वातहृद्दीपनः सरः ॥
शोफव्रणहरः कण्डूकुष्ठप्लीहकृमीञ्जयेत् ॥ १४

अर्कः (Arkaḥ), सूर्याह्वयः (Sūryāhvayaḥ), पुष्पी (Puṣpī), विक्षीरः (Vikṣīraḥ), विकीरणः (Vikiraṇaḥ), जम्भलः (Jambhalaḥ), क्षीरपर्णी (Kṣīraparṇī), आस्फोटः (Āsphoṭaḥ), भास्करः (Bhāskaraḥ), and रविः (Raviḥ) are synonymous.

Arka is pungent in taste, *uṣṇavīrya,* pacifies, *vātadoṣa.*, stimulates digestive capacity, laxative, reduces inflammation and wounds, and is useful in pruritus, disorders of skin, spleen and worms.

राजार्कः Rājārkaḥ (1)
राजार्को वसुकोऽत्यर्को मन्दारो गणरूपकः ॥
एकाष्ठीलः सदापुष्पी स चालर्कः प्रतापनः ॥ १५
राजार्कः कटुतिक्तोष्णो कफमेदोविषापहः ॥
वातकुष्ठव्रणान् हंति शोफकण्डूविसर्पनुत ॥ १६

राजार्कः (Rājārkaḥ), वसुकः (Vasukaḥ), अत्यर्कः (Atyarkaḥ), मन्दारः (Mandāraḥ), गणरूपकः (Gaṇarūpakaḥ), एकाष्ठीलः (Ekāṣṭhīlaḥ), सदापुष्पी (Sadāpuṣpī), अलर्कः (Alarkaḥ), and प्रतापनः (Pratāpanaḥ) are synonymous.

Rājārka is pungent and bitter in taste and pacifies *vātadoṣa* and *kaphadoṣa* . It decreases *meda* and useful in poisons, skin disorders, ulcers, oedema, pruritus and erysipelas.

श्वेतार्कः Śvetārkaḥ (2)
शुक्लार्कस्तपनः श्वेतः प्रतापश्च सितार्ककः ।
सुपुष्पः शङ्करादिः स्यादत्यर्को वृत्तमल्लिका ॥
श्वेतार्कः कटुतिक्तोष्णो मलशोधनकारकः ।
मूत्रकृच्छ्रास्रशोफार्ति व्रणदोषविनाशनः ॥ Raj. ni. Chap. 10

१ 'अध्यर्क' इति पा.

शुक्लार्कः (Śuklārkaḥ), तपनः (Tapanaḥ), श्वेतः (Śvetaḥ), प्रतापः (Pratāpaḥ), सितार्कककः (Sitārkakaḥ), सुपुष्पः (Supuṣpaḥ), शङ्करादिः (Śaṅkarādiḥ), अत्यर्कः (Atyarkaḥ), and वृत्तमल्लिका (Vṛttamallikā) are synonymous.

Śvetārka is pungent and bitter in taste, *uṣṇavīrya,* has purificatory action on *malās*. It is useful in dysuria, pains due to *raktaśopha* and decreases *doṣas* from ulcers.

श्वेतमन्दारः Śvetamandāraḥ (3)
श्वेतमन्दारकस्त्वन्यः पृथ्वी कुरबकः स्मृतः ॥
दीर्घपुष्पः सितालर्को दीर्घात्यर्कः शराह्वयः ॥
श्वेतमन्दारकोऽत्युष्णास्तिक्तो मलविशोधनः ।
मूत्रकृच्छ्रव्रणान् हन्ति कृमीनत्यन्तदारुणान् ॥ Raj. ni. chap. 10

There is an another type of *Arka* called as श्वेतमन्दारक *Śvetamandāraka* of which synonyms are पृथ्वी (Pṛthvī), कुरबकः (Kurabakaḥ), दीर्घपुष्पः (Dīrghapuṣpaḥ), सितालर्कः (Sitālarkaḥ), and दीर्घात्यर्कः (Dīrghātyarkaḥ).

Śvetamandāraka is excessively *uṣṇavīrya,* bitter in taste, and has purificatory action on *malās*. It is useful in dysuria, ulcers and severe infestation by worms.

(Fam. Asclepiadaceae)

I- a- **Calotropis procera** R. Br.*
b Dymock (Pharma. Indica II-428)

II-A-B-a- क्षीरपर्णी (Kṣīraparṇī), क्षीरकाण्डकः (Kṣīrakāṇḍakaḥ), शिवपुष्पकः (Śivapuṣpakaḥ), शुकफलः (Śukaphalaḥ)

A-b (H) Āka; (B) Akanda; (Mar.) Rui; (Tam) Arkam; (Tel.) Jilledu; (Mal.) Erikku Arka = Lilac variety (Roxb.)

B-b Modern names of both the species are the same. (Eng.) Swallow worts.

III.

IV.1) अर्क Arka
.... has two species which are identified with *Calotropis procera* (Ait.) R. Br. *Raktārka* रक्तार्क, and *C. gigantea* (Linn.) R. Br. ex. Ait. *Swetārka*श्वेतार्क (Balawantji p. 23)

2) अलर्क Alarka has always been mentioned with अर्क and not alone. This is usually considered to be bigger and white flowered variety

---

* The current accepted name is -
Calotropis procera (Ait.) R. Br. (U. P.I. p. 98)

C. gigantea R. Br. Ḍalhaṇa also describes it as a tree variety of *Arka* with white flowers (अलर्क श्वेतार्क वृक्षः)
(Balwantji p. 25)

राजार्कः Rājārkaḥ (Fam. Asclepidaceae)

I- a- ***Calotropis gigantea*** R.Br.*
b Kamat

II- a वसुकः Vasukaḥ, मन्दारः Mandāraḥ, एकाष्ठीला Ekāṣṭhilā, अलर्कः Alarkaḥ
b- as in अर्क II b See अर्क IV-2

7 (७) बुकः Bukaḥ

बुको[१] वसुक इत्युक्तः शिवाह्वः शिवशेखरः ।
महापाशुपतश्चैव सुव्रतः शिवमल्लिका ॥ १७
वसुकः कटुतिक्तोष्णः श्लेष्मोद्भूत व्यथापहः ।
व्रणान् समस्तान् हरति प्रलेपादि प्रयोजितः ॥ १८

बुकः (Bukaḥ), वसुकः (Vasukaḥ), शिवाह्वः (Śivāhavaḥ), शिवशेखरः (Śivasekharaḥ),महापाशुपतः (Mahāpāśupataḥ), सुव्रतः (Suvrataḥ) and शिवमल्लिका (Śivamallikā) are synonymous.

Vasukaḥ is pungent and bitter in taste, *uṣṇavīrya*, pacifies disorders caused by *kapha* and by external application it is useful in all types of wounds.

Controversial plant
(Fam. oleaceae)

I- a ***Osmanthus fragrans*** Lour.
b Prof. Balwantji
See IV- 1 below.

II- (a) बुकः (Bukaḥ), वसुकः (Vasukaḥ), बकः (Bakaḥ), महापाशुपतः (Mahāpāśupataḥ), शिवमल्लि (Śivamalli).

III- 1) वसुक (Vasuka) (Su.Sū. 37 & 39)
बुक, वसुक (Buka, Vasuka)
A.H. Sū. 15-5,24.ci. 11.18 etc (Dr. Pendse)
शिवमल्ली - पृथुपुष्पो बकुल विशेष एवेति प्रतिभाति । (A.O.Ni.)

IV- 1) Būka

---

१ वसुर्वसुक इत्युक्तः शिवार्कः शिवशेखरः । इति क्षीः संमत पाठः ।

Note - This may be also a variety of अर्क (Arka). S. D. Kamat.

* *Calotropis gigantea* (Linn.) R. Br. ex Ait. is the current name. (U.P. I.p.98)
Calotropis gigantea (Linn.) Dryand (Comp.p.27)

C.S. Ci. 30-81 (va)
A.H. Su. 15.24; V. 30. 38 (va)
Būka, (बूक)*Baka* (बक) and *Śivamallikā* -(शिवमल्लिका) have been described as synonyms of *Vasuka* - वसुक and have also been called *Bṛhadbakula* बृह्द्बकुल by some. On the basis of comments given by Dalhaṇa, *Śivamallī* appears to be *Osmanthus fragrans* Lour. popularly known as *Bagahula* बगहुल which is an equivalent name for *Bakapuṣpa* -बकपुष्प. It has been found that, *Slianga* सिलंग or *Silangī* सिलंगी is the more common name given to *Osmanthus* by *Garhvālis*. Moreover, it is considered by the local Vaidyas as their *Bakula*. (Balwntji p. 277).

2) *Osmanthus fragrans* Lour.
Syn. *Olea fragrans* Thunb.
O. acuminata Wall.
Vern. silinga, shilinga (kumaon)
A small tree found in the temparate Himalaya,..... sometimes wild, more often cultivated for its sweet scented flowers. It is distributed to China and Japan where it is widely cultivated. The flowers are used in China to flavour tea.
(Watt Dict. "O" p. 654).

3) *Olea fragrans* Linn.
O. fragrans Thunb. (CBC p. 35).

4) बृहद् बकुलः - *Bṛhadbakulaḥ*; बडी मोलसरी *Baḍi molasarī,* शिवमल्ली *'sivamallī,* बक *Baka*, वसु *Vasu.*
Bha. praka. Ni. has recognised two kinds of मोलसरी Molasarī; the larger tree kind is noted as *Baka, Pā'supata* and the smaller kind as *Bakula*. (Bha. Pr. Ni. 494).

8 (८) काकमाची Kākamācī

काकमाची ध्वाङ्क्षमाची काकाह्वा चैव वायसी ।
कट्वी कट्टफला चैव रसायनवरा स्मृता ॥ १९

काकमाची त्रिदोषघ्नी सरा स्वर्या सतित्तका ।
हन्ति दोषत्रयं कुष्ठं वृष्या सोष्णा रसायनी ॥ २०

काकमाची (Kākamācī), ध्वाङ्क्षमाची (Dhwānksamācī), काकाह्वा (Kākāhvā), वायसी (Wāyasī), कट्वी (Kaṭvī), कट्टफला (Kaṭuphalā) and रसायनवरा (Rasāyanavarā) are synonymous.

Kākamācī pacifies all the three *doṣās,* laxative, is beneficial to voice and slighltly bitter in taste.

Kākamācī pacifies all the three *doṣas,* is useful in disorders of skin, is *vṛṣyā, uṣṇavīrya,* and *rasāyana.*

Two varieties of this drug are recognised. The one is A. North-west Himalayan plant and the next is B. Himalayan, extended southwards.

Fam. Solanaceae.

A-a- ***Solanum dulcamara*** Linn

b- R.N. Chopra (Gloss. Ind. Medi. Plants)

B-a- ***Solanum nigrum*** Linn..

Dr. Dymock (Phar. Indi.)

II-A-B- ध्वाङ्क्षमाची (Dhwāṅkśamācī), वायसी (Wāyasī), रसायनवरा (Rasāyanawarā), काकमाता (Kākamātā), बहुतिक्ता (Bahutiktā),

b-a (SK) Kākamācī; (Pun.) Rubābarik; (Bazar) Anab -es-salib.

b-b (SK) Kākamācī; (B) Kamācī, Gurkāmai; (H). Makoi; (Mar.) Kamonī; (Tam.) Manatakali; (Tel.) Kamaneī; (Eng.) Black Night-shade.

III नितत्नि ओषधी "देवी देव्याम्" "या जमदग्निः" इति तृचाभ्यां केशवृद्धिकरणकामः काकमाची फलं जीवन्तीफलं भृंगराजं वा संपात्य अभिमन्त्र्य बध्नीयात् ॥

(Av. Kand VI, Anu. 13, Suk. 13.137)

(Kau. IV-7 See IV-1 infra)

b-1) कामाता काकमाची (Kāmātā Kākamācī), काकमाची तु वायसी इत्यमरः । (Kākamācī tuvāyasī Ityamaraḥ) कालीकामोणीति लोके (Kalikamoṇi ti loke) Rasapaddhati p-1

2) Ast. Hr. Kosh.

3) Harshe.

IV- 1 For the growth of hairs on the head the plant 'Nitanī' is dug out of the ground (6-136-1,3) Jamadagni (6-131-3). Sayan and Kaushika (31-28) prescribe the fruits 'Kākamāchi', Jivantī' and Bhṛṅgaraja should be tied on the head. (Dr. Shende p. 33)

2 See Dr. Kirtikar (II-892 p.)

3 काकमाची (Kākamācī)- (Bha.-Gudu.) *Solanum nigrum, S. dulcamara*. Baḍimakoya is cultivated in Banaras and Lucknow districts. It is called there as *Rasabharī Makoya.* (Ach. Dwivedi)

4. Bitter-sweet - *Solanum dulcamara* Linn. Medical uses (Potter's Cycl. P.40)

5 Balawantji. (pp. 86-87).

6 Black Night-shade.
Solanum nigrum Linn.
In Britain, has earned a bad reputation as a poisonous plant. In West Indies the leaves are used as greens and in parts U.S. America, the fruit is used to make jams. S. nigrum Var. quineensis (Guienensis?) L. cultivated locally under the name Garden Huckleberry. The food value is low and no explanation offered for the contradiction between the European reputation of this plant and its uses on the other side of the Atlantic.
(Prof. Nelson p. 276).

7 *Solanum nigrum* Linn.
Sk. Kākamāchi; B. Kākamāchi; H. Makoi. Berries used in fever, diarrhoea, eye diseases, hydrophobia. Juice of plant hydragouge cath., diuretic, alterative, given in enlargement of liver, in blood spitting, piles, dysentery etc.
Young shoots given in skin diseases and psoriasis ... ... feeding experiments on sheep for toxicity showed negative results. (Chopra)
S. dulcamara Linn.
S. Kākamācī, Pers. Anābesālib
Berries alterative, diur ..... useful in skin diseases, psoriasis, lepra., syphilitic affections, ch. rhumatism, enlargement of the liver etc. Twigs ... narcotic, promote all secretions, used in obstinate cutaneous eruptions, scrofula etc. (Chopra)

8) काकमाची Kākmācī
Solanum nigrum Linn. (Balawantji P. 86)

काकजङ्घा Kākajanghā (4)

काकजङ्घा ध्वाङ्क्षजङ्घा काकपादा तु लोमशा ।
पारावतपदी दासी नदीकान्ता प्रचीबला ॥ २१

काकजङ्घा च तिक्तोष्णा रक्तपित्तज्वरापहा ।
कृमिदोषहरा वर्ण्या विषदोषहरा मता ॥ २२

काकजङ्घा (Kākajanghā), ध्वाङ्क्षजङ्घा (Dhwānksajanghā), काकपादा (Kākapādā), लोमशा (Lomasā), पारावतपदी (Pārāvatapadī), दासी (Dāsī), नदीकान्ता (Nadīkāntā), and प्रचीबला (Prachībalā) are synonymous.

Kākajanghā is bitter in taste, *uṣṇavīrya*, alleviates bleeding disorders and fever, is useful in worms, beneficial to complexion and antipoisonous.

Two kinds of plants are taken for Kākajaṅghā A काकजङ्घा (Kākajaṅghā) accepted by the majority of Kavirajas and the next B- काकजङ्घा (Kākajaṅghā), taken by the Kavirājās of Bengal. Both of them belong to different families.

(For confirmation) (Fam. Acanthaceae)

A-(a) ***Peristrophe bicalyculata*** Nees*

(b) D.K. Kamat IV -1, 2, 3 Below

B-(a) ***Leea aequata*** Roxb. (Fam. Vitaceae)

Syn-*Leea hirta* Roxb.

(b) Dr. W. Dymock (Pharm. indi.).

II (a) A & B काकपादा (Kākapādā), लोमशा (Lomaśā), पारावतपदी (Pārāvatapadī), दासी (Dāsī), नदीकान्ता (Nadīkāntā), प्रचीबला (Pracībalā).

A-(b) (H) Atrilāl; (Bom.) Pitpāpaḍā; (B) Nāsabhaṅgā; (Mar.) Kāṇg; (Guj.) Aghedo, Aghedu.

B-(b)(San.) (H) Kākajaṅghā, (Mar.) Kāng; (Tel.) Surpadi; (Mal.) Kākanāsikā.

III (a) काकजङ्घा - *Leea hitra* (Dr. Ghanekar, Su. Su. 38.5)

(b) काकजङ्घा (Kākajaṅghā) = त्रिधा (Tridhā) (Raj. Ni. Chapter II)

IV 1) (Kākajaṅghā)

Leea hirta Roxb. (Dr. U.C. Datta. Pt. Bhagirath)

2) काकजङ्घा (Kākajaṅghā)

Peristrophe bicalyculata (Ni. Adarash, Ni. Shiromani)

3) काकजङ्घा Kākajaṅghā It has not been identified. In practice, ...two plants i.e. *Peristrophe bicalyculata* Nees, ... *Leea aequata* Linn. are generally used. See synonyms प्रा (प्र) चीबला and वायसजङ्घा (S.Su. 3.20,27, 114 etc. S.Su.21-22, 42.18 etc. A.H. Su. 30.10; U.3.43.) (Balawantji p. 85)

4) प्राचीबला Prācībalā identification most disputed ... both Prācībalā and Kākajaṅghā may be *Vitex peduncularis* Wall. (Balwantji p. 292).

5) See note of Balawantji under Kākanāsā Post No. (5) infra.

काकनासा Kākanāsa (5)

काकनासा ध्वाङ्क्षनासा काकतुण्डफला च सा ।
सुरङ्गी तस्करस्नायुर्ध्वाङ्क्षतुण्डफला मता ॥ २३

* Current accepted name -
P. bicalyculata (Retz.) Nees (comp. p. 116)

काकतुण्डी भवेत्तिक्ता कटूष्णा व्रणशोधिनी ।
[१]अतिबद्धं शोधयन्ती तैलपाके हितावहा ॥ २४

काकनासा (Kākanāsā), ध्वाङ्क्षनासा (Dhwānksanāsā), काकतुण्डफला (Kākatuṇḍaphalā), सुरङ्गी (Surangī), तस्करस्नायु (Taskarasnāyu), and ध्वाङ्क्षतुण्डफला (Dhwānk'satuṇḍaphalā) are synonymous.

Kākatuṇḍī is bitter and pungent in taste, *usṇavīrya,* purificatory of wounds, removes hardened stool and useful for processing (cooking) oils.

(a) Ambiguous

II (a) काकतुण्डी (Kākatuṇḍī), कटूष्णा (Kaṭūsṇā) व्रणशोधिनी (Vraṇa Śodhinī) Dh.Ni., मधुरा (Madhurā), पित्तहारिणी (Pittahāriṇī), रसायनी (Rasāyanī) (Raj. Ni.).

Note - It seems from the medicinal properties of Dh. Ni's and Raj. Ni's plants of काकनासा (Kākanāsā) are different.

गुणाः *काकतुण्डी भवेत्तिक्ता कटूष्णा व्रणशोधिनी ।*
अतिविद्धं शोधयन्ती ॥ (ध. 4.26)

गुणाः –*काकनासा तु मधुरा शिशिरा पित्तहारिणी ।*
रसायनी दार्ढ्यकरी विशेषात्पलितापहा ॥

III 1) काकनासा (Kākanāsā) = Kākatuṇḍī = Vāyasaphalā (Ḍalhaṇa Su. 37)

2) काकनासा (Kākanāsā) = Vāyasaphalam (Cakra. Ca. 31.4.5)
Asclepias curassavica, Linn. Kākatuṇḍī (Chopra)
Pentatropis cynanchoides R. Br.
'Kauāḍoḍi', Śingroṭā (Chopra)

IV 1) काकनासा (Kākanāsā) - Kauaḍoḍī
(1) *Solanum indicum* (2) *Gymnema sylvestre* (3) *Asclepias curassavica* (Vidyotani), Bh. Pr. Ni.)

2) डोडी or कौआडोडी (Ḍoḍī or Kauāḍoḍī) (Guj.)
Leptadenia reticulata Benth.
Pentataropis microphylla, W & A. (Sachitra Ayur. 5.2)

3) Kākanāsā like other drugs have been named after Kāka (Crow) i.e.काकजङ्घा, काकतिक्ता, काकमाची and काकादनी etc. have been identified and the commentators very widely differ .... (Balawantji p. 86)

2) काकनासा It really means those plants whose fruits are just like the beak of a crow. The fruits of many Asclepiadaceae(अर्कादिवर्ग) are very similar to this and so I venture to identifiy काकनासा as कौआडोडी According to the commentator of Sharangadhara काकनासा

---

१ 'अनिविद्धं' इति आनन्दा. पुस्तके पाठः ।

-काकतुंडी सिद्घमंत्र' (सिद्घमंत्र टीका) काकनासा - वायसफला (डल्हण चि. अ. 36)

In Gujarat 'कौआडोडी' is still known by the name डोडी and कौआडोडी being to the same order Asclepiadaceae. डोडी is *Leptadenia reticulata* (Asclepiadacae) and 'कौआडोडी' *Pentatropis microphylla*,

Gujrathi name is शिंगरोटी, the कौआडोडी is काकनासा (B.G.Vaidya Sachi. Ayur. - May 62 p. 944)

3) *Pentatropis microphylla*, W. & A.
H. Ambarvel; S- Singarita; Mar. Shingrota
Plant cooling, alter. W. Peninsula.
Pentatropis cynanchoides R. Br.
P. Vanveri; Bo,. Shingrota; H. Kauathodi.
Sk. Kākāksi.
Dry roots - given in decoction, as astringent, cooling, alterative, used in gonorrhoea. Punjab eastwareds to Jamna, Baluchistan and Sind (Chopra).

काकादनी (Kākādanī) (6)

काकादनी काकपीलुः काकणन्ती च रक्तिका।
वक्त्रशल्या ध्वाङ्क्षनखी दुर्मोहा काकणन्तिका॥ २५

काकणन्ती च तिक्तोष्णा वातश्लेष्महरा मता।
ग्रहदोषहरा केश्या वृष्या चोर्ध्वगदापहा॥ २६

काकादनी (Kākādanī), काकपीलु (Kākapīluḥ), काकणन्ती (Kākaṇantī), रक्तिका (Raktikā), वक्त्रशल्या (Vaktrasalyā), ध्वाङ्क्षनखी (Dhwānksanakhī), दुर्मोहा (Durmohā), and काकणन्तिका (Kākaṇantikā) are synonymous.

Kākaṇantī is bitter in taste, *uṣṇavīrya,* pacifies *vāta* and *kaphadoṣas*, alleviates disorders caused by *Grahās,* is beneficial to hair, is *vṛsya* and useful in the diseases above the sternum (eye, ear, nose etc.).

This plant may be गुञ्जा (Guñjā). The editor of Ānandāśram edition has identified it with गुञ्जा (Guñjā) but Dh. Ni. noted गुञ्जा under the current name चूडामणिः

(a) See Cūdamaṇi (Post No. 7 infra)

III b-1 (Kākajanghā)
Kākādanītyapare गुञ्जेति (Guñjeti) prasiddhā (Dalhan Dr. Ghanekar, Su-Su. Ārgavadhādi p. 278)

2 काकादनी Kākādanī Su. Su. 39 9 etc.
A.H. Ci. 15.78 etc. .... two kinds of काकादनी (Kākādanī) were recognised by Vāgbhat. (Balawantji p. 88)

IV- 1 Kākādanī
S.S. Su. 39.9 Ci. 14.8 etc.
A.H. Ci. 15-78 etc.,
This drug name does not occur in Caraka .... स्थूलकाकादनी ..... two kinds of Kākādanī were recognised by Vāgbhat.
Balwantji p. 88

2 काकादनी (Kākādanī)
Cardiospermum halicacabum Linn. Balwantji p. (VI)

चूडामणिः Cūḍāmaniḥ (7)

चूडामणिः शीतपाकी शिखण्डी कृष्णला मता ।
उच्चटा ताम्रिका गुञ्जा चटकी काकसाह्वया ॥ २७

गुञ्जा रूक्षा तथा तिक्ता वीर्योष्णा च प्रकीर्तिता ।
विषवैषम्य जन्तुघ्नी रोगग्रामभयापहा ॥ २८

चूडामणिः (Cūḍāmaṇiḥ), शीतपाकी (Śītapākī), शिखण्डी (Śikhaṇḍī), कृष्णला (Kṛṣṇalā), उच्चटा (Uccaṭā), ताम्रिका (Tāmrikā), गुञ्जा (Guñja), चटकी (Caṭakī), and काकसाह्वया (Kākasāhvayā), are synonymous.

Guñjā is bitter in taste, *uṣṇasvīrya*, roughning, and is useful in poisons, worms (?antimicrobial) and in various diseases.

Generic name, includes three kinds गुञ्जा (Guñjā) according to the colours of the seeds. A- शीतपाकी काम्भोजी (Śītapākī Kāmbhojī) B- कृष्णला (Kṛṣṇalā), C- ताम्रिका (Tāmrikā). The seeds of this plant are used for decorating चूडा (Cūḍā) bangles by the Adivāsis and such hilly tribes, hence the name Cūḍāmaṇi).

(Fam Leguminosae) Fabaceae

A. see श्वेतकाम्भोजी (Swetakāmbhojī) Post No. 8 infra.

B- ***Abrus precatorius*** Linn.
Black seed, white eye and dark flower plant.

C *A. precatorius* Linn. Red seed with black eye and rose flowered plant. Dr. Roxburgh (Fl. indi.)

II- A See श्वेतकाम्भोजी (Śwetakāmbhojī)
B उच्चटा (Uccaṭā), कृष्णचूडिका (Kṛṣṇa cūḍikā), कृष्णला (Kṛṣṇalā)
(b) (Mar.) Gunja, Gunj; (H.) Gungchi, Rati; (Bom.) Gunja; (SK) Guñjā, Kṛṣṇalā; (Tam.) Gundumanī; (Tel.) Ghenza; (B) Kunch, Gunch, chunhati; (Eng.) Indian or white liquorice.
(c) ताम्रिका (Tāmrikā) रक्त्तिका (Raktikā)
(b) Mordern names as in B-(b) above.

श्वेतकाम्भोजी Śwetakāmbhojī (8)

अपरा श्वेतकाम्भोजी श्वेतगुञ्जा भिराटिका ।
काकादनी काकपीलुर्वक्त्रशल्या सितोच्चटा ॥ २९

गुञ्जाद्वयं च तिक्तोष्णं बीजं वान्तिकरं शिफा ।
शूलघ्नी विषहृत्पत्रं वश्ये श्वेता प्रशस्यते ॥ ३०

The other kind of *Guñjā* is called as श्वेतकाम्भोजी (Śvetakāmbhojī), of which synonyms are श्वेतगुञ्जा (Śvetaguñjā), भिराटिका (Bhirāṭikā), काकादनी (Kākādanī), काकपीलुः (Kākapīluh), वक्त्रशल्या (Vaktraśalyā), and सितोच्चटा (Sitoccaṭā).

Both the *guñjas* are bitter in taste and *uṣṇavīrya,* seeds are emetics, roots relieve colic, and the leaves are antipoisonous. The white one is used in *Vaśīkaraṇa* procedure.

(Leguminosae) Fabaceae.

I (a) White seeds with white flowered *Abrus precatorius* Linn.
(b) Roxburgh (Fl. indi.)
II (a) श्वेतगुञ्जा (Śwetaguñjā), भिराटिका (Bhirāṭikā), काकादनी (Kākādanī), सितोच्चटा (Sitoccaṭā).
II (a) Vernacular names as in चूडामणि (Cūḍamaṇī); (Eng.) Indian or white liquorice.

9 (९) मूलकम् Mūlakam

मूलकं हरिपर्णं मृत्तिकाक्षारमेव च ।
नीलकन्दं[१] महाकन्दं रुचिष्यं हस्तिकन्दकम्[२] ॥ ३१

मूलकं गुरुविष्टम्भि तीक्ष्णमामं त्रिदोषनुत् ॥

१ 'नीलकण्ठं' इति. नि.शे.टीकायाम् २ हस्तिदन्तकम – इति आनन्दा. पाठः ।

तदेव स्विन्नं स्निग्धं च कटूष्णं कफवातनुत् ॥ ३२
त्रिदोषशमनं शुष्कं विषदोषहरं लघु ।[१]

मूलकं (Mūlakam), हरिपर्णं (Hariparṇam), मृत्तिकाक्षारं (Mṛttikākṣāram), नीलकन्दं (Nīlakandam), महाकन्दं (Mahākandam), रुचिष्यं (Rucişyam), हस्तिकन्दकम् (Hastikandakam) are synonymous.

Immature *mūlakam* is *guru,* causes flatulance and is sharp but when the same is processed with oily substances and steamed, pacifies all the three *doṣas.* (otherwise) it is pungent, *uṣṇavīrya* and pacifies *kapha vāta doṣas;* when dried it pacifies three *doṣas,* is antipoisonous and is *laghu.*

Fam. Cruciferae. Brassicaceae.

I - (a) ***Raphanus sativus*** Linn.
(b) Roxburgh (Fl. indica).

II (a) भूक्षारम् (Bhūkshāram), नीलकन्दं (Nīlakandam), हस्तिकन्दकम् (Hastikandakam), सितम् (Sitam).
(b) (H) Muli; (B. Mar.) Muḷa; (Tam, Tel. Mal.) Muḷḷangi; (Eng.) Carrot.

IV Many varieties differ in size shape and colour (Hill).

चाणाख्यमूलकं* Cāṇākhyamūlakam (9)

चाणाख्यमूलकं चान्यच्छालेयं मरुसंभवम् ॥ ३३
शालामर्कटकं मिश्रं विष्णुगुप्तं मतं तथा ॥

चाणाख्यं मूलकं तिक्तं कटूष्णं रुच्यदीपनम् ॥ ३४
कफवातकृमीन्गुल्मं नाशयेद् ग्राहकं परम् ॥

There is an another kind of *mulaka* called as चाणाख्यमूलकं *Cāṇākhyamūlakam* of which synonyms are शालेयं (Śāleyam), मरुसंभवम् (Marusambhavam), शालामर्कटकं (Śālāmarkaṭakam), मिश्रं (Miśram), and विष्णुगुप्तं (Viṣṇuguptam).

Cāṇākhyamūlaka is bitter and pungent in taste, *uṣṇavīrya,* appetizing, stimulates digestive capacity, pacifies *kaphavātadoṣas*, worms, tumors (intestinal diverticulosis) and is good astiringent.

I (a) Variety of ***Raphanus sativus*** Linn.
(b) Kamat.

---

१. S.Su. 46. 241- 42 *'चाणक्य मूलकम्' इति साधु पाठः चौखम्बा मुद्रित पुस्तके ।

II (a) कौटिल्यं (Kauṭilyam), मरुसम्भवम् (Marusambhavam), विष्णुगुप्तम् (Viṣṇuguptakam), शालेयम् (Śāleyam)

(b) Modern names as in मूलकम्

III (b) Sk- चाणाख्यमूलकम् (Cāṇākhyamūlakam), Keral - Valiya mullangi; (Kan) Dodda Mullangi, (Mara.) Thormuḷā (A.O.Ni.)

IV- 1) शालेय Śāleya
C.S.Su. 27-167, Ci.4.75
It is supposed to be a variety of *Mūlaka* known as *Cāṇakyamūlaka* चाणक्यमूलक or जम्बू (Balawantji p. 396).

गृञ्जनम् Gṛñjanam (10)

तृतीयं मूलकं चान्यन्निर्दिष्टं तच्च गृञ्जनम् ॥ ३५
अटवीमूलकं पीतं तच्च नारदकन्दकम् ॥
गृञ्जनं[2] मधुरं तिक्तं विपाके कटुकं तथा ॥ ३६
पित्ताविरोधी कफहृद् गुरु स्याद् वातनाशनम् ॥

The third variety of *mulaka* is called by the name गृञ्जन Gṛñjana, of which synonyms are अटवीमूलकं (Aṭavīmūlakm), पीतं (Pītam), नारदकन्दकम् (Nāradakandakam).

Gṛñjana (*mūlakam*) is sweet and bitter in taste, pungent in *vipāka*, does not aggravate *pitta doṣa*, pacifies *kapha* and *vātadoṣa* and is *guru*.

पिण्डमूलम् Piṇḍamūlam (11)
पिण्डमूलं गजाण्डं च पिण्डकं पिण्डमूलकम् ।
पिण्डमूलं कटूष्णं च गुल्मवातादिदोषनुत् ॥ Raj. ni. chapter VII

पिण्डमूलं (Piṇḍamūlam), गजाण्डं (Gajāṇḍam), पिण्डकं (Piṇḍakam), and पिण्डमूलकं (Piṇḍamūlakam) are synonymous.

Pinḍumūla is pungent in taste, *uṣṇavīrya,* and is useful in tumors (diverticulosis), flatulance etc.

I A variety of *Raphanus sativas* Linn. with round roots.

II - (a) तृतीयं मूलकं + गृञ्जनम् (Tṛtīyam mūlakam + Gṛñjanam), पीतकम् (Pītakam), मधुरम् (Madhuram), स्वाद्ु (Swādu) Dh.Ni.).

---

१ 'पीतक मधुरं स्वाद्ु' इति आनन्दाश्रम पुस्तके पाठः ।
२ 'अटवीमूलकं' इति आनन्दाश्रम पुस्तके पाठः ।

B-(a) शिखिमूलकम् (Śikhimūlakam), यवनेष्टम् (Yawaneṣṭam), वर्तुलम् (Vartulam). (Raj. Ni.)

(b) शलघम् (Śalagham) See III 3 below.

III a) See Rasona - Gṛñjanam.

b) मूलकं पञ्चधा (Mūlakam pañcadhā) (Raj. Ni.)

2) गृञ्जनम् प्रोक्तं लशुने वृत्तमूलके
(Gṛñjanam proktam La'sune Vṛttamūlake) Raj. ni. dway. kosa.26 Śloka 4)

3) गृञ्जनम् (Gṛñjanam) - Sethimula,
(Gaud) Salgham (Pant. Ashutosh Raj. Ni.)
(See -शलघम, रसोनभेद - गृञ्जनम्. पं. भागीरथ)

IV 1) हस्तिगृञ्जनम् (Hastigṛñjanam). Tuber larger than a coconut fruit, containing starch and suger substance.
Beta cyclea,. Mangle wurzil (Hill).

2) *Beta vulgaris* var. *cyclea* ' Chard.' (Hill)
Chard a variety of white beat. (Chem. Dict.)

3) गृञ्जनकGṛñjanaka.
C.S.Su. 27.171, Ci. 12.61 etc.
A.H. Su. 6.128.etc.
This is usually considered to be carrot or turnip ... sometimes allied to *Garlic* (लशुन) or *onion* पलाण्डु such as गन्दना which is *Allium esculentum* Linn. also called one cloved garlic (एकपुतिया लहसुन) (Balwantji)

10 (१०) शिग्रुः Śigruḥ

शिग्रुर्हरितशाकश्च दीर्घको लघुपत्रकः ॥ ३७
अवदंशक्षमो दंशः प्रोक्तो मूलकपर्ण्यपि ॥

शोभाञ्जनस्तीक्ष्णगन्धो मुखभङ्गोऽथ शिग्रुकः ॥ ३८
श्वेतकः श्वेतमरिचो रक्तको मधुशिग्रुकः ॥

शिग्रुस्तिक्तः कटुश्चोष्णः कफशोफसमीरजित् ॥ ३९
कृम्यामविषमेदोघ्नो विद्रधिप्लीहगुल्मनुत् ॥

शिग्रुः (Śigruḥ), हरितशाकः (Haritaśākaḥ), दीर्घकः (Dīrghakaḥ), लघुपत्रकः (Laghupatrakaḥ), अवदंशक्षमः (Avadam'sak'samaḥ), दंशः (Dam'saḥ) and मूलकपर्णी (Mulakaparṇī), शोभाञ्जनः (Śobhāñjanaḥ), तीक्ष्णगन्धः (Tīksṇagandhaḥ), मुखभङ्गः (Mukhabhangaḥ), and शिग्रुकः (Śigrukaḥ), are synonymous. श्वेतकः(Śvetakaḥ), is श्वेतमरिचः (Śvetamaricaḥ), and रक्तकः (Raktakaḥ) is मधुशिग्रुकः (Madhu 'sigrukaḥ).

'Sigru is bitter and pungent, in taste, *uṣṇavīrya,* pacifies *kapha* and *vātadoṣas.* It is useful in oedema (inflammation), worms, *āmadoṣa*, poison, *meda*, abscess, disorders of spleen and tumours (diverticulosis ?).

(Generic name, includes three kinds of tree A.शोभाञ्जनः नील शिग्रुः 'Sobhāñjanaḥ Nīla 'sigrūḥ).B.श्वेतशिग्रुः ('Sweta 'sigruḥ) and the third C रक्त शिग्रुः (Rakta 'sigruḥ), all kinds of the same genus. The same vernacular names are indiscriminately applied to all kinds).

(For confirmation)

(Fam. Moringaceae)

I- A-(a)***Moringa oleifera*** Lam.
Syn. *Guilandiana moringa* Linn.
Moringa polygona DC.
Hyperanthera moringa Willd
(Roxb. Fl. Indi. Edi. Clarke 360)
(b) D.K. Kamat

B-(a) ***Moringa concanensis*** Nimmo
(b) D. K. Kamat

C-(a)Red flowered species. Found in the viscinity of Malda.
(b) Dr. Roxburgh (Fl. indi. p. 360).

II- A-(a) शोभाञ्जनः ('Sobhāñjanaḥ of Raj. Ni.), नील शिग्रुः (Nīla 'sigruḥ), कृष्णशिग्रुः(Kṛṣṇa 'Sigruḥ),जनप्रियः (Janapriyaḥ), मुखामोदः (Mukhāmodaḥ),रुचिरञ्जनः (Ruciranñjanaḥ), स्वादूष्णः ('Swādūṣṇaḥ), पिच्छिलः (Picchilaḥ)
(b)(SK) 'Sobhāñjan; (B) Sajana, Saragavo; (Tam.) Moringai; (Tel.) Sajan Mannaga; (Malbar) Sigru, Murinna; (Mar.) 'Sewagā, 'Segala, Segata; (Bom.) Sargo, Sekato; (Guj.) Saragavo; (Eng.) The indian horse raddish tree.

B-(a) श्वेत शिग्रुः ('Swetasigruḥ) of Raj. Ni.), सुतीक्ष्णः (Sutīksṇaḥ), मुखभङ्गः (Mukhabhangaḥ), सिताह्वयः (Sitāhvayaḥ).
(b)(SK) 'Sweta'sigruḥ;(Bom), Sinjan; (Tel.) Koṇḍa munanga; (Konkan) Rānsegal; (Tam.) Kattu murang.

C-(a) रक्तको मधुशिग्रुकः (Raktakao madhu 'sigrukaḥ), मधुरः (Madhuraḥ), बहुलच्छदः (Bahulacchadaḥ), सुगंधकेशरः (Sugandha Ke'saraḥ), सिंहः (Simhaḥ), मृगारिः (Mṛgāriḥ).

III-a (1) कृष्णगन्धः (Kṛṣṇagandhaḥ)
Ca. Su.I-116-117),
(2) मधुशिग्रुः (Madhu 'sigruḥ)

(3) शिग्रुः (Sigruḥ) - Madhu 'sigru.
(Dalhan Su.su. 46. 221)

(4) मधुशिग्रुः (Madhu'sigruḥ)- Lohit Kusumo Swlpavitapaḥ Sobhañjana Bhedaḥ)

IV 1) *Moringa oleifera* Linn.
Syn. *M. pterygosperma* Gaertn.
(SK.) Shobhāñjan, (Mal.) Sigru; indigenous in the sub Himalayan tract from chamba to oudh, also cultivated throughout India. (Chopra).

2) A red flowered species or variety is found in the viscinity of Malda. Its Sanskrit nameMadu sigru. (Roxburgh).

3) *Moringa concanensis*, Nimmo. Flowers yellowish, little pinkish and reddish ... powerful odour. (Lisboa)

4) *Armoracia lepathifolia* Gilib; native of S.W. Europe. The large white flesh .. roots used as condiment.
... It is similar to mustard oil in its properties. Europe - Horse radish. (Hill).

11 (११) सर्षपः Sarṣapaḥ

सर्षपः शुभ्रगौरस्तु सिद्धार्थो भूतनाशनः ॥ ४०
कटुस्नेहो ग्रहघ्नस्तु कटुको राजिकाफलः ॥
गौरसर्षपकोऽत्युष्णो रक्षोघ्नः कफवातजित् ॥ ४१
कृम्यामकण्डुकुष्ठघ्नः श्रुतिशीर्षानिलार्तिहृत् ॥
तद्वत् रक्तस्तु सिद्धार्थस्तिक्तः स्निग्धोष्णकः कटुः ॥ ४२

सर्षपः (Sarṣapaḥ), शुभ्रगौरः('Subhragauraḥ), सिद्धार्थः (Siddhārthaḥ), भूतनाशनः (Bhūtanā'sanaḥ), कटुस्नेहः (Kaṭusnehaḥ), ग्रहघ्नः (Grahaghnaḥ), कटुकः (Kaṭukaḥ), and राजिकाफलः (Rājikāphalaḥ) are synonymous.

Gaurasarṣpaka is very much *uṣṇavīrya,* antiseptic (destroys *rak'sas*) and pacifies *kaphavātadoṣas*. It is useful in worms, *āmadoṣa*, pruritus, skin disorders, pains in the ear and head due to *vātadoṣa.*

Rakta siddhārtha is similar in properties as above, bitter and pungent in taste, *uṣṇavīrya* and unctuous.

(Generic name, includes two sorts A- सिद्धार्थ गौरसर्षप (Siddhārtha gaura sarṣapa of Dhn. Ni. & Raj. Ni.) B- सिद्धार्थ रक्तः (Siddhārtha raktaḥ of Dh. Ni. only). Both of the same genus. These are the Bhāratīya sorts of सर्षपः -Brassica.)

A-(a) ***Brassica campestris*** Linn. Var. ***glauca*** Sp. Roxb.
Syn. *Sinapis glauca* Roxb.
(b) Kamat D.K.

B-(a) ***B. campestris*** Linn. Var. ***toria*** Duthie & Fuller
syn. *Sinapis glauca* Royle
(b) Kamat D.K.

II- A (a) शुभ्रगौरः (Subhragauraḥ), भूतनाशनः (Bhūtanāsanaḥ), ग्रहघ्नः (Grahaghnaḥ), रक्षोघ्नः (Rakshoghnaḥ), कुष्ठनाशनः (Kuṣṭhanāsanaḥ), सिद्धप्रयोजनः (Siddhaprayojanaḥ).

(b) (H) Sarson, Shetasirasa, Bilā Sarson, Pilīrai; (B) Śwetarāi; (SK) Rājikā, tuwarikā; (Guj.) Raira; (Eng.) White mustard, rape seeds (Indian com. name Bara Ṣarson.)

B- (a) रक्तः (Raktaḥ), कटुः (Katuḥ), सिद्धार्थः (Siddhārthaḥ).

(b) (SK) Tuwarikā; (H) Tori, Khetiya, Lahi, Lai.

III (a) See Āsurī (Pre No. 17)
आबयो अनाबयो रसस्ते उग्र आबयो ।
आबयो रोगनिवृत्यर्थ अद्यमान सर्षपः ।
आवयति अत्तिकर्मा अनाबयो अभक्ष्यमाण सर्षपकाण्ड
(A.V.Kand VI Anu. 2 Su. 3 Sayana)

2) बजस्तान् -तान् सर्वान् बजः श्वेत सर्षपः ।
(A.V. VIII. Anu 3 Su. 6 with Sayana)

3) बजः - पिशङ्गवर्णो बजः सर्षपः ।
(A.V. VIII 3-6 with Sayana)

4) पिङ्गस्तुमुग्रधन्वा - सर्षपाख्यौषधिः ...पिङ्गः गौरसर्षपः । (A.V. VI-3-6 mantra 15 with Syana)

IV 1) See Asuri IV -4 Decandole.

राजक्षवकः (Rājakṡavakḥ) (12)

राजक्षवक इत्युक्तो[1] राजिका कृष्णसर्षपः ।
क्षुधाभिजनकश्चैव[2] स चोक्तो राजसर्षपः ॥ ४२

१ 'इत्यन्यो' इति. नि.शे. टीका संमतः पाठः ।
२ राजक्षवक इत्युक्ता राजिका कृष्ण सर्षपा ।
क्षुधाभिजनका चैव सा चोक्ता राजसर्षपः ॥
इति आनन्दाश्रम मुद्रित पुस्तके पाठ : ।
(अन्यच्च -
राजिका तु कफवातहारिणी रोचकाग्निजननी च कथ्यते ।
कण्ठरुक्कृमिविनाशिनी तथा ऊष्णवीर्यमुपहन्ति शूलिनाम् ॥
कृमिस्निग्धोष्णकुष्ठघ्नः कटुको रसपाकतः ।
तद्गुणा राजिका रुच्या तद्गुणोऽन्योऽपि सर्षपः ॥)

राजिका कटुतिक्तोष्णा कृमिश्लेष्महरा परा ।
रुचिष्या पित्तला प्रोक्ता दृष्टिबस्तिप्रदूषणी ॥ ४३

राजक्षवकः (Rājakṡavakaḥ), राजिका (Rājikā), कृष्णसर्षपः (Kṛṣṇasarṣapaḥ), क्षुधाभिजनकः (Kṡudhābhijanakaḥ), and राजसर्षपः (Rājaṣarṣapah) are synonymous.

Rājikā is pungent and bitter in taste, pacifies *kaphadoṣa* and worms, is *uṣṇavīrya.* It is appetizing, aggravates *pittadoṣa* and is harmful to vison and urinary organs.

(For confirmation)

I (a) ***Brassica juncea,*** Roxb. (Fl. B. Indi. 1-157)*
Syn. *Sinapis ramosa,* Roxb.
S. cuineifolia, Roxb.
S. rugosa, Roxb.
S. juncea Linn.
(b)Kamat (Watt Dic. p. 528)
or

2) (a) ***B. campestris***, Linn. Var. ***dicotoma*** sp. Roxb.
Syn. *S. dichotoma* Roxb.
(b) D.K.Kamat (Watt Dic. I. 523)

II (a) कृष्णसर्षपा (Kṛṣṇasrṣapā), राजिका (Rājikā), राजसर्षपा (Rājsarṣapā)
(1) (b) (H.B) Rāi, Sarson, Barirai; (Kashmir) Asur; (Bom. Mar.) Mohari, Rāi; (Eng.) The rāi or Indian Mustard.
(2) (b) (H) Kāli sarson, Kālirāi,
(B) Kāli sarson, Sadarai;(Mar.) Sirasa, Kalīmoharī; (Tam.) Karuppu-Kadugu; (Tel. Nalla -avalu; (Mal) Karuppa Kaluka; Kāli Sarson (Indian common name).

12 (१२) भूस्तृणः (भूतृणः) Bhūstṛṇaḥ भूतिः (Bhutiḥ)

**भूस्तृणो रोहिषो भूतिर्भूतिकोऽथ कुटुम्बकः ।
मालातृणो प्रलम्बश्च च्छत्रोऽतिच्छत्रकस्तथा ॥ ४४

---

१ 'भूरिः इति नि.शे. टीकासंमतः पाठः ।
२ 'पूतिकोऽथ' इति नि.शे.टीकासंमतः पाठः ।
३ 'मालातृणश्च' इति नि.शे. टीकासंमतः पाठः ।
४ 'पालघ्नं' इति नि.शे. टीकासमतः पाठः ।
५ 'छत्रकश्च्छत्रसंज्ञकः' इति नि.शे. टीकासंमतः पाठः ।
* The current name - *B. juncea* (Linn.) Czern. & Coss. (U.P.I.p. 81)
** भूतृणः इति आनन्दाश्रममुद्रित पुस्तके पाठः ।
D.K. Kamat has followed the same reading. It could be भूस्तृणः

भूस्तृणो लघुरुष्णश्च रूक्षः श्लेष्मामयापहः ।
अस्य प्रयोगः सहसा हन्ति जन्तून् समुद्धतान् ॥ ४५

(अन्यच्च - भूतृणः कटुतिक्तश्च वातसंताननाशनः ।
हन्ति भूतग्रहावेशान् विषदोषांश्च दारुणान् ॥)

भूस्तृण (Bhūstṛna), रोहिषः (Rohiṣaḥ), भूतिः (Bhūtiḥ), भूतिकः (Bhūtikaḥ), कुटुम्बकः (Kuṭumbakaḥ), मालातृणः (Malātṛṇaḥ), प्रलम्बः (Pralambaḥ), च्छत्रः (Cchatrḥ) and अतिच्छत्रः (Aticchatraḥ) are synonymous.

Bhūstṛṇa is *laghu, uṣṇavīrya* and roughening. It pacifies, *kaphadoṣa* and quickly acts on worms (? antimicrobial).

From the other text - *Bhūtṛṇaḥ* is pungent and bitter in taste and pacifies *vātadosa*. It is useful as an antiseptic (*Bhūta*), seizures (*Grahāveśa*) and in poisons.

Under this heading Dh. Ni. has recorded the name of only one plant 'A' भूतृण Bhūtṛṇa but Raj. Ni. adds one more name 'B' सुगन्ध भूतृण (Sugandha Bhūtṛṇa).

(Fam. Graminae) Poaceae.

I- A-a- ***Andropogon schoenanthus*** Linn.*
b- Kamat. See IV - i below.
c- Hotter parts of India wild or cultivated.
B- ***Andropogon citratus*** DC.
b. Kamat (See IV -2 below.
c. Cultivated in gardens, Reported wild in Mysore.

II- A-a- भूस्तृण (Bhustṛṇa) रोहिषः (Rohiṣaḥ), भूतिः (Bhūtiḥ), कुटुम्बक (Kuṭumbaka), मालातृण (Malātṛṇa), च्छत्रः (Chatraḥ) अतिच्छत्रः (Atichatraḥ) (Dh.Ni.)
A-b- (Sans.) Mālāṭṛṇakam Bhustṛṇakam; (Ben.) Gandhabenā.
B-a- सुरसः Surasaḥ, सुरभिः Surabhiḥ, गन्धतृण Gandhatṛṇā. मुखवासः Mukhavāsaḥ.
B-b- (San.) -Bhūstṛṇa; (B.) Gandhabena; (H.) Gandhatṛṇa. (Mara.) Hirwā or olā chā. (Tam.) Vasanappillu. (Tel.) Nimmagaddi (Mal.) Vasanappillai; (Eng.) Lemon grass.

III
b- भूस्तृणम् Bhūstṛṇam
(Mar.) Pāṇyātīl vāḷā; (Kan.) Marimaladar ganjani; *Andropogon martini*
कत्तृणस्य भूतृणस्यापि गुणवीर्यविपाकादिषु किंचित साम्यत्वं विद्यते ।
(Asht. Hr. kosha.)

---

* The current valid name is -
Cymbopogon schoenanthus (Linn.) Spreng.

IV 1) *Andropogon schoenanthus* Linn. Willd; San. Malatrinakanga, Bhustrinanga; Beng. Gandhabena.
Ramaccium. Rheed Hort. Mal. 12 p. 137. T. 72.
The fresh leaves are much used as substitute for tea. The white succulent centre of the leaf bearing culms is often put into curries to give them an agreeable flavour. (C.B.C. p. 92)

2) *Andropogon citratus* DC. (Lemon grass)
Syn. *A. schoenanthus* Roxb.
Ben. Gandhabena; H. Gandhatṛṇa;
Mara. Hirvā or olā chā. San. Bhūstṛṇa.
The vernacular names Gandhabena and Malastrinang, Bhustrinang given to a plant *A. schoenanthus* Linn. This may be probably *A. citratus* DC. but it seems to agree equally well in certain respects with *A. laniger* Desf. (Watt. A p. 242)

3) **भूतृण** Bhūstṛṇa
Andropogon citratus (Vidyotani Bh. Pr.)

4) **भूस्तृण** Bhūstṛṇa
C.S. Su. 169 S.S. Su. 18.17 etc.
A.H. Su. 6.10.106 etc.
This has been identified with a variety of *Gandhatṛṇa* **गन्धतृण** or **द्रोणपुष्प** Droṇapuṣpa. Discussion under **रोहिष** *Rohiṣa* may be consulted. (Balwantji p. 288) .

13 (१३) सुरसा Surasā

सुरसा तुलसी ग्राम्या सुरभी बहुमञ्जरी ।
अपेतराक्षसी[१] गौरी भूतघ्नी देवदुन्दुभिः ॥ ४७

तुलसी लघुरुष्णा च रूक्षा कफविनाशिनी ।
कृमिदोषं निहन्त्येषा रुचिकृद् वह्निदीपनी ॥ ४८

सुरसा (Surasā), **तुलसी** (Tulasī), **ग्राम्या** (Grāmyā), **सुरभी** (Surabhī) **बहुमञ्जरी**(Bahumajñarī),**अपेतराक्षसी** (Apetarākṡasī), **गौरी** (Gaurī), **भूतघ्नी** (Bhūtaghnī), and **देवदुन्दुभिः** (Devadundubhiḥ) are synonymous.

Tulasī is *laghu, uṣṇavīrya,* roughening and pacifies *kaphadoṣa.* It is useful in worms (antiseptic), is appetizer and stimulates digestive capacity.

Fam. Labiatae. Lamiaceae.

१ 'आपीता राक्षसी' इति नि.शे. टीकासंमतः पाठः ।

I
(a) ***Ocimum sanctum*** Linn.
Syn. *O. sanctum* Willd.
(b) Dr. Roxburgh (Fl. indi.)

II (a) तुलसी (Tulasī), ग्राम्या (Grāmyā), सुरभी (Surabhī) बहुमञ्जरी (Bahumañjarī), अपेतराक्षसी (Apetarākṣasī), विष्णुवल्लभा (Viṣṇuvallabhā), हरिप्रिया (Haripriyā), भूतघ्नी (Bhūtaghnī), श्यामा (Śyāmā), तीव्रा (Tīvrā).
(अपेत - deviating from)
(b) (SK) Parṇāsa (As. Res. IV - 188)
(B) Kālā or Kṛṣṇatulasī, Kural.
(H) Kālātulsī, varandā; (Mar.) Kāḷī tuḷasa; (Tel.) Kṛṣṇatulsai, Gaggera cettu; (Tam.) Tulasī; (Kan.) Tulasigida; (Mal. Krsnatulasi, nall tirtta; (Eng.) the sacred basil.

14 (१४) जम्बीरः Jambirah.

जम्बीरः खरपत्रश्च फणी चोक्तः फणिज्जकः ।
मरुत्तको मरुवको मरुर्मरुबकस्तथा ॥ ४९

फणिज्जको हिमस्तिक्तो रूक्षः कफविनाशनः ।
रक्तहारी तथा हन्ति सुघोरं कृत्रिमं विषम् ॥ ५०
मरुबकः कफहरो रुच्यो मुखसुगन्धकृत् ।

जम्बीरः (Jambīraḥ), खरपत्रः (Kharapatraḥ), फणी (Phaṇī), फणिज्जकः (Phanijjakaḥ), मरुत्तकः (Maruttakaḥ), मरुवकः (Maruvakaḥ), मरु (Maru), and मरुबकः (Marubakaḥ) are synonymous.

Phaṇijjaka is *śītavīrya*, bitter in taste, roughening and pacifies *kaphadoṣa*. It is useful in disorders of blood and artificial poisons

Marabaka pacifies *kaphadoṣa*, is appetizing and mouth refreshing.

Generic name includes two plants A.जम्बीरः (Jambīraḥ) and B. मरुबकः (Marubakaḥ).

(Fam. Labiatae) Lamiaceae.

I- A-(a) ***Pogostemon parviflorus*** Benth. and allied species.
(b) Dymock (Pharm. indi.)

B-(a) ***Majorana hortensis*** Moench.
Syn. *Origanum majorana* Linn.

(b) Dymock (Pharm. indi.)

II Syn. *Origanum majorana* Linn.

(a) खरपत्रः (Kharapatraḥ), जम्बीरः (Jambīraḥ), फणिज्जकः (Phaṇijjakaḥ),
(b) (SK) Sugandhika; (Mar.) Phāṅglā, Phāṅgḷi (A strongly scented bush) (a)मरुबकः (Murabakaḥ), मरुवः (Maruvaḥ)
(b) (SK) Maruḥ; (B) Maru; (Bom, Mara, H.) Maravā, Marvā; (Tam.) Maru; (English) Sweet Majorum.

III b 1) द्विधा मरुबकः प्रोक्तो श्वेतश्चैव सितेतरः ।
श्वेतो भिषजकार्ये स्यात् अपरः शिवपूजने ॥

b- 2 फणिज्जकः - फणिज्जक इति लोके अन्ये मरुबकमाहुः । डल्हण सु. सू. ४६. २२१

3 फणिज्जकः (Phaṇijjakaḥ) Ḍalhaṇa Su. Su. 38. 18

4 जम्बीरः (Jambīraḥ) Ḍalhaṇa Su. Su. 46

5 मरिचकः (Maricakaḥ) (Arun, Ast. Hr. Su.)

6 श्वेत मरुबकः (Śweta Marubakaḥ) (Parnāsabhedaḥ) (Chakra, ca. su. 4.4)

7 समीरणो मरुबकः प्रस्थपुष्पः फणिज्जकः । समीरयती 'इर्' गतौ । 'जम्बीरे प्रस्थपुष्पे स्यात् तथा दंतशठे ... इति मेदिनी । पञ्च जम्बीरस्य 'मरुआ' इति ख्यातस्य । भानुजी अमरकोशे ।

IV - 1 Majorum - Sweet majorum. Native of Meditarranean region is an other savory herb of great antiquity. It is a sacred plant of India. (*O. valgare*) (Hill p. 462)

2 फणिज्झकः Phaṇijjhakaḥ
C.S.Su. 2.3,3.3, etc.
S.S.Su. 11.5, 38.18 etc.
A.H.Su. 6.106, 15.30 etc.
. . . .has often been identified with *Ocimum basilicum* Linn. or *Origanum majorana* Linn. But like several others of this group (Surasādigaṇa) it is difficult to specify it botanically with certainty. (Balwantji p. 266).

15. (१५) कुठेरकः (Kuṭherakaḥ)

कुठेरकस्तु वैकुण्ठः क्षुद्रपर्णोऽर्जकस्तथा[१] ॥ ५०
वटपत्रः कुठेरोऽन्यः पर्णासो बिल्वगन्धकः ॥

अर्जकः शीतलस्तित्तः श्लेष्मामयविनाशनः ॥ ५१
द्विविधं च विषं हन्याद् दुष्टरक्तविनाशनः ॥

१ 'क्षुद्रपत्योऽर्जकः सितः' इति क्षी. समंतः पाठः ।

कुठेरकः (Kuṭherakaḥ), वैकुण्ठः (Vaikuṇṭhaḥ), क्षुद्रपर्णः (Kśudraparṇaḥ), अर्जकः (Arjakaḥ),

There is an another type of *kuṭheraka* called by the synonyms वटपत्रः (Vaṭapatraḥ); पर्णासः (Parṇāsaḥ) and बिल्वगन्धकः (Bilvagandhakaḥ).

Arjaka is bitter in taste, *śītavīrya*, and pacifies disorders due to *kaphadoṣa,* and is useful in both types of poisons and disorders due to vitiated blood.

I- Generic name includes two plants

Ambiguous

a) May be of तुलसी गोत्र (tulasī-gotra, Genus Ocimum)

III b 1) कुठेरः (Kuṭheraḥ) सितार्जकनामपर्णासभेदः।कृष्णार्जकाख्य इति क्षीरस्वामी । 'कालमाल कुठेरक' इत्यादि सूत्रवचनान्यप्यत्र संस्मरणीयानि तौ पृथग् पृथगिति । ? (Ah. Hr. Kosh)

IV- 1 कुठेरक Kuṭheraka
C.S.Su. 2.3. 27.99 etc.
S.S. Su. 38. 18 etc.
A.H. Su. 6.106 etc.

This is one of the Surasādi gaṇa ... usually called *Tulasī* varieties. ... it seems difficult to specify them individually ... Similar to this but smaller in size is *Arjak*, which may be identified with *Orthosiphon* species (*O. pallidus* Royle) .... called *Śweta kuṭheraka* (Balwantji P. 103)

शालुकः Śālukaḥ (13)

कुठेरकस्तृतीयोऽन्यः शालुकः कृष्णशालुकः ॥ ५३
कृष्णार्जकः कालमालः करालः कृष्णमल्लिका ॥

त्रयोऽर्जकाः कटूष्णाः स्युः कफवातामयापहाः ॥ *५४
नेत्रामयहरा रुच्याः सुखप्रसवकारकाः ॥

कृत्रिमं च विषं हन्यू रक्तदोषविनाशनाः ॥ ५५

There is a third type of *kuṭheraka* called by the synonyms शालुकः (Śālukaḥ), कृष्णशालुकः (Kṛṣṇaśālukaḥ), कृष्णार्जकः (Kṛṣṇārjakaḥ),कालमालः (Kālamālaḥ), करालः (Karālaḥ) and कृष्णमल्लिका (Kṛṣṇamallikā).

Three types of *Arjakas* are pungent in taste, *uṣṇavīrya* and pacify

---

* कुठेरकाः सुगन्धाः स्युः कटुपाकरसा स्मृताः ।
वातघ्ना लघुरूक्षाश्च तीक्ष्णोष्णाः पित्तवर्धनाः ॥ इति क्वचित् पाठः ।

disorders due to *kapha vātadoṣa,* are appetizing useful for eye diseases and normal labour. These are also useful in artificial poison and disorders due to vitiated blood.

---

ambiguous

I a) May be of Ocimum genus तुलसी गोत्र, (Tulasī gotra.) शालुकः of संहिता is tuberous plant. See Balwantji p. 396

16 (१६) सुमुखः Sumukhaḥ

सुमुखः सुप्रशस्तश्च गरघ्नः कटुपत्रकः ।
दोषोत्क्लेशी सुवक्त्रश्च स्वास्यः सुवदनो मतः ॥ ५६
पित्तकृत् पार्श्वशूलघ्नः सुमुखः समुदाहृतः
कफानिलविषश्वासकासदौर्गन्ध्यनाशनः ॥ ५७

सुमुखः (Sumukhaḥ), सुप्रशस्तः (Supraśastaḥ), गरघ्नः (Garaghnaḥ), कटुपत्रकः (Kaṭupatrakaḥ), दोषोत्क्लेशी (Doṣotkleśī), सुवक्त्रः (Suvaktraḥ), स्वास्यः (Svāsyaḥ), and सुवदनः (Suvadnaḥ), are synonymous.

Sumukhaḥ aggravates *pittadoṣa* and pacifies pains in the sides of the chest (? pleural pain), pacifies *kapha vāta doṣas,* poisons, dyspnoea, cough and foul smell.

Ambiguous

I a) As above वनबर्बरिका Raj. ni.
सुमुखः (Sumukhaḥ),पर्णासभेदः । वनबर्बरिका । ...Basilic-decylon (Fr.); (Eng.) Shruby basil; (Latin) *Ocimum gratissimum* (Ast. Hr. Kosh)

IV-1 सुमुखः Sumukhaḥ
Cakra . . . .one of the पर्णास *Parṇāsa* variety. . . . .Ḍalhaṇa राजिका *Rājikā* or *Vanabarbarikā* (Balwantji P. 437).

17 (१७) आसुरी Āsurī

आसुरी राजिका राजी कृष्णका रक्तसर्षपः ।
तीक्ष्णगन्धा चातितीक्ष्णा क्षुवकः क्षवकः क्षवः ॥ ५८
आसुरी कटुतिक्तगोष्णा कुष्ठघ्नी कफगुल्मजित् ।
निद्राकरी शोफहरी ग्रहकारी[१] च सा स्मृता ॥ ५९

१ 'ग्रहहारी would be a better reading S.D. Kamat.

आसुरी (Āsurī), राजिका (Rājikā), राजी (Rājī), कृष्णका (Kṛṣṇakā), रक्तसर्षपः (Raktasarṣapaḥ), तीक्ष्णगन्धा (Tīkṣṇagandhā), अतितीक्ष्णा (Atitīkšṇā), क्षुवकः (Kšuvakaḥ), क्षवकः (Kšavakaḥ) and क्षवः (Kšavaḥ) are synonymous.

Āsurī is pungent and bitter in taste, *uṣṇavirya,* useful in disorders of skin, tumours due to *kaphadosa,* is soporific, removes inflammation (counter irritant) and alleviates disorders caused by *grahas.*

I Āsurī a vegetable drug of the kind of Indian सर्षप Sarṣapa, wild in the region from Siberia to Europe and now sparingly cultivated in India. The medicinal uses of this drug were not known to vedic priests but were known to Asura women only, from whom the vedic priests, who had happened to come in contact with the Asuras obtained the uses of this drug from these women. From that time the vedic priests stamped the name Āsurī to this kind of Sarṣapa.

But the vedic priests, when and where had come in contact with Asurās is uncertain. According to some historians they had come in contact with the Asuras in central or north westward region of Asia when the vedic people were proceeding Southward from the Arctic region. But it is a conflicting point.

I (a) ***Brassica nigra*** (Linn.) Koch

(b) Kamat (See III, 1,2,3, IV, 1,2, below.)

II (a) आसुरी (Āsurī), राजिका (Rājikā), राजी (Rājī), रक्तसर्षपः (Raktaṣarsapaḥ), मधुरिका (Madhurikā), अतितीक्ष्णा (Atītikṣṇā), क्षुवकः (Kšuwakaḥ).

(b) (B) Rāīsarisa; (H) Asalraī, Tarmirā; (Bom.) Rai; (Tel.) Āwal; (Tam.) Kadugu; (Sk) Madhurikā (Chopra); (Eng.) Black or true mustard.

III See Sarṣapa (Pre No. 11)

(a) श्वेतकुष्ठनाशनम् आसुरी वनस्पति ।
सुपर्णो जातः प्रथमस्तस्य त्वं पित्तमासिथ ।
तदासुरी युधाजीता रुपं चक्रे वनस्पतीन् ॥ १ ॥
आसुरी चक्रे प्रथमिदं किलासभेषमिदत्किलास नाशनम् ॥ â ॥
See below IV 2,3, 4.5 (A.V.i. -24)

(b)1 (Āsurī) (Su. 6) Asuyeteāsurī Āsura Strī Wā. Red Mustard. (Ast. Hr. Kosa)

2 (Āsurī) Rājikā, Maṇḍako Wā. (Dalhana Su. Su. 38)

(c) See current name (I-a) (See watt).

IV The Āsurī Kalpa deals with the

1 black mustard (Āsurī)
(A.V. Parisistha No. 36 Dr. Kārambelkar)

2 Another plant named Āsurī or Śyāmā is also mentioned as a cure against Leprosy (A.V.I.24). This remedy was in possession of an Asura women (A.V. i. 24, 1.2) (A.V 6. 108, 3.2, 3.3. Shende P. 22, 28, 38).

3 Kausika Sutra gives the rite about it.
(30.1.6) as follows ... (Dr. Karambelkar p. 178)

4 आसुरी Āsurī
C.S.Su. 27.98 A.H. Su. 6.106.
At both these places it had been identified with *Brassica nigra* (Linn.) Koch, *Rāi* राई (H) but there appears to be difference in the names आसुरी Āsūrī in C.S. and आसुरी Āsurī in A.H.and also in their properties. (Balwantji) (p.41)

5 See सर्षप Sarṣapa pre. No. 11-III-1 to 5 Supra
All the Brassicas are European and siberian origin and are still to be seen in those regions wild, or half wild in some form or other ... There is no Sanskrit name for these plants but only modern Bengalee names...
There cultivation was diffused in Europe before, and in Asia after the Aryan invasion (A. De candolle P. 36)

6 *Brassica nigra* Koch
(Eng.) Black true mustard; (H) Banarasi-Kali Makrarai; (Sk.) Āsurī, Rājikā, Sarṣapa. Loca.-Cultivated in Bombay state. Distr.-indigenous in Makaronesi and transitation area and Meditarrenean sea. (Agharkar)

*7 It is nowhere extensively cultivated but is met with chiefly on the hills and more than possible that existed on Himalaya from remote times, although unknown to the fathers of Indian botanical science. It is quite likely, however, that the ancient Sanskrit writers had not seen the true and white mustard, and that the word *Rājika* may have originally denoted a form of *B. juncea* and the word *siddhārtha* a form of *campestris*.

8 Touching the question of origin we need not occupy with the botanical limits of the species . . . .

* D.K.Kamat did not intend to include this reference, however, I, have included the same as it is somewhat interestinhg. S.D. Kamat.

Finally, every method, whether botanical, historical or philological leads us to the following conclusion .... There cultivation was diffused in Europe before, and in Asia after the Aryan invasion.

(origin of cultivated plants by De candolle. p. 36)

Suppliment

Foreign Sarṣapa kinds

1) *Brassica alba* (Fl. Br. Indi. I. 157)
White mustard (Watt Dict. P. 520)

2) *B. niger* Koch Black mustard. True Mustard (Watt. Dict. P. 520, 53) आसुरी (Āsurī) (Kamat)

Bhartiya Sarṣapa kinds

1) *B. juncea* (Fl. Br. In. 1.157) Syn. *Sinapis ramosa*, Roxb. The Rai or Indian mustard seeds dark or reddish brown. (Watt. Dict. p. 528) राजक्षवक (Rājak'savaka?)
2) *B. campestris,* Linn. Var. *dichotomos,* Roxb. Syn. *Sinapis dichotomos*, Roxb. Kālīsarsaon Watt. Dict. p. 523) राजक्षवक (Rājak'savaka)?
3) *B. campestris* Linn. Var. *glauca,* Sp. Roxb. Syn. *Sinapis glauca,* Roxb. White sarson (Watt. Dict. Page 524) सिद्धार्थ (Siddhārtha) (Kamat.).
4) *B. campestris* Linn var. *toria,* Duthie & Fuller. Syn. *Sinapis glauca,* Royle सिद्धार्थ (Siddhārthā) (Kamat).

18 (१८) काण्डीरः Kāṇḍīraḥ*

काण्डीरः काण्डकटुको नासासंवेदनः पटुः ।
ऊग्रकाण्डस्तोयवल्ली कारवल्ली सुकाण्डकः ॥ ६०

*हरितो द्विविधः प्रोक्तः काण्डीरस्तत्वदर्शिभिः ।
कटुकः कच्छदेशादौ भक्षयन्त्याममेव तु ॥
द्वितीयस्तूदकोद्भूतः . . . . . सिद्धमन्त्र p. 40 S.D. Kamat

काण्डीरः कटुतिक्तोष्णः सरो दुष्टव्रणार्तिजित् ।
लूतागुल्मोदरप्लीहशूलमन्दाग्निनाशनः ॥ ६१

काण्डीरः (Kāndīraḥ), काण्डकटुकः (Kāṇḍakaṭukaḥ), नासासंवेदनः (Nāsāsamvedanaḥ), पटुः (Paṭuḥ), ऊग्रकाण्डः (Ūgrakāṇḍaḥ), तोयवल्ली (Toyavallī), कारवल्ली (Kāravallī), and सुकाण्डकः (Sukāṇḍakaḥ) are synonymous.

Kāṇḍīra is pungent and bitter in taste, *uṣṇavīrya,* mild laxative and useful in septic wounds, spider poisoning, tumours (diverticulosis), ascites disorders of spleen, colics, and in depressed digestive capacity (anorexia).

Not confirmed

(Fam.Ranunculaceae)

I (a) ***Ranunculus sceleratus***, Linn
Syn. *R. indicus* Roxb. Balwantsimhaji (Gloss. P. 333-334)

II (a) काण्डकटुकः (Kāṇḍakaṭukaḥ), नासासंवेदनः (Nāsāsamvedanaḥ), ऊग्रकाण्डः (Ugrakāṇḍaḥ), तोयवल्ली (Toyavallī), सुकाण्डकः (Sukāṇḍakaḥ).

(b) (Benaras) Devakāndira, Kāndira, Devakāṇḍar; (H) Jal Dhaniyā (Eng.) Water celery.

III -b- 1 400 शाकभिदत्र – समष्टिला । 'गण्डीरो ना समष्ठिले' त्यमरः । 'गाण्डरडूबी इतिख्यातस्यानूपज शाकस्ये ' ति रामाश्रमः । (Harshe)

2 490 समष्टिलेति गण्डीरो गण्डदूर्वा । (Harshe)

3 142 समष्ठिलस्तोयापामार्ग । (Harshe)

4 गण्डीरः समष्ठिलः । Dh. Ni. p. 423

5 गण्डान् ग्रन्थीनीरयति गण्डीरः । सम्यगस्थीनि लाति समष्टिला (ष्ठि) सान्द्रत्वात् समष्ठिला नाम शाकम् यन्माला – गण्डीरो ना समष्टिला । (Ksiraswāmi p.81)

IV - 1 *Ranunculus sceleratus* Linn.
Devakāndar (Ach. Priyavratji)
Habitat - An erect annual 1 -3 feet; met with on river banks in Bengal, Afaganistan, N. India, Himalaya, during cold weather and remains up till the rains.

Medicine - the fresh plant is poisonous and produces violent effect .. the leaves .. to raise blisters.

...Roxburgh remarks that it has no native name, and that its

properties are apparently are unknown. It certainly possesses a very powerful principle.
.... Food - the inhabitants of wallachia use it as a vegetable when boiled, a remarkable fact when it is remembered that it is a poisonous and a harmful vesicant when uncooked. (Watt. Dict.)

2 काण्डीर Kāṇḍīra
C.S.Ci. 3.266 ka. 1. 128. See (Balwantji p. 90)
गण्डीर Gaṇḍīra
C.S.Su. 4.15, 45 etc.
S.S.Su. 45.123, 46-221 etc.
A.H. Su. 15.23.

19 (१९) जलपिप्पली (Jalapippalī)

जलपिप्पल्यभिहिता शारदी तोयपिप्पली ।
मत्स्यादनी मत्स्यगन्धा लाङ्गली शकुलादनी ॥ ६२
जलपिप्पलिका तिक्ता कषाया कफपित्तजित् ।
श्वासास्रविषदाहार्तिभ्रममूर्च्छातृषापहा ॥ ६२

जलपिप्पली (Jalapippalī), शारदी (Śāradī), तोयपिप्पली (Toyapippalī), मत्स्यादनी (Matsyādanī), मत्स्यगन्धा (Matsyagandhā), लाङ्गली(Lāngalī), and शकुलादनी (Śakulādanī) are synonymous.

Jalapippalī is bitter and *kaṣāya* in taste, and pacifies *kapha pitta doṣas*. It is useful in dyspnoea, blood disorders, poisoning, burning sensation, giddiness, syncope and excessive thirst.

I- A controversial plant.

a) 1 ***Commelina silicifolia*** Roxb.*

b) Roxburgh (Fl. indi.)

2 ***Sphenoclea zeylanica*** Willd. (Geart. corp.)**
Syn. *S. pongatium,* Lam.
Gaertnera pangati Retz.

b) Roxburgh.

---

* The current accepted valid name is -
C.longifolia Lamk. (Comp. p. 41)
** *Sphenoclea zeylanica* Gaertn. (U. P. I. p. 592).

3 ***Lippia nodiflora*** Rich. (Chopra)*

b) Kamat (See IV-1,2,3 below)

II a) शारदी (Śāradī), तोयपिप्पली (Toyapippalī), मत्स्यगन्धा (Matsyagandhā), लाङ्गली (Lāngalī),

1) b-(San) Jalapippalī; (B) Panikāncīra; (H) Jalapiplī

2) b- Jeelmarich (Tel.) Neerupipli.

3) b- (H.) Bhuiokra; (Bom. Guj.) Ratolia; (Sans.) Vaśira

III a) वसुक-वशीर (Vasuka Vaśīra),
Jalapippalī (Ast. San. Su. 15.30)

b) 1 शकुलादनी (Śakulādanī)
Jalapippalī (H.) Bhuiokrā
Lippia nodiflora,
Purple Lippia. (Ast. Hr. Kosa)
This plant is Mahārāstrī (महाराष्ट्री) of Raj. Ni.

2 227 तोयपिप्पली (Toya pippalī) (Harshe.)

b-3 H. Bhuiokra, (Bom. Guj.) Ratolia; Sk. Vaśira

IV - 1 जलपिप्पली (Jalapippalī), Purple lippia, *Lippia nodiflora, Commelina ciliciflora* (Ach. Dwivedi Bh. Pr. Ni.)

2. *Lippia nodiflora* Rich.
An evergreen undershrub common in water place throughout India. (Watt. II. 78.)

3 *Lippia nodiflora* Rich.
(Sam.) Vāsīra; (H.) Bhuiokra; (Kan.) Nela Hippali; (Mal) Katutippal (Ni. Adarsha, Desai, Chopra).

4 See शकुलादनी (p. 15)
It has been used as pot herb. (Balawantji p. 15 384)

20 (२०) रसोनः Rasonaḥ

रसोनोलशुनोऽरिष्टो म्लेच्छकन्दो महौषधम् ।
महाकन्दो रसोनोऽन्यो गृञ्जनो दीर्घपत्रकः ॥ ६४

रसोन उष्णः कटुपिच्छिलश्च स्निग्धो गुरुः स्वादुरसोऽतिबल्यः ।
वृष्यश्च मेधास्वरवर्णचक्षुर्भग्नास्थिसंधानकरः सुतीक्ष्णः ॥ ६५

हृद्रोग जीर्णज्वर कुक्षीशूल विबन्धगुल्मारुचिकृच्छ्रशोफान ।
दुर्नाम कुष्ठानलसादजन्तुकफामयान् हन्ति महारसोनः ॥ ६६

* *Phyla nodiflora* (Linn.) Greene (Comp. p. 117)
१ 'रसाख्योन्यो' इति क्षी. संमतः पाठः ।

रसोनः (Rasonaḥ), लशुनः (Laśunaḥ), अरिष्टः (Ariṣṭaḥ), म्लेच्छकन्दः (Mlecchakandaḥ), महौषधम् (Mahauṣadham), are synonymous. There is an another kind of *rasona* called as महाकन्दः (Mahākandaḥ) of which synonyms are गृञ्जनः (Gṛñjanaḥ) and दीर्घपत्रकः (Dīrghapatrakaḥ).

Rasona is *uṣṇavīrya,* pungent and sweet (predominate) in taste, slimy, unctuous, *guru* (heavy to digest), very much strength promoting, *vṛṣya,* improves intellect, voice, complexion, vision and is union promoting in fractures and is very sharp.

Mahārasona is useful in cardiac disease, chronic fevers, pain in abdomen, constipation, tumours (diverticulosis), loss of appetite, dysuria, oedema, piles, disorders of skin, dyspepsia, worms and pacifies disorders due to *kaphadoṣa.*

I Generic name includes two sorts A रसोनः (Rasonaḥ) and B गृञ्जनः (Gṛñjanaḥ). Both of the same genus.

(Fam. Liliaceae) Alliaceae.

A-a- ***Allium sativum*** Linn.
b- Roxburgh (Fl. indi.)

For confirmation.

B-a- ***Allium xiphopetallum*** Ait. & Baker
b- Kamat
Dymock.
See IV below 445.

II- a-A लशुनः (Laśunaḥ), अरिष्टः (Ariṣṭaḥ), म्लेच्छकन्दः (Mlecchakandaḥ) महौषधम् (Mahausadham)

b- (H.) Lasan; (B) Lasūṇ; (Tel. Mal.) Veluli; (Eng.) Garlic.

B-a महाकन्दः (Mahākandaḥ), अन्यरसोनः (Anya rasonaḥ), गृञ्जनः (Gṛñjanaḥ),दीर्घपत्रकः (Dīrghapatrakaḥ)

b- (San) Rakta laśūnaḥ;(Guj.) Rato lasana; (Mar.) Lasuna; (Arab) Thum-el-bari; Wild garlic (Dymock)
Pers. Sir-i-piazak or 'onion garlic'.

III See Gṛñjana

b) 1 रसोनो द्विविधः Two kinds of Rasonaḥ (Raj. Ni. 7.2)
2 गृञ्जनं प्रोक्तं लशुने वृत्तमूलके (Raj. Ni. Dvyath. Kosa)
3 लशुनः (Laśunaḥ) Rasonakaḥ Gṛñjana (Madan. Ni. 74)
4 गृञ्जनकः (Gṛñjanakaḥ) (Su. 6) Rakta laśunaḥ, 'Lohita palāṇḍu' iti Cakrapaṇī Baṣpacandra - Gandhākṛti rasaistulyo Gṛñijanastu

palāṇḍunā Sūkśmanālāgra patratwāt bhidyate sau Palānḍutaḥ iti. (H.) Lāla Lahasan; (Mar.) Rakta Lasuna; (Kan.) Kampina vellulli., (Tam.) Irulli, Vengāya; (Mal.) Cuvannulli ... (Ast. Hr. Kosa)

5 अन्यो रक्त महाकन्दो .... । (Anyo·Rakto mahakando ..) (Saraswati Kosa Ceylon)

IV- 1 गृञ्जन (Gṛñjana) - a sort of Rasona ... Gṛñjana (Śalgam) See also no. 10 गृञ्जन

2 Dr. Desai (Muscat Lasuna)

3 a-*Allium sativum;* The garlic, Lasuna (Common.)

b- *A.ascalonicum* Linn.
The shallot
A hardy bulbous perennial native of palestine ... It is regarded much similar to garlic. Flowers greenish -white or purple white Bulbs - size about a nut, white. It is regarded as much similar to garlic. (Watt. Dict. 'A' Page 168.)

C-. *A. leptophyllum* Wall.
The Himalayan onion ... strong pungency than ordinary onions. Is this the species said to be exported from Lahoul ? (Watt. Dict. 'A' Page 171.)

The greatest possible confusion exists in India regarding the cultivated forms and indeed regarding, the wild forms of the genus Allium and it is probable that ... in addition to many preceeding forms many others are regularly known to natives of India, and even cultivated and sold in our bazar.

(Watt. Dict. 'A' Page -174.)

4 *A. ziphopetalum* Ait. ex Baker
Wild garlic of the Arabs. It has a bulb resembling Badashasalap in shape and appearance, but much smaller, a powerful garlic odour. In punjab it is known as sir-i-piazak or Badshahi garlic ... growing abundantly in Badagis. In Bombay it is best knwon as Maskat garlic. (Dymock Vol. III 492)

5 *Alluim ascalonicum.*
The shallot. It is called by the natives 'Eka-kali-lasun', one cloved garlic and used by them to cure earache. A small piece being placed in the meatus.' (Dymock III 492.)
San. Raktalaśuna; Mar. rānaṭī Lasuna. The clove small and smell like garlic. (Gṛñjan Dr. Desai)

6 Gṛñja, Gṛñjana Gṛñjanaka.

C.C. 27.171 Kal.7.28
S. 36.14 (Gṛñja)
A.H. Su-6-128.

This is usually considered to be a carrot or Turnip (Bh.Pr.) or Palāṇḍu such as Gandhanā which is *Allium ascalonicum* Linn. also called one cloved garlic (Ek putia Lahasun.)

(Balawantji p. 143)

Dr. Desai's and Balvantjis' plants are one cloved (Ekakali Lahasun) but Nighantus Gṛñjana is Mahākanda, महाकन्द.

21. गृञ्जरम् Gṛñjaram

गर्जरं पिङ्गलं मूलं पीतकं मूलकं तथा ।
स्वादुमूलं सुपीतं च नागरं पीतमूलकम् ॥ ६७
गर्जरं मधुरं रुच्यं किंचित् कटु कफापहम् ।
आध्मानकृमिशूलघ्नं दाहपित्तज्वरापहम् ॥ ६८

गर्जरं (Garjaram), पिङ्गलं मूलं (Pingalammūlam), पीतकं मूलकं (Pītakam mūlakam), स्वादुमूलं (Swādumūlam), सुपीत (Supītam), नागरं (Nāgaram), and पीतमूलकं (Pītamūlakam) are synonymous.

Garjara is sweet and slightly pungent in taste and appetizing. It pacifies *kapha doṣa* and is useful in flatulence, colic due to worms, burning sensation and fever due to *pittadoṣa.*

Fam. Umbelliferae. Apiaceae

I (a) ***Daucus carota*** Linn. var. ***sativa*** DC.
(b) Roxburgh (Fl.indi.)

II (a) गर्जरं (Garjaram), पीतमूलं (Pītmūlam), स्वादुमूलं (Swādu mūlam), नागरं (Nāgaram)
(b) (San.) Śikhāmūlam; (H.B. Mar.), Gājara, Shekhakul (Dymock)

IV 1) The carrot -*Daucus carota* Linn. cultivated for over 2000 years ... The numerous varieties of carrots differ in size, shape, colour and quality (Hill p. 361).
2) As. Res. IV 225.
3) The wild carrot is native of ... and in Himalaya, grows to the height of six feet ... Shekhakul, Indian shekhakul (Dymock).

22. पलाण्डुः Palāṇḍuḥ
*23 दुर्द्रुमः

पलाण्डुर्यवनेष्टश्च सुकन्दो[1] मुखदूषकः ।
हरितोऽन्यः[2] पलाण्डुश्च लतार्को दुर्द्रुमः स्मृतः ॥ ६९

पलाण्डुस्तद्गुणैर्न्यूनो विपाके मधुरस्तु सः ।
कफं करोति नो पित्तं केवलोऽनिलनाशनः ॥ ७० Ca.Su. 27

ऊलिः पञ्चरसाऽपि स्यात् गुरूष्णा चाम्लवर्जिता ।
वायुशोफारुचिश्लेष्मकृमिहृद्रोगनाशिनी ॥ ७१

पलाण्डुः कटुको बल्यो गुरुर्वातास्रपित्तजित् ।
अन्यः क्षीरपलाण्डुश्च वृष्यो मधुरपिच्छिलः ॥ ७२

पलाण्डुः (Palāṇḍuḥ), यवनेष्टः (Yavaneṣṭaḥ), सुकन्दः (Sukandaḥ), मुखदूषकः (Mukhadūṣakaḥ), are synonymous. There is an another kind greenish in colour called as हरितः (Haritaḥ) of which synonyms are लतार्कः (Latārkaḥ) and दुर्द्रुमः (Durdrumaḥ).

Palāṇḍu is similar but less in properties to those of *rasona* and sweet in *vipāka*. It neither aggravates *kapha* nor *pitta* and only pacifies *vātadoṣa* .

Ūliḥ is also having five types of tastes and is not sour. It is *uṣṇavīrya* and *guru*. It is useful in oedema due to *vātadoṣa,* loss of apptite, worms due to *kaphadoṣa* and cardiac disorders.

Palāṇḍu is pungent in taste, strengthḥ promoting, *guru* and pacifies *vāta, rakta* and *pittadoṣa*.

There is an another kind of *Palāṇḍu* called as क्षीरपलाण्डु (Kṡīra-palāṇḍu). It is sweet in taste, *vṛṣya* and slimy.

I (Generic name includes two kinds A. Palāṇḍuḥ proper and the B-(Rājpalāṇḍuḥ of Raj. Ni.) of the same genus. रक्त (Rakta), हरित (Harita), and क्षीरपलाण्डु (Kṡirapalāṇḍu) are the names of bulbs with different colours, but now, it seems these kinds of different colours are developing into races and varieties.

A. (Fam. Liliaceae.) Alliaceae

---

१ 'मुकुन्दो' इति. क्षी. संमतः पाठः ।
२ 'हरिणोऽन्यों इति. क्षी. संमतः पाठः ।
* पलाण्डु and दुर्द्रुमः are separately mentioned in Gaṇadravyāvali, while in पर्यायनामद्रव्यावली Paryāyanāmadravyāvali these are mentioned together. Late vd. D.K. Kamat has followed the numbers according to Ānandāsrama edi. The reading उलिःपञ्चरसा to नाशिनी is not found in Chaukhamba editions. S.D. Kamat.

a- ***Allium cepa*** Linn.
d- Watt Dict.

B- for confirmation

a- ***Allium macleani*** Baker
b- Dymock (Pharm. indi.).

23 (२४) कदली Kadalī

कदली सुकुमारा च रम्भा स्वादुफला[1] मता ।
दीर्घपत्रा[2] च निःसारा मोचा हस्तिविषाणिका ॥ ७३

कदली मधुरा शीता रम्या पित्तहरा मृदुः ।
कदल्यास्तु फलं स्वादु कषायं नातिशीतलम् ॥ ७४
रक्तपित्तहरं वृष्यं रुच्यं कफकरं गुरु[3] ।
कन्दस्तु वातलो रूक्षः शीतोऽसृक्कृमिकुष्ठनुत् ॥ ७५

कदली (Kadalī), सुकुमारा (Sukumārā), रम्भा (Rambhā), स्वादुफला (Swāduphalā), दीर्घपत्रा (Dīrghapatrā), निःसारा (Niḥsārā), मोचा (Mocā) and हस्तिविषाणिका (Hastiviṣāṇikā) are synonymous.

Kadalī is sweet in taste, *śitavīrya,* delightful, pacifies *pittadoṣa* and is soft.

The fruit of *kadalī* is sweet and *kaṣāya* and not very much *śitavīrya.* It is useful in bleeding disorders, *vṛṣya* appetizing, aggravates *kapha doṣa* and *guru.* It's bulbous root is *śitavīrya,* aggravates *vātadoṣa,* roughening, and useful in *raktadoṣa,* worms and disorders of skin.

I (Nighaṇṭus have recorded four kinds of Kadalis. Out of them this plant is known as banana kind. The ripen fruits of which are edible.)

(Fam. Musaceae)

a) ***Musa paradisiaca*** Linn. Var. ***sapientum*** Kuntz.
Syn. *Musa sapientum* Linn.
b) Dymock (Pharm. indica)

II a) रम्भा (Rambhā), स्वादुफला (Swāduphalā), मोचा (Mocā)
b) (Sans.) Rambhā; (H.Bom.) Keḷe, Kela

---

१ 'भानुफला' इति. नि. शे. टीका तथा क्षी. संमतः पाठः ।
२ काष्ठीरसश्च'निःसारा मोचा हस्तिबुषा तथा । इति क्षी. संमतः पाठः । 'वारणविषा' इति केषांचित् संमतः पाठः इति क्षी. ।
३ ' रक्तपित्तहरं वृष्यं रुच्यं श्लेष्मकरं गुरुं । इति सुश्रुतपाठः सु.सू. ४६. १८१

B) Kālā (Tam. & Tel.) Kadalī; (Mal.) Kadalum; (Eng.) Banana
See Kāṣṭhakadalī

काष्ठकदली Kāṣṭhakadalī (14)

काष्ठकदली (ध.नि.)
द्वितीया काष्ठकदली श्वेताऽरण्यकदल्यपि ।
विषघ्नी कदली चापि पाषाणकदली तथा ॥ ७८
स्यात् काष्ठकदली रुच्या रक्तपित्तहरा हिमा ।
गुरुर्मन्दाग्निजननी दुर्जरा मधुरा परा ॥ ७८

The other kind of Kadalī is called as काष्ठकदली (Kāṣṭhakadalī) of which synonyms are श्वेता (Śvetā), अरण्यकदली (Araṇyakadalī), विषघ्नी कदली (Viṣaghnī kadalī) and पाषाणकदली (Pāṣāṇakadalī)

Kāṣṭhakadalī is very sweet, *śītavirya*, appetizing., and useful in bleeding disorders.It is *guru,* depresses digestive capacity and difficult to digest.

गिरिकदली **Girikadalī (15) (Raj. ni.)**

गिरिकदली गिरिरम्भा पर्वतमोचाऽप्यरण्यकदली च ।
बहुबीजा वनरम्भा गिरिजा गजवल्लभाऽभिहिता ॥

गिरिकदली मधुरहिमा बलवीर्यविवृद्धिदायिनी रुच्या ।
तृट्पित्तदाहशोषप्रशमनकर्त्री च दुर्जरा च गुरुः ॥ Raj. ni. chap. 11

गिरिकदली (Girikadalī), गिरिरम्भा (Girirambhā), पर्वतमोचा (Parvatmocā), अरण्यकदली (Araṇyakadalī), बहुबीजा (Bahubījā), वनरम्भा (Vanarambhā), गिरिजा (Girijā) and गजवल्लभा (Gajavallabhā) are synonyms.

Girikadalī is sweet in taste, *śītavirya,* promotes strength and potency, is appetizing, pacifies thirst, *Pittadoṣa,* burning sensation and consumption. It is difficult to digest and *guru.*

सुवर्णकदली (रा.नि.) **Suvarṇakadalī (16)**

अन्या सुवर्णकदली सुवर्णरम्भाकनकरम्भा च ।
पीता सुवर्णमोचा चम्पकरम्भा सुरम्भिका सुभगा ॥

हेमफला स्वर्णफला कनकस्तम्भा च पीतरम्भा च ।
गौरा च गौररम्भा काञ्चनकदली सुरप्रिया षड्भूः ॥

सुवर्णमोचा मधुरा हिमा च स्वल्पाशने दीपनकारिणी च ।
तृष्णापहा दाहविमोचनी च कफावहा वृष्यकरी गुरुश्च ॥ Raj. ni. chap. 11

There is an another type of *kadalī* called as सुवर्णकदली (Suvarṇakadalī) of which synonyms are सुवर्णरम्भा (Suvarṇarambhā), कनकरम्भा (Kanakarambhā), पीता (Pītā), सुवर्णमोचा (Suvarṇamocā), चम्पकरम्भा (Campakarambhā), सुरम्भिका (Surambhikā), सुभगा (Subhagā), हेमफला (Hemaphalā), स्वर्णफला (Swarṇaphalā), कनकस्तम्भा (Kanaka stambhā), पीतरम्भा (Pītarambhā), गौरा (Gaurā), गौररम्भा (Gaurarambhā), काञ्चनकदली (Kāñcana kadalī) and सुरप्रिया (Surapriyā).

Suvarṇakadalī is sweet in taste, *śītavīrya,* if taken in small quantity stimulates digestive capacity, relieves thirst and burning sensation, aggravates *kaphadoṣa,* is *vṛṣya and guru.*

(Developed species of wild Musa. Now the fruits are used for vegetable or made into flour. See below IV 1-2)

(Fam. Musaceae)

a) ***Musa paradisiaca*** Linn.

b) Roxburgh (Fl. indi.)

a) काष्ठकदली (Kāṣṭhakadalī), रानकदली (Rāna Kadalī), पाषाणकदली (Pāṣāṇakadalī), शिलारम्भा (Śīlārambhā)

b) (Mar.) Āmbeli keḷen, Lokhandī -Mhaseḷīkeḷen (the fruit), (H) Kelā; (B) Kālā; (Eng.) Plantain.

IV -1) ... I shall therefore confine myself to (which I think), the original wild Musa, from which I conclude all the cultivated varieties of both Plantain and Banana produced, and which I consider as varieties of that one species. (Roxb. Fl.)

2) The plantain (Musa paradisiaca), a close relative of Banana .. ... There are some 75 varieties, all so old, that they have been propogated by seed within recorded times. Plaintain are always eaten cooked or made in flour.

24 (२५) सिन्दुवारः Sinduwāraḥ

सिन्दुवारः श्वेतपुष्पः सिन्दुकः सिन्दुवारकः ।
नीलपुष्पः शीतसहो निर्गुण्डी नीलसिन्दुका ॥ ७८

निर्गुण्डी कटुतिक्तोष्णा कृमिकुष्ठरुजापहा ।
वातश्लेष्मप्रशमनी प्लीहगुल्मारुचीर्जयेत् ॥ ७८

सिन्दुवारः (Sinduvārah), is (of white flowers) श्वेतपुष्पः (Śvetapuṣpaḥ), of which synonyms are सिन्दुकः (Sindukaḥ), and सिन्दुवारकः (Sinduvārakaḥ), and नीलपुष्पः (Nīlapuṣpaḥ) is called as निर्गुण्डी (Nirguṇḍī) of which synonyms are शीतसहः (Śītasahaḥ), and नीलसिन्दुका (Nīlasindukā).

Nirguṇḍī is pungent and bitter in taste, pacifies *vata kapha doṣas* and *uṣṇavīrya*. It is useful in worms, disorders of skin, disorders of spleen, tumours (diverticulosis) and in loss of appetite.

I. Generic name, includes two kinds A- श्वेतपुष्पः (Śwetapuṣpaḥ) and B.नीलपुष्पः (Nīlapuṣpaḥ), both of the same genus.

For confirmation
(Fam. Verbenaceae)

a-A-i) ***Vitex leucoxylon*** Willd.

or

ii) ***Vitex altissima*** Linn. f.

b- Kamat.
(See IV 3, 4 Roxburgh & Cooke)

B- ***Vitex arborea*** Roxb.

b- Kamat
(सिन्दुवार द्रुमेऽपि च Sinduwāra drumepica See III b-1 below)

II A-a सिन्दुवारकः (Sinduwārakaḥ), श्वेतपुष्पः (Śwetapuṣpaḥ),

b (H) Samhālu, Meuḍi; (Mar.) Lingaḍa, Nigaḍa; (B) Niśindā (Tam.) Nocci; (Tel.) Vāvilā; (Kan.) Bilienekki; (Eng.) Five leaved chaste tree, Indian privet.

B-a नीलपुष्पः (Nīlapuṣpaḥ), नीलसिन्दुकः (Nīlasindukaḥ), स्थिरसाधनकः (Sthirsādhanakaḥ), अर्थसिद्धकः (Arthasiddhakaḥ), निर्गुण्डी (Nirguṇḍī)

b as in A above.

III- a- See IV-5 below.

b- 1) सिन्दुवार द्रुमेऽपि च (Sinduwāra drumepica) Maheshwar on Amara 2.4.70

2) 151 निर्गुण्डीति
इन्द्रसुरा - सुरवारुणी । 'ऐन्द्रीत्विन्द्रसुरा चित्रा गवाक्षी सुरवारुणी' ति हृदयदीपकः 'निर्गुण्डीन्द्राणिका नीलशेफाल्यो करहाटके' ति लोचनः । करहाटका- शिफाकन्दः ।सिन्दुकः सिन्दुवारकः सितपुष्पकःशीतसह इति । निर्गुण्डी 'कट्टग्राढकी सन्दला गुल्मगुच्छा व्यक्तसस्या सित' इति । 'मढण्डी'

इति माला । अन्या तादृशी तनुः शेफालि शृंगारहारः-इति वृन्दावनवने प्रसिद्धा ।
Harshe

3) See शेफालिका III-b- 1 & 2

4) अथ सिन्दुवारः (मेउडी) निर्गुण्डी (नीलसम्हालू) सिन्दुवारः श्वेतपुष्पः सिन्दुकः सिन्दुवारकः । नीलपुष्पी तु निर्गुण्डी शेफाली सुवहा च सा ।
(Chuneker Bh. Pr. P. 344)

see IV-8 below.

IV- 1 *Vitex trifolia* Willd.
Flowers small of a lively light blue purple (Roxb.)

2 *V. arborea* Roxb.
Trunk straight high and of a large size... the wood is exceedingly hard and durable.
Flowers numerous, small blue.

3 *Vitex leucoxylon* Willd......
growing to be a tree of very considerable size.
Flowers -numerous, fragrant, pretty larger, of white straw colour. (Roxb. C.B.C.)

4. *Vitex altissima* Linn.
A very large tree .. The wood is hard, weighing 60 lbs. Cu. feet... used for building purpose, furnitures and carts .... Corolla white tinged with blue. (Cooke fl.)

5 सिन्दु (न्ध) वार C.S.Su. 3.27, 4.16, etc.
S.S.Su. 46. 286, Ka. 5.66 etc.
A.H.Su. 7.25, U. 36-57 etc.
Sinduwāra and Nirguṇḍi are usually considered to be two different species of Vitex bearing respectively white and blue flowers. It may be noted that *Vitex negundo* Linn. itself contains forms possessing both white and blue flowers and have 3-5 foliate leaves, although a different species *V. trifoliata* Linn f. is sometimes mentioned to be *Sinduwāra* and the blue flowered form of *V. negundo* is accepted *Nirguṇḍī.* (Balvantji P. 433)

6 सम्हालू-निर्गुण्डी *Vitex negundo* Linn. Eng. Five leaved chaste tree, Indian Privet. It is a shrublike small tree. Flowers (मञ्जरी) white or light blue purple. (Chunekar Bh. Pr. p. 345)

7 निर्गुण्डी Nirguṇḍi *Vitex negundo* Linn. Syn. (Sans.) सिन्दुक, सिन्दुवार. सुवहा

There appears some confusion regarding the diffeent varieties of *Nirguṇḍī* and *Sinduwāra* .... but for all purposes the above mentioned plant may be used for both *Nirguṇḍī* and *Sinduwāra.* .... (Balavantji p. 276)

25 (२५) निर्गुण्डी Nirguṇḍī (शेफालिका Śephālikā)

शेफालिकाऽन्या निर्गुण्डी वनजा नीलमञ्जरी ।
कृष्णसंज्ञो विषघ्नश्च पवित्रो गिरिसिन्दुकः ॥ ७९
शुक्लाऽन्या श्वेतसुरसा भूतकेशी[१] च कथ्यते ॥

There is an another type of निर्गुण्डी (Nirguṇḍī), called as शेफालिका (Śephālikā), of which synonyms are वनजा (Vanajā), नीलमञ्जरी (Nīla mañjarī), कृष्णसंज्ञः (Kṛṣṇa samjñyaḥ), विषघ्नः (Viṣaghnaḥ), पवित्रः (Pavitraḥ), and गिरिसिन्दुकः (Girisindukaḥ). The white flowered variety शुक्ला (Śuklā) has the synonyms श्वेतसुरसा (Śvetasurasā) and भूतकेशी (Bhūtakeśī).

I Generic name includes two plants A नीलमञ्जरी (Nīlamañjarī) and B-श्वेतसुरसा भूतकेशी (Śwetasurasā Bhūtakeśī). The latter is now noted here as it is mentioned by Raj.Ni. He notes it under a separate heading शुक्लांगी (Śuklāṅgī).

For confirmation Fam. Verbenaceae.

I- A-a Blue flowered variety of *Vitex negundo* Linn.
b- Pant. Bhagirath.
B-a White flowered variety of *Vitex negundo* Linn.
b Pant. Bhagirath.
(See below IV -5 Bhagirath and Sinduwāra IV -5 Balwantji)

II A-a निर्गुण्डी (Nirguṇḍī), नीलसिन्दुक (Nīlasinduka), नीलमञ्जरी (Nīlamañjarī)
b As in सिन्दुवारः (Sinduwāraḥ).

II B-a शुक्लाऽन्या (Śuklānyā), श्वेतसुरसा (Śwetasurasā), भूतकेशी (Bhūtakeśī), इंद्राणी (Indrāṇī), नीलिका (Nīlikā)
b As in Sinduwāraḥ.

III - See Sinduwāraḥ
a- शेफाली (Śephālī) A.H.U. 13. 90,
b- 1 त्र्यर्थे सुवहा, रास्ना शेफालिका, गन्धनाकुली (K'śīraswāmi Amar)
2 शेफालिका तु सुवहा निर्गुण्डी नीलिका च सा ।
श्वेताऽसौ श्वेतसुरसा भूतवेश्याऽथ मागधी ॥
Bhūtāni Viśati ālhādayati Bhūtaveśī, Nīlvarṇā (Nīlikā) ...
Śerate śephā alayosyām śephālikā
(K'śīraswāmī, Bhānujī on Amarakośa)

---

१ 'भूतवेशी ' इति. क्षी. नि. शे. टीका संमतः पाठः ।

3 शेफालिका (Śephalikā) - Catwārī Kṛṣṇapuspyā Nirgundyām, निर्गुण्डी नील शेफाल्याम् सिन्दुवार द्रुमेऽपि च। इति मेदिनी-इति भानुजी सिन्दुवारे।
(Maheswara on Amara 2-4-70)

4 Seeसिन्दुवार Sinduwāra III b-2 Harshe

C-1) भूतकेशी (Bhūtakeśī), Śukla nirgundī (A. San. U. 6. 666)

2) शेफालिका - Nirguṇḍi (Rasa P. 154 Ātankāntaka Rasa)

3) शेफालिपत्र (Śephālipatra- Nirguṇḍī patra) (Sharng. M. 2. 84) (Gṛdhrasyām Yogadwayam).

IV- 1 *Vitex negundo* Willd. (San.) Sinduka, Sinduwāra, Nirguṇḍi, Indra Surasā, Indrāṇikā, (H.B) Nisindā.
Flowers small, numerous, most beautiful bluish purple. (Roxb.) नीलशेफालिका.

2 शेफालिका (Śephālikā) - Raktavṛnta Śārada Kusumā (Ḍalhaṇa Su.)

A.8) This interpretation aptly corresponds to पारिजातक (Pārijātaka) Ni. Adarsha.

3 निर्गुण्डी (Nirguṇḍī)

a) Śwetapuspā Sinduwāra.

b) Nīlapuṣpī Nirguṇḍī - Śephalikā; (H.) Sambhālu. (vd. Phadke) शेफाली *Śephālī* leaves have been used and the drug has been identified with blue flowered variety of *Nirguṇḍī* by Bhavmishra. In other Nighaṇṭus (Raj.ni. & Dh. Ni.) *śephālī* is also the name of a variety of *Nirguṇḍi* from the two (white & blue) varieities of *Nirguṇḍī*. It is felt that there is some confusion which can only be cleared if the so called *Śephālī* variety of *Nirgundī* is correctly identified. We have already referred to *Symphorema* species in our comments on *Girikarṇikā* गिरिकर्णिका. This too has leaves nearly resembling the *Śephālikā* leaves in appearance. This has a chance to be considered as this *Śephālī* ...etc.
(Balavantji p. 407 -8)

* This statement of Raj. ni. is mentioned under *Sinduwāra* and not under Śephālī. Probably Prof. Balwantji seems to be misguided by the statement of Raj. Ni. under *sinduwāra,* 'स्थिरसाधनको नेता सिद्धकश्चार्थसिद्धकः।' If that is the cause of doubt then it is totally improper, because there are certain varieties in *Sinduwāra* सिंदुवार which were used for construction of wooden bridges over the small rivers. Similarly, a piller of सिन्दुवार *Sinduwāra* was used to be posted in the centre of tanks. These are aptly mentioned by रा.नि. as स्थिरसाधन, नेता, सिद्धक, अर्थसिद्धक. Such piller posts can be observed in some tanks (rarely) till this time.

*Free & abridged translation of a Marathi note of the author D.K. Kamat.

1) See *Sinduwāra* सिंदुवार IV -5 Balvantji.

5) अपराजिता - शुक्लाङ्गी (Aparājītā Śuklāngī) (Śephalikā Viśesaḥ) हरशृंगार (Haraśṛngāra) has not manjari मंजरी inflorescence of racemose branching). For this (Harasṛngāra) cannot be शेफालिका of Nighanṭus. शेफालिका रक्तवृन्ता...पारिजातक हरश्रृंगार इति प्रसिद्धम्'। Ḍalhaṇa Su. Su. 8 Here Ḍalhaṇa is misleading ... But शेफालिका (*Śephālikā*) must be confirmed with *Nirguṇḍi* which has white and blue inflorescence.

Vitex negundo, V. trifolia (Pant Bhagirath p. 260).

26 अश्वक्षुरकः (Aśwakśurakaḥ)
२७ गिरिकर्णिकाद्वयम् Girikarṇikādvayam

अश्वक्षुरा श्वेतपुष्पी श्वेता च गिरिकर्णिका ॥ ८१
कटभी श्वेतनामा च श्वेतस्पन्दाऽपराजिता ॥
नीलपुष्पीमहाश्वेता गिरिकर्णी गवादनी ॥ ८२
वल्ली चात्युग्रगन्धा च नीलस्पन्दा प्रकीर्तिता ॥

*(गिरिकर्णी हिमा तिक्ता पित्तोपद्रवनाशिनी ।
विषनेत्रविकारांश्च हन्ति कण्ठरुजापहा ॥)

गिरिकर्णीद्वयं तिक्तं पित्तोपद्रवनाशनम ॥ ८३
चक्षुष्यं विषदोषघ्नं त्रिदोषशमनं च तत् ॥

अश्वक्षुरा (Aśvakśurā), श्वेतपुष्पी (Śvetapuṣpī),श्वेता (Śvetā), गिरिकर्णिका (Girikarṇikā), कटभी (Kaṭabhī), श्वेतनामा (Śvetanāmā), श्वेतस्पन्दा (Śvetaspandā), अपराजिता (Aparājitā), are synonyms for white flowered variety, while नीलपुष्पी** (Nīlapuṣpī),महाश्वेता (Mahāśvetā), गिरिकर्णी (Girikarṇī), गवादनी (Gavādanī), वल्ली (Vallī), अत्युग्रगन्धा (Atyugragandhā) and नीलस्पन्दा (Nīlaspandā) are synonymous with blue flowered variety.

(*Girikarṇī* is bitter in taste, *śītavīrya* and alleviates disorders due to *pitta doṣa,* poison, diseases of eye, and diseases of throat.)

Both the types of *Girikarṇī* are bitter in taste, alleviate disorders due to *pitta doṣa*, pacify the three *doṣas,* and are beneficial to eyes and disorders due to poison.

(Generic name, includes two kinds of A-श्वेतपुष्पी (Śwetapuṣpī) and the next B- नीलपुष्पी (Nīlapuṣpī) गिरिकर्णिका (Girikarṇikā). Both are

* This is an additional reading found in Anandasram edition.

** *Nīlapuṣpī Mahāśvetā* can also be a single synonym. S. D. K.

of the same species, and the differance is only in colour of flowers A variety is white flowered plant and B variety is blue flowered plant.)

Fam. Leguminosae. Fabaceae

IA&B-a ***Clitoria ternatea*** Linn.
b Kamat.

II A-a गिरिकर्णिका (Girikarṇīkā), श्वेता (Śwetā), कटभी (Kaṭabhī), अपराजिता(Aparājitā), श्वेतस्पन्दा (Śwetaspandā),
a-b महानीला (Mahānīlā), नीलस्पन्दा (Nīlaspandā), गिरिकर्णिका (Girikarṇikā)
A-b (Sans.) Aparājitā; (H.B.). Aparajit; (Mar.) Pāṇḍharī Gokaṛṇa; (Tel.)Tella dintana.
B. (Mar.) Nili Gokarṇa; (Tel.) Nella dintana (Blue flowered) Roxburgh; अश्वक्षुरः (Aśwakśuraḥ) Girikarṇikā (Ast. San.U.A. 40)
b) 1) अश्वक्षुरः (Aśwakśuraḥ) - Adrikarṇikā, Kaṭabhī, Dadhipuṣpikā, Viṣṇukrāntā + Bhavaprakasake; (Mar.) Pāṇḍharī Gokarṇa. (Ni. Shiroamani - Pade)
2) 48 शङ्खपुष्पी (Śaṅkhapuṣpī), Girikaṃikā Yawatikatā + Sitapuṣpī *Clitoria ternatea* valiya Śaṅkhapuṣpī., (Shree Krishnan A. Manj. No. 48).

27 (२८) जन्तुकारी Jantukārī

जन्तुकारी[१] जन्तुकृष्णा जतुका रञ्जनी[२] स्मृता ॥ ८४
जननी चैव संहर्षा[३] जन्तुका[४] चक्रवर्तिनी ॥
जन्तुका शिशिरा तिक्ता रक्तदोषनिबर्हणी ॥ ८५
पित्तोपशमनी हन्ति विषयोगं प्रयोगतः ॥

जन्तुकारी (Jantukārī), जन्तुकृष्णा (Jantukṛṣṇā), जतुका (Jatukā),रञ्जनी (Rañjanī), जननी (Jananī), संहर्षा (Samharṣā), जन्तुका (Jantukā) and चक्रवर्तिनी (Cakravartinī) are synonymous.

Jantukā is bitter in taste, *śītavīrya*, pacifies *pitta* and *rakta doṣas* and poisons.

I Ambiguous
II जतुका (Jatukā) रञ्जनी (Rañjanī), चक्रवर्तिनी (Cakrawartinī),

---

१ "जन्तुवारा" २ "रजनी" ३ "संस्पर्शा" ४ " जतुका"

तिर्यक्फला (Tiryakphalā), सूक्ष्मवल्ली (Sūkśhmavallī), वृक्षरुहा (Vṛkśaruhā), दीर्घफला (Dīrghaphalā).

28 (२९) पद्मचारिणी Padmacāriṇī

पद्मचारिण्यतिचरा पद्मा पद्मावतीति च ॥ ८६
चारटी गन्धमूला च लक्ष्मीः श्रेष्ठा सुपुष्करा ॥
पद्मा सुगन्धा तिक्ता च मोहापस्मारनाशिनी ॥ ८७

पद्मचारिणी (Padmacāriṇī), अतिचरा (Aticarā), पद्मा (Padmā),पद्मावती (Padmāvaṭī), चारटी (Cāraṭī), गन्धमूला (Gandhamūlā), लक्ष्मीः (Lakśmiḥ),श्रेष्ठा (Śreṣṭhā) and सुपुष्करा (Supaṣkarā) are synonymous.

Padmā is bitter in taste, fragrant and useful in mental confusion and epilepsy.

For confirmation

Fam - Liliaceae.

I a) ***Colchicum luteum*** Baker

b) Kamat (following Dr. Apte, Dymock, Desai).

II a) अतिचरा (Aticarā), पद्मा (Padmā), पद्मवती (Padmavati), चारटी (Cāraṭi), गन्धमूला (Gandhumūlā), सुपुष्करा (Supuṣkarā), अम्बुरुहा (Amburuhā),पुष्करिणी (Puṣkariṇī),पुष्कराद्यपर्णिका(Puṣkarādyaparṇikā), स्थलपद्मी (Sthalapadmī)

b) (SK) Sthalapadmā, Sthalakamal, Hiraṇyathutha, (H.) Hirantutiya; (Kāshmir) Virkam; (Pers.) Surinjan - i- talkh; (Eng.) Meadow Saffron, Bitter Hermodectyl.

III b) (Padmacārini), (Keral-orilattamara), Kalattāmara. Karattamara.अयं प्रायः पद्माकारा स्थले जायमाना च । अस्याः पत्रनालपुष्पकर्णिका पद्मापेक्षया लघुतराकृतयः मूलं च सुगन्धीति भेदः । एषा प्रायः शरदि च जायते । (Tam.) Orillai-Hamarai, (Mar.) स्थलकमलिनी; (Kan.) Kaludavare (A.O.Ni.)

2) पद्मा - See फञ्जी and भाङ्गी (A.H.Su. 15.37) (Balawantji p. 55)

3) 329 अव्यथा पद्मचारिणी । 'अव्यथातिचरा पद्मा चारटी पद्मचारिणी' त्यमरः । Harshe

Colchicum luteum; (SK) Hiranyatuttha. Flowers yellow, two kinds - Surinjan Talkah (Bitter) and the next 'Surinjan Shirin' (Sweet). Su. talkh is used in medicine. (Desai.)

4) *Colchicum luteum* Baker
Flowers golden yellow (Dr. Kirtikar)

IV 1) There are some (aquatic) plants in Kashmir which are known there as ' Sthala kamala'; have yellow or rose coloured flowers. *Colchiucm luteum* Baker स्थलकमल (Apte vol.. p. 88)

2) Colchicum root is the dried corm of meadow saffron (*Colchicum autamnale*) a perenial tuliplike shrub of Europe and Northern Africa. The active principle is an alkaloid colchicin which is used in the treatment of rhumatism and gout. (Hill P. 245)

3) See ऋद्धि Habeneria species. Balawantji p. 53
See वृद्धि Balawantji p. 377
Habeneria commelinfolia Wall. ex Lindle. Fam. Orchidaceae. Western Himalayas, Kumaon, Parasnath, Kokan, W. Ghat, N. Canara, (Chopra).

29 (३०) गृष्टिः Gṛṣṭiḥ (वाराही- Vārahī)

गृष्टिर्विष्वक्सेनकान्ता वाराही गृष्टिका च सा ।
माधवी सौकरी कान्तिः कान्ता च वनमालिनी ॥ ८८

कान्ता सौकरिका तिक्ता कुष्ठकृमिगरार्तिजित् ।
वाराह्याः कफहा कन्दः कटुको रसपाकतः ॥ ८९
हिमः कुष्ठकृमिहरो हृद्यो बल्यो रसायनः ॥

गृष्टिः (Gṛṣṭiḥ), विष्वक्सेनकान्ता (Viṣvaksenakāntā), वाराही (Vārāhī), and गृष्टिका (Gṛṣṭikā) are synonymous. माधवी (Mādhavī), सौकरी (Saukarī) ,कान्तिः (Kāntiḥ), कान्ता (Kāntā) and वनमालिनी (Vanamālinī), are synonymous.

Kāntā saukarikā is bitter in taste, useful in disorders of skin, worms and artificial poisons. *Vārāhī kanda* is pungent in taste and *vipāka*, *śītavīrya* and is useful in skin disorders, and worms, is cordial, strength promoting and *rasāyana*.

I Generic name. The description of the plants stated in Dh. Ni. is some what confusing. But while describing the medicinal properties two different drugs are clearly mentioned. A वाराही (Vārāhī) and the next B. कान्ता सौकरिका (Kantā Saukarikā). Raj. Ni. has given medicinal propertiies of वाराही only. Both plants are of different genera.

Fam. Taccaceae.

A-1a) ***Tacca aspera*** Roxb.*

b) Dymock (Pharm. Indi.)
also

2) ***Tacca pinnatifida*** Willd & Forst.**
Syn. *T. pinnatifolia* Roxb.

a-B (Fam. Dioscoreaceae)
Dioscorea pentaphylla Linn.

b. Kamat. See III, IV below.

II A.a गृष्टिः (Grṣtiḥ), वाराही (Vārāhī), माधवी (Mādhavī), वराहकन्दः (Varāhakandaḥ), ब्राह्मकन्दः (Brāhmakandaḥ),

b (SK) Vārāhi; (Mar.) Ḍukarakanda; (H.B) Vārāhī Kanda; (Pahāḍī) Bhevari ki-vela.

1) (Mar.) Devakāndā, Sarde cāmhāra; (Kokani) Surnū; (Kan) Sūrana; (Santal) Dhai;(Dec.) Barākanda; (Mal.) Canekizhana; (Tam) Karacumai.

B-a विष्वक्सेनकान्ता (Viṣwaksena Kāntā),वनमालिनी (Vanamālinī), क्रोडकन्या (Kroḍakanyā), ब्रह्मपुत्री (Brahmaputrī), वनवासी (Vanawāsī), शबरकन्दकः (Śabarakandakaḥ)

b (Mar.) Ullasi, Sendavela, Sendurvel; (H.) Suaralu; (Mar. Kātkarī) Madācā Kāndā, (b) Kāntālu, Suaralu, (Tam.) Kattu Kilangu; (Tel.) Dukapendalamu; Nākuli Kanda (Sachitra Ayurveda 10-61)

III

1 वाराही ("Vārāhī Kanda evānyascarmakāraluko mataḥ") Bh. Pr. Ni. Abhāve. 47.
तेषां तपस्तपस्यौ शिशिरः, मधुमाधवो वसन्तः (Madhu-mādhavo Vasantaḥ) (Su. Su.14)
चैत्रस्तु .. मधु.. वैशाखो माधवो। भवेद् वसन्तो मधु माधवाभ्याम ।(Caitrastuaḥ) Madhu ... Vaiśākho Madhavo Bhavedvasanto Madhu Mādhavābhyām || Raj. NI. U. 21-46

2 वाराहीकन्दः (Vārahī kanda.)पश्चिमे गृष्टि संज्ञकः
D. sativa = True Vārāhī.
D. bulbifera, Physicians of the west do not accept this (Ciraiyā Kanda, Dehalī) as Varāhī kanda (Vidyotani, Bh. Pr. Ni.)

3 वाराही |Ci 11 | (Vārāhī) ताम्बूलसदृशैः पत्रैः (Ast. hr. kosa)

4 वाराही माधवी गृष्टि ... वनमालिका । (Madan Ni. 1. 221)

5 वाराह कन्दो (Vārāha Kando) ....'Bakālaki' iti Prasidhaḥ ..Grstikā.. (Dalhan Su. Su. 46. 309).

---

* The current valid name is - *T. integrifolia* Ker. - Gawl.

** The present valid name is - *T. leontopetaloides* (Linn.) O. Kuntz. (Comp. p. 148).

6 'ऐन्द्री दूर्वा .. विष्वक्सेना स्थापयेद् गर्भम्' Viṣwaksenā Vārāhī (Ast. sang. referred in A.H. Su. 15-18)

7 वाराही कन्द (Vārāihī Kanda) Abhāve Carmakārāluko mataḥ (Cakradatta abhave Chapt.)

IV (See *Tacca pinnatifida* Willd & Forst.)
Dioscorea bulbifera Linn. (Bom.) Kārindā, Kaḍu Kārindā.(Watt Dict.)

b -1 *Tacca aspera* (Roxb.)
(H.B.S.) Vārāhī Kanda; (Mar.) Dukar Kanda (Chopra)

2 *Dioscorea pentaphylla*, Willd. (B.) Kanta alu. (? Kanta) flower ing rainy season (Roxb.)

2-a) *Tacca aspera,* Roxb.
It blossoms during the hot and rainy season.

2-b) *Tacca pinnatifida* Willd. & Forst.
Sy. *T. pinatifolia*, Gaertn. Flowers June - July (Roxb.)

3 *Tacca aspera* Roxb. Vārāhī kanda of Nighaṇṭus. *T. aspera, T. laevi, T. pinnatifida* ... Starch resembling arrowroot may be obtained. Dymock.

4 वाराही (Vārāhi) The commentator of Cakradatta has given very apt description of ताम्बूल सदृशैः पत्रैः ... किन्तु वाराहीकन्दापेक्षया चर्मकारालुकस्यप्रति हीन गुणत्वेन नास्य तत् प्रतिनिधित्वं युक्तम् ....।
(Sachi. Ayu. 10. 1967)

5 वाराह (Vārāha) Vārāhī Gṛṣtikocyate (Keyadeva). Some people suppose *Kaḍu Kārindā* as *Ḍukara kanda,* but it is not true *Ḍukarakanda* (vd. Bodas)

6 *Tacca pinnatifolia.*
(Mar.) Sardecāmhāra, Devkāndā.
Tuber of this plant is used like *Ḍukarkanda* (Desai)

7 *Tacca pinnatifida*, Forst ... flowering September, Verna. Devakāndā, (Cooke Fl.; Chopra)
.. Root stock globose 6-10 in. diam., rootlets superficial... leaves 1- feet in diam., circular in outline, 3 partiate. The segments variously pinnatifid, margin undulate, petiole 1-3 ft. long; Flowering Sept; Vern. Devakanda ... useful in dysentery. (Cooke fl.)

8 *Dioscorea pentaphylla* Linn.
D. triphylla Linn.
D. jacquemonti Hook f.
Root tubers oblong, very long (5-6 ft. according to Thwaites) .....Male flowers pale greenish, fragrant... The tubers of the wild

plants are eaten ..... the fragrant male flowers are sold in native bazars and eaten as greens .. Flowering September, October ... vern. Shendvel (Cooke Fl.)

9 *Tacca aspera* Roxb.
Root an oblong, curved tuber of meddling size, with wiry fibers, from its sides, inward colour pale yellow . ..Berry oblong flesh. Stems none or very trifling. Leaves radial, oblong, recurved, entire, acuminate, smooth parallel, veins 8 to 16 in. long and 4 to 5 in. broad. ... It blossoms during the hot and rainy season. (Roxb.)

10 B.H.& S: Vārāhīkanda'
Mara. Ḍukarkanda ... Tubers tonic useful in heamorrhagic diathesis, skin diseases and leprosy ... Pahadi Bhevrekā kanda, Sindh: Suvarkanda (Chopra)

11 H. Bom. Kanṭālu; B. Suarālu; Mar. ulsi (Chopra)
Mara. Mħadācā kāndā, šendavel, Sendurvela, Ulasī.
(Dr. Desai)

12 *Diosocroea bulbifera* Linn. (Blue bearing yam; H. Zamikand; Santal -Pisk; Bo. Karindā; Kadu Karindā ... ..
The bulbs on the stems and tubers under ground are used as vegetable. (Watt. Dict.)

13 H. Ratalu; Mar. Karu Karinda; B. Banālu, kukuralu; Tam. Kodihilangu; Tel. Cheddu paddu- dump
D. bulbifera Linn.
Syn. *D. crispata* Roxb.
D. pulchella Roxb.
D. sativa Thunb. non Linn.
D. versicolor Buch. Ham. ex Wall .(Chopra).

30 मांसरोहिणी Māmsarohiṇī

मांसरोहिण्यतिरुहा वृत्ता[१] चर्मकसा[२] च सा ॥ ९०
विकसा मांसरोहा च रुहा रक्ता प्रकीर्तिता ॥

विकसा कटुका तिक्तग तथोष्णा स्वरसादनुत् ॥ ९१
रसायनप्रयोगाच्च सर्वरोगहरा मता ॥

In Dhanvantariya Ni. the synonym रोहिणी (Rohinī) is applied to 'Kāsmarya', 'Jambu', 'Manjiṣṭhā, 'Māmsarohinī. D.K. Kamat.

१ 'वृन्ता' इति नि.शे. टीका. संमतः पाठः ।

२ 'चर्मकशा इति नि.शे. टीका संमतः पाठः ।

कषाया ग्राहिणी वर्ण्या रक्तपित्तप्रसादनी ॥ ९२
*रोहिणीयुगुलं शीतं कषायं कृमिनाशनम् ।
कण्ठशुद्धिकरं रुच्यं वातदोषनिषूदनम् ॥ ९३

मांसरोहिणी (Māmsarohiṇī), अतिरुहा (Atiruhā), वृत्ता (Vṛttā), चर्मकसा (Carmakasā), विकसा (Vikasā), मांसरोहा (Māmsarohā), रुहा (Ruhā) and रक्ता (Raktā) are synonymous.

Vikasā is pungent and bitter in taste, *uṣṇavīrya* and restores normalcy to voice and useful in many diseases by *rasāyana* procedure.

It is *kaṣāya* in taste, astringent, improves complexion and useful in bleeding disorder.

Both types of *rohiṇi* are *kaṣāya* in taste, useful in worms. These pacify *vātadoṣa,* are useful in clearing the throat and appetizing.

I Generic name, includes two plants A चर्मकसा (Carmakasā) and the next B-विकसा (Vikasā)

Controversial - not identified

II A a) अतिरोहिणी (Atirohiṇī), वृत्ता (Vṛttā), चर्मकसा (Carmakasā), सदामांसी (Sadāmāmsī), सुलोमा (Sulomā), लोमकरणी (Lomakaraṇī).

B a) विकसा (Vikasā), रुहारक्ता (Ruhāraktā), मांसरोही (Māmsarohī), ग्राहिणी (Grāhiṇī)

III 1 रोहिणी (Rohiṇī), Ca, Su.-4 Balye Mahākaṣāye Sū. su. Nyagrodhādi gaṇe.

2 रोहिणी (Av. IV. 12 Pant. Satavlekar Part V)

b- 1 मांसरुहा (Māmsaruhā) Vanamāli, dwitiya carmakasā, Rohinī.

2 मांसरोहिणी - के. मांसरोहिणी । विवरणम् - एषा द्विविधा । तत्रैका द्वितीया मांसरोहिणी इति पूर्वमुक्ता । मांसरोहिणी वृक्ष : प्रायः जांगलेषु जायते । अस्य पत्रं कर्णिकारपत्रमिवाल्पाकृतिः । फलं भृशं पिच्छिलं सुगन्धि च । (A.O.Ni.)

IV 1 अरुन्धती (Arundhatī) Rohiṇī or Lākśā (AV IV 12-1. P.16) Arundhati is also called as Rohiṇī and Lākśā (Kausika 28-14) (Dr. Shende Av. IV-12)

2 रोहिणी (Rohini) Creeper or Tiger (Dr. Karambelkar AV. IV. 12-1)

3 *Swietania febrifuga* Willd; (Tel.) Soyamid, (B) Rohan (Vd. Kudtarkar Shastri.)

---

* This reading is found in Anadaśram edtiton and resembles exactly with Raj. Ni's. reading. S.D. Kamat.

4 मांसरोहिणी (Māsmsarohiṇī); (H.) Rohan, Rohin; (B) Rohan; (Santal) Ruben; (Gond) Soimi; (Kan) Swāmimar, Sambi; (Tam.) Semaram; Somadanam (Bom) Rohan.
Soymida febrifuga A. Juss (Dr. Desai, Ach. yadavji, Acha. Priyavrat) Bom Gaze XXV Guj. Trees

5 *Soymida febrifuga* Juss.
.. ... notices are found in some of their books on Materia Medica under the name Rohana (Dymock I-336)

6. 58 मांसरोहिणी *Soymida febrifuga* A. Juss. Ḍalhaṇa has interpreted Rohiṇī as Kaṭukī, Kāyaphal, bitter tumbī (कडवी तुम्बी) and Haritakī variety (Chunekar Bh. Pi. Ni. Page 358)

7 Thus the use of Soymida bark may be tried .... especially when the wound healing properties have been emphasized. (Balawantji 341)
मांसरोहिण्यतिरुहा वृत्ता चर्मकसा वसा ।
प्रहारवल्ली विकसा वीरवल्यपि ॥
.. स्यात् मांसरोहिणी सरा ॥

V 1) 58 *Soymida febrifuga* A. Juss (Chunekar Bh. Pr. P. 358...)
2) मंजिष्ठा . . विकसा . . . योजनवल्ली... वस्त्रभूषणा ... रक्तयष्टिका ...रोहिणी .. कालमेषिका ॥ (Dhn. Ni. P. 10 Plant pre No. 10).

31 (३२) वन्दका Vandakā

वन्दाकः स्याद् वृक्षरुहा शेखरी कामरूपका[1] ॥
वृक्षादनी तरुरुहा कामिनी पद्मरूपिणी[2] ॥ ९४
वन्दाकः शीतलः पाके ग्राही स्याद् व्रणरोपणः ॥

वन्दाकः (Vandākaḥ), वृक्षरुहा (Vṛkṡaruhā), शेखरी (Ṡekharī), कामरूपका (Kāmarūpakā), वृक्षादनी (Vṛkṡādanī), तरुरुहा (Taruruhā), कामिनी (Kāminī) and पद्मरुपिणी (Padmarūpiṇī) are synonymous.

Vandāka is *ṡītavīrya,* after digestion it is astringent and useful for healing wounds.

I (Under this heading, it seems that two kinds of plants are included. The one is A. वन्दका (Vandakā) which is a partial parasitic plant growing on the trees, next B. वृक्षादनी (Vrkṡādanī) entirely parasitic plant growing on the trees.

---

१ 'कामवृक्षकः' इति नि.शे. टीका संमतः पाठः ।
२ 'कामिन्यङ्घ्रिप्ररोहणी' इति नि.शे. टीका संमतः पाठः ।

Fam. Orchidaceae.

I A-a- ***Saccolabium papilosum*** Lindl.*
Dendrobium macraei Lindl.
Vanda roxburghii R. Br.
These and other partial parasitics of the orchidaceae family.
b. Kamat
c. See IV below.

II A-a- वन्दका (Vandakā)
b (H.) Bandā; (B) Bāndā, nādī; (Santal) Derabanki; (Mar.) Rāsnā; (Tel.) Kanapchettu, mardaru.

B-a. ***Loranthus longiflorus*** Desr.**
Viscum album Linn.
These and other allied species of Loranthaceae family.
b. Watt Dict. V-93
c. Tropical Himalaya ... from Oudh to Assam and scattered to Travancore, Ceylon and Malacca. (See IV-1)

II a-b वृक्षादनी (Vṛkšādanī), तरुरुहा (Taruruhā), कामरूपका (Kāmarūpakā), कामिनी (Kāminī), (Dhn. Ni.), शिखरी (Šikharī), केशरूपा (Kešarūpā),
b Santal-Bandā; Tel. Madinika, Yeliga; San. - Vṛkšharuhā, Vrkshādanī (Watt dict. V-99)

II a- See IV-3 below.
b 1) वन्दा वृक्षादनी वृक्षरुहा . . Amar. 2-4-82. जन्मवृक्षमत्ति नाशयति वृक्षादनी । वृक्षे रोहति - वृक्षरुहा । त्र्यर्थे जीवन्ती गुडूची वृक्षरुहा । (Ksīraswāmī)
2) 279 वृक्षवन्दा -वृक्षरुहा ।
'अन्य वृक्षेऽन्यवृक्षऽस्य शिफाया सा च वन्दिका । (Harshe)

IV 1) *Loranthus longiflorus* Desr.
Syn. *L. bicolor* Roxb.
Var.*falcata* Kurz.
Var. *amplexifolia* Thunb.
Var.*pubescence*
The varieties *falcata* Kurz. and *pubescens* are confined to western India and Ceylon.
2) *Viscum album* Linn.
(Unani) Kishmis kāblī from Kashmir to Nepal, parasitic, grows on Akrod (अक्रोड - Walnut) or on Gulab (गुलाब). The fruits are used in medicine. (Chunekar Bh. Pr.)
3) वन्दाक Vandāka Su. Ci. 6.17

---

* The current valid name is *Acampe papillosa* (Lindle) Lindle. (Comp. p. 2)
** The current valid name is *Dendropthoe falcata* (Linn f.) Ettingshausen (Comp. p. 51)

Loranthus longiflorus Desr.
वृक्षरुहा. संहर्षा
.... other epiphytes and semiparasites are also called Bāndā (Balavantji p. 358).

32 (३३) सुवर्चला Suvarcalā.

सुर्वचलाऽऽदित्यकान्ता सूर्यभक्ता सुखोद्भवा ॥ ९५
मण्डूकपर्णी मण्डूकी वरदाऽऽदित्यवल्ल्यपि ॥

आदित्यभक्ता कटुका तथोष्णा स्फोटकापहा ॥ ९६
सरस्वती सरा स्वर्या रसायनविधौ हिता ॥

सुर्वचला (Suvarcalā), आदित्यकान्ता (Ādityakāntā), सूर्यभक्ता (Sūryabhaktā), सुखोद्भवा (Sukhodbhavā), मण्डूकपर्णी (Maṇḍūkaparṇī), मण्डूकी (Maṇḍūkī), वरदा (Varadā) and आदित्यवल्ली (Ādityavallī) are synonymous.

Ādityabhaktā is pungent in taste, *uṣṇavīrya,* and useful in blisters (blebs.) *Saraswatī* is laxative, beneficial to voice and useful in *rasāyana* procedure.

I Confirmed.

Fam. Umbelliferae. Apiaceae.

a- ***Hydrocotyle rotundifolia*** Roxb.*

b- D. K. Kamat

II a- आदित्यकान्ता (Ādityāntā), वरदा (Varadā), सूर्यलता (Sūryalatā), मण्डूकपर्णी (Maṇḍūkaparnī), मण्डूकी (Maṇḍukī), सुखोद्भवा (Sukhodbhawā), सुरसंभवा (Surasambhawā), सरस्वती (Saraswatī), स्वर्या (Swaryā),

b- (H) Kulakuri; (M) Balaikarai; (Mar. & Bom) Bṛāhmī Kaṛivaṇā; (B) Gimsāg.

III a- See Brāhmī, K'sudrapatrā, Ajagandhā

b- 1 सुर्वचला (Suwarcalā), Maṇḍūkaparṇī, Varadā (Abh. Manj.)

2 सुवैचला (Suwarcalā)

a- सुर्वचला (Suwarcalā), वरदा (Varadā), सूर्यावर्ता (Sūryāvartā), सूर्यभक्ता (Sūryabhaktā), हिमा (Himā), स्वादुपाका (Swādupakā),

b- परा ब्रह्मसुवर्चला (Parā Brahmasuvarcalā)

c- अन्या (Anyā), तिक्ता (Tiktā), उष्णा Uṣṇā, कटु (Kaṭu)

* The current valid name is *H. sibthorpioides* Lam. (Comp. p. 80)

d ब्राह्मीनामानि (Brāhmī nāmāni), तद्वन्मण्डूकपर्णिका (Tadwanm-aṇḍūkaparṇikā) (Bh. pr. Ni. shl. 285)

3 मण्डूकपर्णिका (Maṇḍūkaparṇikā) (Vadikhanda v.2)

4 सुर्वचला (Suwarcalā) - Maṇḍūkaparṇikā, Maṇḍūkī. (Shivdas Ast. Hr. U. 1-44)

e- *Hydrocotyle rotundifolia* Roxb.
uses similar to *H. asiatica,* Willd. (Roxb.)

IV

1) *Cleome viscosa* Linn.
Wild Mustard ... The seeds are known in Bazar as (Curī ajwān) (Kannayalal)

2) Suvarcalā, Sūryāvartā (Ast. Hr. Kosa)

3) *Helianthus annuus*, Linn. (Fl. indi. Roxb.)

4) *Crozophora* (*Chrozophora*) *plicata* A. Juss (Watt. Dict.)

5) Brāhmī, Nīrabrāhmī, Maṇḍūkaparṇī (Sachi. ayu. 10-61)

6) Sūryaphūl, Brāhmī (Abhi. Buti Darpan Part 1- 1937) pp. 20, 99)

V b-

1 *Cleome viscosa* Linn.
Ādityabhaktā, Suvarcalā, tilaparṇī, Tiḷawaṇa.

2 *Helianthus annuus* Linn., Sūryaphula

3 *Malva rotundifolia* Linn.
(H.B.) Khubāsi; (Tel.) Tricamalli; (Kan.) Kadukadaligida;

4 *Chrozophora plicata.* A. Juss.
(H) Sadevi, Subali; (SK.) Sūryāvartā

Reasoning -

1) *Cleome viscosa* Linn.
Tilaparṇī, Hurhura, Tilwaṇa.

a- The leaves of Suvarcalā described by our Nighaṇṭus are Maṇḍūki, Maṇḍūkaparnī, (Cordate, rotundus, filiform) while those of Tilaparṇī are oblong, lanceolate, apex pointed.

b- Suvarcalā of Nighaṇṭus is like latā (Sūryalatā), तृणवत तृणक (Tṛṇavat tṛṇaka-Shivkosh), कपोतवेगा (ध.नि.) i.e. a creeping herb, while Tilaparṇī is an erect small shrub.

c- Suvarcalā is cooling (Śiśira Raj. Ni.) while Tilaparṇī is blistering, If its juice is poured into ears, it causes this effect.

d- Suvarcalā clears the throat and vocal cord (Swaryā) and gives clear speech (Śaraswatī Symbolized as the Godess of speech Vāgdevatā).

e- Maṇḍūkaparṇī is used as Brāhmī (H. asiatica) says Dr. roxburgh (above III-F) but Tilaparṇī is not substituted for Brāhmī)

Tilaparṇī is vesicant (Chopra) and it has considerable degree of pungency in taste (Fl. ind. Roxb.)

f- It is वनयवानी (Vanayawānī) of some commentators and अजगन्धा (Ajagandhā) of Dhn. Ni. and अन्या सुवर्चला (Anyā Suvarcalā of Bh. Pr. Ni.) See above III d.

g- The comparison of synonyms mentioned in the enclosed table clearly shows that (Suvarcalā) is the common or generic name and it contains Suvarcalā proper and Suvarcalā Brāhmī.

For these reasons Tilaparṇī *Cleome viscosa* cannot be confirmed with Suvarcalā of our Nighaṇṭus.

2) Sun flower - *Helianthus annuus*

Native of America - Lately introduced into Inida in or after 16th century A.D. i.e. at least about 500 years after Dh. Ni. The plant is erect, small shrub (See Watt. Dict & Fl. Indi Roxb) i.e. not Tṛṇavat Tṛṇaka of Shivakosh. Therefore this plant cannot be confirmed with our Nighaṇṭus 'Suvarcalā'.

3) *Malva rotundifolia* Linn.

A plant of Malvaceae family. Leaves absolutely lobed (Not rotundus, native of Persia, as well as of Europe, annual, leaves are used as potherb (Roxb.). Chopra & Roxburgh do not name it as Maṇḍukaparṇī or Suvarcalā. This plant may have been adopted as 'Sunflower' in its native country and it may have been adopted as 'Sunflower' also by some Indian writers. Be it as it may but it does not correspond to Suvarcalā and is not a native of India. Therefore it cannot be accepted as Suvarcalā of our Nighaṇṭus.

4 The name *Crozophora plicata* A. Juss. is misleading and wrongfully imagined to be 'Sunflower' (See Watt. Dict.)

Suvarcalā

Suvarcalā proper	Brāhmī proper
1. Suvarcalā (Dhn. Ni. Raj. Ni.)	Suvarcalā (Raj. Ni.)
2. Maṇḍūkī (Dhn.. Ni. Raj. Ni.)	Maṇḍūkī (Raj. Ni.)
3. Suvarcalā (Bh. Pr. Ni.)	Brahmasuvarcalā (Bh. Pr.; Dhn. Ni.
4. Maṇḍūkparṇī (Dhn. Ni.)	(Maṇḍūkaprṇī (Dalh. Su. 31.5) (Indu Aṣṭ. san.31. p.205 U. Page 405)
	(Abhi. Man. Mooss)

5. Aparā Suvarcalā, Brāhmī Maṇḍūkparṇī (Mooss,Abhi.Man.)	
6. Kapotavankā (Indu. Ast. San. 28)	Kapota vegā (Dh. Ni. Raj. Ni.)
7. Saraswatī (Dhn. Ni.)	Saraswatī (Raj. Ni.)
8. Swaryā (Dhn. Ni.)	Swaryā (Raj. Ni.)
9. Suvarcalā, Maṇḍūkparṇī Maṇḍūkī (Shivadas A.Hr.U.1-44)	
10. *Hydrocotyl rotundifolia* Roxb.	*Centella asiatica* (L) Urban Syn. *H. asiatica* Linn. Maṇḍūkparṇī (Chopra)
11. ...	Brāhmī (Suvarcalā Viśeṣaḥ) (Dhn. Ni. Anandāśram)

ब्राह्मी (Brāhmī) (18)

ब्राह्मी सौम्या विनिर्दिष्टा दिव्यतेजा महौषधी ॥ ९६
कपोतवेगा त्वष्टा च सैव ब्रह्मसुवर्चला ॥

ब्राह्मी सौम्या रसे तिक्ता शोफपाण्डुज्वरापहा ॥ ९७
दीपनी कुष्ठकण्डूघ्नी प्लीहवातबलासजित् ॥

ब्राह्मी (Brāhmī), सौम्या (Saumyā), दिव्यतेजा (Divyatejā), महौषधी (Mahauṣadhī), कपोतवेगा (Kopotavegā), त्वष्टा (Tvaṣṭā) and ब्रह्मसुवर्चला (Brahmasuvarcalā) are synonymous.

Brāhmī is bitter in taste, *śītavīrya*, useful in oedema, anaemia and fever. It stimulates digestive capacity, pacifies *vātakaphadoṣas* and used in skin disorders and pruritus.

क्षुद्रपत्रा (रा. नि.) (Kśudrapatrā) (19)
ब्राह्मी तु क्षुद्रपत्राऽन्या लघुब्राह्मी जलोद्भवा ।
ब्राह्मी तिक्तरसोष्णा च सरा वातामशोफजित् ॥ Raj. ni. V.

The other type of *Brāhmī* is called as क्षुद्रपत्रा *Kśudrapatrā* of which synonyms are लघुब्राह्मी (Laghubrāhmī) and जलोद्भवा (Jalodbhavā). It is bitter in taste, *uṣṇavīrya* .It is laxative and useful in *vātadoṣa* and *āmaśopha* (or *āmadoṣa* and oedema)

I a- ***Centella asiatica*** Linn.*
Syn. *Hydrocotyle asiatica* Linn.
b- Dr. Dymock (Pharm. Indi.)
II a- सोमा (Somā), कपोतवेगा (Kapotvegā), ब्रह्मसुवर्चला (Brahma-suvarcalā), मेध्या (Medhyā), भारती (Bhāratī), सरस्वती

* The current valid name is *Centella asiatica* (Linn.) Urban. (Comp. p. 33)

(Saraswatī), स्वर्या (Śwaryā), शारदी (Śāradī), मण्डूकी (Manḍūkī), मत्स्याक्षी (Matsyākśhī)

b- (SK), Brāhmī Manḍūkaparṇī; (Mar. & Bom.) Brāhmī, Karivaṇā; (H.) Brāhmamaṇḍūkī; (B) Tholkhuri; (Tel.) Vellarai, Brami; (Mal.) Kutaran, Kulanal.

III See Suvarcalā.

a- 1) AV IV 37, 57, (Pant. Satavalekar)

2) Yaj. V. XX 57 (Vd. Jangale Part II.)
See क्षुद्रपत्रा. द्वितीया ब्राह्मी (Raj. Ni.)

1) श्वेवेकः कपिरिवैकः कुमारः सर्वकेशकः प्रियोदृशः इव भूत्वा गन्धर्वः सच ते स्त्रियस्तस्मितो नाशयामसि ब्रह्मणा वीर्याऽवता ॥ ' (वीर्यवता ब्रह्मण तं इतः नाशयामसि) वीर्ययुक्त ब्राह्मी नामक औषधीने त्यांचा येथून आम्ही नाश करतो अथ. कां. ४३७ पं. सातवळेकर.

2) तनुपा भिषजा सुतेऽश्विनो भा सरस्वती । मध्या रजाँसीन्द्रियमिन्द्राय पथिभिर्वहान् ।

3) इन्द्रायेन्दु सरस्वती नराश सेननग्नहुम् ।
अधातामश्विना मधुभेषजं भिषजं भिषजातु ते ॥
(अपनी विद्यापारंगत वैद्यने सुप्रजाजननके लिये सरस्वती (ब्राह्मी) शहद के साथ मिश्रण . . . देना चाहिये । इ.)
(यजु. अ. २० मं ५७ भा. २)

4) मण्डूकपर्णी - ब्राह्मी । डल्हण सु. सू. ४६. २६२

5) कपोतवंका - ब्रह्मसुर्वचला । (डल्हण । सु.चि. ३१.५)

6) कपोतवंका - सुवर्चला तस्या मूलेन । (इन्दु अ. स. २८ पृ. २०५)

7) ब्राह्मीस्वरसमादाय (मेधायुष्कामीय सु. चि. 28. 4)

8) ब्राह्मी चांगेरी . . . नागवल्लिका मीनाक्षी मण्डूकपर्णिका ॥
(दिव्यौषधी र. रत्ना. वादी उ. ३ä)
(Note - it is to be noted here that ब्राह्मी, मीनाक्षी & मण्डूकपर्णी are all mentioned in the same stanza D.K. Kamat)

9) मीनाख्यां महाराष्ट्र्यां काकमाच्यां मत्स्याक्षी च प्रचक्षते । (Raj. Ni. Chaturtatha - 5)

10) मण्डूकपर्णी ब्राह्मी च । (का. सं. राजयक्ष्मा)

11) ब्राह्मी मत्स्याक्षक ब्राह्मसुवर्चलैः । ब्रह्मसुर्वचला मण्डूकपर्णी । इन्दु अ.सं. उ. पृ. ४०६

12) ब्राह्मी कपोतवङ्का च सोमवल्ली सरस्वती । मण्डूकपर्णी माण्डूकी त्वाष्ट्री दिव्या महौषधी ॥ . . . .
तद्वत् मण्डूकपर्णिका ॥ २८५ (गुडूच्या. भा. प्र)

13) रवेर्वल्ली - मण्डूकपर्णी - 'मण्डूकपर्णी मण्डूकी वरदादित्यवल्ल्यपि' इति निघण्टः । (शिवदास अ. ह. उ. १. ४४)

b-1) मीनाख्यां महाराष्ट्र्यां काकमाच्यां मत्स्याक्षी च प्रचक्षते ।
(Raj. Ni. Chaturtatha -5)

2) ब्राह्मणेति (Brāhmạṇetī) Bhūsaktā, Manḍūkī. (Dr. Harshe)

14) ब्राह्मी - (Brāhmī) - Saraswatī, Manḍūkī, Manḍūkparnī (Bh. Pr. Gudu, P. 285)

15) ब्रह्मसोमा (Brahmasomā) कपोतवङ्का - ब्रह्मसुवर्चला Kapotvankā Brahmasuvarcalā (Shivadas. A.H. v. 47 III 47 ?)

16) *Centella asiatica* Urban.
(Sans.) Mandūkaparṇī, (Mal.) Kutaran, Kulanal; (Tel.) Vallazi.

17) अपरा सुर्वचलाह्वा ब्रह्मी मण्डूकपर्णी च। वरदा सुखोद्भवाऽख्या मण्डूकी स्यान्मुनि ब्राह्मी ॥ अभि. मं. *Centella asiatica* Urban is also known as Brāhmī in some parts of India. It has caused a confusion in respect of real Brāhmī which in *Moniera cuneifolia* Mich. But centella asiatica is considered as a variety of Brāhmī and has been given the name of another Brāhmī.However *Centella asiatica* is neither Brahmi nor is used as Brahmi in Keral. (Mooss).

18) पूर्व भागात - बिहार ओरिसावासी जिला ब्राह्मी मानतात तिला सं. प्रांत पश्चिमोत्तर प्रदेश निवासी 'जलब्राह्मी , जलनीम' नावाने पुकारतात.

19) The Brāhmī of the Bengali Kavirajas is *Bacopa moniera*. It is the नीरब्राह्मी or बाम of Gujarath. How bengali Kavirajas have taken this to be the Brahmi we have no clue.
We in Gujrath know *Centella asiatica* (L) Urban ... to be the Brāhmī. We are using this in nervous weakness, insanity. Nobody will be able to decide the correctness of these two Brāhmīs. So let us accept for the time being Brāhmī to be the *Bacopa moniera* (L) Pennell and *Centella asiatica* (L) Urban. (Sa. Ayu. 1961)

20) *Hydrocotyle asiatica,* Willd; H. Thulkaura ... ...Creeping in shady places, leaves - long petioled, reniform dentate, umbellets, from the joints two or more together, short peduncled. Three or four flowered, involucre two -four leaved ... (Roxburgh.)

21) *Hydrocotyle rotundifolia*, Roxb. ... ... filiform, Creeping leaves long petioled, round lobated, crenate smooth, Umbellets erect, from eight to two (?) flowered, Involucre from three four or more minute leaflets .. .. (Roxb. flora)
Reasoning.
In some parts of India Jalabrāhmī (*Bacopa Monnieri*) is accepted as Brāhmī, but it does not correspond to the Brāhmī of our Nighanṭus for :

1) Brāhmī of our Nighanṭus is कपोतवेगा (Kapotvegā) i.e. movinglike a Kapot; Bhūsaktā (S. Kosa) i.e. creeping, (Tṛṇavat Tṛṇaka) तृणवत तृणक (S. Kosh) a grass like herb, while जलब्राह्मी (Jalabrāhmī) is procumbent, but then erect, herb of 1/2 to 1 ft.height.

2) The leaves of Brāhmī (ब्राह्मी) are मण्डूकपर्णी (rotundus) long petioled, dentate while those of जलब्राह्मी (Jalabrāhmī) are sessile, long (non-round) and entire.
3) (Jalabrāhmī) is not recorded in Dhn. Ni. The omission of Dhn. Ni. is suggestive. From this omission it can be inferred that Jalabrāhmī was not traditional Brāhmī, and was not reckoned as Brāhmī by the Ayurvedic world prior to Dh. Ni.
4) Raj. Ni. has recorded Nīrabhrāhī under the heading ksudrapatrā but he has recorded 'Brāhmī proper first, and below that (Ksudrapatrā) is recorded by him. Medicinal properties of these two plants which are recorded by Raj. Ni., are quite different from each other. Therefore according to Raj. Ni. Jalābrahmi can not be the Brāhmī proper.
5) The synonyms सरस्वती (Saraswatī), सुरेज्या (Surejyā), भारती (Bhāratī), परमेष्ठिनी (Parameṣṭhini), as a token of diginity are applied to Brhāmī proper by Raj. Ni. But to jalabrāhmī as 'Ksudrapatrā' क्षुद्रपत्रा, Laghubrāhmī लघुब्राह्मी.
On these grounds जलब्राह्मी (Jalabrāhmī) cannot be confirmed with Brāhmī of our Nighaṇṭus.

33 नाकुली (Nākulī) (३४) नाकुल्यौ Nākulyau

नाकुली सर्पगन्धा च सुगन्धा भोगिगन्धिका ॥ ९९
सैव सर्पसुगन्धा च तथा चीरितपत्रका[१] ॥

नाकुली कटुरुष्णा स्यात् तिक्तऽपि परिकीर्तिता ॥ १००
मूषिकस्य विषं हन्ति कृमिदोषविनाशिनी ॥

नाकुली (Nākulī), सर्पगन्धा (Sarpagandhā), सुगन्धा (Sugandhā), भोगिगन्धिका (Bhogigandhikā), सर्पसुगन्धा (Sarpasugandhā) and चीरितपत्रका (Cīritaptrakā) are synonymous.

Nākuli is pungent and bitter in taste, *usṇavīrya*. It is useful in rat-bite (poison) and disorders due to worms.

I Controversial -confirmed.

(Fam. Convolvulaceae)

a- ***Merremia vitifolia*** Hallier. *
Syn. *Ipomoea vitifolia* Sweet

b- Kamat.

---

१ 'चिरिजपत्रिका' 'विरिजपत्रिका' इति आनन्दा पुस्तके पाठः ।

* The current accepted name is *Merremia vitifolia* (Burm.f.) Hallier

II a- सर्पगन्धा (Sarpagandhā), विरजपत्रिका (Virajapatrikā), रक्तपत्रिका (Raktapatrikā), ईश्वरी (Īśwarī), सर्पादनी (Sarpādanī), व्यालगन्धा (Vyālagandhā), भोगिगन्धिका (Bhogigandhika)

b- (SK) Nākuḷī.
(Bom), Nāvaḷ, Nāvaḷī, Mungusvel.

III a- 1) नकुलो वेद भेषजम् । . . . हुवे । 23 (A.V.8-7)

2) C.ci.3.266 (with Rāsnā and Gandhanākulī)
Su. Ka. 8-102 (Balavantji)

3) अगरु, रास्ना, रुहा, रोहा. नाकुली, गन्धनाकुली (C.Ci.3.267)
See note on Rāsnā in 1st Chapter.

b- 1) 466रास्नाभित् - 'नाकुली' सर्पगन्धा च सुवहा भोगिगन्धिका । सर्पाक्षी नकुलेष्टा चे' ति नामगुणमाला 'नाइ' इति लोके ।

2) नाकुली सर्पगन्धा च सुगन्धा भोगिगन्धिका सैव सर्पसुगन्धा च तथा चीरितपत्रिका ॥ 103 Dhn. Ni.
. . . रक्तपत्रिका . . . नागगन्धा । . . . चाप्यहिभुक्स्वरसा तथा । 152
सर्पादनी व्यालगन्धा . . . (Raj. Ni. Dhn. P. 154)
अन्या महासुगन्धा च सुवहा गन्धनाकुली । सर्पाक्षी नकुलेष्टा च छत्राकी ॥
105 Dhn. Ni.
सर्पाक्षी फणिहन्त्री . . . अहिभुक् . . ॥ 153 ॥ Raj. Ni. (Dhn. Ni.Raj. Ni. P. 155)

3) नाकुली सुरसा नाग (रास्ना) सुगन्धा । अमर २.४.११
नकुलानाम् प्रिया नाकुली । नागसुगन्धा सर्पगन्धत्वात् । . . . अर्धेन रास्ना अर्धेन सर्पाक्षीति गौडः । वैद्यास्तु नाकुली गन्धनाकुल्यौ . . . भिन्नौ मन्यन्ते ।
आह च - नाकुली सर्पगन्धा च सुगन्धा भोगिगन्धिका ।
सैव सर्पसुगन्धेति । . . छत्राकी विषमर्दिनी ॥ (Ksīraswamī - Amara)

4) अथ (रास्नाभेद) नाकुली नाम गुणानाह
नाकुली सुरसा नागसुगन्धा गन्धनाकुली ।
नकुलेष्टा भुजंगाक्षी सर्पाक्षी विषनाशिनी ॥ (Chunekar Bh. Pr. Ni. p. 82)

5) According to our understanding Nākuli (नाकुली) is Sarpagandhā and is *Rauwolfia serpentina*. (Ach. Dwivedi ... Sachi Ayur. March 1958)

6) Nākulī -धवलबरुआ, सर्पगन्धा *Rauwolifa serpentina* Benth. Shrub high sometimes 3 feet. Leaf 3-7 inches. Flowers white or some what rosy 2-4 inches long. Properties bitter, hypnotic, tonic, cooling, antipyretic. It is known in Bihar as पागलकी दवाइ and also used in other mental diseases. (Abbreviated from Chunekar Bh. P. 82)

7) नाकुली (Nākulī), नाकुली द्वय (Nākulīdwaya), (reference form texts see II- a above)

There is clear mention of this as two kinds of *Nakulī* known as

Nākulī & Gandhanākulī..... *Nākulī* has been used in the texts under the other names such as *Sarpasugandhā* (etc.) especially in Suśṛut Samhitā. It appears that the two kinds are distinguished from each other by the presence or absence of an aromatic smell in them. It is therefore suggested that 1) *Rauwolfia serpentina* Benth ex Kurz. and 2) *Aristolochia indica* Linn. may respectively be called *Nākulī* and *Gandhanākuli*. (Balawantji P. 219)

V) 1) नाकुली (Nākulī) Nakuli kanda, Mungusvel, Sāpsand (Mar.) *Rauwolfia serpentina* (Vidyotanti Bh. Pr. Ni.)

2) नाकुलीकन्द (Nakulikanda)
(H) Nai, Nakulakand; (Guj.) Nolvel; (Mar.) Sāpsan, Munguswel. *R. serpentina* (Ach. Dwivedi Bh. Pr. Ni.)

3) नाकुली, सुरसा. सुगन्धा, रास्ना. नकुलेष्टा । (Nākulī, Surasā, Sugandhā, Rāsnā, Nakuleṣṭā) *Ophiorrhiza mungos* Linn. (Dymock)

4) नाकुली (Nākulī) (Pant. Hariprapannaji Abhi. Buti. Darpan) *

---

* It seems that D.K. Kamat has to say something further about Nākulī as he has noted on a piece of paper in Marathi as follows : (I have not mentioned the names of the local persons whose names have appeared in this note.)

सर्पगन्धा हे नाकुलीचे समानार्थी परंतु गौण नाम आहे. सर्पगन्धा ही नाकुलीची गंधदर्शक बहुव्रीही समासात्मक नामें आहेत.

अमरकोशांत सर्पगन्धा पद नाही त्याऐवजी नागगंधा पद आहे. क्षीरस्वामी सर्पगन्धा भोगीगंधिकाचा अर्थ सैव सर्पसुगन्धेति असा देतात. यावरुन सर्पगन्धा हे पद गन्धदर्शक आहे.
सर्पगन्धा पद गंधदर्शक व हा गंध नाकुलीत उठून दिसतो. रावलफिया हे क्षुप आहे व तिला सर्पगंध नाही. रावलफियाला 'सर्पगन्धा' नांव कोणी दिले याचा इतिहास शोधून निर्णय घेतला पाहिजे. रावलफिया चीरीत पत्रा नाही चीरीत, विरज, वारिज, असे पाठ भेद आहेत.
(रा.नि.) जांबवती हे क्षुप - नागदमनी वृत्तपुष्पा व मदघ्नी हे गुण रावलफियात आहेत. पाने 'दीर्घगोल. नावळी -Ipomea Vitifolia बहुवर्षायु, मौठी चढणारी, द्राक्षाचे वेली प्रमाणे ५ रवाचांची पानें, फुले पिवळी, मोठी व लांब देंठ, कोंकणांत प्रसिद्ध, कोवळया पानांची भाजी करीत असत. पानांचे पृष्ठभागावर लव असते.

नावळीचे वर्णन वरील प्रमाणेच वै. पदे करतात. अलिबाग. आंग्रेबाग. पोयनाड, . .. रोहा. काले खिंड पहा our collection BSI (Pune Division)

'*Sarpagandhā*' सर्पगन्धा is the secondary similitive term of or synonym of Nākuli नाकुली. *Sarpagandhā* which is a compound term suggesting the smell. In Amarkosa there is no such synonym as *Sarpagandhā* but there is *Nāgagandha*. The meaning of Sarpagandhā as mentioned by Ksiraswāmī is *Bhogiganhikā*. It shows that the term *Sarpagandhā* is suggestive of smell. This smell is predominantly found in *Nākulī*. Rauwolfia is a herb and there is no smell; who has given this name sarpandha to Rauwolfia is to be found out. Rauwolfia is not *Cīrit patrā*. Raj-ni's *Jambavati* is herb - *Nagadamani*, *Vṛtta puṣpā* & *madaghnī* etc. synonyms appear.
Navaḷī नावळी is perennial, big climber having leaves like *Drākṣha* with yellow flowers, with long petiole, very frequent in Konkan area. It is a pot herb. vd. Pade also describes it. It is found in Alibag, Angrebag, Poyanad, Roha, Kale Khind. See our collection BSI (Pune division).

(Free tranlsation) S.D. Kamat

34 महासुगन्धा (Mahāsugandhā) गन्धनाकुली (Gandhanākulī)

अन्या महासुगन्धा च सुवहा गन्धनाकुली ॥ १०१
*सर्पाक्षी नकुलेष्टा च च्छत्राकी विषमर्दिनी ॥

सर्पाक्षी कटुका तिक्ता तथा च कृमिरोगजित् ॥ १०२
वृश्चिकोद्भवसर्पादिविषघ्नी व्रणरोपणी ॥

There is an another type of *Nākulī* called as महासुगन्धा (Mahāsugandhā) of which synonyms are सुवहा (Suvahā) गन्धनाकुली (Gandhanākulī), सर्पाक्षी (Sarpākṣī), नकुलेष्टा (Nakuleṣṭā), च्छत्राकी (Cchatrākī) and विषमर्दिनी (Viṣamardinī).

Sarpākṣī is bitter and pungent in taste, it is useful in worms, poisoning due to scorpion and serpent bite etc. and it helps in healing of ulcers.

I (Fam. Rubiaceae)

a- ***Ophiorrhiza mungos*** Linn.
b- Dymock (Pharm Indi.)

II a- सुवहा (Suvahā) गन्धनाकुली (Gandhanākulī), सर्पाक्षी (Sarpākṣī), छत्राकी (Chatrākī), नकुलेष्टा (Nakuleṣṭā), विषमर्दिनी (Viṣamardinī)
b- (SK. Tel.) Sarpakṣī; (H) Sarahaṭṭi; (B) Gandhanākulī; (Mal.) Avilapuri; (Tam.) Kiri, Kiripurandana.

III 1 सर्पाक्षी (Sarpākṣī) - Gandhanākulī (Ast. Sang. Su. 45)

35 (३५) वृद्धदारुकः ** (Vrddhadārukaḥ)

वृद्धदारुक आवेगी जुङ्गको दीर्घवालुकः[१] ॥ १०३
[२]वृद्धः कोटरपुष्पी स्यादजान्त्री[३] छगलान्त्र्यपि[४] ॥

वृद्धदारुः कटुस्तिक्तस्तथोष्णः कफवातजित् ॥ १०४
श्वयथुकृमिमेहास्रवातोदरहरः परः ॥

---

* शोढलेन नाकुल्यानंतरं सर्पाक्षी निर्दिष्टा -
'सर्पाक्षी नकुलेष्टा च छत्रका विषमर्दिनी ।
महावीर्या सुगन्धा च जयन्ती चापराजिता ॥' Sodhal P. 58.
This attracts our attention by the synonyms जयन्ती Jayantī & अपराजिता Aparājitā towards the the Extra chapter plant बलामोटा . S.D. Kamat.

** the pages of comments on this drug by Late Vd. D.K. Kamat are missing from the files, however for the completion of the work I have commented the same. S.D.K.

१ 'दीर्घवालकः' २ 'अन्तः कोटरपुष्पी' इति नि. शे. टीका संमतौ ।
३ 'अजाण्डी' इति नि.शे. टीका संमतः पाठः ।
४ 'छगलाण्ड्यपि' इति नि.शे. टीका संमतः पाठः ।
१ 'जीर्ण वालुकः' इति आनन्दा, पुस्तके पाठभेदः ।

वृद्धदारुक (Vṛddhadāruka), आवेगी (Āvegī), जुङ्गकः (Jungakaḥ),दीर्घवालुकः (Dīrghavālukaḥ), वृद्धः (Vṛddhaḥ), कोटरपुष्पी (Koṭarapuṣpī), अजान्त्री (Ajāntrī) and छगलान्त्री (Chagalāntrī) are synonyms.

Vṛddhadāru is pungent and bitter in taste, *uṣṇavīrya,* pacifies, *kaphavātadoṣas.* It is useful in anasarca, worms, diseases characterized by polyuria, pacifies *rakta doṣa* and abdominal swelling due to *vātadoṣa* (ascites).

वृद्धदारकः (रा.नि.)
जीर्णदारुर्द्वितीया स्यात् जीर्णाफञ्जी सुपुष्पिका ।
अजरा सूक्ष्मपत्रा च विज्ञेया च षडाह्वया ॥

वृद्धादारुद्वयं गौल्यं पिच्छिलं कफवातजित् ।
बल्यं कासामदोषघ्नं द्वितीयं स्वल्पवीर्यदम् ॥ Raj. ni. Chapt. III

The second type of *Vṛddhadāraka* is called by the (Six) synonyms, जीर्णदारुर्द्वितीया (Jirṇadārurdwitiyā) जीर्णा (Jīrṇā), फञ्जी (Phañji), सुपुष्पिका (Supuṣpikā), अजरा (Ajarā) and सूक्ष्मपत्रा (Sūksmapatrā).

Both the *Vṛddhadārukas* are sweet in taste, pacify *kapha vāta doṣas, are* slimy and strength promoting .These are useful in cough.and *āmadoṣa* The second variety is little lesser in quality.

According to Dhn. ni. it seems that only one plant is mentioned, however Raj. Ni. has mentioned the second variety जीर्ण दारुर्द्वितीयः (Jīrṇadārurdwitīyaḥ) and has mentioned the properties of both the varieties.

A- वृद्धदारुः (Vṛddhadāruḥ)
B- वृद्धदारुर्द्वितीय : (Vṛddhadāruḥ dwitīyaḥ)
Both belonging to the same family.

Fam. Convolvulaceae.

Controversial

I- A-a- ***Argyreia nervosa*** (Burm f.) Boj.
Syn. *A. speciosa* Sweet.
Eng. Elephant Creeper (U.P.I. Page. 51)
Syn. *Lettsomia nervosa* Roxb. (Chopra Gloss. p. 24)

b- Roxb. Fl. Ind. Ed. CBC 164.

c- Throughout India (except in dry western regions) up to elevation of 100ft. (Chopra Gloss.) p. 24.

B-a- ***Ipomoea biloba*** Forsk.
Syn. *I. pes caprae* Sw.

b- Roxb. Fl. Br. In. V. II P. 212

c- Throughout India, abundant near sea (Chopra Gloss. p. 142) A & B

II -a वृद्धदारुकः Vṛddhadārukah आवेगी Āvegī दीर्घवालुकः Dīrghavālukaḥ, अजान्त्री Ajāṇtrī Dhn Ni. जीर्णा (Jīrṇā), फञ्जी (Pañjī), अजरा Ajarā, सूक्ष्मपत्रा Sūkšmapatrā.

A-b- Sans.Vṛddhadāru (H.) Samudrašosh, Vidhārā (Mar.) Samudrašoka; (Guj.) Samundar shosha, Vardharo, (Ben.) Bidhatak; (Tel.) Samudrapal; (Tam.) Samudrapacchai.

B- (Sans.)Vṛddhadāru Maryādavalli; (H.) Dopātilatā, Vidhara; (Ben.) Chāgalkhuri; (Mar.) Maryādvela; (Guj.) Marjadvela; (Kan. Tam.) Adumbu.

III - 1) The name Vṛddhadāraka does not appear in Caraka, Susruta & AH.In *Śyāmādi gaṇa* श्यामादि गण of Suśruta, महाश्यामा *Mahāśyāmā* and छगलान्त्री *Chagalāntrī* are mentioned. These are respectively commented as वृद्धदारक Vṛddhadāraka and वृद्धदारकभेदः Vṛdhadārakabhedaḥ.In South India *I. biloba* Forsk is accepted as vidhārā. In Kanpur, and Allahabad and in the forests of Chitrakuta what is obtained as विधारा Vidharā is *Ipomoea petaloidea*, Chois. (Abbreviated from Ni. Ada. Bapalalji P.II p. 92.93).

2) 296 वृद्धदारको - वल्लरी ।
'त्रिकोणकाण्डा सुबहुप्रताना फलेषु पीता कुसुमेषु रक्ता ।
दलैः सुदुग्धैर्मृदुरोमवद्भिः ताम्बूलतुल्यैर्घनमूलकन्दैः । इत्यष्टांगसंग्रहः । (Harshe - Shivakosa P. 123).

36 रक्तपादी (Rāktapādī) (३६) रक्तपाद्यौ (Raktapādyau)

रक्तपादी शमीपत्रा समङ्गाञ्जलिकारिका ॥ १०५
नमस्कारी गन्धकारी स्पर्शसंकोचपर्णिका ॥

रक्तपादी कटुः शीता पित्तातीसारनाशिनी ॥ १०६
शोफदाहश्रमश्वासव्रणकुष्ठकफास्रनुत् ॥

रक्तपादी (Raktapādī), शमीपत्रा (Śamīpatrā), समङ्गा (Samaṅgā) अञ्जलिकारिका (Añjalikārikā), नमस्कारी (Namaskārī), गन्धकारी (Gandhakārī), and स्पर्शसंकोचपर्णिका (Sparṣa sankocaparṇikā) are synonymous.

Raktapādī is pungent in taste, *śītavīrya*, pacifies *kapha* and *rakta doṣas*. It is useful in diarrhoea due to *pitta doṣa*, oedema, burning sensation, fatigue, dyspnoea, wounds and disorders of skin.

वैपरित्या लज्जालुः (रा.नि.)
लज्जालुर्वैपरीत्याऽन्या अल्पक्षुपबृहद्दला ।
वैपरित्यादिलज्जालुर्ह्यभिधाने प्रयोजयेत् ॥

There is an other kind of *Lajjālu* called as वैपरीत्या (Vaiparītyā), It is a smaller herb with bigger leaves. It is called by the synonyms of *Lajjālu* by addition of the term *vaiparītyā.*

I (Generic name -Dhn. Ni. has recorded one plant, and the same by Raj. Ni. which is A. रक्तपादी (Raktapādī) but Raj. Ni. has added one more plant It is B- लज्जालुर्वैपरीत्या (Lajjālurvaiparityā).

Fam. Geraniaceae. Oxalidaceae

A.a- ***Biophytum sensitivam*** (Linn.) DC.
b- Dymock (Pharm. Indi.)

B a- ***Mimosa pudica*** Linn. Fam. Leguminosae. Mimosaceae.*
b- Dymock (Pharm. Indi.)

II A-a- रक्तपादी (Raktapādī), समङ्गा (Samangā), नमस्कारी (Namaskārī), शमीपत्रा (Samīpatrā), रक्तमूला (Raktamūlā). सप्तपर्णी (Saptaparṇī), गण्डमालिका (Gaṇḍamālikā)
b- (SK) Samangā; (B) Vananarānga, Zalai (Datta-Botany); (H) Lajalu; (Konkan), chatrī; (Guj.) Zarer; (Tam.) Toḍḍamaṇi, Thinḍanazhī; (Mal) Tinṭanazki, Mukkuṭṭi; (Eng.) Sensative wood sorrel.

B a- लज्जालुर्वैपरीत्या (Lajjālurvaiparityā), बृहद्दला (Bṛhaddalā), अल्पक्षुप (Alpakśupa).
b- (SK) Varāhakrāntā, Lajjalu; (Guj.) Rīsāmaṇi; (Mar.) Lājari, Lājaḷū; (B) Lājak; (H) Lajāḷu; (Tel.) Peḍḍnidra Kanṭi; (Tam.) Totalwadi; (Mal.) Totalvadi; (Kan) Mudu gudu vare; (Eng.) The Sensitive plant.

III a-1) C.Su. 4-9.
2) S.Su. 37-24.
3) A.H. Su. 15-37, 38.
4) A.H. U. 34-45.

b-1) 349 समङ्गा (Samangā) - Lohita puṣpikā raktakesarā Jāti Karikā, Raktamūl Raktapādī (Abhi. Manj.)
2) 350 नमस्कारी (Namaskārī) अञ्जलिकारि (Añjalikārī), काञ्चनपुष्पी (Kāñcanapuṣpī); (Abhi Manj.)

(Note : The compiler of Abhi. Manjari has altered flowers. His रक्तपादी

---

* There seems some confusion while giving the botanical names to plants A & B. It should have been mentioned reversely. S. D. Kamat.

(Raktapādi) is काञ्चनपुष्पी (Kāncanapuṣpī) while नमस्कारी (Namaskāri = *M. pudica*) is Lohit puṣpikā -raktakesarā)

3) लज्जालुः Lajjāluḥ

a- नमस्कारी Namaskārī Śamīpatrī

b- Samṇgā- Raktapādikā (Madan. Ni. Varga I)

4) Namaskārī Su. 15
See समङ्गा (Samangā) Ast. Hr. Kosa.

5) समङ्गा (Samangā) Su. 15
Sparsarodanikā (Guj.) Risāmaṇi. Lajjāmaṇī; (Kan.) Nacccikegida, Mundalamurikke; (Tam.) Lottar Curunki, Toṭṭal vaṭi, Ttinṭarmaṇi; (Tel.) Munuguḍamaramu; (Eng.) Mimosa pudica (Asta. H. Kosa)

6) लज्जालु, समङ्गा (Lajjālu, Samangā), Raktapādī. *Mimosa pudica* (Vidyotani)

7) अलम्बुषा (Alambuṣā)
Neptunea oleracea acquatic Lajjālu (Vidyotanī)

8) *Mimosa pudica - M. sensitiva* - Lajjālu (Ach. Dwivedi)

9) अलम्बुषा (Ci. 8)
A kind of Lajjālu; (Tam.) Varāḷccunti, Toṭṭarcuṇāki; (Mal.) Mukkutti, Tiṇtanaḷi. A sort of sensitive plant (Bh. Pr. Ni.) - Aṣt.Hr. Koṣa

10) समङ्गा (Samangā) Varahakrānta (Cakra, Ca. su. 4-9)

11) समङ्गा (Samangā) (Lajjālu it loke, Varahakrāntām apare (Dalhaṇa Su. Su 37-24 Sū. Ci. 8-44)

12) समङ्गा - नमस्कारी (Samangā Namaskārī) Namaskārī Raktamūlākhyā, Namaskārī Samangā (Arun) (Samangā - Lajjikā, Namaskārī Lajjikā (Hemadri) (Ast. Hr. Su- 15.37.38)

13) अथ लज्जालुः
लज्जालुः स्याच्छमीपत्रा समङ्गाऽञ्जलिकारिका ।
रक्तपादी नमस्कारी नाम्ना खदिरकेत्यपि ॥
अथ अलम्बुषा
अलम्बुषा खरत्वक् च तथा मेदोगला स्मृता ॥
(Chunekar Bh. Pr.P . 456)

IV 1) समङ्गा (Samangā) - Rakta maṇḍalikā iti Candraḥ.

2) समङ्गा (Samangā)
Mimosa pudica Dr. Ghanekar Su. Su. 38-44

3) रक्तपादी (Raktapādī) Small lajjālu. वैपरित्या लज्जालु (Vaiparityā Lajjālu) Large Lajjalu (Ni. Shiro. Pade)

4) *Biophytum sensitium*
(Eng.) Sensitive wood sorrel

(B) Bun naranga; (M) Mukkutti, Thindanzhi.
(Prof. Datta Botany, Ach. Priyavratji)

5) रीसामणि (Risāmaṇi); (SK.) Lajjālu, Namaskārī ; *Mimosa pudica...* Reasoning : This plant is not included in Caraka & Suśṛuta., It is included in Vāgbhata as Namaskārī ... Kannayalal informs that this plant is the native of Brazil America. (Ni. Adarsha)

6) See N.S. Mooss.
Biophytum sensitivum (L) DC.-A descriptive article on Samaṅgā & 'Namaskārī referring Abhi Manj. and some other books.

7) समङ्गा Samaṅgā
It appears to be *Mimosa pudica* Linn. known as *Lajjalu* ... ... An other little plant *Biophytum sensitium* (Linn.) DC.or the waterplant *Neptunea oleracea* Lour. may be given similar names but *samaṅgā* is none else than *Mimosa.* (Balvantji p. 422, 23).

37 विश्वग्रन्थिः Viśvagranthiḥ

रक्तपाद्यपरा प्रोक्ता विश्वग्रन्थिस्त्रिपाद्यपि ॥ १०६
हंसपादी हंसपदी घृतमण्डलिका च सा ॥

रक्तप्रसादनी शीता दाहवीसर्पनाशिनी ॥ १०७
व्रणप्ररोपणी हंसपदिका हंसपादिका ॥

The another kind of रक्तपादी (Raktapādī) is called as विश्वग्रन्थिः (Viśvagranthiḥ) of which synonyms are त्रिपादी (Tripādī), हंसपादी (Hamsapādī), हंसपदी (Hamsapadī), and घृतमण्डलिका (Ghṛtamaṇḍalikā),

Haimsapādikā is *śitavirya* purifies blood, is useful in burning sensation, erysipelas and healing of wounds.

I Generic name - Dh. Ni. has recorded only one but Raj. Ni. may have recorded more than one, of which is identified and confirmed with Nighaṇṭus is recorded here below.
It is a kind of fern plant.

(Fam. Polypodiaceae) Adiantaceae.

a) ***Adiantum lunulatum*** Burm.* & Species.

---

१ 'विषग्रन्थिः' इति चौखम्बा पाठः ।
२ 'वर्ण प्रारोपणी इति आनन्दाश्रममुद्रित पुस्तके पाठः ।
* The current - valid name is *A. philippense* Linn. (Comp. p. 4)

b) Dymock Vol. III 624.
हंसपादी (Hamsapādī), घृतमण्डलिका (Ghṛtamaṇḍalikā), सञ्चारिणी (Sañcāriṇī), कीलपादिका (Kīlapādikā), गोधापदी (Godhāpadī), धार्तराष्ट्रपदी (Dhārtaraṣṭrapadī).

b) (SK) Hansavatī; (H) Kalizānti; (B) Goyāliata; (Bom) Hansrāj; (Poona) Hansrāj; (Ratnagiri) Kāwalyāce pāya; (Eng.) (A sort of Maiden Hair)

III See Raktapādī

a) हंसपादी (Hamsapādī) Su. su. 38. (Vidāriganạ) (Ast. Hr. Su.15.9) कैडर्य – हंसपादी Ca. Kaṇṭhyādi'gana.

b- 1) हंसपादी (Hamsapādī) - Ci.5 -हंसपादाकार पत्रलता त्रिपादी । (Ref. ḌalhanVidārīgana). Gowāliyā ityakhyāta iti Bhāskaraḥ; (B) Govaliyālata; (Mar.) Hansapadi; (Kan) Naviladi; (Tel.) Hansapadamu; (Mal.) Nilamparaṇṭyā, Panappuḷḷati, Cerupuḷḷati, Motirakkaṇṇippaca; *Adiantum lunulatum*. (Ast. Hr. Kosa)

2) 158 धृतराष्ट्रपदी (Dhṛtarāṣṭrapadī) Sakalā Madhusrava, Tripadika Hansapadi iti. *Vitis pedeta* Nilambaranda (Nilappullandi) (Ceruppulladi) (Shri Krishnan Abhi. Manj)

3) 231 - हंसपदी – मधुस्रवा । हंसपदाकार पत्रा पीतपुष्पा (?) जलमुक्त देशजाता 'हसवा' इति लोके' इति डल्हणः । त्रिपादिका कीटमारी परपर्याया' इति चन्द्रनन्दनः । 'मुलीस' इति लोके । (Dr. Harshe)

IV 1) *Adianutum venustum* Don
Himalaya, Afaganistan, Persia etc. Hansrāj, Mubaraka (Bajar name)
Under the name of (adiondron) a fern is described by Diascoriodes as having leaves serrated at the top like coriander ... This plant was doubtless *Adiantum capillus veneris* .... The western Arabs, however, appear to use. *A. capillus veneris* ..as they call the plant. Kuzburat -el-bir or 'Coriander of the well' ... other arabic names for the genus Adiantum are 'Fairies hair' Hair of the mountain', 'Hairs of omen', 'Black stem' etc. (Dymock III 624).

2) *Adiantum capillus veneris* Linn : हिं. हंसराज Hansarāj
Used as demulcent, expectorant, diuretic, tonic, and febrifuge. common in S. India, in Bombay and Madras state upto 5000 ft. and on the mountain N. India. -Chopra

3) A. *venustum* G. Don
हिं हंसराज, सं. हंसपदी, तमील – मयूरशिखा.
Fronds tonic, resolvent, expectorant, diuretic, astringent. N. Himalayas 3000 to 5000 ft., very common in Simla. Chopra.

4) *A. lunulatum* Linn.
Used in fever, erysipelas; throughout N. India, S. India very gen-

eral on Western side in the plains and lower slopes of Hills. (Chopra)

5) See रक्तपादी IV Balwantji
III -3 Ast. Hr. Kosa

6) हंसपादी (Hansapādī) हंसपंदाकारपत्रा पीतपुष्पा जलमुक्तदेशजाता 'हसपाई इति लोके प्रसिद्धा । (Dalhaṇa)
In Bengal the plant which is known there as 'Goyalilata' is accepted as 'Hansapādī' (Adiantum lunulatum). But is different from Ḍalhaṇa's plant. (Dr. Ghanekar Su. Su. 38.4)

7) त्रिपादी(Tripādī) - Hansapadī Kītamāri kākhyā)
(Arun Ast. Hr. Su. 15.9)

38 (३८) शङ्खपुष्पी Śankhapuṣpī

शङ्खपुष्पी कम्बुपुष्पी शङ्खाह्वा कम्बुमालिनी ॥ १०९
तिलकी शङ्खकुसुमा मेध्या वनविलासिनी ॥
शंखिनी कटुतिक्तोष्णा कासपित्तबलासजित् ॥ ११०
विषापस्मारभूतादीन् हन्ति मेध्या रसायनी ॥

शंङ्खपुष्पी (Śankhapuṣpī), कम्बुपुष्पी (Kambupuṣpī), शङ्खाह्वा (Śankhāhvā), कम्बुमालिनी (Kambumālinī), तिलकी (Tilakī), शङ्खकुसुमा (Śankhakusumā), मेध्या (Medhyā) and वनविलासिनी (Vanavilāsinī) are synonymous.

Śankhinī is pungent and bitter in taste and pacifies *pitta kapha-doṣas.* It is useful in cough, poisoning, epilepsy, and as *bhūtaghna* (microorganisms or evil spiritis causing psycological disorders). It is intellect promoting and *rasāyana.*

I a-1 ***Canscora decussata*** R. & Seb.*
Syn. *Pladera decussata* Roxb.
b Majority of modern writers.
c See IV. 4
a कम्बुपुष्पी (Kambūpuṣpī), शङ्खाह्वा (Śañkhāhvā), शङ्खकुसुमा (Śankhakusumā), सितपुष्पी (Sitapuṣpī), मेध्या (Medhyā), भूलग्ना (Bhūlagnā.)

---

* The current accepted name is -
C. decussata (Roxb.) J.A. Schult. & J.H.Schult. (Comp. p. 28)

b (SK) Śaṅkhapuṣpī; (H) Śaṅkhaphuli; (B) Dānkunī (Kaccha), Śaṅkhapuṣpī; (Mar.) Sānkhavel; (Guj.) Śankhāvalī; (Maly.) Śaṅkhamūlī, Saṅkhāmalarī; *Canscora decussata*,. Adrikarṇī, Keralesceke. (Ast. Hr. Kosa).

III See Viṣnukrāntā

a- 1 प्रतीची सोममसि प्रतिच्युः सूर्यम् ।
Anayā prākṛtā (Ṛca) Saṅkhapuṣpakhyā osadhiḥ stūyate (Sayan AV VII 39)
C.S. S.S. A.H. See below.

a-A2 *Canscroa diffusa* R. Br.
Syn. *Pladera virgata* Roxb.
common throughout India (Watt Dict. II 128) See IV 3 below
2 ब्राह्मी . . . शङ्खिनी (Brāhmī Śaṅkhinī) unmādāpahārakā ...
Medhyā viśeṣeṇatu Saṅkhapuṣpī (Cakra Ca. Ci-1)
See IV -6 Balawantji below.

3 शङ्खपुष्पी (Śaṅkhapuspī)
C.3 Śankhākarā Kusumam Bhūlagnā K'sudralatā Viśeṣaḥ
(Asta Hr. Kosa)

b- शङ्खपुष्पी .. शङ्खपुष्पी सरा मेध्या वृष्या मानसरोगहृत् । रसायनी कषायोष्णा स्मृतिकान्ति बलाग्निदा । दोषापस्मारभूताश्रीकुष्ठकृमिविषप्रणुत् ॥ २७०
(Chunekar, Bh. Ni. p. 454)

2 - 345 मेध्या शङ्खपुष्पी (Medhyā Śankhapuṣpī) Harshe.

IV 1 शङ्खपुष्पी (Śaṅkhapuṣpī): *Pladera decussata* Roxb.(Śuklapuṣpī); *P. sessiliflora,* Roxb. (Raktapuṣpī); *P. virgata*, Roxb. (Śaṅkhapuṣpī).

2 शङ्खपुष्पी (Śaṅkhapuṣpī) *Canscora decussata* (Vidyotani Bh. Pr.)

3. *C. decussata* R. & Seb.
Syn. *P. decussata* Roxb.
(SK) Śaṅkhapuṣpī, daṇḍotpala .. Nervine tonic, used in insanity and nervous debility.
C. diffusa R. Br. Syn. *P. virgata* Roxb. used as substitue for *C. decussata.* (Watt. dict II. 128)

4 159 शङ्खपुष्पी (Śaṅkhapuṣpī)
Convolvulus pluricaulis Choisy
Prostrate.
161 दानकुनी (शङ्खपुष्पी) (B.) Dānkunī; (Mar.) Yavocī.
Canscora decussata Schult.
160 विष्णुक्रान्ता (नीलशङ्खपुष्पी)
Mar. Sankhavel; H. Śankhāhulī. *Evoluvlus alsinoides* Linn.

(Chunekar Bh. Pr. Ni. 454)

5 *Pladera decussata* Roxb.
Flowers white
P. virgata Roxb.
Flowers - rose coloured, corolla - rose coloured.
P. sessiliflora Roxb.
Flowers pale red. Corolla funel shaped (Fl. Indi. P. 139)

6 शङ्खपुष्पी (Śaṅkhapuṣpī) *Canscora decussata* (Desai)

7 शङ्खावली शङ्खपुष्पी (Śaṅkhāvalī, Śaṅkhapuṣpī)
Convolvulus microphylla (Ni. adarsha)
This plant is included in genera विष्णुक्रान्ता (Dhn. Ni.) by the name (Sarpākṣī).

8 *Pladera decussata* Roxb.
B. Dānkunī - Annual erect, four winged branches cross armed. This species resembles *P. virgata*, but is a little more robust and seldom so high. It is a native of same places. Flowering time the same.
Stem 1 ft. high erectly erect, four sided angles, vary shape ..... smooth, ramous, branches always opposite, cross armed in other respects like the stem. Leaves spreading, sessile, lanceolate, sharp pointed, entire, smooth, three nerved, size various, flowers teminal and axillary, peduncled, the terminal flowers three lobed, the axillary single, larger than those of the last species and white. Peduncles four sided like the stem and branches, calyx large four tooth - four sided - four winged.
Coral stamens etc. exactly as in the last species (See IV -5)
(Abbreviated Roxb. C.B.C. p. 135)

9 *Pladera virgata*
Syn. *Gentiana diffusa* Vahl
Stems about a foot or sometimes two feet high erect, four sided, ramous, smooth branches opposite, above alternate.
Leaves - opposite, sessile the lower lanceolate the upper broader,all are pointed and three nerved, entire, smooth shape various.
Flowers-numerous, terminal, peduncled, small rose coloured ++ corolla funnel shaped in the groove is lodged the fourth or large stamen. *Filaments* four inserted into the mouth of the tube, the most longer... and bearing an orange coloured and longer anther, anther, which when shedding its pollen, is bent over the fissures on the stigma, anthers of the other three filaments equal, pale, yellow, style single... Stigma two cleft, segments recurved,

capsule one celled, many seeded. (Roxb. C.B. C. p. 134)

10) शङ्खपुष्पी Śaṅkhapuṣpī
Convolvulus pluricaulis choisy.
Śaṅkhāhulī शंखाहुली and Kauḍenā (H) C.Ci. : 1.1, 46 -56 etc. S.Su. 42. 18 (Va) Sa. 10-6 Ci. 30-24 etc. A.H. Ci- . 127 U. 1. 9 -43 etc.
This drug a well known nervine tonic, is also subject of controversy. *Clitoria ternatea* Linn. has been accepted as *Śaṅkhapuṣpī* by most of the south indian vaidyas, while this is believed to be *Canscora decussata* Schult. by majority of Bengali Kavirajas. These two plants should be treated as शंखिनी and यवतिक्ता may serve as nervine tonics. (Balwantji p. 385).

विष्णुक्रान्ता Viṣṇukrāntā (20)

विष्णुक्रान्ता नीलपुष्पी सतीनच्छदिका तथा ॥ १११
शुक्लपुष्पा भूमिलग्ना ह्रस्वा सा शङ्खपुष्पिका ॥

सूक्ष्मपत्रान्तरा ज्ञेया सर्पाक्षी रक्तपुष्पिका ॥ ११२
विष्णुक्रान्ता कटुस्तिक्ता कफवातामयापहा ॥

विष्णुक्रान्ता (Viṣṇukrāntā), नीलपुष्पी (Nīlapuṣpī), सतीनच्छदिका (Satinacchadikā) are synonymous. शुक्लपुष्पा (Śuklapuṣpā), भूमिलग्ना (Bhūmilagnā), ह्रस्वा शंखपुष्पिका (Rhasvāśankhapuṣpikā), are synonymous and सूक्ष्मपत्रा (Sūkṣmapatrā), सर्पाक्षी (Sarpākṣī), रक्तपुष्पिका (Raktapuṣpikā), are synonymous.

Viṣṇukrāntā is pungent and bitter in taste and pacifies *kapha vāta doṣas.*

I Under this heading the compilers have included three species which are 'A' विष्णुक्रान्ता नीलपुष्पी (Viṣṇukrāntā Nīlapuṣpī), 'B' शङ्खपुष्पा शुक्लपुष्पा (Śankhapuṣpa Śuklapuṣpa), and third 'C' सर्पाक्षी रक्तपुष्पिका (Sarpākṣī Raktapuṣpikā).

(Fam. Convolvulaceae)

I A-a- ***Evolvulus alsinoides*** Linn.*
Syn. *E. hirsutus* Lam. et Willd.

---

* The curent accepted (Valid) name is -
E. alsinoides (Linn.) Linn. (comp.p.63)

b - See Watt Dict. IV-9 and Roxb. IV -1 under

B-a- ***Convolvulus microphyllus*** *

b- Bapalaji (Ni. Adarsh)

c- as I a -A above

C-a- ***Convolvulus pluricaulis*** Choisy.**

b Balawantji see IV-11 under

c- As I-a - A above.

II- A-a- विष्णुक्रान्ता (Viṣṇukrāntā), नीलपुष्पी (Nīlapuṣpī), सतीना(Satīnā), अपराजिता (Aparājitā), नीलक्रान्ता (Nīlakrāntā), छर्दिका (Chardikā)

b (SK) Viṣṇukrāntā; (H) Kawalī; (Guj.) Śankhāvalī; (Mar.) Sankhāvalī, Sāṅkhavela (Tam.) Viṣṇukānti, Viṣṇukarāndi; (Tel.) Viṣhṇukrantamu, Viṣhṇukaranta; (Kan.) Viṣṇukānti; (Mal.) Vitsnaklandi.

B-a- शुक्लपुष्पा (Śuklapuṣpā), भूमिलग्ना (Bhūmilgnā), (ह्रस्वा) (Rhasvā), शंखपुष्पिका (Śaṅkhapuṣpikā) (Mara.) Sānkhvela, Śaṅkhāhulī.

C-a सर्पाक्षी (Sarpākśī), सूक्ष्मपत्रा (Sūkśmapatrā), रक्तपुष्पिका (Raktapuṣpikā)

III See Śaṅkhapuṣpī

a- 1) A.Hr. Su. 6.72

b 1) आस्फोता गिरिकर्णिस्यात् विष्णुक्रान्ताऽपराजिता । चत्वारि विष्णुक्रान्तायाः । (Bhanuji, Amar 2.4 - 114)

2) विष्णुक्रान्तेति । (Viṣṇukrānteti) नीलपुष्पी शङ्खिनी भेदः (Nīlapuṣpī Śaṅkhinibhedaḥ) (Dr. Harshe)

3) सतीना (Satīnā), viṣṇukrāntā (Arun; A. Hr. Su. 6.72).

IV सर्पाक्षी (Sarpākśī) - Lohita puṣpā Śaṅkhapuṣpībhedaḥ (Ḍalhaṇa Kalp. 8) Śaṅkhāvali of Bengalis is different (*Canscora decussata*) This is not Śankhāvalī (N. Adarsha U.P. 679).

2) a- शङ्खावली, शङ्खपुष्पी (Śaṅkhāvalī, Śaṅkhapuṣpī) *Convolvulus microphyllus.*

b) नीलपुष्पी विष्णुक्रान्ता (Nīlapuṣpī Viṣṇukrāntā) *Evolvulus alsinoides.* (N. Adarsha).

3) शङ्खपुष्पी (Śaṅkhapuṣpī) *Evolvulus erecta.*

---

* The curent accepted name - *C. microphyllus* Sieb.ex Spreng. (Comp. p. 42)

** *C. microphyllus* Sieb. ex Spreng. (Comp. 42)

Śaṅkhāhulī, flowers small, colour bright white.
(Br. Ni. Pade p. 172)

4) विष्णुक्रान्ता (Viṣṇukrāntā) (Br. Ni. Pade p. 171).

5) विष्णुक्रान्ता कटुस्तिक्ता कफवातामयापहा । Dhn. Ni. 4 (20)

Note : Bh. Pr. Ni. records Vişhṇukrāntā as nervine tonic but Dhn. Ni. does not record it. (See IV 4 above)

6) विष्णुक्रान्ता (Viṣṇukrāntā) described under *Clitoria ternatea* Linn. (Shri. Mooss)

7) विष्णुक्रान्ता (Viṣṇukrāntā)
Evolvulus alsinoides Linn.
E. hirsutus, Lam.

8) शङ्खपुष्पी (Śaṅkhapuṣpī)
Convolvulus pluricaulis Choisy
(Chopra Handa - Priyavrata)

9) शङ्खपुष्पी (159-Śaṅkhapuṣpī)
Convolvulus pluricaulis Chois.
160 विष्णुक्रान्ता (Nīlaśaṅkhāpuṣpī)
Evolvulus alsinoides Linn. (Chunekar Bh. Pr. Ni. P. 454 & 342)
Evolvulus alsinoides Linn.
E. hirsutus Lam.
E. angustifolius Roxb. (C.B.C. p. 276)
Medicine : Mohameden physicians believe that this plant has the power of strengthening the memory and brain. The other kind blue coloured flowered form is called 'Viṣṇugrandhic; the other kind has white flower and is called Śivagrandic.
Habitat : A prostrate perennial herb with wiry stems and blue or white flowers, found nearly all over India on dryish ground. (Watt Dict. III 305-306).

10) *Evolvulus alsinoides* Linn.
may be treated as *Viṣṇukrāntā* which is usually believed to be a variety of Śaṅkhapuṣpī *Convolvulus pluricaulis* Choisy. Saṅkhapuṣpī (Balawantji pp. 395 & 305).

11) *Convovulus hirsutus* Willd.
Viṣṇukandi Rheed Mal.
Is a native of the various parts of India root... perennial, ..long soft white hairs when young. Stems scarcely any, corolla .. deep bright blue (Roxb. C.B.C. p. 276).

12) See para no. 38 Śaṅkhapuṣpī IV-10 Balawantji.

39 (३८) तण्डुलीयकः Taṇḍulīyakaḥ

तण्डुलीयस्तु उद्दिष्टस्तण्डुलस्तण्डुलीयकः ॥ ११३
भण्डीरस्तण्डुलीबीजो मेघनादो घनस्वनः ॥

तण्डुलीयो विषघ्नश्च रूक्षः शीततरः शुचिः ॥ ११४
मधुरो रसपाकाभ्यां रक्तपित्तापघातकः ॥ S.S.Su. 46.258

तण्डुलीयः (Taṇḍulīyaḥ), तण्डुलः (Taṇḍulaḥ), तण्डुलीयकः (Taṇḍulīyakaḥ), भण्डीरः (Bhaṇḍīraḥ), तण्डुलीबीजः (Taṇḍulībijaḥ), मेघनादः (Meghanādaḥ), and घनस्वनः (Ghanasvanaḥ), are synonymous.

Taṇḍulīyaḥ is sweet in taste and *vipāka* and much *śītavīrya*. It is antipoisonous, roughening, clean and useful in bleeding disorders.

I. Generic name. Three kinds, recorded by Nighaṇṭus are A- तण्डुलीयकः (Taṇḍulīyakḥ) B- तण्डुलीबीजः (Taṇḍulībījaḥ) and the third C-मेघनादः (Meghanādaḥ). But of these the 'A' kind is self sown kind and the other two kinds are cultivated in gardens. Now these kinds are developed into sorts and forms. Some of them can be found in (Dr. Roxburg's fl. indi.)

(Fam. Amaranthaceae)

A-a-1 ***Amaranthus blitum*** Linn.*
2 *A. spinosus* Linn.

B-a ***A. caudatus*** Linn.
Syn. *A. paniculatus* Linn.**
b Watt Dict.

C- 1) ***Amaranthus tristis*** Willd***
2) *A. oleraceus* Willd & varieties
b Roxburgh (fl. Indi)

II A-a तण्डुलीयकः (Taṇḍulīyakaḥ)
b 1) (SK) Alpamārīṣaḥ; (H.B.) Sadanatiya;(Mar.) Cavalāī, Tāndulјā
2) (SK) Taṇḍulīay; (H) Kaṇṭailī Caulāī; (B) Kāte natiya; (Mar.) Kātemāth; (Tam.) Mulluka kirai; (Tel.) Mullaṭoṭakura

B-a) भण्डीरः (Bhaṇḍīraḥ), तण्डुलीबीजः (Taṇḍulībījaḥ),
b- (SK) Rājagiri; (Mar.) Rājgirā; (Bom). Koholbhāji; (Guj) Rājgaro

C- मेघनादः (Meghanādḥ) घनस्वनः (Ghanaswanaḥ), वीरस्तण्डुलः

---

१ 'चण्डाला' इति नि.शे. टीका संमतः पाठः ।
२ 'गण्डीरः इति नि.शे. टीका संमतः पाठः ।
* The current accepted name is *A. lividus* Linn.
** *A. caudatus* & *A. paniculatus* are two distinct species. (see comp. p. 9)
*** *A. tricolor* Linn. *var. tristis* (Willd) Meharotra, Aswal et Bist. (Comp. p. 9).see note.

(Vīrastaṇḍulaḥ), ग्रन्थिलः (Granthilaḥ)

1) (H) Lālsāga; (Tel.) Sīrukuru; (B.) Campānatiya; (SK) Meghanāda; (Mar.) Moṭhā māṭh; (Tam) Sirukirai.

III a 1) See IV a Balawantji

2) Taṇḍula - AV X -9-26
MS i-6-6,
KS XI,
AB i-i, S. Br. i-4-3
Ch.u. iii 14-3
KAS. p. 149 Taṇḍulīyaka.

Dhn. IV -6 Taṇḍulī (Harshe)

b) तण्डुलीय (Taṇḍulīya); Meghanādaḥ Caurāi (Dipika p 254 -280)

IV 1) .. three distinct groups of Amaranthus.

1) Cultivated in gardens.
2) Wild species.
3) Forms cultivated in fields, so as edible forms.
(Amaranthus Com. Pr. of Indi p. 62)

2) तण्डुलीयक Taṇḍulīyaka
Amaranthus spinosus Linn.
Syn. भण्डी and भण्डीर
C.Su. 27.92 etc. Su. Su. 16.27 (10) etc.
A.H. Su. 6.83 etc.
There are different varieties of Caulāi (चौलाई) differing in the presence or absence of spines and colour of leaves i.e. green, red or mixed with blue. (Balwantji p. 174).

40 (३९) कासमर्दः Kāsamardaḥ

कासमर्दोऽरिमर्दश्च कासारिः कर्कशस्तथा ॥ ११५
[१]कालः कनक इत्युक्तः स च स्यात्कासमर्दकः ॥
कासमर्दः सुतिक्तः स्यान्मधुरः कफवातजित् ॥ ११६
विशेषतः पित्तहरः पाचनः कण्ठशोधनः ॥ S.S. Su. 46. 236.

कासमर्दः (Kaśamardaḥ), अरिमर्दः (Arimardaḥ), कासारिः (Kāsāriḥ), कर्कशः (Karkaśaḥ), कालः (Kālaḥ), कनकः (Kanakaḥ), कासमर्दकः (Kāsamardakaḥ), are synonymous.

Kāsamarda is bitter and sweet in taste, pacifies *kapha vāta* and especially *pitta doṣas*, is digestant and clears the throat.

१ कालंकतक' इति चौखम्बा मुद्रित पुस्तके पाठः ।

Leguminosae. caesalpiniaceae.

I a- ***Cassia sophera*** Linn.
b- Dymock in (Pharm. indi.)

II a- कासारिः (Kāsarih) जरणः (Jaraṇaḥ), कालः (Kālaḥ),
b- (SK) Kāsamarda; (H) Kāsundā; (B) Kālā Kāsunda (Mar) Kāsavindā, Rāntākaḷā. (Tam.) Surali; (Tel.) Konda Kasinda.

41 (४०) इक्षुः Ikśuḥ

इक्षुः कर्कोटको वंशः कान्तारो वेणुनिस्वनः ॥ ११७
इक्षुरन्यः पौण्ड्रकस्तु रसालः सुकुमारकः ॥

इक्षुःसरो गुरुःस्निग्धो बृंहणः कफमूत्रकृत् ॥ ११८
वृष्यः शीतःपवनजित् भुक्ते वातप्रकोपनः ॥ A.H. Sū. S. 42

अन्यः खरकशाली स्यादिक्षुयोनीक्षुवालिका ॥ ११९
तथाऽन्यश्चेक्षुगन्धः स्यादिक्षुरः कोकिलाक्षकः ॥
"अतीव मधुरो मूले मध्ये मधुर एव च ॥ १२०
अग्रे[१] त्वचि च विज्ञेय इक्षूणां लवणो रसः ॥ S.S. Su. 45. 155

इक्षुयुग्मं रसे स्वादु पित्तघ्नं वृष्यशीतलम् ॥ १२१

गुडः **(Jaggery)** (21)**
गुडः स्यादिक्षुसारश्च मधुरो रसपाकजः ॥
गुडः समधुरः क्षारो गुरूष्णः कफवातनुत् ॥ १२१

अहितः पित्तरक्ते च जीर्णश्चैव रसायनः ॥

इक्षुः (Ikśuḥ), कर्कोटकः (Kārkoṭakaḥ), वंशः (Vamśaḥ), कान्तारः (Kāntāraḥ) and वेणुनिःस्वनः (Veṇunisvanaḥ), are synonymous. Other kind of *Ikśuḥ* is called पौण्ड्रकः (Pauṇḍrakaḥ), of which synonyms are रसालः (Rasālaḥ) and सुकुमारकः (Sukumārakaḥ).

Ikśu is laxative, *guru*, unctuous, bulkpromoting, aggravates *kapha* and increases the quantity of urine. It is *vṛṣya, śitavirya,* pacifies *vātadoṣa* but if taken immediately after meals it aggravates *vātadoṣa*.

---

* Few modern writers have accepted *Cassia occidentalis* Linn. for *Kāsmarda*. The white & black are two varieties of *Kāsmarda*. The white one is *C. occidentalis* Linn. & the black one is *C. sophera* Linn. S.D. Kamat.

** गुडोऽभिष्यन्दि मधुरो बृंहणः कफकारकः ।
गुरुः शुक्रकरश्चैव पित्तलश्च विशेषतः ।
इत्यधिकः पाठः आनन्दाश्रम पुस्तके दृश्यते ।
सुश्रुतसंहितायां इक्षोर्द्वादशजातयः निर्दिष्टा ।

१ 'अग्रेष्वक्षिषु' इति सुश्रुत पाठः । S.Su. 45. 155

There is an other kind of *ik'su* called as खरकशाली (Kharakaśālī) of which synonyms are इक्षुयोनी (Ikśuyonī) and इक्षुवालिका (Iksuvālikā). The another type of *Ik'su* is called as इक्षुगन्धः (Ikśugandhaḥ) of which synonyms are इक्षुरः (Ikśuraḥ) and कोकिलाक्षकः *Kokilākśakaḥ*.

Ik'su (Cane) is very sweet at its root portion and sweet in central portion, but at its tip and peel, it is salty.

Both types of *Ik'su* are sweet in taste, *'sītavīrya*, pacify *pittadoṣa* and *vṛṣya*.

गुड (Guḍa) Jaggery, इक्षुसारः (Ikśusāraḥ), मधुरः (Madhuraḥ) and रसपाकजः (Rasapākajaḥ) are synonymous.

It is sweet, salty in taste, guru, *uṣṇavīrya* and pacifies *kaphavāta doṣas*, is not beneficial in disorders due to *rakta* and *pitta doṣas*. old Jaggery is *rasāyana*.

I (Generic name, Raj. Ni. notes five kinds according to the colour and taste, but all are of the same species (A). But Dhn. Ni. has noted more one different plant to which he calls B- इक्षुगन्धः कोकिलाक्षः* (Iksugandnaḥ, Kokilākśaḥ; Kokilākśa plant smelling like Ikśu).

(Fam. Graminae) Poaceae.

A a ***Saccharum officinarum*** Linn.

b Roxb. (Fl. ind. p.7a)

B a ***Astercantha longifolia*** Nees.**
syn. *Hygrophila spinosa* T. Anders
Ruellia longifolia Roxb.

b Dymock (Pham. Ind.)

II A a- कर्कोटकः (Karkoṭakaḥ), वंशः (Vamśaḥ), पौण्ड्रकः (Pauṇḍrkaḥ), Five kinds of Raj. Ni. सितः (Sitaḥ), पुण्ड्रः (Puṇḍraḥ), करङ्गेक्षुः (Karangekśuḥ),कृष्णः (Kṛṣṇaḥ), रक्तः (Raktaḥ)

b- (Sans.) Ikśu, Rasāla (The light coloured variety (Roxb.) Kangak (The red -Roxb); (B) IK, Oak, Ak, Kushira; (Tel.) Cheukoo bodi; (Guj.) Sherdi; (Mar. Bom.) Ūsa; (Kan. Mal.) Ikśu; (Tam.) Karumbu.

B-a कोकिलाक्षः (Kokilākśaḥ), इक्षुरः (Ikśuraḥ), पिच्छिलः (Picchilaḥ), इक्षुगन्धः (Iksugandḥ) (Raj.Ni. Pari. varga IV -26)

b (H) Tālamakhānā; (Mar.) Talimakhānā, Koḷsundā, Koḷistā; (Tam.) Nirmalli; (Tel.) Nirguvi veeru.

---

* This may be a kind of Iksuh only belonging to Graminae.

** B-a plant *Astercantha* belongs to Fam. Acanthaceae while A-a plant *Saccharum* belongs to Fam. Poaceae (Graminae).

42 (४१) काशः Kāśaḥ

काशः काण्डेक्षुरुद्दिष्टः काकेक्षुर्वायसेक्षुकः ॥ १२३
इक्ष्वारिकेक्षुकाण्डश्च स चैवेक्षुरकः स्मृतः ॥

श्वेतचामरपुष्पश्च तथेक्षुकुसुमश्च सः ॥ १२४
काशः स्वादु रसे तिक्तो विपाके वीर्यतो हिमः ॥

तर्पणो बलकृद् वृष्यः श्रमशोषक्षयापहः[1] ॥ १२५
काशद्वयं च पित्तास्रकृच्छ्रजिन्मधुरं हिमम् ॥

काशः (Kaśaḥ), काण्डेक्षुः (Kāṇḍekśuḥ), काकेक्षुः (Kākeśuḥ), वायसेक्षुः (Vāyasekśuḥ), इक्ष्वारिका (Ikśvārikā), इक्षुकाण्डः (Ikśukāṇḍaḥ), इक्षुरकः (Ikśurakaḥ), श्वेतचामरपुष्पः (Śveta cāmarapuṣpaḥ), इक्षुकुसुमः (Ikśukusumaḥ) are synonymous for both the kinds of kāśa.

Kāśa is sweet and bitter in taste, (?sweet) in *vipāka, śītavīrya*, nutrient, strength promoting, and *vṛsya.* It is useful in alleviating thirst due to fatigue (exercise) and consumption.

Both types of *kāśa* is useful in bleeding disorders and dysuria sweet in taste and *śītavīrya.*

---

a- ***Saccharum spontaneum*** Linn.
Syn. *S. semidecumbens,* Roxb. (Watt. Dict.)

b Roxburgh (Fl. indi.)

II- a श्वेतचामरपुष्पः (Śwetacāmarapuṣpaḥ), काण्डेक्षु (Kāṇḍekśu), सितपुष्पकः (Sitapuṣpakaḥ), दर्भपत्रः (Darbhapatraḥ), लेखनी (Lekhanī), काण्डकाण्डकः (Kāṇḍakāṇḍakaḥ), गौल्यः (Gaulyaḥ).

b (SK) Kāśa; (H) Kāns, Kāgrā; (Tam.) Nanala; (B) Kāsh; (Mal.) Nannana; (Tel.) Kakīceruka, Relugaddī.
Note : Raj. Ni. has noted अशिरी (Aśirī), a kind of Kāśa which is not identified here.

III a- 1) Kāsa -RV. X-10 -10. VI-9-1 (Harshe No. 22)
2) See IV 3 Balwantji (Below).

b- काशः (Kāśaḥ) Śweta cāmarakaḥ (Arun; Ast. H. Su. 15-25)

IV- 1) काशः (Kāśaḥ) *Saccharum spontaneum* Linn.
culms from 5 to 15 feet high.
(U.C. Datta, Vidyotani Bh. Pr. Ni.)
2) (Kāśa) *S. cylindricum* Lam. (Ach. Dwivedi, Bh. Pr. Ni.)
3) काश (Kāśa)

---

१ 'भयापहः' इत्यानंदाश्रममुद्रित पुस्तके पाठः ।

Saccharum spontaneum Linn.
C. Su. 3.26, 4.17.35 , etc.
S.Su. 6.37, 38.10, 75 etc.
A.H. Su. 6.171, 15.24 etc. (Balwantji p. 96)

43 मुञ्जः Muñjaḥ (४२) दर्भौ Darbhau

मुञ्जः क्षुरः स्थूलदर्भो बाणाह्वो ब्रह्ममेखलः ॥ १२६
मुञ्जोऽनुष्णो विसर्पास्रमूत्रबस्त्यक्षिरोगनुत् ॥

बाणाह्वो मधुरः शीतः पित्तदाहतृषापहः ॥ १२७

मुञ्जः (Muñjaḥ), क्षुरः (Kšuraḥ), स्थूलदर्भः (Sthūladarbhaḥ), बाणाह्वः (Bāṇāhvaḥ), and ब्रह्ममेखलः (Brahmamekhalaḥ), are synonymous.

Muñja is slightly *usṇavīrya* and useful in erysipelas, *raktadoṣa*, disorders of urinary organs and diseases of eyes. *Bāṇa* is sweet in taste, is *sitavīrya,* pacifies *pittadoṣa*, burning sensation and alleviates thirst.

Two kinds A- Muñjaḥ and B- Bāṇaḥ)

I- a- ***Saccharum munja*** Roxb.*
Syn. *S. ciliare* Anders
b- Roxburgh (fl. indi.)

II a क्षुरः (Kšuraḥ), स्थूलदर्भः (Sthūladarbhaḥ), ब्रह्ममेखलः (Brahmamekhalaḥ), तेजनः (Tejanaḥ), वानीरजः (Vānīrajaḥ), दूरमूलः (Dūramūlaḥ)
b- (SK) Muñja; (Tel.) Gundrā, (H) Sarakaṇḍā; (B.Bom) Sara.

III a
1 मुञ्जः Muñjaḥ RV. I-191-3
AV.i-24
TS.V -1-9-4
S.Br. IV-3,3-16
2 See IV-4 Balwantji (below).

IV 1 मुञ्ज (Muñja) 2), भद्रमुञ्ज (Bhadra muñja) are two kinds of muñja
Saccharam sara
S. munja (Ach. Dwivedi Bh. Pr. Ni.).
2 मुञ्ज (Muñja) *Saccharum cilare,* भद्रमुञ्ज (Bhadra Muñja)
S. aurundinaceum. (Vidyatoni Bh. Pr. Ni.)
S. ciliare Anders
Syn. *S. munja* Roxb.

---

* Currently accepted name is
S. bengalense Retz. (Comp. p. 133)

(SK) Gundrā, Tejanak, Śara, (H.) Sara, Muñja; (Santal) Sir Muñjā Leaf. sheaths, Sar-Leaves.
Munja is much valued on account of its strength, elasticity and power of resisting moisture ...
Considerable confusion still prevails as to the particular species of saccharum which should be regarded as having afforded the sacrodotal girdle. (Watt Dict.)

4 शर Śara, सर Sara.
Saccharum munja Roxb.
C. Su. 5.20 (इषिका) 14.22 etc.
A.H. Su. 6.171, 30.42 etc.
See synonyms मुञ्जः and इषिका refer to (Balvantji p. 390)
Note : Balwantji believes *Muñja* मुञ्जः and *Sara* to be the same plant but the compiler of Dhn. Ni. and Raj. Ni. have recorded these two plants under two seperate plant headings. We think there is some confusion among modern writers about these plants. See Śara Pre. No. 45 infra.

44 मृदुदर्भः Mṛdudarbhaḥ (कुशः - Kuśaḥ)

मृदुदर्भः कुशो बर्हिः शुचि[1]चीरः सुवृत्तकः ॥
खरोऽन्यः पृथुलः शीरी[2] गुन्द्रा[3] च नीरजः स्मृतः ॥ १२८

दर्भयुग्मं पवित्रं स्यान्मूत्रकृच्छ्रघ्नशीतलम् ॥
रक्तपित्तप्रशमनं केवलं पित्तनाशनम् ॥ १२९

मृदुदर्भः (Mṛdudarbhaḥ), कुशः (Kuśaḥ), बर्हिः (Barhiḥ), शुचिचीरः (Śucicīraḥ), सुवृत्तकः (Suvṛttakaḥ), are synonymous and for the other kind खरः (Kharaḥ), पृथुलः (Pṛthulaḥ), शीरी (Śirī), गुन्द्रा (Gundrā), and नीरजः (Nīrajaḥ) are synonymous.

Both types of *darbha* are auspicious, *śitavīrya,* pacifiy *pittadoṣa,* and useful in dysuria and bleeding disorders.

I Generic name, includes three kinds of plants, one A कुशः (Kuśaḥ) and the next B शीरी (Śirī) of Dhn. Ni. and C कुशोऽल्पः (Kuśaḥ alpaḥ) of Raj. Ni.

For Confirmation

---

१ 'सूचिवीरस्तु पत्रकः' इति नि.शे. टीका संमतः पाठः ।
२ 'सीरी' इति नि.शे. टीका संमतः पाठः ।
३ ' गुन्द्राह्वो नीरजो निशिः इति नि. शे. टीका संमतः पाठः ।

(Fam. Graminae) Poaceae

A-a- ***Poa cynosuroides*** Linn. & Willd.*
Syn. *Uniloa bipinnata* Linn.

b Roxburgh (F. inid.)

B-a a kind of *Saccharum spontaneum* Beauv.

b Kamat (Following the note given in Kāśa)

C-a- ***Imperata arundinacea*** Cyrill.
Syn. *I. cylindrica* Beauv.
Saccharum cylindrica Linn. (Watt. Dict.)

II A.a कुशः (Kuśaḥ), बर्हिः (Barhiḥ), सितदर्भः (Sitadarbhaḥ), यज्ञीयपत्रकः (Yajñīya patrakaḥ), ब्रह्मपवित्रः (Brahma pavitraḥ), सूचिमुखः (Sūcimukhaḥ).

b (San.) Kuśa, Darbha, (B.) Kusa; (Tel.) Darbha, Dubha, Durpā; (H.) Dābe, Durvā; (Bom.) Darbha.,
(H.) Dāb, Durva; (Bom.) Durbha.

B शीरी (Śirī), गुन्द्रा (Gundrā), खरः (Kharaḥ), पृथुलः (Pṛthulaḥ),

C a - कुशोऽल्पः (Kuśolpaḥ), शरपत्रः (Śarapatraḥ), हरिदर्भः (Haridarbhaḥ), पवित्रः (Pavitraḥ).

b- (SK) Darbha (Datta), Barhiśa (Elliot); (H) Dābh; (B) Ulū; (Tam.) Durbhai pul.

III a-1) 27 Kuśa - S. Br. II-5-2-15.
T. Br. -1- 5-10
M.S. IV. 5-7,
46 Darbha- RV-i-119-3
AV - iii-12-7
TS ii 05-1-4 (Dr. Harshe. S. Kosa)

2) आपस्तम्ब – बर्हिरघे कुशाभावे प्रतिनिधयः । स्मृत्यर्थः काशमयं ग्राह्यं न लभ्यन्ते कुशा यदि । (Prayog Ratnakar Narayan Bhatti)

b 1) कुश (Kuśa) -*Andropogon nardus;* (Mar.) Barik darbha; (H.) Dābh (Vidyotani & Ach. Dwivedi Bh. Pr. Ni.)

2) Thora darbha, Dab-*Poa cynosuroides*
(Vidyotanī -Bh. Pr. Ni.)

3) कुशद्वयम् (Kuśadwayam) - iti Darbha- dwayam.
(Dīpika -Sharn, S.P. 157)

IV - 1 See *Desmostachya bipinnata* Stapf.

The present accepted name is -
* *Desmostachya bipinnata* (Linn.) Stapf
Syn. *Eragrostis cynosuroides* Beauv.
Poa cynosuroides Retz.
Kusa and Darbha are separate grasses. Kusa is *D. bipinnata and Darbha is Imperata cylindrica* Beauv. 'Chunekar'. J. R.I. M & yoga. 1977 (March). pp. 116-121).

Syn. *Eragrostis cynosuroides* Roem & Schult. (Dymock).
Poa cynosuroides Linn. (Chopra)

45 शरः Śaraḥ (४३) शरद्वयम् Śaradvayam.

शरो बाण इषुः काण्डः उत्कटः[1] सायकः क्षुरः ॥
स्थूलोऽन्यः ईक्षुको[2] प्रोक्तः इक्षुरश्चापि[3] नामतः ॥ १३०

शरद्वयं स्यान्मधुरं सतिक्तं
कोष्णं कफभ्रान्तिमदापहारि ।

बलं च वीर्यं च करोति नित्यं
निषेवितं वातकरं च किञ्चित् ॥ १३१

शरः (Śaraḥ), बाणः (Bāṇah) इषुः (Iṣuḥ), काण्डः (Kāṇḍaḥ), उत्कटः (Utkaṭaḥ), सायकः (Sāyakaḥ), क्षुरः (Kśuraḥ) are synonymous. The other kind is called as स्थूलशरः (Sthūla śaraḥ) of which synonyms are इक्षुकः (Ikśukaḥ) and इक्षुरः (Ikśuraḥ).

Both the kinds of *śara* are sweet and slightly bitter in taste, slighlty *uṣṇavīry,* pacify *kapha* and slightly aggravate *vātadoṣa* if used daily (Continyously). These are useful in giddiness and intoxication, and are strength promoting and energizer.

(Generic name, includes two kinds A शरः (Śaraḥ) and B. स्थूलशरः (Sthūlaśarah). Both of the same genus.

(Fam. Graminae) Poaceae

I- A a- ***Saccharum sara*** Roxb. *
b- Roxburgh (Fl. indi.)

(For confirmation)

B a- ***Saccharum exaltum*** Roxb.
b -Kamat (following Fl. Indi.)

II- A a- शरः (Śaraḥ), बाणः (Bāṇaḥ), सायकः (Sāyakaḥ), उत्कटः (Utkaṭaḥ),
b- (SK) Gundrā, Tejanak, Śara; (B) Śara; (H) Śara; (Tel.)Gundrā

B स्थूलशरः (Sthūla Śaraḥ), इक्षुरकः (Ikśurakaḥ), महाशरः (Mahāśaraḥ),

---

१ इक्ष्वटः २ इक्षुरः ३-४ इक्ष्वारश्च पितामहः। नि.शे. टीकायाम

* *Saccharum sara* Roxb.
Syn. *Erianthus munja* Jesw.
See under मुञ्जः (U.P.I.pp.200; 537)

क्षुरपत्रः (Kśurapatraḥ),

b- (Tel.) Kondā manamāu.

III a-1) 114 Sara RV. -I-191-3,
TS VII-12-1,
S.Br. II-5-2-12. (Dr. Harshe S. Kosa)
d,e,f, See current names and Synonyms.

46 (४४) वंशः (Vamśaḥ)

वंशो वेणुर्यवफलः कार्मुकस्तृणकेतुकः ॥[१]
त्वक्सारः शतपर्वा च मस्करः कीचकस्तथा ॥१३२

वंशस्त्वम्लः कषायश्च कटुस्तिक्तश्च शीतलः ।
मूत्रकृच्छ्रप्रमेहार्शः पित्तदाहास्रनाशनः ॥ १३३
*(वंशो व्रणास्रसंहारो भेदनः सकषायकः ।
वंशश्च शूलकफकृद्विष्टम्भी श्लेष्मवातलः ॥)

वंशः (Vamśaḥ), वेणुः (Veṇuḥ), यवफलः (Yavaphalaḥ), कार्मुकः (Kārmukaḥ), तृणकेतुकः (Tṛṇaketukaḥ), त्वक्सारः (Twaksāraḥ), शतपर्वा (Śataparvā), मस्करः (Maskaraḥ), and कीचकः (Kīcakaḥ) are synonymous.

Vamśa is sour, *kaṣāya,* pungent and bitter in taste, *śītavīrya* and pacifies *pitta* and *raktadoṣa.* It is useful in dysuria, disorders characterized by polyuria, piles and burning sensation.

I (Generic name. several kinds and forms are included. But after the writings of our Nighaṇṭus the genera is developed into more races or varieties than before. Therefore some of them, which can be identical with those of our Nighaṇṭus are noted here below.

(Fam. Bambuceae) Gramineae, Poaceae

A-a- ***Bambusa aurundinacea*** Retz.**
Syn. *Arundo bambos* Linn.

B-a- ***B. vulgaris*** Wendle
Syn. *B. arundinacea* Aiton.

b Kamat

B-a ***Bambusa stricta*** Corom Pl. (Roxb.)

---

१ 'कर्मार' इति साधुपाठः । नि. शे. टीका । रा. नि.

* This is an additional reading in Anandasram edition.

** The current accepted name is *B. aurundinacea* (Retz.) Roxb.

Syn. *Dendrocalamus strictus* Nees (W. dict.)

b- Kamat (following fl. indi. of Roxburgh & Watt Dict.).

II A-a- 1 & 2

वंशः (Vaṁśaḥ), यवफलः (Yavaphalaḥ), तृणकेतुकः (Tṛṇaketukaḥ), शतपर्वः (Śataparvaḥ), कण्टकी (Kaṇṭakī), धनुर्द्रुमः (Dhanurdrumaḥ),

b (H) Bānsa, Magarbans; (B) Bāns, Behurbans; (Tam.) Mongal, Velmankil; (Kan.) Bidungulu; (Bom) kaḷaka; (Tel.) Mulkas, Vendru; (Eng.) The spiny Bamboo.

B- a- रन्ध्रवंशः (Randhravaṁśaḥ), वेणुः (Veṇuḥ), त्वक्सारः (Twaksāraḥ), कीचकः (Kīcakaḥ), मस्करः (Maskaraḥ), वादनीयः (Vādanīyah), सुषिरः (Suṣiraḥ),

b- (H.) Bāns. Bāns khūrd; (b) Karail; (Mar.) Bhovarlit; (Bom) Udha, Kaban, Vāsā, Māṇḍagā; (Tel.) Sadanapavudrū; (Eng.) the male Bamboo.

III See Vaṁśāgram, Vaṁśarocanā.

a- 100 Vanśa - R.V.V-10-1,
A.V. iii -12-6,
T.Br. i-2-3-1. (Harshe)

IV 1) Bamboos ... The species are numerous and belongs to Arundinaria, Dendrocalamus, Phyllostachys, and closely allied genera. (Hill, p. 47).

वंशाग्रम् Vaṁśāgram (22)

वंशाग्रं तु करीरः स्याद् वंशांकुरपरुः स्मृतः ।
पित्तास्रदाहकृच्छ्घ्नो रुचिकृत् पर्वनिर्गुणम् ॥ १३४

वंशाग्रं (Vaṁśāgram), the tender sprout of bamboo is called by the synonyms करीर (Karīra) and वंशांकुर (Vaṁśānkura), परुः (Paruḥ), Joint is called as पर्व (Parva).

Vaṁśāgra pacifies *pitta* and *rakta doṣas*. It is appetizing and useful in burning sensation and dysuria. The joint does not have (much) properties.

(Fam. Bambuceae) Poaceae.

I a- Edible young shoots of Bamboo genera. Some of them, the shoots of which are used in food by the Bharatiyas, are *Bambusa aurundinacea, B. tulda, B. vulgaris* and allied species and varieties.

b- Kamat.

II करीरः (Karīraḥ), वंशाङ्कुरपरुः (Vamśākuraparuḥ).
यवफलाङ्कुरः । तस्य ग्रन्थिस्तु परुः पर्व तथा काण्डसन्धिश्च ।
(Yawaphalāṅkuraḥ, tasya Granthistu Paruḥ Parva tatha, Kāṇḍasandhisca)

b (Konkan) kalakace Komba.
(H) bāns kā kulli.

IV - The young shoots of *Bambusa tulda* ... are when about two feet high, tender and very frequently pickled and made excellent one they make, when properly prepared. (Roxb.)

47 (४५) नलः Nalaḥ

नडो नटो नलश्चैव स च पोटगलः स्मृतः ।
धमनो नर्तको रन्ध्री शून्यमध्यो बिभीषणः ॥ १३५

नलः शीतः कषायश्च पित्तमूत्रविनाशनः ॥

नडः (Naḍaḥ), नटः (Naṭaḥ), नलः (Nalaḥ), पोटगलः (Poṭagalaḥ), धमनः (Dhamanaḥ), नर्तकः (Nartakaḥ), रन्ध्री (Randhrī), शून्यमध्यः (Śūnyamadhyaḥ), and बिभीषणः (Bibhiṣaṇaḥ) are synonymous.

Nala is *śitavīrya, kaṣāya* in taste pacifies *pitta* and is useful in urinary disorders.

(Fam. Graminae) (Poaceae)

I a- ***Arundo karka*** Linn. et. Willd.*
Syn. *Phragmites roxburghii* Kunth.

b Roxburgh (Fl. inid.)

II a नडः (Naḍaḥ), नटः (Naṭaḥ), पोटगलः (Poṭagalaḥ), रन्ध्री (Randhrī), शून्यमध्यः (Sunyamadhyaḥ), धमनः (Dhamanaḥ), नर्तकः (Nartakaḥ).

b (SK) Naḍa, Nala, Poṭagala; (B), Nal, Nar; (H.) Narkul; (Kumaon) Karka, nul; (Tel.) Naga-sara, Maitanto.

III 1) केशा नडा इव वर्धन्ताम् । AV-VI-138.

2) Nada (SI) RV-VIII-1-33 (Harshe).

IV 1 Pipes are made of the culms particularly those used by the people who carry about the dancing snake. (Roxb. 1- 348).

2 *Phragmites karka* Trim.

The Current name is-
Phragnmites karka Trim. ex Steud. (U.P.I.p. 449)

Syn. *Arundo karka,* Royle; (Sans.) Nala, Śunyamadhya; (Mar.) Devanaḷa; (Ni. Adarsha, U. C. Datta, Acha. Priyavratji).

3 See (Nala) (Ayur. Patrika 16.4.61)

4 Nala
Phragmites maxima Blatter & McCann
C. Ci. 3-257, 4. 102 etc.
Su. Su. 9-4, 36.9 etc.
A.H. Su 15-24 & etc. (Balavantji p. 267).

महानलः Mahānalaḥ (23)

अन्यो महानलो वन्यो देवनालो नलोत्तमः ॥ १३६
स्थूलनालः स्थूलदण्डः सुरनालः सुरद्रुमः ॥
महानलोऽधिको वीर्ये शस्यते रसकर्मणि ॥ १३७

The other type of *nala* is called as महानलः (Mahānalaḥ), of which synonyms are वन्यः (Vanyaḥ) देवनालः (Devanālaḥ), नलोत्तमः (Nalottamaḥ), स्थूलनालः (Sthūlanālaḥ), स्थूलदण्डः (Sthūladaṇḍaḥ), सुरनालः (Suranālaḥ) and सुरद्रुमः (Suradrumaḥ).

Mahānala is more potent in properties and is useful in the process of mercury.

For confirmation
Fam. Graminae. Poaceae.

I a- ***Arundo donax*** Linn.
Syn. *Donax arundinaceus* Beauv.
Arundo bengalensis Retz.
b- Chopra (Gloss. indi. Medi. plants)

II a- वन्यः (Vanyaḥ), देवनालः (Devanālaḥ), स्थूलदण्डः (Sthūladandạḥ), सुरनालः (Suranālaḥ), सुरद्रुमः (Suradrumaḥ)
b (H.) Barnal; (B.) Ghanal; (P.) Bansi.

48 (४८) दूर्वा Dūrvā

नीलदूर्वा[1] स्मृता शष्पं[2] शाद्वलं हरितं[3] तथा ।
शतपर्वा शीतवीर्या[4] शतवल्ल्यपि[5] शीतला ॥ १३८

१ 'नीली दूर्वा' २ 'शस्या' इति. नि.शे. टीका संमतः ।
३ 'हरिता' क्षी. संमतः पाठः । ४ 'शतवीर्या' इति. क्षी. संमतः पाठः । ५ 'शतवल्ल्यसिता लता' । इति क्षी. संमतः नि.शे. टीकायां च पाठः ।

श्वेतदूर्वा तु गोलोमी श्वेतदण्डा[६] सितालता ।
सहस्रवीर्याऽनन्ता च दुर्मरा भार्गवी रुहा ॥ १३९

गण्डदूर्वा च गण्डाली तीव्रा मत्स्याक्षिकाऽपि च ।
बह्वी[७] नाडीकलापश्च[८] वारुणी[९] शकुलाक्षिका ॥ १४०

दूर्वा शीता कषाया च रक्तपित्तकफापहा ॥

नीलदूर्वा (Nīladūrvā) has the synonyms as शष्पं (Śaṣpam), शाद्वलं (Śādvalam), हरितं (Haritam), शतपर्वा (Śataparvā), शीतवीर्या (Śītavīryā) शतवल्ली (Śatvallī), and शीतला (Śītalā).

श्वेतदूर्वा (Śvetadūrvā), गोलोमी (Golomī), श्वेतदण्डा (Śvetadaṇḍā), सितालता (Sitālatā), सहस्रवीर्या (Sahasravīryā), अनन्ता (Anantā) दुर्मरा (Durmarā), भार्गवी (Bhārgavī) and रुहा (Ruhā) are synonymous.

गण्डदूर्वा (Gaṇḍadūrvā), गण्डाली (Gaṇḍālī), तीव्रा (Tīvrā), मत्स्याक्षिका (Matsyākṣikā), बह्वी (Bahvī) नाडीकलापः (Nāḍikalāpaḥ), वारुणी (Vāruṇī), and शकुलाक्षिका (Śakulākṣikā) are synonymous..

Durvā is *śītavīrya*, *kaṣāya* and pacifies *rakta, pitta* and *kapha-doṣas*.

I. Generic name, includes four kinds A नील (Nila), हरित (Harita), श्वेत (Śweta), and गण्डदूर्वा (Gaṇḍa dūrvā). Raj. Ni. has recorded some more forms but these all kinds, except गण्डदूर्वा (Gaṇḍadūrvā) are of the same species only. The differance is only in their colour and height according to the nature of the soil where they grow. Therefore all these kinds, except 'Gaṇḍadūrvā' are included herebelow in one current name.

(Fam. Graminae)

a- A,B,C, ***Cynodon dactylon (L.)*** Pers.
Syn. *Panicum dactylon* Linn. (Sp. ed. Willd (R.)
Agrostis linearis Linn. (Sp. edi. Willd (R.)
b- Roxburgh (Fl. Indi.)
D गण्डदूर्वा (Gaṇḍadūrvā)
Not identified

II a See Balavantji p. 401, and Chunekar p. 386
A नीलदूर्वा (Nīladūrvā), शष्पम् (Śaṣpam)
B हरितम् (Haritam = Green), शतपर्वा (Śataparvā), शतमूला (Śatamūlā), शिवेष्टा (Śiveṣṭā)
b (SK) Dūrvā, Śataparvā, Bhārgavī, Anantā, (B) Durbā; (Mar.) Dūrvā; (H.) Dūba, Hariyāli; (Tel.) Gherica, Haravali; (Tam.)

---

६ 'श्वेतदण्डा' इति नि.शे. टीकायाम । ७ 'वल्ली' इति नि.शे. टीकायाम । ८ 'कलायश्च' इति नि.शे. टीकायाम । ९ 'धरणी' इति नि.शे.टीकायाम पाठः।

Arugām-pilā, Arugaml pulu; (Eng.) Creeping panic grass, Coach grass.

C a श्वेतदूर्वा (Śweta dūrvā), गोलोमी (Golomī), श्वेतदण्डा (Śweta daṇḍā), सहस्रवीर्या (Sahasravīryā), अनन्ता (Anantā)

b modern names as in b-B.

III a 1) दूर्वाशाला - आयते ते परायणे दूर्वा .... ।
... पुष्पयुक्त कोमला दूर्वा रोहन्तु । (Sāyana) विनियोगः ... (Kausīk. Su. I-3) A.V. VI-1-6

2) सहस्त्रा परमादेवी शतमूला शताङ्कुरा । ... दूर्वा दुःस्वप्ननाशिनी काण्डात् -काण्डात् प्ररोहन्ती परुष परुषस्परि ॥ ॥ या शतेन प्रतनोषि सहस्रेण विरोहसि । ... (Nārayaniyopaniṣad)

3) IV Dūrvā - R- V. i- 191-3 (Harshe)
Misfortunes are prayed to depart like Dūrvā whose seeds fall from the plant (R.V. X 1340 (watt Dict.)

2 *Cynodon dactylon* (L.) Pers.
Two varieties white and green have been recognised and used. All the under mentioned names except *'sādvala* are either (अनेकार्थ) multimeaning or not correctly identified and Dūrvā varieties are used as substitutes in their place.
अनन्ता, अजलोमी, गोलोमी, शतवीर्या, श्वेता, (द्वय) and सहस्रवीर्या
(Balavantji p. 205)

Note- White Dūrvā (श्वेतदूर्वा) is not a variety but green *Dūrvā* हरितदूर्वा when creep more and more the green ends fade into white. *Nīla durvā* is not a variety or sort but grows even on foot height. It does not spread on soil like green Durvā.

3 गण्डदूर्वा (Bh. Pr. Ni. 176 गुडूच्यादि)
It is a sort of *Dūrvā*. It is larger than the *Dūrvā* and grows generally on river banks.
Stems thick and large. Leaves similar to Durvā but rather larger.
(Chunekar Bh. Pr. Ni. 386)

49 पुण्डरीकम् Punḍarīkam

(४७) श्वेतनीलारुणोत्पलम Śvetanīlāruṇotpalam

पुण्डरीकं श्वेतपद्मं सिताब्जं श्वेतवारिजम् ॥ १४१
हरिनेत्रं शरदपद्मं शारदं शम्भुवल्लभम् ॥
पुण्डरीकं हिमं तिक्तं मधुरं पित्तनाशनम् ॥ १४२
दाहघ्नमस्रशोषघ्नं पिपासा भ्रमनाशनम् ॥

पुण्डरीकं (Puṇḍarīkam), श्वेतपद्मं (Śvetapadmam), सिताब्जं (Sitābjam), श्वेतवारिजम् (Śvetavārijam), हरिनेत्रं (Harinetram), शरद्पद्मं (Śaradpadmam), शारदं (Śāradam), and शम्भुवल्लभम् (Śambhuvallabham) are synonymous.

Puṇḍarīka is bitter and sweet in taste, *śītavīrya* and pacifies *pittadoṣa*. It is useful in burning sensation, blood disorders, consumption, thirst and giddiness.

I- a ***Nelumbo nucifera*** Gaertn.
Syn. *Nelumbium speciosum* Willd.

b Watt Dict, V 344 Roxburgh. (Fl. Indi C.B.C 450)

II a श्वेतपद्मम् (Śwetapadmam), शरद्पद्मम् (Śaradpadmam), श्वेतपत्रम् (Śwetapatram)

b (SK) Puṇḍarīka, Śwetapadma; (H) Kanval; (Mal. Tel), Tamārā; (Eng.) The sacred lotus.

III See Padminī

a Puṇḍarīka RV X - 142 -8,
Br. Up ii-3-10,
T.B. 1-8-2-1,
S.Br. V 5-5-6 (Harshe)

IV - 1 There are three varieties of lotus or water lily. The white called *'Puṇḍarīka'*, the red *Kokanada* and the blue *Indīvara*. The entire plant is called *'Padminī'* ... The allusions to the sacred lotus in ancient Hindu literature appear equally to different kinds of Nymphaea' as *Nelumbium speciosum*, which by many authors, has hitherto been regarded as the particular plant referred to. (Nymphaea - Watt Dict V. 437).

2) See Fl. indi. (Roxb.) C.B. Clarke edition pp. 427-428, 540, 647.

3) See Pharm. Indi. :- (Dymock)
Nymphaea and lotus flowers.

4) See Nelumbium in 'Hindu Mat. Medica U.C. Datta.

5) See ibid plant in Vanaushadhi Sangraha of Desai.

6) पुण्डरीक Puṇḍarīka
C.Su. 4.34 etc.
S.Su. 13.13 etc.
A.H. ci. 8.129, Ka 41.17 etc.
It is a variety of Padma described extremely white variety by Dalhaṇa. *Puṇḍarīka* and *Prapauṇḍarīka* प्रपौण्डरीक are definitely two different drugs (See A.H. Ka. 4. 14 But as the latter has not been identified, *Puṇḍarīka* is often suggested as its substitute.

See प्रपौण्डरीक (Balawantji P. 252)

7) See Pre No. 50 सौगन्धिकं IV-1 infra.

50 सौगन्धिकं Saugandhikam

सौगंधिकं नीलपद्मं भद्रं कुवलयं कुजम् ॥ १४३
इन्दीवरं तामरसं कुवलं कुड्मलं मतम् ॥

नीलाब्जं शीतलं स्वादु सुगंधि पित्तनाशनम् ॥ १४४
रुच्यं रसायने श्रेष्ठं देहदार्ढ्यं च केशदम् ॥

सौगंधिकं (Saugandhikam), **नीलपद्मं** (Nīlapadmam), **भद्रं** (Bhadram), **कुवलयं** (Kuwalayam), **कुजं** (Kujam), **इन्दीवरं** (Indīvaram), **तामरसं** (Tāmarasam), **कुवलं** (Kuwalam), and **कुड्मलं** (Kuḍmalam) are synonymous.

Nīlapadma is sweet in taste, *sītavīrya*, fragrant and pacifies *pittadoṣa.* It is appetizing, best as *rasāyana*; provides firmness to body and is beneficial to hair.

Not confirmed.
(Fam. Nymphaceae)

I- a- ***Nymphaea stellata*** Willd.*
b- Roxburgh (Fl. indi.)

II a- **नीलपद्मम्** (Nīlapadmam), **इन्दीवरम्** (Indīvaram), **तामरसम्** (Tāmarasam)
b- (SK) Nīlotpala (Mar.) Niḷen Kamaḷa; (H) Nīlakamal (B) Chota Shālk, (Bom.) Upaliya Kamala; (Tel.) Nilikulav; (Mal.) Sitambel.

III See Padminī, Puṇḍarīka.

IV- 1) Utpala उत्पल
C.Su. 2.20, 9.22 etc.
S.Su. 19.13, 38. 51 etc.
A.H. Su. 3.35, 6, 90 etc.
Although there is considerable confusion in correct identification of the different varieties of *Kamala* (कमल) and *Kumuda* (कुमुद) and a list of names given to them in the literature, *Utpala* उत्पल is considered to be another name for *Kumuda,* and *Nilotpala*

---

* The current accepted valid name is
N. nouchali Burm.f. (comp. 108)

(नीलोत्पल) and identified as *Nymphaea stellata* Willd. (Balawantji p. 51).

2) Varieties of *N. stellata* Willd.

1) *Cyanea* flowers medium sized, blue, scarcely odorous syn. *N. stellata* Willd.

2) *Parviflora* flowers usually smaller, blue, syn. *N. stellata* Willd.

3) *Versicolor* flowers large white blue or purple or flesh colour. Syn. *N. versicolor* Roxb. (Watt. Dict V 438)

3) *N. cynea* Roxb.
(Sans.) *Kalhāra* flowers pale blue condsiderably smaller than either of the former
(*N. Lotus* and *N. versicolor*), petioles from 8 to 12 (Roxb. C.B. C. 428).

51 रक्तपद्मम् Raktapadmam

रक्तपद्मं तु नलिनं पुष्करं कमलं नलम् ॥ १४५
राजीवं स्याद् कोकनदं शतपत्रं सरोरुहम् ॥

वीर्ये रक्तोत्पलं शीतं तिक्तं च मधुरं रसे ॥ १४६
भिनत्ति पित्तसंतापौ ध्वंसयत्यस्रजां रुजम् ॥

रक्तपद्मं (Raktapadmam), नलिनं (Nalinam), पुष्करं (Puṣkaram), कमलं (Kamalam), नलम् (Nalam), राजीवं (Rājīvam), कोकनदं (Kokandam), शतपत्रं (Śatapatram) and सरोरुहम् (Saroruham) are synonymous.

Raktotpala is bitter and sweet in taste, *śītavīrya.* It pacifies *pittadoṣa* and is useful in disorders of blood.

Not confirmed

I (Fam. Nymphaceae)

a- ***Nymphaea rubra*** Roxb.
Syn. *N. lotus* Linn.

b- Roxburgh (Fl. Indi.) Watt Dict. V -436

c- Native of India.

II a- नलिनम् (Nalinam), पुष्करम् (Puṣkaram), कोकनदम् (Kokanadam), शतपत्रम् (Śatapatram),

b- (SK), Rakta Kamala, Aruṇa Kamala; (B) Rakta kambal (H) Chota Kanval; (T) Allitamarai (Tel. Errakalvo; (Mal.) Ampala.

IV 1) *N. lotus* Linn.
A large aquatic herb common throughout warmer parts of India. Flowers- White, pink or crimson, variety of (N. pubescens) with pubescent leaves and smaller flowers also occur. (Watt. Dict. V 436)

2) *N. rubra* Roxb. *
(Sans.) Hallaka and Rakta Kamala; (Tel.) Vera Kalwa, flowers red, stamina from 40 to 50.
There is a small rose coloured variety with 20-25 stamina. (Roxb. C.B.C. 428).

कुमुदम् Kumudam (24)

कुमुदं श्वेतजलजमब्जमम्भोजमम्बुजम् ॥ १४७
पंकजं चारविन्दं च कल्हारं च कुशेशयम् ॥

कुमुदं शीतलं स्वादु पाके तिक्तं कफापहम् ॥ १४८
रक्तदोषहरं दाहश्रमपित्तप्रशान्तिकृत् ॥

कुमुदं (Kumudam), श्वेतजलजं (Śvetajalajam), अब्जं (Abjam), अम्भोजं (Ambhojam), अम्बुजं (Ambujam), पंकजं (Pankajam), अरविन्दं (Arvindam), कल्हारं (Kalhāram) and कुशेशयम् (Kuśeśayam) are synonymous.

Kumuda is sweet and bitter in taste, *śītavīrya* and sweet in *vipāka* pacifies *kapha, rakta* and *pitta doṣas*, and is useful in burning sensation and fatigue.

Not confirmed

I- a- ***Nymphaea lotus*** Willd.
b- Roxburgh (Fl. indi.)

II a- अरविन्दम् (Aravindam), कल्हारम् (Kalahāram), इन्दुकमलं (Indukamlam), शशिकान्तम् (Śaśikāntam), धवलोत्पलं तु कुमुदम् (Dhavalotpalam tu kumudam.)
b- (SK) Koomood (Roxb.); (Tel.) tella Kalva, (H.) Koee (B.) Saluka.

III Note- *N. lotus* Linn and *N. lotus* of Willd. These two plants are different See. *N. rubra* Roxb. Pre. No. 51. The interested readers should read p. 437 of Watt. Dict. Vol.V.

---

* The current accepted name is - *N. rubra* Roxb. ex Salisb. (Comp. p. 108)

IV - 1) *N. lotus* Willd.
It differs from *N. rubra* in colours of flowers. There is a beautiful variety with pink coloured flowers. The white sort is commonly found in ponds of fresh water in every part of India.

क्षुद्रमुत्पलम् K'sudramutpalam (25)

ईषच्छ्वेतं विदुः पद्ममीषन्नीलमथोत्पलम् ॥ १४९
ईषद्रक्तं तु नलिनं क्षुद्रं तच्चोत्पलत्रयम् ॥

उत्पलस्य त्रयं स्वादु कषायं पित्तजिद् हिमम् ॥ १५०

क्षुद्रमुत्पलं (K'sudramutpalam) is of three types (1) ईषत्श्वेतं (Īṣat'svetam) having slightly white coloured flowers is called as पद्मम् (Padmam), (2) ईषन्नीलम् (Īṣannilam) slightly bluish coloured flowers is called as उत्पलम् (Utpalam), and (3) ईषद्रक्तम् (Īṣadraktam) with Slightly red coloured flowers is called as नलिनम् (Nalinam.)

These three types are sweet and *kaṣāya* in taste, *'sītavīrya* and pacify *pittadoṣa.*

I (Generic name includes three kinds A- ईषच्छ्वेतम् (Īṣat'svetam) B-ईषद्रक्तम् (Īṣadraktam) and the third C- ईषन्नीलम (Īṣannīlam.). All of the same family.

(Fam. Nymphaceae)
Not identified

(४८) पद्मिनी -बीज-मृणाल-मूल-केसरम्
Padmini - Bīja-Mṛṇāla-Mūla-Kesaram.

52 पद्मिनी Padminī

पद्मिनी स्यात् पुटकिनी[१] नलिनी च कुमुद्वती ॥
पलाशिनी पद्मवती वनखण्डा[२] सरोरुहा ॥१५१

पद्मिनी शिशिरा रूक्षा कफपित्तहरा स्मृता ॥

पद्मिनी (Padminī), पुटकिनी (Puṭakinī), नलिनी (Nalinī), कुमुद्वती (Kumudvatī), पलाशिनी (Palāsinī), पद्मवती (Padmavatī), वनखण्डा

---

१ 'कुटपिनी' इति नि.शे. टीका संमतः पाठः ।
२ 'वनखण्ड' इति नि.शे. टीका संमतः पाठः ।

(Vanakhaṇḍā), and सरोरुहा (Saroruhā), are synonymous.

Padminī is *śītavīrya,* roughning and pacifies *kapha pitta doṣas.*

I a- The name is alluded to the whole plant of lotus (Watt Dict.)

b- See IV-1 under Puṇḍarīka Pre No. 49. vide supra.

53 पद्मबीजं Padmabījam.

पद्मबीजं तु पद्माक्षं गालोड्यं पद्मकर्कटी ।
भेडः क्रौञ्चादनो क्रौञ्चो नामतश्चैव पद्मकम् ॥ १५२
*(भेडा क्रौञ्चादिनी क्रौञ्चो नापाकश्चैष कन्दली ।)

स्वादु तिक्तं पद्मबीजं गर्भस्थापनमुत्तमम् ।
रक्तपित्तप्रशमनं किंचिन्मारुतकृद् भवेत् ॥ १५३

पद्मबीजं (Padmabījam), पद्माक्षं (Padmākṡam), गालोड्यं (Gālodyam), पद्मकर्कटी (Padmakarkaṭī), भेडः (Bhedaḥ), क्रौञ्चादनः (Krauñcādanaḥ), क्रौञ्चः (Krauñcaḥ) and पद्मकम् (Padmakam) are synonymous.

According to another text - the synonyms are भेडा (Bhedā), क्रौञ्चादिनीः (Krauñcādini) क्रौञ्चः (Krauñca), नापाकः (Nāpakaḥ) and कन्दली (Kandalī).

Padmabīja is sweet and bitter in taste, stabilises foetus well, slightly aggravates *vātadoṣa* and is useful in bleeding disorders.

I a- Seeds of lotus genera

b- Roxburgh (Fl. indi. CBC 450)

II - a- पद्माक्षम् (Padmākṡam), गालोड्यम् (Gālodyam), पद्मकर्कटी (Padmakarkaṭī), कन्दली (Kandalī), श्यामा (Śyāmā),

b- (Mar.) Kamalabīja; (SK) Karṇikā (Watt.)

IV 1) The seeds of *Nelumbium speciosum* Willd. are eaten raw, roasted or boiled (Roxb.)

2) *Euryale ferox* Salisb.
Syn. *Anneslea spinosa* Roxb.
E. indica Planch.
H. Makhānā.
A stemless aquatic plant from Assam, E. Bengal, Manipur, Outh and Kashmir. (Watt. Dict. III 303)

3) *Anneslea spinosa* Roxb.
Native of sweet water lake and pond. Tippra, Eastwards of Calcutta. Flowers-lovely blue-violet. The seeds are farinaceous....

---

* इति पाठः आनन्दाश्रम पुस्तके दृश्यते ।

sold in the public bazars.. The Hindoo physicians consider these seeds to be possessed of powerful medical virtues such as restraining seminal gleet etc. (Roxb. C.B.C. 127)

Note: These seeds are the 'Kamalabīj' sold in Bazars.*

54 बिसम् Bisam. (मृणालम्) Mṛṇālam.

बिसं मृणालं बिसिनी मृणाली स्यान्मृणालिका ॥ १५४
मृणालकं पद्मनालं तण्डुलं नलिनीरुहम् ॥

अविदाही बिसं प्रोक्तं रक्तपित्तप्रसादनम् ॥ १५५ S. Su. 46.303
विष्टम्भि मधुरं रूक्षं दुर्जरं वातकोपनम् ॥

बिसं (Bisam), मृणालं (Mṛṇālam), बिसिनी (Bisinī), मृणाली (Mṛṇālī), मृणालिका (Mṛṇālikā), मृणालकं (Mṛṇālakam), पद्मनालं (Padmanālam), तण्डुलं (Taṇḍulam) and नलिनीरुहम् (Naliniruham) are synonymous.

Bisam is sweet in taste, aggravates *vātadoṣa*, reduces burning sensation in the epigastrium, restores normalcy of *rakta-pitta doṣas*, is constipating, roughning and difficult to digest.

(Fam. Nymphaeaceae)

I a - The stalks of Lotus genera.

b- Roxburgh (Fl. indi.)

II a- मृणालम् (Mṛṇālam), पद्मनालम् (Padmanālam), पद्मतन्तु (Padsmatantu), नलिनीरुहम् (Naliniruham).

b (SK), Mṛṇāla, (Mara.) Bisen.

III 1) The tender shoots of the roots of (Nelumbium Sp.) between the joints are eaten.

2) See lotus flowers (Dymock).

55 पद्ममूलम् Padmamulam

पद्ममूलं तु शालूकं सकलं करहाटकम् ॥ १५६
शालीनं पद्मकन्दं च जलालूकं निगद्यते ॥

अविदाही बिसं प्रोक्तं रक्तपित्तप्रसादनम् ।
विष्टम्भि मधुरं रूक्षं विरसं मारुतावहम् ॥ S. S. Su. 56.363

* At present in northern market roasted seeds are sold as 'Makhānā', while dry seeds of *N. Speciosum* are sold as kamalabīja.

पद्मकंदः कषायः स्यात् तिक्तः स्वादुर्विपाकतः ॥ १५७
शीतवीर्योऽस्रपित्तोत्थं रोगभङ्गाय कल्पते ॥

पद्ममूलं (Padmamūlam), शालूकं (Śālūkam), सकलं (Sakalam), करहाटकं (Karahāṭakam), शालीनं (Śālinam), पद्मकन्दं (Padmakandam), and जलालूकं (Jalālūkam) are synonymous.

Padmakanda is *kaṣāya* and bitter in taste, *śītavīrya*, and sweet in *vipāka*. It is useful in bleeding disorders.

I (Fam. Nymphaeaceae)

a- Creeping roots of lotus genera.

b- Dr. Desai (Oushadhi Sangraha P. 78)

II a शालूकम् (Śālūkam), पद्मकन्दम् (Padmakandam), जलालूकम् (Jalālūkam).

IV 1) (Makhān)

2) Makhan .... dried roots are said "Bhishi' and 'Makhan' to the flour in Bom. Market (Dr. Desai) .

56 पद्मकेसरम् Padmakesaram.

पद्मकेसरमापीतं किञ्जल्कं किञ्जमेव च ॥१५८
मकरन्दं तथा तुङ्गं गौरं काञ्चनकं च तत् ॥
तृषाघ्नं शीतलं रूक्षं पित्तरक्तक्षयापहम् ॥ १५९
पद्ममकेशरमेवोक्तं पित्तघ्नं च कषायकम् ॥ ½

पद्मकेसरं (Padmakesaram), आपीतं (Āpītam), किञ्जल्कं (Kiñjalkam), किञ्जं (Kiñjam), मकरन्दं (Makarandam), तुङ्गं (Tungam), गौरं (Gauram), and काञ्चनकं (Kāñcanakam) are synonymous.

Padmakeśara is *kaṣāya* in taste, *śītavīrya*, pacifies *pittadoṣa* is roughening and alleviates thirst. It is useful in anaemia due to *pittadoṣa*.

I (Fam. Nymphaeaceae)

a- Filaments of lotus genera.

b- D.K. Kamat

II a- किञ्जल्कम् (Kiñjalkam), काञ्चनकम् (Kāñcanakam), परागम

(Parāgam), मकरन्दम् (Makarandam),

b- (Mara.) Kamala kesara.

Note : Nighaṇṭus have included the synonym (Makaranda) in 'Padma Kesara' but 'Makaranda' is the name given to honey formed in flowers.

करवीरादिको वर्गश्चतुर्थः समुदाहृतः ।
नानाव्याधि प्रशमनो नानाद्रव्यसमाश्रयः ॥

And thus had been told the Karavīrādi chapter 4th. In this chapter the various drugs have been mentioned which are useful in alleviation of various diseases.

वर्गेतराणि (Plants not mentioned in the chapter)

१) बलामोटा

बलामोटा सूक्ष्ममूला हरिता च जयावहा ।
विजया च जयन्ती च तथा चैवापराजिता ॥

विषघ्नी तिक्तकटुका कफपित्तसमीरजित् ।
अपराजिता केशरुहा तथा चैव नियोजिता ॥

विजया[१] नागदमनी निःशेषविषनाशनी ।
विषमोहप्रशमनी महायोगेश्वरीति च ॥

बलामोटा (Balāmoṭā), सूक्ष्ममूला (Sūkṣmamūlā), हरिता (Haritā), जयावहा (Jayāvahā), विजया (Vijayā), जयन्ती (Jayantī), and अपराजिता (Aparājitā) are synonymous.

It is bitter and pungent in taste and pacifies *kapha -pitta doṣas.*

(The second kind) is similar in properties and has the synonyms as अपराजिता (Aparājitā), केशरुहा (Keśaruhā), विजया (Vijayā), नागदमनी (Nāgadamanī), निःशेषविषनाशनी (Niḥśeṣaviṣanāśanī), विषमोहप्रशमनी (Viṣamohapraśamanī) and महायोगेश्वरी (MahāYogeśvarī).

It is not mentioned in the Dhn. Ni. However Raj. ni. has mentioned two. types (A) बलामोटा *Balāmoṭa* or जयन्ती *Jayantī* & (B) असिता बलामोटा *Asitā bālāmoṭā*. It is a controversial plant.

F.N. Four plants are described in Anandasram edition as (Vargetarāni) i.e. Not mentioned in the 4th chapter. These are 1) बलामोटा *Balāmoṭa* 2) सोमवल्ली *Somavalli* 3) पोतकी *Potakī* 4) अर्शोघ्नः Arśoghnaḥ. D.K. Kamat has not commented upon these plants. In other chapters he has commented such extra plants. Therefore for the the completion of the work I have conmmented upon these plants. S.D. Kamat.

For. confirmation.

Leguminosae

Fam. (Papilionaceae) (Fabaceae)

I- A-a- ***Sesbania aegyptiaca*** Pers.
Sesbania sesban Merill; Eng. Common sesban (U.P.I.p. 568)

b- Roxburgh F.B. Ind. II. 114

c- Throughout India.

B-a- ***Sesbsania aculeata*** Pers.
Syn. *S. cannabina* (Retz) Pers.
F.B. Ind. II- 114. (U.P.I. 568)

b- Roxbugh. *S. aculeata* Pers. Var. *cannabina* Baker.
Eng. Daincha, Prickly Sesban.

c- Cultivated on the plains of India.

II- A-a- सूक्ष्ममूला Sūk'smamūlā, जयन्ती Jayantī, अपराजिता Aparājitā, नागदमनी Nāgadamanī, महायोगेश्वरी Mahāyoge'swarī

b- कृष्णा (बलामोटा) Kṛṣṇā (balāmotā) Raj. ni.

A-b- H.Jayanti, Jait Jhijan, Janjhan, Raisin., dhandiyan; B Jayanti, Berar- Sarori, sewri , Shewari; Pb.-Jait, Jant, Jaintar; Bom-Sewri, Shevari, Shewari, Jati; Mar.-Sewri, Guj-Raysingni ... Deccan-Shewari, Shezeri. Watt. VI-II-543

B- H. Jayanti, brihat- Chakramed; B.-Jayanti, dhanicha, dhunchi; Pb. Jhigan, Jhanjhan, Jaintar, NWP Dhandain; Bom. Rānshewrā; Mar. Kan. -Sevri, bhuiavali, Ranshevari ... Sans. Jayanti. (Watt. VI-II-542)

III-a- It is not mentioned in the classical books. (Samhitās).

b- जयन्ती तु बलामोटा हरिता च जया तथा ।

1) विजया सूक्ष्ममूला च विक्रान्ता चापराजिता ॥
ज्ञेया जयन्ती गलगण्डहारि तिक्ता कटूष्णाऽनिलनाशनी च ।
भूतापहा कण्ठविशोधनी च कृष्णा तु तत्र रसायनी स्यात् ॥

Raj. Ni. Chap. IV.

2) बलामोटा तु कटुका तिक्तोष्णा मदगन्धिका ।
... ... असिता बलमोटा तु रसायनकरी मता ।
गुणाश्चान्ये जयन्तीवत्स्मृताः पूर्वैर्महर्षिभिः

Nighanṭa Ratnākar.

3) बलामोटा Balāmoṭā 1) नागदवणी Nāgadavaṇī 2) ब्राह्मी Brāhmī 3) शेवरी Sewari (Dictionary appended to Nighanṭu Ratnākar)

4) जयन्ती Jayanti; Mar. Jayantī, Shewarī; Guj. Nahāni Khapat; Kan. Togarse; *Sida humilis*. (Pade. Br. Ni.)

5) विज्ञेया नागदमनी बलामोटा विषापहा ।
नागपुष्पी नागपत्रा महायोगेश्वरीति च ॥
सर्वग्रहप्रशमनी निःशेष विषनाशिनी । Bh. Pr.
Dr. Desai confounds Nāgadavan (Nāgadamanī) with species allied to *Crinum asiaticum* Linn. Some scholars confound to a species of artemisia. Th. Balvant simhaji in Bihar ki Vanaspatiyan points to *Pupalia lappacea* Moq.* (Fam. Amaranthaceae) Chunekar Bh. Pr. 472-473)

6) 341जयन्ती – बलामोटा । 'बलामोटा सूक्ष्मफला जयन्ती विजया जये' ति केयदेवः । सा च पीतरक्त कृष्णगुच्छपुष्पा शिरीषपत्रा शम्बिनीवृक्षः कुल्यादि समीपे जायते । Harshe Shivkosh P. 131

7) .... The Marathas have a superstition that the sight of the seeds will remove the pain of scorpion stings, Watt. VI-II-P. 568
... grown for shed in coffee, turmeric and cotton plantations and for support to betel, pepper and grape vines; seeds used as food in times of scarcity only though they are rich in protein, it is of poor quality due to the presence of canavinine which is an inhibitor of arginine....
Petroleum ether extract and the inorganic fraction obtained from aqueous extract of flowers exhibit antifertitility activity.
(U.P.I.p. 569)

a- *Sesbania aculeata* Pers.
Several varieties of this species are described in the F.B. I.
(Watt. VI. II. 542)

8) Dr. Bhagwandash has confounded it with *Artemisia vulgaris* in Iatro chemistry of Ayurveda but the description there does not corroborate. (P. 397-398-P.496).

२ सोमवल्ली Somavalli

सोमवल्ली यज्ञनेत्री सोमक्षीरी द्विजप्रिया ।
सोमवल्ली त्रिदोषघ्नी कटुस्तिक्ता रसायनी ॥

सोमवल्ली (Somavallī), यज्ञनेत्री (Yajñyanetrī), सोमक्षीरी (Somakśīrī) and द्विजप्रिया (Dwijapriyā), are synonymous.

Somavallī is pungent and bitter in taste and pacifies all the three *doṣas* and is *rasāyana*.

This is also not mentioned either in गणद्रव्यावली *Gaṇadravyāvali* or पर्यायनामद्रव्यावली *Paryāyanāmadravyāvali*. It seems to be copied by some

* *Pupalia lappacea* Juss. (U.P.I. p. 505)

one from भावप्रकाश निघण्टु *Bhāvaprakāśa Nighaṇṭu.*

सोम *Soma* has been described as a divine drug (दिव्यौषधी). In the vedas especially in Ṛgveda much devotion is given to it as it has an important role in the religious rituals or sacrificial rites. Early European scholars on indology have shown much interest in identifying the सोम *soma.* The Parsis were also using this सोम(होम Homa) and it was imported in Mumbai from Persia.

Botanically, it was identified to be *Ephedra girardiana.* The search for the vedic *Soma* has remained a curiosity and a subject of research to modern orientalists up till now. Mr. R. Gordon Wasson* has identified it with a mushroom called Fly agaric and known botanically as *Amanita muscaria* Linn.

Traditionally here, in this part of the country the plants which are used as सोमवल्ली Somavallī are noted here below.

(Fam. Gnetaceae.)

I- a- 1) ***Ephedra gerardiana*** Wall.
Syn. *E. vulgaris* Hook. f (non A. Rich)

2) *E. major* Host.
Syn. *E. nebrodensis* Tineo. etc. (U.P.I.p.197)

b- Roxb. Fl. Br. Ind. V. 640.

C- Drier regions of the temperate and Alpine Himalaya, from western Tibet to Sikkim, ascending to 16000 ft.
(Watt. VI. II-P. 52)

II- a- सोमवल्ली Somavallī यज्ञनेत्री Yajñyanetrī, सोमक्षीरी Somakśirī, द्विजप्रिया Dwijapriyā, सोमलता Somalatā.

b- Amsānia, budshur, chewa. *Ladakah Pb.*
Tse, teapat; Bushar- Rachi, Khandapag; sutlejvalley- Phok; H. Tutgantha; Sans. Soma. Eng. Ephedra, Iran-Hom; Hum.

1) The nineth Maṇḍala of the Ṛgveda describes *Soma* in detail.

III- 2) सोम Soma
C.S.Ci. 1-4-6.
S.S.Ci. 29;30 (whole chapter)
सोमवल्ली Somavallī
C.S.Vi. 8.146.
S.S.K. 1.54; V. 28.7
Cakra has supposed it to be *Somalatā* सोमलता while Dalhana

* The soma of Rigveda; what was it ?" J. Amer. Orien. Soc. Vol. 91/ Num, 2/ April-June 71

thinks it to be *Gudūcī* गुडूची.

(Balavantji, P. 449-456)

Thakur Balavantji has done a very good discussion on सोम *Soma.*

3) Raj. Ni. after describing सोमवल्ली *Somvallī* has mentioned महिषवल्ली Mahiṣavallī or प्रतिसोमा *Pratisomā* having similar properties.

सोम्या महिषवल्ली च प्रतिसोमान्त्रवल्लिका ।
अपत्रवल्लिका प्रोक्ता काण्डशाखा षडाह्वया ॥
रसवीर्य विपाके च सोमवल्लीसमा स्मृता ॥

Raj. Ni. Guḍūcyādi Chapter III

It is botanically identified with *Sarcostemma brevistigma* W.& A.

4) 80 सोमवल्ली धन्वतरुर्यज्ञनेता द्विजप्रिया ।
पक्षपत्रो महार्घोऽन्यो महागुल्मो मखप्रभुः ॥
श्येनाहृतस्तस्यभेदा विंशतिश्चतुरुत्तरा । इति केयदेवः । Harshe P. 82.

5) Vd. Bapalaji vaidya has given an account of Soma in his Nighaṇṭu Adar'sa Vol. II Page 44 to 56 (Hindi Edition).

3 पोतकी Potakī

पोतकी पोतका प्रोक्ता मत्स्या काली सुरङ्गिका ।
पोतकी शीतला स्निग्धा श्लेष्मला वातपित्तजित् ॥

पोतकी (Potakī), पोतका (Potakā), मत्स्या (Matsyā), काली (Kālī) and सुरङ्गिका (Surangikā) are synonymous.

Potakī is *'sitavīrya,* unctuous, aggravates *kaphadoṣa,* pacifies *vāta* and *pitta doṣas.*

Here only one type of पोतकी *Potakī* is mentioned while Raj. Ni. has mentioned four types चतुर्धा उपोदकी (Caturdhā Upodakī) - A) उपोदकी Upodakī B) सूक्ष्मपत्रा उपोदकी Sūk'smapartā Upodakī C) वनजा उपोदकी Vanajā Upodakī D) मूलपोती Mulapoti or क्षुद्रवल्ली K'sudravallī. All belonging to the same genus. In cultivated state it is of white coloured and red coloured stems.

Fam. Basellaceae.

I- a- ***Basella alba*** Linn.
Syn. *Basella rubra* Linn.
Eng. Indian Spinach.

b- Watt. Vol. I.(p. 203.)

c- Cultivated all over India.

II- a- पोतकी (Potakī), मत्स्या (Matsyā), काली (Kālī), सुरङ्गिका (Suraṅgikā),

b- H.B. Mar. - Poi; Tel. Batsala; Kan. Basale; Mal. Basala.

III - उपोदिका Upodikā
Basella rubra Linn.
C.S.Su. 2.32; 26. 116, 27.91. etc.
S.S. Su. 20.13; 46. 259 etc.
A.H. Su. 6.84;Ci. 9.21
Closely allied species *B.alba* Linn. may also be taken as a variety of it. (Balavantji p. 53)

IV- 2) The generic name is said to be the Malabar name of the plant. (Watt. Dict. I.P. 403)

3) Food.The succulent leaves and stems are used as pot herb (made into curry) by natives of all classes.. .. scarcely a village exists in Bengal at least, where a hedge row covered with this favourite pot-herb may not be seen (Watt. I.404)

1) ९४ उपोदका पोतकी ।
उपोदकोर्ध्वगा वल्ली पिच्छिलच्छदना स्थिरा ।
वृत्तपत्रा रक्तदण्डा रक्तबीजरसा च सा । इति ।
Harshe S. Kosha p. 85.

4) Tender stems and leaves ... cousumed as pot herb .. .. Juice of the leaves given to children and pregnant women to remove constipation. (U.P.I.p. 68).

४ अर्शोघ्नः Arśoghnaḥ सूरणः Sūraṇaḥ

अर्शोघ्नः सूरणः कन्दः कन्दार्हः कन्दवर्धनः ।
दुर्नामारिः सुवृत्तिश्च वातारिः कन्दसूरणः ॥

सूरणः कटुको रुच्यो दीपनः पाचनस्तथा ।
कृमिदोषहरो वातशूलगुल्मास्रदोषनुत् ॥
श्वासं कासं च च्छर्दिं च निवारयति सेवितः ।

अर्शोघ्नः (Arśoghnaḥ), सूरणः (Sūraṇaḥ), कन्दार्हः (Kandārhaḥ), कन्दवर्धनः (Kandavardhanaḥ), दुर्नामारिः (Durnāmāriḥ), सुवृत्तिः (Suvṛttiḥ), वातारिः (Vātāriḥ), and कन्दसूरणः (Kandasūraṇaḥ) are synonymous.

Sūraṇa is pungent in taste, appetizer, stimulates digestive capacity and is digestant. It is useful in disorders due to worms, colics, tumours and blood disorders due to *vātadoṣa, it* removes dyspnoea, cough and vomitting.

Here only one kind is noted while Raj. Ni. has noted *Sitasūraṇaḥ vanasūraṇaḥ* which is an uncultivated form. There is also an another species *Amrophophallus sylvaticus* (Roxb.) Kunth. Syn. *Synantherias sylvatica* Schott which is confounded with *Vajrakanda.*

Fam. Araceae.

I- a- ***Amorphophallus campanulatus*** Blume ex Decne.
b- most of the modern writers.
c- Cultivated largely throughout the plains of India. (Chopra).

II- a- अर्शोघ्नः (Arśoghnaḥ), दुर्नामारिः (Durnāmāriḥ), सुवृत्तिः (Suvṛttiḥ) vide above सितसूरणः (Sitasūranaḥ), वन्यः (Vanyaḥ), अरण्यसूरणः (Araṇyasūraṇaḥ) Raj. ni.
b- Sans. Arshoghna; H. Suran kanda, Jami kanda, ola; B. ola; Mar. Suran; Guj. Suran; Kan. Surnagadde; Tel. Kanda, Kandagadda; Tam. Karuna-kalang; Mal. Karuna-kirhanna.

III- 1) सुरेन्द्रकन्द्रः श्लेष्मघ्नो विपाके कटुः पित्तकृत् । सुरेन्द्रकन्दो – वज्रकन्दः । Dalhan S.S. 46.305.स्थूल सूरण माणक प्रभृतयः कन्दाः ईषत्कषायाः कटुका रूक्षा .. ... पित्तहराश्च । S.S.46 306 स्थूलकन्दो – ग्राम्यकन्दः केचित् सकलकन्दं इति पठन्ति तत्रापि स एवार्थः शूरणः स्वनाम प्रसिद्धः माणकं महापत्रं यथापूर्वमधः पत्रत्यागि । Dalhana.

2) Sūrana
Amorphophallus campanulatus (Roxb.) Bl. ex Decne.
Sūraṇa सूरण Jimikanda जिमीकन्द (H.)
S.Su. 46. 306.7. A.H. Su. 6.113 Ci. 8. 21 etc. (Balavantji P. 443)
अमरवरायुधसाह्वय Amaravarāyudhasāhvaya.
S.S. Ci. 17.41
It is another name for *vajrakanda* which too is not specified.
(Balavantji p. 16)
वज्रप्रोक्ता Vaijraproktā
वज्रप्रोता Vajraprotā
S.S.U. 60.40
This is identfied by Ḍalhaṇa with *Vijrakanda* which too is not properly specified .. ... Desai, however, has named two aroids i.e. *Plasmonium* (Arum) ? *margaratiferum* (Roxb.) Schott and *Amrophophallus sylvaticus* (Roxb.) Kunth as *Vijrakanda* .....
(Glossary. Th. Balavantji & chunekar.)

इति करवीरादिश्चतुर्थो वर्गः

Thus ends the Karavīrādi Chapter Fourth.

अथ आम्रादिः पञ्चमो वर्गः ।

ĀMRĀDIḤ CHAPTER V.

१ आम्र : Āmraḥ

आम्रश्चूतो रसालश्च कीरेष्टो मदिरासखः ।
कामाङ्गः सहकारश्च परपुष्टो मदोत्सवः ॥ १

अन्यच्च[१]

आम्रो रसालो माकन्दः कामाङ्गः पिकबान्धवः ।
वनपुष्पोत्सवश्चूतः परपुष्टो मदोद्भवः ॥२

मधुचूतो मधुफलः सुफलो मदिरासखः ।
वसन्तपादपोऽसौ तु सहकारोऽतिसौरभः ॥ ३

बालं कषायं कट्वम्लं रूक्षं वातास्रपित्तकृत् ।
सम्पूर्णमामम्लं च रक्तपित्तकफप्रदम् ॥ ४

हृद्यं वर्णकरं रुच्यं रक्तमांसबलप्रदम् ।
कषायानुरसं स्वादु वातघ्नं बृंहणं गुरु ॥ ५

पित्ताविरोधि संपक्वमाम्रं शुक्रविवर्धनम् ।
मधुरं बृंहणं बल्यं गुरुविष्टम्भ्यजीर्णकृत् ॥ ६ S..S.46. 153-154

सहकाररसो हृद्यः सुरभिः स्निग्धरोचनः ।
त्वङ्मूलपल्लवं ग्राहि कषायं कफपित्तजित् *॥ ७

(A.San.Su.&.186- 88)

आम्रः (Āmraḥ), चूतः (Cūtaḥ), रसालः (Rasālaḥ), कीरेष्टः (Kīreṣṭaḥ), मदिरासखः (Madirāsakhaḥ), कामाङ्गः (Kāmāṅgaḥ), सहकारः (Sahakāraḥ), परपुष्टः(Parapuṣṭaḥ), and मदोत्सवः (Madotsvaḥ), are synonymous for *Āmrah.*

From the other text :

आम्रः (Āmraḥ), रसालः (Rasālaḥ), माकन्दः (Mākandaḥ), कामाङ्गः (Kāmāṅgaḥ), पिकबान्धवः (Pikabāndhavaḥ), वनपुष्पोत्सवः (Vanapuṣpotsavaḥ), चूतः (Cūtaḥ), परपुष्टः (Parapuṣṭaḥ), मदोद्भवः (Madodbhavaḥ), मधुचूतः (Madhucūtaḥ), मधुफलः (Madhuphalaḥ), सुफलः (Suphalaḥ), मदिरासखः (Madirāsakhaḥ),वसन्त पादपः (Vasantapādapaḥ), सहकारः (Sahakāraḥ), (This is attributed to when it is very fragrant.)

Very immature mango fruit is *kaśāya* (astringent), pungent and sour

---

१ अन्यच्च - इ. पाठः आनन्दाश्रम पुस्तके मुद्रितः । अपिच नि.शे. कांड १ श्लोक संख्या १२१- १२२ इत्यत्र (अस्याग्रे)

पक्वाम्रं सकषायाम्लं भेदनं कफवातजित् ।

हृद्यं वर्णकरं रुच्यं रक्तमांसबलप्रदम् ॥ इत्यधिकःपाठः आनन्दाश्रम पुस्तके ।

in taste and roughning. It aggravates *vāta, pitta* and *rakta doṣas*. When it is matured it tastes sour and aggravates *rakta, pitta* and *kaphadoṣas*. Matured mango fruit is sweet in taste with subsidiary taste *Kaṣāya*.

It is cordial, improves complexion of the body, appetiser, and increases blood. It pacifies *vāta,* increases the bulk of the body and is *guru*. Nicely ripened mango fruit is sweet in taste, bulk promoting (of the body), increases *śukradhātu,* does not aggravate *pitta,* is *guru*, strength giving and causes flatulance with indigestion.

The juice of the *sahakāra* mango is cordial, having flavour, is *snigdha* (unctuous), and appetizer.

The root, bark and leaves taste *kaṣāya* and astringent in a action and pacify *kapha* and *pittadoṣas*.

Fam. Anacardiaceae.

I- a- ***Mangifera indica*** Linn.

b- accepted by all modern writers.

c- Probably indigenous in Sikkim,.Assam, Khasia hills, Satpuda ranges, Khandesh and along the western Ghats (Chopra)

Tropical Himalaya. Cultivated in Muscat in all Western Asia and generally in tropics. De candolle writes....native of S. Asia or of the Malaya Archipilago, when we see multitude of varieties cultivated in these countries and number of common names. (Watt Dict. V. 147)

II- a- *cf* आम्र (Āmra)-(Agrawal-p.209-210)
कीरेष्ट (Kīreṣṭaḥ) कामाङ्गः (Kāmāngaḥ), परपुष्टः (Parapuṣṭaḥ), मदिरासखः (Madirāsakhaḥ), कामशरः (Kāmaśaraḥ), कोकिलोत्सवः (Kokilotsavaḥ), वसन्तदूतः (Vasantadūtaḥ)

b- (H) Ām; (B) Ām, Āmbra; (Kol) Uli , Ul; (Santal) (Gond) Marka; (Mar). (Bom.) Āma, Āmbā; (Tam.) Mad, Mangas, Mammarum; (Tel) Elā māru, Mamdi, Mamdi Chettu, mamadimu, Guggu- mamidi; Eng. The Mango tree.

III- a- 1 See IV- 1 below Balvantji.

2 आम्रवण - This is the earlier reference of आम्र (Āmra)- (Agrawal-p.209-210)

b) 1-64 'सहकारफलमति सुरसाम्रफलं । वसन्त दूतमाकन्द साहारपिकबन्ध (?बान्ध)वः ॥ सहकारेऽस्य तु फलं पुण्डरिकमितिरितं' सिंहः ।
(Harshe)

2 क्वचित पुस्तके अपुष्पफलवानाम्रः पुष्पितश्चूत उच्यते । पुष्पैः फलैश्च संयुक्तः सहकारः स उच्यते । इति । Foot note- ed.purandare.IV

1 आम्र Āmraḥ
C. Su. 2.27. 4-10 etc.
Su. Sū 38. 47, 42-16 etc.
A.H. Sū 6. 127, 7. 44 etc.
Synonyms चूत; सहकार (Page 427.) (Balvantji p. 37)

2) *M. indica* Linn.
Syn. *M. domestica* Gaertn.
Cultivated races - cultivated races of mangos, I have collected upwards of 500 and from these I have selected 100 good ones ... The sorts planted were as follows. ...etc.
(Watt Dict, V 147).

क्षुद्राम्रः (Kśudrāmraḥ) (1)

क्षुद्राम्रः स्यात्कृमितरुः लाक्षावृक्षो जतुद्रुमः ।
सुकोशको घनस्कन्धः कोशाम्रश्च सुरक्तकः ॥८
कोशाम्रोऽम्लः कटुःपाके वीर्योष्णोऽथानिलापहः ।
कफपित्तकरो रुच्यः कुष्ठघ्नो रक्तशोधनः ॥९

क्षुद्राम्रः (Kśudrāmraḥ), कृमितरुः (Kṛmitaruḥ), लाक्षावृक्षः (Lākśāvṛkśaḥ), जतुद्रुमः (Jatudṛumaḥ), सुकोशकः (Sukośakaḥ), घनस्कन्धः (Ghanaskandhaḥ), कोशाम्रः (Kośāmraḥ), and सुरक्तकः (Suraktakaḥ) are synonymous.

Kośāmra is sour in taste, *usṇavīrya* and pungent in *vipāka*. It pacifies *vātadoṣa* and aggravates *kapha* and *pitta doṣas*. It is useful as appetizer, in skin disorders, and has purificatory action on blood.

(Fam. Sapindaceae)

I- (a) ***Schleichera oleosa*** (Lour.) Merr.*
Syn. *S. trijuga* Willd.
(b) Chopra
(c) Dry forests of the Sub.Himalayan tract from the Sutlej to Nepal, Central and Southern India, not in Assam.

II- (a) कृमितरुः (Kṛmitaruḥ), लाक्षावृक्षः (Lākśāvṛkśah), जतुद्रुमः (Jatudṛumaḥ), घनस्कन्धः (Ghanaskandhaḥ), कोशाम्रः (Kośāmraḥ).
(b) (H). Kosam; (Santal) Baru; (Mar. Bom.) Kosam, Koshimb; (Tam) Kolam; (Tel). Pasuku; (Kan) Chakota, akota; (Eng.) The lac tree, Kosumbra, The ceylon oak.

---

* The present accepted name *is S. oleosa* (Lour.) Oken

III a See IV 1 bellow.

IV 1) कोशाम्र Kośāmra.
Schleichera oleosa (Lour) Merr.
C.Su . 26. 112, vi. 147 etc. Su. Sū 38.48, 42.18. etc.
A.H. Cī 13. 30 etc (Balvantji p. 122).

2) *S. trijuga* Willd.
It exudes a yellowish resin. The lac produced upon this tree is known as kosum lac and is the most highly prized quality.
(See coccus laca Vol.II- 409) (Watt Dict. p. VII -II 486)

3) *Mangifera sylvatica* Roxb.
(H.) Kosam, (Silhet) Laxmiam, (San) Kośāmra.
(Watt Dict. V. 157).

राजाम्रः Rajāmrah (2)

राजाम्र उक्त आम्रान्तो मन्मथोद्भवनस्तथा ।
टङ्को नीलकपित्थोऽन्यो राजपुत्रो नृपात्मजः ॥१०
राजाम्रयुगुलं चाम्लमुष्णवीर्यं च पित्तलम् ॥

The synonyms for राजाम्र (Rājāmra) are आम्रान्त (Āmrānta), and मन्मथोद्भवनः (Manmathodbhavanaḥ). For other type of *Rājamra* the synonyms are टङ्कः (Taṅkaḥ), नीलकपित्थः (Nīlakapitthaḥ), राजपुत्रः (Rājaputraḥ), and नृपात्मजः (Nṛpātmajaḥ),

Both the types are sour in taste, *uṣṇavīrya* and aggravate *pitta.* This may be a kind of mango tree giving the highly praised fruits.

2. (२) आम्रातकः Āmrātakaḥ

आम्रातकः पीतनकः कपिचूतोऽम्लवाटकः[१] ।
शृङ्गी[२] कपी रसाढ्यश्च तनुक्षीरः कपिप्रियः ॥११
आम्रातकफलं वृष्यं पित्तास्रकफवह्निकृत् ।
शीतं कषायमधुरं किंचिन्मारुतकृद् गुरु ॥१२

आम्रातकः (Āmrātakaḥ), पीतनकः (Pītanakaḥ), कपिचूतः (Kapicūtaḥ), अम्लवाटकः(Amlavāṭakaḥ), शृङ्गी (Śṛṅgī), कपी (Kapī), रसाढ्यः (Rasāḍhyaḥ), तनुक्षीरः (Tanukśīraḥ) and कपिप्रियः (Kapipriyaḥ) are synonymous.

---

१ अम्लपादपः इति शोढल संमतः पाठः । २ तुंगी इति शोढल संमतः पाठः ।

It's fruit is *kaṣāya* (astringent), and sweet in taste. It is *vṛṣya* and aggravates *kapha, pitta, rakta* and *vātadoṣa* to some extent and stimulates digestive capacity and is *guru.*

I- a- 1) ***Spondias mangifera*** Willd.*
Syn. *S. amara* Lamk.
The Hog plum.
b- Watt Dict. VI. (Vol.3)
c- A small deciduous tree found wild or cultivated throughout India.

II a- पीतनकः (Pītanakaḥ), कपिचूतः (Kapicūtaḥ), अम्लवाटकः (Amlawāṭakaḥ), तनुक्षीरः (Tanukśīraḥ).
b (H.B.) Āmrā; (Bom. Mar.) āmbādā, Rān-āmbā; (Tam.) Mari mancedi, Kat mara; (Tel.) Ambāl chettu; (Kan). Ambat mara, Ambte; (Sans) Āmrātak (Watt. Dict.)

3 (३) जम्बीरः Jambīraḥ

जम्बीरो जम्भलो जम्भः प्रोक्तो दन्तशठस्तथा ॥ १३
गंभीरो वक्त्रशोधी च रोचनो दन्तहर्षणः ॥
तृष्णाशूलकफोत्क्लेशच्छर्दिश्वासनिवारणः ॥ १४
वातश्लेष्मविबन्धघ्नं जम्बीरं गुरु पित्तलम् ॥

जम्बीरः (Jambīraḥ), जम्भलः (Jambhalaḥ), जम्भः (Jambhaḥ), दन्तशठः (Dantaśaṭhaḥ), गंभीरः (Gambhīraḥ), वक्त्रशोधी (Vaktraśodhī), रोचनः (Rocanaḥ), and दन्तहर्षणः (Dantaharṣaṇaḥ) are synonymous.

Jambīra aggravates *pitta doṣa* and is *guru.* It is useful in thirst, colic, nausea, sense of regurgitation of *kapha,* vomiting, dyspnoea and in obstruction due *vāta* and *kapha* (in the gastro intestinal canal).

I- a- ***Citrus medica*** var. ***limonum*** sp. Risso*

---

* Curent accepted name- *Spondias pinnata* (Linn..f.) Kurz.
* The present accepted name for *C. medica* var. *limonum* of Watt is *C.limon* (Linn.) Burm f. (U.P.I. p. 128)

b- Watt Dict. II. 351

c- Cultiivated in South of Europe and in India.

II- a- जम्भलः (Jambhalaḥ), दन्तशठः (Dantaśaṭhaḥ), दन्तहर्षणः (Dantaharṣaṇaḥ),

b- (H.) Jambīra, Barānimbu (Mar.) Thor limbū; (Tam). Periya yelumichai pashum; (Tel.) Peda nimma padu; (Kan) Dodda nimba pannu; (San). Maha Jambīra; Eng. The lemon.

c- Cultivated in South Europe and in India.

IV- 1) ... That the wild form of this plant has not as yet been discovered. All the Himalayan and Khasia plants as far as the writer's experience goes, wild forms of the lime, are citron but not of the lemon...Dr. Royle is said to have found the tree growing wild in the north of India... etc. (Watt. Dict. II. 352)

मधुजम्बीरः Madhu Jambīraḥ (4)

अन्यो मधुजम्बीरो मधुजम्बीरफलश्चान्यः ॥ १५
शङ्खद्रावी शर्करकः पित्तद्रावी च षट्संज्ञः ॥

मधुरो मधुजम्बीरो शिशिरः कफपित्तजित् ॥ १६
शोषघ्नस्तर्पणो वृष्यः श्रमघ्नः पुष्टिकारक : ॥

There is other kind of *Jambīra* called as मधुजम्बीरः (Madhujambīraḥ) and मधुजम्बीरफलः (Madhujambīraphalaḥ), शङ्खद्रावी (Śaṅkhadrāvī), शर्करकः (Śarkarakaḥ) and पित्तद्रावी (Pittadrāvī) are its synonyms.

Madhujambīra is sweet in taste, *śitavīrya* and pacifies *kapha* and *pitta doṣas,* it alleviates thirst, is nourishing, *vṛsya* and removes fatigue.

This may be a variety of citrus species.

I- A-a- ***Citrus medica** Var. **limetta*** W& A.*
The Sweet lime of India.

c- Commonly cultivated in most parts in India ....most probably a native of southern India. (Watt. Dict. II. 357)

B- *Citrus medica var.limetta*. W. & A.

---

१ 'वक्त्र बोधी' इति पा.

* The current accepted name for *C. medica* var. *limetta* W. A. of Watt is *C. limettioides* Tanaka (U.P.I. 128)
C. limetta Risso. (Comp. p. 38)

The Sweet lime.

C- This form is very little known in India and occurs only occasionally in gardens. It is probable that with the lemon this is not an Indian form.. (Watt. Dict. II 357)

II- A & B-a

मधुजम्बीरः (Madhu Jambīrah), शङ्खद्रावी (Śaṅkhadrāvī) ,शर्करकः (Śarkarakah), पित्तद्रावी (Pittadrāvi)

A-b-(H) Miṭhā nimbu; (Guj. & Bom.) Mîtha Limbu; (Tam) Elemiterum, (Tel.) Nema pandu; Gajanimma; (Mal.) Eramitechi; (Sans.) Madhu karkaṭika.

B-b-Vern- names - Asian Limetta... (Watt Dict. II. p. 357)

IV 1) *Citrus limettiodes* Tanaka.
Syn. *C. medica* var. *limetta* W. & A.
(B & H.) Mitha nimbu. Commonly cultivated in central and northern part of India. (Chopra)
(Sans) Madhu Jambīra. (Desai & Yadavaji)

4. (४) नारङ्गः Nāraṅgah

नारङ्गस्त्वक्सुगन्धश्च नागरङ्गो[१] मुखप्रियः ॥ १७
स चैरावतिकः प्रोक्तो योगी वक्त्राधिवासनः ॥
अम्लं समधुरं हृद्यं विशदं भक्तरोचनम् ॥ १८
वातघ्नं दुर्जरं प्रोक्तं नारङ्गस्य फलं गुरु ॥ S.S.Sū 46. 161

नारङ्गः (Nāraṅgah), त्वक्सुगन्धः (Twaksugandhaḥ), नागरङ्गः (Nāgaraṅgaḥ), मुखप्रियः (Mukhapriyaḥ), ऐरावतिकः (Airāvatikaḥ), योगी (Yogī) and वक्त्राधिवासनः (Vaktrādhivāsanaḥ) are synonumous.

The fruit of *Nāraṅga* is sweet and sour, cordial, clears the mouth and improves appetite. It pacifies *vātadoṣa* and is *guru.*

I- Modern writers have recorded several species and varieties with different tastes, colours under the name Nāranga. The place of origin of sweet orange is suggested to be china, cochin china (De candolle p. 187-188) while that of bitter orange is sugested by some in Northern India. But after all we have come to the conclusion that the original place of this plant is uncertain till

---

१ सुधातक्राधिवासनः इति क्षी.संमतः पाठः ।
योषित् वक्त्राधिवासनः इति नि.शे. टीका संमतः पाठः ।

now. (See IV-145) The Nighaṇṭus have recorded only two kinds A-अम्लम् (Amlam) and B- मधुरम् (Madhuram).

A-a- ***Citrus reticulata*** Blanco.
Syn. *C. qurantium* Var. *aurantium* proper (in part)
b- Chopra
c- Cultivated

B-a- ***C.sinensis*** (Linn) Osbeck.
Syn. *C aurantium* Linn. & Willd.
b-1) De Candolle c-Cultivated .

II- a- त्वक्सुगन्धः (Twak Sugandhaḥ), ऐरावतकः (Airāvatakaḥ), योगीरङ्गः (Yogīrangaḥ), अम्लम् (Amlam).
b- (B) Kamlā nimbu, Narangī; (H.) Santrā; (Mar.) Santre; (Eng.) Mandarin (Hill).

B-a-नागरङ्गः (Nāgarangaḥ), मधुरम् (Madhuram)
Eng. Sweet orange (Hill).

III-a- 1) See under IV- Naranga Balvantji.
b- 1) 319 नागरङ्गो - नार्यङ्गः । नारङ्गी नार्यङ्गस्तक्रवासनः । ऐरावतश्च सैव' .. इति. सिंहः (Harshe)
2) ऐरावतो नागरङ्गे । (2-4-38) अमरः । इरावत्या विद्युत इवायं रक्तत्वादैरावतः नागस्य सिन्दुरस्येव रङ्गोऽस्य नागरङ्गः । ... आह च नागरङ्गः त्वक्सुगंधो नागरङ्गो मुखप्रियः । स च ऐरावतः प्रोक्तः सुधातक्राधिवासनः ॥ (क्षीरस्वामी)

IV- 1) There seems very probability that this difficult subject when approched in a scientific manner will be radically changed and the account here given may help to direct attention to the point which will be changed earlier investigation while giving popular and commercial information of some practical value. The following anlaysis .... may be found useful.

1. **C. Medica**- A shrub, young shoots purple, petioles more or less naked, petals generally tinged with red, stamens 20- 40, style long, fruit globose, ovoid or long .... rind very thick and rough.

2. **C. Nobilis & C. Limetta** A tree 15-20 ft. in height, petioles short, winged, flowers small white, style long, fruit globose or somewhat oblong, not mamiliate, rind very thin, nearly smooth shining yellow or orange coloured....

3. **C. Hystrix** ....

4. **C. aurantium .** A tree young shoots whitish. petioles more than twice the length of the length of the two preceeding species... stamens 20-30, style long... fruit globose or flattened, pulp sweet

acid or bitter.

C. decumans.
young shoots and under surface of the leaves pubescent.
(Watt. Dict. p. 334. 335) vol. II.

2) The sweet orange
Citrus aurantium Linn.
Var. I *Aurantium proper* (Var. P. dulcis Linn.)
(For Var. 2 see p. 335.) The sweet orange china orange.

History "De-candolle ... The Asiatic names now given to this form more correctly belong to the *Bitter orange* and that the sweet orange is most probably not originally Indian.... Sweet variety of orange came from china and cochin china. It spread towards the beginning of christan era. (Watt. Vol. 2-p. 336).

Dr. Bonavia... seems fully of the opinion that even the sweet orange is indigenous to India.
By some writers:- The sweet and bitter oranges are to be derived from the same stock. The others mentioned say 'Northern India is the native country of the orange tree. In Garhawal, Sikkim and the Khasia Hills, orange which is the supposed parent of the cultivated orange whether "Sweet or Bitter " (Watt. 2. 338)
(See IV-5 below)

Race - 1st Santara rind smooth... ... Vern. Kamalā -moglāi (Sweet orange) 'Nāringhi'

Race-2nd - Nāringhi or keonlā ... rind being rougher or dark colour ... Vernacular name not available. (P. 339)

Race-3rd Malta or blood red orange (Conf. with *C. nobilis* ...) (P.340).

Race 4th Manderine Orange
(Conf. with *C. nobilis*) ...

Having now briefly indicated the chief forms of sweet orange met within India, the present article may be completed giving some idea of the orange industry at the two great commerical centres Sylhet and Nagpur. (Watt. II. 341).

3) *Bitter orange.*
Var. Bigaradia
The Bitter or seville orange,
Syn, *C. vulgaris* Risso.
C. buxifolia Poir.
Flowers very large, strongly scented rind very aromatic, pulp bitter.

Oil of Neroli

Oil & perfumery : Neroli camphor (p. 346. Watt. II)

Var 3. Bargamia. Bargamot orange.

Habitat The Bargamot orange is cultivated near Reggio in South Colabria in Sicily and in the South of France ... rarely met with India.

Bargamon Oil

Medicine The juice of the fruit possesses properties similar to those of Lemon juice (See under *C. medica var. limonum.*) (Watt. II- 345-346).

a) *C. aurantium* Linn.,
C.aurantium Risso.

.. I have sown *pips* of sweet oranges taken from the natural tree; sometimes from oranges grafted on bitter orange trees. The result has always been trees bearing sweet fruit, and the same has been observed for more than sixty years by all the gardeners of Finale.

Gallesio:- There is no instance of a bitter orange tree from seed of sweet orange tree nor of a sweet orange tree from the seed of bitter oranges.

Macfadyn- Fl. Jamaica ... that the seed of sweet orange very frequently grows up into a tree into a bitter fruit ... ... I am not aware, however, that the seed of bitter orange has ever grown up into the sweet fruit variety.

Duchassasing says

The seeds of sweet orange often yield bitter fruit.

Dr. Earnst -They sometimes yield sour but not bitter fruit .*Brandis* Khasia in India ... extensive plantation of sweet oranges are from seed.

These differeances show the variable degree of heredity and confirm the opinion that these two kinds of orange should be considered as two varieties, not two species. (De. Candolle p. 183)

5) Orange bitter - *Citrus aurantium* Linn.
Sub sp. *amara* Eng.
Syn. Seville orange, Bigaradier orange, C. Bigaradia. Naranja
Habitat Originated in Northern India but now cultivated in mediterenean countries.
Description ... .. Orange water is made from flowers ...
Parts used the fruit rind, oil, flowers. ... ...
Orange Sweet -*Citrus sinensis* Linn.
Syn. Portugal orange, China orange .

Habitat The sweet orange peel has less bitterness than that of Seville orange. The flowers of the orange are white etc.

Medicinal properties .... possesses the same properties as bitter orange and used for similar purposes. (Potter's cyclo.)

6) नारङ्ग Nāraṅga

Citrus reticulata Blanco.

S. Sū 46 . 139, 161. see synonym ऐरावत and नागरङ्ग (P. 223)

नागरङ्ग Nāgaraṅga

C.S.Su. 27. 154: (P. 222)

ऐरावत Airāvata

C.S. Sū. 27. 158 etc.

S. S. Sū. 46. 162 etc.

A. H. Sū 6. 138.

Airāvata is a kind of acid fruit, which is according to some a small and more sour variety of orange. Ḍalhaṇa at one place (Su.46-191) has decribed it as blackish red fruit ..... (p.60).

(Balwantji)

5. (५) बीजपूर्णः Bījapūrṇaḥ बीजपूरः Bījapūraḥ

बीजपूर्णो बीजपूरः केशरः[१] फलपूरकः ॥ १९
पूरकः केशराम्लश्च मातुलुङ्गः सुपूरकः ॥

वराम्लो बीजको लुङ्गो रुचको मध्यकेशरः ॥ २०
कृमिघ्नो गन्धकुसुमः केशरी सिन्धुपादपः[२] ॥

'श्वासकासारुचिहरं तृष्णाघ्नं कण्ठशोधनम् ॥ २१
लघूष्णं दीपनं हृद्यं मातुलुङ्गमुदाहृतम् ॥

त्वक् तिक्ता दुर्जरा तस्य वातकृमिकफापहा ॥ २२
स्वादु शीतं गुरु स्निग्धं मांसं मारुतपित्तजित् ॥

मेध्यं शूलार्तिच्छर्दिघ्नं कफारोचकनाशनम् ॥ २३
दीपनं लघु संग्राहि गुल्मार्शोघ्नं तु केशरम् ॥

पित्तमारुतकृद्बल्यं दीपनं बद्धकेशरम् ॥ २४
हृद्यं वर्णकरं रुच्यं रक्तमांसबलप्रदम् ॥

शूलाजीर्णविबन्धेषु मन्दाग्नौ कफमारुते ॥ २५
अपचीश्वासकासेषु रसस्तस्योपयुज्यते ॥ S. S. Su. 46

---

१ 'केशरी' शोढल संमतः पाठः ।

२ 'शीधुपादप' इति नि. शे. टीका संमतः पाठः ।

रसोऽतिमधुरो हृद्यो शुक्रपित्तानिलापहः ॥ २६
कफकृद् दुर्जरा पाके मातुलुङ्गजटा कटुः ॥
मूलं चैव कृमीन् हंति पुष्पं बीजं च गुल्मजित् ॥ २७

बीजपूर्णः (Bījapūrnaḥ), बीजपूरः (Bījapūrah), केशरः (Keśaraḥ), फलपूरकः (Phalapūrakah), पूरकः (Pūrakah), केशराम्लः (Keśarāmlaḥ), मातुलुङ्गः (Mātuluṅgaḥ), सुपूरकः (Supūrakah), वराम्लः (Varāmlaḥ), बीजकः (Bījakaḥ), लुङ्गः (Luṅgaḥ), रुचकः (Rucakaḥ), मध्यकेशरः (Madhyakeśaraḥ), कृमिघ्नः (Kṛmighnaḥ), गन्धकुसुमः (Gandhakusmaḥ), केशरी (Keśarī), and सिन्धुपादपः (Sindhupādapaḥ) are synonymous.

Mātuluṅga is *uṣṇavīrya* and *laghu*. It is appetizer and cordial; useful in thirst and disorders of throat, cough, anorexia, and dyspnoea. Fruit skin (peel) is bitter, difficult to digest is carminative, anthelmintic and pacifies *kaphadoṣa.*(*Māmsa*) pulp of the fruit is sweet in taste, *śītavīrya, guru,* unctuous and pacifies *vāta* and *pitta doṣas,* Its filamentous portion केशरम् (*Keśaram*) is intellect promoting, appetiser, *laghu,* astringent and antiemetic. It is useful in colic, anorexia due to *kaphadoṣa,* tumors (or diverticulosis) and piles.

The matured fruit बद्धकेशरम् (Badhkeśaram), (where the filaments are matured but not fully matured) aggravates *pitta* and *vāta doṣa.* It is cordial, improves complexion, is appetizer and increases blood, flesh (muscular tissue) and strength.

It's juice is indicated in colics, indigestion, constipation, decreased digestive capacity, *apacī* (scrofula), dyspnoea and cough. It pacifies *kapha* and *vāta doṣas.*

The juice which is very sweet (fully ripen fruit) is cordial, and pacifies *vāta piita doṣas* and recduces *śukra dhātu.* Its root is pungent in taste, aggravates *kaphadoṣa* and is anthelmintic Its seeds and flowers are useful in tumors (or diverticulosis).

(Fam. Rutaceae.)

I- a ***Citrus medica*** Linn.
Syn. *C. medica* var. *medica proper.*

b- Watt. (Dict.).

c- Cultivated throughout warmer parts of India, wild in chitgaon, the Khasia and Garo Hills.

II- a मातुलुङ्ग (Mātulunga), बीजपूरः (Bījapūraḥ), केसरी (Kesarī)

b- (H.) Bījapūr Turanga; (Tel .) Lungamu; (B)Bara nimbu (Mara.) Mahaḷunga, Mavḷang; (Mal) Gilam; (Tam.) Kadara marathai; (Eng.) The Citron, Adam's apple.

IV See

(1)Watt. Dict. II. 350. 351.

(2) Roxb. flora Indi. C. B. C. P. 500

2. ... Under the above definitions I mean to comprehend various varieties, if not species, of the sour lemons or limes found in India and as the petioles are very generally winged, I think it is necesary to separate them from the lemons and citrons which have not that mark, or have it in a very trifling degree. (Roxb).

Citrus Medica Linn. (Watt. Dict).

Var. I	Var 2`	Var. 3
Medica proper The Citron	Limonum Sp. Risso The lemon. Jambhra limbu Pahari, Kagri (Much recent origin) (īḍalimbu Dr. Gharpure) Nimbu, Khata Nimbu. abundant acid juice Lemon- De candolle	Acida The Sour lime of India Limbu, Nimbu. Kagji

Var. 4	Var.5
Limetta The sweet lime of India Mitta nimbu. India, Sākhara limbu Kamat- konkan sweet non aromatic.	Lumia The sweet lemon very little known to occurs in garden.

मधु कर्कटी Madhukarkatī (5)

बीजपूरोऽपरः प्रोक्तो मधुरो मधुकर्कटी ।
मधुवल्ली च विज्ञेया वर्धमाना महाफला ॥ २८

मधुकर्कटिका स्वादुः शीता पित्तास्रजिद् गुरुः ।
एषा त्रिदोषजिद् वृष्या रुचिकृच्चैव दुर्जरा ॥ २९

There is an another kind of बीजपूरः (Bījapuraḥ), called as मधुकर्कटी (Madhukarkaṭī), of which synonyms are मधुरः (Madhuraḥ), मधुवल्ली

(Madhuvallī), वर्धमाना (Vardhamānā), and महाफला (Mahāphalā).

Madhukarkaṭī is sweet in taste, *śītavīrya* and *guru.* It pacifies all the three *doṣas* and is *vṛṣya.* It is useful in haemorrhagic disorders, promotes appetite and difficult to digest.

This may be one of the preceding two plants recorded under the heading मधुजम्बीर *Madhujambīra.* There are some wild kinds of बीजपूर *Bījapūra* which are not recorded under botanical names separately. The interested readers may read the subject which is discussed under sweet orange and under *C. medica* in watt's Dict. Vol II 364.

6. (६) अम्लिका Amlikā अम्लीका Amlīkā

अम्लिका चुक्रिका चुक्रा साम्ला शुक्ताऽथ शुक्तिका ।
अम्लीका चिञ्चिका चिञ्चा तिन्तिडीका सुतित्तिडी ॥ ३०

अम्लिकायाः फलं चाम्लमत्यन्तं पित्तकृल्लघु ।
रक्तकृद् वातशमनं बस्तिशुद्धिकरं परम ॥ ३१

पक्वं तु मधुराम्लं च भेदि विष्टम्भवातजित्[१] ।
त्वक्भस्म स्यात् कषायोष्णं कफघ्नं त्वनिलापहम् ॥ ३२

अम्लिका (Amlikā), चुक्रिका (Chukrikā), चुक्रा (Cukrā), साम्ला (Sāmlā), शुक्ता (Śuktā), शुक्तिका (Śuktikā), अम्लीका (Amlīkā), चिञ्चिका (Ciñcikā), चिञ्चा (Ciñcā), तिन्तिडीका (Tintiḍīkā) and सुतित्तिडी (Sutittiḍī) are synonymous.

The fruit of *Amlikā* is very sour in taste and aggravates *pitta* and *rakta doṣa,* is *laghu*, pacifies *vātadoṣa* and has purificatory action on urinary organs; when fully ripe it is sweet and sour in taste, purgative useful in constipation and *vāta*. The ash of the peels is *kaṣāya* in the taste, *uṣṇavīrya* and pacifies *kapha* and *vātadoṣas*.

Fam. Leguminosae. Caesalpiniaceae.

I- a ***Tamarindus indica*** Linn.

b- Watt. Dict.

c- Cultivated and widly grown or self sown.

II- a- चुक्रिका (Cukrikā), चिञ्चिका (Ciñcikā), चिञ्चा (Ciñcā), तित्तिडीका (Tittiḍīkā),

---

१ 'विष्टम्भि' इति मुद्रितपुस्तके पाठः । रा. नि. पाठः 'विष्टम्भ' वातजित् ।

b- (Mar.), Cincā; (Tel.) Amlikā; (H.P.) Imli, Amli; (B). Ambli, Tenluli, (Tam) Amilam; (Mal.) Amlam.

क्षुद्राम्लिका Kśudrāmlikā (7)

क्षुद्राम्लिका तु चांगेरी लोणिका चाम्ललोणिका ।
लोला लोणा चतुष्पर्णी सैव दन्तशठा मता ॥ ३३

चांगेरी कफवातघ्नी ग्राहिण्युष्णा च पित्तकृत् ।
अम्ला क्षुद्राम्लिका प्रोक्ता स्वादूष्णा सकषायका ॥३४

ग्रहण्यर्शो विकारघ्नी सामवातकफे हिता ।

क्षुद्राम्लिका (Kśudrāmlikā), चांगेरी (Cāngerī), लोणिका (Loṇikā), अम्लुलोणिका (Amlaloṇikā), लोला (Lolā), लोणा (Loṇā), चतुष्पर्णी (Catuṣparṇī) and दन्तशठा (Dantaśaṭhā) are synonymous.

Cāngerī pacifies *kapha* and *vātadoṣa* is astringent, *uṣṇavīrya* and aggravates *pittadoṣa*. It is sour, sweet and *kaśāya* (astringent)and useful in *Grahaṇi*, piles and *Āmavata* and *kapha doṣas*.

Fam. Oxalidaceae

I- a- ***Oxalis corniculata*** Linn.

b- Kamat C. Wildly self grown in gardens. Himalaya.

II- a- चांङ्गेरी (Cāngerī), अम्ललोणिका (Amlaloṇikā), चतुष्पर्णी (Catuṣparṇī) दन्तशठा (Dantaśaṭhā).

b- (H). Amrul; (Mar.) Ambuti; (Tam.) Paliyakiri; (Tel.) Pulicinta; (Mal.) Poliyarala.

7. (७) आरुकम् (Ārukam)

आरुकं वीरसेनं तु वीरं वीरारुकं तथा ॥ ३५
विद्याज्जातिविशेषेण तच्चतुर्विधमारुकम् ॥
आरुकाणि च हृद्यानि मेहार्शोनाशनानि च ॥ ३६

आरुकं (Ārukam), वीरसेनं (Vīrasenam), वीरं (Vīram), वीरारुकं

(Vīrārukam), are the four kinds of *Ārukam.*

All these four kinds of *Ārukas* are cordial and useful for disorders characterized by polyuria (including diabetes) and piles.

(Nighaṇṭus have noted only four species from which hundreds of varieties and kinds are developed now, known as 'Apricot' (Zardālu), 'Peach' (Āḍu, Āru), sweet and sour cherry (Ālubālu, Gilās) 'Plum' (Alubukhārā) etc. etc.

Being such circumstances it is difficult to identify from the modern developed varieties, which of them aptly corresppond to those of Nighaṇṭus. But it may be presumed that Nighaṇṭu's four plants are the original source of modern developed kinds and varieties. We are noting some of them herebelow.

IV - See following books.

1) Nelson, Hill - ***Prunus armeniaca*** Linn.
Eng. Apricot, Ūrumāṇa.

2) Nelson, Hill - ***Prunus persica*** Batsch.
Eng. Stone fruit, Peach.

3) Hill
Prunus cerasus Linn.
Sour Cherry.
P. avium Linn.
Eng. sour & sweet cherry.

4) Nelson - ***Prunus domestica*** L. Var. ***communis*** Huds.

5) Nelson, Dymock.
Pyrus communis Linn.
Eng. Pear.

6) Hill, Yadavji, Desai
Malus sylvestrus Mill.
Syn. *Pyrus malus* Linn.
Eng. Apple.

7) Hill
Cydonia oblonga Mill
Eng. Quince.

8) *Āruka is Prunus domsetica* Linn. (H.) Ālubukhāra आलूबुखार, other edible prunus fruits together with *P. persica* Batsch. आड़, Āḍu. Pichesū पिचसू and *Prunus armeniaca* Linn.Khubānī खुबानी, Cola चोला may provide some clues for the identification of Pichu पिचु Nicula, निचुल (Balwantji p. 38.)

8. (८) भवम् Bhavam

भवं भव्यं भविष्यं च भावनं वक्त्रशोधनम् ।
तथा पिच्छिलबीजं च तच्च रोमफलं मतम् ॥ ३७
भव्यमम्लं च वातघ्नं पिच्छिलं वक्त्रशोधनम् ।

भवं (Bhvam), भव्यं (Bhavyam), भविष्यं (Bhaviṣyam), भावनं (Bhāvanam), वक्त्रशोधनम् (Vaktraśodhanam), पिच्छिलबीजं (Picchilabījam), and रोमफलं (Romaphalam) are synonymous.

The *Bhavya* (fruit) is sour in taste, slimy, pacifies *vātadoṣa* and clears the mouth.

(Fam. Dilleniaceae)

I- a- ***Dillenia indica*** Linn.
b- U.C.Dutta c-all over india but rare in South India (?), plentiful from Southern Canara south wards.

II- a- वक्त्रशोधनम् (Vaktraśodhanam), पिच्छिलबीजम् (Picchilabījam), रोमफलम् (Romaphalam), भव्यम् (Bhavyam)
b- (Mar: Bom) Karambela; (H.B.) Mothā Chaltā; (Tam.) Ulva; (Tel.) Pedda kalinga; (Kan.) Betta Kanangala; (Sans.) Bhavya.
Habitat- large evergreen tree of Bengal, central and southern India. Eastern peninsula ... becomes plentiful from south canara southwards.
Medicine - The juice of the fruit ... in fever, bark is used medicinally. The Fruit is large about- 4,6 inches in diameter and surrounded by accrescent calyces, which when the fruit is fully grown (in February) have an agreeable acid taste and are eaten by the natives either raw or cooked ... and also made into a pleasant jelly. (Watt. III. 13)
There is also a tree of the same modern name identified as *D. pentagyna* Roxb. but it may not have been used for medicinal purpose. The leaves of which are used as dishes and thatching houses. The berries are acid taste. It is a deciduous tree while (Bhavam) (I-a above) is an evergreen tree.

9. (९) तिन्दुकः Tindukaḥ

तिन्दुको नीलसारश्च कालस्कन्धोऽतिमुक्तकः ॥ ३८
स्फूर्जकः स्फूर्जनस्तुष्टः स्पन्दनो रामणो रवः ॥

द्वितीयस्तिन्दुकः काकतिन्दुर्मर्कटतिन्दुकः ॥ ३९
काकेन्दुकश्च विख्यातः कपीलुः काकतिन्दुकः ॥

आमं कषायं संग्राहि तिन्दुकं वातकोपनम् ॥ ४०
विपाके गुरु संपक्वं मधुरं कफपित्तजित् ॥ S.Sū. 46. 168

तिन्दुकः (Tindukaḥ), नीलसारः (Nīlasāraḥ), कालस्कन्धः (Kālaskandhaḥ), अतिमुक्तकः (Atimuktakaḥ), स्फूर्जकः (Sphūrjakaḥ), स्फूर्जनः (Sphurjanaḥ), तुष्टः (Tuṣṭaḥ), स्पन्दनः (Spandanaḥ), रामणः (Rāmaṇaḥ), and रवः (Ravaḥ) are synonymous.

There is an another kind of *Tindukaḥ* called as काकतिन्दुः (Kākatinduḥ) and मर्कटतिन्दुकः (Markatatinduḥ), काकेन्दुकः (Kākendukaḥ), कपीलुः (Kapīluḥ), and काकतिन्दुकः (Kākatindukaḥ), are its synonyms.

The unripe fruit of *tinduka* is *kaṣāya* (astringent) in taste and astringent in action and aggravates *vāta doṣa.* When the fruit is fully ripe it is sweet in taste, and *guru* after *vipāka,* and pacifies *kapha* and *pitta doṣas.*

(Under this heading are included two kinds, one of it is A-नीलसारः (Nīlasārah) and the next is B काकतिन्दुकः (Kākatindukaḥ)

Fam. Ebenaceae.

I- A-a- ***Diospyros melanoxylon*** Roxb.

b- Watt Dict. (See bellow IV -2)

A-a2) ***D. peregrina*** Gurke*

Syn.

D. embryopteris Pers.

D. malabarica Desr. (Chopra)

D. glutinefera Roxb.

D. glutinosa Koen.

(Watt. 'D' 141)

b- Kamat, Ni. Adarsha.

c- See below IV 3

B-a- *Diospyros tomentosa* Roxb.* *

b- Roxburgh (C.B.C. edi. p. 419) and watt. Dict. Vol III -155

c See below IV 4 watt Dict.

II- A-a- नीलसारः (Nîlasāraḥ), कालस्कन्धः (Kālaskandhaḥ), स्पन्दनः (Spandanaḥ).b-A-1) (H.B.) Tendu; (Bom. Mar.) Temburni; (Tam.) Karuthumb; (Tel.)Timmuri , Damdoli; (Kan) Balai; (Sans) Kenduk

---

* The current name for *D. peregrina* Gurke is *D. malabarica* (Desr.) Kostel.

** The current accepted name for *D. tomentosa* Roxb. is *D. exculpta* Buch.-Ham.

(Eng.) Coromondel Ebony. (Watt, III. 147)

A-b-2) Gāb; (Tel.)Tinduki; (Kan). Bandar mar; (Tam) Tumbi; (Mar. Bom.) Temburnui. (Watt. Dict.) III. 141

B-a तिन्दुक : (Tindukaḥ), *Kākatindukaḥ, Markat tindukaḥ*

b- (H.) Mithā tendu; (Tel.) Chilta Timiki (San) *Kakatinduka.* (Watt. Dict. III. 155)

III a- 1 See below IV Balwantji

b- 1) 29स्फूर्जः- कालस्कन्धा कालसारा तनुका दीर्घनख्ययोः । स्पन्दिता स्फूर्जनः स्फूर्जो लोके 'तन्दू' इति विश्रुतः । इति । (Harshe)

2) 23-काकतिन्दुकः कपीलुः
'कपीलुः कुलकः काकतिन्दुकः काकपीलुकः ।
काकेन्दुर्विषतिन्दुश्च लोके तु 'कुचिला'ऽभिधः ।
पादपो विषतिन्द्वाख्यो दीर्घशेलुदलः कटुः ।
तद्बीजं वृन्तकठिनं शाणिकं पाण्डुलोमश' मिति ॥
(Harshe)

Note- In this reference two plants are recorded काकतिन्दुक, विषतिन्दुक i.e. कुचिला

IV 1) तिन्दुक (Tinduka)
तिन्दुकी
Diospyros tomentosa Roxb.
D. melanoxylon Roxb.
D. embryopteris Pers.
केन्दु, तिरला and मकरतेन्द (H.)
Syn.कालस्कन्धः विरला, and स्फूर्जक
C.S.Sū 4.43; 25. 139 49; etc.
S.Sū. 12-26; 38-48; 42-18 etc.
A.H.Ci. 12-12; 14-117; etc

These species yield fruits which are edible when ripe. *D. montana* Roxb. is called विषतेन्द (Viṣatenda) (Balwantji p. 182)

Note- About the fruit of *D. montana* Roxb. there are conflicting remarks about the posion. It is recorded in Watt. Dict. (III-151-52). The authour of शिवकोश notes विषतिन्दुक as लोके कुचिला ' *

2) *D. melanoxylon* Roxb.
Coromondel ebony.
Habitat- A large tree .. height of 60 to 80 ft. ceylon, malabar, Coromondel.orissa (Roxb.), western representative first as *D.*

* Here is a reference which shows how one plant name is identified by another plant in the later period कुचिला (Kucilā) is *Strychnos nuxvomica.* Linn. S.D. Kamat.

tomentosa might be said to be the eastern and western Indian form.

Structure of the wood

Hard, of a light pink colour ... It is used for building shoulder poles and carriage shafts, and ebony for all purposes, for carving purposes..... (Watt. Dict. III 149)

3) *D. embryopteris* Pers.

(Syn. *D. peregrina* see above I- a-A2 chopra)

Habitat- A dense evergreen small tree with dark green foilage and long shining leaves common throughout India and Burma except arid and dryzones of Punjab.

Distributed to Ceylon, Siam, and the Malayan Peninsula.

Structure of the wood

Grey, moderately hard, close grained .... used for building pur poses. Also the masts and yards of country vessels are made from the tree in Ceylon.

Domestic uses. The carpenters of the Malabar coasts use the juice of the fruit as an excellent glue. (Watt. III 143- 43)

4) *D. tomentosa* Roxb. (See above I-a-B)

Kakenduka (San.)

Habitat -A small crooked tree found in the northern parts of Bengal, Behar, Chutia Nagpur, Bundelkhand and extended to the tract of Punjab.

Food When ripe the berries are yellowish and are filled with a soft yellowish, sweetish astringent pulp, eaten by natives.

Structure of the wood

....Black hard and heavy and is in short the ebony of Bengal ... It carves well. (Watt. III 155)

10. (१०) विकङ्कतः Vikaṅkataḥ

विकंकतो मृदुफलो ग्रन्थिलः स्वादुकण्टकः ॥ ४१
गोपकण्टः काकपादो व्याघ्रपादोऽथ किंकिणी ।

गोपकण्टः[१] रसे तिक्तः शीतलः शोफनाशनः ॥ ४२
हन्ति श्लेष्माणत्युग्रमुद्रत्तं हन्ति योगतः ।

विकंकतः (Vikaṅkataḥ), मृदुफलः (Mṛduphalaḥ), ग्रन्थिलः (Granthilaḥ),

१ 'गोपघोटः' । इति आनन्दा. पाठः ।

स्वादुकण्टकः (Swādukanṭakaḥ), गोपकण्टः (Gopakanṭaḥ), काकपादः (Kākapādaḥ), व्याघ्रपादः (Vyāghrapādaḥ), and किंकिणी (Kinkiṇī) are synonymous.

Vikankata is bitter in taste, *śītavīrya* and useful in oedma. It pacifies *kapha doṣa* and by proper use is useful in severe haemorragic disorders.

(Fam. Flacourtiaceae)

I- a- ***Flacourtia indica*** Merr.*
Syn. *F. ramontchi* L'Herit.
b- Balwantji
c- See - IV- below.

II- a- स्वादुकण्टकः (Swādu kanṭakaḥ), मृदुफलः (Mṛuduphalaḥ), किङ्किणी (Kinkiṇī), गोपघोटः (Gopaghoṭaḥ), (Dhn. ni.) स्रुवद्रुमः (Sṛuvadrumaḥ), यज्ञीयः (Yajñīyaḥ), ब्रह्मपादपः (Brahmapādapaḥ).

b) (H) Bilangra, Bhanker; (B)Katai, Tāmbal; (Bom.) Swādu kanṭaka Tambat; kaikiṇī, Bhaikal; (Mar.) Pahār, Bhekal Aturṇi; (Mahirwal) kaikan; (Tel.) Kanergu, Pedda Kanru. (Watt. III. 399) Eng. Governor's plum.

III 1) See below IV -1 Balwantji
2) वैकङ्कती -यज्ञीयपात्रम् । (Nārāyanbhatti)
3) वैकङ्कती स्रुवा भवति -खदिरः स्रुवा भवति । (S.K.S. p.3)
4) इध्म-पलाश, वैकंकत (शतपथ ब्रा. दर्शपूर्णमास (१.३.४. ४.) referred in S. K. S. p. 192.

b-1) विकङ्कते प्रसरति विकङ्कतः ककि गत्यर्थः ।,
स्रुवा स्रुक् सा हि वैकङ्कती आम्नाता । (Ksiraswami Amar 2-4-36)
2) 209 स्रुवोद्रुमः 'व्याघ्रपादः स्रुवतरुः स्वादुकण्टो विकङ्कते ।'इति केयदेवः ।
'वृक्षकण्टकारी' ति डल्हणः । (Harshe)

IV- 1) विकङ्कत (Vikankata)
Flacourtia indica Merr.
Syn. *Flacourtia ramontchi* L'Herit
कटाय, कवैया (H.); बैच्या (B.)
C. S. 27. 142; Vi 8-150 etc.
S.S. Cī- 11-9 etc.
A.H. Ci 3-135 V. 3 7-82 वैकङ्कती
Some have however attempted to identify it with *Gymnosporia*

---

* The current accepted name is *F. indica* (Burm.f.) Merr. (Comp.p. 66)

spinosa (Forsk) Fiori having some what similar names.Bopadeva has mentioned कण्टकी *kaṇṭakī* and कण्टकारिका *kaṇṭakarikā* tobe synonyms of कण्टकारी Solanum speices.

(Balvantji. p. 368)

2) *Flacorutia ramontchi* L. Herit
Syn. *F. sapida* Roxb.
Governor's plum.
Habitat - A small thorny deciduous tree met within dry hill throughout India.
Food & Fodder The fruit and the leaves are eaten, the former is the size of the plum, has a sharp but sweetish taste and is used either raw or cooked . The leaves are used as cattle fodder.

(Watt III 399)

3) *Flacourtia indica* Merr.
F. ramontchi L' herit.
Eng. Governors plum.
Considerable confusion exists regarding the nomenclature of this species. It has been included along with *F . sepiaria* under *F. indica.* Indian workers prefer to keep these two separately.

(Wealth of India)

4) *Flacourtia sapida* Roxb. (?)
विकङ्कत (Dr. Raghuivr IV. 3-14).

11. (११) मधूकः Madhūkaḥ

मधूको मधुवृक्षस्तु मधुष्ठीलो मधुस्रवः ॥ ४३
गुडपुष्पो लोध्रपुष्पो वानप्रस्थोऽथ माधवः ।

मधूकं मधुरं शीतं पित्तदाहश्रमापहम् ॥ ४४
वातलं न तु दोषघ्नं वीर्यपुष्टिविवर्धनम् ।

बृंहणीयमहृद्यं च मधूककुसुमं गुरु ॥ ४५
वातपित्तोपशमनं फलं तस्योपदिश्यते । S.S. Su 46. 186

मधूकः (Madhūkaḥ), मधुवृक्षः (Madhuvṛkaśaḥ), मधुष्ठीलः (Madhuṣṭ-hīlaḥ), मधुस्रवः (Madhusravaḥ), गुडपुष्पः (Guḍapuṣpaḥ), लोध्रपुष्पः (Lodhrapuṣpaḥ), वानप्रस्थः (Vānaprasthaḥ), माधवः (Mādhavaḥ), are synonymous.

Madūka is sweet in taste, *śītavīrya,* it pacifes *pitta,* is useful in burning sensation, removes fatigue.It does not pacify *doṣās* but aggravates *vāta*. It is energizer and nourishing.

The flowers of *Madhūka* are body promoting, non cordial and *guru*.

Its fruit pacifies *vāta pitta doṣas*.

(Fam. Sapotaceae)

I- a- ***Madhuca indica*** J. F. Gmel.*
Syn. *M. latifolia* (Roxb.) Macbride
Bassia latifolia (Roxb.)
(Chopra)

b- Roxburgh C- See bellow IV- 1

II- a मधुवृक्षः (Madhuvṛkṡaḥ), मधुष्ठीलः (Madhuṣṭhīlaḥ), मधुस्रवः (Madhusravaḥ), गुडपुष्पः (Guḍapuṣpaḥ) माधवः (Mādhavaḥ).

b- (H) Mahuā; (B) Mavhā; (Mar.) Moha, Mohata; (Tam.) Kattiluppai; (Tel.) Madhukamu; (Mal.) Irippa; (Eng.) Illipa Butter.(Hill).

IV- 1) ***Bassia latifolila*** Roxb.
The Butter or Mahua tree.
Habitat. A large deciduous tree .... indigenous ... C. P., Kangra, Komaon, and oudh, western Ghat, plentiful in the part of Bombay Presidency. (Watt. Dict. I- 406)

2) मधूक Madhūka.
Madhuca indica J. F. Gmel.
C.Sū. 3.20. 4.32 etc.
S.S. Sū 2.4. 16.45 etc.
A.H.Sū 6-110; 9-26; 10.24 etc.
The synonym मधु may be used for Madhuka or Madhūka.
(Balwantji p. 296).

3) मधूकपुष्पी – (Madhūkapuṣpī)
C.S. IV. 8-146.
Other species of Madhūka i.e. *M. butyracea* (Roxb.) Macbride etc.may be substituted for *Madhuka* and called *Madhukapuspi*.
(Balvantji p. 296)

4) *Bassia butyracea* Roxb.
The Indian butter tree. (H.) Phalwar or Phulwārā.

---

* The current accepted name is *Madhuca longifolia* (Koen.) Macbride.
M. indica & *M. longifolia* listed as two distinct species, are now treated as one species.मधूक Madhūka & दीर्घपत्रक मधूक Dīrgha patraka madhūka are mentioned separately in Dhn. ni. see the next plant S. D. Kamat

The butter from the fruit is called chaurā -ke- pinā (Almora) and Phulel or Phalwārā (in the plains)
Habitat -A deciduous tree of the sub Himalayan tract from konkan to Bhutan. (Watt. I-405)

जलदः Jaladaḥ (8)

मधूकोऽन्यो द्वितीयस्तु जलदो दीर्घपत्रकः ॥ ४६
ह्रस्वपुष्पो फलस्वादुः गौडिकोऽथ मधूलिका ।

(अन्यो जलमधूकस्तु मधुपुष्पो जलाख्यकः ॥
रसपुष्पो दीर्घपत्रो गोरङ्को मधुपुष्पिकः ।) *

ज्ञेयो जलमधूकस्तु मधुरो व्रणनाशनः ।
वृष्यो वान्तिहरः शीतो बलकारी रसायनः ॥ ४७

There is an another type of *Madhūka* called as जलमधूक (Jalamadhūka) of which synonyms are जलदः (Jaladaḥ), दीर्घपत्रकः (Dīrghapatrakaḥ), ह्रस्वपुष्पः (Rhasvapuṣpaḥ), फलस्वादुः (Phalaswāduḥ), गौडिकः (Gauḍikaḥ) and मधूलिका (Madhūlikā).

According to different version mentioned in Anandāsram edition follwoing synonyms are noted जलमधूकः (Jalamadhūkaḥ), मधुपुष्पः (Madhupuṣpaḥ), जलाख्यकः (Jalākhyakaḥ), रसपुष्पः (Rasapuṣpaḥ), दीर्घपत्रः (Dīrghapatraḥ), गोरङ्कः (Gorankaḥ) and मधुपुष्पिकः (Madhupuṣpikaḥ)

Jalamadhūka is sweet in taste, *śītavīrya,* useful in wound *healing, vṛṣya,* antiemetic, strength promoting and *rasāyana* (rejuvinating).

I-(Under this heading two species are included. One of them is 'A' जलदः Jaladaḥ and the next is 'B' जलमधूकः (Jalamadhūkaḥ). Both of the same family.)

Fam. Sapotaceae.

A-a- ***Madhuca longifolia*** (L) Macbride.**
Syn. *Bassia longifolia* willd (Watt Dict.)

b- Kamat.

c- See below IV-1

---

* इत्यधिकः पाठःआनन्दा. मुद्रित पुस्तके दृश्यते ।

** Some authors have merged *M. indica* J.F. Gmel and *M. longifolia* (Koenig) Macbr. under the latter name, distinguishing var. *longifolia* and var. *latifolia* (Roxb.) Chewal. (U.P.I. p. 347)

II A-a जलदः (Jaladaḥ), दीर्घपत्रकः (Dīrghapatrakaḥ), ह्रस्वपुष्पः (Rhaswapuṣpaḥ), गौडिकः (Gauḍikaḥ), मधूकोऽन्योद्वितीयः (Madhūkonyo dwitīyaḥ).

A-b (Bom. H.) Local names as in Madhūka proper.

B-a अन्यो जलमधूकः (Anyo Jalamadhūkaḥ), मधुपुष्पः (Madhupuṣpaḥ), मधुपुष्पिकः (Madhupuṣpikaḥ) (Dhn. Ni.)

B-b Modern names as Madhūka proper (I-a-A) मधूकपुष्पी (Madhūkapuspī) see मधूक (Madhūka) S. No. pre (II-IV-3 Supra)

IV- 1) *Bassia longifolia* Willd.
The Mowa or Mauha tree of South India (Tam.) Illupi, Iruppai; (Mar.) Mohāche Jhāda; (H) Moha, Mahuwa
Habitat. A large evergreen tree of south India and ceylon common in Canara, Mysore, Malabar and circars.
Food - Economic use of this tree in the south are similar to those of *B. latifolia* in the central table land of India.
(Watt,. Dict. I-416)

2) *Bassia malabarica* Bedd.
A middle sized tree native of south Canara, Malabar and Annamallaya.
A very nearly allied species to the Ceylons.
B. nerifolia Moon (Watt. Dict. 416)

12. (१२) पीलुः Pīluḥ

पीलुः शीतः सहस्रांशी धानी गुडफलोऽपि च ॥
विरेचनफलः शाखी श्यामः करभवल्लभः ॥४८

रक्तपित्तहरः पीलुः फलं कटुविपाकी च ।*
अर्शोघ्नं बस्तिशमनं सस्नेहं कफवातजित ॥४९
(पीलुजं च रसे स्वादु गुल्मार्शोघ्नं तु तीक्ष्णकम ।) S.Sū.46

पीलुः (Pīluḥ), शीतः (Śitaḥ), सहस्रांशी (Sahasrānśī), धानी (Dhānī), गुडफलः (Guḍaphalaḥ), विरेचनफलः (Virecanaphalaḥ), शाखी (Śākhī), श्यामः (Śyāmaḥ), and करभवल्लभः are synonymous.

Pīluḥ is useful in haemorrhagic disorders (see the differance in F.N.) Its fruit is pungent in *Vipāka.* It is useful in piles, disorders of urinary tract,

* 'तिक्तं' पित्तकरं तेषां सरं कटुविपाकी च । 'S.Sū.46. 195.

slightly unctuous and pacifies *kapha* and *vāta doṣas.*

(According to bracketed version -the fruit is sweet in taste and useful in tumors (or diverticulosis) , piles and is *tīkṣṇa* (sharp).

बृहत्पीलुः Bṛhat Pīluḥ (Raj. ni.)

अन्यच्चैव बृहत्पीलुर्महापीलुर्महाफलः ।
राजपीलुर्महावृक्षो मधुपीलुः षडाह्वयः ॥

मधुरस्तु महापीलुर्वृष्यो विषविनाशनः ।
पित्तप्रशमनो रुच्यः आमघ्नो दीपनीयकः ॥ Raj. Ni. Chap. 11

There is an another kind of पीलुः (Pīluḥ), called as बृहत्पीलुः (Bṛhatpīluḥ) of which synonyms are महापीलुः (Mahāpīluḥ), महाफलः (Mahāphalaḥ), राजपीलुः (Rājapīluḥ), महावृक्षः (Mahāvṛksaḥ), and मधुपीलुः (Madhupīluḥ) (total names six).

Mahāpīluḥ (?fruit) is sweet in taste *vṛsya,* antidote to poisons and pacifies *pittadoṣa.* It is appetizer, pacifies *āmadoṣa* and stimulates digestive capacity.

I (Under this heading Dhn. Ni. notes one but Raj. Ni. notes two kinds of plants A- (Pīluḥ) & B- (Bṛhatpīluḥ)

Fam. Salvadoraceae.

A-a-***Salvadora oleoides*** Decne.
b- Chopra
c- See below IV-1
B-a-***Salvadora persica*** Linn.*
b-Chopra c-See below IV

II- A-a- धानी (Dhānī) ,गुडफलः (Guḍaphalaḥ), विरेचनफलः (Virecanaphalaḥ), शाखी (Śākhī), श्यामः (Śyāmaḥ), करभवल्लभः (Karabhavallabhaḥ),
b- (Mar), Pīlu, Khākani, Kinkan, Sārī; (H). Bahaphal; (Tam) Kalav.
B-a- बृहत्पीलुः (Bṛhatpīluḥ), महापीलुः (Mahapīluḥ),महाफलः (Mahāphalaḥ), मधुपीलुः (Madhupīluḥ).
b- (Bom) Pilu; (Mar.) Rānmiri; (Tam) Perungoli; (Tel.) Gogu.

IV- 1) *Salvadora oleoides* Don.

---

* Current name for *Salvadora persica* Linn. is *Salvadora persica* Linn. var. *wightiana* (Planch ex Thw.) Verdc.

(Mar) Khakin, Pilu (Oil) Kinknel.

Habitat - A large evergreen shrub or tree of the arid tracts of Sind, Punjab, and Rajasthan. It extends to trans Himalaya Hills.

Food- The fruits are eaten by the natives, large number of whom go out to collect in the season. (Watt. Dict. IV. 448)

2) *Salvadora persica* Linn.

The tooth brush (tree), Mustards tree (Royle); (H.) Pilu (or chota Pilu); (Bom.) Pilu, khakan; (Tam.) opa, Karkol, Kabariva; (Tel.) waragu venki, shunia.

Habitat. - A small evergreen tree in drier parts of India from Punjab, Sind to Patna, Southward to Konkan, Persia, Syria, Arabia and East Africa.

Food - The fruits (or small berries) are eaten by natives of India. They have a strong aromatic smell and a pungent taste like mustard or garden cresses and are not very much appreciated as article of diet.

13. (१३) खर्जूरी Kharjūrī

खर्जूरी तु खरस्कन्धा कषाया मधुराग्रजा ।
दुष्प्रधर्षा दुरारोहा निःश्रेणी स्वादुमस्तका ॥५०

क्षतक्षयापहं हृद्यं शीतलं तर्पणं गुरु ।
रसे पाके च मधुरं खर्जूरं रक्तपित्तजित् ॥ ५१

खर्जूरी (Kharjūrī), खरस्कन्धा (Kharaskandhā), कषाया (Kaṣāya), मधुराग्रजा (Madhurāgrajā), दुष्प्रधर्षा (Duṣpradharṣā), दुरारोहा (Durārohā), निःश्रेणी (Niḥsreṇī), and स्वादुमस्तका (Swādumastakā) are synonymous.

Kharjūra (the fruit) is cordial, consumption due to injury (or pulm. cavities) *śitavirya,* sweet in taste and in *vipāka* and *guru*. It is useful as satiating and in haemorrhagic disorders.

Fam. Palmae

I- a- ***Phoenix sylvestris*** Roxb.*

b- Roxburgh C) All over India wild and cultivated for Tāḍī (Toddy) (ताडी)

II a- खरस्कन्धा (Kharaskandhā), दुरारोहा (Durārohā), निःश्रेणी (Nihśreṇī), स्वादुमस्तका (Swādumastakā)

b- (Mar.) Khajūrī, sindi, god-sindi; (Mal) Kalinta; (Tel) Pedda

* The current name is *P. sylvestris* (Linn) Roxb.

yetoo; (Eng.) The Wild date, Date sugar Palm.

III- See Dīpyā, Pālewata.

IV- 1) *Phoenix sylvestris* Roxb.

.... produce an inferior yellowish or reddish fruit eaten by native boys and the poor classes .... extensive utilisation of its sap in making sugar. (Watt. Dict. VI. 1 209).

2) see Roxb Fl. indi, CBC p. -122-23.

दीप्या Dīpyā

दीप्या[1] च पिण्डखर्जूरी स्थलपिण्डा मधुस्रवा ।
फलपुष्पा स्वादुपिण्डा हयभक्षा रसाभिधा[2] ॥ ९४

दीप्या (Dīpyā), पिण्डखर्जूरी (Piṇḍakharjūrī), स्थलपिण्डा (Sthalapiṇḍā), मधुस्रवा (Madhusravā), फलपुष्पा (Phalapuṣpā), स्वादुपिण्डा (Swādupiṇḍā), and हयभक्षा (Hayabhakṡā), these seven are synonymous.

(The plants noted by the Nighaṇṭus under this heading are the species of phoenix genus. Dhn. ni. notes only one kind but Raj. ni. has noted three to four kinds more. Raj. Ni's plants are not identified here but only Dhn. Ni's plant is noted here below)

I- a- ***Phoenix dactylifera*** Linn.

b- c-

II- a- पिण्डखर्जूरी (Piṇḍakharjūrī), स्थलपिण्डा (Sthalapiṇḍā), फलपुष्पा (Phalapuṣpā), स्वादुपिण्डा (Swādupiṇḍā).

b- (H.B. Mar.) Khajur; (Tam.) Parichum; (Tel.) Khajuram; (Sans.) Piṇḍa Kharjūrī; (Eng.) The edible date.

III- a- See below IV -1 Balwantji.

IV 1) खर्जूरी Kharjurī.

C.S.Sū. 4-40, 23-37 etc.

S.S. Sū. 42-18, 45-174 etc.

A.H. Su . 5-72, 6-109 etc.

Kharjura is the name of the fruit. *Kharjūrī* is the source plant and *Kharjura mastaka* खर्जूर मस्तक, *Kharjūramadhya* खर्जूरमध्य and *kharjūra majjā* is the edible growing point of the stem. Different kinds of kharjūrī belong to differnet species of Phoneix

---

१ परद्वीपात समागता इति व्यवहारात् द्वीप्या इति साधु पाठः । S.D. Kamat.
२ 'स्वराभिधा' इति रा. नि. पाठः । साधु च ।

i.e. *P.sylvestris* Roxb, *P.dactylifera* Linn. (The true Arabian date palm); *P. acaulis* Buch.- Ham. but the fruits of former two only are used. The edible growing end of the stem especially the pith appears to have been used under the name *kharjura mastaka*.It may be interesting to note that some professional people are seen selling small pieces of the decorticated and big reddish tuberous structure which they call Mūlakanda मूलकन्द or Rāmakanda . रामकन्द (Balwantji p. 131).

---

14. (१४) द्राक्षा Drākṡā

द्राक्षा चारुफला कृष्णा प्रियाला तापसप्रिया ।
काश्मीरिका विनिर्दिष्टा रसाला करमर्दिका ॥ ५३

द्राक्षा हृद्यरसा स्वर्या मधुरा स्निग्धशीतला ।
रक्तपित्तज्वरश्वास तृष्णादाहक्षयापहा ॥५४

द्राक्षा (Drākṡā), चारुफला (Cāruphalā), कृष्णा (Kṛṣṇā), प्रियाला (Priyālā), तापसप्रिया (Tāpasapriyā), काश्मीरिका (Kāṡmīrikā), रसाला (Rasālā), and करमर्दिका (Karamardikā) are synonymous.

Drākṡa is cordial, improves voice, is sweet in taste, and *sītavīrya*. It is useful in haemorrhagic disorders (*Raktapitta*), fevers, dyspnoea, thirst. burning sensation and consumption.

(Fam. Vitaceae)

I- a- ***Vitis vinifera*** Linn.
b- c- Cultivated.

II- a- कृष्णा (Kṛṣṇā),काश्मीरिका(Kāṡmīrikā), करमर्दिका (Karamardikā)
b- (H.B.D.) Angūra, Darāk; (Bom. Mar.), Drākṡa, Manukā (dried); (Tel.) (Kan.) Drākṡā; (Tam) Kottani; (Mal.) Gostani.; (Eng.) Wine grape.

उत्तरापथिका Uttarāpathikā (10)

उत्तरापथिका प्रोत्ता कपिला सा फलोत्तमा ।
स्वादुपाका मधुरसा मृद्वीका गोस्तनी स्मृता ॥५५

मृद्वीका मधुरा स्निग्धा शीता वृष्यानुलोमनी
रक्तानिलश्वासकासभ्रमतृष्णाज्वरापहा ॥ ५६

उत्तरापथिका (Uttarāpathikā) a type of *Drāks'ā* has synonyms as कपिला (Kaphilā), स्वादुपाका (Swādupākā), मधुरसा (Madhurasā), मृद्वीका (Mṛdvīkā) and गोस्तनी (Gostanī).

Mṛdvīkā is sweet in taste, unctuous and *s'ītavīrya, vṛṣya* and mild laxative. It is useful in pacifying *rakta* and *vāta doṣas*, dyspnoea, cough, giddiness, thirst and fevers.

(Under this heading Dhn. Ni. notes a black coloured kind of northern (uttarāpathikā) region, but Raj. Ni. has recorded more two 'हरिता' (Haritā) and काकली (Kākalī).

I- a- Indian developed kinds of wine grape.
b- Kamat c-Cultivated.

II- a- कपिला (Kapilā), गोस्तनी (Gostanī), हरिता (Haritā), हारहूरा (Hārahūrā), काकली निर्बीजा (Kākalī nirbījā).
b- Modern names as in (Vide pre No. 14 Supra)
कपिला ((Kapilā) is known as काळी द्राक्ष (Kāḷidrāks'a), गोस्तनी(Gostanī) is oblong black drāks'ā, काकली (Kākalī) small sweet yellow *draks'ha* which has no seeds known as बेदाणा (Bedaṇā) in Maharashtra, हरिता (Haritā) may be round greenish bigger *drāks'ā.*

15. (१५) अक्षोडः Aks'odaḥ

अक्षोडः पार्वतीयश्च फलस्नेहो गुडाश्रयः[1] ।
कीरेष्टः कर्परालश्च[2] स्वादुमज्जा[3] पृथुच्छदः[4] ॥ ५८
अक्षोडकः स्वादुरसो मधुरः पुष्टिकारकः ।
पित्तश्लेष्मकरो बल्यः स्निग्धोष्णः गुरुबृंहणः ॥ ५९

अक्षोडः (Aks'odaḥ), पार्वतीयः (Pārvatīyaḥ), फलस्नेहः (Phalasnehaḥ), गुडाश्रयः (Guḍās'rayaḥ), कीरेष्टः (Kīreṣṭaḥ), कर्परालः (Karparālaḥ), स्वादुमज्जा (Swādumajjā), and पृथुच्छदः (Pṛthucchadaḥ) are synonymous.

---

१ 'गुहाश्रयः' इति नि.शे.टीका।
२ 'कन्दरालश्च' इति नि.शे. टीका।
३ 'स्वादुमज्जो' इति नि.शे. टीका।
४ 'मृदुच्छदः' इति नि.शे. टीका।

Ak̓soḍa is sweet in taste and in *vipāka*, *uṣṇavīrya*, *guru* and unctuous. It aggravates *pitta kapha doṣas*. It is nourishing, strength promoting, and bulk promoting.

(Fam. Juglandaceae)

I- a- ***Juglans regia*** Linn.

b- Chopra c- Wild and cultivated , temp. Himalaya, Khassi Hills, Baluchistan.

II- a- पार्वतीयः (Pārvatīyaḥ),

b- (Mar.) Akroḍa; (H.B.) Akrot; (Tam. Tel.) Akrottu; (Eng.) The Walnut tree; Persian Walnut.

III-a- See below IV 2- Balwantji.

IV- 1) *Juglans regia* Linn.
Syn. *J. regia* var. *kumaonica* DC.
Habitat. Wild and cultivated in the temparate Himalaya and Western Tibet ... distributed to Northern Persia etc.
(Watt. Dict. I. 162.)

2) अक्षोटAk̓soṭa, अक्षोड Ak̓soḍa
Juglans regia Linn. अखरोट (H.)
C.S. Sū. 13. 9, 26-112 (etc.)
Su. S. Sū 45-120. 46- 187 (etc.)
A.H. Sū. 6. 120, 10-22 (etc.)

3) Brandis mentions three varieties.

a) Tenera - (thin shelled)

b) Brandistana, c) Kamaonia.
at Chamba and Kashmir a superior quality is grown which is characterised by having a soft shell.
(Watt. Dict. IV. 550)

4) Walnuts - Number of species in the genus Juglans are included as walnuts. The most important is *Persian* (English) walnut (*J. regia* Linn.) a high source of vit C. The other species of Juglans ... do not show high vit C. (Nelson).

Wild Akrods

Fam. Euphorbiaceae.

1) ***Aleurites moluccana*** Willd.
Syn. *A. triloba* Forst.
The Belgum or the Indian Walnut. The Candle nut.
(B.H.) Akrot; (Sans,) Ak̓sota; (Mar. G.) Jophal, Akrot; (Tam.) Nattu Akrottu Kottai; (Tel.) Natu akrottu, Vittu; (Kan.) Natakrodu. (Watt. Dict. I- 163).

16.(१६) परुषकः Parūṣakaḥ

परुषकं परु प्रोक्तं नीलवर्णं परावरम् ॥
परिमण्डलमल्पास्थि[१] परुषं चापि नामतः॥ ६१

परुषकफलं चाम्लं वातघ्नं पित्तकृद् गुरु ।
तदेव पक्वं मधुरं वातपित्तनिबर्हणम् ॥ ६२

परुषकं (Paruṣakam),परु (Paru), नीलवर्णं (Nīlavarṇam), परावरम् (Parāvaram),परिमण्डलमल्पास्थि (Parimaṇḍalamalpāsthi) and परुषं (Paruṣam), are synonymous.

The fruit of *Paruṣaka* is sour in taste, pacifies *vātadoṣa* and aggravate *pittadoṣa* and is *guru.* But the same when fully ripe is sweet in taste, pacifies *vāta* and *pitta doṣas.*

(Fam. Tiliaceae).

I- a-***Grewia asiatica*** Linn.
b- Desai (Page 151) c- Cultivated
The wild state unknown.

II- a-नीलवर्ण or नीलपर्ण (Nīlavarṇa or Nīlaparṇa), परिमण्डल मध्यास्थि (Parimaṇḍala madhyāsthi), गिरिपीलु (Giripīlu).
b- (Mal, H.B.) Phālasā; (Tam) Palisa; (Tel.) Peddajana.

III a- C. Sū 27. 125, 129.
S. Sū 38. 43
A. H. Sū. 15-13
b- 1) परुषकः धन्वनपत्रकः पसिद्धः । स द्विविधः मधुराम्ल भेदेन ।
Cakra Su. 27. 43.
2) द्विधा वृक्ष विटपभेदात् । (Ḍalhaṇa Sū 38-43)
3) परुषकम् - मृदुफलं धन्वनच्छदः । (Aruna Su. 15-13)

17. तूलम् - (तूदं) Tūlam (Tūdam)

तूदं तूलं च यूपं च क्रमुकं ब्रम्हकाष्ठकम् ।
ब्रम्हदारु ब्राम्हणेष्टं[२] ब्रम्हण्यं ब्रम्हचारिणम्[३] ॥ ६३

---

* The current name for *G. asiatica* Linn. is *Grewia subinaequalis* DC.

१ 'माल्यास्थि' इति शोढल संमतः पाठः ।
'मध्यास्थि' इति आनन्दाश्रम पुस्तके ।
२ 'ब्रम्हनिष्ठं' इति नि.शे. टीकासंमतः पाठः ।
३ 'ब्रम्हचारि च' इति नि.शे. टीकासंमतः पाठः ।
'तथा ब्रम्हनाम च' इति शोढल पाठः ।

तूदं तु मधुराम्लं स्याद् वातपित्तहरं सरम् ।
दाहप्रशमनं वृष्यं कषायं कफनाशनम् ॥ ६२
(तूलस्य च फलं स्वादु बलवर्णाग्निवृद्धिकृत् ।)

तूदम् (Tūdam), तूलं (Tūlam), यूपं (Yūpam), क्रमुकं (Kramukam), ब्रह्मकाष्ठकम् (Brahmakāṣṭhakam),ब्रह्मदारु (Brahmadāru), ब्राह्मणेष्टम् (Brāhmaṇeṣṭam), ब्रह्मण्यं (Brāhmaṇyam), and ब्रह्मचारिणम् (Brahmacāriṇam) are synonymous.

Tūdam the fruit is sweet, sour and *kaṣāya* in taste, pacifies *vāta, pitta* and *kaphadoṣas* and is laxative. It alleviates burning sensation and is *vṛṣya*.

(It's fruit is sweet in taste and promotes strength, complexion and improves digestive capacity).

(Fam. Moraceae) (Chopra)
(Urticaceae) (watt.)

I- a- ***Morus indica*** Linn.
Syn. *Morus alba* var. *indica* Bureau
M. parvifolia Royle
M. acidosa Griff.
M. cuspidata Wall.
M. alba var. cuspidata Bureau

b- Watt. Dict. V. 281.

c- See IV- 1 below.

II- a- तूलम् (Tūlam), तूदम् (Tūdam), यूपम् (Yūpam), ब्रह्मदारु (Brahmadāru), ब्राह्मणेष्टम् (Brāhmaneṣṭam)(Dhn.Ni.) नीलवृन्तकम् (Nīlavṛntakam), क्रमुकम् (Kramukam), मृदुसारम् (Mṛdusāram) (Raj. Ni.).

b- (H.) Tut, tūtri (B.) Tut; (Bom) Tut, tutri, ambor Tula; (Mar.) Tut., (Tam). Kambili, pūch, Mush Kattai; (Tel.)Kambali būchi; (Kan). Hippal - nerali; (Sans) Shalmali vṛikshaḥa, Tuda. (Watt. II-281)

III-a- 1) See below IV -1 Balwantji

b- 1) 442 तूल इति ।
'पुंलिंगस्तु पिचौ तूलः क्लीबं स्यात् ब्रह्मदारुणि । इति रुद्रः । बह्मदारु ब्रह्मकाष्ठं' तूतं इति लोके । (Harshe)

IV 1) *Morus indica* Linn.
Habitat A moderate sized deciduous tree or shrub found in

The current name for *Morus. indica* Linn is *M. australis* Poir.

the temparate and subtropical Himalaya from kashmir to sikkim. Also met with wild and cultivated for silk worm feeding in Bengal, Assam and Burma. Distributed to China & Japan.

Food The fruit is inferior to that of *M. alba* (p. 281). The Indian white mulberry .... The fruit varies greatly in different localities ... *Brandis* writes there are many varieties sweet and acid and of all shades of colour from white to black purple.

2) See Hill p. 404 and As. Res. IV. 225.

3) तूद Tūda
Morus indica Griff
C.S. Sū. 27-132
A.H. Sū. 6-138
See क्रमुक, तोदन and पूग (Balvantji p. 189)
Note - Raj. Ni. has recorded a species of morus having fruits of नीलवृन्तक. This plant may be *Morus nigra* Linn. (Chopra) Hill notes it by the name 'Black mulberry'

18. (१८) पालेवतम् Pālevatam

पालेवतं रैवतकं ज्ञेयमारेवतं तथा ।
महापालेवतं चोक्तं रक्तपालेवतं तथा ॥ ६३
पालेवतं सितं पुष्पैस्तिन्दुकाभफलं मतम् ।
अन्यन्माणवकं ज्ञेयं महापालेवतं तथा ॥ ६४
पालेवतं तु मधुरं स्निग्धं हृद्यं समीरजित् ॥

पालेवतं (Pālevatam), रैवतकं (Raivatakam), आरेवतम् (Ārevatam), महापालेवतं (Mahāpālevatam), and रक्तपालेवतं (Raktapālevatam) are synonymous (in general).

White flowered and having the size of *tinduka* fruit is *Pālevatam; Mahāpālevatm* and *Māṇavakam* are other kinds.

Pālevatam is sweet in taste, unctuous and cordial. It pacifies *vātadoṣa*.

Under this heading the compiler of Dhn. Ni. has recorded four kinds which are 'A'पालेवतम् (Pālevatam), 'B' महापालेवतम् (Mahāpālevatam), 'C' रक्तपालेवतम् (Raktapālevatam), 'D' माणवकम् (Māṇavakam); Raj. Ni. records the following kinds 'E' पारेवतम (Pārevatam), 'F' महापारेवतम

(Mahāpārevatam) ,स्वर्णपारेवतम् (Swarṇa pārevatam), 'G' साम्राणिजम् स्वस्तिकं च रक्तपारेवतम् हि तत् ' H' बृहत् पारेवतं प्रोक्तं द्वीपज्जं द्वीपखर्जुरी ।

From the above description it can be summarized as follows.

i) Dhn. Ni.s' 'A' Pālevata and Raj. Ni's 'E' Pārevata are the same plants.

ii) Dhn. Nis 'B' Mahāpālevata and Raj. Nis. Mahāparevatam are the same plants.

iii) Dhn. Ni's 'C' Rakta pālevatam and Raj. Ni's 'G' Raktapārevatam are the same plants in which he includes 'Sāmrāṇijam' and kharjura kind. These two kinds seem to be edible date palms of India and Arabia.

iv) Raj. Ni's 'G' Mahāpārevata and 'H' Bṛhatpārevata may be the same plants to which he notes द्वीपी (Dwīpī) i.e. foreign plants. The name ' Sāmrāṇi' which includes in Raktakharjūra is also a foreign name.

From the above discussion it will be found that only four kinds 'A' 'E' Pālevata, 'B' 'F' Mahāpālevatam, 'C' 'G' Raktapālevatam and the fourth 'C' Māṇavaka (of Dhn. Ni. only) remain for identification and confirnation with the Nighaṇṭus recorded above and for the identification of above plants we have accepted family 'Palmae'

(Fam. Palmae)

I- A & E-a-***Phoneix pussilla*** Gaertn.
Syn. *P. farinifera* Roxb.
b- Chopra & watt Dict. VI-1
a- 'B' & 'F' species and varieties of trees those produce highclass fruits of edible dates of India and of foreign countries.
a- 'C' & 'G' may be black red coloured khārika (खारीक)
a- D- Not identified . (See III b-1)

II- a- 'A' and 'E' पाले or पारेवतम् (Pāle or Pārevatam), रैवतकम् (Raivatakam), आरेवतम् (Ārevatam), मधुकफल अमृत फलाख्यम् (Madhukaphala Amṛtaphalākhyam).
b- A and E (H.) Pālevata; (Tel.) chittaoita, It-kayyā; (Tam.) Etcham-Chatiu, Kassange; (Kan.) schal; (Mal.) chitintab (Watt. Dict. VI I. 207).
a- B and F महापालेवतम (Mahā pālevatam), स्वर्णपारेवतम् (Swarṇa pārevatam).
b- B and F modern names may be those of the best kinds of edible

date fruit of India and foreign (Dwīpī. द्वीपी)

a- C and G रक्तपालेवत (Raktapālevata), साम्राणि(Sāmrānī), रक्तरैवतकम् (Raktaraivatakam), खारीकम् (Khārikam)

b- As in Mahāpālevatam

a- 'C' माणवकम् (Māṇavakam)

b- Not known. (See III b-6)

II a- 1) See below IV Balwantji.

b- 1) 100 माणवकं पालेवतम् । तद् द्विविधं स्वाद्वम्लम् । यथा सिद्धमन्त्रप्रकाशे बोपदेव : -
'पारेवतं' मधुरमम्लमिति द्विधा स्यात् तत् तिन्दुकाकृति फलं लघुपाण्डुपुष्पं नीलच्छदा हि गदितं तु पारेवताख्यं ।
तत्पुष्कराश्रमसमीपवने प्रसिद्ध मिति । (Harshe)

IV 1) *Phoenix farinifera* Willd.

Roxb. Fl. Indi. CBC p. 722.

H. Palāvat

Habitat A considerable amount of confusion regarding this species appear to exist amongst Botanists ... According to *Roxburgh* it is a dwarf species with scarcely any stem.

Food -The fruit has small quantity of pulp but it is sweet and mealy, is said to have the flavour of chestnut and is eaten by the natives... According to a writer in Indian forester, the cabbage or young top of leaf buds, is eaten similarly to that of *P. dactylifera.*

(Watt. Dict. VI- I- 206 7)

2) *P. pusilla* Gaertn.

(H.) Palawat; (Kan.) Ichalu; (Mal.) Chit tinial; (Tam.) Kalangei; (Tam). Kalangei.

Coromondal coast not far long from the sea, in the northern part of Ceylon in dry forest. (Chopra p. 190)

3) पारावत (Pārāvata)

It is said to be a kind of acid fruit , sweetish in the taste and reddish gray in the colour when ripe. According to Ḍalhaṇa, it is found in *kāmarūpa* (Assam), Some believe it to be the guava fruit *Psidium gujava* Linn. -Amrūd (H.)which is of exotic origin.

C.S.Sū 26 112 27, 131

S.S, Sū-42-18; 46-139; 158

See पालेवत (Pālevata)

पालेवत Pālevata

A.H.Su. 6.135, 10 26

See पारावत (Balvantji p. 246)

19. तालः Talaḥ

तालो ध्वजद्रुमः[१] प्रांशुर्दीर्घस्कंधो दुरारुहः ॥ ६५
तृणराजो दीर्घतरुर्लेख्यपत्रो द्रुमेश्वरः ॥

फलं स्वादुरसं पाके तालजं गुरु पित्तजित् ॥ ६६
तद्बीजं स्वादुपाकं तु मूलं स्याद् रक्तपित्तजित् ॥ S. Su.46. 179.

तालः (Tālaḥ), ध्वजद्रुमः (Dhwajadrumaḥ), प्रांशुः (Prāṁśuḥ), दीर्घस्कंधः (Dīrghaskandhaḥ), दुरारुहः (Durāruhaḥ), तृणराजः (Tṛṇarājaḥ), दीर्घतरुः (Dīrghataruḥ), लेख्यपत्रः (Lekhyapatraḥ), and द्रुमेश्वरः (Drumeśvaraḥ), are synonymous.

The fruit is sweet in (taste) and *vipāka*, *guru* and pacifies *pittadoṣa* (The seeds are sweet in *vipāka*), and the roots are useful in haemorrhagic disorders.

(Fam. Palmae) Arecaceae.

I- a- ***Borassus flabellifer*** Linn.
Syn. *B. flabelliformis* Roxb.

b- Roxburgh

c- all over India near seashore, Bihar, Bengal, Thana, Surat.

II- a- ध्वजद्रुमः (Dhwajadrumaḥ), लेख्यपत्रः (Lekhyapatraḥ),मदाढ्यः (Madādhyaḥ),दीर्घपत्रः (Dīrghapatraḥ), आसवद्रुः (Āsavadruḥ)

b- (B.) Tāla; (H. Bom. Mar.) Tāḍa; (Tam.) Pamai, Tālai; (Tel.) Tādi chettu; (Mal.) Pana; (Eng.) The palmyra palm; Bear Palm.

III-a 1) See below IV -1 Balvantji.

b- 1) तृणराजस्य तृणद्रुममध्ये मुख्यत्वात् । तलति प्रतितिष्ठति मूलत्वात् तालः । (Kśiraswami, Amar 2-4. 169)

3) 441- तालो लेख्यपत्रः प्रसिद्धः । 'तृणराजो दीर्घतरुः लेख्यपत्रो द्रुमेश्वरः इति नाममाला - (Harshe).

IV- 1) ताल Tāla
Borassus flabellilfer Linn.
(H.) ताड Tāḍa.
C.S. Sū, 25-49; 27. 113 etc.
S.S. Sū, 20-12; 38. 11 etc.
A.H. Su,. 3.33. 39 6-119 etc.
The growing stem apex is called Tāla mastaka तालमस्तक and its pith-mastaka majjā मस्तकमज्जा (Balvantji p. 178)

2) *Borassus flabellifer* Linn.

---

१ 'चंडद्रुमः' इति शोढल संमतः पाठः ।

The palmyra Palm, The Bear Palm.
Habitat - Cultivated throughout India and beyond the tropics in Bengal and Southern parts of the Northwest provinces ... It extends up both sides of the Persian gulf attaining about the same altitude as in North west india.
Synopsis of the Economic uses
Every part of this plant is made use of in some way or the other. A tamil poem enumerates some 800 uses in which the various parts are put.
The gum.
Fibre
Medicinal - Juice stimulant, when fresh drawn it is exceedingly sweet. *Special opinions* ....The juice slightly fermented is used in diabetes. (p. 456)

Food Juice, Toddy and Sugar. (p. 497)
Domestic and *sacred uses.* (p. 503)
Sacred uses (p. 504)
(Watt. Dict. Page 495-504).

माडः Māḍaḥ (13)

माडो माडद्रुमो दीर्घो ध्वजवृक्षो वितानकः ॥ ६७
मद्यद्रुमो मोहकारी मद्यद्रुऋजुरङ्कधा ॥
माडस्तु शिशिरो रुच्यः कषायः पित्तदाहनुत् ॥ ६८
तृष्णापहो मरुत्कारी श्रमहच्छ्लेष्मकारकः ॥

माडः (Māḍaḥ), माडद्रुमः (Māḍadrumaḥ), दीर्घः (Dīrghaḥ), ध्वजवृक्षः (Dhwajavṛkṣaḥ), वितानकः (Vitānakaḥ), मद्यद्रुमः (Madyadrumaḥ), मोहकारी (Mohakārī), मद्यद्रुः (Madyadruḥ), and ऋजुः (Ṛjuḥ) are synonymous.(Nine synonyms).

Māḍa is *śītavīrya, kaṣāya* in taste, appetizer, pacifies *pitta* and aggravates *kapha* and *vātadoṣas.* It is useful in burning sensation, thirst and in removing fatigue.

Fam. Palmae. Arecaceae

I- a- ***Caryota urens*** Linn.
b- Chopra. C- See bellow IV -1

The same synonyms and properties are mentioned in Raj. ni. The synonyms are restricted by the term 'अङ्कधा' (i.e. 9).

II- a- माडः (Māḍaḥ), ध्वजवृक्षः (Dhwaja vṛkśaḥ), वितानकः (Vitānakaḥ), मद्यद्रुमः (Madya drumaḥ), मोहकारी (Mohakārī).

b- (San) Dhwajvṛkśa; (B) Bhirlimāḍ; (H.) Māri; (Tam.) Irambunai, Tippili; (Tel.) Jilaguttu; (Mal.) Auapanga. (Chopra) (Eng.) Toddy palm (Hill.); (Bom.) Hill Palm, Sagopalm (Watt. Dict.)

IV- 1) *C. urens* Linn.

Freshly drawn Toddy laxt. Fresh juice of the palm contians 13.6% sucrose and a trace of reducing Sugar. While fermentated juice or toddy contains 1 % reducing sugar, 3-4.5% alcohol and 0-3% acetic acid. (chopra p. 53).

20. (२०) प्रियालः (Priyālaḥ)

प्रियालोऽथ खरस्कन्धश्चारो बहुलवल्कलः ॥ ६९
स्नेहबीजश्चापवटो ललनस्तापसप्रियः ॥
वातपित्तहरं वृष्यं प्रियालं गुरु शीतलम् ॥ ७०
चारस्य च फलं पक्वं स्वाद्वम्लं दुर्जरप्रियम् ॥
चारमज्जा समधुरा वृष्या पित्तानिलापहा ॥ ७१

प्रियालः (Priyālaḥ), खरस्कन्धः (Kharaskandhaḥ), चारः (Cāraḥ), बहुलवल्कलः (Bahulavalkalaḥ), स्नेहबीजः (Snehabījaḥ), चापवटः (Cāpavaṭaḥ), ललनः (Lalanaḥ), and तापसप्रियः (Tāpasapriyaḥ) are synonymous.

The fruit (seeds) of *Priyāla* is sweet and sour in taste when ripe. It pacifies *vāta* and *pitta doṣas,* is *guru* and *śītavīrya.* It is difficult to digest and is cordial. The seed is sweet in taste, *vṛṣya* and pacifies *pitta* and *vāta doṣas*.

Fam. Anacardiaceae

I- a- ***Buchanania lanzan*** Spreng.
Syn. *B. latifolia* Roxb.

b- Roxburgh c-See below IV -2

II- a खरस्कन्धः (Kharaskandhaḥ), चारः (Cāraḥ), बहुलवल्कलः (Bahulawalkalaḥ), स्नेहबीजः (Snehabījaḥ), तापसप्रियः (Tāpasapriyaḥ),

१ 'पियाल' इति क्षीर. पाठः । २ 'सन्नकद्रुः' इति क्षीर. पाठः ।
३ प्रियालमज्जा मधुरो वृष्यः पित्तानिलापहः । S.Su.46.205

b- (H.B.) Cironjī, Piyal; (Mar, Guj. Bom.) Cāra, Cāroḷī; (Tam.) Mudaima; (Tel.) Sārā (Sans) Piyālaka (Chopra)

III a-1 See bellow IV - 3 Balvantji.

IV- 1) *Buchanania latifolia* Roxb.

(H.) Peeyar, Peeyal; (B). Piyal, Chironjī the name of the fruit (S) Chirica. The name of the fruit (Tel.) chiroo, Mamudca. Drupe, oblong, villous, tapering equally towards each end.Seed lanceolate., it is a native of mountainous parts of India. (Roxb.fl.II385)

2) *Buchanania latifolia* Roxb.

(San) Piyal, chare, chirica; (Tam), Momda or kalimargo maṙum, katmaa kat- mā maram; (The plant) Kat māmayam (The kernel), Tel. Chru. charu, chara mamdi, charaendi, chara pandu (the tree)' Chara puppu (the kernel); (Kan,) Maskul- Nurkalu; (Mar.) Piyal Char; (Mal.) Kāla Maram.

Habitat - A tree .... found in the sub Himalayan tract from sutlej eastward throughout India and Burma. Common in the hotter and drier parts of the empire and frequently associated with the sāl, the mahua and the dāk.

Food The kernel is the common substitiue for almond amongst the natives, It is largely used in sweet meats. In flavour it is described as between that of the pistachio and the almond. It is eaten roasted with milk. (Watt. Dict. I- 545)

3) प्रियाल Priyāla

Buchanania lanzan Spreng.

C. S. Sū. 3.20, 4-40 , 43 etc.

S.S. Sū 38-48, 42-18 etc.

A.H. Su 6-121, 124, 15-41 etc.

(Balvantji p. 264).

21. (२१) नारिकेलः Nārikelaḥ

नारिकेलो[१] रसफलः सुतुंग : कूर्चशेखरः[२] ।
तालवृक्षो[३] दृढफलो लाङ्गली दाक्षिणात्यकः ॥ ७२

नारिकेलं गुरु स्निग्धं पित्तघ्नं[४] स्वादुशीतलम् ।
बलमांसप्रदं वृष्यं बृंहणं बस्तिशोधनम् ॥ ७३ S .Su.46.180

नारिकेलः (Nārikelaḥ), रसफलः (Rasaphalaḥ), सुतुंगः (Sutuṅgaḥ),

१'नालिकेर' इति. नि. शे. टीका संमतः पाठः । २ 'कूर्च केसरः ' इति नि.शे. टीका संमतः पाठः ।
३'लता वृक्षो' इति शोढल पाठ : ।
४ 'पित्तकृत' इति । चौखाम्बा पाठः

कूर्चशेखरः (Kurcaśekharaḥ), तालवृक्षः (Tālavṛkśaḥ), दृढफलः (Dṛḍhaphalaḥ), लाङ्गली (Lāṅgalī), and दाक्षिणात्यकः (Dākśiṇātyakaḥ), are synonymous.

Nārikela (fruit) is sweet in taste, *śītavīrya, guru* and unctous (*Snigdha*). It promotes strength and *māmsa* (helps to promote muscular tissue), is *vṛṣya*, promoting body weight and has purificatory action on urinary organs.

(Fam. Palmae) Arecaceae

I- a- ***Cocos nucifera*** Linn.

b- Roxburgh c- Cocus islands, cultivated all over india,

II- a- कूर्चशेखरः (Kūrcaśekaraḥ), दृढफलः (Dṛḍhaphalaḥ), तालवृक्षः (Tāla-vṛkśaḥ), त्र्यम्बकफलः (Tryambakaphalaḥ), तालवृक्षः (Tāla vṛkśaḥ), लाङ्गली (Lāṅgalī), दाक्षिणात्यकः (Dākśiṇātyakaḥ).

b- (San.) Nārikela,, śrīphala; (H). Nāriyal; (Mar.) Nāraḷa; (B) Dub, Nārikel; (Tam.) Ṭamkai, Tenga; (Tel.) Nārikelamu; (Mal.) Nārikelam; (Eng.) Coconut tree.

III- a- 1) See below Iv -1, (Balvantji).

b- 1) नलिकान्नलयुक्तान्पुष्पादीनीरयति नालिकेरः ।
हलाकारपत्रशाखत्वात् लांगली । (Ksīraswami 2.4-16a)

2) 427 नालिकेरस्त्रिनेत्रः । ... बाह्यास्थि किं मदाहर नालिकेरमिति विदग्धमुखमण्डने ।' ना अलिकेअर' इति छेदः । ... (Harshe)

3) 391 सदाफल इति । नालिकेरस्त्रिनेत्रः । (Harshe).

IV 1) नारिकेल - Nārikela.
Cocos nucifera Linn.
Syn. नालिकेर
C.S. Su. 26. 112., 27. 127. etc.
S.S.Su. 20. 3, 42-18 45-120 etc.
A.H. Su. 5-19; 6-119; etc. (Balvantji p. 223)

2) *Cocos nucifera* Linn.
The cocount palm.
(Tam.) Tenna, Tengā, khobari Tennaun Chedi, Tennamaram; (Tel.) Nari Kadam, Tenkaiā, Kobbari, goburi kaya; (Kan.) Tengina gida, Theginna cippu; (Mal.) Tengam, Ten marum, Kalapa, Kalambir; (Sans.) Narikel, Naliker.
Dry kernel - Copra (Kopra)
Water- Yella nir; (Tel.) yella nīru.
Toddy - (H.) Narel; (Tam). Tenga kallu; (Tel.) Tenkāy nūne,

Tenkāy Kallu; (Mala.) Tenna enna Minak, Kalap, Minnuknur; (Kan.) Tenginā Yanne, Kobri.

Habitat on the eastern and western coast it is particularly abundant more towards the South ... Decandolle states briefly the arguments in favour of an American as well as those of an Asiatic origin for this tree and concludes by expressing the opinion that it must probably belongs to the "Indian Archipelago. The introduction into Ceylon, India and China he states does not date further back than three thousand years "but the transport by sea to the coasts of America and Africa took place perhaps in a more epoch although posterior to those epochs when geographical and physical conditions were different from those of our day. "

(Watt. Dict. II- 416).

22. (२२) वटः (Waṭaḥ)

वटो रक्तफलः शृङ्गी न्यग्रोधः स्कन्धजो ध्रुवः[1] ।
क्षीरी वैश्रवणावासो बहुपादो वनस्पतिः ॥७४

वटः शीतः कषायश्च स्तम्भनो रूक्षणात्मकः ।
तथा तृष्णा छर्दिमूर्च्छा रक्तपित्तविनाशनः ॥७५

वटः (Vaṭaḥ), रक्तफलः (Raktaphalaḥ), शृङ्गी (Śṛṅigī), न्यग्रोधः (Nyagrodhaḥ), स्कन्धजः (Skandhajaḥ), ध्रुवः(Dhruvaḥ), क्षीरी (Kśirī), वैश्रवणावासः (Vaisravaṇāvāsaḥ), बहुपादः (Bahupādaḥ), and वनस्पतिः (Vanāspatiḥ) are synonymous.

Vaṭa is *kaṣāya* (astringent) in taste, *śitavīrya, stambhana* (astringent), *rūkśaṇa* (roughning). It is useful in thirst, emesis, syncope, and *raktapitta* (haemorrhagic disorders).

(Fam. Moraceae)

I- a- ***Ficus benghalensis*** Linn.
Syn. *F. indicus* Linn. (Kirtikar).
b- Roxburgh
c- throughout India wild and cultivated.

II- a- रक्तफलः (Raktaphalaḥ), शृङगी (Śṛṅgī), न्यग्रोधः (Nyagrodhaḥ), वैश्रवणावासः (Vaiśravaṇāwāsaḥ), यक्षावासः (Yakśāvāsaḥ), यक्षतरुः (Yakśataruḥ).

---

१ जटी इति शोढल पाठः ।

b- (H.) Bad; (B) Bod; (Mar.) Vaḍa; (Tam.) Puḍavam; (Tel.) Peḍḍamaṭṭi; (Eng.) Banyan.

IV 1) *Ficus benghalensis* Linn.
The Banyan tree.
Syn. *F. indica* Linn.
(Tam.) Ala (Tel.) Mari, Peddi mari, (Kan.) Aloda, Ala, Alava, Alhada, (Sans.) Vaṭa (H.) Ber, Bar.
In the Poona Gazeteer (Vol. XVIII, p.1.p.54), Banyan is spoken in the Andhra valley so large as to afford of shade to 20,000 people. *Forbes* describes as circumference as of 2000 ft.and its overhanging branches beyond the daughter stems as stretching over a much larger area. It had about 120 large trunks and over 3000 smaller and was capable of sheltering 7000 men. High floods have however since carried away portions of the islands of this great tree. (Watt. Dict. I.343)

2) *Ficus indica* Linn.
A large spreading tree of Burma & Andaman islands. It seems probable that some of the economic information recorded under *F. benghalensis* may probably refer to this species ..... as a synonym for *F. benghalensis.*

23. (२३) पिप्पलः Pippalah

पिप्पलः केशवावासश्चलपत्रः पवित्रकः ।
मङ्गल्यः श्यामलोऽश्वत्थो बोधिवृक्षो गजाशनः ॥ ७६

(श्रीमान् क्षीरद्रुमो विप्रः शुभदः श्यामलच्छदः ।
पिप्पलः गुह्यपत्रस्तु सेव्यः सत्यः शुचिद्रुमः ॥
चैत्यद्रुमो धर्मवृक्षः[१] चन्द्रकरमिताह्वयः ।)

अश्वत्थोऽपि स्मृतस्तद्वद् रक्तपित्तकफापहः ॥

पिप्पलः (Pippalaḥ), केशवावासः (Keśavāvāsaḥ), चलपत्रः (Calapatraḥ), पवित्रकः (Pavitrakaḥ), मङ्गल्यः (Maṅgalyaḥ), श्यामलः (Śyāmalaḥ), अश्वत्थः (Aśvatthaḥ), बोधिवृक्ष (Bodhivṛkśaḥ) and गजाशनः (Gajāśanaḥ) are synonymous.

(श्रीमान् (Śrīmān), क्षीरद्रुमः (Kśīradrumaḥ), विप्रः (Vipraḥ), शुभदः (Śubhadaḥ), श्यामलच्छदः (Śyāmalacchadaḥ), पिप्पलः (Pippalaḥ), गुह्यपत्रः (Guhyapatraḥ), सेव्यः (Sevyaḥ), सत्यः (Satyaḥ), शुचिद्रुमः (Śucidrumaḥ), चैत्यद्रुमः

१ 'वन्यवृक्षः' इति पा. 'श्रीमान् क्षीरद्रुमः इत्यादारभ्य चन्द्रकरमिताह्वयः' इति पाठः रा. नि. तः प्रतिलिपिं कारयित्वा समाविष्टः इति मन्ये । तदेतत् रा.नि. पाठ. आनन्दाश्रम मुद्रित पुस्तके न तु चौखम्बा पुस्तके दृश्यते । स.दि.का.

(Caityadrumaḥ), धर्मवृक्षः (Dharmavṛkśaḥ), are synonymous.) (This reading seems to be copied from Raj. ni.)

Aśvatthaḥ is similar in properties to that of *vaṭaḥ* and pacifies *raktapita* (haemorrhagic disorders) and *Kaphadoṣas*.

Under this heading Dhn. Ni. notes only Pippala but Raj.Ni. notes A-पिप्पलः (Pippalaḥ proper) and B-अश्वत्थी (Aśvatthī)

(Fam. Moraceae).

A-a- ***Ficus religiosa*** Linn.

b- Roxburgh c- throughout India, wild and cultivated.

B-a- Not identified.

Note Raj. Ni. has noted medicinal properties of this plant.

II- A-a- चैत्यद्रुमः (Caityadrumaḥ), केशवावासः (Keśawāvāsaḥ), याज्ञिकः (Yājñikaḥ), पवित्रकः (Pavitrakaḥ), चलपत्रः (Calapatraḥ), बोधिवृक्षः (Bodhivṛkśaḥ).

b- (Sans.) Aswattha; (B.) Aswattha; (H) Pippal; (Mar.) Pimpaḷa; (Tel.) Pippali; (Tam.) Arus.

a- B-अश्वत्थी (Aśwatthī), लघुपत्रिका (Laghupatrikā), पवित्रा (Pavitrā), ऱ्हस्वपत्रिका (Rhaswapatrikā), पिप्पलिका (Pippalikā), वनस्था (Vanasthā), अश्वत्थसंनिभा (Aśwattha sannibhā).

III a- 1) See below IV- Balwantji.

IV- 1) अश्वत्थ Aśwattha.

Ficus religiosa Linn.

C.S.Sū. 4.33, 5-18; 25. 40 etc.

S. S. Sū. 38-48; Ci 3-6. etc.

A.H. Sū 21-16, 25-35 etc.

(Balwantji p. 29).

24. प्लक्षः Plakśaḥ

प्लक्षः कपीतनः शृङ्गी सुपार्श्वश्चारुदर्शनः ॥ ७७
प्लवको गर्दभाण्डश्च कमण्डलु वटप्लवः ॥

प्लक्षः कटुकषायश्च शीतलो रक्तपित्तजित् ॥ ७८
मूर्च्छाश्रमप्रलापांश्च हरेत्प्लक्षो विशेषतः ॥

प्लक्षः (Plakśaḥ), कपीतनः (Kapītanaḥ), शृङ्गी (Sṛṅgī), सुपार्श्वः (Supārśvaḥ),

चारुदर्शन : (Cārudarśanaḥ), प्लवकः (Plavakaḥ), गर्दभाण्डः (Gardabhāṇḍaḥ), कमण्डलुः (Kamaṇḍaluḥ) and वटप्लवः (Vaṭaplavaḥ) are synonymous.

Plakśa is pungent and *kaśaya* (astringent) in taste, *śītavīrya* and pacifies *rakta* and *pitta doṣas* (haemorrhagic disorders). It is useful in syncope, fatigue and delirium.

Under this heading two plants are included A-प्लक्षः (Plakśaḥ) and पिप्परिः (Pippariḥ).

confirmed.
(Fam. Moraceae)

I- A-a- ***Ficus infectoria*** Willd.*
b- Kamat c-Northern India, Bengal, Madars.
B-a- ***Ficus retusa*** Linn.**
Syn. *F. benanjamina* Willd. (Non Linn.).
b- Kamat c- Nagpur , Bihar, Madhy. Bharat, Southern India, Konkan.

II- a- A-शृङ्गी (Sṛṅgī), चारुदर्शन : (Cārudarśanaḥ), कमण्डलुः (Kamaṇḍaluḥ) वटप्लवः (Vaṭaplavaḥ), दृढप्ररोहः (Dṛḍhaprarohaḥ).
b- (Sans.) Plakśāḥ; (B) Pakar; (Mara,) Mothi Pāyar.
a- B-(Sans) ह्रस्वप्लक्षः (Rhaswaplakśaḥ),सुशीतः (Suśītaḥ), महाप्ररोहः (Mahāprarohaḥ),मंगलच्छायः (Mangalacchāyaḥ), पिप्परी (Pipparī).
b- (Konkan) Pāyar; (Bom) Pilāl, (Poona), Nāndarukha (B.H.) Kāmrup; (Tel.) Yerajuvi; (Sans.) Laghu plakśa .
(Br.Ni. Pade).

III- a 1) 73 Plakśa - AV- V-5
T.S. VI 3.10 2; Vii 4-12-15.
M.S. iii) -12 (Harshe)
2) शमी पलाश न्यग्रोध प्लक्ष..... । यज्ञियः । (Narayan Bhatti)
1) प्लक्ष्य अधोगच्छति मूलैः .... । पर्कटी प्लक्षः (Kshiraswami)
2) प्लक्ष Su. 15 प्लक्ष्यते कीटैः । प्लक्षत्यधो गच्छति मूलैः वा ।
F. tsiela, Thespepsia populnea (Vaidya)

IV 1) प्लक्षः 365 कपीतनः गर्दभाण्डः सुपार्श्व चारुदर्शनः । (Abhi. Manji.)
Ficus infectoria (?) (Krishnan)
2) शृङ्गी -प्लवाख्य : । (Arun Sū. 15-41)
3) *Ficus infectoria* Willd. IV-1136, Leaves ovate, oblong, acute, placksha (Plucksha) As. Res. IV- 310

---

* The current accepted name for *F. infectoria* Willd. is *F. virens* Aiton.
** The current accepted name for *F. retusa* Linn. is *F. microcarpa* Linn. f.

Tsejkela - Rheed. Mal. iii + 64
F. Tsjakela Burm Fl. indi. 227.
A large and most beautiful tree with a far most extended numerously dense head, a native of Bengal. I never met with it on the Coromondal coast. The trunk is large and irregular like that *F. religiosa*. Sometimes drooping roots of considerable magnitude from the trunk and branches.Fruit paired, axillary, sessile, the size of a pea, roundish, pretty smooth, when ripe white.
(Roxb. Fl. indi.)

4) *Ficus retusa* Linn.
Syn. *F. benjamina* Willd.
Nāndarukh (Cooke)
ऱ्हस्वप्लक्षः - लघुपिप्परी (Pade Br. Ni.)

5) *F. tsjakela.* Burm. (Fl. indi. 227)
Syn.*F. infectoria* Willd
A large glabrous tree without aerial roots, leaves for a time during the dry season. (Cooke II - 650- old).

6) *F. infectoria* Roxb. (Fl. indi. 3-551)
(exclude syn. Rheed.)
F. lacor Buch.- Ham.
A large spreading deciduous tree.

Note- The oldest name of this plant is. *F. lacor* Buch.-Ham. (1825) for although *F. infectoria* as a species in Hor. Beng. (1814 - page 66) He has there founded the species on Rheed Hort. Mal. (Vol.3-64) which is *F. tsjakela.*
(Cooke II 550) (p. 651 Old)

V- 1) प्लक्ष (Plakśa)
Ficus lacor Buch.- Ham.
पकडी Pakaḍī and पाकड Pākaḍa
Syn. पर्कटकी Parkaṭakī
C.S.Su. 4.33, 5.18 etc.
Su.S. Su. 121, 124 etc.
Other species of Ficus such as
F. arnottiana Miq.
F. rumphii Blume and *F. talboti* G. King have been given the same name in other parts of the country (Balvantji P. 263)

2) प्लक्षप्ररोह इव सौधतलं विभेद । रघु ८-९३ प्लक्षान् प्ररोह जटिला नियमन्ति वृद्धा । रघु १३.७१

In Sanskṛt literature प्लक्ष Plaksha is interpreted as वट(Vata) But वट (Vaṭa) and प्लक्ष (Plakśa) are two different trees. प्लक्ष Plakśa) is now identified as *Ficus lacor* Buch.- Ham. It is commonly known as पाखर Pakhara, of medium height with

densely branched evergreen tree. (Uniyal - Kalidas)
(Sachi. Ayu 4. 1976).

3) ... (Several geographical forms) A large deciduous tree found in Suleman, Salt ranges ... Commonly planted, rarely met wild.
(Watt. Dict.)

4) *F. tsiela* Roxb.
(Tel.) Joovee or Pedda Joovee.
No roots from the trunk nor from branches.
(Roxb III 550, chopra, Cooke).

5) *F. talboti* G. King
(Sans.) Plaksha (Chopra) apparently endemic
(Cooke II 647 old).

6) *F. arnottiana* Miq:.
(Sans.) Plaksha (Chopra) (Cooke).

Note - As to *Ficus lacora* Buch.- Ham. in Cooke's flora we find some coufusion about this tree name. Once the author gives a synonym to *F. tsjakela* Burm. and also to *F.infectora* Roxb. But morphologically these two plants are quite different (see. V. 3-4 above), These two trees as recorded by cooke do not have aerial roots and are deciduous and as *F.lacora* Buch Ham is given as a synonym of these two trees, it may be also deciduous and without having aerial roots, and if it is so this tree *(F. lacora)* can not be accepted as (Pluksa) of our Nighaṇtu.
Dr. Roxburgh has recorded Willd's *F. infectoria* willd and has given *F. tejkela* Burm as its synonym and also has given its full descriptiopn wherein we find that Willd's tree has ariel roots and is also an evergreen plant.. Dr. Roxburgh has not given *F. lacora,* Buch. -Ham. as a synonym to Willd's *F. infectoria* (IV -3).

Discussion on Plakśa

Plakśa is a controversial plant name several botanical names under *Ficus genus* are recorded as *Plakśa* (See Chopra under ficus). But now some modern writers have identified it as follows : -

A. *Ficus infectoria* Roxb. (Fl.Ind.V.3. 551)
Synonym *F. lacor* Buch.- Ham. (Cooke II 550) see V-3 a)

B. *Ficus lakor* Buch.- Ham. (See V- 2 and 3)

C- *Ficus infectoria* Willd Plukśa As.- Res IV-3-310)
Synonyms *F. tejakala Rheed* (Mal. III to 68)
F. tsjakela Burm. (fl. ind. 227).
Out of these three names we have accepted the thrird name *F- infectoria* Willd. as Plaksa of our Nighaṇtus for the following

reasons : -

1) Our Nighaṇṭu's tree has drooping roots.
2) Its head is like a Kamaṇḍalu,(कमण्डलु)
3) and it is (चारुदर्शनः) A beautiful tree.

The compiler has put the equivalent कमण्डलु Kamaṇḍalu to have exact idea of the head of this tree and holy water pot made up of a roundnecked white gourd *Alābu* (*Lagenaria species*) which is kept always by Hindu संन्यासी sanyasis and योगी Yogis. This equivalent gives exact idea of the shape of the head of compiler's tree. Wanderer tribes, carry out their pretty business camps under the shed of this ever green tree for two to three months in winter and in hot season.

The compiler remarks his tree with the equivalent *cārudarśanaḥ* (II-a-A) which shows as a most beautiful tree. (H.14. 3)

From the description as given above it would be found that compiler's प्लक्ष Plakśa must have drooping root from its trunk and branches. (IV-3-5 above.)

Branching must be of numeroulsy dense head (Iv-3 above) The tree must be चारुदर्शनः *cārudarśanah* i.e. beautiful in appearance. (Iv-3 above.)

This description aptly correspond to the Roxburgh's *F. infectoria* Willd. and therefore, we have confirmed it as compilers Plakśa (I-a-A).

As to *Ficus lacor* Buch.- Ham. this tree species is accepted by majority of modern writers as प्लक्ष Plaksa but we think without comparing morphologically with classical Ayurvdic books they might have accepted this name.

In Cookes flora this plant name is recorded as a synonym of *F. infectoria.* Roxb. (See above v.) which is noted as without aerial roots and is deciduous. He further notes that original name of this tree was as *Ficus lacor* Buch.- Ham. If this informationm would be correct then it follws that the tree of these two different names is the same and one plant and as it is without aerial roots and is deciduous it cannot be accepted as प्लक्ष Pluksa of our Nighaṇṭus.

For these reasons as discussed above either *F. infectoria* Roxb. or *F. lacor* Buch.- Ham. cannot be accepted for the present as प्लक्ष Plaksa of our Nighaṇṭus.

25. (२५) जम्बूः Jambūḥ

जम्बूः सुरभिपत्रा च राजजम्बूर्महाफला । ७९
सुरभिः स्यान्महाजम्बूर्महास्कन्धा प्रकीर्तिता ॥

वेतसी काकजम्बूश्च नादेयी शीतवल्लभा ॥ ८०
भ्रमरेष्टा नीलवर्णा द्वितीया जम्बूरुच्यते ॥

जाम्बवं वातलं ग्राहि स्वाद्वम्लं कफपित्तजित् ॥ ८१
हृत्कण्ठघर्षणं चान्यत्कषायं क्षुद्रजाम्बवम् ॥ S.S.Su. 46.166

जम्बूः (Jambuḥ), सुरभिपत्रा (Surabhipatrā), राजजम्बूः (Rājadambūḥ), महाफला (Mahāphalā), सुरभिः (Surabhiḥ), महाजम्बूः (Mahājambhuḥ), महास्कन्धा (Mahāskandhā) are synonymous (Rāja Jambuḥ).

वेतसी (Vetasī), काकजम्बूः (Kākajambuḥ), नादेयी (Nādeyī), शीतवल्लभा (Śītavallabhā), भ्रमरेष्टा (Bhramareṣṭā), and नीलवर्णा (Nīlavarṇā), are synonymous for the second kind of *Jambuḥ*.

The fruit of *Rāja Jambuḥ* is sweet and sour in taste, astringent and pacifies *kapha, pitta doṣas* but aggravates *vātadoṣa.* The second type *Kśudra Jambu* fruit is of *kaṣāya* taste and has constricting action on throat and heart (stomach.)

Under the name जम्बू (Jambu) having different taste, size of their fruits and habitat, many species are recorded by the modern writers and botanists but our Nighaṇṭus have recorded only three kinds which are A- राजजम्बूः (Rājjambūḥ), काकजम्बूः (Kākajambūḥ), and c- भूमिजम्बूः (Bhūmi Jambūḥ) all of the same family.

(Fam. Myrtaceae)

I- A-a-1) ***Eugenia jambolana*** Lam.*
Syn. *Syzygium jambolanum* DC.
S. cumini (L) Skeels (Chopra)
b- Watt,Dict, & Chopra
c- See below IV- 1 watt Dict.

A-a-2) ***Eugenia operculata*** Roxb.**
Syn. *E. cerasoides* Roxb.
b- Watt. Dict.
c- below IV-2

---

* The present accepted name for *Eugenia jambolana* Lam. is *Syzygium cumini* (Linn.) Skeels
** The present accepted name is *Syzygium operculatum* (Roxb.) Gamble

B-a- ***E. heyneana*** Wall. (Fl. Indi.)*

b- watt. Dict C- Bombay Ghats and in the beds of the rivers in Berar.

C-a- ***E. zyelanica*** Wight**

b- Watt. Dict,. c-a small shrub Orissa, Konkan and South wards.

II- A1 & A2 a- महाजम्बूः (Mahājambūḥ), राजजम्बूर्महाफला (Rājajambūr-mahāphalā), राजार्हा (Rajarhā), महास्कन्धा (Mahāskandhā), मेघमोदिनी (Meghamodinī)

A1 b-(H.) Jāmun; (B.) Jam, Kala jam; (Mar.) Jāmbhūḷa; (Tam.) Nāval, navar, naga; (Tel.) Naredu, rāch naredu, Pedda nerudu (large fruit variety), nāgar, nasedu; (Kan) Naral, Nerlu, Neral; (Sans.) Jambū, (Eng.) Black plum.

A 2a- (H) Raijaman, dugdukiya

B-a- वेतसी (Vetasī), काकजम्बू (Kākajambūḥ), भ्रमरेष्टा (Bhramareṣṭā) काकफला(Kākaphalā),नादेयी (Nādeyī)

b- (Mar.) Pan Jāmbul.

C-a- भूमिजम्बू (Bhūmi Jambūḥ), ह्रस्वफला (Hrswaphalā), भ्रमरेष्टा (Bhramareṣṭā), काष्ठजम्बूः (Kāṣṭha Jambūḥ).

b- (Mar.) Bhedas; (Kan.) Neral. (Watt. Dict.)

III-a-1) See below IV- 2 Balvantji.

b-1) बार्हतं च फले जम्बवा ... जम्बू जाम्बवम् । (Ama. 2-4-19) बृहत्या फलं बार्हतम्. फलति फलं फलनिष्पत्तौ । जम्बवा (सू.) इत्याणि जाम्बवम् । (Ksiraswāmi Amar.)

2) 203...'काकजम्बूः क्षुद्रफला नादेयी गन्धपल्लवे' ति । केयदेवः । (Harshe)

3) 320 जम्बूभिदत्र महाजम्बूः - जम्बूः सुरभिपत्रा च राजजम्बूर्महाफला । सुरभी च महास्कंधा महाजम्बूर्निगद्यते । (Harshe)

4) 485जम्बूल इति । श्यामपत्रः -जम्बू विटपः । (Harshe)

IV- 1) राजजम्बू-तन्नामानि - फलेन्द्रा कथिता नन्दी राजजम्बूर्महाफला । तथा सुरभिपत्रा च महाजम्बूरपि स्मृता । राजजम्बूफलं स्वादु ।
Eugenia jambolana Lam.

2) जम्बू Jambū जाम्बव Jāmbava
Syzygium cumini (L.) Skeels
C.S.Su. 2.27, 4.28 etc.
Su. S. Su 20.2, 12 36.47 etc.
A.H. Sū 6-127; 15-41 etc.

---

* The present accepted name is *Syzygium zeylanicum* (Linn.) DC. (U. P. I. 614.)

** The present accepted name *Syzygium heyneanum* Wall. ex Gamble (Roxb.)

Jāmbava is the name of the fruit of Jambū. Other speices distinguished by काकजम्बू (Kāka Jambū), नदीजम्बू (Nadī Jambū), and क्षुद्रजम्बू etc. have also been mentioned. *Eugenia operculata* Roxb. known as Topākuḍā (टोपाकुडा) in the forests of Bihar appears to be a medicinally important plant. It is a common item in the prescription of tribal Vaidyas in singbhum. Bihar.

(Balvantji p. 164)

3) *Eugenia jambolana* Lam.
Black plum.
Habitat : a moderate sized tree, found wild, cultivated over the greater part of India from the indus eastwards and to the exterme south of the Madras Presidency.
Food : The fruit which is sometimes as large as a pigeon's egg and of a purple colour is eaten by all classes of people ... In Goa, a wine, faintly rsembling a port is prepared from the ripe fruit. (Watt. Dict . III. 284-86).

4) *E. operculata* Roxb.
Habitat : A moderate sized or even large evergreen tree, met with the sub Himalayan tract from Jammu to Assam up to 2000 ft.in the forest of Chitgong, Burma, the western Ghats and in Ceylon. Brandis says that under favourable conditions it grows to one of the largest and most handsome trees of the genus.The leaves turn bright red before falling.
Var.-obovata Kurz
Food: It yields an edible fruit which ripens towards the end of the hot season.

5) *E. heyneana* Wall.
Habitat : A shrub or small tree, found in the Bombay ghats and in the beds of river in Berar and Cenrtal provinces

(Watt. III. 283)

6) *E. zeylanica* Wight
Habitat : A small myrtle like shrub of the shruby forests of Orissa. A shrub or small tree in Concan and northwards, also in Syelhet... In Kanara it is used for building purpose.(Watt. III 290).

26. (२६) उदुम्बरः Udumbaraḥ

उदुम्बरो क्षीरवृक्षो हेमदुग्धः सदाफलः॥ ८२
अपुष्पफलसंबंधो यज्ञाङ्गः शीतवल्कलः ॥

उदुम्बरं कषायं स्यात् पक्वं तु मधुरं हिमम् ॥ ८३
कृमिकृत् पित्तरक्तघ्नं मूर्च्छादाहतृषाहम् ॥

उदुम्बरः (Udumbaraḥ), क्षीरवृक्षः (Kśīravṛkśaḥ), हेमदुग्धः (Hemadugdhaḥ), सदाफलः (Sadāphalaḥ), अपुष्पफलसंबंधः (Apuṣpaphalasambandhaḥ), यज्ञाङ्गः (Yajñyāṅgaḥ), and शीतवल्कलः (Śītavalkalaḥ) are synonymous.

Udumbara fruit is *kaṣāya* (astringent) in taste, and when ripe is sweet and *śitavīrya*. It is helminth promoting and pacifies *pitta* and *raktadoṣa* and is useful in fainting, burning sensation and thirst.

Under this heading two kinds of Udumbara are included 'A' उदुम्बर (Udumbara proper) and 'B' लघूदुम्बरिका (Laghūdumbarikā).

Fam. Moraceae

I- A-a- ***Ficus racemosa*** Linn.
Syn. F. glomerata Roxb.

b- Roxburgh c-wild and cultivated all over india.

c- See below Iv- 2
For confirmation.

B-a- ***Ficus heterophylla*** Linn. var. *F. rep.* Willd.
F. heterophylla Linn. var. *F. scabrella*. Roxb.
F.heterophylla Linn. Var. *aquatiloba* Mic.

b- Roxburgh & Watt. Dict.

C- See below VI -3

II- A-a क्षीरवृक्षः (Kśīravṛkśaḥ), हेमदुग्धः (Hemadugdhaḥ), यज्ञाङ्गः (Yajñyāṅgaḥ), अपुष्प फल संबंधः (Apuṣpaphala sambandahaḥ) शीतवल्कलः (Śītavalkalaḥ).

b- (H.) Gular; (Mar.) Umbar; (B) Jagya-dumar;(Tel.Tam. mal.) Atti.

B-a- नदीदुम्बरिका(Nadīudumbarikā), लघुपत्रः (Laghupatraḥ), लघुहेमदुग्धा (Laghu hemadugdhā), लघुउदुम्बर (Laghu udumbara)

b- (B.) Bhui umbara; (S) Trayamaṇa; (Mar.) Dātir; (Tam) Kodigatti; (Mal.) Vallilerakam (chopra).

III- See kākodumbara.

b- 1) 419 उदुम्बर इति । हेमदुग्धः 'उदुम्बरो हेमदुग्धो हरिताक्षो वसुद्रुम' इति केयदेवः । (Harshe)

IV- 1) उदुम्बर Udumbara
Ficus racemosa Linn.
C.S. Sū. 4-33; 5.18 etc.

S.S.Sū. 38-47; ci. 3-6 etc.
A.H. Sū 10-32 21 16 etc.
H. Gūlar Dūmar (Balvantji p. 51)

2) *Ficus glomerata* Roxb.
Syn. *F. racemosa* Wall (non Roxb.)
F. gulereea Roxb.
(H.) Gular, Umbar; (B) Jagya dumar; (Bom. Mar.) Umbar; (Tam.) Atti; (Tel.) Moyadi, Atti; (Kan.) Kulla Kith,atti; (Sans) Udumbara.
Habitat A large tree of the Salt Range and Rajputana along the sub Himalayan tract to Bengal,. central and south india.
(Watt. Dict. III. 254)

3) *Ficus heterophylla* Linn.
B.Bhui dumar; (Tel.) Bur-ani; (Maly.) Valli.-Teragam; (Sans) Trāyamāṇā
Hibitat : A creeping pubesecent shrub along the banks of large rivers. Throughout the hotter parts of India.*Medicine* : The juice of the root of this shrub is internally administered in colic pains and the juice of the leaves mixed with milk in dysentery. The bark of the root, which is very bitter, pulverized and mixed with coriander seed is considered a good remedy in cough and asthma.
Food : The fruit of scrabrella (see above I-a-B)Var. scrabrella is eaten by the natives of Chitegong in curries (Roxb.)
(Watt. Dict. III. 355).

27. (२७) काकोदुम्बरिका Kākodumbarikā (फल्गुः Phalguḥ)

काकोदुम्बरिका फल्गू राजिफल्गुः शिवाटिका ॥ ८४
फाल्गुनी फलसंभारी मलयूश्चित्रभेषजा[१] ॥

काकोदुम्बरिका श्वित्र[२]कण्डूकुष्ठव्रणापहा ॥ ८५
रक्तपित्तहरा शोफपाण्डुश्लेष्महरा च सा ॥

काकोदुम्बरिका (Kākodumbarikā), फल्गुः (Phalguḥ), राजिफल्गुः (Rājiphalguḥ), शिवाटिका (Śivāṭikā), फाल्गुनी (Phālgunī), फलसम्भारी

Laghudumbarikā has been recorded by Rāj.Ni. under the heading
नद्युदुम्बरिका (लघ्वाद्युदुम्बराह्वा) S.D. Kamat

१ 'श्वित्र' भेषजम् इति नि.शे. टीका ।
२ 'ग्राही' इति आनन्दा. मुद्रित पुस्तके पाठः ।

(Phalasambhārī), मलयूः (Malayuḥ), and चित्रभेषजा (Citrabheṣajā).

Kākodumbarikā pacifies *kaphadoṣa.* It is useful in leucoderma, pruritus, skin disorders including leprotic ulcers, haemorrhagic disororders (*Raktapitta*), oedema and anaemia.

Fam. Moraceae.

I- a- ***Ficus hispida*** **Linn.** (f).
Syn. *F. oppositifolia* Willd.

b- Roxb. C- Below IV

II- a- फल्गू(Falgū), राजिफल्गूः (Rājifalgūḥ), शिवाटिका (Śivāṭikā), मलयू (Malayū) (Dhn. Ni.); कृष्णोदुम्बरिका (Kṛṣṇoḍumbarikā), कठिना (Kathinā), कुष्ठघ्नी (Kuṣṭhaghnī), चित्रभेषजा (Citrabheṣajā).

b- (H) Kaṭ-gularia; (B.) Dumar, kaokodumr; (Bom). Rambal, dumar,. dhedu; (Mar,) Kāḷāumbar, Bokheḍā; (Tel.) Bod- mamadi, Velliyatti; (Kan) Advi atti; (Mal & Tam) Peyatti.

III-a- See below IV - 1 Balwantji.

b- 1) काष्ठोदुम्बरिका 'कडुबरी' शब्द वाच्या । (Dipika p.264 Rasamarana)

2) काष्ठोदुम्बरिका- 'लोके कट गूलरी' शब्द वाच्या
(Dipika p. 276 Udayadi Rasa)

3) अञ्जीरं मज्जलं ज्ञेयं काकोदुम्बरिका फलम् -। (Madan Ni. 6.66)

4) काकोदुम्बरिका 191स्वनामख्याता । *Ficus oppositifolia* अञ्जीरं इत्येके।(Vaidya)

5) विष्टम्भि मधुरं स्निग्धं फल्गुजं तर्पणं गुरु ।
अञ्जीरं विष्टम्भजनकं मधुरं स्निग्धं तृप्तिकारकम् ।
(Dr. Ghanekar Sū 46-171)

IV- 1) काकोदुम्बरी Kākodumbarī
Ficus hispida Linn. f.
C.S. Vi. 8-150 ; ci 7-169 etc.
S. S. Ci. 9-10; 25 etc.
A.H. Ci. 19-36
Phalgu and *Malayu* are said to be two varierties of it. *Ficus cunia* Ham. & Roxburgh may be one of the two.
(Balvantaji p. 89)

2) *Ficus hispida* Linn.
Syn. *F. oppositifolia* Willd. (Roxb. corum)
(Bom.) Dumbar, Dheda;(Mar.) Kharoti, (Panchamahal) Dhedumbar; (Tam). Pe-attis; (Tel.) Bad-mamasto, Bomma-medi, Brahma-medi, Karosang; (Mal) Pe-yatti, Paraka; (Kan.) Advai-.

atti; (Sans) Kakodumbar.
Habitat - A moderate sized tree or shrub, common throughout the outer Himalaya, Bengal, Central and South India, Malacca, Ceylon, China and Australia. (Watt. Dict. III. 345).

28. (२८) क्षीरी (राजादनः) Kśirī (Rājādanaḥ)

क्षीरी चोत्तरस्तु राजन्यः सक्षीरशुक्लको नृपः ॥ ८६
राजादनो दृढस्कन्धः कपीष्टः प्रियदर्शनः ॥

राजादनो रसे स्वादुः पाकेऽम्लः शीतलस्तथा ॥ ८७
रुचिकारी भवेद्वातनाशनश्च प्रकीर्तितः ॥

क्षीरी (Kśirī), राजन्यः (Rājanyaḥ), क्षीरशुक्लकः (Kśiraśuklakaḥ), नृपः (Nṛpaḥ), राजादनः (Rājādanaḥ), दृढस्कन्धः (Dṛḍhaskandhaḥ), कपीष्टः (Kapīṣṭaḥ), and प्रियदर्शनः (Priyadarśanaḥ) are synonymous.

Rājādana is sweet in taste, *śītavīrya* and sour in *vipāka*. It is appetizer and pacifies *vātadoṣa*.

(Fam. Sapotacea)

I- a- ***Mimusops hexandra*** Roxb.*

b- Watt. Dict. c-upper gangetic plain, C & S , India, Konkan, Khandesh, Colaba Dist.

II- a- राजादनः (Rājādanaḥ), प्रियदर्शनः (Priyadarśanaḥ), राजफलः (Rājaphalaḥ), क्षीरवृक्षः (Ksīravṛkśaḥ), निम्बबीजः (Nimbabījaḥ),

b- (Sans) Rājādana; (Bom) Rānjaṇa; (H.) Khirnī; (B) Khir Khajur; (Tam. Tel. & Malya.) Pale.

b-1) 'राजादनः फलाध्यक्षः क्षीरिकायामथद्वयोः ।
–क्षीरिका क्षीरस्वादत्वात्, आद्ये तु मिष्टान्नत्वान्नामानि ।
आह च' 'क्षीरिकोत्तरा च राजन्यः क्षीरी मृत्सूपको नृपः । राजादनो दृढस्कन्धः कपीष्टः प्रियदर्शनः ।' (Kśiraswāmī- Amar 2-4 -46)

2) 16 राजादनो दृढस्कन्धः । 'राजादनतरुः क्षीरी बालबिम्बफलं मधु । पक्वं पीतं कृष्णबीजं विशेषात् वानरप्रियम्' इति । राजादन इति च 'खिरणी' इति लोके । (Harshe)

IV- 1) क्षीरिका Kśirikā

---

* The current accepted name for *M. hexandra* Roxb. is *Manilkara hexandra* (Roxb.) Dubard
क्षीरी चोत्तरा तु राजन्या क्षीरभृद् रूपको नृपः (नि.शे. टीका)

C.S.Ci. 2-3-8,
According to Ḍalhaṇa it is *(Mimusops hexandara* Roxb.) called Khiranī (H).
See synonyms राजादन and क्षीरिणी (Balvantji. p. 126)
राजादन, राजाह्व
C.S. Su. 25-49, 27-14 0 etc.
S.S. Su. 38-43; 42-18 etc.
A.H. Su. 6.119; 10-23 15.13
(राजाह्व) 29-78
Rajādana is considered to be a syn. of both *Kśīrikā* (*Mimusops hexandra* Roxb.) खिरनी and *Priyāla* प्रियाल. (Balvantji. p. 336)

2) *Mimusops hexandra* Roxb.
Syn. *M. indica* A. DC. (Non Linn.)
M. kauki Wall.
(H.) Kshiri, Khirni; (Bom.) Rayan, Kirni, Raini; (Gond) Raini; (Mar.) Rayan; (Tam.) Palla, Kanna Palle; (Tel.) Pala, Palle, Palla-pandu; (Sans.) Rājādani, Kśiriṇi.
Habitat : A large tree found in the mountains of south India North of the Godavari, wild in Ceylon.
Food :- Produces an olive shaped yellow berry which is eaten. (Watt. Dict. V. 259)

3) *Mimusops kauki* Linn.*
The obtuse leaved Mimusops.
(Bom. H.) Khirni; (Mar) Kauki
Habitat ..It may be mentioned .. that *M. manilkara* Don (=*Achrus sapota* Linn.) a tree cultivated in Bengal for its fruits.(Watt.V.252)
Manilkara kauki Don
Syn. *Mimusops kauki* Linn.
(H.) (Panj.) (Bom.) Khirni; (Tam.) Pallai; (Mar.) Kauki; (Mal.) Manilkara (Chopra p. 161).

29. श्लेष्मातकः Śleṣmātakaḥ

श्लेष्मातकः कर्बुदारः पिच्छिलो लेखसारकः[१] ॥ ८८
शेलुः शैलुर्बहुवारः शापितो द्विजकुत्सितः ॥

श्लेष्मातको हिमो स्वादुः स्याद्रूक्षः पिच्छिलः शुचिः ॥ ८९

* The present accepted name is *Manilkara kauki* (Linn.) Dub.
१ 'लेखशाटकः' इति आनन्दा. पुस्तके पाठः ।

श्लेष्मातकः (Śleṣmātakaḥ), कर्बुदारः (Karbudāraḥ), पिच्छिलः (Picchilaḥ), लेखसारकः (Lekhasārakaḥ), शेलुः (Śeluḥ), शैलुः (Śailuḥ), बहुवारः (Bahuvāraḥ), शापितः (Śāpitaḥ), द्विजकुत्सितः (Dwijakutsitaḥ).

Śleṣmātaka is *śītavīrya* and sweet in taste. It is *rukṣa* (roughning), slimy and holy.

The modern writers differ in giving the local names which would imply the reverse.

Fam. Boraginaceae.

I- A-a- ***Cordia myxa*** Linn.*
b- Watt. Dict. II- 563 C- below Habitat
B-a- ***Cordia wallichi*** G. Don*.
Syn. *C. obliqua* Willd var. *Wallichi* (Chopra)
C. latifolia Roxb. (Watt. Dict.)
C- See below Habitat.

II- A &Ba- कर्बुदारः (Karbudāraḥ), शेलुः (Śeluḥ), भूतद्रुमः (Bhūtadrumaḥ), पिच्छिलः (Picchilaḥ), द्विजकुत्सितः (Dwijakutsitaḥ), गन्धपुष्पः (Gandhapuṣpaḥ), बहुवारः (Bahuvāraḥ).

A-b-(H.) Lasorā, Bhokar; (Bom) Gondan, Semar, Pistan; (Mar.) Bhokar, moṭha bhokar, Lasura, Gundo, Raigundo, Lapistan; (Tam.) Vidi, Varsu; (Tel.) Pedda boku , Makera, Irki, Peda-baketu;(Kan.), Chotte-chollutimar, chalemara;(Sans) Bahuwaraka (According to *Fleming*), Būkampadāruka (According to *Ainsli.*) (Watt. Dict.)
(H) Lasora, Chota Lasora; (B.) Bohodari; (Bom.) Gondan (Tam.) Naru-vili; (Tel.) Chinna nakkera (Chopra).

Note- See the remark noted under the heading *C. obliqua* in Watt. Dict.

B-b- (H.) Chhotā Lasora; (Bom.) Chhota bohnari; (Tam.) Bargūnā, Sirunaruvti; (Tel.) Chinna-botuga, Chinna-meker-chettu. (Watt. Dict.)

Modern names, noted by chopra are as above.

Habitat:

A. *C. myxa.* A moderate size deciduous tree ... salt ranges, sub Himlalayan tract from the Chenab to Assam, Bengal, Sind, western (North Canara), Central and South india.

B- Found in western India from the Punjab and Hindustan to

---

* The current accepted name for *C. myxa* Linn. is *C. dichotoma* Forst. and *C. wallichi* G. Don is *Cordia obliqua* Willd var. *tomentosa* (Willd.) Kazmi (comp. p. 43. see the note)

Ceylon. The variety, *C.wallichi* (The Dhaivan of Bombay) differs only in the degree of stellate tomentum on the leaves. (Watt., Dict.)

Medicine

A- According to Sanskrit writers the bark is useful in calculus affections, strangury and catarrh. The ripe fruits are sweet, cooling and demulcent. (U.C. Dutt)

B- The fruit in its raw state contains a gum used beneficially in gonorrhoea. (T. N.Ghose)

Food A- The fruit grows in clusters and consist of a drupe, the pulp of which is soft and clammy.

The fruit when ripe is eaten by the natives and also pickled ... The fruit which contains a great deal of mucilage is eaten by the natives.

B- The fruit is eaten and in the Deccan is generally known as bhokar. (Watt. Dict. II- p. 564-65).

IV- 1) *Cordia obliqua* Willd.

This is a large sebestan according to stocks, Dymock, Birdwood etc. *C. myxa* being the lesser, but the vernacular names given would imply the reverse to be the case. (Watt. II. 565).

2) श्लेष्मातक Ślesmātaka,

श्लेष्मातकी Śleṣmātakī

Cordia myxa Roxb. Lasodha लसोढा (H.) San. कर्बुदारः (?) and शेलुः C.S. Su. 4.16. 27. 158 etc.

Su. S. Su. 46. 193 (फल) etc.

A,H. 6-120 Ci. 18-16 etc.

Some other species of cordia such as *C. rothii* Roem. & Schult. and *C. wallichii* G. Don may also be used in its place. (Balvantji p. 413).

30. (३०) शमी Śamī

शमी शङ्कुफला तुङ्गा केशहन्त्री शिवाफला ॥
ईशानी शङ्करी लक्ष्मीर्मंगल्या पापनाशिनी ॥ ९०
शमीफलं गुरु स्वादु रूक्षोष्णं केशनाशनम् ॥

शमी (Śamī), शङ्कुफला (Śankuphalā), तुङ्गा (Tungā), केशहन्त्री (Keśahantrī), शिवाफला (Śivāphalā), ईशानी (Īśānī), शङ्करी (Śankarī), लक्ष्मीः (Lakśmīḥ), मंगल्या (Mangalyā), and पापनाशिनी (Pāpanāśinī) are synonymous.

The fruit of śamī is sweet in taste, *uṣṇavīrya, guru, rūkṣa* (roughning) and has depilatory properties.

Two plants are included under the heading 'A' शङ्कुफला (Śaṅkuphalā Dhn. Ni. & Raj. Ni. And 'B' अपराजिता (Aparājitā) (Raj.Ni.).

Fam. Leguminosae (Mimosaceae)

I- A-a- ***Prosopis spicigera*** Linn. & Willd.*

b- Roxburgh C-Punjab, Rajputana, Maharastra, Baluchistan.

B-a- ***Acacia suma*** Buch.- Ham.**

Syn. *Mimosa suma* Roxb.

Acacia polycantha Willd.

b- Roxburgh C- Common tree about calcutta and over Bengal; rare about Ambegaon forest, in Peth Dist. Nasik.

II- A-a-लक्ष्मी (Lakśmī), शङ्कुफला (Śaṅkuphalā), केशहन्त्री (Keśahantrī)

b- (H) zāṇḍ; (B) Śamī; (Guj.) Khijado; (Mar.) Śamī, soundal; (Tel.) Jammi; (Tam.) Kalisam; (Mal.) Paramppu.

B- शमी (Śamī), शान्ता (Śāntā), शुभा (Śubhā), भद्रा (Bhadrā), अपराजिता (Aparājitā).

III-a 1) केशवृद्धिकरणकामा... शमी (Sayan AV. Vi. 30)

2) Any offence against 'Shami causes the fall of hair making the head bald. (Shende Vi. 30; ii-3 p.35).

3) A person, who has come in contact with 'Shami tree' is called 'Shamiluma' and he was supposed to be in danger of suffering from injuring to his head. (See Kau. 31-1 Karambelkar)

4) See below IV-5,6,7 Balvantji.

5) 70 कदरः । सितखदिरः । 'कदरः खदिरे सिते सोमवल्केऽपि' त्यमरः । (Harshe)

6) 110 सोमवल्कलः कट्फलः । (Harshe)

7) सोमवल्को कण्टकित्वात् - शुक्लत्वाद् वा । आह च कदरः श्वेतसारोऽन्यः सोमवल्कः पथिद्रुमः । त्र्यर्थे सोमवल्कः खदिरः कट्फलम् . करञ्जश्च । (Ksīraswami-Amar 2-4-51)

IV- 1) *Mimosa suma* Roxb.

A. suma Buch.- Ham.

A. polycantha Wlld.

(Sans.) Shamee, (B). Sial -kanta

---

* The current accepted name is *Prosopis cineraria* Druce

** The current accepted name is *Acacia polycantha* Willd. (Comp. p.2)

A very common tree about calcutta and over Bengal.
Arboreous with remarkably white bark. (Roxb. CBC 423)

2) *A .suma* Kurz
(Mara.) Son khair; (Kan,) Bannimara (Bom. gaz. III 175)

3) *A. suma* Buch.- Ham.
Wood black (Lisboa)

Note - This tree may be 'Soma valkaḥ śyāmasraḥ of Dhn. Ni. who has not noted here under Śamī. Only Raj. Ni. notes it, we have found it on the bank of the Pāra river (पारनदी) near Ambegaon in Peth Taluka Dist. Nasik.

4) -शमी Śamī
Prosopis spicigera Linn.
C.S. Su. 25. 49; 27-157 etc.
S.S. Su. 48-123; Ci. 1-106 etc.
A.H. Su. 6-130 Ci. 8-18 etc. (Balwantji 390)

5) कदर Kadara
C.S. Su. 4-43; 25-49 etc.
S.S. Su. 38-12; Ci. 11-8
A.H. Su. 15-19
According to Dalhan it is like *khadira* with yellow wood (आपीतसार खदिराकारः) but it is usually said to be श्वेत खदिर *śveta khadira* which may be other species of Acacia such as *A. suma* Buch.- Ham.
See सोमवल्क (Balwantji p.70)
Somavalka is usually accepted as a synonym for 1) Khadira खदिर or श्वेत खदिर Śveta khadira and 2) Kaṭphala कट्फल
(Balvantji p. 456)

6) See सोमवल्क Post No. Guḍūcyādi Chapater 1.

7) *Acacia suma* Kurz.
Syn, *Mismosa suma* Roxb.
Baneswara - Dhaula khajra (White acacia) (Mar. Pāṇḍharākhair.)
Dang- Son Khair; Tel. Tella sundra.
Habitat Common in Bengal, Behar, the western Peninsula.
Botanic diagnosis .... (Watt. Dict. I-60)

8) खदिरः सोमवल्कोऽन्यः कदरः सोमवल्कलः । ..Safed Khair (i.e. white khair); (H.) Paparia Khair, safed khair; (Mar.) Pāṇḍharā Khair, Lat. *Acacia suma* Kurz.
There is an another species of white khair *Acacia ferruginea.*
(Chunekar Bh. Pr, Ni. 526).

31. (३१) बदरं Badaram (कोलम्) (Kolam)

बदरं कोलकं कोलं सौवीरं फेनिलं कुहम् ॥ ९१
कर्कन्धुकं गुडफलं बालेष्टं फलशैशिरः ॥

कर्कन्धुकोलबदरमम्लं वातकफापहम् ॥ ९२
पक्वं पित्तानिलहरं स्निग्धं च मधुरं रसे ॥

पुरातनं तृट्शमनमामघ्नं दीपनं लघु ॥ ९३
सौवीरबदरं स्निग्धं मधुरं वातपित्तजित् ॥

बदरं (Badaram), कोलकं (Kolakam), कोलं (Kolam), सौवीरं (Sauvīram), फेनिलं (Phenilam), कुहम् (Kuham), कर्कन्धुकं (Karkandhukam), गुडफलं (Guḍaphalam), बालेष्टं (Bāleṣṭam) and फलशैशिरः (Phalaśaiśiraḥ) are synonymous.

Karkandhu, Kola and *Badaram* when unripe is sour and pacifies *vātakapha doṣas;* when it is full ripe it pacifies *pitta* and *vātadoṣa,* is sweet in taste and *snigdha* (unctuous). The oldish one pacifies thirst, *āmadoṣa*, stimulates digestive capacity and is *laghu.*

Sauvīrabadara is sweet in taste, *snigdha* (unctuous) and pacifies *vāta* and *pitta doṣas.*

Under this heading three to four kinds are recorded by the Nighaṇṭu but rather difficut to identify and confirm them from modern kinds which are developed in several kinds by natural and cultivation processes. Our Nighaṇṭus record three kinds 'A' कोलम् (Kolam), 'B' कर्कन्धुकम् (Karkandhukam), 'C' सौवीरं बदरं (Sauvīram badaram). These are the only three edible kinds of Nighantu's.

Fam. Rhamnaceae (Chopra)
Rhamneae (Watt. Dict)

I- A-a- ***Zizyphus jujuba*** Lam.*
The indian jujuba or chinese date.
Syn. *Rhamnus jujuba* Linn.
b- Watt. Dict . See below IV-1
B-a- ***Zizyphus nummularia*** W & A.**
Syn. *Z. microphylla* Roxb.
(Watt. Dict.)
b- Chunekar Bh. Pr. Ni. P. 573
c- See below IV-2

---

* The current accepted name for *Z. jujuba* Lam.is *Z. mauritiana* Lam.

** The current accepted name is *Z. nummularia* (Burm. f.) wight & Arn.

C-a- *Zizyphus vulgaris* Lam.*
The common jujube
Syn. *Z. nitida* Roxb,
Z. sativa Gaertn.
b- Chunekar (Bh. Pr. Ni.) p. 572
c- See below IV -3

II- A-a- बदरम् (Badaram), कोलकम् (Kolakam) कोलम् (Kolam)
b- (H) Ber, badar; (B.) Kulber; (Mar.) Bor, Borīce zād; (Tam.) Ilande (Tel.) Regu cettu; (Eng.) Plum (Chunekar); (Tam.) Ilandai; (Tel.) Gangarena; (Mal.) Badaram; (Kan.) Bore;(Chopra) (Mar.& Bom.) Bor, Bordi, Burmi; (Sans.) Badari, Kola, Badara. (Watt. Dict.).

B-a-कर्कंधुकम् (Karkandhukam),गुडफलम् (Guḍaphalam) बालेष्टम् (Baleṣṭam) फलशैशिरः (Phalasaiśirah)
(H.) Jarberi, (Bundelkhand) Kānṭāber; (Kan.) Parpali gidda. (Watt.Dict).
(H.) zad ber; (Mar.) Jangali bor; (Guj.) Caniabor, Canibor, (Lat) *Zizyphus nummularia* W. & A.**
(Tam.) Koragoai; (Tel.) Neluregu; (Kan.) Pur pulli; (Chopra).

C-a- सौवीरं फेनिलम् (Sauvīram phenilam), स्निग्धं (Snigdham),मधुरम् (Madhuram), (Dhn. Ni.) गुडफलः (Guḍaphalaḥ), नृपबदरः (Nṛpabadaraḥ) राजकोलः (Rājakolaḥ) (Raj. Ni.)
b- (Sans.) Sauvīra, Rājabadara; (H,) Unnāb; (Eng.) Jujube.
Lat . *Zizyphus sativa* Gaertn.
Z. vulgaris Lam. (Chunekar)
(H.) Kandihari; (Bom.) Unnab. (Chopra)
(H.) Kaniari, Pitini or Pitniber; (Bom). Unnab, Ranbor. (Watt. Dict.)

III-a- 1) See below IV Balvantji`
b- 1) कर्को लोहितोन्धुः कर्कन्धु..... । बदति बदरी, बद् स्थैर्ये । ...
सुवीरदेश भवं सौवीरम् । (Kṣīraswāmi 2-4-37)

IV- 1) *Zizyphus jujuba* Lam.
The Indian jujube or chinese date.
Habitat. A small tree wild and extensively cultivated throughout India ... According to De Candolle the great numbers of known cultivated races indicate an ancient domestication ..an interesting paper written by *Babu Radhakant Deb.* .... in that article we read " According to Purānās, there was in former times, a

---

* The current name for *Z. vulgaris* Lam. is *Z. jujuba* Mill.
Zizyphus = Ziziphus

** The current name is - *Ziziphus nummularia* (Burm.f.) W. & A. (Comp. p. 162) celebrated place of pilgrimage 'Badaricāshrama' (The Badrinath of modern travellers) a town and a temple on the west bank of the Alacananda river in the province of shrinagar, which abounded with the badari or jujube trees.... is supposed to have been introduced more generally into other parts of India. Cultivation by selection and grafting has very much imporved the wild jujube fruit in India and as a natural consequence many kinds exist, which differ from each other in size. shape and flavour.

(Watt. Dict . VI- 4 -369 70)

2) *Zizyphus nummularia* W. & A.

Habitat : A prickly shrub found in the Punjab ... , North west provinces, Sind and Baluchistan, in Gujarat and the western Peninsula from the Deccan and Konkan southwards.

Food : The fruit is small, round, acid and much inferior to the preceding ... it is sweet acidulous and not unplesant flavour.

(Watt. Dict VI -4-370 -71)

3) *Zizyphus vulgaris* Lam.

Syn. *Z. sativa* Gaertn. The common jujube

Habitat : A shrub or small tree with rigid branches ... wild and cultivated in the Punjab ... North western frontier ... De Candolle expresses the belief that it is not truely wild in India ... but simply an escape from cultivation. ... 'It appears to me that the species is of North china, but it was introuduced in the west of Asia after the epoch, the epoch of Sanskrit language perhaps two thousand five hundred or three thousand years ago.

Food : The fruit is very similar in every way to that of *Z. jujuba* being an oval pulpy drupe about the size of a plum. It varies much and can be greatly improved ...... when fresh it is rather acid but when dried is much sweet. (Watt. VI- 4-373-74)

4) बदर Badara, बदरी Badarī

Zizyphus jujuba Lam.

C.S. Su. 4-10; 22, 24 etc.

S.S.Su. 38-47; 39-7 etc.

A.H. Su. 6-120; Ci. 1-33-35 etc.

The tree is called Badarī and the fruit is Badara. Kola कोल, कर्कन्धु Karkandhu, सौवीर Sauvīra are all various species of *zizyphus* out of which the first three only are edible.. The so called other Badara varieties as सिंचितिका *Sincitikā* and कुवल *Kuvala* have different botanical source. (Balvantji p. 268)

There are about fifty species found in tropical Asia and America. In India some eighteen to .....species are recorded, out of them our Nighaṇṭus have recorded three species as edible and medicinal kinds.

32. (३२) करीरः Karīraḥ

करीरो गूढपत्रश्च शाकपुष्पो मृदुफलः ॥ ९४
ग्रन्थिलस्तीक्ष्णसारश्च क्रकचस्तीक्ष्णकंटकः ॥

वातश्लेष्महरं रुच्यं कटूष्णं गुदकीलजित् ॥ ९५
करीरमाध्मानकरं रुचिकृत् स्वादुतित्तक्म् ॥

(अन्यच्च)
करीराक्षक पीलूनि त्रीणि स्तन्यफलानि च[१] ।
स्वादु तीक्ष्णकटूष्णानि कफवातहराणि च ॥१००

S. S.Su. 46. 194

करीरः (Karīraḥ), गूढपत्रः (Gūḍhapatraḥ), शाकपुष्पः (Śākapuṣpaḥ), मृदुफलः (Mṛduphalaḥ), ग्रन्थिलः (Granthilaḥ), तीक्ष्णसारः (Tīkṣṇasāraḥ), क्रकचः (Krakacaḥ), and तीक्ष्णकंटक : (Tīkṣṇakanṭakaḥ) are synonymous.

Karīra (Fruit) pacifies *vāta* and *kapha doṣas*, is pungent in taste and *uṣṇavīrya* and useful in piles.

Karīra causes flatulence. It is appetiser, sweet and bitter in taste. The fruits of *karīra*, *Akṣaka* and *pīlu* are sweet, pungent, *uṣṇavīrya* and *tīkṣṇa*. These pacify *kapha* and *vāta doṣas*.

Fam. Capparidaceae

I- a- ***Capparis decidua*** Edgew.
Syn. *C. aphylla* Roth.

b- Dymock c- More or less all over India, but not to the Eastern Indian coast.

II- a- गूढपत्रः (Gūḍhapatraḥ) शाकपुष्पः (Śakapuṣpaḥ) तीक्ष्ण कंटकः (Tîkṣṇakanṭakaḥ) मृदुफलः (Mṛduphalaḥ)

b- (H) Karer; (Bom) Kārī; (Poona) Neptī, Neptād; (Tel.) Kariramu; (Tam & Mal.) Sengam.

III- a See below IV 1 Balvantji
2) 19 Karira TS ii-4-9-2

---

१ तृणशून्य फलानि च इति सौश्रुतः साधु पाठः ।

* The current accepted name is *C. decidua* (Forsk). Edgew.

S.Br. ii-5-2-11 (Harshe)

IV- 1) करीर Karīra.
Capparis decidua Edgew.
C.S. Su. 27.139 etc.
S.S. Su . 8-15 etc.
A.H.Su. 6-77 etc. (Balwantji p. 78).

33. (३३) करमर्दकम् Karamardakam

करमर्दकमाविग्नं सुषेणं पाणिमर्दकम् ॥ ९६
कराम्लं करमर्दं च कृष्णपाककलं मतम् ॥
अम्लं तृष्णापहं रुच्यं पित्तकृत्करमर्दकम् ॥ ९७
पक्वं तु मधुरं शीतं रक्तपित्तहरं मतम् ॥

करमर्दकम् (Karamardakam), आविग्नं (Āvignam), सुषेणं (Suṣeṇam), पाणिमर्दकम् (Pāṇimardakam), करासूं (Karāmlam), करमर्दं (Karamardam) and कृष्णपाककलं (Kṛṣṇapākaphalam) are synonymous.

(when uripe) the fruit of *Karamadaka* is sour in taste, appetizer, alleviates thirst and aggravates *pitta,* when ripe it is sweet in taste, *śitavīrya* and useful in haemorrhagic disorders (*raktapitta*).

Fam. Apocynaceae.

I- a- ***Carissa carandas*** Linn.

b- Chopra c- wild throughout India in dry regions.

II- a पाणिमर्दकम् (Pāṇimardakam), कराम्लम् (Karāmlam), सुषेणम् (Suṣeṇam), कृष्णपाकफलम्. (Kṛṣṇapākaphalam), आविग्नम् (Āvignam).

b- (S.) Kāncuka; (B) Karamech; (Mar.) Karawand; (Tel.) Vaka; (Tam). Kalakkay; (Mal.) Karakka.
ii) (S) karamardikā; (Tel.) Kalivi; (Tam.) Ciree; (Kashmir) Karavand

III- a- 1) See below IV- 1 Balvantji.

b- 1) कृष्णं पाकं फलमस्य । आविजेरमाविग्नः । सुषेणक कपिमुखाभः । करेण मृद्यते करमर्दः. कराम्लोऽपि । ... (Ksriraswami 2-4-68 Amar)

IV 1) करमर्दक Karamardāka
C.S. Su . 4.10 26-112 etc.

---

* The current accepted name is *C. congesta* Wight

S.S.Su. 38-73 42.18 etc.

Karamarda is known as *Carissa carandas* Linn. *Karaunda* H. and its wild kind called *karamardikā* करमर्दिका (Raj. Ni) is *C. spinarum* Linn. करौंदी (H). (Balvantuji p.76)

2) *Carissa carandas* Linn.

(H.) Karaunda or Karonda; (Ben.) Kārumia , Kāramchi; (Mar.Bom.) Karavanda, karānda; (Sans.) Karamarda (the tree,) Karamardaka, Aving (the fruit) (Tam.) Kalak; Kalapa (Tel.) Kulini Kāya, Waaka; (Kan) Kara kai. heggarjige.

Habitat : A dichotomously branched bush, cultivated for its fruit in most parts of India, said to be wild in Oudh, Bengal and south India, in Punjab and Gujarat it frequents hedges and forms spiny low dense bushes .... It flowers from February to April and produces a small fruit which is grape green when young, white and pink when approaching maturity and nearly black when ripe The fruit ripes in July to August.

Food : The fruit is made into pickle just before it is ripe .... when ripe it makes a very good jelly .. foı which it is cultivated in gardens owned by Europeans.

Structure of the wood : White , hard smooth, close grained.

Domestic uses : Strong fences. (Watt. Dict. II. 165 - 66)

There are twenty species African, Asiatic and Australian. Sir J.D. Hooker remarks five Indian species that they are probable mere forms of one or two variable plants but only four are recorded. these are :

a) *Carissa carundas* Linn.

Syn. *C. congesta* Wight

b) *Carissa diffusa* Roxb.

Syn. *C. spinarum* A. DC.

C) *C. macrophylla* Wall.

Syn. *C. lanceolata* Dalz.

Deccan peninsula, Coorg, Konkan at Ramghat ... The fruit is eaten size of a plum ripens in May ... Superior to that of *C. carandas*.

Habitat : A large shrub with very strong curved thorns.

d) *C. spinarum* A.DC.

Syn. *C. diffusa* Roxb.

The flora of Br. indi.regards this species as probably only a state of *C. carandas* concurring in his opinion with Dr. Brandis. It is nearly distinguished by its being a smaller plant with shorter and more slender spines, more acute leaves and a smaller berry.

Var. hirsuta is more pubescent than the type condition, it is *C. villosa* Roxb. edi. Carry & Wall. and also of Wight ... a form which Roxburgh regards it a quite different from the others..... described by him and of *'little economic value'* H. Karaund; Sans. Karamardica. Tel. Wakoilu.

Habitat : Wild in most parts of India especially in drier regions and in the plains of Punjab, the sub Himalayan tract ....

Birdwood views it introduced into Bombay and not indigenous, *Roxburgh* says it is a native of Ganjam district and from thence northward to the Hugali. (*C.diffusa*).

Food : The fruit is used generally in tarts . fenses.. (Watt. Dict .)

Domestic uses : Largely used for dry fenses.... excelleut fuel.

From the above information we come to know that in India only 4 to 5 species are recorded by botanists but it would be proper to say that of these four, *C.carands* Linn. and *C. spinarum* A.D C.may be common or original source of the re maining races or varieties.In Watt. Dict. and in Chopra's glossary medicinal uses are given only of *C. carandas* and *C.spinarum* but those of *C.carandas* are more extensive (Watt) and generally all the modern writers have accepted it to be the Karamarda करमर्द (*C.carandas*Linn. I-a above) of Sanskṛt books. Bhavamishra has recorded two kinds of *Karamarda* and notes the fruits of which are smaller is *karmardikā*. (Chunekar Bh. Pr. Ni.574-75)

This may be *C. spinarum* A.DC.

34. (३४) (कदम्बौ) (Kadambau) कदम्बः Kadambaḥ

कदम्बो वृत्तपुष्पश्च नीपस्तु ललनाप्रियः ॥ ९८
कादम्बर्यङ्कवृक्षोऽन्यः सुवासः कर्णपूरकः ॥

धाराकदम्बः प्रावृष्यः कादम्बर्यो हरिप्रियः ॥ ९९
नीपो धूलिकदम्बोऽन्यः सुवासो वृत्तपुष्पकः ॥

कदम्बस्तु कषायः स्यात् रसे शीतो गुणेऽपि च ॥ १००
व्रणसंरोहणश्चापि कासदाहविषापहः ॥

कदम्ब (Kadamba), वृत्तपुष्पः (Vṛttapuṣpaḥ), नीपः (Nīpaḥ), ललनाप्रियः (Lalanāpriyaḥ), कादम्बर्य (Kādambaryaḥ), अङ्कवृक्षः (Ankavṛksaḥ), are synonymous. The other type is having सुवासः (Suvāsaḥ), and कर्णपूरकः

(Karṇapūrakaḥ) धाराकदम्बः (Dhārākadambaḥ), प्रावृष्यः (Prāvṛṣyaḥ), कादम्बर्यः (Kādambaryaḥ), हरि (लि) प्रियः (Hari(li) priyaḥ),नीपः (Nīpaḥ) are synonymous,. There is an another type of Kadamba called as धूलिकदम्बः (Dhūlikadambaḥ)of which synonyms are सुवासः (Suvāsaḥ) and वृत्तपुष्पकः (Vṛttapuṣpakaḥ).

Kadamba is *kaṣāya* in taste, and *śītavīrya*. It is useful in woundhealing, cough (*kāsa*), burning sensation and in poisons.

Under this heading four plant names are recorded. These are 'A' कदम्ब (Kadamba) proper, 'B' धूलिकदम्ब (Dhūli kadamba), 'C' धाराकदम्ब कादम्बर्य (Dharākadamba, Kādambarya) and the fourth 'D'भूमि (मी) कदम्ब (Bhumi (ī) Kamdmba) which is included by Raj. Ni.

I- A-a-***Mitragyna parvifolia*** Korth.*
Syn. *Stephegyne parvifolia* Korth
Nauclea parvifolia Willd.
b- Chopra, Watt Dict.
c- See blelow IV -3 Watt Dict.
B-a- ***Anthocephalus indicus*** A. Rich,**
Syn. *A. cadamba* Miq.
Nauclea cadamba Roxb. (Chopra)
A. *cadamba* Benth. & Hook f.
b- Watt Dict. Chopra.
c- See below IV- 4 Watt Dict.
C-a- ***Adina cordifolia*** (Roxb). Benth. & Hook. f.***
b- Watt. Dict. c-See below IV- 5
D-a- ***Sphaeranthus indicus*** Linn. and its allied varieties.
(see chapter 1 Plant No. 49)

II- A-a- वृत्तपुष्पः (Vṛttapuṣpaḥ), सुरभिः (Surabhiḥ), (Raj. Ni.)
b- (H) Kadam; (Bom. & Mar.) Kaḷamba; (Tam.) Kadambai, (Tel) Nirukadami; (Mal.) Sira Kaṭam.
B-a- नीपः (Nīpaḥ), धूलिकदम्ब (Dhūlikadmba), सुवासः (Suvāsaḥ), वृत्तपुष्पः (Vṛittapuṣpaḥ), क्रमुकप्रसूनः (Kramukaprasūnaḥ) परागपुष्पः (Parāga puṣpaḥ), मकरन्द वासः (Makaranda vāsaḥ), रेणुकदम्बः (Reṇukadambaḥ)
b- (H.) Kadamba; (Bom. Mar.) Niva; (B). Kadam; (Tam.) Vellai

---

* The current name is
Mitragyna parvifolia (Roxb) Korth.
** The current accepted name is
Anthocephalus chinensis (Lamk.) A. Rich. ex. Walp.
*** The current name is
Adina cordifolia (Willd ex. Roxb.) Hook f.ex. Brandis.

Kadamba; (Tel.) Kadambamu; (Kan.) Kadavailu, Kadab, Kadval.

C-a- कादम्बर्यः (Kādambaryaḥ),सिन्धुपुष्पः (Sindhupuṣpaḥ), मदाढ्यः (Madādhyaḥ), कर्णपूरकः (Karṇapūrakaḥ), धाराकदम्बः (Dhārākadambaḥ), हरिप्रियः (Haripriyaḥ), पुलकी (Pulakī)

b- (Sans.) Dhārākadamba; (H.) Haladu; (B) Kelikadam; (Tam. & mal.) Manja Kadamba; (Tel.) Pasapu Kadamba; (Mar. Bom.) Heda, Hedu.

D-a- भूमि कदम्बः (Bhūmikadambaḥ), भूनिम्बः (Bhūnimbaḥ),भूमिजः (Bhūmijaḥ), वृत्तपुष्पः (Vṛtta puṣpaḥ),व्रणहारकः (Vraṇahārakaḥ) त्रिकदम्बा कटुर्वर्ण्या etc.

Note - Compiler of Dhn. ni. notes medicinal uses of कदम्ब Kadamba but that of Raj. Ni. has recorded those of कदम्ब (Kadamba) proper and also those of three other Kadambas without mentioning their names.

They may be *kadamba* (I-A-a), *Nīpa* (I-B-a) and third *Dhārādkadamba* (I-D-a above), *Bhūmikadamba* which is recorded by him, seems to be excluded. from them.

III- a- 1) See below IV- 1 Balvantji.

b- 1) चतुर्विधः कदम्बोऽथ -॥ (Raj. Ni. -9)

2) अन्यो धूलिकदम्बः स्यात् नीपो राजकदम्बक : । (Madanapala Ni.)

3) नीपं दृष्ट्वा हरितकपिशं केसरैरर्धरुढम् -। (Pūrva Megha)

4) त्यक्त्वा कदम्ब कुटजार्जुनसर्जनीपान् । (Ri. Sam. 3-13)

5) हरिद्रुः पीतदारुः कदम्बकः सुपुष्पश्च ।
....सुराह्वः पीतकद्रुमः ॥...... (Raj. Ni. Dhn. Ni. P. 366)

6) महाश्रावणिका... कदम्बपुष्पा...भूकदम्बः । (Raj. Ni. Dhn.Ni, p. 38)

Note :- Kalidas mentions Nīpa and Kadamba as two distinct tree species (See III -3, 4 above)

7) नयति सुखं नीपः । प्रीणाति प्रियकः । के दाम्यति कदम्बः । हलिनः प्रियः सुगंधि वासनात् । धाराकदम्बो राजकदम्बश्चासौ । धूलिकदम्बोऽन्यः । आह च 'कदम्बः प्रावृषेण्यः कादम्बर्यो हलिप्रियः । नीपो धूलिकदम्बोऽन्यः सुवासो वृत्तपुष्पकः ।' (Kṣīraswāmi; Amar 2-4- 42)

8) 303 कदम्बः कुत्सिताम्बः । 'वृत्तपुष्पः प्रावृषेण्यो हरिद्रुश्च हरिप्रियः'। इति हारावली । (Harshe)

9) 368 हरिप्रियमिति 'हरिप्रियं' कालसारं तथा कालानुसार्यकं कालंबक इति ख्यात चन्दनजाती । कदम्ब प्रावृषेण्यः । (Harshe)

10) 365 हरिप्रियः - कदम्बः 'मर्कट नीपयोः ।' (Harshe)

IV- 1) कदम्ब (Kadamba)

Anthocephalus indicus A. Rich
C.S.Su. 4.20, 47, etc.
S.S. Su. 6-33 38-13 etc.
A.H. Su. 10-32; 15-41 etc.
See कुत्सिताम्ब, नीप and प्रियक

कुत्सिताम्ब Kutsitāmba
A.H. Su. 15-26
See synonym कदम्ब

नीपः Nīpaḥ
C.S. Su. 4.23; 27-142 etc.
S.S.Su. 6-33; 46-139 etc.
A.H.Ci. 19-81, 20-30 etc.

Nīpa has been addressed by Ḍalhaṇa as *Dhūlikadamba* or *Mahākadamba* This may be the *Nīpa* variety of *Kadamba* although it may also be used as a synonym of Kadamba where edible fruit has been described under the name of *Nīpa;* an other kind of *kadamba* is *Mitragyna parvifolia* Korth which we have accepted as *Girikadamba*. Thus *Adina cordifolia* Benth. and Hook. F. which has been described in Raj. Ni. as Haridru may be Nīpa variety and *Anthocephalus cadamba*. Miq., Syn. *A. indica* A. Rich may be kadamba proper. See कदम्ब (Kadamba)
(Balwantji p. 228).

2) "Sweet heart how I am bewitched by the kadamba blossom all the other flowers together have not such a power. Variely kāma wields nowadays a bow armed with honeyball of Kadamba. (Dymock See Ayu. Patrikā 16-10-62 p. 225, *A. indica* A. Rich.).

3) *Stephegyne parvifolia* Korth.*
Syn. *Nauclea parvifolia* Willd.
N. parviflora Pers.
Cephalanthus pilulifer Lam.
(H.) Kadamba, Kalamba; (Mar. Bom.) Kadamba, Kalam, Kadam; (Tam.) Buta-Kadamba; (Tel.) Mir kadambe, Bata ganapu; (Kan) Kongu, Hedu Kadani.
Habitat : A large deciduous tree found in the dry forests of tropical Himalayas .. .. and throughout the drier parts of India, Burma and Ceylon.
Domestic The timber is used in planking and hermitura.
(Watt. Dict. VI. 3 p. 360)

4) *Anothocephalus cadamba* Miq. (See Vol. V. 343).

* The current accepted name is *Mitragyna parvifolia* (Roxb.) Korth.

Syn. *A. cadamba* Benth. & Hook f.
Nauclea cadamba Roxb. (Vol. I. 266)
(H) Kadaṃba; (Bom) Kadam, Nhyee; (K.) Niva; (Mar.) Kadam, Nhiv, Niva; (Tam.) Velutta kadamba; (Tel.) Kadamba, Rudraksa Kadamba; (Kan.) Kadaga, kadwal, Kaad vailu.

Habitat :
A large deciduous tree, wild in the Northern and Eastern Bengal, Pegu and the western coast. It grows very fast.

Food: The fruit is eaten and the foilage some times used as fodder for cattle.

Domestic uses : The flowers are offered at Hindu shrines, They are sacred to Śiva, often cultivated for ornament and for the greatful shed its large close foilage offers. (Watt. I. 266)

5) *Adina cordifolia* Benth. & Hook. f.
Syn. *Nauclea cordifolia* Roxb.
(H) Haldu, kadāmi; (Ben.) Kelikadam, Petpuria; (Tam.) Manjakadambe; (Tel.) Dudagu , Paspu Kandi, Paspu; (Kan.) Hedde, Yettega -pettig, Arsanategu;, (Mar.) Hedu; (Guj.) Heldhawan; (Sans) Dhārākadamba.

Habitat. A large deciduous tree, found in the sub Himalayan tract from Jamna ..... extending throughout the moist regions of India, Burma and Ceylon. It is common in the western peninsula ... especially in the forest of Ratnagiri and in the Thana districts in the Konkan, Surat, Baroch ... South in the forests of Mysor, upper Godavari.

Structure of the wood yellow moderately hard, No heartwood ... good polished, and is durable, furniture, agricultual impliments. (Watt. I. 114-15)

6) See Chunekar (Bh. Pr. Ni.) P. 495

7) See चन्दन Candana.
Chapter III हरिचन्दन (Haricandana) etc.

35 (३५) करञ्जौ Karañjau- करञ्जः Karañjaḥ

करञ्जो नक्तमालश्च पूतिकश्चिरबिल्वकः ॥ १०१
घृतपर्णः करञ्जोऽन्यः प्रकीर्यो गौर एव च ॥

करञ्जश्चोष्ण तिक्तः स्यात् कफपित्तास्रदोषजित ॥ १०२
व्रणप्लीहकृमीन् हंति भूतघ्नो योनिरोगहा ॥

१ 'चिरबिल्वः' करञ्जोऽन्यः प्रकीर्यो गौर एव च । इति शोढल पाठः ।

चिरबिल्वः करञ्जश्च तीव्रो वातकफापहः ॥ १०३

करञ्जः (Karañjaḥ), नक्तमालः (Naktamālaḥ), पूतिकः (Pūtikaḥ) and चिरबिल्वकः (Cirabilvakaḥ) are synonymous. There is an another type of *Karañja* called as घृतपर्ण करञ्जः (Ghṛtaparṇa karañjaḥ) of which synonyms are प्रकीर्यः (Prakiryaḥ) and गौरः (Gauraḥ).

Karañja is bitter in taste, *uṣṇavīrya* and pacifies *kapha pitta* and *rakta doṣas*. It is useful in wounds, disorders of spleen, helminths, as antiseptic and in disorders of female genital tract.

Cirabilva karañja is sharp in action and pacifies *vāta* and *kapha doṣas*.

करञ्ज Karañja as a generic compound word is applied to plant names of some species by some Sanskṛt writers. But the compiler of Dhn. ni. included only three plant species namely 'A' करञ्जः (Karañjaḥ) proper, 'B' चिरबिल्वः (Cirabilvaḥ) and the third 'C' घृतपर्णः करञ्जः (Ghṛtaparṇaḥ Karañjaḥ). He noted medicinal uses of करञ्जः (Karañja) and चिरबिल्व (Cirabilva) only. but Raj. Ni. notes also those of घृतपर्णः करञ्जः (Ghṛtaparṇaḥ Karañja). In Gaṇadravyāvalī the first part of this book are noted करञ्जौ (Karañjau i.e. two Karañjas -see. IV- 5).

Fam. Leguminosae

I- A-a- ***Pongamia pinnata*** Merr. *
Syn. *P. glabra* Vent (Chopra)
b- Watt. Dict. & Roxburgh
c- See below IV-8 Watt.Dict.

Fam. Urticaceae. Ulmaceae

I- B-a- ***Holoptelea integrifolia*** Planch **
The Entire leaved Elm.
Syn. *Ulmus integrifolia* Roxb. (Watt. Dict)
b- Chopra.
c- See below IV -7

For Confirmation

Fam. Leguminosae Caesalpiniaceae

I- C-a- ***Caesalpinia digyna*** Rottl.
b- Desai C-See below IV-9

II - A -a- करञ्जः (Karañjaḥ), नक्तमालः (Naktamālaḥ)
b- H. Karañja, Kiramāl; B. Dahur Karanja; Bom. Mar. Karanja;

---

* The current accepted name is *Derris indica* (Lam.) Bennet.

** The current accepted name is *Holoptelea integrifolia* (Roxb.) Planch.

Mal. Punnu; Tam. Pungu; Tel. Kranuga.

II- B-a- पूतिकः (Pūtikaḥ); चिरबिल्वः (Cirabilvaḥ)

b- Sans. *Chirabilva* (Chopra); H. Pāpri Karanji, Chilbil; Mar. Vāvali; Tam. Aya, Tum-karhi-maram; Tel. Nemli, Naveli; Kan. Rasbija.

C-a- घृतपर्ण करञ्जः (Ghṛtaparṇa Karañjaḥ), प्रकीर्यः (Prakīryaḥ) गौर (Gaura)

b- H. Vākeri-mūla; B.Umūl, Kūchi; Tel. Nāni gutcha; Mar. & Bom. Vākeriche bhāte, Vākeri mūla.

The compiler of Dhn. Ni. has not recorded the medicinal uses of this plant species (घृतपर्ण करञ्ज) but Raj. ni. records them., as follows.

अन्यो घृतकरञ्जः स्यात् प्रकीर्यो घृतपर्णकः ।
स्निग्धपत्रस्तपस्वी च विषारिश्च विरोचनः ॥
घृतकरञ्जः कटूष्णो वातहृत् व्रणनाशनः ।
सर्वत्वग्दोषशमनो विषस्पर्शविनाशनः ॥

The synonyms घृतपर्ण करञ्जः Ghṛtaparṇa Karañjaḥ or घृतकरञ्जः Ghṛta Karañja प्रकीर्य Prakīryaḥ followed in the both Nighaṇṭus seem to be of the same and one plant.

III- a-1) See below IV-1 Balwantji.

b-1) चिरि (र) बिल्वो नक्तमालः करजश्च करञ्जके ।
प्रकीर्यः पूतिकरजः पूतिकः कलिमारकः ॥
करञ्जभेदा षड्ग्रन्थो मर्कट्यङ्गारवल्लरी ।

अमर ४.४८

चिरिणं बिलति भिनत्ति चिरबिल्वः । नक्तं रात्रावालमस्मान्नक्तमालो भूताश्रयत्वात् रक्तमाल इत्येके । कं रञ्जयति करञ्जः (करजश्च) । प्रकीर्यते प्रकीर्यः । पूतिको दुर्गन्धः । कलेर्मारकः कलहहृत् यदिन्दुः "करञ्जो रक्तमालश्च पूतिकश्चिरिबिल्वकः । घृतपर्ण करञ्जोऽन्यः प्रकीर्यो गौर एव च ॥"
पूतिकरञ्जःसुमनास्तथा कलहनाशनः ।द्व्यर्थे करजः करञ्जो नखश्च ।

(Kshīraswami Amar 2-4-48).

2) करञ्जः षड्विधः ।

(Raj. Ni. Chap. Dh. Ni. P.364)

3) चिरबिल्वः -वृद्धकरञ्जः 'चिरिहिली' इति लोके।

(Ḍalhaṇa. S. Sū.37.10)

पूतिकरञ्जः । (Arun A.H.Su. 6. 98.)

4) पूतिकः चिरबिल्वः कण्टकी विटप करञ्जः ' इत्येके ।

Ḍalhaṇa S. Sū, 38.8

5) करञ्जौ च । (Gaṇadravyāvali First part of this book.)

Note - This reference mentions two karañjas.

6) करञ्जद्वयम् - एकः पूतिकरञ्जः चिरिबिल्वाख्योऽपरो नक्तमालश्च ।
(Arun A.H. Sū. 15-19)

7) द्वौ करञ्जौ - करञ्जश्च पूतिकरञ्जः ।
(Kāsyap. sam. Mūtrakṛchra)

8) पूतिकारग्वधयोः पत्राणि । पूतिकः चिरबिल्वः । (Dalhan. 39.4)

9) चिरबिल्वः मरा. घाणेरा करंज, मल्या. आविल, कोंकण - वावळी *Eleocarpus serratus* (A.H.Kosh.)

10) नतमाल - पूतिकः । नक्तमालः बृहत् करञ्जः पूतिकः चिरबिल्वः ।
(Dalhan, S.Su. 38.8.10)

11) प्रकीर्यः - पूतिकरञ्ज दुर्गन्धी करञ्जः । (Amar MṢS)

IV- 1) करञ्जः Karañjaḥ.

Three plant species have been accepted under the name of Karañja and its several synonyms mentioned below. Seeds, seed oil, bark and leaves are the parts which have been recommended for use. But there seems to be much confusion regarding actual plant species which should be accepted under particular synonyms mentioned below. The three plant species are

(1) *Pongamia pinnata* (Linn.) Merr. Ḍahara Karañja डहर करञ्ज B; Ḍiṭhoharī डिठोहरी H; (2) *Caesalpinia crista* Linn Nāṭā Karañja B. Kāṇṭā नाटा करञ्जः NaṭaKarañja करञ्जः H.

2) *Holoptelea integrifolia* Planch, Pāprī पाप्री, Cilbil चिलबिल H. In Su 1.81and 114 Caraka hasmentioned the first two species under the names of *Udakīrya* उदकीर्य and *Prakīrya* among the purgative fruit drugs (Virecaka Phalinis विरेचकफलिनी) and Pūtika पूतिक as purgative (Virecaka) tree bark ..In spite of these clear indications it is suprising that *Pūtika* or *Pūtikarañja* has been identified with Kāntā karañja which in none of its parts appears to have any smell as the name appears to indicate. It is, therefore, suggested that *Cirabilva* (*H.integrifolia*) may be accepted under the name of *Pūtika* etc. and the first two may be accepted under *Karañja Dwaya,* while *Karañjikā* and *Naktamāla* may be equated with Pongamia. It might be noted that *Karañja* has been mentioned in the pungent group *(Kaṭu skandha*) and *Naktamāla* in the bitter group (*Tikta skandha*) .... see synonyms उदकीर्य, करञ्जिका, चिरबिल्व, नक्तमाल, नक्तगहव and प्रकीर्य.

C.S.Su.3-2, 12, 13, 14, etc.
S.S. Su. 36.32, 38. 5, 15, etc.
A.H. Su. 2.2, 15. 1, 17, 25, 45, etc. (Balwantji pp. 74.76)

i) पूतिक, पूतीक Pūtika, Pūtīka.
C.S.Su. 1.14. 115 etc.
S.S.Su. 11.11, 19; 16.27 etc.
A.H. Su. 30.9, 21 etc.
See करंज, चिरबिल्व, पूतिकरञ्जः (Balwantji p. 256)

ii) नक्तमाल Naktamāla
C.S.Su. 4.14, 17 etc.
S.S.Su. 11.11, 14.36 etc.
A.H. Su.10.29; 30.9 etc. (Balwantji p. 214)

iii) पूतिकरञ्जः Pūtikarañja
C.S. Ci. 26.12
S.S. Su. 46.27 8 etc.
Ḍalhaṇa appears to believe that *Pūtika* or *Pūtikarañja* is *Cirabilwa* चिरबिल्व and others think it to be *Kaṇṭaki karañja* (Bonduc nut) which does not have any Pūti (bad smell) in any of the part except in its seed oil. (Balwantji p. 257)

iv) चिरबिल्व Cirabilwa
Holoptelea integrifolia Planch.
Cilbil चिल्बिल् H; पापडी Pāpaḍī; Garhwal.
C.S.Su. 4.3, 4. etc.
S.S.Su. 36.10 ci. 2.89 etc.
A.H.Su. 6.98 ci. 8.16 etc.

In Caraka Samhita ci. 13. 166 there is a suggested change in the version (पाठ) wherein *Cirabilwa* has been replaced by *Pūtika* पूतिक. It may also be noted that its young leaves (पल्लव)or (अंकुर) have been often used as vegetable. It has been previously shown that *Cirabilva* and *Pūtika* should be considered synonyms. (Balwantji p. 158)

2) See Chunekar Bh. Pr. Ni. p. 348. 354.

3) पूतिक (Pūtikā), पूतिकरञ्ज (Pūtikarañja), लता करञ्ज (Latā Karañja).
Caesalpinia bonducella
चिरबिल्व (Cirabilva), पूतिकरञ्जपत्रक (Pūtikarañja Patrak), पूतिगन्ध (Pūtigandha) *Holoptelea integrifolia* .(Ni. Adarsha)

4) 501 महाकरञ्ज (Mahākarañja)
Mara. Thora Karañja; Konkan वावळा (Vāvaḷā), पापडी (Pāpadī) (Br. Ni. Pade)

5) 500 घृतकरञ्ज – Mara. Copadā karañja; Kan. Tapasiya.
(Br. Ni. Pade)

6) *Holoptelea integrifolia* Planch.
H. & B. Papari; Mar. Vāvaḷā; Sans, Chirabilva (Chopra)

7) *Holoptelea integrifolia* Planch.
The entire leaved elm.
Syn. *Ulmus integrifolia* Roxb.
H. Papri, chilbil; Mar. vāvaḷī; Tam. Aya; Tambachi-maram; Tel. Mamli, Namba; Kan. Raebija.
Habitat : A large spreading deciduous tree, met with the outer lower ranges of Himalayas from Jamna to Oudh .... Behar to Travancore. (Watt. Dict. IV. 261)

8) *Pongamia glabra* Vent.
Syn. *Galedupa indica* Lam.
G. arborea Roxb.
Dalbergia arborea Willd.
H. Karañja, Papar, Kirmal; Mar. Karanj; Tel. Karug, Kagger Sans. Karañja, Naktamala.
Habitat : A tall erect tree or climber, met with all over India from the central and eastern Himalaya to Ceylon & Malacca.
Watt. Dict. VI. 332.

9) *Caesalpinia digyna* Rottl.
Syn. *C. oliosperma* Roxb.
Hibitat : A prickly tree of the eastern Himlalaya, eastern and Western Peninsulas, Ceylon.
Oil : Roxburgh says that an oil is expressed from the seeds which is used for lamps.
Medicine : The root is prescribed in native practice and has marked astringent properties (....) Dr. Dymock (....) says it is given in pthisis and scrofulous affections, when sores exist it is applied externally as well, a kind of tuberous swelling which is found on the root is preferred. (Watt. Dict. II -9)

10) *Caesalpinia digyna* Rottle
Root ....given internally in phthisis, scrofulus affections and diabetes .... bitter substance bonducin,. saponin. (chopra p.44).

V 1) अथ कण्टककरञ्जघृतकञ्जौ
करञ्जो नक्तमालश्च करजश्चिरबिल्वकः ।
घृतपूर्ण करञ्जोऽन्यः प्रकीर्यो पूतिकोऽपि च ॥
स चोक्तः पूतिकरञ्जः सोमवल्कश्च स स्मृतः ।
Bh. Pra. Nī. Chunekar. p. 350.

करञ्ज (वृक्ष करञ्ज) (Tree)

Pongamia glabra Vent.
करञ्ज (कंटकरञ्ज) (spiny)
Sans. Pūtikarañja पूतिकरञ्ज, Latā karañja लता करञ्ज
Kaṇṭakīkarañja कण्टकी करञ्ज
Caesalpinia bonducella Fleming
Chunekar Bh. Pr. Ni. p. 352.

2) लता करञ्जः Lata Karañjaḥ (Raj. Ni.)
Medicinal uses.
लता करञ्जपत्रं तु कटूष्णं कफवातनुत् ।
तद्बीजं दीपनं पथ्यं शूलगुल्मव्यथापहम् ॥
(Raj. Ni. Dhn. Ni. p. 358)

3) स्रंसनमित्यादि
पूतिकरञ्जः कण्टकीकरञ्जः अन्ये तु पूतिकरञ्जश्चिरबिल्वकः ।
(Ḍalhaṇa Su. su. 46. 278)

4) पूतिकरञ्ज - कुबेराक्ष
Caesalpinia crista
श्वसनं कटुकं पाके लघुवातकफापहम् ।
शोथघ्नमुष्णवीर्यं च पत्रं पूतिकरञ्जजम् ।
(Yadavji, S. Su. 46)

5) प्रकीर्य - कण्टकी विटपकरञ्ज
(Dalhaṇa Su. Su. Du. 39.9).

उदकीर्यः (ध.नि) Udakīryaḥ (15)

उदकीर्यस्तृतीयोऽन्यः षड्ग्रन्थो हस्तिचारिणी ॥[१]
मदहस्तिनिका रोही हस्तिरोहणकः प्रियः ॥ १०४

There is a third type of *Karañja* उदकीर्य (Udakīrya) synonyms of which are षड्ग्रन्थः (Ṣaḍgranthaḥ), हस्तिचारिणी (Hasti cāriṇī), मदहस्तिनिका (Madahastinikā), रोही (Rohī), हस्तिरोहणकः (Hastirohaṇakaḥ) and प्रियः (Priyaḥ).

Ambiguous

The compiler of Dhn. ni. has not recorded medicinal uses of this plant species and editor Purandare has not recorded Raj. ni.s' plant of this name under this heading. He notes a different plant species namely प्रकीर्य (Prakīrya) under this heading which should have a special heading.

---

१ 'उदकीर्योऽथ षड्ग्रंथा घृतपर्णः प्रकीर्तितः इति शोढल पाठः
"महाकरञ्जस्तिक्तोष्णः कटुको विषनाशनः ।
कण्डूविचर्चिकाकुष्ठ त्वग्दोषव्रणनाशनः ॥" Chaukhamba edition P.167) (Sharma)

Compiler of Dhn. Ni. seems silent about Prakīrya which is a synonym of various plants. (See Anandashrama Dh. ni. index page 86.)

IV- 1 C.S. Su. 1.81; 2.8 vi 8-144 si. 10.24
S.S.Su. 39.8 Ci. 12.5
A.H. Su. 15.38
See Karañja करञ्ज (P.51)
In su.1.81 and 114 Caraka has mentioned first two species under the names Uadkīrya उदकीर्य and Prakīrya प्रकीर्य among the purgative fruit drugs (virecana phalini) and Pūtika पूतिक as purgative (Virecana) tree bark (Balwantji p. 75 करञ्ज).

अंगारवल्लिका (ध. नि.) Angāravallikā (16)

अङ्गारवल्लिकाऽम्बष्ठा काकघ्नी काकभाण्डिका ।।
वायव्या काल्मिकाभेदा काकवल्ल्यपि चोच्यते ।। १०५

अङ्गारवल्लिका (Angāravallikā), अम्बष्ठा (Ambaṣṭhā), काकघ्नी (Kākaghnī), काकभाण्डिका (Kākabhāṇḍikā), वायव्या (Vāyavyā), काल्मिकाभेदा (Kālmikābhedā) and काकवल्ली (Kākavallī) are synonymous.

In Chaukhamba edition the medicinal properties of *Mahākarañja* are noted under *Udakīrya* while in Raj.ni. the synonyms of *Udakīrya* and *Angāravallī* are mentioned together.

Ambiguous.

Compiler of Dhn. ni. recognises अङ्गारवल्लिका (Angāravallikā) as महाकरञ्जः (Mahākarañjaḥ) and notes medicinal uses of it under अङ्गारवल्लिका The editor Purandare has recorded Raj. ni's plant महाकरञ्जः Mahākarañjaḥ and अंगारवल्लि Angāravalli under Dhan.'s अंगारवल्लिका. But it seems that Raj. ni's synonyms do not corroborate with those of Dhn.ni. Medicinal uses given by Raj. ni. of his plants are as if a copy of those of Dhn. ni. It should be noted that the equivalents of Dhn. Ni. उदकीर्य (Udakīrya) and those of Raj. ni's महाकरञ्जः seem similar. Such is the controversy about उदकीर्य (Udakirya) and अंगारवल्लिका (Angāravallikā).

36. शिरीषः Śirīṣaḥ

शिरीषो मृदुपुष्पश्च भण्डिकः शंखिनीफलः ।।
कपीतनः शुकतरुः श्यामवर्णः शुकप्रियः ।। १०६

'भण्डिलः' इति शोढल पर्यायः ।

तिक्तोष्णो विषहा वर्ण्यस्त्रिदोषशमनो लघुः ॥
शिरीषः कुष्ठकण्डूघ्नस्त्वग्दोषश्वासकासहा ॥ १०७

शिरीष (Śirīṣa), मृदुपुष्पः (Mṛdupuṣpaḥ), भण्डिकः (Bhaṇḍikaḥ), शंखिनीफलः (Śankhinīphalaḥ), कपीतनः (Kapītanaḥ), शुकतरुः (Śukataruḥ), श्यामवर्णः (Śyāmavarṇaḥ) and शुकप्रियः (Śukapriyaḥ) are synonymous.

Śirīṣa is bitter in taste, *uṣṇavīrya*, antipoisonous, improves complexion, pacifies all the three *doṣas* and is *laghu.* It is useful in disorders of skin, pruritus, skin diseases, dyspnoea and cough.

Fam. Leguminosae (Mimosaceae)

I- a- ***Albizia lebbeck*** Benth.*

b- Watt. Dict. See below IV -2

II- a- मृदुपुष्पः (Mṛdupuṣpaḥ), शंखिनीफलः (Śankhinīphalaḥ), कपीतनः (Kapītanaḥ), शुकतरुः (Śukataruḥ), श्यामवर्णः (Syāmavarṇaḥ), शुकप्रियः(Śukapriyaḥ), विषहा (Viṣahā).

b- Sans. Śirīṣa; H,. B. & Bom. Sirisa; Tam. Vagai; Tel. Dirsan.

III-a- 1) See below IV-I

2) विषकुष्ठविनाशनः । Su. Su. 38.1

IV 2) शिरीष Sirīṣa

C.S.Su.2.4; 3.3. 27.28 etc.

S.S.Su. 36.33, 30.12 etc.

A.H. Su. 10.31 15.4; 17.3 etc.

See क्षीरी, किणिही and गण्डीर

1) *Albizia lebbeck* Benth. सिरस (H.)*

2) *A. odoratissima* Benth. सिरस (H.)**

3) *A. procera* (Roxb.) Benth. किनई (Mar.)

Synonyms कटभी, किणिही, भण्डी & शुकतरु (Balwantji p. 399)

IV- 2) *Albizia lebbeck* Benth.

The Siris tree.

Syn. *Acacia sirissa* Ham.

Mimosa sirissa Ham.

H. Siras; Tam. Vaghe, kot vaghe; Tel. Dirsan, Darshan; Kan. Kalbaghi, Goddhunshe; Mar. Motha siras, chichol; Bom. Shirisha, Siras; Sans. Pīt Sirisha

---

1) * The current accepted name is 1) *Albizia lebbeck* (Linn.) Willd.

2) ** *A. odoratissima* (Linn.f) Benth.

3) Albizzia -erroneous.

Habitat : A large deciduous spreading tree found wild or cultivated in most parts of India ... sub Himalayan tract from the Indus East wards, in Bengal, Burma, Central and South India.

(Watt. Dict. I.157)

There are some 30 species in the family Leguminosae and the sub. family Mimosaceae distributed through the tropical old world, but the following plant species are in practice for medicinal uses.

1) *Albizia amara* Boivin.
   Sans. Kṛṣṇa Siriṣa.

2) *A. julibressin* Durazz.
   used as A. lebbeck

3) *A. lebbeck* Benth.
   The Siris tree
   Antidote to poison and used in various diseases of the eyes.

4) *A. odoratissima* Benth.
   Is considered eficacious in leprosy etc.

5) *A. procera* (Roxb.) Benth.
   H. safed siris; Mal. & Bom. kinai, kinhai. (Watt. & chopra).

37 (३७) अर्जुनः Arjunaḥ

अर्जुनः ककुभः पार्थश्चित्रयोधी धनंजयः ॥
वीरान्तकः किरीटी च नदीसर्जोऽपि पाण्डवः ॥ १०८

ककुभस्तु कषायोष्णः कफघ्नो व्रणनाशनः ॥
पित्तश्रमतृषार्तिघ्नो मारुतामयकोपनः ॥ १०९

अर्जुनः (Arjunaḥ), ककुभः (Kakubhaḥ), पार्थः (Pārthaḥ), चित्रयोधी (Citrayodhī), धनंजयः (Dhananjayaḥ), वीरान्तकः (Vīrāntakaḥ), किरीटी (Kirīṭī), नदीसर्जः (Nadisarjaḥ) and पाण्डवः (Pāṇḍavaḥ) are synonymous.

Arjuna is *kaṣāya* in taste, *uṣṇavīrya,* pacifies *kapha* and *pitta doṣas* and aggravates the disorders caused by *vātadoṣa*. It is useful in healing of wounds,and removing tiredness and thirst.

Under this heading name two plant species are included., A-अर्जुनः (Arjuna proper) and B- ककुभः (Kakubha) both of the same genus.

Fam. Combretaceae

I- A-a- ***Terminalia arjuna*** Bedd. *
Syn. *Pentaptera arjuna* Roxb. (Watt. Dict.)
b- Roxburgh c- see bleow IV-3 Watt. Dict.

I- B-a- ***Terminalia tomentosa*** W. & A; *T. glabra* Var. *tomentosa* Dalz. & Gibs., *Pentaptera tomentosa* Roxb.
b- Roxburgh (CBC p. 383 Watt. Dict.)
c- See below IV -2

II- a- नदीसर्जः (Nadīsarjaḥ)
b- Sans. Arjuna; H. B. & Bom. - Arjun; Guj. Arjunsadara; Tam. Marudu; Tel. Tella maddi; Mal. vella marudu. (Chopra p. 241)

II- B-a- (Kakubhaḥ)
H. & P.Asana; B. Piasal; Tam. Karuppu marudu; Tel. Nella madu; Mal. Pavu; Assam. Amari. (Chopra)
Bom. & Mar. Āyan (Asana), Ayan sajda, Kahuwā (=Kakubha) कउवा Kauvā, Kala Arjuna; Kan. Karematen. (Bom. Gaz. III)

III-a 1) See below IV-1.
2) बभ्रवः अर्जुन काण्डः (AV. il -8-VIII-7)
3) सर्जार्जुन (Ast. san. V.A.32)
4) करहाटकार्जुन ककुभ सर्जः (Ast. San. Su. Kṣārāgada.)
5) कदम्बोदुम्बराश्वत्थ सर्जार्जुन । (Ast. San. U.Bhagnapratiśedha A.)
6) जम्बीरः स्यान्मरुबके गुच्छे चार्जुनयुग्मके । (Raj. ni.Caturarthāḥ Dh.ni. P.430)
7) अर्जुन C. Ci. 13.13.
Su. V. 45.23. Rakta pitta
A.H.U. 32.16
8) ककुभ C.Ci. 9.214; Ci. 7.126; A.H.Ci.
11.37 Mutrāghāta Sā. 2.44
9) ककुभः - Ast. San. U.A. 32 Sadyovraṇa
10) ककुभः -A.H. Kalp. 6.9
11) ककुभः -Su. S. Sālasārādi gaṇa, & Nyagrodhādi gaṇa.
12) ककुभपुष्पम् Su. Sū. 16.27,

b- 1) क्षयकासे अर्जुनत्वक् ।
ककुभपिष्टे वासकरसभावितं मूत्ररोधे च उदावर्ते
(Bh. Pr. ref. Ni. Adarsha)
2) हृदामये अर्जुनत्वक् हृद्रोगाधिकारे. दीर्घायुष्ये ककुभः । उदावर्ते -ककुभः (Vṛnda ref. in. Ni. Adarsha)
3) ककुभ महातैल (Gadanigraha)

* The current accepted name is *Terminlia arjuna* (Roxb.) Wight & Arn.

4) साजडो वनजो वृक्षः कृष्णत्वक् श्यामसारकः ।
धाराफलः ....॥
Terminalia glabra a kind of a Arjuna; H. Kauhā; Mar. Ayan, Ain; Guj, Sājadā (Shaligr. Ni.)

5) वीरतरुरर्जुननाम साम्यात् । ककुभः सन्त्यस्य दिग्व्यापकत्वात् ककुभः ।
(Kṡīraswāmī. Amara P. 61)

IV- a) अर्जुन Arjuna
Terminalia arjuna W. & A.
C.S. Su. 3.4; 4.43 etc.
S.S. Su. 14.36; 38 12 etc
A.H. Su. 15.41; 29. 12 etc.
Synonyms ककुभ, धनञ्जय (Balwantji p. 24.)

b) ककुभ Kakubha
C.S. Su. 5.70; 7.128 etc.
S.S.Su. 38-48; Ci. 3-6 Ka 6.3 (together with अर्जुन)etc.
S.H. Su. 2.2; Sa 2.44 etc.
Its occurence together with Arjuna as a separate substance does indicate that besides Arjuna, this is also a name for another drug as Ḍalhaṇa has clearly stated in his comments on Ārtagala आर्तगल (Balwantji pp.24.61.)

2) *Terminalia tomentosa* Bedd.
Synonyms see above II-a-Ḃ.
H. Sājā, Āsan, Āssanai, ain; Bom. Ain, Sādadā; Mar. Ain, Sādaḍā; Sans. *Asana.*
A large deciduous tree attains a height of 90 to 100 feet, common throughout the moist regions of India. Gum -P.39, Dye and tan (P.39) Medicine P. 41. Watt. Dict . Vol VI pp. 37.42.

3) *Terminalia arjuna* Bedd.
Syn. *Pentaptera arjuna* Roxb.
H. Arjan, Arjun Kahava.
Habitat : A large deciduous tree common throughout the Sub-Himalayan tracts of North-west provinces, the Deccan, Southern Behar, Burma & Ceylon.. (Watt. Vol. VI.32-34).

4) *Penataptera arjuna* Roxb.
Bark smooth, branches horizontal, leaves sub-opposite, linear, oblong... having two sessile glands underneath the base and not visible when looking at the surface of the leaf. A. stout quick growing timber tree . Native of various parts of India ((Roxb. CBC 382).

5) *Terminalia tomentosa* Roxb.
Bark deeply cracked; Leaves ... some ....glands on the rib near the base.

Sans. Usan; Ben. Peeasal or Asana; Tel. Nella- madoo. (Roxb. CBC 383).

6) ककुभ *Terminalia tomentosa*
(Dr. Ghanekar Su. Sū. p. 292)

7) असन *Terminalia tomentosa* (Dr.Ghanekar Su. Su. Veeratarvādi)

8) कुकुभ (ककुभ) *Terminalia arjuna*
(Bapalalji contro. plants J.R.I.M.V. 1-1970)

The reference given above (III-a, 3, 4,6,8,9,10,11,12, IV-b 2,4; ib 4,5,6,7) clearly indicate that Arjuna and Kakubha ककुभ Syn.असन are two separate tree species.

38 (३८) वेतसः Vetasaḥ

वेतसो निचुलः प्रोक्तो वञ्जुलो दीर्घपत्रकः ॥
कलनो मञ्जरीनम्रः सुषेणो गन्धपुष्पकः ॥ ११०

नादेयी मेघपुष्पोऽन्यो जलकामो निकुञ्जकः ॥
जलौकःसंवृतश्चैव विदुलो जलवेतसः ॥ १११

वेतसस्य द्वयं शीतं रक्षोघ्नं व्रणशोधनम् ॥
रक्तपित्तहरं तिक्तं सकषायं कफापहम् ॥ ११२

वेतसः (Vetasaḥ), निचुलः (Niculaḥ), वञ्जुलः (Vañjulaḥ), दीर्घपत्रकः (Dīrghapatrakaḥ), कलनः (Kalanaḥ), मञ्जरीनम्रः (Mañjarīnamraḥ), सुषेणः (Suṣeṇaḥ) and गन्धपुष्पकः (Gandhapuṣpakaḥ) are synonymous. There is an another type of *vetasa* of which synonyms are नादेयी (Nādeyī), मेघपुष्पः (Meghapuṣpaḥ), जलकामः (Jalakāmaḥ), निकुञ्जकः (Nikuñjakaḥ), जलौकःसंवृतः (Jalaukaḥ samvritaḥ), विदुलः (Vidulaḥ), and जलवेतसः (Jalavetasaḥ).

Both the types of *Vetasa* are *kaṣāya* and bitter in taste and pacify *kaphadoṣa.* These are *sītavīrya*, destroying *rakṣas* (microbes or evil spirits or antiseptic.) and purifier of wounds.

वेतस *Vetasa* is a family or group name and generally the name is confounded with the name of the varieties containing the group. But some modern writers have recognised it as a specific name. The Vetasa group is now recognised and identified as Salix species or a group of Salix genus. only one or two species of Salix are now identified but the remaining are not recognised and identified. Under this heading name the compiler of Dhn. ni. has noted three plant names, but if Vetas (वेतस) would be accepted as a special name these would be four as below.

'A' वेतस (Vetas) when specific name is accepted, 'B' निचुलः (Nicula) 'C' वञ्जुल (Vañjula) and 'D' विदुल (Vidula) all of the same Salix genus. The Ni. has noted the medicinal uses of two plants only but without mentioning their names.

Fam. Salicaceae (Chopra)
Salacinae (Watt Dict.)

I- A-a- ***Salix caprea*** Linn.
The sallow.

b- Balwantji's glossary (see below IV-1)

c- See below IV-3

B-a- *Nicula* not identified.

C-a- Vañjula not identified.

D-a- Vidula see Amlavetasa under the heading Amlaḥ (Chap. II. Serial no .pre. 38 p. 89 of Dhn. ni.)

II- A-a- वेतसो निचुलः प्रोक्तो (Vetaso Niculaḥ prokto)

Note - The word *Vetasa*, it seems is applied to *Nicula* to denote the family name of *Nicula* and is not used as a specific name.

B-a-b.Nicula
No synonyms are given; modern names are not known.

C-a- वञ्जुलः (Vañjulaḥ), दीर्घपत्रकः (Dīrghapatrakaḥ), कलनः (Kalanaḥ), मञ्जरीनम्रः (Mañjarī namraḥ), सुषेणः (Suṣeṇaḥ), गन्धपुष्पकः (Gandhapuṣpakaḥ).

b- Modern names not known.

D-a- विदुलः (Vidulaḥ) नादेयी (Nādeyī), मेघपुष्पोऽन्यो (Meghapusponyaḥ), जलकामः (Jalakāmaḥ), निकुञ्जकः (Nikuñjakaḥ), जलौकःसंवृतः (Jalaukāḥsamvṛtaḥ), जलवेतसः (Jalavetasaḥ)
If it would be अम्लवेतस Amlavetasa (*Salix tetrasperma Roxb.*) of Dhn. ni. the modern names would be the same i.e. of *Amlavetasa*.

III-a-

1) See bleow IV-1

2) 110 Vetasa R.V.IV.-58-5; A.V.X-7-47; V.S.XVII-6;
T.S. V.3-12-2 (Harshe)

b- 1) वेतसे ॥ २९
रथाभ्रपुष्प विदुलशीतवानीरवञ्जुलाः ।
द्वौ परिव्याध विदुलौ नादेयी चाम्बुवेतसे ॥ ३० Amar 2.4. 29.30

Commentery
वेत्यम्भोनुवर्तते । वितस्यत वा वेतसः । रमन्तेऽस्मिन् रथः । अभ्राणि पुष्पाण्यस्याभ्रपुष्पः । विदोल्यते वेगेन विदुलः । शीतो वीर्येण

लेपाद्दाहशमनात् । वनति भजत्यम्बु वानीरो वञ्जुलश्च । परिव्याध्यते
ऽम्भसा परिव्याधः । नद्या भवा नादेयी .... । चन्द्राद्या विभागेनाहुः -
"वेतसो विदुलो नम्रो वञ्जुलो दीर्घपत्रकः ।
नादेयी गन्धपत्रश्च जलौकाः संभृतस्तथा ॥
नदीकूलप्रियस्त्वन्यः सुशीतो घनपुष्पकः ।
जलजातस्तोयकामो विदुलो जलवेतसः ।
निचुलो वेतसादन्यो वक्ष्यते (स्थलवेतसः) ॥

K'sīraswamī

b- 2) 208 व्याधिघात इति । आरग्वधः शम्पाकः । आम्लवेतसः इज्जलः । 'व्याधिघातः प्रग्रहे जलवेतस' इत्यभिधानचूडामणिः । Harshe

3) 474 विदुल इति । आम्लवेतसः वेतसाम्लः । 'वेतसो नम्रकः । 'विदुलस्तु भवेदम्लवेतसे वेतसेऽपि च' ति शाश्चतः । Harshe

4) 473 'वेतसो नम्रकः प्रोक्तो वानीरो वञ्जुलस्तथे' ति 'वंजुलो वेतसाशोकति-निशोष्वि' ति विश्वः । Harshe

5) वानीरो वृत्तपुष्पश्च शाखालो जलवेतसः ।
व्याधिघातः परिव्याधो नादेयो जलसम्भवः ॥ Raj. ni. Dhn. ni. p. 365

6) हिज्जुलोऽथ नदीकान्तो जलजो दीर्घपत्रकः ।
नदीजो निचुलो रक्तः कार्मुकः कथितश्च सः ॥ Raj. ni. Dhn. ni. p. 363

7) See अम्ल Pre no. 38 of Śatapuṣpādi Chapter II of Dhn. ni.

IV- 1) Amlavidula

a) A.H.Ci. 8-149
This is also split up to mean two substances i.e. अम्ल (अम्लवेतस) and विदुल (Balwantji p.20).

b) वेतस Vetasa *Salix caprea* Linn.
(Balwantji p. 224).

c) निचुल Nicula
Barringtonia acutangula (Linn.) Gaertn. (Balvantji P 324)
Nicula has been identified as *Hijjala* हिज्जल, Vetasa वेतस and Jalavetasa. These names refer to two different tree genera belonging to *Salix* and *Barringtonia.* Where *Nicula phala* or *Niculāni* (Pleural form of *Nicula*) are mentioned the Barringtonia fruits are intended. Vetasa, Vañjula and Jalavetasa are undoubtedly salix Species which are either *Jalaja* (aquatic) or *Sthalaja* (terrestrial). Barringtonia grows near water course, and its root bark has properties similar to that of Salix. Both being *Śitavīrya* and emetic can serve as substitutes of each other. But the Barringtonia fruits are *usṇavīrya*, bitter in taste, emetic and laxative and should only be used when specially mentioned ... . (Balwantji p. 225)

विदुल Vidula,
C.S.Su. 4.23; Vi. 8.143 etc.
S.S.Su. 39.3, Ci. 1-95 etc.
A.H. Su. 15-1 Ci-8 149 etc. (Balavantjit p. 225)

d) वानीर Vānīra
C.S. Ci. 3.275 with वेतस; 4.101 ka. 1.8; Si 10. 20
It is said to be another kind of *Vetasa,* a Salix species. Vañjula वञ्जुल and Vānira वानीर in C.S. ka. 8.1 have been described as inhabiting river banks and therefore, they appear to be those Salix species only which are found usually in such places. *Vetasa* वेतस proper may be *Salix caprea* Linn. known as Vedamuṣka, while *Vañjula* may be *Salix tetrasperma* Roxb.,also known as Jalavetasa जलवेतस. It appears that Cakra was not aware of the identity of *Vetasa* and its varieties . He has therefore supposed them to be Usira उशीर varieties (Balwantji p.364)

e) Vañjula
C.S.Su. 4.47 etc.
S.S.Su. 38.47 etc.
A.H.Su.15.41
Also a synonym of अशोक *Asoka* and *Tinisa.*
(Balvantji p. 356)

2) इज्जलो हिज्जलश्चापि निचुलश्चाम्बुजस्तथा ।
जलवेतसवद्वेद्यो हिज्जलोयं विषापहः ॥
64 इज्जल (समुद्रफल) H.-Ijjala, Hijjala, Samudraphal;
Mara. Satphal, Samudraphala. *Barringtonia acutangula* (Linn). Gaertn. (Chunekar Bh. pr. Ni. 363-364).

3) *Salix alba* Linn
White or Hutingdon willow.
A large tree cultivated in the North west Himalaya, distributed to Europe and Northern Asia (Watt.Dict. VI-II-388).

4) *Salix caprea* Linn.
The Sallow.
Habitat : Cultivated in North West Himalaya, distributed to Europe and Northern Asia. It is abundant at Peshawar and Lahor, introduced from Kasmira after the conquest of that country by Ranjitsing. (Watt. Dict. VI II-389).

DISCUSSION

Vetasa is a generic or group name of a family which is now identified as *Salix* species. In this family containing about 150 species, 26species of which are found in the Indian Peninsula, but out of them only 4 to

5 kinds are recorded as medicinal plants in Ayurvedic books. From these species two are indentified botanically.

In बृहत्त्रयी Bṛhattrayi 5 or 6 species are found recorded as medicinal plants (See IV-a above) . In अमरकोश Amrakosa 4 to 5 kinds or species are recorded under the name वेतस vetasa (See III-b-1 Ksīraswāmī Tīka above)

The compiler of Dhn-ni. records three species under the heading name वेतस Vetasa, but if Vetasa is accepted as a specific name one plant name would be more. Raj-ni has copied under this heading the plant name of Dhn-ni but under it he has recorded two plant names (1) वानीर Vānīra and हिज्जल Hijjala (see III-5,6 above) These are not included in Dhn's Vetasa heading.

Compiler of Bh-Pr-Ni records the same plant names noted in the text of Dhn. ni. but he also records वानीर Vānīra and हिज्जल Huijjala (See Chunekar Bh.Pr. Ni. pp. 361, 369).

But as the plant names वानीर Vānira and हिज्जल Hijjala are not noted in Dhn. ni's text and as our study is limited to the plants recorded in Dhn-ni we need not discuss them here. In some books निचुल Nichula is recognised as having two species one of them is an aquatic (जलज Jalaja) and the next स्थलज (Sthalaja-terrestrial). (See III-b. 1 Ksīraswāmī निचुलो वेतसादन्यो वक्ष्यते स्थलवेतस IV-3 above). The स्थलज Sthalaja species is now identified as *Barringtonia species* समुद्रफल Samudraphala but निचुलजलज Niculajalaja is not identified (see above IV-1 discussion on Nicula by Balvantji). Raj. ni. records समुद्रफल Samudra-phala under separate heading name (See Dhn ni p. 343) but as the compiler of Dhn. ni. has not mentioned two species of Nicula we also avoid to discuss about this doubtful identification though we know the medicinal use of समुद्रफल Samudraphala. The various plant names recorded in above work seem similar in their names but their morphological descriptions given there are contrary to the same name of other books or that the plant name in one book may not be the same plant of other book. In such difficulty we have to follow only to the text given in Dhn. ni. The compiler of Dhn.ni. has recorded three plant names under this heading (See above). If वेतस Vetasa would be accepted as a specific name then they would be four, but medicinal uses are given of only two plants. (वेतसस्य द्वयं शीतम्) without mentioning their names. It is a point for discussion why should he omit other plants noted by him in his text. We think the compiler may have omitted two names namely वेतस Vetasa and विदुल Vidula. He may have acccepted वेतस Vetasa as a family or group name of *Vetasa* species and विदुल Vidula may have accepted as अम्लवेतस Amalvetasa (See 1 III -B,3, b-1) which he has included under the heading name अम्ल Amlaḥ (see :

chap. II plant No. 38 Dhn. ni-p.89)

Some modern writers have accepted वेतस Vetas as a specific name and identified it as *Salix caprea* Linn. but writers of Nighaṇṭus and Kośas have treated the word वेतस Vetasa as a group name (See Amarakośa वेतस Vetasa i.e. vetasa group) Compounded the name विदुल as वेतस विदुलः (III-b-1) and शिवकोश mentions also विदुल as अम्लवेतस, वेतसाम्ल (III-b-3) such are several compound words of such kinds.

The etymology of Vetasa given by Kṣīraswāmī as "Those grow in or near water source" and all the Vetasa species recorded in Ayurvedic basic books are aquatic plants (जलज Jalaja). The omitted next plant विदुल *Vidula* is recorded by Nighaṇṭus and *Kośas* as अम्लवेतस Amlavetasa (III-b-3) which is now identified as *Salix terasperma* Roxb. After discussing the reason why the complier should have omitted the name वेतस Vetasa and विदुल Vidula, we conclude that the given medicinal uses are of the unmentioned names निचुल Nicula and वञ्जुल Vañjula which also are not recognised and identified by modern scientists and if our conclusion would be found acceptable the botanical name *Salix caprea* Linn., now applied to वेतस would not be tenable. It is not a native of India and is not found recorded as an aquatic plant. Ayurvedic varieties of Vetasa family are aquatics. Some modern writers without authority have recorded *Garcinia pedunculata* Roxb. as Amlavetasa अम्लवेतस. But this is now substituted for Cakotrā (of Nepal) which is included under the heading अम्लः Amlaḥ and is said to be a fruit of a *Citrus species*. (See chapt II *Śatapuṣhpā* Pre. No. 38.) It is said to be फलाम्लवेतस Phalamlavetasa of Raj. Ni.

39. (३९) वरुणः Varuṇaḥ

वरुणः श्वेतपुष्पश्च तिक्तशाकः कुमारकः ॥
श्वेतद्रुमो गन्धवृक्षस्तमालो मारुतापहः ॥ ११३

वरुणः शीतवातघ्नस्तिक्तगे विद्रधिजन्तुजित् ॥
तथा च कटुरुष्णश्च रक्तदोषहरः परः ॥ ११४

वरुणः (Varuṇaḥ), श्वेतपुष्पः (Śvetapuṣpaḥ), तिक्तशाकः (Tiktaśākaḥ), कुमारकः (Kumārakaḥ), श्वेतद्रुमः (Śvetadrumaḥ), गन्धवृक्षः (Gandhavṛksaḥ), तमालः (Tamālaḥ) and मारुतापहः (Mārutāpahaḥ) are synonymous.

Varuṇa is bitter and pungent in *taste*, *uṣṇavīrya* and pacifies *raktadoṣa*. It is *śītavātaghna* and useful in abscess and *Jantu* (microbes).

Fam. Capparidaceae. Capparaceae

I- a- ***Crataeva nurvala*** Buch.-Ham. (Chopra)
syn. *C.religiosa* Forst.
C. nurvala Ham.
Capparis trifoliata Roxb. (Watt. Dict.)

b- Roxburgh (Fl. indi. CBC 426)

c- श्वेतपुष्पः (Śwetapuṣpaḥ), तिक्तशाकः (Tiktaśākaḥ), कुमारकः (Kumārakaḥ), श्वेतद्रुमः (Śwetadrumaḥ), गन्धवृक्षः (Gandhavṛksaḥ), तमालः (Tamālaḥ), मारुतापहः (Mārutāpaḥ).

d- San. -Varuṇa, Tiktashaka; B. -Huroona; Tel.-Tella woolee mara (Roxb.); Mar. Bom.- Vāya varnā; Tam. Maralingam, Narval; Tel. Mugalingam; H.B. - Barna, Barun; Sans -Varuna, Ashmarighna. (Watt. Dict.)

1. वरुण Varuna,
Crataeva nurvala Buch.- Ham.
C.S.Ci. 19-69; 29.92 etc.
S.S.Ci. 7-10; 15-44 etc.
A.H.Su. 20.37; Sa. 2.50; etc. (Balvantji p. 360).

40. (४०) शिंशपा Śimśapā

शिंशपा तु महाश्यामा कृष्णसारा स्मृताऽगुरुः[1] ॥
कुशिंशपाऽन्या कपिला भस्मगर्भा[3] वसादनी ॥ ११५

शिंशपायुगुलं वर्ण्यं हिक्काशोफौ विसर्जयेत् ॥
पित्तदाहप्रशमनं बल्यं रुचिकरं परम् ॥ ११६

*(कटूष्णं कण्डुदोषघ्नं बस्तिरोगविनाशनम् ।)

शिंशपा (Śimśapā), महाश्यामा (Mahāśyāmā), कृष्णसारा (Kṛṣṇasārā) and अगुरुः (Aguruḥ), are synonymous. There is an another kind called as कुशिंशपा (Kuśimśapā) of which synonyms are कपिला (Kapilā), भस्मगर्भा (Bhasmagarbhā) and वसादनी (Vasādanī)

Both of these are useful in improving complexion, hiccup, odema. These pacify *pitta doṣa,* alleviate burning sensation, are strength promoting and promoting desire for food.

१ 'स्मृता गुरुः' इति आनन्दा,मुद्रित पुस्तके पाठः। २ 'कृष्णसारः स्मृतोऽगरुः इति क्षीर संमतः साधु पाठः ।
३'भस्मगर्भा च सादिनी' इति क्षीर.संमतः पाठः ।
* कोष्ठकान्तर्गतः पाठः आनन्दाश्रम मुद्रित पुस्तके दृश्यते ।

(***From other books*** - Both of these are bitter in taste and useful in pruritus, and diseases of urinary organs.)

Under this heading compiler of Dhn. ni. has recorded two tree species 'A' महाश्यामा कृष्णसारा (Mahāśyāmā Kṛṣṇasārā) and the next 'B' कुशिंशपा भस्मगर्भा (Kuśimśapā bhasmagarbhā). Both of the same genus.

Fam. Leguminosae. Fabaceae

I- A-a- ***Dalbergia sissoo*** Roxb.*
The sissoo.
b- Roxburgh (Fl. ind. C.B.C. 533)
c- See below IV-2

B-a- ***D. latifolia*** Roxb.
The blackwood or Rosewood of southern India.
Syn. *D. emarginata* Roxb. (Watt. Dict)
b- Kamat, C-See IV3-below.

II- A-a- महाश्यामा (Mahāśyāmā), कृष्णसारा (Kṛṣṇasārā), गुरुः (Guruḥ) (अगरुः)
b-. San. Singshupa; (Roxb.)
H. Sisam, Kapilvarna Śisam; B. Sisu; Mar. Sisavā, Sisam, Sissa; Kann. Agaru didda; Siridi, Chisambage; Tam; yette, Nukka Kaṭtai; Tel-Sissu-Kora, Sissu; Sans. Simshapa.

B-a- कुशिंशपा (Kuśimsapā), कपिला (Kapilā), भस्मगर्भावसादनी (Bhasmagarbhāvasādanī); Medi. uses शिंशपा युगुलं वर्ण्यं ... ॥ (Simsapā yugulam (both) varṇyam...) etc.

Note - Medi. uses of the both trees are recorded together.

II-A-b- Hindi, Bengāli, Guj. and marathi names are the same as those of above. South Indian names: Tam.Iti, Erimadi, Tātkatti, Yerugudu; Tel. Irungudu, Viragadu; Kan. Biti, Thodgatti. (Watt. Dict.).

III-a-1) See IV-1 below.

b- 1 .... पिच्छिलागरु शिंशिपा ॥ अमरः २.४.६३
....चन्द्रनन्दनस्तु शुकमालकमाह । अगुरुतुल्य सारा शिंशपा अगरु शिंशपा । यदाह –
शिंशपा तु महाश्यामा कृष्णसारः स्मृतोऽगरुः ।
अगुरुर्धूपद्रव्यं शिंशपासारं चाहुः । ....कुशिंशपान्या कपिला भस्मगर्भा च सादिनी ... । (Kśiraswāmī 2-4.63)

---

* The current accepted name is *D. sissoo* Roxb. ex.DC.

IV- 1) शिंशपा Śiṁśapā
Dalbergia sissoo Roxb.
C.S. Su. 25-49; Vi, 9-151 etc.
S.S.Su. 38-12; 20 etc.
A.H.Su. 15-19, 32 etc.

2) *D.sissoo* Roxb.
The Sissoo
Habitat : A large deciduous tree of the sub Himalayan tract from the Indus to Assam .... found throughout India.
(Watt. vol. III-13)

3) *D. latifolia* Roxb.
Syn. *D. emarginata* Roxb.
Habitat : A deciduous tree attaining a large size in South India ..Eastern Bengal and central India .... Common throughout Western India. The tree grows extensively and vigorously in Deccan, Konkan and Gujarat forests. (Watt. Dict. III-8)

4) *Dalbergia latifolia* Willd.
Tel. Birugudu charwa B. Sitsal; Eng. blackwood tree.
.... Leaves alternate 6 - to 9 in. long ... flowers small white... The wood of the centre of the trunk is called black wood ... used for making furniture, its colour is greenish black..... It is rather heavy sinking in water .... and admitting of the finest polish.
(Roxb. CBC 532).

5) *D. sissoo* Roxb.
Sans. Singshapa; H. Sissoo.
... Colour light greenish brown with darker coloured veins, Flowers small of a yellowish white colour.

6) *D.emarginata* Roxb.*
Native of Andamans.
...Flowers pure white .... In habit it resembles *D. sissoo* Roxb. Fl. Ind. CBC 533

7) *D. sissoo* Roxb; H. Sisam.
There is another species of this tree namely *D. latifolia* Roxb; Eng. Rosewood.
The heart wood of this tree is used for furniture. (Chunekar Bh. Pr. 22)

8) *Dalbergia emarginata* R.

The current name is *D. latifolia* Roxb. (comp. p 49)

Kṛsṇasimsapā
D.sissoo R., (Eng.) Rosewood. (Nadkarni)

9) *D.emarginata* R.; See
D.latifolia Roxb.
Sans. Shimshap; B. Sitsal; Eng. Rosewood (Hill), Sisam (Birdwood).

41 (४१) सर्जकः Sarjakaḥ

सर्जको बस्तकर्णश्च[1] कषायश्चिरपत्रकः[2] ॥
सस्यसंवरकः शूरः सर्जोऽन्यः शालं[3] उच्यते ॥ ११७

कुष्ठकण्डूक्रिमिश्लेष्मवातपित्तरुजो जयेत् ॥
सर्जयुग्मं कषायं स्यात् वर्ण्यं रूक्षं कफापहम् ॥ ११९

सर्जकः (Sarjakaḥ), बस्तकर्णः (Bastakarṇaḥ), कषायः (Kaṣāyaḥ),चिरपत्रकः (Cirapatrakaḥ), सस्यसंवरकः (Sasyasamvarakaḥ), and शूरः (Sūraḥ) are synonymous. There is an another type of सर्जः (Sarjaḥ) called as शालः (Śālaḥ).

Both of these types are *kaṣāya* (astringent) in taste, pacify *kapha* and *vāta pitta doṣas,* are *rūkṣa* (causing dryness) and improve complexion. These are useful in disorders of skin, pruritus and worms.

Under this heading the compiler has recorded two or three species. 'A' सर्जकः (Sarjakaḥ proper) and the next 'B' शाल (Śāla) and medicinal uses are given of both trees, while Raj. ni. records one more namely 'C' अजकर्ण (Ajakarṇa). This is not recorded by the compiler of Dhn. ni. under this heading. However, we have recorded it here below.

Fam. Dipterocarpaceae.
Dipterocarpae.

I- A-a- ***Vateria indica*** Linn.
The white Damer of South India, Piney Varnish or Indian copal.
Syn. *V. malabarica* Blume.

b- Balvantji (See IV-1 below)

---

१ 'सर्जकश्चाश्वकर्णश्च कषायी दीर्घपत्रकः । सस्यसंवरणः शूरः सर्जकः साल उच्यते ॥' इति क्षीर. संमत पाठः ।

२ 'चीरपत्रक' इति चौखम्भा मुद्रितपुस्तके पाठः ।
अश्वकर्णः इति क्षी. संमतः पाठः । 'असनो बीजकः शालः सर्जः शालं सर्जं च सूरय' इति हलायुधः ।

c- See below IV-4

B-a- ***Shorea robusta*** Gaertn.

See राला Rālā Pre-no 47 in chapter III candanādi Page 119 of Dhn. ni.

C-a- ***Dipteropcarpus turbinatus*** Gaertn.

b- Balvantji P. 6

c- Assam and Andamans.

II- A-a- सर्जकः (Sarjakaḥ), बस्तकर्णः (Bastakarṇaḥ), चिरपत्रकः (Cirapatrakaḥ), सस्यसंवरकः (Sasyasamvarakaḥ), सर्जोऽन्यः शाल उच्यते (Sarjonyaḥ śala ucyate) Dhn. Ni.

b- Safed damar, Sandras; Deccan, Safed Dāmar; Bom. Rāla; Tam. vellai; Kunrukam, Pinay maram, Kundricum, Dhup-maram; Kan. Dupa Dāmaru, Teka-dāmaru; Maly. Dupa damara, Vella Kunturukkam, Painy marum. (Watt. Dict.)

B-a & b See note under I-B-a--above.

C-a- अजकर्णकः(Ajakarṇakaḥ), बस्तकर्णः (Bastakarṇaḥ), ललनः (Lalanaḥ), गन्धवृक्षकः (Gandhavṛksakaḥ).

B-b- Teli garjan, Assam-Gurjun, Kuroisal. (Chopra)

III-a-1) सर्ज Sarja; सर्जनाम Sarjanāma.
C.S.,Su. 3.4; vi 8-151 etc.
S.S.Su. 6.33 14.37 etc.
A.H. Ci. 1-163 11. 16. 24. 25 etc. (Balwantji p. 424).

b- 1) सर्जरसः Su.29 राल इति प्रसिद्धः । Yellow resin-*Mimosa rubricaulis* or *M. mutabilis.* 'रालस्तु सर्जनिर्यासः तथा सर्जरस स्मृतः । देवधूपो यक्षधूपः तथा सर्जरसश्च सः ।' भा. प्र (Ast. Hr. Kosha)

2) ...साले तु सर्ज. ॥ ४५
स्यति सालः । कृश्यति कार्श्यः । अश्वकर्णाभपत्रकः (अश्वकर्णकः) सस्यं फलं संवृणोति सस्यसंवरः । आह च सर्जकावश्वकर्णश्च'
(Ksiraswāmī. Amar 2.4.45)

IV- 1) सर्ज Sarja सर्जनाम Sarjanāma
Sarja is believed to be *Vateria indica* Linn. which is found in Western India. But it may be noted that many tree species characterized by resinous exudations especially those belonging to the families of Dipterocarpaceae and Combretaceae are given names such as *Laghusarja* लघुसर्ज, *Mahāsarja* महासर्ज, *Nadisarja* नदीसर्ज, *Nīlasarja* नीलसर्ज and *Sarjaka* सर्जक. Thus it may be presumed that *Sarja* could better be a group name for all such trees showing resinous exudations (सृजति इति सर्जः सृज विसर्गे) In popular usage also *Loka* names such as sajā साजा (for

Terminalia tomentosa W. & A.) and Sarjam सर्जम् (for *Shorea robusta* Gaertn.) are prevalent in some tribal areas of U.P. and Bihar. It may also be noted that for the *Sarjarasa* of the texts *śālarasa* शालरस is being acutally used by the Vaidyas. Inspite of what has been said above, it is very clear that *Sarja* has been accepted in the text as a specific tree different from *Aśwakarṇa* अश्वकर्ण, *Ajakarṇa* अजकर्ण;and Śāla शाल, and may be identified with *Vateria indica* Linn. See अजकर्ण, अश्वकर्ण, शाल and सर्जरस (Balwantji P. 424)

Note - सर्ज-सज्ज (Prākṛta), साज-साजडा (Khandesh, Marathwada), नदीसर्ज (for अर्जुन) नदीसाजडा *Nadisājada* (Kathiawad), असन *Asana* (For *Terminalia tomentosa* W. & A.), असन Asana, अयन Ayan, आयन Āyana, ऐन * Ain (Marathi)

2) अजकर्ण, Ajakarṇa
Dipterocarpus turbinatus Gaertn. **
C.S.Vi. 8.151
S.S.Su. 38.12 Ci. 9.14 etc.
The identities of अजकर्ण *Ajakarṇa* and अश्वकर्ण Aśwakarṇa have been discussed under *Aswakarṇa* अश्वकर्ण (Balvantji p. 6)

Note - see Aśwakarṇa under the heading name जरणद्रुम Jaraṇadruma recorded by Raj.ni. in his प्रभद्रादिवर्ग Prabhadrādi Chapter IXS. No.3.Dhn. ni. p. 364 It is not mentioned by Dhn. ni. but Balvantji's discussion under this heading (Aśwakarṇa) is sheding much light and disclosing morphlogical confusion regarding the oleoresin yielding trees in old Ayurvedic (Sanskṛt) and modern books.

3) अश्वकर्णAśwakarṇa.
C.S. Su. 4.43; 14.45 etc.
S.S.Su. 11.11; 36.28 etc.
A.H. Su. 15.19; 30. 28 etc.
Aswakarṇa अश्वकर्ण and Ajakarṇa now appear to be identified with the oleoresin yielding tree of the family *Dipterocarpacae* Shri Yadavji identified *Aśvakarṇa* with *Dipterocarpus alatus* Roxb. which is known as Garjana गर्जन, Jayan जयन or Jaraṇadruma जरणद्रुम (Rajanighaṇṭu) all allied names and the other synonyms such as Kusikataru कुशिकतरु (Gum yielding tree), Sasyasamavaraṇa सस्यसंवरण (fruit covered by accrescent calyx lobes) and cīraparṇaḥ चीरपर्ण (Calyx lobes looking like wings of birds and helping in fruit dispersal by wind) are exactly applicable to it. The names *Aśvakarṇa* and *Ajakarṇa* also seem to

---

* अश्वकर्णः सस्यसंवरः ऐन इति प्रसिद्धः । बोपदेवः सिद्धमंत्रप्रकाश p. 26 (S.D.K.)

* * The current name is *D. turbinatus* Gaertn. f.

imply that out of five, only two calyx lobes become wing like or like the earlobes of Ajā or Aśva. This is so in *D. alatus* and other Dipterocarpus species, such as *D. turbinatus* Gaertn. f. (F.B.I. in part). Thus *Ajakarna* may better be identified with the latter than *Vateria indica* Linn. (Balvantji p. 28).

4) *Vateria indica* Linn
Habitat : A large evergreen tree of western Peninusla from Kanara to Travancore.
Resin : This tree yields of true resin of considerable value, known as white damar. (Watt. Dict. VI-222)

Note - The Dipterocarpaceae family includes about 50 species native of tropical east Asia ... of these India possesses 17 of which 6 occur in India proper. Besides the above noted species there are some other species which yield white damar resembling with that of *Vateria indica* Linn. e.g. See *Hopea odorata,* Watt Dict. IV.p. 272 para 365 and Roxb. Fl. indi. CBC p. 438.

अशनः (ध. नि.) Aśanaḥ (19)

अशनस्तु महासर्जः सौरिर्बन्धूकपुष्पकः ॥
प्रियको बीजकः श्यामः सुनीलः प्रियशालकः ॥ ११९
बीजकः सकषायश्च कफपित्तास्रनाशनः ॥

अशनः (Aśanaḥ), महासर्जः (Mahāsarjaḥ), सौरिः (Sauriḥ), बन्धूकपुष्पकः (Bandhūkapuṣpakaḥ), प्रियकः (Priyakaḥ), बीजकः (Bījakaḥ), श्यामः (Śyāmaḥ), सुनीलः (Sunīlaḥ) and प्रियशालकः (Priyaśālakaḥ) are synonymous.

Bījakaḥ is *kaṣāya* (astringent) in taste and pacifies *kapha, pitta* and *rakta doṣas.*

Fam. Leguminosae. Fabaceae.

I- a- ***Pteropcarpus marsupium*** Roxb.
b- Roxburgh (Fl. indi. CBC. p. 536)
c- See below IV- 2

II- a- अशनः (Aśanaḥ), महासर्जः (Mahāsarjaḥ) बन्धूक पुष्पकः (Bandhūka puṣpakaḥ), बीजकः (Bījakaḥ), श्यामः (Śyāmaḥ), प्रियशालकः (Priyaśālakaḥ).

b- H. Bījā, Bijasāl; B.Pitsāl; Bom. Biblā, bija; Mar. Bivḷā, Dhorbivala; Āsan, Huni; Tam. -Vengai maram, vengai; Tel. Peddagi, yeengai, yengi; Kan.-Benga, Hunne, Bibla; Maly.-Karinthagara, Venna. (Watt. Dict.)
Tel. Yennga-sha; Beng.-Peetsal; (Roxb.)
Eng. East Indian Kino tree, Madras Kino, Kochin Kino tree.

III- a
1) See IV below

b- 1) अशनः पीतशालाख्यः । (Aruṇa 15-19)
2) अथ पीतसालके । सर्जकासन बंधूक जीवकः ।
पीतसारोऽस्य; रलयो एकत्वम् । .... प्रियकः पीतसारके विजयसारस्य । (Bhānuji-Amara)
3) साले तु सर्ज काश्यो ... ॥ (Amar 2.4.44)
पीतवर्णः सालः (पीतसालः) । सृजति निर्यासं सर्जः । अस्यत्यसनः ।
बन्धूकस्येव रक्ताणि पुष्पाण्यस्य बन्धूकपुष्पः काम्यत्वात् प्रियत्वात् प्रियकः । जीवयति जीवकः । बीजक इति तु निघण्टुः 'संज्ञया बीजको ज्ञेयो बीजपूरस्तथासनः "॥ आहुश्च
बीजकस्त्वसनः काम्यः सौरिः कृष्णलव (क) प्रियः ।
तिष्यपुष्पः पीतसालः प्रियकः प्रियसालकः ।
सुगन्धिनीलनिर्यासस्तथा बन्धूकपुष्पकः ।
.... महासर्जश्च नामतः ॥ (K'siraswāmī 2.4.44)

IV- 1) बीज Bīja, बीजकः Bījakaḥ
C.S.Ci. 16. 106 etc.
S.S.Ci. 6. 19 9.50 etc.
A.H. Ci. 3-134 etc.
This is the name of *Pterocarpus marsupium* Roxb. See Synonyms असन *Asana* and *Bījak* बीजक
It is wrong to think that *Asana* and *Bijaka* are two different plants.(Balvantjī p. 276)

2) असन
Pterocarpus marsupium Roxb.
C.S.Su. 4.43; 5.70 etc.
S.S.Su. 6.37; 38.12 etc
A.H.Su. 15;7; 19 etc.
सालसारादि *Sālasaradi* or असनादि *Asanādi* group of drugs which is exclusively a group of wood drugs used in *kustha* and *meha*. (Balvantji P. 31)

3) *Pterocarpus marsupium* Roxb.
The Indian Kino tree.
H. Bīja, Bijasāl.
Habitat : A large deciduous tree of central and South India and

Ceylon, extending north west as far as Banda dist. of the north-west provinces.

Gum: The species yields the gum, kinio of European materia medica. The gum as it exudes has the appearance of red currant jelly. (Watt. VI. I. 357).

42. (४२) शाल्मली Śālmali

शाल्मली रक्तपुष्पा तु कुक्कुटी चिरंजीविका ॥१२०
पिच्छिला चूलिनी मोचा कण्टकाद्या सुपूरणी ॥

शाल्मलीवेष्टकः पिच्छा निर्यासः स च शाल्मलः ॥१२१
मोचस्त्रावो मोचरसो मोचनिर्यासकस्तथा ॥

शाल्मली शीतला स्निग्धा शुक्रश्लेष्मविवर्धनी ॥ १२२
कषायस्तद्रसो ग्राही पुष्पं तद्वत्तथा फलम् ॥
(शाल्मली पिच्छला वृष्या बल्या मधुरसा तथा ।
तद्रसस्तद्गुणो ग्राही स च मोचरसस्तथा ॥)

शाल्मली (Śālmalī), रक्तपुष्पा (Raktapuṣpā), कुक्कुटी (Kukkuṭī), चिरजीविका (Cirajīvikā), पिच्छिला (Pichcilā), चूलिनी (Cūlinī), मोचा (Mocā), कण्टकाढ्या (Kaṇṭakāḍhyā) and सुपूरणी (Supūraṇī) are synonymous.

The exudate from *śalmalī* is शाल्मलीवेष्टक (Śālmalī veṣṭaka), शाल्मलपिच्छा (Śālmalapicchā) शाल्मल निर्यासः (Śālmalaniryāsaḥ), मोचस्त्रावः (Mocasrāvaḥ), मोचरसः (Mocarasaḥ) and मोच निर्यासकः (Mocaniryāsakaḥ) are its synonyms.

Śālmalī is *śitavīrya, snigdha* (unctuous), and increases *śukra* and *kapha*. Its sap is astringent. Its flowers and fruits are having similar properties.

[*Śalmalī* is *picchila* (slimy), *vṛṣya*, promotes strength and is of sweet taste, its exudate (sap) is of similar properties and is astringent. It is called as *Mocarasa*.]

Fam. Bombacaceae
Malvaceae (Watt. Dict.)

I- a- ***Salmalia malabarica*** Schott & Engl. *

---

१ 'स्थिरजीवितां' इति क्षी. संमतः पाठः ।
( )कोष्टकान्तर्गतः पाठः आनंदाश्रम पुस्तके दृश्यते ।
* The current accepted name is *Bombax ceiba* Linn.

Syn. *Bombax malabaricum* DC. *B. ceiba* Linn...
Silk Cotton tree. (Chopra).

b- Watt. Dict. Vol. I.487

c- See IV 2 below.

II- a- वेष्टकः (Veṣṭakaḥ), पिच्छा (Picchā), रक्तपुष्पा (Raktapuṣpā), चिरजीविका (Cirajīvikā), चूलिनी (Cūlinī), मोचा (Mocā) कण्टकाढ्या (Kaṇṭakāḍhyā), सुपूरणी (Supūraṇī), मोचनिर्यासकः (Mocaniryāsakaḥ), (Dhn. ni.) यमद्रुमः (Yamadrumaḥ), चिरजीवी (Cirajīvī) (Raj. ni.).

b- Sans. Śālmalī; Mar. Sāwar, Sewar; B.Rakto Simul; Konkan-Sewar; H. Simul or shembal; Tel. Mundla-buraga chettu; Tam. Mulilava, Mul-elva-maram Pula; Maly-Mulila pula, Pul-maram; Kan. Mulu-beraga-mara. (Watt. Dict.)

III-a- 1) See IV- 1 below

b- 1) पिच्छिला पूरणी मोचा स्थिरायुः शाल्मलिर्द्वयोः ।
पिच्छा तु शाल्मलीवेष्टे रोचनः कूटशाल्मलिः ॥ (अमर २.४.४७)
पिच्छा अस्त्यस्याः पिच्छिला । पूरयति पूरणी । मुञ्चति रसं मोचा ।
स्थिरायुः कालसहस्रत्वात् । शालते दैर्घ्याच्छलति वा शाल्मली शाल्मलिश्च ।
आह च ... ॥ रोचते रोचनः शाल्मलिविशेषः । कूटेन कुत्सितत्वं द्योत्यते.
दुर्गादिर्हि परसैन्यदलनार्थे सा क्षिप्यते । .....
(Kṣīraswāmī Amar 2. 4.47)

2) 100 चिरायुः-शाल्मली । षष्ठिवर्षसहस्राणि वने जीवति शाल्मली ।(Harshe)

Note - कूटशाल्मली Kūṭaśālmalī is found included in Rohitak. It is also known as Śweta śālmalī श्वेतशाल्मली; Mar. Pāṇḍharī Sāwar; H. Safed Sāwar and identified with *Ceiba pentandra.* (L.) Gaertn. Syn. *Eriodendron anfrctuousm* DC.
Kapok tree, Cotton tree of Tropical america, Asia & Africa.

IV- 1) शाल्मल Śālmala.
शाल्मली Śālmalī.
Salmalia malabarica Schott & Endl.
Syn. *Bombax ceiba* Linn.
Syn. मानद्रुम, मोच and मोचका
C.S.Su. 4.32, 27. 97 etc.
S.S.Su. 14.36. 46. 249 etc.
A.H.Sa 2.25 27. etc.

2) *Bombax malabaricum* DC.
The cotton tree.
H. Semul; Sans. Śālmalī, Mocā
Habitat : A very large deciduous tree, with branches in whorls..

met with throughout hotter forests of India & Burma. (It is abundant on the Eastern side of India. It is the largest and most characteristic of the eastern Rajputana. (Watt. Vol. I).

43. (४३) मुष्ककः Muṣkakaḥ

मुष्कको मोक्षको मुष्टिर्मूषको मुञ्चकस्तथा ॥ १२३
क्षारश्रेष्ठो गोलकश्च द्विविधः श्वेतकृष्णकः ॥
वातश्लेष्महरः क्षारश्रेष्ठो ग्राही च गुल्मनुत् ॥ १२४

मुष्ककः (Muṣkakaḥ), मोक्षकः (Mokśakaḥ), मुष्टिः (Muṣṭiḥ), मूषकः (Mūṣakaḥ), मुञ्चकः (Muñcakaḥ), क्षारश्रेष्ठः (Ksārasreṣṭhaḥ) and गोलकः (Golakaḥ), are synonymous. It is of two types (1) श्वेतः (Svetaḥ) and (2) कृष्णः (Kṛṣṇaḥ).

It is the sourcc of best क्षार (Kśāra) alkali. It pacifies *vāta* and *pittadoṣas* and is useful in tumors (intestinal diverticulosis).

Under this heading two tree species are included 'A' श्वेत (Śweta) and the next 'B' कृष्ण (Kṛṣṇa).

Fam. oleaceae

I- A-a- ***Schrebera swietenioides*** Roxb.
b- Watt.Dict. VI-II. 488
c- See IV-2 below.

Fam. Celastraceae

B-a- ***Elaeodendron glaucum*** Pers. *
b- Priyavrat Sharma., Balavantji
c- See IV 3 below.

II- A &B- a- मुष्ककः (Muṣkakaḥ), मोक्षकः (Mokśakaḥ), मुष्टिर्मूषकः (Muṣṭirmuṣakaḥ), मुञ्चकः (Muñcakaḥ), द्विविधः श्वेतकृष्णकः (Dwividḥ śwetakṛṣṇakaḥ) of two types white & black (Dhn. ni.) गोलीढः (Goliḍhaḥ), मोहनः (Mohanaḥ), पाटलिः (Pāṭaliḥ), जटालः (Jaṭālaḥ), श्वेतकृष्णश्च स द्वेधा (Śweta kṛṣṇasca sa dwedhā) of two types White & Black.

---

१ 'घण्टा इति क्षी. संमतः पाठः। २ 'रञ्जकस्तथा' इति क्षी. संमत पाठः
३ 'गोलिहः' इति क्षी. संमतः पाठः।
* The present accepted name - *Cassine glauca* (Rottb.) Kuntze. (Comp. p. 31)

A-b- H. Mokhā., Bunpalās; B. Ghaṇṭā pārul, Bundel-Ghantapatali; Muskaka, Ghanta Patali. (Watt. Dict.)

B-b-C.P -Kālā mukhā; Mara. Bhūtapala; Kokan -Burkan. (Watt. Dict.)
H. Bakra; Bom. Bhūtpala; B. Chikyeng; Tam. Karuvali, Pujari; Tel. Nirija. (chopra)
Peth - Barhe, Nasik -Bhutiyāche zād,

III-a- 1) See IV- 1 below

b- 1) गोलिहो झाटलो घण्टापाटलिर्मोक्षमुष्ककौ ॥ Amar II-IV-P. 40
गोभिर्लिह्यते गोलिहः गोलीढोऽपि । झाटं संघातं लाति झाटलः । हन्यते घंटा । पाटं विस्तारं लाति पाटलिः । मोक्ष्यति सहते मोक्षः । मुष्णाति रोगान् क्षारकत्वात् मुष्ककः । आह च-
(Kṣiraswāmī, Amar 2.4.40)

IV- 1) मुष्कक Muṣkaka.
C.S. Ci. 15-189 etc.
S.S. Su. 11.11 (असित मुष्ककः)
38.20; 46. 284; Ci. 7-11
A.H. Su. 15.7; 32; 39. 12 13 etc.

2) *Schrebera swietenioides* Roxb.
H. Ghaṇṭā घण्टा, Ekasirā एकसिरा
Syn. श्वेतमोक्षकः
Elaeodendron glaucam Pers.
H.Kālā mokhā कालामोखा, Jamrāsī जमरासी, Ratangarūr रतनगरूर
Syn. असित मुष्कक (Balvantji p. 312)
Interested readers, may go through the original discussion by Tha. Balvantji.

3) *Schrebera swietenioides* Roxb.
H. Mokhā; Sans. Muṣkaka, Ghaṇṭā Paṭalī
Habitat : A deciduous tree, 40 to 50 feet high found in the tropical Himalaya of Komaon and in the central and southern India. The leaves were eaten as vegetable in the Nasik district during the famine of 1877-78 (Watt. VI.II. 488)
Mokhā, Mokhiri, Goki, (Cooke II-117)

4) *Elaeodendron glaucum* Pers.
Syn. *E. paniculatum* W. & A.
Neerija paniculata Roxb.
Habitat : A moderate sized tree or occassionaly only a shurb, occuring throughout the hotter parts of India and Ceylon,outer parts of Himalaya.
According to Sakharam Arjun the leaves dried and powdered acts as a sternutatory and are used as fumigatory to rouse women from hysterical fits.

A snuff of the leaves is also employed to relieve headaech.
(Watt. Dict. III-275)

Note- The powder of leaves is a powerful sternutatory substance which we have experienced it ourselves.
If used once it makes to sneeze several times, up to 50 times or more; to stop sneezing ghee should be used.

रोहितकः Rohitakaḥ (21)

रोहीतको रोहितको रोही दाडिमपुष्पकः ॥
कुशाल्मलिः शाल्मलिको रोचनः कूटशाल्मलिः ॥१२५
रोहितको यकृत्प्लीहगुल्मोदरहरः सरः ॥
श्वेतो[१] रोहितकश्चान्यः कटूष्णमुभयं स्मृतम् ॥१२६
कर्णरोगहरं चैव विषवेगविनाशनम् ॥

रोहीतकः (Rothītakḥ), रोहितकः (Rohitakaḥ), रोही (Rohī), दाडिम पुष्पकः (Daḍimapuṣpakaḥ), कुशाल्मलिः (Kuśālmalih) शाल्मलिकः (Śālmalikaḥ), रोचनः (Rocanaḥ), and कूटशाल्मलिः (Kūṭśalmaliḥ) are synonymous.

Rohitaka is mild laxative and useful in disorders of liver, spleen tumors (diverticulosis) and abdominal swellings or ascites.

There is an another type of *Rohitaka* called as *Śveta rohitaka.*

Both the types of *Rohitaka* are pungent in taste, *uṣṇavīrya* and useful in the diseases of ear and antipoison.

Under this heading various plants are recorded by modern writers. The bark of this tree is used in medical practice as Rohitak bark. The compiler's description is clear. He records two tree species. The one is 'A' रोहीतक दाडिमपुष्पकः (Rohitaka dāḍimapuṣpakaḥ) and the next is 'B' कूटशाल्मलिः रोचनः (Kūṭāśalmalih Rocanaḥ) (See note under Śālmaliḥ). Raj. Ni. has noted the plants of the same names of Dhn. ni. but has added one more plant namely 'C' श्वेतरोहितः (Śwetarohitaḥ). The compiler of Dhn. ni. has recorded uses of रोहीतक Rohītaka only. He might have excluded कुशाल्मलिः Kuśālmalīḥ. Raj. ni. notes medicinal uses of both the two trees, रोहीतकौ (Rohitakau)

Fam. Bignoniaceae.

I- A-a- ***Tecomella undulata*** (G. Don) Seem. *

---

१ श्वेतों इत्यत्र शुष्कों इति पाठः आनन्दाश्रम पुस्तके दृश्यते। The Ananda. edition was used by D.K. Kamat therefore he has to use Raj. ni. for 3 rd i.e.'C' plant.

* The current accepted name is *Tecomella undulata* (Sm.)Seem.

b- Chopra C- see IV-2 below

Fam. Bombaceae

B-a- ***Ceiba pentandra*** (Linn.) Gaertn.
Syn. *Eriodendron anfractuosum* DC.

b- Chopra C-See IV-3 below.

Fam. Meliaceae

C-a- ***Aphanamixis polystachya*** (Wall.) Parker.
Syn. *Amoora rohituka* W & A.
Andersonia rohituka Roxb. (Watt. I.224)

b- Roxburgh C-See IV-6 below

II- A-a- रोहितकः (Rohitakaḥ), रोहीतकः (Rohītakaḥ),रोही (Rohī), दाडिमपुष्पकः (Dāḍimpuṣpakaḥ)

b- H. Bom. Ragatrorā; Mar. Rakta rohaḍā; Sans; Rohī (Chopra)

B-a- कुशाल्मलिः (Kuśālmaliḥ), रोचनः (Rocanaḥ) कूटशाल्मलिः (Kūṭaśalmaliḥ), शाल्मलिकः (Śālmalikaḥ).

B-b- B. Shweta Simul; Bom. Safed Sāvar; Mal. Mulli lava; Tam. Havum; Sans. Shweta Śālmalī. (Chopra)
Eng. Kapok Cotton tree (Hill)

III-a-1) See below IV-1

b-1) रोहीतः दाडिमपुष्पः कूटशाल्मलिः । (Madan. Ni. I-300)

2) दाडिमपत्र प्लीहघ्नो रोहिणो 'गणनामके'।
(Ni. Shiromani p. 124)

3) रोहि रोहितकः ... दाडिमपुष्पकः ॥ ४९ Amar 2.4. 49
रोहयति रोहितः रोहतीति लोके छिन्नरूढत्वात् ।
'रोहितको रोचनकः प्लीहघ्नो रक्तपुष्पकः ।
रक्तघ्नो रोहितो रक्तो रोही दाडिमपुष्पकः ।
(Ksiraswami. Amar. 2.4.49)

4) रोहितको ... दाडिमस्य पुष्पमिवपुष्पमस्य । (Bhanuji. Amar. 2.4.49)

5) 195 रोही वनतिक्तः । (Harshe)

6) 182 रक्तइति – रोहितकः ।
'रोहीतको दीर्घपत्रो द्रुमो गिरौ ।
पीतारुणैर्दाडिमाभैः पुष्पैर्द्धः फलशङ्किकैरिति । (Harshe)

7) रोहीतको रोहीतकः रोहीतश्च कुशाल्मलिः ॥ सदाप्रसूनश्च कूटशाल्मलिश्च विरोचनः ॥ ५६ (Ni. Shiromani P. 124)

8) रोचते रोचनः शाल्मलिविशेषः आह च – 'कुशाल्मलिः शाल्मलिको रोचनः कूटशाल्मलिः । (Ksiraswami. Amar. 2.4.47)
(See Śālmali III b-1 Pre no. 42 Supra)

IV- 1) रोहितक Rohitaka, रोहीत Rohīta, रोहीतक Rohītaka.

Tecomella undulata (G. Don) Seem.
C.S.Ci. 6.34; 7.128 etc.
S.S.Ci. 10.4; 11.7 etc.
A.H.Ci. 6.53; 12.16 etc.

The indentiy of *Rohitak* is clearly indicated in its rural and descriptive names such as *Roherā* रोहेरा (Cakra), *Dāḍimacchada* दाडिमच्छद and *Dāḍimapuṣpaka* दाडिमपुष्पक (leaves and flowers like those of *Dāḍima*) which are undoubtedly applicable to *Tecomella*. But, probably due to its distribution limited to the western parts of the country and Deccan, other plants such as *Aphanamixis polystachya* (Wall.) Parker, Syn. *Amoora rohituk* W. & A. have been used in the Eastern parts of this country. Again, the bark of *Erythrina* has also been found to be used as *Rohitaka* since the time of Bopadeva who has mentioned *Pārijāta* as its synonym. It appears that *Śālmalika* mentioned as a synonym of *Rohitaka* acutally refers to Erythrina. (Balvantji P. 341.42)

2) *Tecoma undulata*. G. Don
Syn. *T. glabra* (?) D.C.
Bignonia undulata Smith
B. glauca Dcne.
T. undulata Seem.
H. Raktarora; Bom. Roira; Mar. Rakta reora.
Habitat : A shrub or small tree, wild in Sindha, Punjab, Gujarat and Rajputana, distributed to Baluchistan, and Arabia ... culti vated in gardens on account of its beautiful orange flowers. *Structure of the wood.:* Bark greyish or yellowish brown.
(Watt. Dict. VI.IV.1)

3) *Eriodendron anfractuosum* DC.
The white silk cotton tree, Kapok floss.
Syn. *Bombax pentandrum* Linn.
B. orientale Spreng.
Ceiba pentandra Gaertn.
H. Hattian, Safed semal; Tam. Havam; Tel. Buruga, Buraza Shānn; Mar. Pāṇḍharī Sāwar, Shalmali; Kan. Billi burga, Billi burlu.
Habitat : A tall tree with straight trunk, prickly when young... Flowers dirty white and much smaller than those of Bombax... According to flora of British India the tree occurs in the forest throughout the hotter parts of India and Ceylon. Distributed to south America, west Indies and tropical Africa. Although occassionally met with districts of India in only a few localities.
(Watt. Dict. Vol. III-259).

4) *Tecomella undulata* Seem.
Syn. *Tecoma undulata* G. Don
Rakta Rohida. Lohero; Corolla orange yellow. (Cooke Fl. p. 328)

5) *Rakta rohido, Rohitaka, Dāḍimapuspaka; Tecoma undulata*
A tree with drooping branches like weeping willow, showy flowers...The true Rohitaka is *T. undulata.* (Ni. Adarsha)

6) *Andersonia rohituka* Roxb.
Sans. Rohitaka; Beng. Tiktaka; Male tree flowers sessile, small white inodorus, *Hermophrodite* tree - Flowers sessile, small, numerous, cream coloured (Roxb. Fl. Ind., CBC.p. 311)

V. Plant species used as *Rohitaka* रोहीतक in some parts of the country but not corresponding to those mentioned by the compiler of Dhn. Ni.

1) रक्तःस्तु रक्तपुष्पश्च रक्तघ्नः पारिजातकः ।
(Keyadeva, Ni. Siromani p. 124)

2) पारिजात रोहीतक रोहडा (Kashyap sam. p. 182)
White flowered varities

3) *Maba nigrescens* Dalz.
Corolla white (Cooke Fl. Part- II97)
This is also known in Southern Bombay as Raktarora.
(Watt. Dict. V. 102)

4) *Rhamnus wightii* W. & A.
Corolla greenish yellow. (Dr. Desai)
Rakta rohida.
The bark is highly esteemed in the wesern Peninsula. (Dymock)
(Chopra, Watt Dict. VI-1-443)

5) *Chloroxylon swietenia* DC.
A native of western peninsuala yields an astringent bark which is prescribed under the name of *Raktaroda.* The wood is satin wood (Dymock -The Indian Satin Wood) (Watt. Dict. II-270)

DISCUSSION

The tree species पारिभद्र *Pāribhadra* is not recorded by compiler of Dhn. ni. but by that of Raj. ni. (Dhn. Ni. -p-375) who has not noted शाल्मलीक *śālmalīka* as a synonym of पारिभद्र *Pāribhadra* (Erythrina). Bhavamisra does not include शाल्मलीक *Śālmalīka* in the text as a synonym of पारिभद्र *Paribhadra* (Chunekar Bh-Pr-Ni.p.334)

It is true in some books the equivalent *Rohitaka* is applied to *Pāribhadra* (See V-e above) which is not appearing in the Nighaṇṭus mentioned above.

The true name शाल्मली Śālmalī which is identified for *Bombax malabarica* DC. is recorded as a valid name under the same heading nameशाल्मली Śālmalī (See Pre No. 42 supra).

The true name कुशाल्मली *Kuśālmalī* - synonyms कूटशाल्मली *Kutaśālmalī* and शाल्मलीक *Śālmalīka* is occured under the heading name रोहितक *Rohitaka* as a next kind of रोहितक in Nighaṇṭu and is identified now as *Ceiba pentandra* Gaertn.

From the above discussion it clearly appears that according to above Nighaṇṭus, पारिजात *Pārijāta* cannot be accepted as *Rohitaka* रोहितक species and शाल्मलीक *Śalmalīka* is not the synonym of पारिजात *Pārijāta* but that of *Rohitaka.* This is our conclusion, about the controversy of the names पारिभद्र - पारिजात *Pāribhadra -Pārijāt* and शाल्मलीक *Śalmalīka.*

The flowers of शाल्मली are pure red colour but those of रोहितक *Rohitaka* are orange yellow (see above IV-4 Cooke) or दाडिमपुष्पक *Dāḍimpuṣpaka* i.e. similar to those of *Punica granatum* Linn.

44. (४४) *इरिमेदः Irimedah. (अरिमः) (Arimaḥ)

इरिमेदोऽरिमेदश्च गोधास्कन्धोऽरिमेदकः ॥ १२७
अहिमेदोऽहिमारश्च पूतिमेदोऽहिमारकः ॥
मुखरोगहरः शीतो रक्तगमस्तम्भकारकः ॥ १२८

इरिमेदः (Irimedaḥ), अरिमेदः (Arimedaḥ), गोधास्कन्धः (Godhāskandhaḥ), अरिमेदकः (Arimedakaḥ), अहिमेदः (Ahimedaḥ), अहिमारः (Ahimāraḥ), पूतिमेदः (Pūtimedaḥ) and अहिमारकः (Ahimārakaḥ) are synonymous.

Irimeda is *śītavīrya,* styptic and causes holding back of *āma*. It alleviates the diseases of mouth.

Fam. Leguminosae. Mimosaceae.

I- a- ***Acacia farnesiana*** Willd.**
Syn. *Mimosa farnesiana* Linn.

---

* 'अरिमः' इति गणद्रव्यावल्यां पाठः । 'अरिम' पदेन' अरिमेदः-इरिमेदः' गृह्यते ।
'प (अ) रिमेदोऽरिमेदश्च गोधास्कन्धोऽरिमेदकः ।
अहिमेदोहिमारश्च रिमः पूत्यरिमेदकः ॥ " इति क्षीर. संमत पाठः ।
१ 'अरिमेदोऽरिमारश्च' इति पाठभेदः आनन्दा. पुस्तके ।
२ 'पूतिश्च मेदः प्रत्यरिमेदकः इति पाठभेदः आनन्दा., पुस्तके ।
* The present accepted name is *Acacia farnesiana* (Linn.) Willd.

Eng. Cassia flower, spongy tree, Stinging Acacia.

b- Roxburgh. Fl. Ind. CBC p. 421

c- See below IV 8, 9, 10

II- a- इरिमेदः (Irimedaḥ), अरिमेदः (Arimedaḥ), गोधास्कन्धः (Godhāskandhaḥ), अरिमेदकः (Arimedakaḥ), अहिमारः (Ahimāraḥ), पूतिमेदः (Pūtimedaḥ), अहिमारकः (Ahimārakaḥ).

b- Sans. Arimeda (Chopra); H.Pissibābūl; Guj. Kikar, Ganda-bābul, Vilayati bābul; B-Guya-bābul; Santal-Gabur; Mar. Guya-bābūl; Tam.-Vedda-Vala, Kampu-tamma; Tel.Maurki-tumma; Naga tumma, Kampu-tamma; Kan-Jāli. (Watt. Dict.); Bom. Devabābul (Chopra)
Guj. Gandhelo-khair; Kokan-Kusti-zada, Kankri; Mal.-Karivelam.

III-a-1) See IV-below.

b-1) अरिमेदो विट्खदिरे Amaraḥ 2.4.50 P. 62 अरिर्दुःसहोमेदः सारः स्रावो-स्यारिमेदः - विड्गन्धिखदिरः पूतिखदिराऽख्यः ।
(Kṣīraswāmī. Amar 2.4.50 P. 62)

2) अरिमेदः । ३.२२ । अरिरिव मेदः स्नेहोऽस्य । विट्खदिरवृक्षः । ते. नुगतुम्म कस्तुरी केम्पु; क. कमजाली, किरिजाली, करि कस्तुरी, सण्णजाठि; कों कुस्री झाड; ता. पिक्करवेल; मला. करिवेलं पौवेलं (लिनारी इति केचित्) *Acacia farnesiana* (Ast. Hr. Kosha)

3) 1113* अरिमेदो भवेद्वेलो मुखरोगरिपुर्हिमः (Abhi. manj.)

4) 1114 अरिमेदो द्वितीयः स्यात् प्रत्यक्पुष्पप्यहिमारकः ।
महामेदः कृष्णपक्षः पुन्नागः पुष्पहन्तृकः ॥ (Abhi. manji.)

5) इरिमेदो विट्खदिरः 'रेउज' शब्दवाच्यः । (Dipika-Irimedali Tail)

6) इरिमेदो विट्खदिरः 'अरिमेदक' । (Bh. Pr. Ni. Vaṭādi chapter)

7) इरिमेदः विट्खदिरः 'ओज' शब्द वाच्यः । (Dipika - Kāsisadi Taila.)

9) 'पूत्यरिभेदः' दुर्गन्धोऽहिमारकः । (Ast. Sang. Su. 15)

IV- 1) अरिमेद *Arimeda*
Acacia leucophloea Wlld
Revān रेवाँ, *Remajā* रेमजा (H.)
Syn.अहिमार
C.S.Ci. 4.43. 48; 25. 49 etc.
S.S.Su. 19.28; 39.3 etc.
A.H.U. 22. 90; 96.106 etc
This has been mentioned by Ḍalhaṇa as *Arimajja* अरिमज्ज and *Rāmaka* रामक and विट्खदिर *Viṭkhadira* by later writers.
(Balvantji p. 22)

---

* वेळुत्तवेलम् । (Vd. Mrs. Chitra K.)

2) कालस्कन्ध Kālaskandha
It is mentioned in *Śālasarādi Gaṇa* of S.S. and may be any of विट्खदिर, तिन्दुकभेद or तमाल. (Balvantji p. 94.)

3) इरिमेदः
(17) दुर्गन्धखैर (Durgandha Khair i.e. foetid *Khaira*)

Acacia farnesiana Willd.
It produces unagreeable foetid smell from its bark hence the name *Viṭkhadira*. (Chunekar Bh. Pr. Ni. P. 527)

4) दुर्गन्ध खदिर (रोहिजे)
Acacia farnesiana (Vidyotini)

5) इरिमेद - विट्खदिर (Irimeda-Viṭkhadira)
Acacia farnesiana. (Ach. Priyavratji Sharma)

6) *Acacia farnesiana* Willd.
Sans., Arimedaḥ (Chopra)

7) *Mimosa farnesiana* Linn.
Syn. *A. farnesiana* Willd.
Sans. urimeda., Viṭkhadira
Tel. Kusturi. Piktoomee.
Ben. Guvā babula (Roxb. C.B.C. p. 421)

8) *Acacia farnesiana* Willd.
Syn. *Mimosa farnesiana* Linn.
The cassia flower.
Habitat : The fl.of British India regards this small tree as Indigenous to India " Cosmopolitan in the tropics, but often cultivated:" It is common everywhere in India and Burma growing freely by selfsowing. Its strong scented yellow flower heads perfume the atmosphere very pleasantly. Cultivated in Europe.
Botanic diagnosis :An erect shrub or low tree with straight spines ... etc.
Gum: The gum is collected in Sind (Bom. Gaz. part I.p.60)... says the gum exudes from the trunk in considerable quantities... superior to gum arabic and as a medicine.
Medicine. It is very desirable that its peculiar properties should be investigated, a fair substitute for gum arabia. Decoction may be used in diarrhoea.
Dye & Tan. : ... The plant wild in most parts of Bengal ... may be used as a hedge plant. (Watt. Dict. I.p.48)

9) *Acacia farnesiana*
Thorny shrub, native of the west Indies but it occurs spontaneoulsy in many tropical and sub-tropical countires (Hill)

10) *Acacia farnesiana* Willd.
A small tree known in Europe as cassia flower, curioulsy enough in India as *'Kikar' 'Babul'* or *'Kankar'* .... indigenous in America, largely cultivated in France for rich perfume obtained from the flowers. (Comm. Prod. of India by Sir G. Watt.)

11) *A. farnesiana.* Willd.
Arimedakaḥ (Chopra Handa 1958 p. 492)

12) दुर्गन्धखैर (Durgandha khair)
Acacia farnesiana Willd.
Eng. cassia flower.
It is also said *Viṭkhadira* (Vit-foetid) due to foetidous smell of the wood and bark, especially in the root.
(Chunekar Bh. Pr. Ni. p. 527)

V- 1) इरिमेद (Irimeda)
Acacia leucophloea.
Etymology अरिमेदः । अरिः द्धःसहो मेदः स्त्रावोऽस्य इति । विट्खदिरः विष्ठावत् दुर्गन्धित्वात् विट्खदिरः । (स्वल्पखदिर विशेषः)
Ca. Vi. 8. 165
तुलां खदिरसारस्य द्वितुलामरिमेदस्य ।
Su. Su. 14. 47 क्षारागद. A.H. U. 22. 96. अरिमेद गुटिका ।
(Bapalaji 1968 p. 512). (Ni. Adarsha)

Tree species suggested by some writers not corresponding to our accepted plants. see Balwantji IV 1 above
Acacia leucophloea Willd.
Sans. Sweta barbura vṛksah (Modern Sanskrit)
H. Safed kikar; B. Safed Babul; C.P. & Mar. Hevar, Pāndharā Babhaliche zad. Compare with *A. arabica.* Gum-obtained from this species used in the native medicine.
Medicine : On an official correspondence with the Government of India, it is recommended that this drug should be excluded from further trial.
Botanic diagnosis : A large deciduous tree, short straight white spines ... flowers in small round yellow heads. (Watt. Dict. I-52)

45. (४५) मल्लिका Mallikā

मल्लिका शीतभीरुश्च मदयन्ती प्रमोदनी ॥
मदनीया गवाक्षी च भूपद्यष्टपदी[१] तथा ॥ १२९

---

१ 'अष्टपदी' इति शोढल पाठः ।

मल्लिकोष्णा कटुः स्वादुर्दारयत्यास्यजान् गदान् ॥
संत्रासयति नेत्रोत्थरुजः पित्तसमीरजित् ॥ १३०

मल्लिका (Mallikā), शीतभीरुः (Śītabhīruḥ), मदयन्ती (Madayantī), प्रमोदनी (Pramodanī), मदनीया (Madaniyā), गवाक्षी (Gavākṣī), भूपदी (Bhūpadī) and अष्टपदी(Aṣṭapadī) are synonymous.

Mallikā is pungent, *uṣṇavīrya* and sweet in taste. It is useful in the disorders of mouth and eyes. It pacifies *vāta* and *pitta doṣas*.

The heading name मल्लिका (Mallikā) is a plant species included in *Jasminum* a genus of scandant or erect shrub belonging to the family (N.O.) Oleaceae and comprising species distributed over tropical or warm temperate parts of the old world. Of these some 40 to 49 are natives of India. Under the heading the compiler has recorded only one plant species namely 'A' मल्लिका मदयन्ती (Mallikā-madayantī) but, Raj. ni. has recorded one more namely 'B' वटपत्रा अन्या मल्लिका (Vatapatrā anyā mallikā) both of the same genus. Really stating the plant species of Jasminum genus are not recognised and identified. It is seen that the same plant names are named to different botanical (species) names. *Navamallikā, vanamallikā* etc. are of this sort. (See watt. Dict. Roxburgh's fl. indi. and Chopra.)

Fam. Oleaceae

I- a-I) ***Jasminum sambuc*** Ait.*
The Arabian Jasmine.
Syn. *J. undulatum* Willd.
J. zambac Roxb.
J. pubescens Watt. (Not of Willd.)
Mogorium sambuc Lamk.
Var. 1. Sambuc proper
Var. 2 Hyneana
(See Watt Dict, Roxburgh Fl. indi. and Chopra.)

A.II) ***Jasminum angustifolium*** Vahl
b- Watt. Dict. IV.5 41-44
c- See below IV-2

B-a- A double flowered sambuc; Arabian tuscan Jasmine.
b- Cooke flora Part II-111
Roxb. Fl. Ind., CBC p. 30
c- See IV

II- a-AI & AII

---

१ 'स्वादे' हरत्यर्शादिका व्यथाः इति पाठः क्वचित

* The current accepted name is *Jasminum sambuc* (Linn.) Ait.

शीतभीरुः (Śītabhīruḥ), मदयन्ती (Madayantī), मोदनी (Modanī), मदनीया (Madanīyā), गवाक्षी (Gavākṣī) Dhn. ni. भद्रवल्ली (Bhadravallī), वनचंद्रिका (Vanachandrikā), नारीष्टा (Nārīṣṭā), गिरिजा (Girijā)

AI & AII-b-
H. Bānmallika, Mogra; B. Bela, Nava mallikā, Mogra; Bom. Mara... Mogri Mogrā; Tam. Mallippu, Malligaippu; Tel. Boddu Malle, Navamllka; Kan. Mallige; Sans-Vana mallikā, Navamallikā, Vārṣikī, Āsphotā (Watt. Dict.)

B-a- मोदिनीचान्या (Modinīcānyā) वटपत्रा (Vaṭapatrā), कुमारिका (Kumārikā), सुगन्धाढ्या (Sugandhāḍhyā), वृत्तपुष्पा (Vṛttapuṣpā), वृत्तमल्लिका (Vṛttamallikā)

B-a- Mar. Bom. Baṭmogrā H. Motiyāmogrā (Cooke II-111)

III-a-1) See IV 1 below.

b-1) मल्लिका । भूपदी शीतभीरुश्च ...
आस्फोता वनोद्भवा ॥ ७० ॥ अमरः 2.4 70 p. 65
मल्ल्यते मूर्ध्नि मल्लिका । भुवि पदमस्या भूपदी । शीतभीरु ग्रैष्मकत्वात् । आह च ... । Kśīraswāmī 2.4.70.p.65

2) 344 मल्लिका वार्षिकी (Harshe)

3) मल्लिका वार्षिका जाती वासन्ती ग्रैष्मचम्पकाः ।
तरुण्यौ यूथिका कुन्दा शतपत्रातिमुक्तकैः ॥
बकुलः किणिरातश्च तिलकाशोककिंशुकाः ।
पुष्पाण्येतानि धार्याणि वृक्षसौगन्ध्यमिच्छता ॥
(Dhn. ni. Gaṇadravyāvali pp. 5.6)

IV 1) मल्लिका Mallikā
Jasminum sambac Ait.H. बेला
S.S.Su.41.286 A.H. Su. 3-40, 24.21 Ci. 7.82
See मदयन्ती Madayantī (Balvantji p. 300)
C.S.Ci. 8.129; 10.21 etc.
S.S.Ci. 2.91; 9,34 etc.
A.H.Ci. 2.27, V.7.22 etc.
Mallikā मल्लिका which is usually considered to be a Jasminum species.
See नवमल्लिका, मदनक and मोदयन्ती (Balvantji p. 292)
नवमल्लिका Navamallikā
C.S.Ci. 26.184
S.S.Sa 10.57
It is said to be what is also known as वासन्तीपुष्प Vāsantīpuṣpa

which too is unidentified. *Vāsantī, Navamallikā* नवमल्लिका and Nepālī नेपाली known as Newārī नेवारी are considered by many to be the names of a variety of *kunda* कुन्द identified as *Jasminum arborescens* Roxb.

मदनकः Madanakah

C.S.Ci. 28.252(मदनपल्लवैः ।) A.H.Ci. 21.79

This synonym does not occur in मल्लिका of Dhn. ni.

2) *Jasminum sambac* Ait.
Habitat : A fragrant climbing shrub common throughout India, extensively cultivated in the tropics of both hemispheres.
(Watt. Dict. IV-544)

3) *J. sambac* Ait.
A suberect shrub, scarcely climbing...flowers white, very fragrant...usually in 3 flowered (many flowered in cultivation)...Flowers more or less throughout year. Vern. Butmogra ... is known as *Arabic* or *Tuscan* Jasmine (Cooke II-118)

4) 732 *J. sambac* Ait.
Syn. *J. Zambac* Roxb.
Uses... insanity, weakness of sight and affections of mouth (Baden Powell) (Kirtikar p.761)

5) *Jasminum zambac* Willd.
Syn. *Mungorium sambac* Lam.
of this we have varieties, viz.-
1st single flowered *Arabian Jasimine* which I suppose to be *J. undulatum* Willd; Ben. -Banmallikā or Deshimallikā.
2nd -Double flowered -*Arabian Jasmine*
3rd -Great double *Arabian* or *Tuscan Jasmine*
All varieties flowers chiefly in rains. (Roxb. Fl. Ind. CBC.p.30)

46. (४६) वार्षिकी Vārṣikī

वार्षिकी सुपुटा[१] त्र्यस्रा सुरूपा सुभगा प्रिया ॥
श्रीम्मती षट्पदानन्दा सुवर्षा मुक्तबन्धना ॥ १३१

[२]वार्षिकी शिशिरा हृद्या सुगंधा पित्तनाशिनी ॥

वार्षिकी (Vārṣikī), सुपुटा (Suputā), त्र्यस्रा (Tryasrā), सुरूपा (Surūpā),

१ 'त्रिपुटा इति आनन्दा. मुद्रितं पुस्तके पाठः ।
२ 'श्रीमती षट्पदानन्दा सुगन्धा पित्तनाशिनी ।' इति. आनन्दा. मुद्रित पुस्तके पाठः ।

सुभगा (Subhagā), प्रिया (Priyā), श्रीमती (Śrīmatī), षट्पदानन्दा (Ṣaṭpadānandā), सुवर्षा, (Suvarṣā), मुक्तबन्धना (Muktabanbhanā) are synonymous.

Vārṣikī is *śītavīrya,* cordial, fragrant and pacifies *pitta doṣa.*

Some modern writers have recognised this as a synonym of *Mallikā* मल्लिका, but it is recorded under a separate heading by the compilers of the both Nighaṇṭus. In Bh. Pr. Ni., *Mallikā* मल्लिका and *varṣikī* वार्षिकी are recorded under two separate headings. We assume मल्लिका and वार्षिकी are two separate plant species or two varieties of a *mallikā* common. Dr. Roxburgh has recorded 3 varieties of *Mallikā*. *Vārṣikī* may be one of them which flowers only in *Varṣāṛtu* i.e. in rainy season but we have not recorded its botanical name as it is remained unidentified.

I- a- Not recognised.

II- a- त्रिपुटा (Tripuṭā), सुभगा (Subhagā), त्र्यस्रा (Tryasrā), श्रीमती (Śrīmatī), षट्पदानन्दा (Ṣaṭpadānandā), मुक्तबन्धना (Muktabandhanā)

47. (४७) जाती Jātī

जाती मनोज्ञा सुमना राजपुत्री प्रियंवदा ॥ १३२
मालती हृद्यगन्धा च चेतिका[1] तैलभाविनी[2] ॥

मालती कफपित्तास्यरुक्पाकव्रणकुष्ठजित ॥ १३३
चक्षुष्यो मुकुलस्तस्यास्तत्पुष्पं कफपित्तजित्[3] ॥
सुगन्धि च मनोज्ञं च सर्वश्रेष्ठतमं मतम् ॥ १३४

जाती (Jātī), मनोज्ञा (Manojñā), सुमना (Sumanā), राजपुत्री (Rājaputrī), प्रियंवदा (Priyamvadā), मालती (Mālatī), हृद्यगन्धा (Hṛdyagandhā), चेतिका (Cetikā), and तैलभाविनी (Tailabhāvinī) are synonymous.

Mālatī pacifies *kapha pitta doṣas* and is useful in the diseases of mouth like glossitis and ulcers. It is also useful in disorders of the skin. It's flowerbud is beneficial for eyes and the flower pacifies *kapha -pitta doṣas,* is fragrant, and is the best amongst the flowers.

Fam. Oleaceae

I- a- ***Jasminum grandiflorum*** Linn. (Fl. Br. Ind. III. 603)
The spanish Jasmine.

---

१ 'वैदिका' इति क्षी. संमतः पाठः 'वेशिका' इति शोडलः ।
२ 'तिलभाविनी इति क्वचित् पाठः आनन्दा पुस्तके । ३ 'कफवातजित् इति पाठभेदः आनन्दा. पुस्तके ।

Syn. *Jasminum aurum* Don

b- Watt Dict. IV-542, Cooke fl. II-115

II- a- जाती (Jātī), मनोज्ञा (Manojñā), राजपुत्री (Rājaputrī), मालती (Mālatī), हृद्यगन्धा (Hṛdyagandhā), तैलभाविनी (Tailabhāvinī) Dhn. ni. संध्यापुष्पा (Sadnhyāpuṣpā), तैलभाविनी (Tailabhāvinī)

b- *Chamelī* H. Jātī, Tel. - Jāti; Guja & Bom.- Chambeli; Mar. -Jaī; Sans. Jāti.

III-a- 1) See below IV -1

b- 1) मालयत्यामोदैर्मालती । जायतेऽनया प्रीतिर्जातिः । (Kṡīraswāmī, Amara; 2.4.73 P. 66)

IV- 1) *Jasminum grandiflorum* Linn.
H. Chameli. Syn. Mālatī; मालती and Sumanā सुमना
C.S.Sū. 4.13 etc.
S.S. Su. 36.16 (जाती कल्प) etc.
A.H. Ci. 1.57, 69 etc. (Balwantji p. 166)

2) *J. grandiflorum* Linn.
A. large scandent glabrous shrub found in the sub. tropical North-west Himalaya-often cultivated throughout India.
Oil : The fragrant flowers are used in India for preparing scented oil. (Watt. Dict. IV. 542)

3) See Roxb. Fl. Indi. CBC. P. 34.
Sans... Jātī, Mālatī

4) See Cooke Fl. II.115
Jasminum grandiflorum Linn. sp. Pl.
ed. 2. (1762) P.9
Spanish Jasmine.
In Cook's fl. (II-113) two plant species are recorded under the name *Jāī,* जाई one of it, we have accepted *Jāti* जाती (See I-a-above) the Spanish Jasmine and the next recorded by him is *Jasminum auriculatum* Vahl...Jāī जाई. It seems that the latter plant species is not included in Watt. Dict. It may be called as *Jāī* जाई in some parts of the country but Roxburgh has noted its Sanskrit name as *Yūthikā* यूथिका (See plant name no. 53 infra).

5) जाई, चमेली *Jasminum grandiflorum*
Eng. Catalonian, Spanish Jasmine; Guj.Chambeli; H. Chambeli; Kan. Ajjiege, Anamallige.,
Jaimalle; Sk. Chambeli
Charcters : A large scandent shrub, leaflets 7-11, terminal rather large, fl. 3.8 cm across, white often tinged with pink outside,

fru.-ripe carpels 2; fl. time July Sept.
Distri: Cultivated throughout India wild in subtropical Himalayas, salt range, Kumaon, Rajputana.
Oil The fragrant flowers are used in India for preparation of a scented oil ... In Europe the flower is very highly esteemed... (Mah. State Gaz.p. 132).

48. (४८) वासन्ती Vāsantī

वासन्ती प्रहसन्ती स्यात् सुवसन्ती वसन्तजा ॥
शोभना शीतसंवासा सेव्या भ्रमरबान्धवा ॥ १३५
वासन्ती शीतला हृद्या सुगन्धा स्वेदनाशिनी ॥

वासन्ती (Vāsantī), प्रहसन्ती (Prahasantī), सुवसन्ती (Suvasantī), वसन्तजा (Vasantajā), शोभना (Śobhanā), शीतसंवासा (Śītasamvāsā), सेव्या (Sevyā), and भ्रमरबान्धवा (Bhramarabāndhavā) are synonymous.

Vāsantī is *śītavīrya,* cordial, fragrant and anti diphoretic.(reduces perspiration).

49. (४९) ग्रैष्मी Graiṣmī

ग्रैष्मी तु सुरभिः कान्ता सुगन्धा वनमालिनी ॥ १३६
सुकुमारा शिखरिणी च नेपाली वनमालिका ॥

नेपालिका रसे तिक्ता वीर्ये चोष्णा प्रकीर्तिता ॥ १३७
वातपित्तरुजां नेत्ररोगाणां नाशिनी मता ॥

ग्रैष्मी (Graiṣmī), सुरभिः (Surabhiḥ), कान्ता (Kāntā), सुगन्धा (Sugandhā),वनमालिनी (Vanamālinī), सुकुमारा (Sukumārā), शिखरिणी (Śikhariṇī), नेपाली (Nepālī) and वनमालिका (Vanamālikā) are synonymous.

Nepālikā is biitter in taste, *uṣṇavīrya* and pacifies *vāta pitta doṣas.* It is useful in diseases of the eye.

Vāsantī वासन्ती and ग्रैष्मी *Graiṣmī* are not found recorded and

* Śodhala mentions वासन्तीग्रैष्मचम्पकौ *Vāsantī Graiṣma Campakau* in his *Ganadravyāvalī* गणद्रव्यावली (P.6) and mentions synonyms of *Nepālī* नेपाली only. (p.69)

identified, but the names suggest, their flowering seasons which are from March to June. There are some plants species of *Jasminum,* those flower in these season. Out of these two plant species we have recorded herebelow.

Fam. Oleaceae.

I- a- वासन्ती Vāsantī
Jasminum malabaricum Wight.
J. arborescens Wooder.
J.latifolium Grah.
Kusar कुसर (Cooke fl. II. III)

a- ग्रैष्मी Graiṣmī
J. roxburghianum Wall.
J. arborescens Roxb. (Cooke Fl. II.119)

II- a- वासन्ती (Vāsantī), वसन्तजा (Vasantajā), शीतसंवासा (Śitasamvāsā), Dhn. ni.; माधवी (Mādhavī), वसन्त दूती (Vasantadūtī) Raj. Ni.

b- कुसर Kusar (Cooke)

a- ग्रैष्मी (Graiṣmī), नेपाली (Nepāli), वनमालिका (Vanmālikā),ग्रीष्मोद्भवा (Grīṣmodbhavā), सप्तला (Saptalā).

The name (Nepālī) is recorded as a synonym of ग्रैष्मी (Grāismī) by Dhn. ni.but the compiler of Bh. Pr. Ni. has (also?) given this name and Dr. Chunekar has identified it with *J.arborescens* Roxb.

b- H. Nevārī, Vāsantī, Camelī; B. Bara kunda; Bom.kusara; Tam. Nagmatti. (Chunekar Bh.Pr. P. 489)

नेवारी Nevārī; Mar. नेवाळी (ली), Nevālī is wild in the hill slopes near Maval Junnar of Poona Dist. (Dr. Balasaheb Joshi of Junnar, now in W. Mulund, Bombay.)

IV- 1) नवमल्लिका Navamallikā
C.S.CI. 26. 184, S.S. Su. 10.57
It is said to be what is known as *Vāsantī puspa* वासन्तीपुष्प which too is unidentified *Vāsantī, Navamallikā* and *Nepālī* नेपाली known as Nevārī are considered by many to be names of a variety of *Kunda* कुन्द identified as *Jasminum arborescens* Roxb.

(Balvantji p. 218.)

50. (५०) चम्पकः Campakaḥ

चम्पकः सुकुमारश्च सुरभिः शीतलश्चः सः ॥ १३८
चाम्पेयो हेमपुष्पश्च काञ्चनः षट्पदातिथिः ॥

चम्पकः कथितः शीतो वीर्येऽति कटुको रसे ॥ १३९
हृद्यः सुगन्धिर्विषहा कफपित्तविनाशनः ॥

चम्पकः (Campakaḥ), सुकुमारः (Sukumāraḥ), सुरभिः (Surabhiḥ), शीतलः (Śītalaḥ), चाम्पेयः (Cāmpeyaḥ), हेमपुष्पः (Hemapuṣpaḥ), काञ्चनः (Kāñcanaḥ), and षट्पदातिथिः (Ṣaṭpadātithiḥ) are synonymous.

Campaka is pungent in taste, *śitavirya,* cordial, fragrant, antipoisonous and pacifies *kapha pitta doṣas*

Fam. Magnoliaceae

I- a- ***Michelia champaca*** Linn.
b- Roxburgh Fl. inidi. CBC, 453
c- See IV-b-1 below.

II- a- चम्पकः (Campakaḥ), सुरभिः (Surabhiḥ), हेमपुष्पः (Hemapuṣpaḥ), काञ्चनः (Kāñcanaḥ), षट्पदातिथिः (Ṣaṭpadātithiḥ), Dhn. ni; भृङ्गमोही (Bhṛngamohī) Raj. ni.
b- H.B. champā, Mar. -Pivaḷāchāphā, Soncāphā, Tam. Shempang. Tel. Shemangamu, Kanchanmu, Shampngipuv, shampangi; Malay. Jampaca, Champkam. (Watt. Dict.).

III- See IV 1 below.

IV- 1 चम्पकः Campaka
Michelia champaca Linn.
S.S.Su. 28.11. 45.12 etc.
2. A large evergreen tree with yellow sweetly scented flowers cultivated throughout India, wild in Nepal, Bengal., ... Assam, Nilgiri and in the forests of Western Ghats as far as Kanara. There are two other tree species under the name campā. These are
1) *Michelia excelsa* Blume
White magnolia
Nepal-Bara chapa, safed chapa.
Temparate Himalaya from Nepal to Bhutan and in the Khasia Hills.
2) *M. nilagirica* Zenk.

---

१ 'चम्पकः कटुकः शीतः कफपित्त विषापहः। हृत्सुगन्धिश्च पित्तघ्नो विशेषाद् राजचम्पकः॥ इति पाठभेदः आनन्दाश्रम मुद्रित पुस्तके दृश्यते।

This different reading has some importance as it differentiates the varieties as 1)चम्पकः *Campakaḥ*, 2) राजचम्पकः *Rājaampakaḥ* & 3) क्षुद्रचम्पकः *Kśudra campakah* of Raj. Ni. S.D.K.

H. Pilā Champā.
A tall tree or shrub found in the higher forests of western Ghats and Ceylon. (Watt. Dict. V. 241-242).

51. (तरुण्यौ Taruṇyau), तरुणी Taruṇī

तरुणी[1] रामतरुणी कर्णिका[2] चारुकेसरा ॥ १४०
सहा[3] कुमारी गन्धाढ्या द्विरेफगणसंमता ॥
तरुणी श्लेष्मपित्तघ्नी ग्राहिणी शीतलाऽग्निजित् ॥ १४१

तरुणी (Taruṇī), रामतरुणी (Rāmataruṇī), कर्णिका (Karṇikā), चारुकेसरा (Cārukesarā), सहा(Sahā), कुमारी (Kumārī), गन्धाढ्या (Gandhāḍhyā) and द्विरेफगणसंमता (Dwirepha gaṇasammatā) are synonymous.

Taruṇi pacifies *kapha* and *pitta doṣas,* is *śītavīrya,* astringent in action and depresses digestive capacity (decreases burning sensation.)

A controversial plant name. Some modern writers have identified it as अबोली *Abolī* (Marathi name) but it is doubtful. We only note it here below without accepting identification of modern writers.

Fam. Acanthaceae

I- ***Crossandra undulaefolia*** Salisb. *
Syn. *C. axillaris* Nees
Ruellia infundibuliformis Roxb. Var. *aboli* (Cooke fl. II-378)

II- a- तरणी (Taraṇī), रामतरणी (Rāmataraṇī), कर्णिका(Karṇikā), चारुकेसरा (Cārukesarā), सहा (Sahā), कुमारी (Kumārī), गन्धाढ्या (Ganḍhād yā), ग्राहिणी (Grāhiṇī) Dhn.Ni.; सुदला (Sudalā), बहुपत्रा (Bahupatrā), भृङ्गेष्टा (Bhṛṅgeṣṭā) Raj. ni.
Raj. ni. records in the text a different plant name, the synonyms of which are: महती तु राजतरणी (Mahatī tu Rājataraṇī), महासहा (Mahāsahā), वर्ण्यपुष्पकोऽम्लानः (Vaṇyapuṣpakoamlānaḥ) सुवर्णपुष्पश्च (Suvarṇa puṣpaśca)
Medicinal uses given by Raj. ni. of *Taraṇī* तरणी and राजतरणी *Rājataraṇī* are different. Medicinal uses of *Rājataraṇī* are noted as कफकारिणी Kafakāriṇī, चक्षुष्या Cakṣuṣyā, हर्षदा Harṣadā, सुरभिः

---

१ 'तरणी रामतरणी' इति आनन्दाश्रममुद्रित पुस्तके पाठः । In गणद्रव्यावली Gaṇadravyāvalī the reading is तरुण्यौ Taruṇyau suggesting two kinds.
२ 'वार्षिका इति शोढल पाठः । ३ 'महाकुमारी इति शोढल पाठः ।
See - Chopra -Gloss. p. 81 mentions 'Priya-darsa' as its bazar name.
* The current accepted name is *Crossandra infundibuliformis* (Linn.) Nees

Surabhiḥ, सुरवल्लभः Suravallabhaḥ.

III-a-1) See IV 1 below.

b-1) सहा कुमारी तरणिरम्लानस्तु महासहा । 'सहते परिमलं सहा । कु भूमिष्टान् मारयति कुमारी। कुत्सितो मारोऽस्या इति वा जरां न यातीत्येके । तरत्यनया (दुःखं) तरणिः । ... कुरण्टको हि म्लानिं न गच्छति तेनाम्लानः यन्माला - अम्लानस्तु कुरण्टकः त्र्यर्थे सहा मुद्गपर्णी वचा तरणी च ।

(K'siraswāmī Amar. 2.4.74 partly)

IV- 1) तरणी Taraṇī

C.S. Vi. 8.151; Si. 10.30

S.S.Su. 46.249

It is considered to be Rose (*Rosa centifolia* Linn.); Gulāba गुलाब H. (Balvantji p. 175)

2) *Crossandra undulaefolia* Salisb.

Leaves 4 to 6 whorl .. inserted close to one another .... *Flowers* numerous axillary *Corolla* orange yellow, very common in gardens, often planted about temples rarely found wild. *Dist*. India. (W. Peninsula), Ceylon. (Cooke Fl. II. 378)

Taranī तरणी is *Sahā* सहा and Rājataraṇī राजतरणी is *Mahāsahā*. The synonym *Mahāsahā* also occurs in the text of कुब्जक *Kubjaka.Abolī* अबोली is the only species of Crossandra in India.Watt also did not mention it. Again the colour of the flower of Raj. nis's Rājtarṇī राजतरणी is yellow while that of the Crossandra is orange, therefore it cannot be confounded with *Rājataraṇī*.राजतरणी. If these are accepted as rose species. *Rosa gigantea* Collet (Watt. Dict.VI-I-867) may be confounded with *Rājtaraṇī* राजतरणी. of Raj. ni. तरणी Taraṇī, कुब्जक Kubjaka, भद्रतरणी Bhadaratarnī of Dhn. ni. & शतपत्री (Satapatri) seem to be belonging to a group. Out of these राजतरणी does not seemto be considered by the modern scholars. However, it should be a species of Rose (गुलाब Gulāba) only.

52. कुब्जकः Kubjakaḥ (Dhn. ni.)*

कुब्जको भद्रतरुणी बृहत्पुष्पाऽतिकेशरा ॥
महासहा कण्टकाढ्या नीलालिकुलसंकुला ॥ १४२

कुब्जकः सुरभिः स्वादुः कषायस्तु रसायनः ॥ १४३
त्रिदोषशमनो वृष्यः शीतः संग्रहणोपरः ॥

* It is not mentioned in Gaṇadravyāvalī.

कुब्जकः (Kubjakaḥ), भद्रतरुणी (Bhadrataruṇī), बृहत्पुष्पा (Bṛhatpuṣpā), अतिकेशरा (Atikeśarā), महासहा (Mahāsahā), कण्टकाढ्या (Kaṇṭakāḍhyā) and नीलालिकुलसंकुला (Nīlālikulasamkulā) are synonymous.

Kubjaka is fragrant, sweet and *kaṣāya* (astringent) in taste and *rasāyan* (rejuvinating). It pacifies all the three *doṣas* and is *vṛṣya, śītavīrya* and astringent in action.

The plant name कुब्जक *Kubjaka* is said to be a species of Rosa family. A synonym महासहा Mahāsahā occured in Dhn. ni is also seen in Amarakosha and Kśīraswāmī in his comments interpreted it as *Kuranṭaka* कुरण्टक. But the synonyms बृहत्पुष्पा *Bṛhatpuṣpā* अतिकेशरा *Atikeśarā* नीलालिकुलसंकुला *Nīlālikulasamkulā* are not applicable to कुरण्टक *Kurantaka*. For the present we also accept it as a species of *Rosa* Family.

Fam. Rosaceae.

I- a- ***Rosa moschata*** Herrm. *
R. moschata Mill. (Watt. Dict.)
Syn. *R. recurva* Roxb. (CBC 407)

II- a- कुब्जकः (Kubjakaḥ), भद्रतरुणी (Bhadrataruṇī), बृहत्पुष्पः (Bṛhatpuṣpaḥ), अतिकेशरा (Atikeśarā), महासहा (Mahāsahā), कण्टकाढ्या (Kaṇṭakāḍhyā), सुरभिः (Surabhiḥ), स्वाद्वः (Swāduaḥ), रसायनः (Rasāyanaḥ) Dhn.ni.
वृत्तपुष्पः (Vṛttapuṣpaḥ), रक्तपित्तकफापहः (Raktapittakaphāpaḥ),पुष्पं तु शीतलम् (Puṣpam tu śītalam), दाहघ्नम् (Dāhaghnam).

b- H. Kuji, Karer, Kujā; Kashmir - Phulwari, chal. (Watt. Dict. VI. I.563)
Sans. Kubjaka; H. Kujai; B. Kuja. (Chopra)

III-a-1) See IV-1 below.

b-1) 106 कुब्ज इति कुब्जो बृहत्पुष्पः शतपत्रिका भेदः । (Harshe)

IV- 1) कुब्जक Kubjaka
S.S. Ci. 7.6; V.17.8
A species of Rosa called *Rosa moschata* Herrm. (Balvantji p. 105)

2) *Rosa moschata* Mill.
The musk rose, *The moisette Rose* is a hybrid between this and *R. indica.*
Habitat : A large thorny climbing shrub found in the North west Himalaya from Afaganistan to Nepal, ascending to 11000 feet. Most elegant as it is the most abundant of the North

---

* The current acceptped name is *R. brunonii* Lindl.

west Himalayan Roses. The neighbourhood of Simla in spring, is literally perfumed with the odour of this elegant and copiously flowering rose.

Domestic : The wood is used in the Himalaya for making walking sticks. (Watt. Dict. VI.I 569).

3) 206 तरुणी कुल (Taruṇī kula)
कुब्जक (Kubjaka), wild Gulab जंगली गुलाब
Rosa involucrata Roxb.
Wild climbing rose ... mostly on river bank, flowers white diameter 2 inches ... In some parts it is called *Kūjā* कूजा or *Kūjoi* कूजोई. It is possible of being कुब्जक *Kubjaka* of Nighaṇṭus. (Tha. Balwantji - Behar - Translated).

53. (५२) यूथिका Yūthikā

यूथिका बालपुष्पा तु पुष्पगन्धा[१] गुणोज्ज्वला ॥
गणिका चारुमोदा च शिखण्डी स्वर्णयूथिका[२] ॥ १४४
सुवर्णयूथी हरिणी पीतिका पीतयूथिका ॥
प्रोक्तान्या शङ्खधवला नामतः शङ्खयूथिका ॥ १४५
यूथिका युगुलं स्वादु शर्कराघ्नं सुगन्धि च ॥

यूथिका (Yūthikā), बालपुष्पा (Bālapuṣpā), पुष्पगन्धा (Puṣpagandhā), गुणोज्ज्वला (Guṇojjvalā), गणिका (Gaṇikā), चारुमोदा (Cārumodā), शिखण्डी (Sikhaṇḍī), are synonyms of *Yūthikā.* The another type of it is called स्वर्णयूथिका (Swarṇayūthikā) the synonyms of which are सुवर्णयूथी (Suvarṇayūthī), हरिणी (Hariṇī), पीतिका (Pītikā), and पीतयूथिका (Pītayūthikā). There is a third type called as शङ्खयूथिका (Sankhayūthikā) the synonym for which is शङ्खधवला (Sankhadhavalā).

Both the types are sweet in taste, fragrant and useful in urinary gravels.

Under this heading the compiler has recorded more than two plant names, but medicinal uses are given of two plants which are 'A' यूथिका बालपुष्पा (Yūthikā Bālapuṣpā) and the next 'B' is हेमयूथिका (Hemayūthikā). Raj. ni, records रस (Rasa), वीर्य (Vīrya), and विपाक (Vipāka) of all varieties and mentions that *suvarṇa yūthikā*

---

१ 'पुण्यगन्धा इति शोढल पाठः । २ 'कृष्णयूथी' इति शोढल पाठः । शोढले तु कृष्णयूथिका, पीतयूथिका, शंखयूथिका इति त्रिप्रकारा (Sodhal p. 69.) (ध.नि. पर्यायेष्वपि अन्या शङ्खयूथिका निर्दिष्टा । S.D. Kamat.

सुवर्णयूथिका is (Viśeṣa) विशेष i.e. having distinguished properties.

Fam. Oleaceae.

I- A-a-***Jasminum auriculatum*** Linn. *

b- Roxburgh fl. indi. CBC P. 33

c- See below IV-2

B-a- ***Jasminum humile*** Linn.

Syn. *J. chrysanthemum* Roxb.

b- Roxburgh Fl. indi CBC P. 33

c- See IV-3 below

II- a- A, बालपुष्पा (Bālapuṣpā), गणिका (Gaṇikā), शिखण्डी (Śikhaṇḍī), भृङ्गानन्दा (Bhṛṅgānandā)

b- Sans. Māgadhī, Gaṇikā, Yūthikā

(Roxb. Fl. indi. C.B.C. 33)

Sans. Kan. & Tel. Mādhavi; Tam. digal; Maly. Bolodda. (Chopra)

a-B- अन्यायूथी (Anyā yūthī), सुवर्णाह्वा (Suvarṇāvhā), हेमयूथिका (Hemayūthikā)

b- Sans. Hemapuṣpikā (Roxb.) H. ... Pitmalli; B. Swarṇajui; Tel. Pacha, Advimalla; Tam. Semmalligai; Malya -Mulla. (Chopra)

III-a-1) see IV-1 below

IV- 1) यूथिका Yūthikā

Jasminum auriculatum Vahl

C.S.Ci. 1.1.56; 8. 128 etc.

S.S.Su. 46.249; Ci. 11.9 etc.

A.H. Su. 26.24; Ci. 9.24 (Balvantji p. 331)

2) *J. auriculatum* Vahl

Deccan, carnatic, Western peninsula (Chopra p. 144)

3) *J. humile* Linn.

Syn. *J. chrysanthemum* Roxb.

J. bignoniasceum Wall.

Habitat : A small erect rigid shrub; Native of the sub. tropical Himalaya from Kashmir to Nepal, found also in South India. (Watt. Dict. IV. 543).

54. (५३) कुन्दः Kundaḥ

कुन्दः सुमकरन्दश्च सदापुष्पो मनोहरः ॥ १४६
अट्टहासो भृङ्गसुहृत् शुक्लः शाल्योदनोपमः ॥

* The current accepted name is *Jasminum auriculatum* Vahl (comp. p. 85)

कुन्दस्य कुसुमं हृद्यं स्वल्पगन्धि मनोहरम् ॥ १४७

कुन्दः (Kundaḥ), सुमकरन्दः (Sumakarandaḥ), सदापुष्पः (Sadāpuṣpaḥ), मनोहरः (Manoharaḥ), अट्टहासः (Aṭṭahāsaḥ), भृङ्गसुहृत् (Bhṛṅgasuhṛt), शुक्लः (Śuklaḥ) and शाल्योदनोपमः (Śālyodanopamaḥ) are synonyms.

The flower of *Kunda* is cordial, having little fragrance and charming.

Fam. Oleaceae.

I- a- ***Jasminum multiflorum*** Andr. *
Syn. *J. pubescens* Willd. (Chopra)

b- Roxburgh (C.B.C. P. 31)

c- See below IV-2

II- a- कुन्दः (Kundaḥ), सदापुष्पः (Sadāpuṣpaḥ), शुक्लः (Śuklaḥ), मकरन्दः (Makarandaḥ).

b- H. Kundaphul, Kunda; B. Kunda; Sans. Kunda; Tam. Magarandam; Tel. Kundamu; Malya. Kundam.

III-a- 1) See below IV-1

IV- 1) कुन्द Kunda
Jasminum multiflorum Andr.
S.S.U. 7:30; 51.37 etc.
A.H.Su. 3.30; 19.72 etc.
H.Kunda कुंद (Balvantji p. 105)

2) *J. pubescens* Willd.
Habitat : A large tomentose shrub common thoughout India. (Watt. Dict. IV .544)

3) *J. pubescens* (Linn.) Willd.
Sans. Māghyam, Koondam, Ben. Koonda. A very ramous shrub ...umbels terminal, sessile, tending to be trichotomous, containing from ten to thirty sessile flowers, downy in all parts, flowers large, pure white, fragrant ...

---

* The current accepted name is *J. multiflorum* (Burm. f.) Andr. (Comp. p. 85)
Soḍhala in his Gaṇadravyāvali has mentioned अमिलातः Amilātaḥ after कुन्दः Kundaḥतरुणी यूथिका कुन्दः सामिलातोऽतिमुक्तकैः । (P.6) and has mentioned the synonyms of अमिलातः Amilātaḥ only (P.70). Kṣīraswāmī in Amarakosh while commenting on ... अम्लानस्तु महासहा has quoted a reading by mentioning आह च –
'अविम्लानोऽपरिम्लानस्तथैवाम्लानकः स्मृतः । Kṣīrswamī has mentioned Dhn. ni. reading only whenever he states आह च । Śodhala reading.:
'अमिलाते परिम्लानस्तथैवाम्लानको मतः ।
चोरटश्च समाख्यातो वर्णपुष्पस्तथैव च ॥ Soḍhal p.70. Possibly the MSS in front of Kṣīraswamī & Śoḍhala might have the similar reading in Gaṇadravyāvali & Paryānāmadrayāvali.

Its numerous pure white fragrant flowers opening in succession makes it very desirable. (Roxb. C.B. ed p. 31).

55.(५४) शतपत्री Śatapatrī

शतपत्री तु सुमना सुशीता शिववल्लभा ॥
सौम्यगन्धा शतदला सुवृत्ता शतपत्रिका ॥ १४८

शतपत्री हिमा तिक्तग कषाया कुष्ठनाशिनी ॥
मुखस्फोटहरा रुच्या सुरभिः पित्तदाहनुत् ॥ १४९

शतपत्री (Śatapatrī), सुमना (Sumanā), सुशीता (Suśītā), शिववल्लभा (Śivavallabhā), सौम्यगन्धा (Saumyagandhā), शतदला (Śatadalā), सुवृत्ता (Suvṛttā), and शतपत्रिका (Śatapatrikā) are synonyms.

Śatapatrī is bitter and *kaṣāya* in taste, and *śitavīrya*. It is useful in skin disorders, mouth ulcers, is fragrant and pacifies the burning sensation due to *pittadoṣa*.

Fam. Compositae; Asteraceae

I- A-a- ***Chrysanthemum coronarium*** Linn.
Eng. Chrysanthemum.

b- Kamat. c-IV 1 below

B-a- ***Chrysanthemum indicum*** Linn.
Eng. The common garden chrysanthemum of India.

b- Desai C-See IV 2 below.

II A-B-a शतपत्री (Śatapatrī), सुमना(Sumanā), शिववल्लभा (Śivavallabhā),सौम्यगन्धा (Saumyagandhā), सुवृत्ता (Suvṛttā), कुष्ठनाशिनी (Kuṣṭhanāśinī), रुच्या (Rucyā), सुरभिः (Surabhiḥ), तिक्तग (Tiktā).

b- Sans. Shevantikā, chandramallikā; H. Gulchini, Gul-dāudi; Assam. Pitna garkah; Punjab-zanil, Bagaur; Bom. seoti; Mar. Tursiphal, Sevati; Tam. Shemantip -pu; Tel. chemanti; B. Guldāudī. Pers. Gul.-Daudi. Gulchini is also applied to *Plumeria acutifolia* Poir (Fam. Apocynaceae) (Watt. Dict. II-272)

Note- *Plumeria acutifolia* Poir. is Khad-chāphā., Khairchāphā of Bombay and Marathi.
See note on *Matricaria bauna* in IV-1 below.

IV-B-b- H. Guldāudi; Bom. Sevati, Akur Kura; Mar. Sevanti; Tam.

Akkarkartam; Tel. Chemanti (Watt. Dict. II-272).

IV- I- *Chrysanthemum coronarium* Linn.

Chrysanthemum

Habitat- A native of Mediterranean region, only known in India under cultivation as an ornamental garden plant ...several varieties some large other small flowers and white yellow or orange coloured. Two of the coarser forms seem almost naturalised in India.

Medicine : The flowers are stated by Dalzell & Gibson to form a substitute for chamomile for medicinal purpose.

Sacred uses: The beautiful yellow fragrant flowers of this plant are made into garlands and are offered at the shrines of Viṣṇu and Śiva." (Watt. II-272.273)

2) *C. indicum* Linn.

The common garden chrysanthemum.

Habitat : Commonly cultivated in Indian gardens and are in part only known in garden state. (Watt. II.272-73)

Note - 1) Chamomile

Matricaria chamomilla Linn.

German chamomile or Persian Chamomile, the true medicinal chamomile being *Anthemis nobilis* Linn. (Watt. Dict. I. 264)

H. Bābunhā

Habitat : A much branched herb found in the upper ganegtic plain and distributed to Northern Asia and Westwards to Atlantic. *Medicine* ..... (Watt. Dict. 1 V. 103.4)

बाबुन्हा Bābunhā

Matricaria chamomilla (Desai)

Punjab, Northern tract of Gangetic valley and Iran. Flowers yellow, similar to शेवन्ती Śevantī, śatapatrī but small. Medicinal substances similar to those of शतपत्री Śatapatrī.

Note -2

But in Konkan a plant namely सुरपिण *Surapiṇa* which may be सुरपर्ण Suraparṇa of Raj.ni. and identified as *Artemisia vulgaris* Linn. by Dr. Desai is used for the same purpose mentioned for शतपत्री (Śatapatrī). It is usually planted with Tulasi (*Ocimum sanctum* Linn.)

3) शतपत्री (Śatapatrī) Mar. शेवन्ती (Śevantī) Kan. शेवन्तिगे (Śevantige) (Ashubodh Raj. ni.)

V- 1) शतपत्री (Śatapatrī), तरुणी (Taruṇī)
Rosa centifolia Linn.
Whether the name तरुणी (Taruṇī) is for Gulaba or any other plant is doubtful. (Chunekar Bh. Pr. p. 488)

2) *Rosa centifolia* Linn.
Habitat : A native or Caucasus assyria, cultivated in India. This with *R. damascene* and *R. gallica* constitute the group of cultivated roses known as the *Galliceae.* The group is most likely confused with Caninae the species of which are *R. indica* and *R. microphylla.* (p. 560)
N.O. Rosaceae comprising about thirty distinct species, nine species occuring as wild in India. (Watt. Dict. VI-I-P.554-60)

56. (५५) अतिमुक्तकः *Atimuktakaḥ

अतिमुक्तः कार्मुकश्च मण्डनो भ्रमरोत्सवः ॥ १५४
अविमुक्तो माधवी च सुवसन्तः पराश्रयः ॥
अतिमुक्तः सुगन्धि स्यात् हृद्यमुक्तं सुमण्डनम् ॥ १५५

अतिमुक्तः (Atimuktaḥ), कार्मुकः (Kārmukaḥ), मण्डनः (Maṇḍanaḥ), भ्रमरोत्सवः (Bhramarotsavaḥ), अविमुक्तः (Avimuktaḥ), माधवी (Mādhavī), सुवसन्तः (Suvasantaḥ), and पराश्रयः (Parāśrayaḥ) are synonymous.

Atimukta is fragrant, cordial and having handsome appearance.

Fam. Malpighiaceae

I- a- ***Hiptage benghalensis*** Kurz **
Syn. *H. madablota* Gaertn. (Chopra)
b- Asiat. Res. 4.282

II- a- अतिमुक्तः (Atimuktaḥ), कार्मुकः (Kārmukaḥ), मण्डनः (Maṇḍanaḥ), भ्रमरोत्सवः (Bhramarotsavaḥ), माधवी (Mādhavī), सुवसन्तः (Suvasantaḥ), पराश्रयः (Parāśrayaḥ).

---

* Kṣīraswāmī (Amara. 2.4. 72 P. 66) while commenting on अतिमुक्त (Atimukta) mentions the reading "अतिमुक्तो माधवी च सुवसन्तो वनाश्रयः ।
अतिमुक्तः कामुकश्च मण्डको भ्रमरोत्सवः ॥ This can be compared with sodhal's
अतिमुक्तः माधवी च सुवसन्तः पराश्रयः ।
अविमुक्तः कार्मुकश्च मंडनो भ्रमरोत्सवः ॥ Sodhal P. 70

* *The current acceptped name is *Hiptage benghalensis* (Linn.) Kurz

b- *Atimukta* Asi. Res.
B. Mudhuva luta (Roxb.); H. Mādhavī; B. Mādhavī latā;
Mar. Madhu mālatī, Haladavel.
Eng. Clustered Hiptage. (Chunekar Bh. Pr. 497)
Tel. Vadalayerala; Tam. Adigum. vasandī (Chopra)
B. Madhublahata, Basanti; Mar. Haladavel., Sing, Atimuktamu.
(Watt. Dict.)

III-a-1) See IV 1 below.
b-1) अतिमुक्तः पुण्ड्रकः स्याद्वासन्ती माधवी लता । Amara.
अतिक्रान्तो मुक्तान्विरक्तानतिमुक्तः । पुण्ड्रदेशे भवः पुण्ड्रकः । मण्डकोऽयमिति निघण्टुश्च । मधो वसन्ते भवा माधवी ।
(Kṡīraswāmī - Amar 2.4.72 p. 66)

IV- 1 अतिमुक्तकः Atimuktakaḥ.
Hiptage benghalensis Kurz
Syn. माधवी
S.S.Sū. 45. 120; ci. 31.5.etc.
A.H.U. 13.90 (Balvantji p. 11)
2 See Chunekar Bh. Pr. Ni. p. 497.
3) *Hiptage madablota* Gaertn.
A common climbing shrub with beautiful and fragrant flowers found in the hotter parts of India, Burma and Ceylon.
(Watt. Dict. IV-252)
Flowers uncommonly beautiful and exceedingly fragrant.
(Roxb. Fl. Indi. CBC P. 366)
The stems of this climber are yellow inside like दारुहरिद्रा Dāruharidrā (*Berberis aristata* DC) hence the Marathi name हळदवेल Haḷadvel i.e. the colour of the wood is like Haridrā (*Curcuma longa* Linn).

57. (५६) बकुलः Bakulah

बकुलः सीधुगन्धश्च मद्यगन्धो विशारदः ॥ १५१
मधुगन्धो गूढपुष्पो शीर्षकेसरकस्तथा ॥ *

"मधुरं च कषायं च स्निग्धं संग्राहि बाकुलम् ॥
स्थिरीकरं च दन्तानां विशदं तत्फलं गुरु ॥१५२ S.S.Sū. 46. 169.

---

* 'बकुलोदभवपुष्पं च सुपक्वं च सुगन्धि च ।' इत्यधिकः पाठः आनन्दाश्रमपुस्तके दृश्यते । पुष्पवर्गान्तर्गतभूतत्वात् । 'मधुरं च कषायं च ..' इत्यादयः बाकुलफल गुणकर्माणि इत्यवधेयम् । शिम्बी केसरकस्तथा । 'इति क्षीरस्वामी संमतः पाठः । अमरः 2.4. 65. P. 65

बकुलः (Bakulaḥ), सीधुगन्धः (Sīdhugandhaḥ), मद्यगन्धः (Madyagandhaḥ), विशारदः (Viśāradaḥ), मधुगन्धः (Madhugandhaḥ), गूढपुष्पः (Gūḍhapuṣpaḥ), and शीर्षकेसरकः (Śīrṣakesarakaḥ) are synonymous.

(The fruit of) *Bakula* is sweet and *kaṣāya* in taste. It is unctuous (*snigdha*), astringent in action, nonslimy (clearing) and provides stability of teeth.

Fam. Sapotaceae.

I- a- ***Mimusops elengi*** Linn.

b- Asi. Res. IV P. 278 (Roxb.CBC 318)

c- See below IV-2

II- a- बकुलः (Bakulaḥ), सीधुगन्धः (Śīdhugandhaḥ), गूढपुष्पः (Gūḍhapuṣpaḥ), Dhn.ni; मधुपुष्पः (Madhupuṣpaḥ), शारदिकः (Śāradikaḥ), मद्यामोदः (Madyāmodaḥ), स्थिरकुसुमः (Sthirakusumaḥ),

b- Sans. Bakula; H.& B. Bakul; P. Moulsari; Malya. Bakulam; Tam. Magilam; Tel. Vakilamu; Bom. Bolsari maram; Tel. Pagada, Pagadamau; Kan. Boklu, Pogada. (Watt. Dict.)

III-a-1) See IV-1) below

1) बकुलः Bakulaḥ

IV- *Mimusops elengi* Linn.
बोलसरि Bolsari and मौलसिरी Maulasiri (H.)
C.S.Vi. 7.22, 8.150 etc.
S.S.Su. 6.28., 42.18 etc. (Balvantji p. 267)

2) A large evergreen tree, frequently cultivated in India, wild in the Deccan and Malaya Peninsula. (Watt. Dict. V. 259)

58. (५७) किंकिरातः Kinkirātaḥ

किङ्किरातः किङ्किराटः पीतकः पीतभद्रकः ॥ १५३
हेमगौरो विप्रलम्भी षट्पदानन्दवर्धनः ॥

किंकिरातोद्भवं पुष्पं सुगन्धि हर्षपुष्टिदम् ॥ १५४

(सुरङ्गी च भवेदुष्णा तित्तग कफविनाशिनी ।
अर्शसां निचयं हन्ति शोफसंघातनाशिनी ॥) *

किङ्किरातः (Kimkirātaḥ), किङ्किराटः (Kimkirāṭaḥ), पीतकः (Pītakaḥ), पीतभद्रकः (Pītabhadrakaḥ), हेमगौरः (Hemagauraḥ), विप्रलम्भी

---

* कोष्ठकान्तर्गतः पाठः आनन्दाश्रम मुद्रित पुस्तके दृश्यते

(Vipralambhī), षट्पदानन्दवर्धनः (Ṣaṭpadānandavardhanaḥ).

The flowers of *Kimkirāta* is fragrant, producing joy and is nourishing.

(*Surangī* is bitter in taste, *uṣṇavīrya* and pacifies *kaphadoṣa*. It is useful in piles and oedema.).

Fam. Guttiferae.clusiaceae

I- a- ***Ochrocarpus longifolius*** Benth. & Hook f. *
Syn. *Calophyllum longifolium* Wall.

b- Kamat - C-See-IV-2 below.

II- a- किंकिरातः (Kinkirātaḥ), मधुपुष्पः (Madhupuṣpaḥ), हेमगौरः (Hemagauraḥ), विप्रलम्भी (Vipralambhī), सुरङ्गी (Surangī).

Note - Raj. ni's text of this name is not recorded under this heading and also is not in परिशिष्ट (Pariśiṣṭa)

b- H & B Nāgakesar; Bom. Surangi; Kan. Surangi; Maly. Surampunna; Tam. Surabunnai (Chopra)
Mal.Sātvin, Surangi,Hadakaya (Birdwood) **
H. Nāgakesara Kiphul; Bom. Tāmbaḍā nāgakesar, Surangi; Mar. Surangi, Rānundi; Tam. Nagap.-pu; Nagkesarpu (Flowers) Nagashap-pu; Tel. Suraponna; Kan. wanai, laringi (male), pune (female) Suringi, Gardundi; Sans. -Nāgakesaram-puspam.
(Watt. Dict. V-439).

IV- 1 पुन्नाग Punnāga
S.S. Su. 6.24; 38.24, 45 etc.
A.H. Su. 15. 37, 43
Calophylm inophyllum Linn.and *Ochrocarpus longifolius* Benth & Hook. f., the south Indian plants belonging to the Nāgakeśara family (*Mesua ferrea*) may be called *Punnāga* and *Surapunnāga* respectively. Their flowerbuds are at present being used in place of real Nāgakeśara.

---

* The current accepted name is *Mammea suriga* (Ham. ex. Roxb.) Kosterm.

** Local names given by Birdwood do not seem to be reliable (S.D.Kamat.)

* I think the inferance drawn by Late Vd. D.K. Kamat is based on the synonym सुरङ्गी Surangī. This is found only in Anandasram edi.(आनन्दाश्रमपुस्तके) Neither Raj. ni. nor Sodhal mentions Surangī the name of *Surangī* as a synonym of किंकिरात Kinkirāta. The Anandasram edition was only available to him. The Chaukhamba editions (2) Raj. nighantu (By Dr. Indradeva Tripathi) and Śodhal nighantu were published later on. The stanza 'सुरंगी च भवेदुष्णा' etc. seems to be an interpolation by some one where सुरंगी Surangī is very common & famous (Konkan area). सुरंगी Surangī seems to be a corruption of सुरपुन्नाग Surapunnāga which is mentioned by Raj. ni. S. D. Kamat.

See- तुङ्ग Tuṅga (Balvantji p. 187)
तुङ्ग Tuṅga
C.S.Su. 3.25; 4.8,47 etc.
S.S.Ci. 11.9; ka. 8.108
Though *Tuṅga* is a synonym of *Punnāga* it is said to be another name for नारिकेल Nārikela as well.
(Balvantji p. 187)

पुन्नागः पुरुषस्तुङ्गः पाटला पुमान् ।
रक्तपुष्पो रक्तरेणुः (Raj. ni. Dhn. ni. p. 368)
(see Amarakosha p. 57.25.)
Ochrocarpus longifolius Benth. & Hook. f.
A large deciduous tree found in the forest of Western Peninsula from Kanara to Konkan. (Watt. V-440)

2) पुन्नाग (Punnāga)
Calophyllum inophyllum (A.M.P.M.P. page 523 uniyal)

Note- Some modern writers have confused this tree with पुन्नाग (Punnāga) *Calophyllum inophyllum* Linn.by naming it as पुन्नाग Punnāga; but the synonym सुरंगी Suraṅgī makes it clear that पुन्नाग Punnāga and सुरंगी Suraṅgī are two separate plants. In Bombay and also other parts of India the garlands of the flowers of this tree are used by ladies for hair dresing.
See -1) Ni-Adarsha New Ed. pp. 144-15
2) Chunekar Bh. Pr. Ni. 230-232
3) Desai pp. 126,127.

59. (५८). तिलकः

तिलकः पूर्णकः[१] श्रीमान् क्षुरकश्छत्रपुष्पकः[२] ॥ १५९
मुखमण्डनको रेची पुण्ड्रश्चित्रो[३] विशेषकः ॥

तिलकत्वक् कषायोष्णा पुंस्त्वघ्नी दंतरोगजित ॥ १६०

तिलकः (Tilakaḥ), पूर्णकः (Pūrṇakaḥ), श्रीमान (Śrīmān), क्षुरकः (K'surakaḥ), छत्रपुष्पकः (Chatrapuṣpakaḥ), मुखमण्डनकः (Mukhamaṇḍanakaḥ), रेची (Recī), पुण्ड्रः (Puṇḍraḥ), चित्रः (Citraḥ), and विशेषकः (Viśeṣakaḥ) are synonymous.

The bark of *tilaka* is *kaṣāya, uṣṇavīrya,* useful in dental diseases and destroys virility.

---

१ 'पुष्पक.' इति क्वचित् पाठभेदः आनन्दाश्रम पुस्तके । 'पुंड्कः' इति शोढल पाठः ।
२ 'शतपत्रक' इति शोढल पाठः । ३ 'बिन्दु चित्रो' इति शोढल पाठः ।

A controversial plant name, we only note the plant names identified by some modern writers without accepting the identity.

Fam. Rubiaceae

I- A-a- ***Wendlandia exserta*** DC.

b- Thakur Balwantsinghji (Gloss.p. 182)

c- See below IV-2

I- B-a- *Viburnum prunifolium*

b- Priyavrata Sharma

c- See below IV-3

II- A &Ba- तिलकः (Tilakaḥ), श्रीमान् (Śrīmān), क्षुरकः (Kśurakaḥ), छत्रपुष्पकः (Chatrapuṣpakaḥ), मुखमण्डनकः (Mukhamaṇḍanakaḥ), रेची (Recī), पुण्ड्रः(Puṇḍraḥ), Dhn.ni.; स्थिरपुष्पः (Sthirapuṣpaḥ), छिन्नरुहः (Chinnaruhaḥ), दग्धरुहः (Dagadharuhaḥ), मृतजीवी (Mṛtajīvī), वासन्तः (Vāsantaḥ), सुन्दरोभीष्टः(Sundarobhīṣṭaḥ).

A-b- H. Chaulai, Chilka, Tela, Tilki, Tilai; Santal.-Hundro. Picharibah, Nepal- Tilki; Baigas in Mundla.-Tilliah; Pa. Pundhārā, Chilkiā

(Watt. Dict. VI 4. 302)

B-b- भूतनोई (Bhūtnoī), रिसनोई (Risnoī) (Balvantji -Bihar 144, 247) This plant name is not included in Watt. Dict. & Chopra's Glossary.

III-a-1) See IV-1 below.

b-1) तिलकः क्षुरकः ...॥ (Amarah 2.4.40)

तिलाभपुष्पस्तिलकः । क्षुरति परुषत्वात् क्षुरकः ।

(Kśiraswāmī -2.4.40 P.60)

2) 30 श्रीमान् तिलकः । 'वासन्तः सुन्दरः श्रीमानिति धर्मिष्टः । (Harshe)

III-a- 3) 42 Tilwaka - S.Br. XIII -8.1.16

4 स्राक्त्य Srāktya -Commentators say that srāktya or srākti is the Tilaka tree A.V. IV.40 (Karambelkar p. 101)

IV- 1) तिलकः Tilaka

Wendlandia exserta DC.

Tilaka तिलक H., *Huṇḍra* हुण्ड्र Bihar

Syn. पुण्ड्र

C.S.Ci. 30.72 (Va)

S.S.Ka.6.30 (Va)

A.H.U.38.30

This is one of the दोहदवृक्ष *Dohad vṛksa* of Sanskrit and Hindi poets. It was wrongly identified with Lodhra but decidedly proved* by us.

---

* It was again confirmed that *Tilaka* is *Wendlandia, Tilwaka* is *Viburnum* species and *Lodhra* is *symplocos* (M.D. thesis by R. K. ojha. B.H.U. 1976.)

Discussion on *Puṇḍra*, *Tilvaka* and तिलपर्णी *Tilaparṇī* may be consulted (Balvantji P. 83.84)

Note - Without examining the medicinal * uses noted by Raj. ni. and without finding the results similar to those of Raj. ni. it cannot be accepted as our Nighaṇṭus plant.

2) *Wendlandia exserta* DC.
Syns. *W. sinerea* DC; *Rondeletia exserta* Roxb; *R. sinerea* Wall.
Habitat : A small deciduous tree of the sub Himalayan tract from the Chenab eastwards to Nepal and Sikkim, also found in Oudh, Bengal, ... central and southern India. (Watt. Dict. VI-4-302)

Note - Medicinal uses are not recorded in Watt. Dict. In the Watt Dict. there appears a plant name *W. tinctroia* DC. the regional names of which are the same as *W. exserta* DC. such as Tilai Santal & Kol; *Kuni* - Nepal; *Telli*-oriya. The description of it is recorded there in as "A small elegant tree, with large crowded panicles of *small white* sweet scer.ted flowers terminating the boughs; common in the forests of the tropical Himalayas from Garhwal east wards Assam, Bengal" etc.
Bark is used as a dye and medicine **

The morphological description of *W. tinctoria* DC. noted in Watt Dict. seems more applicable to *Tilaka* of Raj. ni. and it may be accepted as the plant of our Nighaṇṭu.

3) तिलक Tilaka
रघु. ९.४१. ४४, कुमारसं. ३. ३० मालविका., ३.५.४२ अलिभिरञ्जन बिन्दुमनोहरे ... ।
न खलु शोभयति स्म वनस्थली, न तिलकस्तिलकः प्रमदाविव । रघुः ६.४१
सद्यशकान्तिरलक्ष्यत मञ्जरी तिलकजालक जालक मौत्तिर्गभिः । रघु. ६.६४.

4) Th. Balvantsinghaji has identified तिलक *Tilak as Wendlandia exserta* DC.
Tilaka medium sized tree, Sivalik forests, Madyapradesh, Bihar, inflorescens white, beautiful. (Uniyal, Kalidas, S. Ayu. Jan.76)

---

* Medicinal uses mentioned by Raj. ni. are as follows :

तिलको मधुरः स्निग्धो वातपित्तकफापहः ।
बलपुष्टिकरो हृद्यो लघुर्मेदो विवर्धनः ॥
तिलकत्वक् कषायोष्णा पुंस्त्वघ्नी दन्तदोषनुत ।
कृमिशोफ व्रणान् हन्ति रक्तदोषविनाशिनी ॥ Karavīrādi chapter X th

Sodhal (The present available ed.) does not mention the medicinal uses.

** *W. tinctoria* DC. Ben. -Tula -lodh; Oriya - Telli,... etc.
Bark used as a mordant in dying. An application prepared from the bark is used for cramps in cholera patients. (Useful plants of India Page 688)

60. (५९) अशोकः Aśokaḥ

अशोकः शोकनाशश्च विचित्रः कर्णपूरकः ॥ १५६
विशोको रक्तको रागी चित्रः षट्पदमञ्जरी ॥

अशोकः शीतलश्चार्शः कृमीन् हन्ति प्रयोजितः ॥ १५७
अपचीं नाशयत्येव सर्वव्रणविनाशनः ॥

अशोको मधुरो हृद्यः संधानीयः सुगन्धिकः ॥ १५८

अशोकः (Aśokaḥ), शोकनाशः (Śokanāśaḥ), विचित्रः (Vicitraḥ), कर्णपूरकः (Karṇapūrakaḥ), विशोकः (Viśokaḥ), रक्तकः (Raktakaḥ), रागी (Rāgī), चित्रः (Citraḥ), and षट्पदमञ्जरी (Ṣaṭpadamañjarī) are synonymous.

Aśoka is sweet in taste, *śītavīrya,* cordial, useful for union promoting, and fragrant (? flowers). It is used in piles, helminthic infestations, *apacī* (scrofula), and in all types of wounds.

Fam. Leguminosae; Caesalpiniaceae

I- a- ***Saraca indica*** Linn.
Syn. *Jonesia asoka* R.

b- Asiat. Res. 4. 355 (C.B.C. 312)

c- See IV - 2 below

II- a- अशोकः (Aśokaḥ), कर्णपूरकः (Karṇapūrakaḥ), रक्तकः (Raktakaḥ), रागी (Rāgī), Dhn. ni.; वञ्जुलद्रुमः (Vañjuladrumaḥ), कङ्केलिः (Kankeliḥ), स्मराधिवासः (Smarādhivāsaḥ), रामावामाङ्घ्रिघातकः (Ramāvāmāṅghrighātakaḥ) (Raj. ni.)

b- H & B Ashok; Bom. & Mar. Ashok, Asugī ; Jāsundi; Tel. Ashok, kankeli; Kan.- Ashoge, Ashok; Maly. Asok; Tam. Asoka.

IV- 1) अशोक Aśoka
Saraca indica Linn. Syns. गतशोक & वञ्जुल (?)
C.S.Su. 4.47. etc.
S.S. Su. 6.28; 38.13 etc.
A.H. Ci. 3.10 etc. (Balvantji p. 26)
Habitat :Central and Eastern Himalayas, E. Bengal and western Peninsula, (Chopra)

2) A tree *Polyalthia longifolia* Benth. is also called अशोक Aśoka in some parts of India. It is called (Khoṭā Aśoka-pusudo Aśoka) in Mahārāṣṭra . It is not the true Aśoka of Nighaṇṭus.

---

* *S. asoca* (Roxb.) de Wild (*S. indica* auct. non Linn.) is sometimes considered to be the correct name of this plant. (Comp. p. 136)

3) See Ashoka Bapalaji - Contro. plants J.R.I.M. 1970 p. 143 V.1
4) *Polyalthia longifolia* Benth. & Hook. f.
   खोटा अशोक Khoṭā Aśoka
   Bapalaji J.R.I.M. Vol. 1.1970
5) *Polyalthia longifolia* Benth. & Hook. f.*
   H. Devdar; Bom. - Asok; Kan. Putranjivi; M. Nallilingam; Mal. Ashokam; Tam. Asagam; Tel. Asokamu.(Chopra Handa 1958 P. 520).
6) अशोक Aśoka Two kinds असली Asali (i.e.true) and कमअसली Kamasalī (i.e.false) (V. Chandro. Part p. 94)
7) अशोक *Aśoka*
   Two kinds रक्त Rakta and पीत Pīta. *Saraca indica* Linn. रक्त Rakta
   P. longifolia Benth. & Hook. f.
   Two tree species are found under the name of अशोक Aśoka. One is known as रक्त अशोक Rakta Aśoka, सीतेचा अशोक Aśoka (Wife of Dasharathi Rāma described in Wālmikī Rāmayaṇa). Bengali Aśoka, आसुगी (Āsugī) and is identified by scientiests as *saraca indica* Linn. It is the drug of Indian Materia Medica. While the next Aśoka tree known as देशी अशोक (Deśi Aśoka) (Khoṭā Aśoka-Maraṭhi) i.e.false Aśoka is identified as *Polyalthia longfolia* Benth. & Hook.Flowers of *S. indica* Linn. are redish white those of *P. longifolia* are yellowish. Following books may be referred.

1) Chunekar, Bha. Pr. P. 500)
2) Bapalaji vaidya, Ni. Adarsha Purvardah 484-85
3) Vano. chandrodaya Part 1 p. 84
4) Chopra Handa p. 401
5) S. Ayurveda. April 1970

०१. (६०) किंशुकः Kimśukaḥ

किंशुको वातपोथश्च रक्तपुष्पोऽथ याज्ञिकः ॥
त्रिपर्णो रक्तपुष्पश्च पूतद्रुर्ब्रह्मवृक्षकः ॥ १५९

क्षारश्रेष्ठः पलाशश्च बीजस्नेहः समिद्वरः ॥
* (त्रिवृन्तास्यो ब्रह्मवृक्षः खरपर्णः त्रिपर्णकः ॥

( )कोष्ठकान्तर्गतः पाठः नि.शे. टीकासंमतः ।
* The current accepted name for this plant is *Polyalthia longifolia* (Sonn) Thw. (Comp. p. 122)

क्षारश्रेष्ठः कृमिघ्नश्च संग्राही दीपनः सरः ॥ ।१६०
प्लीहगुल्मग्रहण्यर्शो वातश्लेष्मविनाशनः ॥

किंशुकस्यापि कुसुमं सुगंधि मधुरं च यत् ॥
बीजं तु कटुकं स्निग्धमुष्णं कृमिबलासजित् ॥ १६१

किंशुकः (Kimśukaḥ), वातपोथः (Vātapothaḥ), रक्तपुष्पः (Raktapuṣpaḥ), याज्ञिकः (Yājñikaḥ), त्रिपर्णः (Triparṇaḥ), रक्तपुष्पः (Raktapuṣpaḥ), पूतद्रुः (Pūtadruḥ), ब्रह्मवृक्षकः (Brahmavṛkśakaḥ), क्षारश्रेष्ठः (Kśārasreṣṭhaḥ), पलाशः (Palāśaḥ), बीजस्नेहः (Bījasnehaḥ), समिद्वरः (Samidvaraḥ), [त्रिवृन्तास्यः (Trivṛntāsyaḥ), ब्रह्मवृक्षः (Brahmavṛkśaḥ), खरपर्णः (Kharaparṇaḥ), त्रिपर्णकः (Triparṇakaḥ)] are synonymous.

Palāśa is anthelmintic, astringent, stimulates digestive capacity, *sara*, and pacifies *vāta kapha doṣas*. It is useful in disorders of spleen, tumours, diseases of *Grahaṇī* (characterised by chronic diarrhoea), and piles.

Its flowers are fragrant and sweet and the seeds are pungent in taste *uṣṇavīrya*, pacify *kapha doṣa* and are anthelmintic.

Under this heading the compiler of Dhn. ni. has recorded one plant name A किंशुको रक्तपुष्पकः (Kimśuko Raktapuṣpakaḥ) but Raj. ni. records रक्तः (Raktaḥ), पीतः (Pītaḥ), सितः (Sitaḥ), and नीलः (Nīlaḥ). As a medicinal plant he prefers 'B' सितः (Sitaḥ i.e. white flowered *kimśuka*) which we have recorded herebelow.

Fam. Leguminosae

I- A-a- ***Butea monosperma*** (Lam.) Kuntze *
Syn. *B. frondosa* Koen. ex. Roxb. (Chopra)
B. frondosa Roxb,
Butter gum, Bengali Kino; sometimes called the Bastard Teak. (Watt. I.548)

b- Roxburgh (fl. indi. CBC 540)

c- IV-2 below

B-a- ***Butea parviflora*** Roxb.

b- Kamat C-See IV-43 below.

II- A-a- किंशुकः (Kimśukaḥ), वातपोथः (Vātapothaḥ), रक्तपुष्पः (Raktapuṣpaḥ), याज्ञिकः (Yājñikaḥ), त्रिपर्णः (Triparṇaḥ), वक्रपुष्पः (Vakrapuṣpaḥ), ब्रह्मवृक्षकः (Brahmavṛkśakaḥ), क्षारश्रेष्ठः (Kśārasreṣṭhaḥ), पलाशः (Palāśaḥ).

---

* The current accepted name *Butea monosperma* (Lam.) Taub.

b- H. Ḍhāk, Palās, Kankrel; Mar. Kākrachā Jhāḍ, Paḷasāce Jhād; Tam.Palāsham, Parasan, Parasa, Purasha; Tel. Palās, Marag, mardulu. Palashmu, Kimshukamu; Kan. Matuga, Thorda, Mattuga gida; Sans. Kimśhuka, Palasha; Mal. Marukka maram;. Plach-cha.

B-a- (Sito Vijñyānadaḥ), सितो विज्ञानदः

b- * Plant name is not recorded in Watt. Dict. and Chopra. Roxburgh has not recorded modern names (local names) of this plant species. (B. parviflora R.)

III-a- 1) See IV 1 below.

2) तलाशवृक्षाणामिवहं भूयासमुत्तमः । (AV VI. 2-3)

b- 1) पलाशः किंशुकः ।(Amaraḥ 2.4.30)

... प्रशस्तानि पलाशानि सन्त्यस्य पलाशः, पलमश्नुते रक्तपुष्पत्वाद् वा किंचिच्छुको नीलः किंशुकः । वातं पोथयति वातपोथः ।

(Kśīraswāmī, Amaraḥ 2.4.29)

2) श्वेतपलाश पंचांगं चूर्णितं मधुना सह । (Rasaratnakar, Amarah 2.4.29)

3) अन्ये योगाः ...ब्रम्स्वृक्षस्य ये गुणाः तथैव श्वेत पलाशे भवेयुः साधकस्य वै ।

(Rasaratnakar, Rasāyan khaṇda)

IV- 1) पलाश Palāsa.

Butea monosperma (Lam.) Kuntze.
H. Palās पलास Ṭesū टेसू and Ḍhāk - ढाक
Synonyms किंशुक & वातपोथ
C.S.Su. 2.12; 3.15 etc.
S.S.Su. 2.3.11.11 etc.
A.H.Su. 15.19; 26 32 38 etc. (Balvantji p. 241)

2) *Butea frondosa* Roxb.
Habitat : A moderate sized deciduous tree, found throughout India, extending to North west Himalaya as far as the Jhelum... most beautiful tree of the plains and lower hills of India ... comparatively neglected. *Gum.:* known as 'Kamarkas' in the Bazars of the Northwest Provinces, The gum 'Bengal kino', 'Khakar gond' in Bombay , *chinya gond, kinya-gond* Madras ... largely used in native medicine as substitute for *true kino.* chemical composition etc. (Watt. Dict. vol. I)

3) *Butea parviflora* Roxb.
Copious panicles of small white flowers. In other respects simi-

* *B. parviflora* Roxb. Syn. *Spatholobus roxburghii* Benth, some record is available (UPI)
* Very rarely a Palāsa tree having yellow coloured flowers पीतकुसुम is also said to be present in Karjat (Dist Raigad Maharastra) and certain forests in Madhya Pradesh. (S.D. Kamat)

lar to *Butea superba* Roxb. Fl. Indi. CBC. P. 549)

Plant names of other किंशुक (Kiṁśuka) species noted by Raj. ni. and others are as noted herebelow but the identity of them is doubtful.

1) रक्त -Rakta This is I-a-A of Dhn. ni. recorded above.

2) नील - Nīla (may be called कृष्ण kṛṣṇa i.e. black.
Ougeinia dalbergioides Benth.
Sans. -Tinisa; Mar. & C.P. Kāḷā Paḷas, Tivas (Nadkarni and Watt. Dict. V. 656)

3) कण्टकी पलाश Kaṇṭakī Palāsa
Erythrina indica Lam.
Sans & Beng. Palit mandāra H. Pāṅgārā.

आम्रादिरयमुद्दिष्टो वर्गःश्रेष्ठस्तु पञ्चमः ।
हर्षणो गन्धसौरभ्य फलत्वक् पुष्पसंश्रयः ॥

Thus the Āmrādi fifth and the most improtant chapter has been told. Here the plants having fruits with pleasing odour, barks of क्षीरीवृक्ष, (latex or sap containing plants) and flowers having fragrance are mentioned.

वर्गेतराणि Vargetarani

१ केतकीद्वयम् Ketakīdwayam.

केतकी सूचिकापुष्पो जम्बूकः क्रकचच्छदः ।
सुवर्णकेतकी चान्या लघुपुष्पा सुगन्धिनी ॥

केतकी कटुका पाके लघु तिक्तग कफापहा ।

केतकी (Ketakī), सूचिकापुष्पः (Sūcikāpuṣpaḥ), जम्बूकः (Jambūkaḥ), क्रकचच्छदः (Krakacacchadaḥ), are synonymous. The another type is called as सुवर्णकेतकी (Suvarṇa ketakī) of which synonyms are लघुपुष्पा (Laghupuṣpā) and सुगन्धिनी (Sugandhinī)

Ketakī is bitter and pungent in taste and in *vipāka,* and is *laghu.* It pacifies *kaphadoṣa.*

(Plant names which are not included in this chapter are recorded by the Editor Purandare see introduction by the Editor p.3)

Under the heading two plant names are included (A) केतकी Ketakī & (B) सुवर्णकेतकी Suvarṇa Ketakī,

II- A-a- केतकी (Ketakī), सूचिकापुष्पः (Sūcikāpuṣpah), क्रकचच्छदः (Krakacachadaḥ), Dhn. ni.; कण्टकदला (Kaṇṭakadalā), शिवद्विष्टा (Shivadwiṣṭā) दलपुष्पा (Dalapuṣpā), इन्दुकलिका (Indukalikā). Raj. ni.

B- सुवर्णकेतकी(Suvarṇa ketaī)तीक्ष्णपुष्पा (Tīk'sṇapuṣpā) कनकप्रसवा (Kanakaprasavā), हैमी (Haimī) छिन्नरुहा (Chinnaruhā)

I- A & B-a

Pandanus tectorius Soland. ex Park.
Syn. *P. odoratissimus* Roxb.
P. fascicularis Lam.
Syn. *P. odoratissimus* (Willd) Roxb.

b- Roxburgh Fl. indi. CBC 707
In Konkan two kinds or varieties are found; one is shrub like plant which grows on river banks, or near sweet water courses (nearly an aquatic), spadix golden yellow, & fragrant. It is called locally as सोन केवडा (Sonkewaḍā) or सोन केतकी (Sonketakī) while the next variety grows near seashsore and grows about 30 feet high, spadix white, odourless and is not used as a fragrant flower. This plant is called as केंडा (Keṇḍā) केवड (Kevaḍa) or पांढरा केवट (Pāṇdharā kevaṭa).

2. गणेरुका Gaṇerukā

गणेरुका कर्णिकारः कर्णिश्च गणिकारिका ।
गणेरुः शोधनी शोफश्लेष्मास्रव्रणकुष्ठजित् ॥

गणेरुका (Gaṇerukā), कर्णिकारः (Karṇikāraḥ), कर्णिः (Karṇiḥ), गणिकारिका (Gaṇikārikā), are synonymous.

Gaṇeru is purificatory and pacifies *kaphadoṣa.* It is useful in bleeding disorders, wounds and disroders of skin.

Plant name is not found recorded and identified in modern books. *

3 सागः (शाकः) Sāgaḥ (Śākaḥ)

सागः करच्छदो[१] भूमिसहो दीर्घच्छदो मतः ।
सागः श्लेष्मानिलास्रघ्नो गर्भसंधानदो हिमः ॥

* In chapter 1 on page 65 It has been suggested to be *Pavetta indica* Linn. following the opinion of Pdt. Bhagirath. S.D. Kamat.

१ 'खरच्छदः' इति साधु पाठः ।

सागः (Sāgaḥ), करच्छदः (Karacchadaḥ), भूमिसहः (Bhūmisahaḥ), and दीर्घच्छदः (Dīrghacchadaḥ) are synonymous.

Sāga pacifies *kapha -vāta* and *rakta doṣas*. It is *śitavīrya* and useful for maintainence of pregnancy.

Fam. Verbenaceae.

Tectona grandis Linn.

शाकः (Śākaḥ), क्रकचपत्रः (Krakacapatraḥ), दीर्घपत्रः (Dīrghapatraḥ), श्रेष्ठकाष्ठः (Śreṣṭhakāṣṭhaḥ), गृहद्रुमः (Gṛhadrumaḥ).

4. धवः Dhavaḥ

धवः नन्दितरुर्गौरी शकटाक्षो धुरन्धुरी ।
धवः शीतः प्रमेहार्शः पाण्डुपित्तकफापहः ॥

धवः (Dhavaḥ), नन्दितरुः (Nanditaruḥ), गौरी (Gaurī), शकटाक्षः (Śakaṭākśaḥ), धुरन्धुरी (Dhurandhurī) are synonymous.

Dhava is *śītavīrya* and useful in diseases characterised by polyuria (including diabetes) and piles, it pacifies *pitta* and *kaphadoṣas* and useful in anaemia

---

Fami. Combretaceae

Anogeissus latifolia Wall.

नन्दितरुर्गौरी (Nanditarurgaurī), शकटाक्षः (Śakaṭākśaḥ), धुरन्धुरी (Dhurandhurī), शुक्लवृक्षः (Śuklavṛkśaḥ), धवलः (Dhavalaḥ)

इति आम्रादिः पञ्चमो वर्गः ।

Thus ends the Āmrādi Chapter Fifth.

अथ सुवर्णादिः षष्ठो वर्गः
SUVARṆADIḤ CHAPTER VI
१ सुवर्णम् Suvarṇam (Gold)

सुवर्णं कनकं रुक्मं शातकुम्भं च काञ्चनम् ।
जाम्बूनदं जातरूपं हिरण्यं हेम हाटकम् ॥ १

चामीकरं चारुरत्नं तपनीयं च पीतकम् ।
श्रीकेतनं भूषणार्हं चारुरूपं च तत्स्मृतम् ॥२

वीर्यं विधत्ते हरते च रोगान्करोति सौख्यं प्रबलेन्द्रियत्वम् ।
शुक्रस्य शुद्धिं बलवर्णवीर्यमोजश्च पुष्टिं प्रददाति हेम ॥ ३

"बलं च वीर्यं हरते नराणां रोगव्रजान् पोषयतीह काये ।
असौख्यदं तच्च सदैवमेवं रुक्मं सदोषं मरणं करोति ॥ ४

(Rasa R. Samu. 5.20)

सुवर्णम् (Suvarṇam), कनकं (Kanakam), रुक्मं (Rukmam), शातकुम्भं (Śātakumbham), काञ्चनम् (Kāñcanam), जाम्बूनदं (Jāmbūnadam), जातरूपं (Jātarūpam), हिरण्यं (Hiraṇyam), हेम (Hema), हाटकम् (Hāṭakam), चामीकरं (Cāmīkaram), चारुरत्नं (Cāruratnam), तपनीयं (Tapanīyam), पीतकम् (Pītakam), श्रीकेतनं (Śrīketanam), भूषणार्हं (Bhūṣaṇārham), चारुरूपं (Cārurūpam) are synonymous.

Gold increases energy, and is useful in various diseases of the body, gives happiness, increases the power of organs of perception, has purificatory action of *'sukra,* increases strength, complexion, energy, *oja* and nourishment of the body.

Impure gold decreases energy and strength of the body causes various diseases, unhappiness and even death.

2 रौप्यम् Raupyam (Silver)

रौप्यं सौधं सितं तारं रजतं तप्तरूपकम् ।
शुभ्रं कुप्यं वसुश्रेष्ठं रुचिरं श्वेतकं मतम् ॥ ५

चन्द्रहासं चन्द्रवपुश्चन्द्रभूति महावसु ।
वाक्यलं श्रेष्ठमिच्छन्ति रश्मिजालं तथाऽपरम् ॥ ६

तारं च तारयति रोगसमुद्रपारं देहस्य सौख्यकरणं पलितं वलिं च ।
वर्ण्यं विषघ्नममलं हरति प्रसह्य वृष्यं पुनर्नवकरं कुरुते चिरायुः ॥ ७

अपक्वतारं प्रकरोति तापं विड्बन्धनं यच्छति शुक्रनाशम् ।
अपाटवं वीर्यबलग्रहाणि महान् गदान् पोषयति प्रसिद्धम्॥ ८

रौप्यं (Raupyam), सौधं (Saudham), सितं (Sitam), तारं (Tāram), रजतं (Rajatam), तप्तरूपकम् (Taptarūpakam), शुभ्रं (Śubhram), कुप्यं (Kupyam), वसुश्रेष्ठं (Vasuśreṣtham), रुचिरं (Ruciram), श्वेतकं (Śvetakam), चन्द्रहासं (Candrahāsam), चन्द्रवपुः (Candravapuḥ), चन्द्रभूतिः (Candrabhūtiḥ), महावसु (Mahāvasu), वाक्यलं (Vākyalam), रश्मिजालं (Raśmijālam) are synonymous.

Silver removes various diseases of the body, causes happiness, removes (untimely) graying of hair and wrinkles of the body. It improves complexion and is antipoisonous. It is *vṛsya, rasāyana* (rejuvenating) and increases longevity.

Impure and unprocessed silver produces burning sensation in the body, causes constipation, reduces *śukra,* causes laziness, diminishes energy and strength and gives rise to serious diseases.

3 ताम्रम् Tāmram (Copper)

ताम्रं म्लेच्छमुखं शुल्बं रक्तकं रक्तधातुकम् ।
उदुम्बरं त्र्यम्बकं च विद्यात् त्वाष्ट्रञ्च नामतः ॥ ९

गुल्मं च कुष्ठं च गुदामयं च शूलानि शोफोदरपाण्डुरोगान् ।
उत्क्लेदभेदभ्रममोहदाहान् निहन्ति सम्यङ्मृतमेव शुल्बम् ॥१०

शुल्बं तनौ नयति शेषमशेष धातून्
रोगान् करोति विविधांश्च निहन्ति कान्तिम् ।
कुष्ठं रुजं च विषमं कुरुते विशेषात्
पाकेन हीनमिह वान्तिविरेककारि ॥ ११

हन्त्यायुरुच्चैः कुरुतेऽतितापं मूर्च्छां विधत्ते हरते च शुक्रम् ।
नाना गदानां च सहायकर्ताऽशुद्धश्च शुल्बोऽत्र च जीवहर्ता ॥१२

ताम्रं (Tāmram), म्लेच्छमुखं (Mlecchamukham), शुल्बं (Śulbam), रक्तकं (Raktakam), रक्तधातुकम् (Raktadhātukam), उदुम्बरं (Udumbaram), त्र्यम्बकं (Tryambakam), त्वाष्ट्रं (Twāṣtram) are synonymous.

Nicely processed and reduced to *bhasma* form of *Tāmra* is useful in tumors (diverticulosis), skin disorders, and diseases like, piles, colics, oedema, ascites, anaemias, nausea, diarrhoea, giddiness, syncope, and burning sensation.

Improperly processed *Tāmrabhasma* reduces all the tissues of the body, causes various diseases, decreases complexion, causes various skin disorders and other obstinate diseases, vomitting and purgation.

Impure - unprocessed *Tāmra* reduces the life span, causes great burning sensation and syncope, reduces *śukradhātu*, helps to produce various diseases and even causes death.

4 त्रपु Trapu (Tin) (वङ्गम् -Vangam)

त्रपु त्रपुकमानीलं रङ्गं वङ्गं च पिच्चटम् ।
गुरुश्रेष्ठं सलवणं सुरटी नीलिका घनम् ॥ १३

त्रपु सतिक्तमुष्णं च रूक्षं श्लेष्मविघातकृत् ।
पित्तप्रकोपशमनं विकारं कृमिजं जयेत् ॥ १४

पाकेन हीनौ खलु नागवङ्गौ दुष्टानि गुल्मानि तथा विकोष्ठम् ।
पाण्डुप्रमेहापचिवातशोफ भगन्दरश्वित्रकिलासकुष्ठम् ॥ १५

मेहाश्मरीविद्रधिमुख्यरोगानतीव नित्यं कुरुते बलादौ ।
विषोपमौ रक्तविकारवृन्दं क्षयं च कृच्छ्राणि कफज्वरं च ॥ १६

त्रपु (Trapu), त्रपुकम् (Trapukam), आनीलं (Ānīlam), रङ्गम् (Rangam), वङ्गम् (Vangam), पिच्चटम् (Piccaṭam), गुरुश्रेष्ठं (Guruśreṣṭham), सलवणं (Salavaṇam), सुरटी (Suraṭī), नीलिका (Nīlikā), घनम् (Ghanam) are synonymous.

Trapu is bitter in taste, *uṣṇavīrya*, *ruksa* (drying), pacifies *kapha* and *pitta doṣas* and worms.

Improperly processed *Vanga* and *Nāga* (Lead) *bhasmas* cause tumours (diverticulosis), disorders of gastrointestinal tract, anaemia, urinary disorders characterised by polyuria (including diabetes), scrofula, oedema due to *vatadosa*, fistula in ano, leucoderma, white spots and other skindisorders, calculus and abscess. Both of these reduce the strength of the body, serious blood disorders, consumption, dysuria and fever due to *kaphadoṣa*.

5 रीतिका Rītikā (Brass) - Bell metal पित्तलम् - Pittalam

रीतिका काकतुण्डी* च द्विविधं पित्तलं भवेत् ।
रीतिस्तु लोहकः पिङ्गः कपिलोहं सुवर्णकम् ॥ १७

आरं सैंहलकश्चैव निष्ठुरो दारुकण्टकः ।
राजरीतिः स्मृता राज्ञी राजपुत्री महेश्वरी ॥ १८

---

* After heating it should be immersed in kāñjī (vinegar). If it becomes coppery in colour, then it is called *Rītikā* and if by doing so, it becomes black in colour, then it is called *kākatuṇḍikā*.

ब्रह्माणी ब्रह्मरीतिश्च कपिला पिङ्गलाऽपि च ॥ ½

रीतिद्वयं सकलपाण्डुसमीरणघ्नं रूक्षं सरं कृमिहरं लवणं विषघ्नम्।
वृष्यं वलीपलितनाशनमुग्रमायुर्वृद्धिं करोति सहसा च
रसायनाग्र्यम् ॥१९

Bell- metal is of two types A) रीतिका (Rītikā) and B) काकतुण्डी (Kākatuṇḍī), The synonyms for *Rītiḥ* are लोहकः (Lohakaḥ), पिङ्गः (Pingaḥ), कपिलोहम् (Kapiloham), सुवर्णकम् (Suvarṇakam), आरं (Āram), सैंहलकः (Saimhalakaḥ), निष्ठुरः (Nisṭhuraḥ), and दारुकण्टकः (Dārukanṭakaḥ). A different type of *Rītiḥ* is राजरीतिः *Rājarītih*, the synonyms for it are राज्ञी (Rājñī), राजपुत्री (Rājaputrī), महेश्वरी (Maheśvarī), ब्रह्माणी (Brahmāṇī), ब्रह्मरीतिः (Brahmarītih), कपिला (Kapilā) and पिङ्गला (Pingalā).

Both the types of *Rītiḥ* are *rūkṣa* (roughening), mild laxative, salty in taste and are useful in all types of anaemias, *vātadosa,* worms and poisons. These are *vrsya*, reduce wrinkles and gray hair, increase life span and are *rasāyana* (rejuvenating).

6 सीसकम् Sīsakam (Lead)

सीसकं नागमुरगं कृष्णोरगभुजंगमाः ।
यवनेष्टं विशिष्टं च योगीष्टं चीरपिष्टकम् ॥ २०
नागो हि नागसममेव बलं ददाति
व्याधीन् विनाशयति चाऽऽयुरलंकरोति ।
सद्यो विवर्धयति सोऽपि प्रधानधातुं
मृत्युं निवारयति चापि भुजंगराजः॥ २१

नागं (Nāgam), उरगम् (Uragam), कृष्णोरगम् (Kṛṣṇoragam), भुजंगम् (Bhujangam), यवनेष्टं (Yavaneṣṭam), विशिष्टं (Visiṣṭam), योगीष्टं (Yogīṣṭam), चीरपिष्टकम् (Cīrapiṣṭakam)are synonyms for सीसकम् (Sīsakam).

Nāga (lead) bhasma endows a person with great strength (of an elephant), is useful in various disorders, increaases *sukradhātu* and keeps the death away.

7 कांस्यम् Kāmsyam (Eng. Bell metal)

कांस्यं लोहं निजं घोषं प्रकाशं कांस्यकं बलम् ।
घोषपुष्पं च पठितं शब्दैः पर्यायवाचकैः ॥ २२

कांस्यं तिक्तोष्णरूक्षं च लघुलेखि प्रकीर्तितम् ।
अञ्जनादि प्रयुक्तं च दिव्यदृष्टिप्रदायकम् ॥ २३

(अन्यच्च)
निःसंशयं हन्ति समस्तरोगान् घोषं नृणां स्यात् दृढदेहकर्तृ ।
कामस्य वृद्धिं कुरुते बलासं यकृन्निहन्त्याशु बलं करोति ॥ २४

कांस्यम् (Kāmsyam),लोहम् (Loham), निजं (Nijam), घोषं (Ghoṣam), प्रकाशम् (Prakāsam), कांस्यकम् (Kāmsyakam), बलम् (Balam), घोषपुष्पम् (Ghoṣapuṣpam) are synonyms.

Kāmsya is bitter in taste, *usṇavīrya, rūksa* (roughening), *laghu lekhana* (slimming) and by collyrium it is beneficial for good vision.

According to another text - it is useful in all diseases, makes the body strong, increases sexual appetite, is useful in *kaphadoṣa*, disorders of liver and gives strength.

8 लोहम् Loham (Iron)

लोहं शस्त्रं घनं पिण्डं तीक्ष्णं पारशवं मतम् ।
अयः कृष्णायसं वीरं भ्रमरं कृष्णलोहकम् ॥ २४

मुण्डं तीक्ष्णं च कान्तं च त्रिप्रकारमयः स्मृतम् ।
मृदु कण्टं कडारं च त्रिविधं मुण्डमुच्यते ॥ २५

खरसारं च हर्तालं तालं वल्लं च वज्रजम् ।
काललोहाभिधानं च षड्विधं तीक्ष्णमुच्यते ॥ २६

भ्रामरं चुम्बकं चैव रञ्जकालोचके तथा ।
एवं चतुर्विधं कान्तं रोमकान्तं च पञ्चमम् ॥ २७

कषायं शोफशूलार्शः पाण्डुकुष्ठप्रमेहजित् ।
लोहं तिक्तोष्णरूक्षं स्यात् पाण्डुरोगहरं परम् ॥ २८

कफपित्तापहं पुंसां रसायनमनुत्तमम् ॥ ½

(अन्यच्च)
आयुःप्रदाता बलवीर्यकर्ता रोगापहर्ता मदनस्यकर्ता
अयःसमानो नहि कश्चिदन्यो रसायनं श्रेष्ठतमं वदन्ति ॥

दोषाः
दोषकारि गदकारि चाऽऽयसं चेदशुद्धमसंस्कृतं ध्रुवम् ।
पाटवं न तनुते शरीरके दारुणां हृदि रुजं करोति च ॥ २९

लोहम् (Loham), शस्त्रं (Śastram), घनं (Ghanam), पिण्डम् (Piṇḍam), तीक्ष्णं (Tîkshṇam), पारशवं (Pāraśavam), अयः (Ayaḥ), कृष्णायसम् (Kṛṣṇāyasam)

वीरं (Viram), भ्रमरं (Bhramaram), कृष्णलोहकम् (Kṛṣṇalohakam) are synonymous.

It is considered to be of three types (a) मुण्डं (Muṇḍam), (b) तीक्ष्णं (Tīkṣṇam), and (c) कान्तं (Kāntam).

(a) मुण्डं Muṇḍam is of three types (1) मृदु (Mṛdu), (2) कण्टं (Kaṇṭam) and (3) कडारं (kaḍāram).

(b) तीक्ष्ण (Tīkṣṇa) is of six types (1) खरसार (Kharasāra), (2) हर्ताल (Hartāla), (3) ताल (Tāla), (4) वल्ल (Valla) (5) वज्रज (Vajraja), and ` (6) काललोह (Kālaloha).

(c) कान्तलोहं (Kāntaloha) is of 5 types (1) भ्रामर (Bhrāmara), (2) चुम्बक (Cumbaka), (3) रञ्जक (Rañjaka), (4) आलोचकम् (Ālocaka), and (5) रोमकान्त (Romakānta).

Loha is *kaṣāya* (astringent) and bitter in taste, *uṣṇavīrya* and pacifies *kahpa* and *pitta doṣas.* It is useful in oedema, colic, piles, anaemias, disorders of skin and disorders characterized by polyuria (including diabetes). It is a good antianaemic and *rasāyana* (rejuvenating).

According to another text -*Loha* increases span of life, energy, strength, removes many diseases, improves virility and a good *rasāyana* (rejuvenating).

Impure and unprocessed *Loha* aggravates, the *doṣas,* causes various diseases, *apāṭava* (unsharp reactions to external stimuli due to lack of energy), laziness and epigastric (precordial) pain.

वर्तलोहम् Vartaloham (1)

वर्तलोहं वट्टलोहं वर्तकं लोहमेव च ।
वर्तुलोहं च विख्यातं पञ्चलोहं च नीलिका ॥ ३०

वर्तलोहं हिमं विद्यादम्लं कटुकमेव च
रूक्षं कफविकारघ्नं हन्यात्पित्तोद्भवां रुजाम् ॥ ३१

वर्तलोहम् (Vartaloham), वट्टलोहम् (Vaṭṭaloham), वर्तकलोहं (Vartakaloham) वर्तुलोहम् (Vartuloham), पञ्चलोहम् (Pañcaloham) and नीलिका (Nīlikā), are synonymous.

Vartaloham is *śītavīrya* has sour and pungent taste, *rūkṣa* (roughning)

मुण्डलोहम् - Wrought iorn तीक्ष्णलोहम् - Cast iorn कान्तलोहम् - Magnetic iorn कडारम् - Brittle iorn मृदुलोहम् - Soft iorn.

and pacifies the diseases caused by aggravated *kapha* and *pitta*.

लोहोच्छिष्टम् (मण्डूरम्) Lohocchiṣṭam (Maṇḍūram)

लोहोच्छिष्टं च मण्डूरं किट्टं चैव मलोद्भवम् ।
लोहोत्थं लोहनिर्यासमयःशिष्टं च कीर्तितम् ॥ ३२

आमवातहरणं च शोभनं पाण्डुमेहगदनाशनाग्रजम् ।
दुष्टकुष्ठपवनास्रवातजित् स्यात् जराकृतवलीविनाशनम् ॥३३

लोहोच्छिष्टं(Lohocchiṣṭam), मण्डूरं Maṇḍūram, किट्टं (Kiṭṭam), मलोद्भवम् (Malodbhavam), लोहोत्थं (Lohottham), लोहनिर्यासं (Lohaniryāsam), and अयः शिष्टम् (Ayaḥśiṣṭam) are synonymous.

Mandūra is useful in *āmavāta* (Rhumatoid arthritis), anaemia, diseases characterised by polyuria including diabetes, skin disorders, gout, *vātadosa,* and wrinkles and gray hairs due to old age.

9 पारदः Pāradaḥ Eng. Mercury

पारदः रुद्ररेतश्च रसलोहं महारसम् ।
रसेन्द्रं चपलं सूतं पारदीयं रसोत्तमम् ॥ ३४

पारदः कृमिकुष्ठघ्नः आयुष्यो दृष्टिदः परः ।
सुबल्यः सकषायश्च मूर्च्छितोऽसौ गदापहः ॥ ३५

संस्कार हीनं खलु सूतराजं सेवेत यस्तस्य करोति बाधाम् ।
देहस्य नाशं विदधाति नूनं कुष्टादिदोषान् जनयेन्नराणाम् ॥ ३६

पारदः (Pāradaḥ), रुद्ररेतः (Rudraretaḥ), रसलोहं (Rasaloham), महारसः (Mahārasaḥ), रसेन्द्रः (Rasendraḥ), चपलः (Capalaḥ), सूतः (Sūtaḥ), पारदीयमः (Pāradīyam), रसोत्तमः (Rasottamaḥ) are synonymous.

Pārada is *kaṣāya* in taste and when it becomes *mūrchita* (lit. killed, bhasma or calcined) it is useful in many diseases. It is used in worms, skin disorders, increases life span, is beneficial to eyes and gives good strength.

If it is not processed properly as mentioned in the books, and if it is used internally it definitely causes harmful effects on the body, skin disorders .

हिंगुलः (Hingulaḥ) (3)

हिंगुलं दरदं म्लेच्छं हिङ्गूलं चूर्णपारदम् ।
मणिरागकरं चान्यन्नाम्ना चर्मानुरञ्जनम् ॥३७

हिंगुलं कटुकं पाके वीर्ये चोष्णं प्रकीर्तितम् ।
विषकुष्ठविसर्पादित्वग्दोषदलनं स्मृतम् ॥ ३८

हिंगुलं मधुरं तिक्तमुष्णं वातकफापहम् ।
त्रिदोषद्वन्द्वदोषोत्थं ज्वरं हरति सेवितम् ॥ ३९

(ग्रन्थान्तरे)

हिंगुलः सर्वदोषघ्नो दीपनोऽतिरसायनः ।
सर्वरोगहरो वृष्यो जारणे लोहमारणे ॥

हिङ्गुलम् (Hingulam), दरदम् (Daradam), म्लेच्छम् (Melccham), हिङ्गूलम् (Hingūlam), चूर्णपारदम् (Cūrnapāradam), मणिरागकरं (Manirāgakaram) चर्मानुरञ्जनम् (Carmānurañjanam) are synonymous.

Hingula is pungent in *vipāka* (final transformation after digestion), *usṇavīrya*. It is useful in poisons, skin disorders, erysipelas etc.

Hingula is sweet and bitter in taste, *usṇavīrya* and pacifies *vāta* and *kaphadoṣas*. It is useful in fevers due to vitiation of all the *doṣas* and due to vitiation of two *doṣas*.

According to another text - Hingula pacifies all the three *doṣas*, stimulates digestive capacity, *rasāyana* (rejuvinating), useful in all diseases, *vṛsya* and used in *Jāraṇā* and *Māraṇa* processes of metals.

10 वैक्रान्तम् Vaikrāntam (Tourmaline)

वैक्रान्तं क्रान्तसंज्ञं स्याद् वज्रो भूमिरजस्तथा ।
गोनसं क्षुद्रकुलिशं जीर्णवज्रं तु वज्रकम् ॥ ४०

तत्तु सप्तविधं प्रोक्तमनेककर्मकारकम् ।
षट्कोणं तीक्ष्णधारं च स्वच्छमिन्द्रधनुश्छवि ॥ ४१

तदुत्तमं तु वैक्रान्तं हितं प्रोक्तं रसायने ॥
मेहषाण्डयाशुवार्धक्य क्षयग्रहणिकासजित् ॥४२

वृष्यो रसायनो बल्यो वैक्रान्तो वह्निदीपनः ॥ ½

"आयुष्प्रदश्च बलवर्णकरोति वृष्यः
प्रज्ञाप्रदः सकलदोषगणापहारी ।

दीप्ताग्निकृत् पविसमान गुणस्तरस्वी
वैक्रान्तकः खलु वपुर्बललोहकारी ॥ ४३ R.R. Sam. 2. 54.
अशुध्दवज्रं गुरुपाण्डुताप हृत्पार्श्वपीडाऽरुचीकुष्ठकारी ।
शुध्दं मृतं सौख्यबलप्रदं स्यात् वैक्रान्तभस्मापि रसायनं च ॥ ४४

वैक्रान्त (Vaikrānta), क्रान्त (Krānta), वज्र (Vajra), भूमिरजः (Bhūmirajaḥ), गोनसं (Gonasam), क्षुद्रकुलिशं (K'sudrakuli'sam), जीर्णवज्रम् (Jirṇavajram), and वज्रकम् (Vajrakam) are synonymous.

It is of seven types and used for various purposes. The *Vaikrānta* which has six angles and sharp edge and having the colour resembling the rainbow is supposed to be the best for rejuvenation (*Rasāyana*).

Vaikrānta is useful in the diseases of *Meha* (diseases characterized by polyuria), impotency, early ageing, consumption, *Grahaṇī* (ग्रहणी) and cough. It is *Vṛsya,* rejuvenating, strength promoting and stimulates the digestive (and assimilative) capacity.

Vaikrānta increases *longevity,* gives strength, improves complexion and is *vṛsya*, it improves intellect and is useful in pacifying all the *dosas*. and increases the digestive (and metabolizing) capacity and just like diamond it makes the body strong like iron.

Unprocessed *vaikrānta* causes obstinate anaemia, burning sensation, chest pain, pain in the chest wall, anorexia, and skin disorders and killed *vaikranta* (*Bhasma*) is rejuvenating, and gives strength and happiness.

11 गारुत्मतम् Gārutmatam (Emerald)

गारुत्मतं मरकतं रौहिणेयं हरिन्मणि : ।
सौपर्णं गरुडोद्गीर्णं बुधरत्नाश्मगर्भजम् ॥ ४५
गरलारिर्वायवालं गारुडं रुद्रसंमितम् ।
रौहिणेयं विषघ्नं च शीतलं मधुरं रसे ॥ ४६
अम्लपित्तहरं वृष्यं पुष्टिदं भूतनाशनम् ॥

गारुत्मतं (Gārutmạtam), मरकतं (Marakatam), रौहिणेयं (Rauhiṇeyam), हरिन्मणिः (Harinmaṇiḥ), सौपर्णं (Sauparṇam), गरुडोद्गीर्णं (Garudodgīrṇam), बुधरत्नं (Budharatnam), अश्मगर्भजं (A'smagarbhajam), गरलारिः (Garalāriḥ),

1 रुद्रसंमितम् This style to restrict the numbers of synonyms is of Raj. Ni. and seems to be a later additon. Here it indicates 11 synonyms

वायवालं (Wāyavālam) and गारुडं (Gāruḍam) are synonymous. (which are eleven in number.)

Gārutmatam is sweet in taste, *śitavirya* and antipoisonous .It is useful in hyperacidity, is *vṛsya,* nourising and antiseptic.

12 हीरकम् Hīrakam (Diamond)

हीरकं भिदुरं वज्रं सद्रत्नमशनिः पविः ॥ ४७
सूचिवक्त्रं वराहं च कुलिशं भार्गवं स्मृतम् ॥ çâ

अभेद्यमशिरं रत्नं दृढं भार्गवकं स्मृतम् ॥ ४८
षट्कोणं बहुधारं च शतकोट्यब्धिभूमिजम् ॥ ½

रुजां समूहं हरते नराणां बलं सुरूपं विदधाति युक्त्या ।
देहस्य सौख्यं च सदा करोति चिरं तथाऽऽयुः पलितं च हन्ति ॥४९

"आयुष्प्रदं झटिति सद्गुणदं च वृष्यं दोषत्रयप्रशमनं सकलामयघ्नम् ।
सूतेन्द्रबन्धवधसद्गुणकृत् प्रदीपं मृत्युञ्जयं तदमृतोपममेव वज्रम्"। ५०

R. Ras. samu.4

पीडां विधत्ते विविधां नराणां कुष्ठं क्षयं पाण्डुगदं च दुष्टम् ।
हृत्पार्श्वपीडां कुरुतेऽतिकृच्छ्रामशुद्धवज्रं गुरुतापकारि ॥ ५१

हीरकं (Hīrakam), भिदुरं (Bhiduram), वज्रं (Vajram), सद्रत्नम् (Sadratnam), अशनिः (Aśaniḥ), पविः (Paviḥ), सूचिवक्त्रं (Sūcivaktram), वराहं (Varāham), कुलिशं (Kuliśam), भार्गवम् (Bhārgavam), अभेद्यं (Abhedyam), अशिरं (Aśiram), रत्नं (Ratnam), दृढं (Dṛḍham), भार्गवकं (Bhārgavakam), षट्कोणं (Ṣaṭkoṇam), बहुधारं (Bahudhāram), शतकोटि (Śatakoṭi), अब्धिभूमिजम् (Abdhibhūmijam) are synonymous.

Diamond is useful in various diseases of the body, gives strength and having good appearance, increases happiness, longevity and is useful in untimely graying of hairs.

According to another text - It gives longevity and virtues. It is *vṛsya* pacifies all the three *doṣas,* useful in all diseases. It is useful in processing the mercury in bandhana (binding), reducing to bhasma form, and is comparable to *Amṛt* (nectar)

Impure and unprocessed thouroughly, *Vajra* causes various disorders in the body and causes diseases of skin, consumption, anaemia, precordial pain and obstinate pain in the sides of the chest, and causes severe burning.

राजावर्तः Rājāvartaḥ (4)

राजावर्तश्च राजा च नीलाश्मा तु नृपोपलः ।
सुवर्णधातू राजाद्री राजप्रस्तर एव च ॥ ५२

राजावर्तः कटुः स्निग्धः शिशिरः पित्तनाशनः ।
सौभाग्यं कुरुते नृणां भूषणेषु प्रयोजितः ॥ ५३

राजावर्तः (Rājāvartaḥ), राजा (Rajā), नीलाश्मा (Nīlāśmā), नृपोपलः (Nṛpopalaḥ), सुवर्णधातू (Suvarṇadhātū), राजाद्री (Rājādrī), and राजप्रस्तर (Rājaprastara) are synonymous.

Rājāvarta is pungent, unctuous, *śītavīrya*, pacifies *pittadoṣa*, causes good fortune if used in ornament.

13 मौक्तिकम् Mauktikam (Pearl)

मौक्तिकं शुक्तिकं स्फोटशुक्तिजं शुक्तिसंभवम् ।
भूषणार्हतमं श्रेष्ठं शौक्तिकं भौतिकं तथा ॥ ५४

मौक्तिकं मधुरं शीतं सरं दृष्टिभवं गदम् ।
उन्मीलयति[२] पित्तं च हारालिङ्गेन दाहहत् ॥ ५५

मौक्तिकं (Mauktikam), शुक्तिकं (Śuktikam), स्फोटशुक्तिजं (Sphotaśuktijam), शुक्तिसंभवं (Śuktisambhavam), भूषणार्हतमं (Bhūṣan-arhatamam), श्रेष्ठम् (Śreṣṭham), शौक्तिकं (Śauktikam), and भौतिकं (Bhautikam) are synonymous.

Pearl is sweet in taste, *śītavīrya, sara* (mild laxative) and useful in diseases of the eye. It pacifies *Pitta* and by the use of its garlands etc. it alleviates burning sensation of the body.

14 प्रवालम् Prawālam (Coral)

प्रवालं विद्रुमं रक्तं भूषणार्हं सुवल्लिजम ।
सामुद्रजं महारक्तं वल्लीपाषाणसंभवम् ॥ ५६

पक्वबिम्बीफलच्छायं वृत्तायनमवक्रकम् ।
स्निग्धमव्रणकं स्थूलं प्रवालं सप्तधा शुभम् ॥ ५७

२ 'उन्मूलयति' इति साधु । S.D. K.

पाण्डुरं धूसरं रूक्षं सव्रणं कण्डरान्वितम् ।
निर्भारं शुभ्रवर्णं च नेष्यते सप्तधा त्विदम् ॥ ५८

प्रवालकं सरं शीतं वातपित्तत्रिदोषनुत् ।
दृष्टिदोषविघाताय विषनाशाय चेष्यते ॥ ५९

"क्षयपित्तास्रकासघ्नं दीपनं पाचनं लघु ।
विषभूतादिशमनं विद्रुमं नेत्ररोगनुत् ॥ ६० R.Ras. 4.20

प्रवालं (Pravālam), विद्रुमं (Vidrumam), रक्तं (Raktam), भूषणार्हम् (Bhūṣaṇārham), सुवल्लिजम् (Suvallijam), सामुद्रजं (Sāmudrajam), महारक्त (Mahāraktam), वल्लीपाषाण संभवम् (Vallīpāṣāṇasambhavam) are synonymous.

Characteristics of good Prawāla

The coral having following seven qualities : 1) In colour it resembles the colour of ripe *Bimbī* fruit, 2) roundish, 3) elongated, 4)uncurved,5) unctious 6) free from cracks, and 7) thick (heavy) is supposed to be auspicious.

Characteristics of bad Prawala

The coral which is (1) pale in colours (2) grayish, (3) rough, (4) with cracks (5) with *kandarās* (linings or striations), (6) light wieght, and (7) whitish.

Prawāla is mild laxative, *sītavīrya* and pacifies *vāta, pitta* and also *kaphadoṣa*. It is useful for diseases of eyes and in poisons.

According to another text

Prawāla stimulates digestive capacity and is *Laghu*. It is useful in poison and as an antiseptic (*bhūtaghna*) and in eye diseases.

धान्यवर्गः (Dhānyavargaḥ)

15 शालिः (Śāliḥ)

रक्तशालिर्महाशालिः सुगन्धप्रसवस्तथा।
वृन्दारको मुष्टिकश्च शालीनां प्रवरास्तथा ॥ ६१

शाबरः कृष्णशालिश्च हासो वृन्तक एव च ।
कृष्णशालिश्च गौरश्च शालयो विविधाः स्मृताः ॥ ६२

श्वेतशालिर्महाशालिः स चोत्तगो वर्णपूरक ।
खरशूकश्च काकश्च स च सूकरवालकः ॥ ६३

* अरण्यधान्यनामा च जलजः सप्रसादकः । ½

* अरण्यधान्यनामा च जलजः सप्रसादकः seems to be of कुधान्य -तृणधान्य group.

१ 'कृष्णव्रीहिः' इति चौखम्बा मुद्रित पुस्तके पाठः ।

Śāliḥ (शालिः) is a generic name which includes various forms. However the compiler has mentioned 4-5 special types 1) महाशालिःवर्णपूरकः 2) सूकरबालकः, 3) अरण्यधान्यनामा, 4) जलजः, 5) सप्रसादकः; of these the 1st seems to be cultivated while the remaining, the synonyms of which are suggestive of non- cultivated forms.

रक्तशालिः (Raktaśāliḥ), महाशालिः (Mahāśāliḥ),सुगन्धप्रसवः (Sugandhaprasavaḥ), वृन्दारकः (Vṛndārakaḥ), and मुष्टिकः (Muṣṭikaḥ) are amongst the best of the varieties of rice (*śāli*) (paddy).

शाबरः (Śābaraḥ), कृष्णशालिः (Kṛṣṇaśāliḥ), हासः (Hāsaḥ), वृन्तकः (Vṛntakaḥ), कृष्ण शालिः (Kṛṣṇa śāliḥ), गौरः (Gauraḥ) are some of the varieties of paddy.

श्वेतशालिः (Śvetaśāliḥ), महाशालिः (Mahāśāliḥ) and वर्णपूरकः (Varṇapūrakaḥ) are synonymous. खरशूकः (Kharaśūkaḥ), काकः (Kākaḥ) and सूकरवालकः (Sūkaravālakaḥ) are synonymous.

अरण्यधान्य (Araṇyadhānya), जलजः (Jalajaḥ), and प्रसादकः (Prasadakaḥ) are uncultivated varieties.

I a *Oryza sativa* Linn. (Graminae) (Poaceae)

b Roxb. (Fl. indi.)

c Widely cultivated. One of the oldest food crop. Staple diet of over a third of world's population (U.P.I.)

अरण्यधान्यनामा (Araṇyadhānyanāma) probably नीवारः (Nīvāraḥ) *Hygroryza aristata* Nees mentioned further under Pre. No. 26. uncultivated, जलजः (Jalajaḥ) uncultivated.

प्रसादकः (Prasādakaḥ), probablyप्रशान्तिका or प्रशातिका (Prasātikā) see Ḍalhaṇa III (b).

b) (H.) (B.) Chaval, Dhān; (Mar.) Tānduḷa; (Tam.) Arishi; (Tel.) Dhanyamu; (Mal.) Ari (Bom.) Bhāt; (Sans) Shāli, Dhanya; (Guj.) Chokhā. Chopra Gl. p. 182

III a) 1) C.S. Su. 4.17, 27. 3,8,11,259 etc.

S.S. Su. 12.24, 46.3, 332 etc.

A.H. Su. 6.1 to 5, Ci. 1.72 (Raktaśāliḥ).

2) See IV. Balvantji

b) 1) देशे देशे शूकधान्येषु संख्या ज्ञातुं शक्या नैव तद्दैवतैर्वा ॥

(It is not possible to know the varieties and kinds of (śūkadhānya = awned cereals.) Rāj. Ni. Sālyādivarga

2) इत्याद्यः शालय : सन्ति बहवो बहुदेशज : ।
ग्रन्थविस्तरभीतेस्ते समस्ता नात्र भाषिता : ॥

(There are various forms and kinds of (Śāli) in various regions).
Bh. Pr. chapt.9.6

2) नीवार- उलिकाधान्यं - तद्विविधम् -एकं धान्यसदृशं* विटपं धान्यक्षेत्रजम्, द्वितीयं महादलकाण्डं तु सलिलजं ,तत्र सलिलजं सलिलवृद्धिमात्रस्तम्बप्ररोहं रक्तशूकं च, तदेव 'प्रशान्तिका' इति तन्त्रान्तरेऽपि पठ्यते ।

Dalhaṇa S.S.Su. 46. 21

3) 'रक्तो महान् सकलमस्तूर्णकः शकुनाहतः ।
'शकुनाहतो - यो मगधेषु बुध्दोत्पादकाले उत्तरकुरुभ्यो हंसैरानीतो भृङ्गारपात्रे विशारवाख्यया वापितो विस्तरं गतः ।अत एव शकुनिनाऽऽहृतः शकुनाहत इत्यन्वर्थाऽस्य संज्ञा । Aruna A.H. Su. 6-1
"द्वीपान्तरात्समानीतो गरुडेन महात्मना ।
शकुनाहतः स शालिः स्याद्रूडापरनामकाः"॥ इति वृद्धवैद्याः । Dalhaṇa.

The statement seems to have some historical importance as it states that it was brought by हंस (Hansa) or गरुड(Garuḍa) (Eagle) and was sown in भृङ्गारपात्र (Bhṛṅgārapātra) by विशारवा (Visākhā). This विशारवा (visākhā) maybe a name of a person.

4) अत्र च शालिर्हैमन्तिकं धान्यं, षष्टिकादयश्च ग्रैष्मिकाः व्रीहयः शारदा इति व्यवस्था । चक्र. च. २७.८ इत्यत्र ।
वार्षिका कण्डिताः शुक्ला व्रीहयश्चिरपाकिनः । भा.प्र. धान्यवर्ग.८
'कण्डित शुक्लत्वेन शालित्वमुच्यते तत् षष्टिकेषु व्रीहिषु नाभिहितत्वात् सकलशाल्यव्यापकत्वाच्च न युक्तम् ॥

Cakra Bhanu. Com S. S. 46

IV (1)..... ...Earliest mention of rice cultivation is connected with China. According to *Stanislas Julien,* a ceremony was established in that country about, by the Emperor Chin-nung, in which the sowing of five kinds of grain is the chief observance. The reigning Emperor himself has to sow the rice, but he may delegate the sowing of the other four kinds to the princes of his family.

(Watt V. P. 512)

(2) शालि - *Oryza sativa* Linn.

शालि The sāli variety of paddy is called Haimanta हैमन्त or Jaḍahana जडहन or Agahani अगहनी because they are ready to be harvested in the winter season. The grains are with white, (शुक्ल) husk The text have mentioned a very large number of sub varieties ... (Balwantji p. 395).

(3) "The three principle classes of Rice are *Śālī,* or that reaped in the cold season, *Vrīhī,* or that ripening in the rainy season and shastika or that grown in the hot weather in low lands" (from U.C. Dutt's Materia Medica of the Hindus) ....

(Watt. V. p. 512-13)

* मल्या : 'किलिकारिचेन्नेल्' Abhi. Manj. 415 Devanagari version Vd. Mrs. Chitra krishnan (Personal correspondence)

The most general vernacular name for wild rice is, however, *Uri* and the plant occurs plentifully in Madras, Orissa, Bengal, Cachar, Burma, Cochin-China and Ceylon. It has also been found at numerous isolated localities throughout the more northern tracts since rice often persists self sown in swampy lands under such conditions as to be readily mistaken plant. In fact it may be said that the undoubted wild habitat is within the region where the word *Uri* occurs in greatly diversified tounges as its most general name."

Watt. Vol. II. p. 513-514

... It may be repeated that the chief wild habitat of the plant is, roughly speaking, from Southern India to Cochin China. That belt of land has often vast marshy expanses with low intervening mountains, possesses a tropical climate, as also a strong periodic seasons of rain fall. ... .. its cultivation appears to have spread from thence eastward to China, perhaps 3000 years before the Christian era, and at perhaps a slightly more recent date, westward and northward, throughout India to Persia, Arabia and ultimately Egypt and Europe. An enlightened people like Chinese might be supposed to have more readily realised the importance of rice cultivation than would be the aboriginal tribes on the hills and swamps of lower India, where a sufficiently abundant supply for their wants could be gathered from the wild plant. " Watt-V- p. 519

... In other words the red rices have probably come from *O. rufipogon* and the blackish coloured forms from *O. abuensis,* but both these forms must have yielded to cultivation and produced also the higher class beardless white rices, ...

. Watt. Vol. V p.506. .

... It must, in fact, be admitted that we have to fall back on *Dr. Buchanan - Hamilton's* idea that the chief differences between the thousands of forms of cultivated rices, hinge on their properties and pecularities under cultivation ... ... These pecularities, the Indian cultivator, through the time honoured practices of his ancestors, is able to recognise far more accurately than botanical science has as yet been able to explain. ... .."

Watt. V-p. 506.

16 व्रीहिः Vrīhiḥ

षष्टिकस्तु महाव्रीहिः कृष्णव्रीहिस्ततोऽनु च ॥ ६४
यवकश्चैव पाक्यश्च रक्तसारमुखस्तथा ॥

शालिव्रीहिगुणाः
शीतो गुरुस्त्रिदोषघ्नो मधुरो गौरषष्टिक ॥ ६५
किंचिद्धितो गुरुस्तस्मादपरो रसपाकतः ॥
महाशालिः परो वृष्यः कलमः श्लेष्मपित्तहा ॥ ६६
"मधुरश्चाम्लपाकश्च व्रीहिः पित्तकरो गुरुः ॥"
अत्युष्णो बहुनिष्यन्दी पाटलस्तु त्रिदोषकृत ॥ ६७
"बहूष्मा बहुविण्मूत्रो व्रीहिराशु त्रिदोषलः ॥ C. Sū. 27.14

Amongst the better qualities of व्रीहिः (Vrihiḥ), षष्टिक (Ṣaṣṭika) is the best and is followed by महाव्रीहिः (Mahāvrihiḥ), कृष्णव्रीहिः (Kṛṣṇavrihiḥ), यवकः (Yavakaḥ), पाक्यः (Pākyaḥ) and रक्तसारमुखः (Raktasāramukhaḥ) (in the descending order).

Properties of śāliḥ & vrihiḥ
Gauraṣaṣṭika is sweet in taste, *śītavīrya,* pacifies all the three *doṣas* and is *guru.* The other varieties are slightly *guru* (heavy to digest) in *rasa* and *vipāka* (final tranformation after digestion.) *Mahāśāliḥ* is the best *vṛṣya* amongst them. *Kalama* pacifies *kapha* and *pitta doṣas. Vrīhi* is sweet in taste but sour after *Vipāka*. It aggravates *pittadoṣa* and is *guru* (heavy to digest).

Pāṭalā generates heat in high degree, causes more secretion of mucus and aggravates three *doṣas*. *Āśuvrīhī* generates more heat, more quantity of urine and faeces and aggravates three *doṣas*.

Fam. Graminae (Poaceae).

a) ***Oryza sativa*** Linn.
See Pre. No. 15 शालिः (Śālih).

17 यवः Yavaḥ

अक्षतास्तीक्ष्णशूकाश्च यवाश्चैव तु नामतः ॥ ६८
"रूक्षः शीतो गुरुः स्वादुः सरो विड्वातकृद्यवः ॥
वृष्यः स्थैर्यकरो मूत्रमेदःपित्तकफाञ्जयेत् ॥ ६९
पीनसः श्वासकासोरुस्तम्भकण्ठत्वगामयान् ॥"
C.S. Su. 27.19 A.H. Su. 6.13-19

अक्षताः (Akśatāḥ), तीक्ष्णशूकाः (Tīkśnaśūkāḥ) and यवाः (Yavāḥ) are synonymous.

Yava is sweet in taste, *śītavirya*, *guru* (difficult to digest) and produces more faeces and *vāta* and is mild laxative.

It is *vṛsya,* provides stability, causes lesser quantity of urine, and *meda* (fat) and pacifies *pitta* and *kapha doṣas*. It is useful in sinusitis, dyspnoea, cough, *ūrustambha* (? Thrombosis of femoral artery), diseases of the throat and skin diseases.

I The other Nighaṇṭuṣ esp. Bh. Pr. has mentioned three kinds 1) सितशूकः यवः (Śitaśūkaḥ - Yavaḥ), 2) निःशूकः–अतियवः (Niḥśūkaḥ - Atiyavaḥ), 3) हरितः - स्वल्पः - तोक्यः (Haritaḥ - greenish coloured, Swalpaḥ - smaller in size is called as तोक्यः (Tokyaḥ). All belonging to the same species.

Fam. Graminae (Poaceae)

a) ***Hordeum vulgare*** Linn.
Syn. *H. sativum* Pers.

b) Roxburgh, Watt dict.

c) Cultivated chiefly in North India and upto 13,000 ft. in the Himalayas (Chopra)

II a) अक्षतः (Akśataḥ), तीक्ष्णशूकः (Tīkśṇaśūkaḥ), कञ्चुकी (Kañcukī) (R. Ni.), तुरगप्रियः (Turagapriyaḥ).

b) (Sans.) Yava; (H.) Jau, Jav; (B.) Jab, Jau; (Mar.) Java; (Guj.) Jau, Jav, Yamvah; (Tel.) Barlibiyam, Yavaka; (Tam.) Barliyarisi; (Kan.) Javegodhi; (Mal.) Yavam.

III 1) न्यूना यवादनुयवः ।अ.ह. सू. ६.१५
निःशूको यवो - अनुयवः । - हेमाद्रिः
This seems to be the अतियवः of Bh. Pr. (See - I).

2) अतियवा निःशूकाः कृष्णारुणयवा एव । . . . . तत्र यविका निःशूका स्वल्पा । Ḍalhaṇa Su. Su. 46.43

3) यव Yavaḥ
C. S. Su. 26.17, 46, 148, 282, 27. 26 etc.
S. S. Su. 14.37, 46.16 etc.
A. H. Su. 6.13, 8.42, 47etc.

4) सितशूकस्तीक्ष्णशूको यवो वाजिप्रियः शुचिः ।
निःशूकोऽतियवो ज्ञेयस्तोक्यस्तु हरितो यवः ॥ Kaiyadeva Ni.

IV 1) Watt has mentioned few varieties of this species out of which *H. hexastichum* Linn. is the barley, par excellence, of India, and is almost only cultivated form in India.

2) Little is known regarding its introduction or the origin of its cultivation in the country. ..... It is probable that it was also grown at least in the north of India in very remote times. The supposition is confirmed by the intimate connection of the grain with several of

the rites and beliefs of the Hindu religion. Thus the God Indra is called "He who ripens Barley" and the grain is employed in the ceremonies attending the birth of child, weddings, funerals and in certain sacrificial rites. It is further supported by the antiquity of the Sanskrit name *Yava* which in the earliest times was probably applied as a general term to any grain, or corn yielding plant. ...

Watt Vol. IV Page 277.

3) "...खराब जौ को यवानी कहते थे। ...भाष्यमें अयव और सुयव शब्द आये हैं, जो सम्भवतः उस प्रदेशोंके लिये है, जिनमें यव नहीं होता था या खूब होता था....जौ को पुरानी फारसी में यओ (Yao)कहते थे। यव विश्वकी प्राचीनतम उपजोंमेंसे है। ऋग्वेद में भी इसका उल्लेख मिलता है। (Patañjali Kālin Bhārat By Prabhudayāl Agnihotrī P. 263-64).

18 मुद्गः Mudgaḥ

वासन्ताः कृष्णमुद्गाश्च शारदा हरितास्तथा ॥ ७०
मुद्गानां नामतश्चोक्ताः सूपश्रेष्ठा रसोत्तमाः ॥

(मुद्गः किलाटो माङ्गल्यो हरितः शारदोऽपि च ॥
पित्तप्रसेको वसुको माधवः प्रवरोऽसितः ॥)

मुद्गो रूक्षो लघुर्ग्राही कफपित्तहरो हिमः ॥ ७१
स्वादुरल्पानिलो नेत्र्यो वन्योऽप्येतद्गुणः स्मृतः ॥

(हरितः प्रवरस्तेषां तच्छाकं तिक्तमुत्तमम् ॥
कृष्णमुद्गस्तु वरको राजमुद्गस्तु खण्डकः) ॥

कृष्णमुद्ग (Kṛṣṇamudga), is called as वासन्त (Vāsanta) and हरितमुद्ग (Haritamudga) is called as शारद (Śārada). *Mūga* is supposed to be the best for culinary purpose and has a good taste.

According to another text.

मुद्गः (Mudgaḥ), किलाटः (Kilāṭaḥ), माङ्गल्यः (Māṅgalyaḥ), and शारदः (Śāradaḥ) are synonymous with हरितः (Haritaḥ) and the synonyms for कृष्णमुद्गः (Kṛṣṇamudgaḥ) are पित्तप्रसेकः (Pitta prasekaḥ), वसुकः (Vasukaḥ) and माधवः (Mādhavaḥ). Out of these *kṛṣṇamudgaḥ* is better for culinary purspose.

Mudga is *rūkśa* (roughening), *laghu,* astgringent, *śītavīrya* and pacifies *kapha pitta doṣas*. It is sweet in taste, aggravates *vātadoṣa* slightly and is beneficial to eyes. वन्यमुद्ग *(Vanyamudga)* (uncultivated variety) has the similar properties.

(out of these हरितमुद्‌ग (Haritmudga) is the better or beneficial to human body and as a vegetable it is bitter and good. कृष्णमुद्‌गः (Kṛṣṇamudga) is also called as वरकः (Varakaḥ) and राजमुद्‌गः (Rājamudgaḥ) as खण्डकः (Khaṇḍakaḥ).

I The compiler has mentioned the types according to the colour of the seeds and which are supposed to be of better quality. While mentioning the properties he has mentioned another kind that is वन्यमुद्‌गः (Vanyamudgaḥ) (uncultivated). Both belonging to the same species.

Fam. Leguminosae. Fabaceae

I- A-a ***Vigna radiata*** (Linn.) Wilczek var. *radiata* verdcourt
syn. ***Phaseolus radiatus*** Linn. (Comp. p. 158)
b Roxb.
c Extensively cultivated all over India.

B वन्यमुद्‌गः (Vanyamudgaḥ)

II a) वासन्ताः कृष्णमुद्‌गाः (Vāsantāḥ Kṛṣṇamudgāḥ), शारदा हरिताः (Śāradā Haritāḥ)

b) (Sans.) Mudga; (H.) Mung, Pessara; (B) Mung; (Mar.) Muga (Guj.) Mag; (Tel.) Uthulu, Patchapessalu; (Tam.) Pasi-payaru, Putcha-payaru; (K.) Hesaru; (Mal.) Cherupayara.(U.P.I.p. 677) (चेरुपयर - अभि.मं Cherupayara.)

III 1) C.S. Su 5.3,9, 27.22, Vi. 1.21 etc.
S.S. Su 15.38, 21.18, 46.27, 28,29, 33.. etc.
A.H. Su 3.51, 4.28, 6.17, 18, 33 etc.

2) वनमुद्‌गः (Vanamudgaḥ) is separately mentioned (See under Pre. No. 24) different from वन्यमुद्‌ग (Vanuyamudga) Bh. Pr. has accepted the same synonyms. See IV. (Pre No. 24)

IV I) This pulse is a native of India, and has been cultivated for at least 3000 years. It is met with, both wild and cultivated, throughout the plains..

Duthie and Fuller write - "There are three well marked varieties, having respectively green, yellow and black seeds". The green seeded is the typical and commonest variety (harri-mung), that with yellow seed (Sona mung) has been described as *Phaseolus aureus,* while that with black seeds (Krishna mung) has also been described by Roxburgh as distinct under the name *Phaseolus max.* " (Watt. Vol.VI.1 p. 188)

19 राजमाषः Rājamāsah.

माषो बीजवरो घारीश्चवलो राजमाषकः ॥ ७२
राजमाषो नीलमाषो नृपमाषो नृपोचितः ॥

कफपित्तहरो रुच्यो वातकृद् बलदायकः॥ ७३
¹राजमाषो सरो वृष्यः कफपित्तास्रशुक्रनुत् ॥

सुस्वादुः शीतलो रूक्षः कषायो विशदो गुरुः ॥७४ C.Su.27.25

माषः (Māṣaḥ), बीजवरः (Bījavaraḥ), घारीः (Ghāriḥ), चवलः (Cavalaḥ) राजमाषकः (Rājamāṣakaḥ), राजमाषः (Rājamāsaḥ), नीलमाषः (Nīlamāṣaḥ), नृपमाषः (Nṛpamāṣaḥ), and नृपोचितः (Nṛpocitaḥ) are synonymous.

Rājamaṣa is sweet and *kaṣāya* (astringent) in taste, *śītavīrya*, *rukṣa* (roughening), cleansing, *guru* (heavy for digestion) and pacifies *kapha* and *pitta doṣas,* is appetizer, increases *vāta*, gives strength and decreases *śukradhātu.*

Fam. Leguminosae. Fabaceae

I. ***Vigna unguiculata*** (Linn.) Walp. ssp. cylindrica (Linn.) Van Esettine
Syn. *V. catjang* Walp.
V. cylindrica Skeels (comp p. 158)

b) Roxb. Fl. Indi.

c) Extensively cultivated

II माषः (Māṣaḥ) This name is used for (a) *Phaseolus mungo* Linn. (Pre NO. 28)

(b) राजमाषकः (Rājamāṣakaḥ),चवलः (Cavalaḥ) (Dh. Ni.); दीर्घशिम्बिकः (Dīrghaśimbikaḥ) (Raj. Ni.)

(c)(Mar.) Cavaḷi, Aḷasunde; (H) Lobiya, Rājamāṣa; (B.) Barbati Kalaya, Barbati; (Gu.) Cola; (Kan.) Aḷasande; (Tel.) Boberlu (Chopra), Alasandalu (Chunekar); Boberulu, dantupesalu (U.P.I.); (Tam.) Karamani, (U.P.I.) (Mal.) Kottapayaru, Vellapayaru (U.P.I.)

III 1) राजशिम्बा महाराजमाषाख्या राजशिंबिका ।
दीर्घशिम्बा राजशमी शमीका कथ्यते बुधैः ॥ ४५७ अभि.मं.
(Maly.) Perumpayaru पेरुंपयरु (vd. Nalini K. Personal Correspondence).

III 2) राजमाष

C.S. Su. 27.24

---

१ राजमाषो सरो रुच्यः कफशुक्राम्लपित्तनुत ॥
तत्स्वादुर्वातलो रूक्षः कषायो विशदो गुरुः।
च.सु. २७.२५ किंचित परिवर्तितः अत्र दृश्यते ।

A.H. Su. 6.19
S.Su. 46.35 अलसान्द्र.

IV 1) Several races exist, which differ in the colour of the flower and seeds. (Watt Dict. VI-IV P. 236-37)

20 कोद्रवः Kodravaḥ

कोद्रवः कोरदूषः स्यादुद्दालो वनकोद्रवः ।
कोद्रवः शीतलो ग्राही विषपित्तकफाञ्जयेत् ॥ ७५

कोद्रवः (Kodrava) has the synonym कोरदूषः (Koradūṣaḥ) and उद्दाल (Uddāla) is वनकोद्रवः (Vanakodravaḥ)

Kodrava is *śitavīrya*, astringent and pacifies *pitta* and *kaphadoṣas* and is useful in poison.

I The compiler has mentioned two plants here (A) कोद्रवः (Kodravaḥ) & (B) उद्दालः (Uddālaḥ) but the properties of the 1st are only mentioned. `B' is a wild form,.

Fam. Graminae.Poaceae

a) ***Paspalum scrobiculatum*** Linn.
Syn. P. commersonii Lam.
P. scrobiculatum Var. *commersonii* Stapf.
P. scrobiculatum Var. *frumentaceum* Stapf. (U.P.I. p. 433)

b) Roxb. Fl. Indi. C.B.C. 93

c) Throughout hotter parts of India, wild or cultivated.

II A-a) कोद्रवः (Kodravaḥ),कोरदूषः (Koraduṣaḥ) (Dhn.Ni.)
मदनाग्रजः (Madanāgrajaḥ) (Raj. Ni.)

B उद्दालः (Uddālaḥ), वनकोद्रवः (Vanakodravaḥ)

b) A.B.
Sans. A Kodrava; (B) Uddāla;
(H) kodo; (B) Kododhan; (Mumbai)
Kodra; (Tam. & Maly.) Varaga; (Tel.) Kiraruga;
(Mar.) Kodra, Harik; (Kan) Harak; (Guj.) Kodro,Menya.

III कोद्रवः- कोरदूषः

1) C.S. Su. 21.24, 27.16. etc.
S.S. Su. 46.21, 46.23, ci. 4.36, 17.37 etc.
A.H. Su. 6.11, 13.26. Ni. 7.76 रक्तपित्तनि. also etc.

2) उद्दालकस्तु वीर्योष्णो लेखनो वातलो लघुः ॥
रूक्षः स्वादुः कषायश्च कफजिद्बध्दमूत्रविट ॥ (Śoḍhala p. 172)

3) मदोत्पादका कोद्रवाः मदनकोद्रवाः । Ḍalhaṇa. Kodrava sometimes develops narcotic properties and may then be called 'मदनकोद्रव' (S. S. Ci. 17.37)

4) कोद्रवः कोरदूषश्च कोद्दारुष उदाहृतः ।
438 मदनः चमरीरूषस्तथा मर्षण फेनिलः ॥
436 उद्दालको भिषग्भिः कथितः काकेष्टपर्णीति ।
उद्दालः शूकभवः शुकप्रियः पुंजशूकश्च ॥
438 (केरली) वरकु (Abhi. Mamj.)

IV 1) *Habitat & Cultivation :*

A native of India and extensively cultivated in parts of the country during rainy season.

In the Bombay Presidency several varieties are recognised by the natives, the differences probably resulting from the nature of the soil, the method of cultivation. Two sorts are however, wellknown viz. the wholesome and the unwholesome. The grain of the former is smaller and paler, and is known by the name of *Pechadi* or *Harkin* in the Kokan. In the Goa it is called *Pakad*. The unwholesome variety is called *dhone* or *majori-harik* in the Konkan, and mana kodra in Gujarat . ... The grain is the only poisonous part of the plant. All the varieties are, as a matter of fact more or less poisonous. *Harik* is one of the principal crops of the Ratnagiri District. (Watt. Vo; VI-1 Page 112).

21 नीवारः Nīwārah

नीवारः तापसश्चैव मुनिभक्तः प्रसादकः[१] ।
अरण्यधान्यनामा च रसिकश्च प्रकीर्तितः ॥ ७६

नीवारः मधुरः स्निग्धः पवित्रः पथ्यदो लघुः ।

नीवारः (Nīvāraḥ), तापसः (Tāpasaḥ), मुनिभक्तः (Munibhaktaḥ), प्रसादकः (Prasādakaḥ), अरण्यधान्यनामा (Araṇyadhānyanāmā), and रसिकः (Rasikaḥ) are synonymous.

Nīvara is sweet in taste, unctuous, auspicious, *laghu* (easy to digest and assimilate) and beneficial for diet.

Fam. Graminae. (Poaceae)

I a) ***Hygroryza aristata*** (Retz.) Nees ex Wight & Arn.
Syn. *H. aristata* Nees

'१ प्रसादितः' इति आनन्दा. मुद्रित पुस्तके पाठ ।

b) Roxburgh (Fl. Indi.)

c) Upper and Lower Gangetic plain, Assam, Chittagong and the Deccan. (Chopra)

II नीवारः (Nīwāraḥ), अरण्यधान्य (Araṇyadhānya), a) (Dh.Ni.), मुनिधान्यं (Munidhānyam) Raj. Ni.

b) (H.) Tīni, Tīnni, Jangli Dal; (B) Uridhan; (Mar.) Deobhat; (Guj.) Vanti; (Tam.) Vallipullu; (Kan.) Jyarahumedhe; (Mal.) Nirvvallipullu (Assam) Phutki, putidal. (U.P.I.)

III 1) C.S. Su. 27.16, Ci 4.36.
S.S. Su.20.4, 46.21, 23
A.H. Su. 6.11

2) नीवारः शुक्रघ्नो ऋषिशुक्रविनाशनश्च तनुशूकः।
तापससेव्योऽभिहितः पर्यायैस्तापसाहारः॥ Abhi. Manji. (Kerli - Varinelli)

3) नीवार उड्डिका तृड्डी वनव्रीहिर्मुनिप्रियः ॥१०३॥ (Kaiyadev Ni).

22 श्यामाकः Śyāmākaḥ

श्यामाकस्तृणबीजश्च मुनिभक्ष्यो गवांप्रियः ॥ ७७
सुकुमारो राजधान्यं तृणबीजोत्तमश्च सः ॥

श्यामाको मधुरः स्निग्धः कषायो लघुशीतलः ॥ ७८
वातहृत्कफपित्तघ्नः संग्राही विषदोषनुत् ॥

श्यामाकः (Śyāmākaḥ), तृणबीजः (Tṛṇabījaḥ), मुनिभक्ष्यः (Munibhaksyaḥ), गवांप्रियः (Gawāmpriyaḥ), सुकुमारः (Sukumāraḥ), राजधान्यं (Rājadhānyam), and तृणबीजोत्तमः (Tṛṇabījattomaḥ) are synonymous.

Śyāmāka is sweet and *kasāya* (astringent) in taste, *śītavīrya*, unctuous, *laghu*, pacifies *vāta, pitta* and *kapha doṣas*, is astringent and antipoisonous.

Fam. Gramineae. Poaceae.

I a) ***Echinocloa frumantacea*** Link.
Syn. *E. crusgalli* (Linn.) Beauv. Var. *frumentacea* Wight
Panicum frumentaceum Roxb. (Comp p.57)

b) Roxb. (Fl. indi. CBC)

c) Cultivated over the greater part of India and on the Himalayas upto 6,500 ft. (Chopra)

a) श्यामाकः (Śyāmākaḥ), तृणबीजः (Tṛṇabījaḥ)

b) (H.B.) Sānwā; (SK) Shāmaka; (Tel.) Chamalu; (P) Sanwak; (Tam.) Kudraivali pillu; (Mar.) Samul (Chopra)

III C.S. Su. 27.15.17, Ci. 4.36, etc.

1) S.S. 46.21.23; 21.9. etc.
A.H. Su. 6.11, Ci. 3.22
Another species *E. crusgalli* Beauv. may be Ambhaḥ Śyāmāka.

2) *श्यामाकस्तृण बिन्दुर्याज्ञीयः श्यामको मुनीष्टः स्यात् । ४४० (Abhi Manj.)

3) हस्तिश्यामाक नीवार तोयपर्णी गवेधुका : ।
प्रशान्तिकाम्भः श्यामाक . . . . च. सु. २७.१७
हस्तिश्यामाक श्यामाकभेद एव ।अम्भःश्यामाका जलजा ओडिका लोके 'डे' इत्युच्यते । (Cakraḥ)

4) सु. सू. ४६.२१ कुधान्य विशेषाः ।
श्यामाकस्त्रिविधः - श्यामाकः उष्ट्रश्यामाकः, हस्तिश्यामाकश्चेति, श्यामाकशब्देन तोयश्यामाक उच्यते, उष्ट्रश्यामाकः, स्थूलश्यामाकः, हस्तिश्यामाकः श्यामिकेति लोके । Dalhan

IV 1) *Panicum colonum* Linn.
(H) Sānwak ; (NWP) Sāwan, Janglisānwak, Shāmak (Kumaon) Sānwak, Jangli Sāmak ...; (Pb) Sanwak, Jangli Samak .... ; (Sind) Shamakh; (Bom.) Borrur ....
Panicum crusgalli Linn.
(H)Sanwak (NWP) Jal Sanwak ....
Panicum frumentaceum Roxb.
(See II) (Sans) Śyamak, Shyāmak (Watt. VI-1 p. 7-9)

23 कङ्गुः । प्रियङ्गुः Kaṅguḥ ; Priyaṅguḥ

प्रियङ्गुः कङ्गुकश्चैव चीनकः पीततण्डुलः ॥ ७९
अस्थिसम्बधनश्चैव कङ्गुनी षट् च कथ्यते ॥

प्रियङ्गुर्मधुरो रुच्यः कषायः स्वादुशीतलः ॥ ८०
वातकृत्पित्तदाहघ्नो रूक्षो भग्नास्थिबन्धकृत् ॥

प्रियङ्गु (Priyaṅguḥ), कङ्गुकः (Kaṅgukaḥ), चीनकः (Cīnakaḥ), पीततण्डुलः

---

*तोयश्यामाकोऽन्यो मुनीप्रियश्चाणुरित्युक्तः । ४४१
श्यामाकस्तु तृतीयोऽन्यो हस्तिश्यामाक उच्यते ।
गजभक्षः श्यामिकश्च श्यामा च तृणषण्डकी ॥ ४४२ अभि. मं.
४४० - (मल्या.) श्यामकम् Śyāmakam
४४१ - (मल्या.) चाम Cāma
४४२ - (मल्या.) पुल्चाम Pulcāma (Miss. Nalini k. personal correspondence)

(Pītataṇḍulaḥ), अस्थिसम्बधनः (Asthisambandhanaḥ) and कङ्गुनी (Kanguni) are (six) synonymous.

Priyangu is sweet, *kaṣāya*, *śītavīrya* and appetiser. It aggravates *vāta* and pacifies *pitta,* burning sensation, is *rūkṣa* (roughening) and union promoting in fractures.

I Two plants are mentioned by the compiler (A) कङ्गुकः (Kangukaḥ) (B) चीनकः (Cīnakaḥ)

II (A) कङ्गुकः (Kangukaḥ), प्रियङ्गुः (Priyanguḥ)

(B) चीनकः (Cīnakaḥ), पीततण्डुलः (Pītataṇḍulaḥ)

(A) ***Setaria italica*** Beauv.

(B) ***Panicum miliaceum*** Linn.

III प्रियङ्गुका

1) *Setaria italica* Beau.
2) *Callicarpa macrophylla* Vahl फूलप्रियंगु and दइआ Kumaon.

Setaria species is the source of food grain different from drug *Priyangu* and they may be called *Dhānya Priyangu* and *Auṣadha* (Drug) *Priyangu* respectively. (Balwantji p. 263)

कंगु -Kangu कंगुक - Kanguka

III C.S. Su. 26.112

S.S. Su. 36.28, Ci. 31.5

A.H. Su. 6.11, 7.32, U. 23.23

See प्रियङ्गु (Candanādi Chapter III)

४३७ कंगुर्वानरपुच्छश्च प्रियंगुः कंगुकः स्तनिः ।
शीतसारो भवेत् पीततण्डुलः शीर्षमण्डनः ॥

Abi Man.(Maly.) (कैरली)तिन (Vd. Miss Nalini K.)

III 1) (a) स्त्रियां कङ्गु प्रियङ्गु द्वे कृष्णारक्ता सिता तथा ।
पीता चतुर्विधा कङ्गुस्तासां पीता वरा स्मृता ॥

Bhav. Pr. 8.76.77

(b) चीनाकः काककङ्गुश्च सुश्लक्ष्णः श्लक्ष्णकः स्मृतः
चीनाकः कङ्गुभेदोऽस्ति स ज्ञेयः कङ्गुवद्गुणैः ॥ भा.प्र.वर्ग.

Bhav. Pr. 8.76.78

III 2) कृष्णा रक्ताश्च पीताश्च श्वेताश्चैव प्रियङ्गवः ।
यथोत्तरं प्रधानाः स्युः रूक्षाः कफहराः स्मृताः ॥ Su.Su. 46.24

IV (A) प्रियङ्गु *Setaria italica* Beauv.

Both Dr. Watt and Mr. J. F. Duthie state that it occurs wild in India on parts of Himalayan region, but De candolle appears to doubt whether it has yet been found truely wild anywhere. The last named author, ... comes to the conclusion, however, that the species existed before all cultivation, thousands of yerars ago,

(Garalarih), in China, Japan and Indian Archipelago." .... Mr. Duthie says it is "both wild and cultivated in India and largely grown in other warm countries. "
"The Sanskrit name *Kangu* indicated its antiquity as a cultivated plant in India." Watt. Page 547.

(B) *Panicum milliaceum* Linn.
It is supposed to have been introduced originally from Egypt or Arabia, but its cultivation in India probably dates from a very early period (Watt Vo. VI-1).

24 वनमुद्गः (मकुष्ठकः) Vanamudgaḥ

मकुष्ठको निरूढश्च वनमुदगः कृमीलकः ॥ ८·१
मकुष्ठो वातलो ग्राही कफपित्तहरो लघु ॥

मकुष्ठकः (Makuṣṭhakaḥ), निरूढः (Nirūḍhaḥ), वनमुद्गः (Vanamudgaḥ) and कृमीलकः (Kṛmīlakaḥ) are synonymous.

Makuṣṭha pacifies *kapha pitta doṣas,* aggravates *vātadoṣa,* is astringent and *laghu* (light to digest).

Fam. Leguminosae. Fabaceae.

I ***Vigna aconitifolia*** (Jacq.) Marechal Syn. *Phaseolus aconitifolius* Jacq.
Moth bean or Mat bean, Aconite bean
(U.P.I.p 676)

b) Roxb. Fl. Indi.

c) Cultivated all over India.

II (A) मकुष्ठकः (Mukuṣṭhakaḥ), वनमुद्गः (Vanamudgaḥ), कृमीलकः (Kṛmīlakaḥ)

(B) (Sans.) Makuṣṭhak; (H) Moth, Bhringga; (B) Kheri; (Mar.) Math, Matki; (Guj.) Mat, math; (Tel.) Kuncumpe-salu; (Tam.) Tulukkapayir; (Kan.) Madike; (D.) Moth, bhioni; (Santal) Birmung, Moch, birmoch; (Mundari) Mugirambara. (U.P.I.p. 676)

III

IV 1) *Phaseolus aconitifolius* Jacq.
De Candolle remarks that the absence of a Sanskrit name (by which he probably means an ancient Sanskrit name) and the variety of names in modern Indian languages, point to a recent cultivation. Watt Vol VI I. p. 103.

2) मकुष्ठो वनमुद्गः स्यात् ... ... (Bh. Pr. Chunekar P. 646).

25 आढकी (Āḍhakī)

आढकी तुवरी तुल्या करवीरभुजा तथा ॥ ८२
वृत्तबीजा पीतपुष्पा श्वेता रक्ताऽसिता त्रिधा ॥

आढकी कफपित्तघ्नी किञ्चिन्मारुतकोपनी ॥ ८३
कषाया स्वादुसंग्राही कटुपाका हिमा लघुः ॥

मेदःश्लेष्मास्रपित्तेषु हिता लेपोपसेकयोः ॥ ८४

(See. C.S. Su. 27.33)

The synonyms for आढकी (Āḍhakī) are तुवरी (Tuwarī), करवीरभुजा (Karavīrabhuja), वृत्तबीजा (Vṛttabījā) and पीतपुष्पा (Pītapuṣpā) are synonymous. *Āḍhakī* is of three types 1) श्वेता (Śvetā), 2) रक्ता (Raktā) and 3) (Asitā).

(These three types are mentioned according to the colour of the seeds.)

Āḍhakī is *kaṣāya* (astringent) and sweet in taste, *śītavīrya*, pungent in *vipāka*, *laghu* (light in digestion), pacifies *kapha* and *pitta doṣas*, astringent in action and slightly aggravates *vātadoṣa*. It is beneficial externally in *meda, kapha* and bleeding.

आढकी (Āḍhakī) and तुवरी (Tuwarī) are two varieties of the same species respectively 1) Var. *bicolor* & 2) Var. *flavus*. The second variety ripens earlier. The variety which ripens earlier in the nature is also easily digestible and more (beneficial) during convalescence.

Cajanus cajan (Linn.) Millsp.
Syn. *Cajanus indicus* Spreng.

I a) आढकी *C. indicus* var. *bicolor;* तुवरी *C. indicus* var. *flavus.*
b) Roxb. Fl. indi.
c) cultivated all over India.

II a) वृत्तबीजा (Vṛttabījā), पीतपुष्पा (Pītapuṣpā)

III आढकी *Cajanus cajan* (Linn.) Millsp.; अरहर (H.) Syn. तुवरी
C.S. Su. 21.25, 27.32 etc.
S.S. Su. 20.4, 46.27, 332 etc.
A.H. Su..6.15, Ci 6.73 etc.

IV See Bhavaprakash (Chunekar) (p. 648)
1) The flora of British India regards this bush as doubtfully wild in India, and De Candolle, in his origin of cult. plants views it as more probably a native of tropical Africa, introduced perhaps 3000

years ago into India. Watt.. II p. 2. 13

2) There are two chief varieties : *C. flavus* with the standard or upper petal plain yellow (known in the vernacular as thur); and *C. bicolor* with the standard veined with purple (the arhar). The latter is the most commonly cultivated in the North west provinces and Oudh while in the Central provinces and the Deccan the thur takes the place of arhar. .... Watt.Vo. II p. 13

26 मसूरिका Masūrikā

मसूरा मधुरा सूप्या पृथवः पित्तभेषजम्* ।
मसूरो मधुरः शीतः संग्राही कफपित्तहा ॥ ८५
वातामय**करश्चैव मूत्रकृच्छ्रहरो लघुः ॥

मसूरः (Masūraḥ), मधुरः (Madhuraḥ), सूप्यः (Sūpyaḥ), पृथुः (Pṛthuḥ) and पित्तभेषजम् (Pittabhesajam) are synonymous.

Masūra is *sītavīrya*, astringent in action, pacifies *kapha* and *pitta doṣas*, causes diseases due to *vātadoṣa*, is *laghu* (light in digestion) and useful in dysuria.

I a) ***Lens culinaris*** Medik. (Medic.)
Syn. *L. esculenta* Moench
Ervum lens Linn. (Chopra Gloss p. 152)

b) Roxb. (Fl. indi) Ed. CBC 567)

c) A cold weather crop throughout India.

II a) मसूरः (Masūraḥ), सूप्यः (Sūpyaḥ), मङ्गल्यः (Maṅgalyaḥ), (Raj. Ni.)

b) (H. B. Mar. & Guj.) Masur, Masser, Masūri; (Tel.) Misurpapu, Chrisanagalu; (Kan.) Massur, Chanangi; (P.) Masur, Malka masur, Musri, (Assam) Masurmoha. (U.P.I. p. 322)

III 357 मसूरः– द्वित्रिवर्णः । शिम्बिधान्यप्रसिध्दः ।

१) वेश्यायां व्रीहिभेदे च मसूरा मसुरा स्त्रियाम् ।
मसूरमसुरौ पुंसि द्वावेतावपि चैतयोः ॥ इति रभसः । (Harshe)

२) 450 मसूरी चणकी पीतकलायश्चणको भवेत् ॥ ***Abhi. Manj.

३) मसूरा द्विविधाः –कृष्णा पाण्डुराश्च तत्र कृष्णवर्णा मसूराभिधानाः
पाण्डुवर्णा मङ्गल्यकाभिधानाः । Ḍalhaṇa - S.S.Su. 46.27.

---

* 'अस्याग्रे 'हरेणवः सतीनाश्च चणकाश्चाकरालकाः'।
इत्यधिकः पाठः आनन्दा. पुस्तके पठितः। तत्तु न पठनीयः असंगतत्वात् ।

१ 'सतिनामा च', 'सभ्यनामा च' इति पाठभेदौ आनन्दा. पुस्तके।

'मसूरः' पथ्यतर धान्येषु पठितः इति संस्मरणीयम् । *: करुन्तकटलक्क

IV 1) ...."From a consideration of Sanskrit, Persian and arabic names of the lentil and the evident connection of most local Indian names with these, *De candolle* arrives at the opinion that the plant was not known to India before the invasion of the Sanskrit speaking races. " Watt. Vol. Page 621.

27 गोधूमः Godhūmah

गोधूमा यवकश्चैव हुडुम्बो म्लेच्छभोजनः ॥ ८६
गिरिजः सत्यंनामा च रसिकश्च प्रकीर्तितः ॥
"वृष्यः शीतो गुरुः स्निग्धो जीवनो वातपित्तहा ॥ ८७
संधानो बृंहणो बल्यो गोधूमो स्थैर्यकृत्सरः ॥"A.H.Sū.6.15

गोधूमः (Godhūmaḥ), यवकः (Yavakaḥ), हुडुम्बः (Huḍumbaḥ), म्लेच्छभोजनः (Mlecchabhojanaḥ), गिरिजः (Girijaḥ), सत्यनामा (Satyanāmā), and रसिकः (Rasikaḥ) are synonymous.

Godhūma is *śītavīrya, guru* (heavy to digest), unctuous, vitalizer and pacifies *vāta* and *pitta doṣas*.It is union promoting, body promoting, strength promoting, *vṛṣya* and gives stability to the tissues of the body; and is laxative.

The compiler seems to have perhaps mentioned four kinds of Godhūma (1) यवकः (Yavakaḥ) grains having some similarity with यव (Yavaḥ), (2) हुडुम्बः (Huḍumbaḥ - Mlecchabhojanaḥ) (Perhaps related to or brought by Mohamedans, (3) गिरिजः (Girijaḥ) relates to the cultivation in mountainous area and (4) रसिकः (Rasikaḥ) a very fine variety. All belonging to the same species.

a) ***Triticum sativum*** Linn.

b) Roxb. fl. indi.

c) Cultivated extensively in Northern India and Deccan.

II a) गोधूमः (Godhūmaḥ), यवकः (Yavakaḥ), हुडुम्बः (Huḍumbaḥ), गिरिजः (Girijaḥ), रसिकः (Rasikaḥ), बहुदुग्धः(Bahudughaḥ) Raj.Ni.

b) (H) Gehu; (B.) Gam; (Mar.) Gahu; (Kan.) Godhi; (Tel.) Godumelu; (Tam.) Gadumai (Eng.) Wheat

III. Raj. Ni. has mentioned two varieties 1) गोधूमः (Godhūmaḥ) & (2) लघुगोधूमः (Laghugodhūmaḥ)

१) स्निग्धोऽन्यो लघुगोधूमःगुरुर्वृष्यः कफापहः । Raj. Ni. Varga 9

२) नान्दीमुखी मधूली च मधुर स्निग्धशीतले । C.S.Su. 27-22
नन्दिमुखी यविका, मधूली गोधूमभेद : । Cakraḥ

३) सुश्रुतस्तु कुधान्यवर्गे 'मधूली नन्दीमुखी' पठितवान् ।
यव गोधूम अतियवादिस्तु वैदले ।

४) सुमन इति- 'गोधूमको यवनक : सुमनश्चमठो मत : । इति केयदेवः । 'गोधूमसुमनौ समौ' इति रभस : । (Harshe p. 119)

IV .... "There is thus very nearly as strong presumptive evidence in favour of India being the home of some of the forms of wheat as can be shown for any other part of the globe . ...

It can also be abundantly demonstrated that most of these (i.e. forms of wheat) have been grown for countless ages on very nearly the same fields as they are to be found at the present day."

As in the case of rice, very numerous races of Wheat occur in India distinguished by variation in the colour of the grains, by being "bearded" or beardless" and by many other characters ....

Watt Vol. VI-IV p. 96.

28 माषः – धान्यमाषः Māṣaḥ - Dhānyamaṣaḥ

धान्यमाषस्तु विज्ञेयः कुरुविन्दो वृषाकरः ॥ ८८
मांसलश्च बलाढ्यश्च पित्र्यश्च पितृजोत्तमः ॥

स्निग्धोष्णो मधुरो वृष्यो मेदोमांसबलप्रदः ॥ ८९
वातनुद् बृंहणो बल्यो माषो बहुमलो गुरुः ॥

धान्यमाषः (Dhānyamāṣaḥ), कुरुविन्दः (Kuruvindaḥ),वृषाकरः (Vṛṣākaraḥ), मांसलः (Māmsalaḥ), बलाढ्यः (Balāḍhyaḥ), पित्र्यः (Pitryaḥ), and पितृजोत्तमः (Pitṛjottamaḥ) are synonymous.

Māṣa is unctuous, sweet in taste, *uṣṇavīrya, vṛṣya,* increases *meda* (fatty tissue), *māmsa* (muscular tissue) and gives strength. It pacifies *vātadoṣa*, is body promoting, heavy to digest and increases the quantity of faeces.

Fam. Leguminosae. Fabaceae

I a) ***Vigna mungo*** (Linn.) Hepper
Syn *Phaseolus radiatus* Roxb. non Linn.
P. mungo Linn. non Roxb. & auct.
Eng. Black gram (U.P.I.p. 677)

b) Roxburgh (fl. Indi.); Dymock (Pharm. indi.)

c) Cultivated all over India.

II a धान्यमाषः (Dhānyamāṣaḥ), कुरुविन्दः (Kuruvindaḥ), वृषाकरः (Vṛṣākaraḥ), पित्र्यः (Pitryaḥ).

b) (Sans.) Masha; (H.) Urd; (B.) Mashakalai; (Guj.) Adad, arad ; (Mar.) Udid, muga; (Tel.) Minimulu, Karu minimulu, nallaminimula; (Tam) Ulundu; (Kan.) uddu; (Mal.) Uzunnu.

III 1) माषः Māṣaḥ उरद (Urad)
C.S. Su. 2.27, 26. 107, 111-12., 27.3.23, etc.
C.S. Su. 14.36, 46.34 etc.
A.H. Su. 6.21, 22, 92 etc. (Balvantji)

2) ४५४ माषमाहुर्महामुद्गं धान्यमाषं मनीषिणः ।
कुक्कुण्डं वृष्यमुद्गाख्यं वातभेषजमित्यपि ॥
(Malya) उळुन्नु, Abhi. Manj.

IV Urd has two distinct cultivated forms, one with large black seeds, which ripens in August and September, the other with smaller green seeds, ripening in October and November. Both are however, sown at the commencement of the rains, but may also be occasionally grown as a spring crop in low wet fields, in which case it is sown in February and reaped in May."

Watt. Vol. VI 1 p. 192

29 चणकः Canakaḥ

हरिमन्थाः सुगन्धाश्च चणकाः' कृष्णकञ्चुकाः ॥ ९०
कफास्रपित्तपुंस्त्वघ्नाश्चणका वातला हिमाः ॥

लघवो भृष्टचणका श्रमक्लमहराः पराः ॥ ९१
छर्दिघ्ना रोचना शुष्कास्तेजोवीर्यबलप्रदाः ॥

हरिमन्थः (Harimanthaḥ), सुगन्धः (Sugandhaḥ), चणकः (Caṇakaḥ), कृष्णकञ्चुकः (Kṛṣṇakañcukaḥ) are synonymous.

Harimantha pacifiies *kapha, rakta* and *pitta doṣas,* and virility and aggravates *vātadoṣa* and is *śitavīrya.*

Parched (fried) *Caṇaka* removes fatigue and malaise, and is useful in emesis, is appetising, drying in nature and gives power, energy and strength.

I The compiler seems to have mentioned two types (1) सुगन्धः (Sugandaḥ) and (2) कृष्णकञ्चुकः (Kṛṣṇakañcukaḥ) while Raj. NI. has mentioned (1) कृष्णचणकः (Kṛṣṇacaṇakaḥ) and (2) श्वेतचणकः (Śweta caṇakaḥ)

Fam. Leguminosae. Fabaceae.

a) ***Cicer arietinum*** Linn.

b) Roxb. (fl. Indi. CBC Ed.) Yadavji and most of the modern writers.

c) Extensively cultivated all over India esp. in the northern provinces.

II a) हरिमन्थः (Harimanthaḥ), चणकः (Caṇakaḥ), कृष्णकञ्चुकः (Kṛṣṇakañcukaḥ)

b) (Sans.) Chanaka; (H.) But, chanā, chunnā, (B) cholā, but; (Guj.) Chanā, chania; (Mar.) Harabarā, chaṇe; (Tam.) Kadalai; (Tel.) Sanagalu; (Kan.) Kodale; (P.) Chole; (Eng.) Gram, Bengal gram, Chick Pea.

III 1) The varieties grown in North-Western provinces are classed as large grained and small grained, the former of a reddish and the latter of a light brown colour. There are also a black grained variety and a white grained known as "Cabuli". watt. vol. II. 275

२) चनेके रंग तथा नापके अनुसार कई भेद किये गये हैं जिनमे मुख्य दो वर्ग है। प्रथममें सभी रंगोंके चने आते हैं। दूसरे में काबुली आते हैं जो सफेद एवं बहुत बडे होते हैं। कुछ विद्वानोंनें काबुली क्षुप को भिन्न जातीका (Species) माना है।

(K. C. Chunekar Bh. Pr. NI. p. 649)

3) C.S. Su. 27.27, Ci. 3.189, 4.37 etc.
S.S. Su. 20.4, 46.27, 32 etc.
A.H. Ni. 7.46, Ci. 1.72 etc. (Balvantji).

IV 1) ...Its introduction into India is of more early date, for there is San skrit name and several other names in modern Indian languages. ... "The Western Aryans carried it into India. Its area may have extended from Persia to Greece, and the species now exists only in cultivated ground, where we do not know whether it springs from a stock originally wild or from cultivated plants." (De Candolle) (Watt. Vol. II. p.275).

30 वर्तुलः (चणकः) Vartulaḥ

कलायो मुण्डचणको हरेणुश्च सतीनकः ॥ ९२
त्रासनो नलकः कण्ठी हरेणुर्वर्तुलः स्मृतः ॥

वर्तुलः शीतलो ग्राही कफपित्तहरो लघुः॥ ९३
विपाके मधुरो रूक्षो वातलो भक्षणप्रियः ॥

कलायः (Kalāyaḥ), मुण्डचणकः (Muṇḍacaṇakaḥ), हरेणुः (Harenuḥ), सतीनकः (Satīnakaḥ), त्रासनः (Trāsanaḥ), नलकः (Nalakaḥ), कण्ठी (Kaṇthī), हरेणुः (Hareṇuḥ) and वर्तुलः (Vartulaḥ) are synonymous.

Kalāya is *śītavirya* and pacifies *kaphapitta doṣas,* aggravates *vāta doṣa,* astringent in action, *laghu* (easy to digest), sweet in *vipāka* (final transformation after digestion), *rukṣa* (roughening), and tasty

Fam. (Papilonaceae) (Leguminosae) Fabaceae.

I कलाय (Kalāya) has been used as a generic name,.

a) ***Pisum sativum*** Linn.
Syn. *P. arvense* Linn.

b) Roxb. (Fl. Indi. C.B.C.); most of the modern writers.

c) Cultivated generally.

II. a) कलायः (Kalāyaḥ), मुण्डचणकः (Muṇḍacaṇakaḥ), सतीनकः (Satīnakaḥ), वर्तुलः (Vartulaḥ).

b) (H) Matar, Mattar; (B.) Matar; (Mar.)Vāṭāṇe; (Guj.) Mataṇa, Vataṇā; (Kan.) Vatani; (Tel.) Gundusanagalu, Patnalu; (Tam.& Maly.) Pattani; (Eng.) Field Pea, Garden pea.

III. 1) C.Su. Su. 27.28, Ci. 20.36 etc.
S.S. Su. 19.16, 46.27, 221, 248, 277 etc.
A.H. Su. 6.18, 19.14 etc.

2) सतीनो वर्तुलकः; स्वल्पाः त्रिपुटाः; हरेणुः स्वल्पः वर्तुलः Dalhana
S. Su. 46.27.

3) Kalāya has been confused with सतीन Satina, Tripuṭa त्रिपुट and हरेणु Hareṇu. It appears that *Kalāya* has been used as a generic name for all the above in so much so that near about Varanasi the name *Kerāva* केराव (Kalaya) is given to *Satina* (Maṭara मटर) as well. ..... (Balwantji Page 84)

4) a) सतीनको वर्तुलको हरेणुः स्वल्पवर्तुलः।
सतीनो मधुरः पाके रसे रूक्षो हिमो लघुः ॥

b) हरेणुको हिमो रूक्षः ग्राही समधुरो लघुः ।

c) कलायः खण्डिको ज्ञेयः त्रिपुटः क्षुद्रखण्डिकः ।
कलायो मधुरस्तिक्तः सकषायो विरूक्षणः ॥
तद्वत् त्रिपुटकस्तेषां शाकं पित्तबलासजित् ॥ (Kaiyadeva Ni. p. 313)

This shows that Kaiyadeva has mentioned १) सतीनक Satinaka, २) हरेणुः Hareṇuḥ, ३) कलायः (खण्डिकः) Kalāyaḥ (Khaṇḍikaḥ) & ४) त्रिपुटः (क्षुद्रखण्डिकः) Tripuṭaḥ (Kṣudra khaṇḍikaḥ) separately.

5) .....खण्डिका त्रिपुटकलायः हरेणुः वर्तुलकलायः । कलायो वातलः इति त्रिपुटकलायः C.S. Su. 27.28 Cakrah

6) 166 'त्रिपुटः खण्डिकः साल्पा वज्रबीजा कलापि (य) का ।
श्यामोऽतिवर्तुलः सस्यादङ्कटः स हरेणुक ।' इति सिंह : ।
'कलापे (ये) ऽ पि हरेणुर्ना रेणुकायां स्त्रियां भवेत्' इति रुद्र : ।
कलाप (यः) स्त्रिकटः (त्रिपुटः) प्रोक्तः सतीनो वर्तुलो मतः ।
हरेणुरङ्कटो ज्ञेय'। (हरेणुः खण्डिको ज्ञेय) इति व्याडिः । (Harshe)

7) कलायचणको वातसखा गांगो गभंगिमः ।
शीतेश्वरो महारूक्षो लंका चेति प्रकीर्तितः । ४९१ Abhi. Manj.
कैरली - लङ्कै कटल

8) कलाय, त्रिपुट, खण्डिका- सतान- हरेणु सुश्रुतने वैदलोमें इन चारोंका पृथक् उल्लेख किया है ।
(सु. सू. ४६.२७) Ach- Priyavratji.

IV 1) *Pisum arvense* Linn
Mutter, Mattar, Rewari, Kulon, Desi matter (H.) ..etc.Vernacular names.
Habitat : .. According to De candolle wild in Italy where it grows in hedges and near cultivated ground but also in forests and wild mountainous districts. ... Royle appears to be the only Anglo Indian botanists who has considered the plant to be indigenous to India, and from philological and other evidences, there would seem to be little doubt, not only that it is always cultivated or spontaneous in this country, but that is of comparatively recent introduction. .... It is considered by many botanists to be the wild parent of the cultivated *Pisum satium*, and by Roxburgh is treated as a variety of that species. .... the two crops are generally treated as one. .... (Watt Vo. p. 227).

2) Food and fodder : This pea produces a small, round, compressed, greenish and marbled seed, which is generally eaten as dāl by natives. .... It must be carefully distinguished from kesāri dāl (*Lathyrus sativus*), which it considerably resembles both in the apperance of the grain and in the mode of cultivation ....
(Watt. VI - 1)

3) Vern. Bara matter, bathana, wattahna, gol mutter, battani chola, buttani (H.) .... etc.
Habitat : The garden pea had probably a more southern and more restricted original wild area. According to DeCandolle it has not hitherto found wild ...certain botanists have regarded as probably but a cultivated race, variety or at most subspecies of *P. arvensi,* but further observation and experiment is required.....
(Watt Vol. (VI - 1) p. 227-28).

31 कुलत्थः Kulattaḥ

कुलत्थास्ताम्रवर्णाश्च कलावृत्तानिलापहाः ॥ ९४
कर्षणा पीतमुदगाश्च अलिर्स्कन्धाः[१] सुराष्ट्रकाः ॥ ½

---

१ त्वलिस्कन्धाः इति चांखम्बा मुद्रित पाठः ।

"उष्णः कुलत्थो रसतः कषायः कटुर्विपाके कफमारुतघ्नः ।
शुक्राश्मरी गुल्मनिषूदनश्च संग्राहकः पीनसकासहन्ता ॥९५
आनाहमेदोऽरुचिकीलहन्ता श्वासापहः शोणितपित्तकृच्च ।
बलासहन्ता नयनामयघ्नो विशेषतो वन्यकुलत्थ उक्तः ॥"९६

(S.S.Su. 46. 37. 38)

कुलत्थः (Kulatthaḥ), ताम्रवर्णः (Tāmravarṇaḥ), कलावृत्तः (Kalāvṛttaḥ), अनिलापहः (Anilāpahaḥ), कर्षणः (Karṣaṇaḥ), पीतमुद्गः (Pītamudgaḥ), अलिस्कन्धः (Aliskandhaḥ) and सुराष्ट्रकः (Surāṣṭrakaḥ) are synonymous.

Kulattha is *kaṣāya* in taste, *uṣṇavīrya* and pungent in *vipāka* (final transformation after digestion) and pacifies *kapha* and *vāta doṣas.* It is useful in *śukrāśmarī*, tumour (diverticulosis), as an astringent, in rhinitis, cough, tympanitis, obesity, anorexia piles, dyspnoea and it may cause bleeding disorders. *Vanyakulattha* is especially useful in the diseses of the eyes and pacifies *kaphadoṣa.*

वन्यकुलत्थ (Vanya Kulattha) has been already mentioned in the Chapter III under the heading चक्षुष्या (Cakśuṣyā).

The compiler of Dhn. Ni. has not clearly mentioned but Raj. Ni. has mentioned three types (a) ताम्रबीजः (Tāmrabījaḥ) (b) श्वेतबीजः (Swetabījaḥ), and c) सितेतर बीजः (Sitetarabījaḥ).

Fam. Leguminosae. Fabaceae

a) ***Dolichos uniflorus*** Lamk.

b) 1) Roxburgh (Fl. Indi.)

2) Most of the modern writers.

c) Himalayas to Ceylon, cultivated and wild.

II a) कुलत्थः (Kulatthaḥ), ताम्रवर्णः (Tāmravarṇaḥ), कलावृत्तः (Kalāvṛttaḥ), पीतमुद्गः(?) (Pītamudgaḥ), कर्षणः (Karṣaṇaḥ).

b) (Sans.) Kulattha; (H.) Kulthi; (b.) Kurtikalai; (Mar.) Kuḷith, Kulathi; (Guj.) Kalathi, Kulit; (Mal.) Muthiva, Muthera; (Tel.) Ulavalu; (Tam.) Kollu; (Kan.) Hural; (Eng.) Horsegram.

III 1) C.S. Su 26.112, 27.25. Ci. 3 188 etc.
S.S. Su. 19.16, 46.37, 366, etc.
A.H.Su. 6. 19.33 7:32 etc.
A. H. Su. 6.19, 33, 7.32 etc.

2) 'कुलित्थस्ताम्रबीजश्च श्वेतबीजः सितेतरः । Raj. Ni

IV 1) According to the flora of British India there are two forms of this plant. (*D. uniflorus*), a suberect annual, and (*D. biflorus*) a more or less twining plant. The habitats of these forms are not sepa-

---

**Dolichos uniflorus* Lamk.
Syn. *D. biflorous* auct. (non Linn.) (Comp. p. 55).

rately recorded. ... In popular works on Economic products the Horse gram of Madras is viewed as *D. uniflorus*, and under either of these names (*D. biflorus or D. uniflorus*)a pulse is described as grown, one might almost say, in every dist. of India, but chiefly in Madras and Bombay . ....

2) ......Roxburgh refers to two forms, one with grey, the other with black seeds both of which he implies are cultivated in Bengal and Madras. ... (Watt. Vol. III- Page. 175-176).

जूर्णा Jūrṇā (7*)

जूर्णाह्वा योनला प्रोक्ता यावनाला युगन्धरा ।
कफपित्तहरा वृष्या मृदवो गुरवो हिमाः ॥ ९७
रूक्षा विष्टम्भिनश्चैव न पथ्या गुदरोगिणाम् ॥

जूर्णाह्वः (Jūrṇāhavaḥ), योनलः (Yonalaḥ), यावनालः (Yāvanālaḥ), युगन्धरः (Yugandharaḥ), are synonymous.

Jūrṇā is *śitavīrya,* pacifies *kaphapitta doṣas, guru* (heavy to digest), soft, *vṛṣya*, roughening, constipating and is not beneficial to those having diseases of anus (anal canal).

I. The compiler of Dh. Ni. has not mentioned the kinds of *Jurṇā* while Raj. Ni. has mentioned (a) धवलो यावनालः (Dhavalo yāvanālaḥ - white grained), (b) रक्तयावनालः (Rakta - Yāvanālaḥ) both belonging to the same species.

Fam. Poaceae

a) ***Sorghum bicolor*** (Linn.) Moench
Syn. *S. vulgare* (Linn.) Pers.
Andropogon sorghum Brot.

b) Roxburgh

c) Widely cultivated in India.

II. a) जूर्णाह्वा (Jūrṇāhvā), यावनालः (Yāvanālaḥ).

b) (Sans.) Dirgham(n)āla; (H.P.B &Bom.) Joar, Jowar; (Tam.) Cholam; (Tel.) Jonalu; (Mal.) Chavela; (Kun.) Jolah (Chopra Gloss. p. 231)

III 1) The Śodhala Nighaṇṭu has mentioned some other varieties of जूर्णा(Jūrṇā)

* शोढल (Sodhala) has mentioned जूर्णावर्ग (Jūrṇā class) separately and has given some importance to it. It seems by his time *Jurṇā* had become a staple food of the people of the Deccan. Ach. Priyavratji Sharma has placed Śodhala in the later part of the 12th Century.

ललिता क्रोष्टुपुच्छा च श्रीखंडी च सुगंधिका ।
कृष्णा भाद्रपदी चान्या श्वेता मंटाऽथ जूर्णका ॥
रक्तिका कुक्षिकाद्याश्च बह्व्यो जूर्णाह्वजातयः । (Śodhala p. 172).

IV 1) Juar takes the first place as the staple of Indian diet and ranks a long way before wheat, barley, or Indian corn. The millon of the population of India live far more on millets and pulses than rice, wheat and barley. The chief millets are *Juar* and *Bajra,* but of the former there are numerous varieties and races and even (according to some botanists) several species. ...
(Watt. Vol. VI. Part 3).

2) Dr. Roxburgh at the beginning of this *century, referred the Indian forms to Andropogon and described five species under the section, now isolated as the genus sorghum .....
(Watt Vol. VI Part 3 Page 277).

3) Grains from various spp. used as a cereal, is known as Jowar, fodder obtained from Sorghums is also known by the same name. Mary derivatives and adjectival modifications of this name as well as some other regional names are common, especially in South India. Tel. & Oriya-*Jonna;* Tam. & Mal-*Cholam*; Kan.-*Jola*. Regional names are confusing and cannot be easily related to correct botanical names of species, several sorghum varieties with juicy and palatable stalks have been developed and grown exclusively for fodder purposes. (U.P.I. Page 586)

4) (Dalzell & Gibson) These authors tell us that in Western India it is known as *Shallū* (Eastern Deccan & Gujarat) and they add, "The stalks, as forage for cattle is unsurpassed, it contains a great deal of a saccharine matter and is thus very nutritive. ....
(Watt Vo. VI Part 3 p. 282)

5) Raj. Ni. notes a kind of sugar obtained from यावनाल (Yāvanāla) under a heading यावनाली (Yāvanālī.)
यावनाली हिमोत्पन्ना हिमानी हिमशर्करा ।
क्षुद्रशर्करिका क्षुद्रा गुडजा जलबिन्दुजा ॥ Raj. Ni. Chapter 15th

6) स्याद् यावनाल रसपाकभवो गुडोऽयं क्षारः कषायमधुरः कफवातहारि ।
पित्तप्रदः सततमेव निषेव्यमाणः कण्डुकुष्ठजननोऽस्रविदाहदायी ॥
भोजकुतूहल.

Here are mentioned the properties of Jaggary (Gur) obtained from the stalks of Jowar.

7) Śodhala mentions about the sugar obtained from the leaves of जूर्णा (Jurṇā). जूर्णापत्रोद्भवा किञ्चित् गुणैर्न्यूना भवेदिह ।
Śodhala Ni. 164.

* i.e. at the beginning of the 19th Century.

This reminds us the sugar obtained known as यासशर्करा (Yāsaśarkarā) or तुरंजबीन (Turanjabīn).

करटः Karaṭaḥ (8)

करटाश्च करालाश्च त्रिपुटा खण्डिका मताः ॥ ९८
करालः कफपित्तघ्नो ग्राही शीतोऽतिवातलः ॥
त्रिपुटोऽपि गुणैरेवं तच्छाकं कफपित्तजित् ॥ ९९

करटः (Karaṭaḥ), करालः (Karālaḥ), त्रिपुटः (Tripuṭaḥ) and खण्डिकः (Khaṇḍikah) are synonymous.

Karāla is *śītavīrya*, pacifies *kapha* and *pitta doṣas* and aggravates *vātadoṣa*.

Tripuṭa is having the similar properties and its vegetable pacifies *kapha* and *pitta doṣas*.

I. The compiler has mentioned here two kinds (a) कराल (Karāla) and (b) त्रिपुट (Tripuṭa). We have discussed already about कलायः (Kalāyaḥ) Pre. NO. 30 III 3 & 4.

a) ***Lathyrus sativus*** Linn.

b) Roxburgh (Fl. Indi.) & modern writers.

c) It is cultivated all over India.

II a) करालः (Karālaḥ)त्रिपुटः (Tripuṭaḥ), खण्डिकः (Khaṇḍikaḥ) लङ्का (Lankā) (Raj. Ni.)

b) (Sans.) Khandika, tripuṭi; (H.) Khesari, Latri, Tiuri, Kassar (B.) Khesari; (Mar.) Lakh, Lankh; (Guj.) Lang; (Oriya) Khesra; (Assam) Khesari, teora; (Bihar) Kesari, Kansari, batura; (P.) Chural, Karal, Karil; (Nepal) Kesari.

III 1) See Pre. No. 30. III 3 & 4.
सतीनक (Satīnaka), हरेणुः स्वल्पवर्तुलः (Hareṇuḥ swalpa vartulaḥ,) कलायः खण्डिकः (Kalāyaḥ Khaṇḍikaḥ) त्रिपुटः क्षुद्रखण्डिकः (Triputaḥ Kśudrakhaṇḍikaḥ)

2) कलायचणको वातसखा गांगो गभंगिमः ।
शीतेश्वरो महारूक्षो लंका चेति प्रकीर्तितः । ४५१(Abhi Manj.)

IV 1) An annual herb, indigenous according to De Candolle in the region extending from the South of the caucasus, to the North of India.

It has spread as a weed from its original home. It is cultivated all over India...... (Watt Vo. IV. p. 591)

निष्पावः Niṣpāvaḥ (9)

निष्पावा श्वेतशिम्बाश्च पालकाख्या मुखप्रियाः ।
निष्पावोऽनिलपित्तास्रमूत्रस्तन्यकरः सरः ॥१०३
विदाह्युष्णो गुरुः शोषशोफकृच्छुक्रनाशनः ।

निष्पावः (Niṣpāvaḥ), श्वेतशिम्बः (Śvetaśimbaḥ), पालकाख्यः (Pālakakhyaḥ), and मुखप्रियः (Mukhapriyaḥ) are synonymous.

Niṣpāva aggravates *vāta, pitta* and *raktadoṣas*, is galactogogue, mild laxative, *vidāhi* (causing regurgitation with hyperacidity and poor digestion), *uṣnavīrya, guru* (heavy to digest), causes consumption, oedema and decreases *śukra.*

I.. Though the compiler of the Dhn. Ni. has not clearly mentioned that it is a generic name but according the S. Samhita and other Nighaṇṭus it seems to be a generic name. Thus Raj. Ni. has mentioned along with (a) श्वेतशिम्ब orनिष्पाव the other kind. (B) कट्टनिष्पाव or नदीनिष्पाव

Fam. Fabaceae

a) ****Lablab purpureus*** (Linn.) sweet
Syn. *Dolichos lablab* Linn.

b) Roxb. (fl. indi. C.B.C.)

c) Cultivated and wild all over India, ascending in the Himalayas to 6-7 thousand feet.

II निष्पावः (Niṣpāvaḥ), श्वेतशिम्बः (Śwetasimbaḥ), पालकाख्यः (Pālakākhyaḥ), मुखप्रियः (Mukhapriyaḥ) (Dh. Ni.) कट्टनिष्पावः (Katuniṣpāvaḥ) नदीनिष्पावः (Nadīniṣpāvaḥ) (Raj. Ni.).

b) (H.)) Sem (B.) Shim (Guj.) val (Mar.)Pāvaṭā (Vāla) (tel.) Chikkudu (Tam.) Avarai (Kan.) Chapparada avare (Mal) Avara (U.P.I. p. 182)

१) सितासिताः पीतक रक्तवर्णा भवन्तियेऽनेकविधास्तु शिम्बाः ।
यथादितस्ते गुणतः प्रधाना ज्ञेयाः कटूष्णा रसपाकयोश्च ॥
सु. सू. ४६.४५.४६

२) सस्नेहा बलिभिर्भोज्या विविधाः शिम्बिजातय : । C.S.Su.27.31

---

* *Dolichos lablab* var. *typicus* Prain
Dolichos lablab Var. *lignosus* Prain (U.P.I.p. 182)

विविधाः शिम्बिजातयः इति कृष्णपीतरक्तश्वेतकुशिम्बी भेदाः ..
निष्पावो वल्लः । (Cakraḥ vide above)

३) निष्पाव एलकाख्यो मुखप्रियो मायुगण्डूषः ।
मलकृद्बलहः शिम्बी प्रमाह्वयो श्रीक उच्यते सद्भिः ॥४५२
वननिष्पाविकी शिम्बी कण्टकी वनरंजिनी ।
अगमा च त्रिपर्णीति राजनिष्पाविकी भवेत् ॥४५३ Abhi. Manj.
निष्पाव- अवर । वननिष्पाविकी- काट्टवर

IV. 1) The final conclusions which the writer has arrived at regarding the word *Lobiya* may be expressed briefly: (1) It is incorrectly applied to any species of *Dolichos* or *Phaseolus;* (2) It is of persian origin and may by adaptation have been assigned by the early Persian and Mogul conquerers of India to *Vigna catiang*, but (3) as used by the Indian market gardners of the present day, it is a generic name for any introduced pulse or bean and is no way specific. (Watt. Vol. III p. 186)

2) *Dolichos lablab*

...... The existance of it as a wild plant,combined with the extensive series of vernacular names especially those of lower, eastern and southern India, leave no room for doubt as to its being a native of India indicated as the area of its indigenous habitat. (Watt Vol. III. p. 186).

मेथिका Methikā (14)

मेथिका दीपनी चोग्रा कुञ्चिका बहुपत्रिका ॥ १०१
मल्लिका शीतवीर्या[१] च ज्योतिष्का वल्लरी शिखी ॥

मेथिका कटुरुष्णा च रक्तपित्तप्रकोपनी ॥ १०२
अरोचकहरा दीप्तिकरी वातप्रणाशिनी ॥

मेथिका (Methikā), दीपनी (Dīpanī), उग्रा (Ugrā), कुञ्चिका (Kuñcikā), बहुपत्रिका (Bahupatrikā), मल्लिका (Mallikā), (अ) शीतवीर्या (Śītavīryā), ज्योतिष्का (Jyotiṣkā), वल्लरी (Vallarī), and शिखी (Śikhī) are synonymous.

Methikā is pungent in taste, *uṣṇavīrya* and pacifies *vātadoṣa.* It aggravates *raktapitta* (bleeding disorders.) . It is antianorexic and stimulates digestive capacity.

Fam. Leguminosae. (Papilionaceae). Fabaceae.

a) ***Trigonella foenum-graecum*** Linn.

---

१ 'मल्लिकाऽशीतवीर्या' इतिसाधुपाठः भविष्यति ।

b) Roxburgh (Fl. Ind. CBC).

c) Wild in Kashmir, the Punjab and the upper Gangetic plain, widely cultivated in many parts of India (Watt.)

II a) मेथिका (Methikā) उग्रा (Ugra), बहुपत्रिका (Bahupatrikā), ज्योतिष्का (Jyotiṣkā), वल्लरी (Vallarī),

b) (Sans) Methika, Chandrika; (H)Methi; (B) Methi, Methishak; (Mar) Methi; (Guj). Methi, Methini Bhahji; (Tel.) Mentikoora (Herb) Mentulu (Seed); (Tam.) Vendayam; (Kan.) Menthya, Mentesoppu, Mente; (Mal.) Uluva, Venthium.

III तन्त्रान्तरे माथिका हिस्पित्थयोः पृथग्गुणनिर्देशः कृतः
'वातपित्तहरा तिक्ता लघ्वी श्लेष्माविरोधिनी ।
मेथिका तत्समं किंचिद् हिस्फित्थं पुष्टिदं गुरु ॥ '

Ḍalhaṇa S. S. Su. 46.256.

वनमेथिका Vanamethikā (15)

मेथिका* वास्तिका सेलुः हिस्पित्थो[१] वनमेथिका ॥ १०३
हिस्फित्थो[२]ऽल्पगुणस्तस्या वाजिनां स तु पूजितः ॥

मेथिका (Methikā), and वास्तिका (Vāstikā), are synonymous and सेलुः (Seluḥ), हिस्पित्थ (Hisphittha) and वनमेथिका (Vanamethikā) are synonymous.

Hispittha is little less in potency and beneficial to the horses.

The compiler probably desires to include two plants A) मेथिका (Methikā), वनमेथिका (Vanamethikā), B) हिस्पित्थ (Hispittha).

I A-a- ***Melilotus indica*** (Linn.) All.
Syn. *M. parviflora* Desf.
Trifolium indicum Linn.

B -a ***Medicago sativa*** Linn.

A&B

b Roxburgh (Fl.Indi)A Chunekar (Bh.Pr.), Gloss. chopra (p. 248)

c Bombay Presidency, Bengal, North West provinces and Punjab, Cultivated or found as cultivation weed. (Watt.)
Tropical zone of India. (Gloss. Chopra p. 164)

B. Persia, Afganistan, Buluchistan, Kashmir. (Watt)

A&B

---

* Methikā proper has been already mentioned under, मेथिका. Here it is mentioned again and should be understood for (Vanamethikā)

१ 'अहित्थो' २ 'अहित्थो' इति आनन्दाश्रममुद्रित पुस्तके ।

II मेथिका (Methikā), वास्तिका (Vāstikā), सेलुः (Seluḥ), हिस्फित्थः (Hispitthaḥ), वनमेथिका (Vanamethikā).

b (A)(Sans.) Banmethikā; (H.B.) Bammethi; (P. Delhi, Bihar, Bengal) Senji, Metha, Banmethi; (Orissa), Banmethi, huringupu. (Bom.) Vanmethica, ranmethi, Jhir, Zir (U.P.I. p.362)

(B) (H.) Wilayatigawuth, Lasunghās; (Mar.) Vilayatīgavat (Guj.) Vilayatighās; (Kan.) Vilayatihullu; (Ladakh) Hol; (Punjab) Lusun. (U.P.I. p.359)

अश्वबला तुरुष्कदेशे बृहत्पत्रा मेथिकाभेद एव 'हिस्पित्थ इति लोके । तन्त्रान्तरे मेथिका हिस्पित्थयोः पृथक्गुणनिर्देशः कृतः "वातपित्तहरा तिक्ता लघ्वी श्लेष्माविरोधिनी ।
मेथिका तत्समं किंचित् हिस्पित्थं पुष्टिदं गुरु ॥'इति ।

Ḍalhaṇa, S.S.Su. 46.256

अश्वबला हिस्पित्थो मेथिकाभेद : (Su. Ci. 6.5)

ब्रह्मदेवस्तु अश्वबला यवनभूमौमेथिकाकारबीजा भवतीत्याह ।

Ḍalhaṇa S.Ci. 1.183

नारी नामौषधि : 'अश्वबला इति विज्ञायते या बल्वज सदृशपत्रा'C.Ci. 1.4.7.

'अश्वबलेति ज्ञायते इति ऋषिभिरेवानेन नाम्ना ज्ञायते, न लौकिकः लोकाप्रसिद्धत्वात् ।'Cakraḥ

अश्वबला बृहत्पत्रा मेथिका ।'S.S. 46. 256. Cakraḥ (Bhanumati)

IV *Medicago sativa* Linn.
Lucerne or Purple Lucerne.
Some difference of opinion prevails as to the botanical position to be assigned.....
Fodder : A common weed, collected frequently for fodder .....
Vern : Wilayatki gawuth; (H.); Vilayati ghas; (Guj.) Alfalfa .. fisfisat (Arab.); Isfist (Pers.) (Watt. Vol V p. 199)

अतसी Atasī (16)

प्रतरीर्कतमा प्रोक्ता रुद्रपत्नी सुवल्कला ॥ १०४
उमा सुनीलपुष्पा च वसुतर्का क्षुमाऽपि च ॥

शीता तैलफला चेव पालिका पूतिपूरकः॥ १०५
रुद्रपत्नी तु मधुरा स्निग्धा च बलकारिका ॥

कफवातकरी चेषत्पित्तहृत् कुष्ठवातजित् ॥ १०६

(अन्यच्च)

अतसी नीलपुष्पी च पार्वती स्यादुमा क्षुमा ।

प्रतरीर्कतमा (Pratarīrkatamā), रुद्रपत्नी (Rudrapatnī), सुवल्कला (Suvalkalā), उमा (Umā), सुनीलपुष्पा (Sunīlapuṣpā), वसुतर्का (Vasutarkā), क्षुमा (Kśumā), शीता (Śītā), तैलफला (Tailaphalā), पालिका (Pālikā), पूतिपूरकः (Pūtipūrakaḥ are synonymous.

Rudrapatnī is sweet in taste, aggravates *kapha vāta doṣas* and slightly pacifies *pitta.* It is unctuous, strength promoting, and useful in disorders of skin and *vātarakta*. (?).

According to another text:

अतसी (Atasī), नीलपुष्पी (Nīlapuspī), पार्वती (Pārvatī), उमा (Umā) and क्षुमा (Kśumā) are synonymous.

According to D. K. Kamat (See Introduction to Vol.1) two plants are recorded by the Compiler. (A) उमा (Umā) and (B) क्षुमा (Kśumā) belonging to different families.

(Fam. Linaceae)

I A-a ***Linum usitatissimum*** Linn.
B ***Boehmeria nivea*** Gaud (Fam.urticaceae)

A-b Roxburgh (Fl. Indi.)
B Roxburgh (Fl. Indi.)

A-c Cultivated throughout India upto 6000 ft.
B Cultivated Assam, eastern and northern Bengal etc. (Watt.)

II A & B

प्रतरीर्कतमा (Pratarīrkatamā), सुवल्कला (Suvalkalā), उमा (Umā), सुनीलपुष्पा (Sunīlapuṣpā), क्षुमा (Kśumā)

A) (SK & Tel) Atasi; (H) Alsi; (B) Masina, Tist; (Bom.) Alasi; (Tam.) Alshi; (Mal.) Cheruchanavittintevilta.

B) Schou or Schu or Tehou (the plant), Schou ma (Fibre of Schou) (Watt. vol II. p. 468)

China Grass, Rhea, Ramie.

(Beng.) Kankura; (Assam) Rhea.

III 1) कौटिलीय अर्थशास्त्र २.१२.१६ (Kautilīya Arthashastra 2.12.16)

2) व्रण बन्धन द्रव्याणि क्षौमम् . . . . अतसी तन्तुभिर्व्यूतं अन्ये वस्त्रान्तर- माहुः । क्षौमम्. Cloth woven by the fibres of Atasī, but some others call it as a cloth prepared by different fibres.

Ḍalhaṇa S. S. Su. 14.36.

3) The writer (**Buchanan & Hamilton**) has repeatedly urged, in this work, that the mere existence of Sanskrit names, which by present universal admission allude to a certain plant, should not unreservedly be accepted, as De Candolle very frequently does, to prove ancient cultivation in India. ... Watt. Vol. V. Page 7

4) .... Kshuma, the name which of all others would carry the Asiatic knowledge in linen furthest back, is by some writers supposed to denote silk, indeed, its resemblance to chuma, the chinese for grass cloth, has been suggested as worthy of consideration. Watt V. Page 5.

5) Source of an excellent, lustrous, strong and durable fibre, used for fabrics, plushes and knit material and paper. Gas mantles of good quality are made from it. Ramie is generally used mixed with wool, silk and cotton, its special use being in the manufacture of lustrous, non creasable fabrics (U.P.I. Page 76)

कुसुम्भम् Kusumbham (17)

कुसुम्भं पावकं पीतमलक्तं वस्त्ररञ्जनम् ।
कौसुम्भं स्यात वह्निशिखं वस्त्ररञ्जकसंज्ञितम् ॥१०७

तद्बीजं कीलता लट्वा शुद्धा पद्मोत्तरा तथा ।
कुसुम्भं वातलं रूक्षं रक्तपित्तकफापहम् ॥१०८

कुसुम्भं (Kusumbham), पावकं (Pāvakam), पीतं (Pītam), अलक्तं (Alaktam), वस्त्ररञ्जनं (Vastrarañjanam), कौसुम्भं (Kausumbham), वह्निशिखं (Vahniśikham), वस्त्ररञ्जकं (Vastrarañjakam), are synonymous.

Its seeds are called as कीलता (Kīlatā), लट्वा (Laṭvā), शुद्धा (Śuddhā), पद्मोत्तरा and (Padmottarā).

Kusumbha aggravates *vāta* and pacifies *kapha doṣa,* it is roughening and useful in bleeding disorders.

The compiler of Dhn. Ni. has mentioned only कुसुम्भम् (Kusumbham) while Raj. Ni. has mentioned अरण्यकुसुम्भम् (Araṇya Kumsumbham).

I ***Carthamus tinctorius*** Linn.

A-a- Eng. Safflower.

B- ***Carthamus oxycantha*** Bieb.
Eng. Wild safflower.

A-b- Roxburgh (Fl. Indi.) .

B- Roxburgh (Fl. Indi.)

A-c- Cultivated throughout a large part of India.

B Wild in the arid tracts of Punjab, Baluchistan, N.W.F. province, a troublesome weed.

II a) वस्त्ररञ्जनम् (Vastrarañjanam), वह्निशिखम् (Vahniśikham)

कुसुम्भम (Kusumbham), पीतम (Pītam)

b) अरण्यकुसुम्भम् (Araṇyakusumbham) (R. Ni.)
(b) (A) (Sans.) Kusumbha; (H.) Kusum, Karrah; (B) Kusumphul; (Guj.) Kusumbo; (Mar.) Kardai, Kardi; (Tam.) Sendurakam; (Tel.) Kushumbo;(Kan.) Kusambe, Kusume; (B) (Punjab) Kantiari, Poli, Poliyan, Kasar.

III See IV-1

IV 1) कुसुम्भ Kusumbha
Carthamus tinctorius Linn., Barre बर्रे, Syn.लट्वा
C.S. Su. 13.9, 27.98, 107, 288. etc.
S.S. Su. 45.115, 119, 46.48, 272. etc.
A.H. Su. 5.61, 6.24, 101, 7.33 etc. (Balwantji)

2) *Carthamus oxycantha* Bieb.
Habitat wild in North West Provinces and the Punjab ... Mr. C. B. Clarke thinks this may be the wild form of Safflower.
Watt. Vol. II P. 183

3) ... It has never been found in a wild state, but botanists assign to it an origin in India, Africa or Abyssinia. ... Watt. Vol. II. Page 184.

खस्तिलः Khastilaḥ (18) खस्तिलवल्कलः Khastilavalkalaḥ (19) अफूकम् Aphūkam

खस्तिलस्तिलभेदस्तु शुभ्रपुष्पो लसत्फलः ।
वृष्यो बल्यश्च खस्तिलः श्लेष्मघ्नो वातजिद् गुरुः ॥१०९

वल्कलस्तत्फलो ज्ञेयो रूक्षो ग्राहि विशोषणः ।
अफूकं तद्द्रवीभूतमहिफेनमफेनकम् ॥११०

अफूकं शोषणं ग्राही श्लेष्मघ्नं वातपित्तलम् ॥

खस्तिलः (Khastilaḥ), is a type of *tila* of which synonyms are शुभ्रपुष्पः (Śubhrapuṣpaḥ), and लसत्फलः (Lasatphalaḥ).

Khastila pacifies *vāta* and *kapha doṣas*, is *guru*, *vṛṣya* and strength promoting.

The capsule of the fruit (Phalavalkalaḥ), is roughening, astringent and drying.

Aphūkam -opium (milky sap) obtained from it is called by synonyms अहिफेनं (Ahiphenam) and अफेनं (Aphenam).

Aphūkam pacifies *kaphadoṣa,* aggravates *vāta* and *pitta doṣa.* It is astringent and drying.

I a) ***Papaver somniferum*** Linn.

b) Roxburgh (Fl. Indi.)

c) Cultivated in Uttar pradesh, E. Punjab, (Jullandar and shiarpur), various parts of Rajputana and Madhyabharat.

II a) The seeds खस्तिलः (Khastilaḥ), शुभ्रपुष्पः (Śubhrapuṣpaḥ); लसत्फलः (Lasatphalaḥ) Poppy, फलवल्कलः (Phalavalkalaḥ). The milky sap obtained by scratching the unripe fruit अफूकं (Aphūkam), अहिफेनम् (Ahiphenam).

IV I) That the followers of the faith of Islam proclaimed the properties of opium to the people of India there can be no doubt, since the Sanskrit and all the vernacular names in this country are traceable to the Semetic corruption ... *Afyun.* Thus its best known Sanskrit name is *Ahiphena* and its Hindi Afim. But direct historic records exists which also leave no room for doubt that poppy was not known to the people of India prior to the Arab influence. ....

Interest in the oil yielding seeds and the medicinal capsules had thus been fully aroused in Asiatic countries anterior to the introduction of opium. It is therefore, not difficult to understand the existence of names for these parts of the plant that are undoubtedly more ancient than the word opium.

(Watt. Vol VI. Part I Page 24)

तिलः Tilaḥ (21)

तिलस्तु होमधान्यं स्यात्पवित्रः पितृतर्पणः ॥ १११
पापघ्नः पूतधान्यश्च जर्तिलस्तु वनोद्भवः ॥

तिलो रसे कटुस्तिक्तो मधुरस्तुवरो गुरुः॥ ११२
विपाके कटुकः स्वादुः स्निग्धोष्णः कफपित्तनुत् ॥

बल्यः केश्यो हिमस्पर्शस्त्वच्यः स्तन्यो व्रणे हितः ॥ ११३
दन्त्योऽल्पमूत्रकृद्ग्राही वातघ्नोऽग्निमतिप्रदः ॥

तिलः (Tilaḥ), होमधान्यं (Homadhānyam), पवित्रः (Pavitraḥ), पितृतर्पणः (Pitṛtarpaṇaḥ), पापघ्नः (Pāpaghnaḥ), and पूतधान्यः (Pūtadhānyaḥ) are synonymous.जर्तिलः (Jartilaḥ) is (an uncultivated) wild form.

Tila is pungent, bitter, sweet and *kaṣāya* in taste and *guru,* pungent and sweet in *vipāka, uṣṇavīrya*, unctuous and pacifies *kapha pitta doṣas,* strength promoting, beneficial for hair, cool to touch, beneficial to skin, breast milk, and wounds, beneficial to teeth, decreases the quantity of urine, is astringent, pacifies *vātadoṣa* and decreases digestive capacity.Two kinds are mentioned 1) कृषित (Cultivated) and वनोद्भवः (Wild)

Fam. Pedaliaceae.

I a) ***Sesamum indicum*** Linn.

b) Roxburgh (Fl. Indi.)

c) Cultivated all over India.

I a) होमधान्यं (Homadhānyam), पवित्रः (Pavitrah), वनोद्भवः जर्तिलः (Vanodbhavaḥ Jartilaḥ) = a wild kind.

b) (Sans.) Tila; (H. & Mar.) Til; (Guj.) Tal; (Tel.) Nevvulu; (Tam.) & (Kan.) Karuthellu; (Oriya) Khasa, rasi; (Punjab) Til, Tilli.

III 1) C.S. Su. 2.25, 27, 26, 107. 116, 27.29, 106, 225, 265, 282. etc.
S.S. Su. 11.11, 21, 22, 44.74, 46.40. etc.
A.H. Su. 6.23, 7.41, etc.

IV *Races or varieties of sesamum.*

.... Sesamum may be viewed as indigenous in India, if indeed, it cannot be regarded as occuring at the present day in a truely wild state . ...

The information such as it exists, leads forcibly to one conclusion, viz. that sesamum has been cultivated in India from as a remote a period as rice. .... (Watt . VI Part II Page 504. 05).

2) There are two varieties White (श्वेत) and Black (कृष्ण) of Tila mentioned and used in the texts, where only *Tail* (तैल) (oil) has been mentioned without specifying the source, *Tilataila* (Tila oil) is intended. (Balvantji 183)

द्रवद्रव्याणि (Liquid substances)

32 तैलम् (Tailam) (Oil) oil group.

तैलं स्नेहोत्तमं प्रोक्तं तिलजं तिलसम्भवम् ॥ ११४
अभ्यञ्जनं म्रक्षणञ्च तच्च मर्दनकं स्मृतम् ॥

सकषायं रसे स्वादु सूक्ष्ममुष्णं व्यवायि च ॥ ११५
पित्तलं बद्धविण्मूत्रं न च श्लेष्मविवर्धनम ॥ Ca. Su. 27. 286

तैलम् (Tailam), स्नेहोत्तमं (Snehottamam), तिलजं (Tilajam), तिलसम्भवम् (Tilasambhavam), अभ्यञ्जनं, (Abhyañjanam), म्रक्षणम् (Mrakṣaṇam), मर्दनकं (Mardanakam) are synonymous.

Tailam is *kaṣāya* and sweet in taste, *uṣṇavīrya,* aggravates *pittadoṣa* and does not increase *kapahadoṣa,* enters the fine channels of the body, rapidly spreads (*vyavāyī*) and causes binding of faeces and urine.

Properties and actions of various oils.

तिलतैलम् (Tilatailam) (Seasamum oil) (22)

स्नानाभ्यङ्गावगाहेषु तिलतैलं विशिष्यते ॥ ११६
तद्वत् वस्तिषु पानेषु नस्यकर्णाक्षिपूरणे ॥ Su. Sū. 45.113

अन्नपानविधौ चाऽपि प्रयोज्यं वातशान्तये ॥ ११७
छिन्नभिन्नच्युतोत्पिष्टमथितक्षतपातिते ॥

भग्ने स्फुटितविद्धाग्निदग्धविश्लिष्टदारिते ॥ ११८
भयाभिहतनिर्भुग्ने मृगव्यालादिभक्षिते ॥

तैलयोगश्च संस्कारात्सर्वरोगापहो मतः ॥११९

Tila taila is specifically indicated for bath, massage and immersion of the body. Similarly, it is used in बस्ति (*Basti*- process), instillation into nose, ears, eyes and in the processing of food to pacify the *vātadoṣa.*

It is specially useful in various types of injuries of the body like excision, incision, dislocation, crushed, fractured, churned, wounded, fallen, broken, torn, punctured, burnt by fire, loosened, frightened, bent and torn from the assult by wild animals.

By various methods of processing *taila* is useful in various types of diseases.

अतसीतैलम् (oil obtained from Atasi seeds) (23)

वातघ्नं मधुरं तेषु क्षौमं तैल बलासकृत्[१] । S.S. 45. 116

Out of these, *Atasitaila* is sweet in taste, pacifies *vātadosa* and aggravates *kapha doṣa.*

१ 'बलापहम्' इति सुश्रुतः ।

सर्षपतैलम् Sarṣapa tailam (24)

कटुपाकमचक्षुष्यं स्निग्धोष्णं कफनाशनम् ॥ १२०
कृमिघ्नं सार्षपं तैलं कण्डूकुष्ठापहं लघु ॥

Sarṣapataila is pungent in *vipāka* (final transformation after digestion), *uṣṇavīrya*, *laghu* and pacifies *kaphadoṣa*. It is harmful to eyes, unctuous, and useful in worms, pruritus and disorders of skin.

(Kāśyap Samhitā has mentioned a separate chapter on कटुतैलम् Kaṭutailam).

एरण्डतैलम् (Castor Oil) (25)

तैलमेरण्डजं बल्यं गुरूष्णं मधुरं सरम् ॥ १२१
कफमेदोऽनिलहरं लेखनं कटु दीपनम् ॥

हृद्बस्ति पार्श्वजानूरुत्रिकपृष्ठास्थिशूलिनाम् ॥ १२२
आमदोषेषु वातासृक् प्लीहोदावर्तशोफिनाम् ॥

हितं वातामयस्याग्र्यं ग्रन्थिब्रध्नविकारिणाम्[1] ॥ १२३
तिक्तोष्णं पित्तलं विस्रं रक्तैरण्डोद्भवं भृशम् ॥

A.H.5..58

Eranḍa taila is sweet and pungent in taste, *uṣṇavīrya*, pacifies *vāta* and *kapha doṣas*, reduces fat (*meda*), strength giving, *guru*, purgative, scarificient and stimulates digestive capacity. It is useful for pains in precordium, urinary bladder and kidney, sides of the chest, knee joints, thighs, bones of the back and sacral region, in *āmadoṣa, vātarakta* (gout), disorders of spleen, flatulence and odema. It is the best medicine for disorders caused by *vātadoṣa*, tumours (diverticulosis) and (inguinal) hernia.

Oil of *Rakta eranḍa* is bitter in taste, *uṣṇavīrya* aggravates *pitta doṣa* and has extreme fishy smell.

कुसुम्भतैलम् Kusumbha tailam (26)

कुसुम्भतैलमुष्णं च विपाके कटुकं गुरु ॥ १२४
विदाही च विशेषेण सर्वदोषप्रकोपणम् ॥

Kusumbha tailam is *uṣṇavīrya*, pungent in *vipāka* and *guru,* it aggravates all the *doṣas* and produces burning with hyperacidity.

---

१ 'बन्धविकारिणाम्' इति आनन्दाश्रम-चौखम्बा पाठः । अत्र संशोधितः अ. हृ. संहिताधारेण ।

कोशाम्रतैलम् Kośāmratailam (27)

सरं कोशाम्रजं तैलं कृमिकुष्ठविषापहम् ॥ १२५

Kośāmra tail is laxative and useful in worms, skin disorders and in poisons.

आत्मगुप्तातैलम् Ātmaguptā tailam (28)

गुरूष्णं स्निग्धमधुरं कषायं चाऽऽत्मगुप्तजम् ॥
तैलं बल्यं च वृष्यं च बृंहणं वातजित्परम् ॥१२६

The oil obtained from *Ātmaguptā*' seeds is sweet and *kaṣāya* (astringent) in taste, increases the strength. It is *vṛṣya*, body promoting and best pacifier of the *vātadoṣa*.

निम्बतैलम् Nimbatailam (29)

नात्युष्णं निम्बजं तैलं कृमिपित्तकफापहम् ॥
वातपित्तप्रशमनं मदालक्ष्मी ज्वरापहम् ॥ १२७

The oil of neem seeds is not very *uṣṇavīrya* and pacifies *kapha pitta* and *vāta pitta doṣas*. It is useful in intoxications, fevers, and adversity (uncleanliness).

अक्षतैलम् Akśatailam (30)

आक्षं स्वादु हिमं केश्यं गुरुपित्तानिलापहम् ॥

Ākśataila is sweet in taste, *śītavīrya*, beneficial for hairs, is *guru* and pacifies *vāta* and *pitta doṣas*.

तैलविशेषाः **(Taila Viśesāh)**
(certain oils from other sources)

This heading does not appear in Anandāśram edition but appears in Chaukhamba edition. The verses are taken from Aṣṭangsamgraha Su.6.99 to 102.Some of the plants are not mentioned in the text of Dhn. Ni. and seems to be a later insertion.

---

२ 'मदारुग्मी रुजापहम् 'इति आनन्दा. पाठ.

दन्तीमूलकरक्षोघ्न करञ्जारिष्टशिग्रुजम्।
सुवर्चलेङ्गुदी पीलु शंखिनी नीपसंभवम्॥ १

सरलागरु देवाह्व शिंशपासारजन्म च।
तुवरारुष्करोत्थं च तीक्ष्णं कट्वस्रपित्तकृत्॥ २

अर्शः शुक्रकृमिश्लेष्मकुष्ठ मेदोऽनिलापहम्॥

करञ्जारिष्टके तिक्ते नात्युष्णे तत्र निर्दिशेत्॥ ३॥

कषायं तिक्तकटुकं सारलं व्रणशोधनम्।

भृशोष्णे तिक्तकटुके तुवरारुष्करोद्‌भवे॥ ५
विशेषात्कृमिकुष्ठघ्ने तथोर्ध्वाधोविरेचने।

अक्षातिमुक्तकाक्षोड नारिकेल मधूकजम्॥ ६
त्रपुसोर्वारुकूष्माण्ड श्लेष्मातक प्रियालजम्।
वातपित्तहरं केश्यं श्लेष्मलं गुरु शीतलम्॥ ७

सतिक्तं सहकारस्य तैलं सुरभिरोचनम्।
यवतिक्तोद्‌भवं तैलं सतिक्तं रेचनं तथा॥ ८

दन्ती (Dantī chapter 1), मूलकः (Mūlakaḥ Chapter IV 1), रक्षोघ्न (सर्षप Sarṣapa) (Chapter IV), करञ्ज (Karañja Chapter V), निम्ब (Nimba, Chapter 1), शिग्रु (Śigru Chapter IV), सुवर्चला (Suvarcalā, Chapter IV), इंगुदी (Ingudī), not in Dhn. ni. पीलु (Pīlu, Chapter V), शंखिनी (Śankhinī Chapter 1), नीप (Nīpa Chapter V), सरल (Sarala,. Chapter III), अगरु (Agaru, Chapter III), देवदारु (Devadāru Chapter I) शिंशपा (Śimśapā, Chapter V) तुवरक (Tuwaraka, Not mentioned in Dhn. ni.) अरुष्कर (Aruṣkara, Chapter III). The general properties of oils obtained from *Dantī* to *Aruṣkara* are : Sharp and pungent in taste, and aggravate *rakta* and *pitta doṣas.* These are useful in piles, disorders of *śukra,* worms, *kaphadoṣa,* disorders of skin, *meda dhātu* and *vātadoṣa.*

करञ्ज (Karañja), अरिष्ट-निम्ब (Nimba) : The oils obtained from *Karañja* and *Ariṣṭa* are bitter in taste and not excessively *uṣṇavirya*. सरल (Sarala): Oil obtained from *Sarala* is *kaṣāya,* bitter and pungent. It is useful for purification of wounds. तुवरक (not mentioned in Dhn. ni.) तुवरक (Tuwaraka), अरुष्कर (Aruṣkara): Oils obtained from these two are excessively *uṣṇavīrya*, bitter and pungent. These are specifically useful in worms, disorders of skin and in the procedure of emesis and purgation. अक्ष (Akśa)-बिभीतक(Bibhītaka) has been also already mentioned above. अतिमुक्तक (Atimuktaka, Chapter V). अक्षोड (Akśoḍa, Chapter V), नारिकेल (Nārikela, Chapter V), मधूक (Madhūka, Chapter V), त्रपुस (Trapusa, Chapter I), उर्वारु (Urvāru, Chapter I), कूष्माण्ड (Kūṣmāṇḍa, Chapter I), श्लेष्मातक (Śleṣmātaka, Chapter V), प्रियाल (Priyāla, Chapter V), Oils obtained from *Akśa, Atimuktaka* etc. to *Prīyala* pacify *vāta pitta doṣas,* are beneficial to hairs, aggravate *kaphadoṣa,* are *guru* and *sītavīrya.*' सहकार (आम

Āmra, Chapter V): Oil obtained from it is bitter, sweet smelling and appetizing. यवतिक्ता (Yavatiktā, Chapter I). Oil obtained from this is bitter and purgative.

घृतवर्ग

33 घृतम् (Ghṛtam-Ghee-Clarified butter).

घृतमाज्यं हविः सर्पिः पवित्रं नवनीतजम् ॥ १२८
अमृतं चाभिधारश्च जीवनीयं प्रकीर्तितम् ॥

घृतं (Ghṛtam), आज्यं (Ājyam), हविः (Haviḥ), सर्पिः (Sarpiḥ), पवित्र (Pavitram), नवनीतजम् (Navanītajam), अमृतं (Amṛtam), अभिधारः(Abhidharaḥ), जीवनीयं (Jīvanīyam) are synonymous.

गोघृतम् Goghṛtam. Clarified butter made of cow milk.(32)

"शस्तं धीस्मृतिमेधाग्निबलायुःशुक्रचक्षुषाम ॥ १२९
बालवृद्धप्रजाकान्तिसौकुमार्यस्थिरार्थिनाम् ॥
क्षतक्षीणपरीसर्प शस्त्राग्निग्लपितात्मनाम् ।" १३०

A.H.Sū.5.37.38.

"विपाके मधुरं शीतं वातपित्तविषापहम् ॥
चक्षुष्यं बल्यमग्र्यं च गव्यं सर्पिर्गुणोत्तरम् ॥" १३१

S.Sū.45.97.

Gavya ghṛta (cow's ghee) is beneficial to intellect, memory, intelligence, digestive capacity, strength, longevity, *śukra,* and eyes. It is useful for children and old people, progeny, complexion, softening (of the tissues), for the preservation of the perceptive capacity (or stability of the tissues), to those who are weakened by wounds, erysipelas, languor due to attacks of weapons and fire.

Gavya ghṛta is the best in qualities of all the ghees. It is sweet in *taste* and *in vipāka, sitavīrya*, pacifies *vāta* and *pitta doṣas*, antipoisonous, beneficial to eyes (vision) and the best strength promoting.

महिषीघृतम् । Ghee prepared from the milk of she Buffalo. (33)

"मधुरं रक्तपित्तघ्नं गुरु पाके कफावहम् ॥
वातपित्तप्रशमनं सुशीतं माहिषं घृतम् ॥" १३२

S.Sū.45.98.

Mahiṣī ghṛtam is sweet in taste, *sitavīrya, guru* after *vipāka,* aggravates *kapha doṣa* and pacifies *vāta* and *pitta doṣas* and useful in bleeding disorders.

अजाघृतम् । Ghee prepared of milk of she goat.(34)

"आजं घृतं दीपनीयं चक्षुष्यं बलवर्धनम् ।
कासे श्वासे क्षये चापि पथ्यं पाके च तल्लघु ॥" १३३

S.S ū.45.98.

Ajāghṛta is *laghu* after *vipāka.* It stimulates digestive capacity, is beneficial to eyes, and strength promoting. It is useful in cough, dyspnoeas and consumption.

आविकघृतम् Ghee prepared of milk of a ewe. (35)

"पाके लघ्वाविकं सर्पिर्नच पित्तप्रकोपणम् ॥
कफेऽनिले योनिदोषे शोफे कम्पे च तद्धितम् ॥" १३४

S.S ū.45.101.

Āvika ghṛta is *laghu* after *vipāka*, does not aggravate *pitta doṣa,* pacifies *kapha vāta doṣas* and is useful in disorders of female genital organs, oedema and shaking (parkinson's disease ?).

उष्ट्रीघृतम् Ghee made of milk of she Camel. (36)

"औष्ट्रं कटुरसं पाके शोफकृमिविषापहम् ॥
दीपनं कफवातघ्नं कुष्ठगुल्मोदरापहम् ॥"१३५

मूर्च्छामेहोन्मादगरज्वरापस्मारनाशनम् ॥

Uṣṭrīghṛtam is pungent in taste and in *vipāka,* pacifies *kapha* and *vāta doṣas*, stimulates digestive capacity and is useful in oedema, worms, poision, disorders of skin, tumours (diverticulosis), ascites, fainting, urinary disorders characterised by polyuria, psycholgical disorders (*unmāda*), artificial poison, fever and epilepsy.

अश्वाघृतम् Ghee made of milk of she Mare. (37)

अश्वासर्पिस्तु कटुकं मधुरं च कषायकम् ॥ १३६
ईषद्दीपनकं मूर्च्छाहारि वातात्पदं गुरु ॥

A'svāsarpiḥ is pungent sweet and *kaṣāya* in taste, slightly aggravates *vātadoṣa*, is *guru,* stimulates digestive capacity slightly and is useful in syncope.

गर्दभीघृतम् Ghee made from the milk of a she ass (38)

घृतं गार्दभिकं बल्यं दीपनं मूत्रदोषनुत् ॥ १३७
पाके लघूष्णवीर्यं च कषायं कफनाशनम् ॥

Gardabhī ghṛtam is *kaṣāya* in taste, *laghu* after *vipāka*, *uṣṇavīrya* and pacifies *kaphadoṣa*. It is strengthening, stimulates digestive capacity and eliminates disorders of urine.

हस्तिनीघृतम् Ghee made of milk of she Elephant. (40)

'कषायं बद्धविण्मूत्रं तिक्तमग्निकरं लघु ॥ १३८
हन्ति कारेणवं सर्पिः कफकुष्ठविषक्रिमीन् ॥
S.S.45.104

Hastīni ghṛtam is *kaṣāya* and bitter in taste and *laghu* (in *vipāka*) and pacifies *kapha doṣa.* It is constipating, decreses urine and stimulates digestive capacity. It is useful in disorders of skin, poison and worms.

स्त्रीघृतम् Ghee made of human milk. (41)

'चक्षुष्यमग्र्यं स्त्रीणां तु सर्पिः स्यादमृतोपमम् ॥ १३९
वृद्धिं करोति देहाग्न्योर्लघु पाके विषापहम् ॥"
S.S.45.103

Streeghṛtam is best for vision and is like a nectar or elixir of life, *laghu* in *vipāka*, pacifies *kapha doṣa* stimulates digestive capacity and is antipoisonous.

पुराणघृतम् *Purāṇa* (old) ghee. (42)

'सर्पिः पुराणं तिमिरश्वासपीनसकासनुत् ॥ १४०
मूर्च्छा कुष्ठविषोन्मादग्रहापस्मार नाशनम् ॥
S.S. 45.108

योनि कर्णाक्षिशिरसां शूलघ्नं शोफजित्परम् ॥ १४२
हन्ति दोषत्रयं भेदि व्रणशोधनरोपणम् ॥

उग्रगन्धि पुराणं स्यात् दशवर्षोषितं घृतम् ॥ १४३
लाक्षारसनिभं शीतं तद्वत् सर्वग्रहापहम् ॥
तद्वच्च घृतमण्डोऽपि रूक्षस्तित्तःस्तनुश्च सः । १४६

Old ghee (*ghṛtam*) pacifies three *doṣas*, and is *bhedī*. It is useful in *timira* (eye disease), dyspnoea, ch. cold (sinusitis), cough, syncope, disorders of skin, poison, *unmāda* (a psychological disorder), *graha,* epilepsy, pains in female genital organs, ears, eyes, and head, oedema (inflammation), purification and healing of wounds.

Ten years old ghṛta having strong smell is called *Purāna* (old). It is reddish in colour like *Lākṣārasa* and is *sītavīrya*. It alleviates disorders by all *Grahas.*

The upper thin stratum of the *ghṛtam* is bitter, thin and *rūk'sa* (roughening).

दुग्धम् Dugdham- (Milk) Milk group-दुग्धवर्गः

दुग्धं क्षीरं पयः स्वादुः रसायनसमाश्रयम् ॥
सौम्यं प्रस्रवणं स्तन्यं बालसात्म्यं च जीवितम् ॥१४४

दुग्धम् (Dugdham), **क्षीरं** (Kśīram), **पयः** (Payaḥ),**स्वादुः** (Swāduḥ), **रसायनसमाश्रयम्** (Rasāyana-Samāśrayam), **सौम्यं** (Saumyam), **प्रस्रवणं** (Prasravaṇam), **स्तन्यं** (Stanyam), **बालसात्म्यं** (Bālasātmyam), **जीवितं** (Jīvitam),are synonymous.

Types (according to the source animals)

गव्यमाज्यं तथौरभ्रं माहिषं कारभं च यत् ॥
अश्वायाश्चैव नार्याश्च हस्तिनीनां च यत्पयः ॥१४५

According to the source animals following types of milk are described 1) cow milk, 2) The milk of a she goat, 3) The milk of a ewe, 4) The milk of a she buffalo, 5) The milk of a she camel, 6) The milk of a mare, 7) The Human milk and 8) The milk of a she elephant.

Genesis, & General Properties, of the milk

तदनेकौषधिरसं प्राणिनां प्राणदं गुरु ॥
मधुरं पिच्छिलं स्निग्धं शीतं सूक्ष्मं सरं गुरु ॥१४६

---

१ अस्याग्रे-
'तर्पणं नेत्ररोगघ्नं दाहनुत् पयसो हतम्' इति आनन्दा पाठः ।

Milk is the essence of various plants (ingested by the animal), gives strength, and is *guru*, sweet in taste, slimy, unctuous, *'sītavīrya*, entering the channels, mild laxative, and *guru*.

गोदुग्धम् Cow- milk (43)

पथ्यं रसायनं बल्यं हृद्यं मेध्यं गवां पयः ॥
आयुष्यं पुंस्त्वकृद् वातरक्तपित्तविकारनुत् ॥१४७
गवां सितानां वातघ्नं कृष्णानां पित्तनाशनम् ।
कफघ्नं रक्तवर्णानां गोदुग्धं च त्रिधा स्मृतम् ॥१४८
गोक्षीरमनभिष्यन्दि स्निग्धं गुरु रसायनम् ।
'रक्तपित्तहरं शीतं मधुरं रसपाकयोः ॥१४९
जीवनीयं तथा वातपित्तघ्नं परमं स्मृतम् ।

S.S.45.50

Cow's milk is beneficial to the body, *rasāyana* (rejuvenating), cordial, beneficial to the retaining capacity of memory, (or good for intelligence), longevity and virility. It is useful in diseases caused by *vāta, rakta* and *pitta doṣas*.

The milk of a white coloured cow is useful in *vātadoṣa,* the same of a black coloured is useful in *pitta doṣa* and that of reddish coloured cow is useful in *kaphadoṣa*. This way the milk is of three types.

The cow's milk is not *abhiṣyandī* (causing obstruction in the channels due to excessive secretion of *doṣas*), unctuous, *guru* and *rasayana* (rejuvenating). It is useful in bleeding disorders. *'sītavīrya*, sweet in taste and *vipāka.* It is the best pacifier of *vāta* and *pitta doṣas* and is vitalizer.

अजापयः The milk of a she goat (44)

"छागं कषायं मधुरं शीतं ग्राहितरं लघु ॥१५०
रक्तपित्तातिसारघ्नं क्षयकासज्वरापहम् ॥
अजानां लघुकायत्वाद् नानाद्रव्य निषेवणात् ॥१५१
नात्यम्बुपानात्[१] व्यायामात्सर्वव्याधिहरं पयः "॥

S.S u. 45.52.53

Goat-milk is *kaṣāya* and sweet in taste, *'sītavīrya,* more astringent and *laghu*. It is useful in bleeding disorders, diarrhoea (with blood and of chronic in nature), consumption, cough and fever (chronic).

१ 'अत्यम्बुपानात' इति आनन्दा. तथा चौखम्बामुद्रित पुस्तके पाठः ।

Goat-milk is useful in all types of diseases because it's body is light (small), living upon various types of plants (including bitter and pungent in taste), comparatively drink less amount of water and do more exercise (agile habits).

औरभ्रपयः The milk of a ewe (45)

औरभ्रं मधुरं स्निग्धमुष्णं तिक्तं कफापहम् ॥१५५
गुरु शुद्धानिले पथ्यं शोफे चानिलशोणिते ॥

(Ref. S. Sū. 45. 54.)

The milk of a ewe is sweet and bitter in taste, *uṣṇavīrya,* pacifies *kaphadoṣa* and is *guru*. It is beneficial in isolated *vātadoṣa* disorders, anasarca and *vātarakta* (gout).

महिषीपयः The milk of a she buffalo (46)

'महाभिष्यन्दि मधुरं माहिषं वह्निसादनम् ॥१५३
निद्राकरं शीतकरं गव्यात्स्निग्धतरं गुरु ।

S.S ū.45.55

The milk of a she buffalo is sweet in taste, *sītavīrya*. It is extremely *abhisyandī* and depresses digestive capacity, causes sleep (hypnotic). It is more unctuous than the milk of cow.

उष्ट्रीपयः The milk of a she camel (47)

रूक्षोष्णं क्षीरमुष्ट्रीणामीषत्सलवणं[१] लघु ॥१५५
शस्तं वातकफानाहकृमिशोफोदरार्शसाम् ॥

The milk of a she camel is slightly salty in taste, *usnavīrya, rūk'sa*, and *laghu*. It pacifies *vāta* and *kapha doṣās* and is useful in tympanitis, worms, anasarca, ascites and piles.

अश्वापयः The milk of a mare (48)

अश्वाक्षीरं स्मृतं साम्लं लवणं दीपनं लघु ॥ १५८
देहस्थैर्यकरं बल्यं गौरवकान्तिकृत सरम्[२] ॥

१ ईषत् 'स्वादु' इति सुश्रुतः ।
२ 'अस्याग्रे श्वास वातहरं साम्लं लवणं रुचिदीप्तिकृत' । इति आनन्दाश्रम मुद्रित पुस्तके पाठः ।

The milk of a mare is sour and salty in taste, stimulates digestive capacity, and is *laghu.* It causes stability of the body (tissues), is strength promoting, increases weight, complexion and as a laxative.

गर्दभीपयः The milk of a she ass (49)

कासश्वासहरं क्षीरं गार्दभं बालरोगनुत् ॥१५६
मधुराम्लरसं रूक्षं लवणानुरसं लघु ॥

The milk of a she ass is sweet and sour in taste with salty subsequent taste roughening and *laghu*. It is useful in cough, dyspnoea and diseases of children.

मानुषीपयः Human milk (51)

स्निग्धं स्थैर्यकरं चापि चक्षुष्यं बलवर्धनम् ॥१५७
जीवनं बृंहणं सात्म्यं स्नेहनं मानुषीपयः ॥
नावनं[1] रक्तपित्ते च तर्पणं चाक्षिशूलनुत् ॥१५८

Human milk produces stability of the body (tissues), promotes strength, is vitalizer, body promoting, *sātmya* (beneficial) and unctuous. It is useful as a nasal medication in bleeding (epistaxis) disorders, as a *tarpaṇa* (bath) in painful eyes.

हस्तिनीपयः The milk of a she elephant (52)

"हस्तिन्या मधुरं वृष्यं कषायानुरसं गुरु ॥
स्निग्धं शीतकरं चापि चक्षुष्यं बलवर्धनम् "॥ १५९
S.S u.45.58.59

The milk of she elephant is sweet in taste, *kaṣāya* is subsidiary taste, *sītavirya, vṛsya, guru,* unctuous, beneficial for eyes and strength promoting.

पयः सामान्यगुणदोषाः Properties, merits and demerits of milk.

विवत्सा बालवत्सानां पयो दोषलमीरितम् ॥
पिण्याकाम्लाशिनीनां च गुर्वभिष्यन्दि तद् भृशम् ॥१६०

The milk of an animal whose calf is not alive, and of which calf is

---

१ 'शमनं रक्तपित्तस्य' इति चौखम्बा मुद्रित पुस्तके पाठः ।

very young, that milk will aggravate the *doṣas*. The animals fed on oil cakes and on sour food is extremely *guru* (difficult to assimilate) and *Abhiṣyandi*.

जांगलानूपदेशेषु चरन्तीनां यथोत्तरम् ॥
पयो गुरुतरं स्नेहो यथा चैषां विवर्धते ॥१६१

कृष्णायाः कृष्णवत्सायाः शुक्लायाश्च परं पयः ।
सुखोष्णं कफवातघ्नं श्रृतशीतं च पित्तजित् ॥१६२

आमवातकरं चापि धारोष्णममृतं पयः ।
सुश्रृतं च पयः पीतं पीयूषादपि तद् गुरु ॥१६३

कूर्चिकाश्च किलाटाश्च गुरुवः श्लेष्मवर्धनाः ।
तर्पणाः प्रीणना बल्याः बृंहणा मारुतापहाः ॥१६४

दीप्ताग्नीनामनिद्राणां व्यवाये चापि पूजिताः ।
"अनिष्टगन्धमम्लं च विवर्ण विरसं च यत् ॥१६५

वर्ज्यं सलवणं क्षीरं यच्च विग्रथितं भवेत् ॥

धारोष्णममृतं पथ्यं धाराशीतं त्रिदोषलम् ॥ १६६

श्रृतशीतं त्रिदोषघ्नं श्रृतोष्णं कफवातजित् ।" ½ S.S. 46. 64

जीर्णज्वरे किन्तु कफे विलीने स्याद्दुग्धपानं हि सुधासमानम् ।
तदेव पीतं तरुणज्वरे च निहन्ति हालाहलवन्मनुष्यान् ॥१६७

नवज्वरे च मन्दाग्नौ ह्यामदोषेषु कुष्ठिनाम् ।
शूलिनां कफदोषेषु कासिनामतिसारिणाम् ॥१६८
पयःपानं न कुर्वीत विशेषात् कृमिदोषतः ॥

मुहूर्तपञ्चकादूर्ध्वं क्षीरं भवति विकृतम् ॥१६९
तदेव द्विगुणं काले विषवद्धन्ति मानवम् ॥

The milk of animals roaming in *Ānupa* region is more *guru* than those of *Jāṅgala* region as its fat content increases.

The milk of black coloured cow having black coloured calf and the same of white coloured cow is considered best.

The agreeably hot milk (warm) pacifies *kapha* and *vāta doṣas* and boiled cool milk pacifies *pittadoṣa*.

The warm milk drawn directly from the cow, even it is considered as a nectar causes *āmavāta*, Milk boiled for a long time becomes *guru* (heavier) than *Pīyūṣa*.

Kūrcikā and *kilāṭa* (obtained from processing milk) are *guru* (heavy to digest) and aggravate *kaphadoṣa.* These are satiating and nourishing, strength promoting, increase tissues of the body and pacify *vātadoṣa.* These are useful to those who have strong digestive capacity, who get less sleep and who are engaged in sexual excesses.

The milk which emits undesirable smell, has aquired an acid taste, has become discoloured, undesirable taste, saline in taste, looks shreddy and curdled should be regarded as unwholesome.

The warm milk immediately after milching is just like a nectar and wholesome, but the same after becoming cool aggravates three *doṣas.* Boiled milk pacifies the three *doṣas,* while boiled and warm pacifies *kaphavāta doṣas.*

In chronic fevers when the *kaphadoṣa* is decreased milk is useful like nectar, while in early stage of fever (toxic condition) the same is as a toxic poison like a *hālāhala.*

Milk should not be used in the early stage of a fever, when digestive capacity is poor, in *āmadoṣa,* skin disorders, in colics, cough, (early stage of) diarrhoea and especially in infestations by worms.

(If not preserved properly by boiling etc.) the milk becomes unwholesome after 5 *muhurta,* (about 4 hours). After double this time it beocme poisonous and may kill the human being.

35 दधि तक्रं च Dadhi & Takram

(Curds & Butter milk group)

दधि (Dadhi - curds) (53)

तक्रजन्मं पयोहेतुर्नवनीतोद्भवं दधि ॥ १७०

अम्लं स्वादुरसं ग्राहि गुरूष्णं दधि वातजित् ॥
मेदःशुक्रबलश्लेष्मरक्तपित्ताग्निशोफकृत् ॥ १७१

A. Sam. 6. 62

तक्रजन्म (Takrajanma), पयोहेतुः (Payohetuḥ), नवनीतोद्भव (Navanītodbhava) are the synonyms for *Dadhi* (दधि)

Curds is sour and sweet in taste, *uṣṇavirya,* astringent, *guru* and pacifies *vātadoṣa.* It increases, fat, *'sukra*, strength, *kaphadoṣa,* blood, *pittadoṣa,* digestive capacity and oedema.

मथितदधि-

(Churned curds, its properties and actions) (54)

मथितं गोरसं घीलं द्रवमम्लं विलोडितम् ॥१७२
श्वेतं दण्डाहतं सान्द्रं दध्यम्लं नामतः स्मृतम् ॥

वातदोषहरं ह्लादि मथितं कफपित्तकृत् ॥ १७३

मथित (Mathita), गोरसं (Gorasa), घोल (Ghola), द्रवमम्ल (Dravamamla), विलोडित (Viloḍita), श्वेत (Śveta), दण्डाहत (Daṇḍāhata), सान्द्रं (Sāndram), दध्यम्ल (Dadhyamla) are all synonymous.

Churned curds pacifies *vātadoṣa,* it produces pleasure and aggravates *kapha* and *pitta doṣas.*

पशुविशेषेण दधिगुणाः

Properties and actions of curds of various animals.

गोदधि (Curds from the milk of a cow) (55)

"स्निग्धं विपाके मधुरं दीपनं बलवर्धनम् ॥
वातापहं पवित्रं च दधि गव्यं रुचिप्रदम् ॥"१७४

S .S.Su.46.68.

Curds from the milk of a cow is sweet in vipāka, unctuous, stimulates digestive capacity, is strength promoting, pacifies *vātadoṣa,* clean and appetizing.

अजादधि (Curds from the milk of a she goat) (56)

"दध्याजं कफवातघ्नं लघु पाके क्षयापहम् ॥ १७५
दुर्नामश्वासकासेषु हितमग्नेश्च दीपनम् ॥"

S.Sū. 45. 72.75

Curds from the milk of a she goat pacifies *kapah* and *vāta doṣas,* is *laghu* in *vipāka.* It is useful in consumption, piles, cough, dyspnoea, wholesome and stimulates digestive capacity.

आविकं दधि (Curds from the milk of a ewe) (57)

कोपनं कफवातानां दुर्नाम्नां चाऽविकं दधि'॥ १७६
विपाके मधुरं वृष्यं रक्तपित्तप्रसादनम् ॥

S.S.Su. 45.69.

Curds from the milk of a ewe aggravates *kapaha-vāta doṣas,* causes piles.It is sweet in *vipāka, vṛṣya* and clears impurities of *rakta* and *pitta doṣas.*

महिषीदधि (Curds from the milk of a she buffalo) (58)

'बलासवर्धनं स्निग्धं विशेषान्माहिषं दधि ॥ १७८
महाभिष्यन्दि मधुरं बलमेदोविवर्धनम् ॥

S.S. Su. 45.70

Curds from the milk of a she buffalo is sweet in taste, aggravates *kaphadoṣa*. It is extremely *abhiṣyandī* (causing obstruction in the channels due to excessive secretion of *doṣas*), strength promoting and increases *medodhātu* (fat).

उष्ट्रीदधि (Curds from the milk of a she camel). (59)

विपाके कटु सक्षारमम्लं स्यादौष्ट्रकं दधि ॥ १७९
वातमर्शांसि कुष्ठानि कृमीन्हन्त्यूदराणि च ॥

S.S.45.70

Curds from the milk of a she camel is sour and salty in taste and pungent in *vipāka.* It pacifies *vātadoṣa,* and is useful in piles, disorders of skin, worms and ascites.

अश्वादधि (Curds from the milk of a mare) (60)

दीपनीयमचक्षुष्यं वातलं दधि वाडवम् ॥ १७९
रूक्षमुष्णं कषायं च कफमूत्रापहं च तत् ॥

S.S.Su.45.73

Curds from the milk of a mare is *kaṣāya* in taste, *uṣṇavīrya, rūk'sa* (roughening), and aggravates *vātadoṣa.* It stimulates digestive capacity, not beneficial to eyes and decreases *kaphadoṣa* and urine.

गर्दभी दधि (Curds from the milk of a she ass) (61)

गर्दभी दधि रूक्षोष्णं लघु दीपनपाचनम् ॥
मधुराम्लरसं रुच्यं वातदोष विनाशनम् ॥ १८०

Curds from the milk of a she ass is sweet and sour in taste, *uṣṇavīrya, rūkṣa* (roughening), *laghu,* stimulates digestive capacity and is digestant appetizer and pacifies *vātadoṣa.*

हस्तिनीदधि (Curds from the milk of a she elephant) (62)

लघु पाके बलासघ्नं वीर्योष्णं पत्तिग्नाशनम्॥
कषायानुरसं नाग्या दधि वर्चोविवर्धनम् ॥ १८१

S. S. Su. 45.74.75

The curds obtained from the milk of a she elephant is *laghu* in *vipāka,* pacifies *kapha doṣa, uṣṇavīrya* and depresses the digestive capacity. Its subsidiary taste is *kaṣāya* and increases the quantity of faeces.

स्त्रीदधि (Curds from the milk of a woman) (63)

स्निग्धं च मधुरं बल्यमुष्णं संतर्पणं गुरु ॥
चक्षुष्यमग्र्यं दोषघ्नं दधि नार्या गुणोत्तरम् ॥ १८२

S. S. Su. 45.73

The curds from the human milk is sweet in taste, *uṣṇavirya,* strength promoting, nourishing and *guru.* It is extremely beneficial to eyes and decreases *doṣas.*

सामान्य दधिगुणाः

General properties and actions of the curds.

कफपित्तकृदम्लं स्यादत्यम्लं रक्तदूषकम् ॥
विदाहि सृष्टविण्मूत्रं मधुरं तत् त्रिदोषनुत् ॥ १८३

दध्नस्तु यदधस्तोयं तन्मस्तु परिकथ्यते ॥
शृतात्क्षीराच्च यज्जातं गुणवद्दधि तत्स्मृतम् ॥ १८४

'वातपित्तहरं रुच्यं धात्वग्निबलवर्धनम् ॥
द१ध्यसरं च रुक्षं च ग्राहि विष्टम्भिवातलम् ॥" १८५

S.S. Su. 45.79.

सरं स्निग्धं गुरु वृष्यं कफमेदो विवर्धनम् ॥
बृंहणं मारुतघ्नं च बलासचयकृत्परम् ॥ १८६
कफवातहरं भेदि मस्तु स्त्रोतोविशोधनम् ॥

पीनसे चातिसारे च शीतके विषमज्वरे ॥ १८७
अरुचौ मूत्रकृच्छ्रे च कार्श्ये च दधि शस्यते *॥

The curds is of three types 1) *Sour,* 2) *Very sour,* and 3) *sweet. sour curds* aggravates *kaphapitta doṣas,* very sour curds vitiate blood and causes burning with hyperacidity and poor digestion and *sweet curds* is diuretic and laxative and pacifies all the *doṣas*.

Thin watery part under the curds is called as *mastu.* The curds prepared from boiled milk is considered possessing good qualitities. It pacifies *vāta* and *pitta doṣas,* is appetizing, useful for increasing the tissues, stimulating digestive capacity and strength promoting.

The curds from which the cream is removed is *rūkśa,* astringent, constipating and aggravate *vātadoṣa.*

Cream of the curds is *guru* (heavy to digest), *vṛṣya,* pacifies *vāta doṣa,* aggravates *kaphadoṣa* and increases *medodhātu* (fatty tissue), is body promoting and accumulates *kapha doṣa.*

Mastu pacifies *kapha* and *vāta doṣa*, is laxative and purifies minute channels of the body.

Curds is indicated in chronic coryza, diarrhoea, malarial fevers, anorexia, dysuria and emaciation.

ऋतुविशेषेण दध्नो गुणाः

Seasonal and general recommendations for the use of curds.

"शरद्ग्रीष्मवसन्तेषु प्रायशो दधि गर्हितम् ॥१८८
हेमन्ते शिशिरे चैव वर्षासु दधि शस्यते ॥" S.S. Su.45.80.

---

१ ' दधि सारं ' इति आनन्दा पुस्तके पाठः ।
* "सरसं निर्जल घोलं तक्रं पादजलान्वितम् ।
अर्धौदकमुदश्विच्च मथितं जलवर्जितम् ॥
वातपित्तहरं घोलमुदश्वित् श्लेष्मलं भवेत् ।
त्रिदोषशमनं तक्रं मथितं श्लेष्मपित्तकृत ॥"
इत्यधिकः पाठः आनन्दाश्रम पुस्तके । साधु च । S.D.Kamat.

रक्तपित्तकफोत्थेषु विकारेषु हितं न तत् ।
"विज्ञेयमेषु सर्वेषु गव्यमेव गुणोत्तरम् ॥ १८९
वातघ्नं कफकृत् स्निग्ध बृंहणं न च पित्तकृत् ।"१९०

S.S. Su.45.75.

'न नक्तं दधि भुञ्जीत न चाप्यघृतशर्करम् ॥
नामुद्गसूपं नाक्षौद्रं नोष्णं नाऽऽमलकैर्विना ॥१९१
ज्वरासृक्पित्तवीसर्पकुष्ठपाण्ड्वामयभ्रमान्'॥

A.H.Sū.5.31.

प्राप्नुयात् कामलां चोग्रां विधिं हित्वा दधिप्रियः ॥ १९२

C.S.Sū 8.62

The use of curds is generally prohibited in *Vasanta* (spring), *Grīṣma* (summer) and *'Sarad* (autumn), whereas it is recommended during *Hemanta* (winter), *'Si 'sira* (cold season proper) and *Varṣā* (rains). It is also prohibited in diseases caused by *rakta, pitta* and *kapha doṣas.*

Of all the types, the curds prepared from cow milk is superior in qualities. It pacifies *vāta,* aggravates *kapha*, but does not aggravate *pitta* and is unctuous and body promoting.

Curds should not be taken at night time, it should not be taken without ghee, sugar, soup of *mudga,* honey and emblica (*Āmalakī*) and after warming (heating).

Those who are fond of taking curds without following the instructions mentioned above will have fever, bleeding disorders, erysipelas, disorders of skin, anaemias, vertigo and severe jaundice.

तक्रम् Takram - (Buttermilk)

तक्रं श्वेतपयः सात्म्यं छच्छिका चैव कीर्तितम् ॥

तक्रं (Takram), श्वेतपयः (Śvetpayaḥ), सात्म्यं (Sātmyam), छच्छिका (Chacchikā) are synonyms.

तक्रभेदाः Types of Buttermilk

द्विगुणाम्बु श्वेतपयस्त्वर्धोदकमुदश्वितम् ॥ १९३
तक्रं त्रिभागभिन्नं तु केवलं मथितं स्मृतम् ॥
तक्रस्योपरि यत्तोयं तदुदश्वित् प्रकीर्तितम् ॥ १९४

Depending upon the addition of water while churning of curds, *Takram* becomes of various types. If double the water to curds is added in it is called as *'svetapayaḥ;* if half water is added then it is called as *Uda'svit*, if curds is churned alone it is called as *Mathitam*. The fluid substance above the *takram* is called as *Uda'svit.*

तक्रस्य सामान्यगुणाः

General properties and actions of Butter milk.

'तक्रं लघु कषायोष्णं दीपनं कफवातजित् ॥
शोफोदरार्शोग्रहणीदोषमूत्रग्रहारुचीः ॥१९५
गुल्मप्लीहघृतव्याधि[1]गरपाण्डवामयान् जयेत् ॥"

A H.Su.5.33.34.

Takra is *kaṣāya* (sour) in taste, *usṇavīrya,* stimulates digestive capacity and pacifies *kapha and vāta doṣās.* It is useful in anasarca, ascites, piles, ch. diarrhoeal diseases, suppression of urine, loss of appetite, tumors, (diverticulae), disorders of spleen, disorders due to excessive ghee, artificial poison and anaemias.

समुद्धृतघृतंतक्रमर्धोद्धृतघृतं च यत् ॥ १९६
अनुद्धृतघृतं च स्यादित्येत् त्रिविधं मतम् ॥

पूर्वं लघू च पथ्यं च गुरु वृष्यतरं परम् ॥ १९७
अतःपरं वृष्यतमं यथाक्रममुदीरितम् ॥

अम्लं चात्यम्लमेवान्यत् कषायं स्वादु चापरम् ॥ १९८
तनु सान्द्रं सान्द्रतरं गुरु विद्याद्यथोत्तरम् ॥

तत्र यदुद्धृतस्नेहं साम्लं च मधुरं च यत् ॥ १९९
कषायानुरसं स्वादु नातिसान्द्रं प्रशस्यते ॥

गरोदरार्शोग्रहणीपाण्डुरोगे ज्वरेऽरुचौ ॥ २००
वर्चोमूत्रग्रहप्लीहस्नेहव्यापदि मेहिषु ॥

कषाय[2]शीतमधुरं तक्रं श्रेष्ठतमं मतम् ॥२०१
तर्पणं प्रीणनं बल्यं हृद्यं पित्ताविरोधि च ॥

तक्रं केवलमम्लं च श्लेष्मानिलहरं लघु ॥ २०२
लेखनं दीपनीयं च रक्तपित्तप्रकोपनम् ॥

१ 'घृतव्यापद' इति अ.हृ. पाठः ।
२ 'कषायाशीत मधुर' इति चौखम्बा पाठः ।

तक्रमामं कफं कोष्ठे हन्ति कण्ठे करोति च ॥ २०३
पीनसश्वासकासादौ सिद्धमेव तदिष्यते ॥

Depending upon the quantity of fat contents removed, the *takra* becomes of three types 1) *Takra* from which all the ghee (fats) are extracted, 2) *Takra* from which half the quantity of *ghee* (butter, fats) are extracted, and 3) from which ghee (butter -fats) are not extracted.

The first type is *laghu* and wholesome, the second type is *guru* and more *vṛṣya* and the third type is most *vṛṣya.*

Takra may be if 1) Sour in taste, 2) Very sour in taste; and 3) Sweet and *kaṣaya* in taste. Again it may be 1) Thin or fluid; 2) Thick; and 3) Very thick.

The first one out of these is *laghu*, the second one is *guru* and the third one is more *guru.*

Of all these kind of *takra* from which fats are removed, and which is sour, sweet in taste, having subsidiary taste as *kaṣāya* and which is not very thick is beneficial.

Takram is useful in artificial poison, ascites, piles, diseases characterized by chronic diarrhoea, anaemia, fever, anorexia, constipation, obstruction to urinary flow, disorders of spleen, disorders caused by excess of oleation therapy and in disorders caused by polyuria (including diabetes).

Takram which is *kaṣāya*, sweet and cool is supposed to be the best. It is satiating, nourishing, strength promoting, beneficial for heart and does not aggravate *pitta doṣa.*

Takram which is only sour in taste pacifies *kapha* and *vāta doṣas,* is *laghu*, slimming, stimulates digestive capacity and aggravates *rakta* and *pittadoṣas. Āmatakra* (unprocessed) aggravates *kaphadoṣa* in the throat and pacifies the same *doṣa* in gastrointestinal tract. It should be always used processed in chronic coryza, dyspnoea and cough.

तक्रनिषेधः Contraindications for Butter Milk.

तक्रं नैव क्षते दद्यान्नोष्णकाले न दुर्बले ॥ २०४
न मूर्च्छा भ्रमदाहेषु न रोगे रक्तपैत्तिके ॥ S.S. Su. 45. 86.

The use of *takra is* prohibited to one who is suffering from wounds, in the hot season, to a weak person, in cases of syncope, vertigo, burning sensation of the body and haemorrhagic disorders.

तक्रसेवनम् Indications for butter milk

शीतकालेऽग्निमान्द्ये च कफोत्थेष्वामयेषु च ॥ २०५
मार्गावरोधे दुष्टे च वायौ तक्रं प्रशस्यते ॥

S.S. Su. 45.87.

The use of *Takra* is recommended during cold seasons, in disorders caused by *kapha* and *vāta doṣas* due to obstruction in the minute channels.

दोषविशेषेण तक्रगुणाः

वातेऽम्लं सैंधवोपेतं स्वादु पित्ते सशर्करम् ॥ २०६
पिबेत्तक्रं कफे चापि व्योषक्षारसमायुतम् ॥

Takra should be used with rocksalt in disorders caused by *vātadoṣa*, with sugar in disorders caused by *pittadoṣa* and with *trikaṭu* (7th chapter) and *Yavakṣāra* (2nd chapt.) in disorders caused by *kaphadoṣa*.

तक्रकूर्चिका (Takrakūrcikā)

ग्राहिणी वातला रूक्षा दुर्जरा तक्रकूर्चिका ॥ २०७

S.S. Su. 45.90

Takrakūrcikā aggravates *vātadoṣa;* it is *rūkṣa*, (roughening) and difficult to digest.

मण्डः (Maṇḍaḥ)

तक्राल्लघुतरो मण्डः पुंस्त्वनिद्राप्रदः स्मृतः ॥ S.S.Su.45.91

Maṇḍa (*Takramaṇḍa*) is more *laghu*, virilizing and sleep promoting.

पीयूषमोरटौ (Pīyuṣa mortau)

मधुरो बृंहणौ वृष्यौ तद्वत् पीयूषमोरटौ ॥ २०८

S.S. Su.45.95

Pīyūṣa and *Moraṭa* are sweet in taste, body promoting and *vṛsya*.

नवनीतम् (Navanītam - butter) (64)

नवनीतं दधिभवं घृतहेतुः शिशुप्रियम् ॥
दधिमण्डोद्भवं चैव मन्थनोद्भवमेव च ॥ २०९

नवनीतं नवं हृद्यं ग्राहिरोचनदीपनम् ॥
क्षयारुच्यर्दितप्लीहग्रहण्यर्शोविकारनुत् ॥२१०

चक्षुष्यं शिशिरं स्निग्धं वृष्यं जीवनबृंहणम् ॥
क्षीरोद्भवं हिमं ग्राहि रक्तपित्ताक्षिरोगनुत् ॥ २११

स्मृतिक्षुधाग्निशुक्रौजःकफमेदोविवर्धनम् ॥
वातपित्तविषोन्मादशोफालक्ष्मी जरापहम्[१] ॥ २१२

सर्वस्नेहोत्तमं शीतं मधुरं रसपाकयोः॥

नवनीतं (Navanītam), दधिभवं (Dadhibhavam), घृतहेतुः (Ghṛtahetuḥ) शिशुप्रियं (Śiśupriyam), दधिमण्डोद्भवम् (Dadhimaṇḍodbhavam), मन्थनोद्भवम् (manthanodbhavam) are synonyms.

Navanīta (fresh butter) is palatable (cordial), astringent, appetizing, stimulates digestive capacity. It is useful in consumption, loss of appetite, facial palsy, disorders of spleen, (*Grahaṇī;* disorders charcterized by chronic diarrhoea) and piles.

It is beneficial for the eyes, *sītavīrya,* unctuous, *vṛsya,* vitalizer and body promoting.

Butter extracted from milk is *śitavīrya*, astringent and useful in bleeding disorders and in disorders of eyes.

It is also useful for memory, appetite, digestive capacity, and aggravates *kaphadoṣa* and increases *meda* (fatty tissue).

It pacifies *vāta* and *pitta doṣas* and is useful in poisons and psychological disorders, oedema, unauspiciousness. It is sweet in taste and in *vipāka* and one of the best in fatty substances.

36 क्षौद्रम् Kśaudram (Honey) (मधु- Madhu).

मधु क्षौद्रं तु माक्षीकं माक्षिकं कुसुमासवम् ॥ २१३
पुष्पासवं सारघं च तच्च पुष्परसं स्मृतम् ॥

मधु (Madhu), क्षौद्रं (Kśaudram), माक्षीकं (Mākṣîkam), माक्षिकम्

१ 'ज्वरापहं' इति पाठः ।

(Mākṡikam), कुसुमासवम् (Kusumāsavam), पुष्पासवं (Puṣpāsavam), सारघं (Sāragham), पुष्परसं (Puṣparasam) are synonyms.

मधुजातयः Madhujātayah - Types of Honey

माक्षिकं भ्रामरं क्षौद्रं पौत्तिकं छात्रकं तथा ॥ २१४
आर्घ्यमौद्दालकं दालमित्यष्टौ मधुजातयः ॥ S.S.45.133

'माक्षिकं तैलवर्णं स्यात्क्षौद्रं तु कपिलं भवेत् ॥ २१५
पौत्तिकं घृतवर्णं तु श्वेतं भ्रामरमुच्यते ॥'
Ca. S. S. Su.27. 244.

आपीतवर्णं छात्राख्यं पिङ्गलं चार्घ्यनामकम् ॥ २१६
औद्दालं स्वर्णसदृशं दालं च पाटलं स्मृतम् ॥

माक्षिकं (Mākṡikam), भ्रामरं (Bhrāmaram), क्षौद्रं (Kṡaudram), पौत्तिकं (Pauttikam), छात्रकं (Chātrakam), आर्घ्यम् (Arghyam), औद्दालकं (Auddālakam), दालम् (Dālam). These are the eight types of Honey.

Mākṡika resembles in colour with oil, *kṡaudram* is of brown colour, *pauttikam* resembles in colour with *ghee* and *Bhrāmara* is of white colour.

Chātra is yellowish in colour, the colour of *Ārghya* is slightly yellowish, *Auddāla* is golden in colour and *Dāla* is reddish in colour.

सामान्य मधुगुणाः General Properties of Honey.

कषायानुरसं रूक्षं शीतलं मधुरं मधु ॥ २१७
दीपनं लेखनं बल्यं व्रणरोपणमुत्तमम ॥
सन्धानं लघु चक्षुष्यं स्वर्यं हृद्यं त्रिदोषनुत् ॥ २१८
छर्दिहिक्काविषश्वासकासशोषातिसारजित् ॥
रक्तपित्तहरं ग्राहि कृमितृण्मोहहृत्परम् ॥ २१९

Honey is sweet in taste and has *kasāya* as subsidiary taste, is roughening and *sītavīrya.* It pacifies all the three *doṣas.* It stimulates digestive capacity, is slimming, strength promoting and is good for wound healing. It is useful for fermentation, is *laghu,* beneficial to eyes, voice and is cordial.

It is useful in emesis, hiccup, poison, dyspnoea, cough, consumption, diarrohoea, bleeding disorders, as an astringent, in worms, thirst and fainting.

विशिष्टमधुगुणाः

(Properties of certain types of Honey)

भ्रामरमधु Bhrāmara Madhu

पैच्छिल्यात् स्वादुरूपत्वात् भ्रामरं गुरूसंज्ञितम् ॥
भ्रामरं कुरुते जाड्यमत्यन्तं मधुरं च तत् ॥ २२०

Because *Bhrāmara madhu* is sweet in taste, slimy and *guru,* causes extremely heaviness in the body (malaise).

क्षौद्रमधु Kṣaudra madhu

क्षौद्रं विशेषतो ज्ञेयं शीतलं लघु लेखनम् ॥

S.S. Su. 45.135

K'saudra madhu is especially *'sītavīrya, laghu* and slimming.

माक्षिकमधु Māksika madhu

तस्माल्लघुतरं रूक्षं माक्षिकं प्रवरं स्मृतम् ॥ २२१

S.S. Su. 45.136

Māk'sika madhu is more *laghu,* roughening and is the best amongst all the types of hoeny (mentioned above).

उष्णैर्विरुध्यते सर्वं विषान्वयतया मधु ॥
उष्णार्तमुष्णमुष्णैर्वा तन्निहन्ति यथा विषम् ॥ २२२

S.S. Su. 45.144

On account of its poisonous contact in its origin, honey is opposite to heating. It is injurious to health similar to poison (greatly harmful) to those who are heated (eg. in hot season), when used or combined with heated substances.

तत्सौकुमार्यच्च तथैव सेव्यं वनौषधीनां रससम्भवाच्च ।
उष्णैर्विरुध्येत विशेषतस्तु तथाऽन्तरिक्षेण जलेन वाऽपि ॥२२३

S.S. Su. 45.145

Madhu is especially opposed to heating and heated substance due to its soft nature, and being collected from the sap of variety of flowers. Similarly, it should not be used with atmospheric water.

माध्वी सिता Mādhvī sitā (sugar of honey)

माध्वी सिता मधूत्पन्ना मधुजा मधुशर्करा ।
माक्षीकशर्करा चैषा क्षौद्रजा क्षौद्रशर्करा ॥२२४

यद्गुणं यन्मधुप्रोक्तं तद्गुणास्तस्य शर्करा ।
विशेषाद् बल्यवृष्याश्च तर्पण्यः क्षीणदेहिनाम् ॥२२५

माध्वी सिता (Mādhvī sitā), मधूत्पन्ना (Madhūtpannā), मधुजा (Madhujā), मधुशर्करा (Madhuśarkarā), माक्षीकशर्करा (Māksikaśarkarā), क्षौद्रजा (Ksaudrajā), क्षौद्रशर्करा (Ksaudraśarkarā) are synonymous.

The properties of honey sugar are similar in those of that particular type of honey. The sugar from honey is strength promoting, *vṛsya* and satiating to the weak persons.

37 शुक्तम् * (Śuktam).

शुक्तं सहस्रवेधं च रसाम्लं चुक्रमेव च ।
मुक्तसारं तथा चोक्तं दहनं नीलकारकम् ॥२२६

शुक्तं (Śuktam), सहस्रवेधं (Sahasravedham), रसाम्लं (Rasāmlam), चुक्रं (Cukram), मुक्तसारं (Muktasāram), दहनं (Dahanam) and नीलकारकम् (Nīlakārakam) are synonymous.

रक्तपित्तकरं शुक्तं सद्यो भुक्तविपाचनम् ।
जरणं भेदनं पाण्डुकृमिरोगहरं लघु ॥२२७
तीक्ष्णोष्णं मूत्रलं हृद्यं कफघ्नं कटुपाकि च ।
तद्वत्तदासुतं सर्वं रोचनं तु विशेषतः ॥ २२८

S.S. Su. 210-211

Fermented liquors known as the *śukta* (treacle, honey, fermented rice gruel and watery substance above the curds kept in a new and clean

---

* 'सूक्तं' इति पा. ।

१ 'तद्वत्तदाश्रितम् इति पाठ.

vessel underneath a bushel of paddy for three consecutive days -Ḍalhaṇa) causes aggravation of *rakta pitta* and digests the food immediately. It is digestant, *bhedana* and *laghu*. It is *tīkṣṇa, uṣṇa,* diuretic, cordial, pacifier of *kaphadoṣa* and pungent in *vipāka*. Bulbs and roots, pickled in śukta acquire the properties of the latter. These possess a good appetizing property.

38 काञ्जिकम् (Kāñjikam)

काञ्जिकं चैव सौवीरं कुल्माषाभिषुतं तथा ।
अवन्तिसोमं धान्याम्लमारनालं महारसम् ॥२२९

दाहज्वरापहं स्पर्शात्पानात् वातकफापहम्
विबन्धघ्नमवस्रंसि दीपनं चाम्लकाञ्जिकम् ॥२३०

C.S.Su.27.192

काञ्जिकं (Kāñjikam), सौवीरं (Sauvīram), कुल्माषाभिषुतं (Kulmāṣābhiṣutam), अवन्तिसोमं (Avantisomam), धान्याम्लं (Dhānyāmlam), आरनालं (Āranālam) and महारसम् (Mahārasam) are synonymous.

Dhānyāmlam, the fermented (sour) gruel, by external application removes burning sensation in fevers and orally it pacifies *vāta* and *kapha doṣas*. It is deobstruent, laxative and stimulates digestive capacity.

सौवीरकं, तुषोदकम् (Sauvīrakam & Tuṣodakam) (65)

सौवीरकं सुवीराम्लं यवगोधूमसंभवम् ।
यवाग्रजं यवोत्थं च तुषोदं च तुषोदकम् ॥२३१

जरणीयं च हृत्पाण्डु कृमिरोगविदाहनुत् ।
ग्रहण्यर्शोहितं भेदि सौवीरं च तुषोदकम् ॥२३२

Ca. Su. 27.191.

गौडानि रसशुक्तानि मधुशुक्तानि यानि च ।
यथापूर्व गुरुतराण्यभिष्यन्दकराणि च ॥२३३

S.S.Su 45.122

यन्मस्त्वादि शुचौ भाण्डे सगुडक्षौद्रकाञ्जिकम् ।
धान्यराशौ त्रिरात्रस्थं शुक्तं चुक्रं तदुच्यते ॥२३४

सौवीरकम् Sauvīrakam, सुवीराम्लं (Suvīrāmlam), यवगोधूमसंभवम् (Yavagodhūmasambhavam), यवाग्रजं (Yavāgrajam), यवोत्थं (Yavottham) are synonymous. तुषोदं (Tuṣodam), and तुषोदकं (Tuṣodakam) are synonyms.

Sauvīram and Tuṣodakam : The fermented rice and wheat gruel, are digestants and are efficacious in cases of heart disease, anaemia, worms in the intestines, heartburn, *Grahaṇī* (diseases charaecterized by ch. diarrhoea) and piles. *Sauvira* and *Tuṣodaka* are *bhedi* (purgatives).

Guḍa 'sukta (prepared with treacle), *Rasa śukta* (prepared with juice of sugar cane), and *Madhu'sukta* (Prepared with honey) are *gurutaraṇi* (heavier to digest and assimilate), and *abhiṣyandi* (causing obstruction in the channels due to excessive secretion of *doṣas*), following it in the reverse order of enumeration.

When *śūkta* parepared with *mastu,* jaggery, honey, *kāñjikam* in a clean vessel for three nights in a heap of paddy, then it is called as *cukra.*

मद्यवर्गः Madyavargaḥ (Wines and Spirits.)

39 सुरा Surā

सुरा मद्यं प्रसन्ना स्यान्मदिरा वारुणी रसा ।
वरा मण्डा मदकरी माधवी वरुणात्मजा ॥ २३५

इरा कादम्बरी हाला जगलो मेदको मता ।
सौरेयी मधुमैरेयी सुरा सुरभवा स्मृता ॥ २३६

महासुरा च विज्ञेया त्रिविधाऽपि सुरा मता ।
सर्व मद्यं सुसञ्जातं मधूलकमितिस्मृतम् ॥ २३७

सुरा (Surā), मद्यं (Madyam), प्रसन्ना (Prasannā), मदिरा (Madirā), वारुणी
(Vāruṇī), रसा (Rasā), वरा (Varā), मण्डा (Maṇḍā), मदकरी (Madakarī), माधवी (Mādhavī), वरुणात्मजा (Varuṇātmajā), इरा (Irā), कादम्बरी (Kādambarī), हाला (Hālā), जगलः (Jagalaḥ) मेदकः (Medakaḥ). These are some of the types of सुरा (Surā).

मधु मैरेयी (Madhumaireyī), सुरा (Surā) and महासुरा (Mahāsurā) are also three types of सुरा (Surā). सौरेयी (Saureyī) is the synonym of मधुमैरेयी (Madhumaireyi) and सुरभवा (Surabhavā) is the synonym of सुरा (Surā). The alcoholic beverage (मद्य) nicely prepared is called as मधूलक (Madhulaka).

मद्यसामान्यगुणाः General properties and actions.

दीपनं रोचनं मद्यं तीक्ष्णोष्णं तुष्टिपुष्टिदम् ।

सकषायं स्वरारोग्यप्रतिभावर्णकृल्लघु ॥
नष्टनिद्रातिनिद्रेभ्यो हितं पित्तास्रदूषणम् ॥ २३९
कृच्छ्रशूलहितं[१] रूक्षं सूक्ष्मं मूत्रविशोधनम् ।
वातश्लेष्महरं युक्त्या पीतं विषवदन्यथा ॥ २४०

A.H. S.Su. 5.62-64.

Madya is sweet, bitter, pungent, sour and *kaṣāya* in taste and *amla* (sour) in *vipāka* (final transformation after digestion). It stimulates digestive capacity, promotes desire for food, is sharp, *usnavīrya,* provieds contentment and nourishment.

It is beneficial for voice, health, inspires new ideas, improves complexion and is *laghu.* It is beneficial for those who have insomnia or hypersomnia and causes vitiation (aggravation) of *pitta* and *rakta doṣas.*

It is useful in renal colic, *rūk'sa* (roughening), enters the minute channels and has purificatory action on urine.

It pacifies *vāta* and *kapha doṣas* if used with proper application, if not it acts as a poison.

सुरा Surā

कासार्शो ग्रहणीश्वासप्रतिश्यायविनाशिनी ।
स्वेदमूत्रकफस्तन्यरक्तमांसकरी सुरा ॥२४१
[२]कासार्शो ग्रहणीदोषमूत्राघाताऽनिलापहा ।
स्तन्यरक्तक्षयहिता सुरा बृंहणदीपनी ॥२४२

Surā is useful in cough, piles, *Grahaṇī* (diseases characterized by ch. diarrhoea), dyspnoea and rhinorrhea. It increases perspiration, urine output, *kaphadoṣa,* breast milk, blood and *māmsa* (muscular tissue).

Surā is useful in cough, piles, diseases of *Grahaṇī* (characterized by chronic diarrhoea), suppression of urine, and pacifies *vātadoṣa*. It is body promoting, stimulates digestive capacity and is beneficial to increase the breast milk and blood.

प्रसन्ना Prasannā, its properties and actions.

छर्द्यरोचकहृत्कुक्षितोदशूलप्रमर्दिनी ।
प्रसन्ना गुल्मवातार्शोविबन्धानाहनाशिनी ॥२४३

---

१ 'कृशस्थूलहितं' इति अ. हृ. पाठः ।
२ ग्रन्थान्तरेषूद्धृतः अन्यः पाठोऽयं दृश्यते । गुणकर्मणां पौनरुक्त्याद् ।

Prasannā is useful in emesis, anorexia, pains in stomach, and intestinal and other colics. It is also useful in tumours (diverticulosis), piles due to *vātadoṣa,* constipation and flatulence.

यवसुरादयः Yavasurā and other kinds.

पित्तलाऽल्पकफारूक्षा यवैर्वातप्रकोपनी ।
विष्टम्भिनी सुरा गुर्वी श्लेष्मला तु मधूलिका ॥२४४
रूक्षा नातिकफा वृष्या पाचनी चाक्षिकी सुरा ।

S.S.Su.45.178.79.

Yavasurā aggravates *vāta* and *pitta doṣas* and slightly pacifies *kaphadoṣa*. It is roughening in quality. *Madhūlikā* is constipating, *guru* and aggravates *kaphadoṣa.*

Āk'sikī surā is *ruk'sa* (roughening), does not aggravate *kaphadoṣa* much, is *vṛṣya* and digestant.

सीधुभेदाः Types of Sīdhu.

सीधुरामण्डवासः स्याच्छीतपक्वरसस्तथा ।२४५

आमण्डवास (*Āmaṇḍavāsa,)* शीतरस (*'sītarasa)* and पक्वरस *(pakvarasa)* are the types of *sīdhuḥ.*

मधूकसीधूः Madhūkasīdhuḥ and its properties .

सीधूर्मधूकपुष्पोत्थो विदाह्यग्निबलप्रदः ।
रूक्षः कषायः कफहा वातपित्तप्रकोपणः ॥ २४६

(S.S. Su 45.191)

Sīdhuḥ prepared from the flowers of *madhūka* is *vidāhi* (causes burning with hyperacidity and poor digestion), strengthens the digestive capacity), is *rūk'sa*, *kaṣāya* in taste, pacifies *kapha doṣa* and aggravates *vāta pitta doṣas.*

रसासवः Rasāsavaḥ

बल्यः पित्तहरो वर्ण्यो मृद्वीकेक्षुरसासवः ॥ (S.S. Su. 45.190)

---

१ 'हृद्यश्चेक्षु' इति सौश्रुतः पाठः ।

Āsava prepared from juices of cane sugar and grapes gives strength, pacifies *pittadoṣa* and improves complexion of the body.

कोहलो जगलश्च Kohalaḥ and Jagalaḥ Properties and actions.

त्रिदोषो भेद्यवृष्यश्च कोहलो वदनप्रियः ॥२४७
ग्राह्युष्णो जगलः पत्तग रूक्षस्तृट्कफशोफकृत् ॥

हृद्यः प्रवाहिकाटोपदुर्नामानिलशोषजित् ॥ २४८

S.S.Su.45.180.

Kohala aggravates three *doṣas,* is *bhedi,* opposite to *vṛṣya* and is palatable. *Jagala* is astringent, *uṣṇavīrya,* digestant, *rūkṣa,* causes excessive thirst, oedema due to *kapha doṣa* and is cordial. It is useful in dysentery, tympanitis, piles, *vātadoṣa* and consumption.

बक्कसः Bakkasaḥ - properties and actions

बक्कसो हतसारत्वात् विष्टम्भी वातकोपनः । S.S. Su. 45.181

The *Bakkasa* (the residue) as there is no essence, causes flatulance and aggravates *vātadoṣa.*

मार्द्वीकम् Mārdwīkam - Properties and actions.

मधु मद्योत्तमं हृद्यं मार्द्वीकं कथितं तथा ॥२४९
सरमभिषवक्रान्तं कामिकान्तं मदोत्कटम् ॥

मार्द्वीकं लेखनं हृद्यं नात्युष्णं मधुरं सरम् ॥ २५०
[1]अल्पपित्तानिलः पाण्डुमेहार्शः कृमिनाशनम् ॥

A. Hr. Sū 5.72.

मधु (Madhu), **मद्योत्तमं** (Madyottamam), **हृद्यं** (Hṛdyam), **मार्द्वीकं** (Mārdwīkam), **सरम्** (Saram), **अभिषवक्रान्तं** (Abhiṣavakrāntam), **कामिकान्तं** (Kāmikāntam), **मदोत्कटम्** (Madotkaṭam) are synonyms.

Mārdwīkam is *lekhana* (emaciating), cordial (or useful to heart) not very excessively *uṣṇavīrya* and is sweet and *sara* (laxative). It does not aggravate *pitta vāta doṣas* much and is useful in anaemia, *meha* (polyuria including diabetes), piles and intestinal worms.

---

१ 'अल्पपित्ता' इ. अ.सं., अ.हृ. ५. ७२ पाठः ।

खार्जूरम् Khārjūram - its properties and actions.

'तस्मादल्पान्तरगुणं[1] खार्जूरं वातलं गुरु ।'२५१
दीपनं सृष्टविण्मूत्रं विशदाल्पमदं मतम् ॥ A. Sang. Su. 6.121.

Khārjūra is slightly less in qualitiy and slightly differes in properties from the above, it is *guru* and aggravates *vātadosa,* stimulates digestive capacity is diuretic and laxative, non slimy and less intoxicant.

गौडसीधुः शार्करसीधुश्च
Properties and actions of Gauḍa Sīdhuḥ and Śārkāra Sīdhuḥ.

कषायो मधुरः सीधुः गौडः पाचन दीपनः ॥ २५२
शार्करो मधुरो रुच्यो दीपनो बस्तिशोधनः ॥
वातघ्नो मधुरः पाके हृद्य इन्द्रियबोधनः । S. S. Su. 45. 182. 183

Gauḍa sīdhuḥ is *kaṣāya* and sweet in taste and stimulates digestive capacity and is digestant. *Śārkara sīdhuḥ* is sweet in taste, appetising, stimulates digestive capacity and has purificatory action on urinary organs. It pacifies *vāta doṣa,* is sweet in *vipāka*, cordial and stimulates sense organs.

शीतरसिकः Śītarasikaḥ - properties and actions.

कर्षणः शीतरसिकः श्वयथूदरनाशनः॥ २५३
वर्णकृज्जरणः स्वर्यो विबन्धघ्नोऽर्शसां हितः ॥ S.S. Su. 45.185

Śītarasikaḥ is useful for emaciating, anasarca and ascites. It improves complexion, it is digestant, beneficial for voice, removes constipation (deobstruent) and is useful for those who have piles.

40 आसवम् - तद्भेदाश्च Āsavam and its kinds.
मध्वासवः 'Madhwāsavaḥ - properties and actions.

छेदी मध्वासवस्तीक्ष्णो मेदःपीनसकासजित् ॥ २५४
A.S. Su. 6.124

Madhvāsava is sharp and channel cleansing and useful in (reduction of) *meda,* chronic coryza and cough.

---

१ 'अस्मादल्पान्तर इति. अ.सं. अ. ह. सू. ५.७३ इत्यत्र पाठः ।

शार्करो माधवश्च

Śārkaraḥ and Madhavaḥ - properties and actions.

शार्करः सुरभिः सौम्यो माधवो रूक्षणात्मकः ।
आसवो मुखवासश्च सुकुमारः सुयोजितः ॥२५५

Śarkara is fragrant and mild while *Mādhava* is roughening. Both are mild (soft) and used as mouth refreshing.

सुरासवः Surāsavaḥ - properties and actions.

सुरासवस्तीक्ष्णमद स्वादुस्तृष्णानिलापहः ॥ A. S. Su. 6.124

Sūrāsava is strongly intoxicating, sweet in taste, alleviates thirst and pacifies *vāta doṣa*.

मैरेयः Maireyaḥ - properties and actions

तीक्ष्णः कषायो मदकृद् दुर्नामकफगुल्महृत् ॥ २५६
कृमिमेदोऽनिलहरो मैरेयो मधुरो गुरुः ॥ S.S. Su. 45.189.

Maireya is sweet, *kaṣāya* in taste, *guru*, sharp and intoxicating. It is useful in piles, tumours (diverticulosis) due to *kaphadoṣa*, worms and reduces fat and *vātadoṣa*.

आक्षिकसीधुः Akṡika Sīdhūh - properties and actions.

आक्षिकः पाण्डुरोगघ्नो व्रण्यः संग्राहको लघुः ॥ २५७
कषायो मधुरः सीधुः पित्तघ्नोऽसृक्प्रसादनः ॥ S.S. Su.45.186

Ākṡika sidhu is *kaṣāya* and sweet in taste, vulnerary, astringent and *laghu*. It pacifies *pitta doṣa*. purifies blood and useful in anāemia.

जाम्बब सीधुः

Jāṁbava Sīdhuḥ and others and their properties.

जाम्बवो बध्दनिष्यन्दस्तुवरो वातकोपनः ॥२५८
निर्दिशेत् रसतश्चान्यान् कन्दमूलफलासवान् ॥ S. S.Su.4 5.187.

Jāmbavasīdhu is *kaṣāya* in taste, aggravates *vāta doṣa* and reduces the quantity of urine.

The other types of *sīdhus* and *āsavās* prepared from tubers, roots and fruits should be determined by their tastes (etc.).

अरिष्टः Ariṣṭaḥ - properties and kinds.

अरिष्टो द्रव्यसंयोगसंस्कारादधिको गुणैः ॥ २५९
बहुदोषहरश्चैव दोषाणां शमनश्च सः ॥

दीपनः कफवातघ्नः सरः पित्तविरोधनः ॥ २६०
शूलाध्मानोदरप्लीहज्वराजीर्णार्शसां हितः ॥

पिप्पल्यादिकृतो गुल्मकफरोगहरः स्मृतः ॥ २६१
चिकित्सितेषु वक्ष्यन्तेऽरिष्टाः रोगहराः पृथक् ॥

S.S. Su. 45.194. 197

अरिष्टासव सीधूनां गुणान्कर्माणि चाऽऽदिशेत् ॥
बुद्धया यथास्वं संस्कारमवेक्ष्य कुशलो भिषक् ॥ २६२

S.S. Su. 45.197-98

The *Ariṣṭa* is more efficacious owing to the combination of drugs and processing. It is useful in various conditions and pacifies all the *doṣas*.

It stimulates digestive capacity, pacifies, *kapha* and *vāta doṣas* and not hostile to *pitta doṣas* and is laxative. It is useful in colics, flatulence, ascites, disorders of spleen, fevers, indigestion and piles.

The *ariṣṭa* prepared from *pippalī* etc. is useful in tumours (diverticulosis) and disorders caused by *kapha doṣa.* The different types of *ariṣṭas* will be described in *cikitsā sthāna.* (of Suśrta Samhitā)

The intelligent physician can understand the properties and actions of different types (for different diseases) of *ariṣṭas*, *āsavas* and *sīdhus* according to the drugs entering into their composition and the processing method adopted there in.

नवजीर्णमद्यगुणाः

Properties of Madya. - immature & mature

नवं मद्यमभिष्यन्दि गुरु वातादिकोपनम् ॥ २६३
अनिष्टगन्धं विरसमहृद्यमविदाहि च ॥

सुगंधि दीपनं हृद्यं रोचिष्णु कृमिनाशनम् ।२६४
स्फुटस्रोतस्करं जीर्णं लघु वातकफापहम् ॥

Immature *madya* is *abhiṣyandi, guru,* aggravates all the three *doṣas*, bad smelling, does not have proper taste, non cordial and does not cause burning with hyperacidity.

Mature *madya* is aromatic, stimulates digestive capacity, is appetizing, destroys worms, dilates the minute channels of the body, is *laghu* and pacifies *vāta* and *kaphadoṣas*.

वर्ज्यमद्यम् Properties of alcoholic beverages which should be avoided.

सान्द्रं विदाहि दुर्गन्धं विरसं कृमिलं गुरु ॥ २६५
अहृद्यं तरुणं तीक्ष्णमुष्णं दुर्भाजनस्थितम् ॥

अल्पौषधं पर्युषितमत्यच्छं पिच्छिलं च यत् ॥ २६६
तद्वर्ज्यं सर्वदा मद्यं किंचिच्छेषं तु यद् भवेत् ॥

S.S. Su. 45-198-199.

तत्र यत्स्तोकसम्भारस्तरुणं पिच्छिलं गुरु ॥ २६७
कफप्रकोपि तन्मद्यं दुर्जरं च विशेषतः ॥

पित्तप्रकोपि बहलं तीक्ष्णमुष्णं विदाहि च ॥२६८
अहृद्यं फेनिलं पूति कृमिलं विरसं गुरु ॥

तथा पर्युषितं चापि विद्यादनिलकोपनम् ॥ २६९
सर्वैदोषैरुपेतं तु सर्वदोषप्रकोपणम् ॥ S.S. Su. 45.200-203.

The following kinds of *madya* should always be rejected viz. very viscous (thick), causing burning, bad smelling, having improper taste, full of worms, *guru,* unpleasant (non cordial), newly prepared (immature), sharp in taste, hot, preserved in improper vessel; prepared with a comparatively lesser number of ingredients, or have become stale, very clear, slimy and having very small residual portion is remained.

The *madya* prepared from a comparatively lesser number of ingredients, immature, *slimy* and *guru* aggravates *kaphadosa* and is difficult to digest.

The *madya* which is very viscous, sharp, hot and acidic in taste (causes burning sensation), and aggravates *pitta doṣa.*

Non cordial, frothy, having putrid odour, marked by germination in it, has lost its natural taste, *guru* and which has become stale aggravates *vātadoṣa.*

Madya having all the above defects aggravates all the three *doṣas.*

(मद्यप्रभावः) (Madyaprabhāvaḥ)

मद्यं कथं कार्यं करोति ? Mode of action of Madyam

तस्यानेक प्रकारस्य मद्यस्य रसवीर्यतः ॥ २७०
सौक्ष्यादौष्ण्याच्च तैक्ष्ण्याच्च विकासित्वाच्च वह्निना ॥

समेत्य हृदयं प्राप्य धमनीरूर्ध्वमागतम् ॥ २७१
विक्षोभ्येन्द्रिचेतांसि वीर्यं मदयतेऽचिरात् ॥

चिरेण श्लेष्मिके पुंसि पानतो जायते मदः ॥ २७२
अचिराद् वातिके दृष्टः पैत्तिके शीघ्रमेव तु ॥ S.S.Su. 45.204-206.

The various types of alcoholic beverages, due to its *rasa* (taste) and *vīrya*, capacity to enter the fine channels, *uṣṇavirya* property, *tīk'sṇaguṇa*, (permeation), *vikāsī* guṇa (forcible entrance into channels) and due to heating property (of the body) (*vanhī*) it enters the heart and through the upward channels of the heart (i.e. arteries), and then due to its own potency de-thrones the power of organs of perception and mind and intoxicates (the individual) immediately.

An individual of *kaphaprakṛti* can bear the alcoholic beverages well and symptoms of intoxication usually appear later in him. An individual of *vātaprakṛti* gets intoxicated inmmdiately, while the man of *pitta prakṛti* gets intoxicated easily.

प्रकृत्यनुसारेण मद्यपरिणामाः

Effects of *Madya* according to the psychological setup of the individual

सात्विके शौचदाक्षिण्यहर्षमण्डनलालसः ॥ २७३
गीताध्ययनसौभाग्य सुरतोत्साहकृन्मदः ॥

राजसे दुःखशीलत्वमात्मत्यागं ससाहसम् ॥ २७४
कलहं सानुबन्धं तु करोति पुरुष मदः ॥

अशौचनिद्रामात्सर्यागम्यागमनलोलताः ॥ २७५
असत्यभाषणं चापि कुर्याद्धि तामसे मदः ॥

An individual of a *Sātvika* frame of mind exhibts under the influence of alcoholic beverages a predilection for purity, competancy, desire to decorate his body with fine dress and joyfullness.

An individual of *Rājasika* frame of mind beocmes melancholic, of wild daring to the extent of getting killed himself or in such acts which will result in quarreling.

An individual of *Tāmasika* frame of mind shows tendency for uncleanliness, sleep, envy and envinces a desire for women with whom connection is forbidden and speaks untrue.

41 मर्जिका Marjikā*

मर्जिका शिखरिण्युक्ता रसाला सुरभिस्तथा ॥ २७६
उल्बणी खाण्डवरसा चातुर्जातकसंगता ॥

मर्जिकाया गुणा ज्ञेया बीजद्रव्यगुणैः समा ॥२७७

मर्जिका (Marjikā), शिखरिणी (Śikhariṇī), रसाला (Rasālā), सुरभिः (Surabhiḥ), उल्बणी (Ulbaṇī), खाण्डवरसा (Khāṇḍavarasā), चातुर्जातकसंगता (Cāturjātakasangatā) are synonymous.

The properties of *marjikā* are to be understood according to the components entering into·it..

42 जलम् Jalam जलवर्गः Jalavargaḥ

In this class, the synonyms of water its general properties, sources, properties and actions, the nature of wholesome and unwholesome water etc. are mentioned.

पानीयम् Pāniyam (water group) जलवर्ग

पानीयमापः कीलालं नीरं कं सलिलं जलम् ।
अमृतं वारुणं तोयं वार्यम्भोऽम्बूदकं पयः ॥२७८

पानीयं (Panīyam), आपः (Āpaḥ), कीलालं (Kīlālam), नीरं (Nīram), कं (Kam), सलिलं (Salilam), जलम् (Jalam), अमृतं (Amṛtam), वारुणं (Vāruṇam), तोयम् (Toyam), वारि (Vāri), अम्भः (Ambhaḥ), अम्बु (Ambu), उदकम् (Udakam), पयः (Payaḥ), are synonymous.

साधारण गुणकर्माणि General properties and actions.

साधारणं जलं रुच्यं दीपनं पाचनं लघु ।
श्रमतृष्णापहं वातकफमेदोघ्नपुष्टिदम् ॥२८०

---

* Marjikā has been mentioned in *Gaṇadravyāvali.* However it is not found in both the chaukhamba published editions but found in Anandāsram edition. There are various types of रसाला (Rasālā) or शिखरिणी (Śikhariṇī). One is found in seventh chapter again. This is the only representative of the कृतान्नवर्ग (Kṛtānna varga) of the Samhitās and other Nighaṇṭus.

पानीयं मधुरं हिमं च रुचिदं तृष्णास्यशोषापहम् ।
मोहभ्रान्तिमपाकरोति कुरुते भुक्तान्नपत्तिं परम् ॥२८०

निद्रालस्यनिरासनं विषहरं भ्रान्तार्तसंतर्पणम् ।
नृणां धीबलवीर्यवृद्धिजननं नष्टाङ्गपुष्टिप्रदम् ॥२८१

Water, in general is appetizing, stimulates digestive capacity, digestant and *laghu.* It alleviates fatigue, thirst, pacifies *vāta* and *kapha doṣas*, decreases fat *(meda)* and is nourishing.

Water is sweet in taste, *śītavīrya,* appetizing, alleviates thirst, dryness of mouth, fainting and vertigo. It assists in digestion of food.

It is useful in alleviating excessive sleep and lethargy, poison and satiating to persons having pain and fainting.

It is useful in restoring mental capacity, is strength promoting, potentiating and nourishing to the weakned body.

गगनाम्बु Gaganāmbu.

गगनाम्बु त्रिदोषघ्नं गृहीतं यत्सुभाजने ।
बल्यं रसायनं मेध्यं पात्रापेक्षि ततःपरम् ॥ २८२

S.S. Su.45. 26.

Gaganāmbu (rain water directly coming from the sky) collected in a good pot pacifies *three doṣas,* is strength promoting, *rasāyana,* intellect promoting and then afterwards the properties depend upon the pots in which it is preserved.

अनार्तवादि भेदाः

Non seasonal rain water and other types with properties and actions.

अनार्तवं विमुञ्चन्ति वारि वारिधरास्तु यत् ।
तत्त्रिदोषाय सर्वेषां देहिनां परिकीर्तितम् ॥२८३

दिव्यवाय्वग्निसंयोगात्संहता खात्पतन्ति याः ।
शिलाप्रकरबद्धास्ताः करका अमृतोपमाः ॥२८४

अपि नद्याः समुद्रान्ते बहिरापस्तदुद्भवाः ।
धूमावयवनिर्मुक्तगस्तुषाराख्यास्तु ताः स्मृताः ॥२८५
प्राक् समुद्राम्बुसपर्कसमीरणसमन्विताः ।

Clouds bring out rain sometimes apart from the usual seasons, such unseasonal rain water aggravates all the *doṣas.*

By the combination of divine *vāya, agnī* and *āpa* sometimes water solidifies and fall from the sky like stones (hailstone), those are known as *karakā,* which are nectar like in properties.

Moist vapour that arises from the river when they reach the sea, the water above the surface of these rivers looking like smoke particles is called *tuṣāra* (spray dew). It is intermingled with the water of eastern sea (Bay of Bengal) and eastern wind.

अंशूदकम् Amśūdakam

दिवा सूर्यांशुसंतप्तं निशि चन्द्रांशुशीतलम् ॥२८६
कालेन पक्वं निर्दोषमगस्त्योदय निर्विषम् ॥

अंशूदकमिति ख्यातं शारदं विमलं शुचि ॥२८७
स्नानपानावगाहेषु शस्यते तद् यथाऽमृतम् ॥

The water which gets the light of the sun in the day and becomes cool by the moonrays, which is ripen by time, becomes devoid of defects (*doṣa*) and becomes nontoxic due to the rising of the *Agastya Nakśatra* in the *Śarad ṛtu* (autumn), and which is clean and auspicious is called *Amśūdakam.* It is useful for bathing, drinking, swimming and is like a nectar.

[It is the same which is mentioned in A. H. by the name हंसोदकम् (Hamsodakam)].

चन्द्रकान्तजलम् Candrakānta Jalam

चन्दकान्तोद्‌भवं वारि पित्तघ्नं विमलं स्मृतम् ॥२८८

The water from the gem *candrakānta* pacifies *pitta doṣa* and is clean.

नादेयादिजल गुणाः

Properties of the river water and other types of water.

नादेयं वातलं रूक्षं दीपनं लघु लेखनम् ।
तदभिष्यन्दि मधुरं सान्द्रं गुरु कफापहम् ॥२८९
Su. Sū. 45. 31.

तृष्णाघ्नं सारसं बल्यं कषायं मधुरं लघु ।
ताडागं वातलं स्वादु कषायं कटुपाकि च ॥२९०
Su. Sū. 45. 32.

वातश्लेष्महरं वाप्यं सक्षारं कटु पित्तलम् ।
सक्षारं पित्तलं कौपं श्लेष्मघ्नं लघु दीपनम् ॥२९१
Su. Sū. 45. 33.

चौण्ड्यमग्निकरं रूक्षं मधुरं कफकृन्न च ।
कफघ्नं दीपनं हृद्यं लघु प्रस्रवणोद्भवम् ॥२९२ Su. Sū. 45. 31

मधुरं पित्तशमनमविदाह्यौद्भिदं स्मृतम् । Su. Sū. 45. 31.

कैदारं मधुरं पाके गुर्वभ्यभिष्यन्दि दोषलम् ॥२९३
तद्वत् पाल्वलमुद्दिष्टं विशेषात् दोषलं तु तत् । S.S.Su. 45.36

सामुद्रमुदकं विस्रं लवणं सर्वदोषकृत् ॥ २९४ S.S.Su. 45.37

नद्यः पाषाणविच्छिन्न विक्षुब्धाभिहतोदकाः ।
हिमवत्प्रभवाः पथ्याः पुण्या देवर्षिसेविताः ॥२९५

C.S.Su..27. 210 .

Nādeya jala (river water) is *rūksa* (roughening), stimulates digestive capacity, *laghu* and slimming. It is sweet in taste, causes excessive secretion of *doṣas* and obstruction in the channels, viscid, *guru* and pacifies *kaphadoṣa.*

Sārasa jala (Water of natural lakes) pacifies thirst is strength promoting, *kaṣāya,* sweet in taste and *laghu* (easy to digest).

Tāḍāga jala (water of ponds) aggravates *vātadoṣa,* is sweet and *kaṣāya* in taste and pungent in *vipāka.*

Vāpya jala (water from the wells with steps) is salty and *pungent* in taste, pacifies *vāta* and *kapha doṣas* and aggravates *pitta.*

Kaupa jala (water from the well) is salty in taste, aggravates *pittadoṣa* and pacifies *kapha doṣa,* is *laghu* and stimulates digestive capacity.

Chauṇḍya jala (water from pits in rocks) stimulates digestive capacity, is roughening, sweet in taste and does not aggravate *kaphadoṣa.*

Prāsravaṇa jala (water from the fountain) pacifies *kaphadoṣa,* stimulates digestive capacity, is cordial and *laghu* (easy to digest.).

Audbhida jala (water from the springs) is sweet in taste, pacifies *pitta doṣa* and is *avidāhi* (pacifies burning and hyperacidity.)

Kaidāra jala (water from cultivable fields) is sweet in taste, *guru* in *vipāka,* causes excessive secretion of *doṣās* and obstruction in the channels and aggravates *doṣas.*

Pālvala jala (water of small pool) is similar in properties to that of *kaidāra jala* but it especially aggravates the *doṣas.*

Sāmudra jala (sea water) is salty in taste, smells fishy and aggravates all the *doṣas.*

The rivers originating from Himālaya, the waters of which have been agitated, smitten and interrupted by stones, are beneficial and utilised by *Devarṣis* (sages).

The differences of opinon regarding the water from the rivers originating in the Himalayas between the texts of *Caraka* and *Susrata* has been clarified by Cakrapanidatta as follow :

. . पाषाणैर्विच्छिन्नं विक्षुब्धमभिहतं चोदकं यासांस्तास्तथा एतेन अधित्यकाप्रभवा एव हिमालये नद्यः पथ्या उक्ता भवन्ति, यतोऽधित्यका प्रभवास्वेव पाषाणविच्छिन्नत्वादि; अतश्च सुश्रुते यदुक्तं 'हिमवद्प्रभवा ह्द्रोगादीन् जनयन्ति' (सु,सू,अ. ४५) इति तदुपत्यकाभिप्रायेणेति न विरोधः । . . .C.S. Su. 27.210 H.) S.D. K.

पारियात्रभवा याश्च विन्ध्यसह्यभवाश्च याः ।
शिरोहृद्रोगकुष्ठादि हेतुस्ताः श्लीपदस्य च ॥२९६
चन्द्रार्करसंस्पृष्टं वायुनाऽऽस्फालितं बहु ।
पर्वतोपरि यद्वारि समं पौरन्दरेण तु ॥ २९७

तस्यानुगुणमुद्दिष्टं शैलप्रस्रवणोद्भवम् ।
लेखनं दीपनं रूक्षं किञ्चित् वातप्रकोपनम् ॥ २९८

The water of the rivers which arise in *Pāriyātra* mountain and the same of the river which arise in *vindhya, sahyādri* mountains produce diseases of the head, heart disease, skin disorders and elephantiasis.

The water in the table land of a mountain gets the light of the sun, the rays of the moon and which is agitated by force of strong wind is similar in properties to *gaganāmbu.* (*Paurandara jala*)

Following the above mentioned, the properties of the spring water of the mountains should be understood. It is slimming, stimulates digestive capacity, is roughening and slightly aggravates *vāta doṣa.*

आनूपदिदेशभेदेन जलभेदाः

Types of water according to Ānūpādi regions.

आनूपदेशजं वारि तत्सान्द्रं गुरुपिच्छिलम ।
प्रमेहश्लीपदच्छर्दिगलगण्डास्यशोषकृत् ॥ २९९
विपर्ययं जाङ्गलं च समं साधारणं स्मृतम ।

The water from *Ānupadesa* is viscid, *guru* and slimy. It causes disorders characterized by polyuria, elephantiasis, vomiting, goitre and dryness of mouth. The water from *Jāngala deśa* has the opposite properties to the above. The water from *Sādhāraṇa desa* possesses common properties.

ग्राह्याग्राह्य जलस्वरूपाणि

(Nature of wholesome and unwholesome water)

अगन्धमस्पष्टरसं सुशीतं तृड्विनाशनम् ॥३००
अच्छं लघु च हृद्यं च तोयं गुणवदुच्यते ॥

पिच्छिलं कृमिलं क्लिन्नं पर्णशैवालकर्दमैः ॥ ३०१
विवर्णं विरसं सान्द्रं दुर्गन्धं न हितं जलम् ॥

दिवाऽर्ककिरणैर्जुष्टं निशायामिन्दुरश्मिभिः ॥३०२
अरूक्षमनभिष्यन्दि तत्तुल्यं गगनाम्बुना ॥ S.S.Su. 45. 25

Good drinking water is that which has no smell, no perspicuous taste, is cool, relieves thirst, *laghu* (easily digestible) and cordial.

Water which is slimy, having worms in it, moistened with leaves, algae and mud, with various colours, tasteless, viscid and of bad smell is unwholesome (and should be avodied).

Water exposed to the rays of the sun during day time and to the rays of the moon during night time and which is not roughening, not *abhiṣyandī* is equal in properties of *Gaganāmbu.*

श्रृतादिजलभेदाः गुणकर्माणि

(Boiled water its properties and certain other instructions for the use of water)

कफमेदोऽनिलामघ्नं दीपनं बस्तिशोधनम् ॥ ३०३
कासश्वासज्वरहरं पथ्यमुष्णोदकं सदा ॥

भिनत्तिश्लेष्मसंघातं मारुतं चापकर्षति ॥३०४
अजीर्णं जरयत्याशु पीतमुष्णोदकं निशि ॥

मद्यपानसमुद्भूते रोगे पित्तोद्भवे तथा ॥३०५
सन्निपातसमुत्थे च श्रृतशीतं प्रशस्यते ॥

पक्वं त्रिभागार्धहीनं पादहीनं तु हैमने ॥३०६

शिशिरे च वसन्ते च ग्रीष्मे चार्धावशोषितम् ॥
विपरीतमृतुं दृष्ट्वा पादांशं चाष्टभागिकम् ॥३०७

यत् क्वाथ्यमानं निर्वेगं निःफेनं निर्मलं भवेत् ।
चतुर्भागावशेषं तु तत्तोयं गुणवत् स्मृतम् ॥३०८
S.S.Su. 45. 40

तत्पादहीनं वातघ्नमर्धहीनं च पित्तजित् ।
कफघ्नं पादशेषं तु पानीयं लघु दीपनम् ॥३०९

धारापातेन विष्टम्भि दुर्जरं पवनाहतम् ।
श्रृतशीतं त्रिदोषघ्नं बाष्पान्तर्भावशीतलम् ॥३१०
दिवा श्रृतं तु यत्तोयं रात्रौ तदगुरुतां व्रजेत्
रात्रौ श्रृतं दिवा चैव गुरुत्वमधिगच्छति ॥३११
मूर्च्छापित्तोष्णदाहेषु विषे रक्ते मदात्यये ।
भ्रमक्लमपरीतेषु तमके वमथौ तथा ॥३१२
ऊर्ध्वगे रक्तपित्ते च शीतमम्भः प्रशस्यते ।
पार्श्वशूले प्रतिश्याये वातरोगे गलग्रहे ॥३१३
आध्माने स्तिमिते कोष्ठे सद्यः शुद्धे नवज्वरे ।
हिक्कायां स्नेहपीते च शीताम्बु परिवर्जयेत् ॥३१४
अरोचके प्रतिश्याये प्रसेके श्वयथौ क्षये ।
मन्दाग्नावुदरे कुष्ठे ज्वरे नेत्रामये तथा ॥३१५
व्रणे च मधुमेहे च पानीयं मन्दमाचरेत् । S.S.Su. 45. 46.

नद्यः शीघ्रवहा लघ्व्यः प्रोक्ता याश्चामलोदकाः । ३१६
गुर्व्यः शैवालसंछन्नाः कलुषा मन्दगाश्च याः ॥ S.S.Su. 45.22.

प्रायेण नद्यो मरुषु सतिक्ता लवणान्विताः । ३१७
ईषत्कषायमधुरा लघुपाका बले हिताः ॥ S.S.Su. 45. 23.

Hot water pacifies *kapha* and *vāta doṣas*, decreases fat (*meda*) and *āma,* stimulates digestive capacity, clears the urinary organs, alleviates cough, dyspnoea, and fever. It is wholesome (beneficial) all the time.

Hot water taken at night liquifies *kapha doṣa,* pushes the *vātadoṣa* in its natural course and digests the food immediately.

Boiled and cooled water is indicated in the disorders caused by alcoholism and *pitta doṣa* and in the (undigested) disorders caused by *sannipāta*.

Water, boiled down to one third, half and quarter parts of its original quantity should be used in *Hemanta*, *Śiśira* and *Vasanta ṛtu* respectively. In *Grīṣma* it should be used boiled half. If there is unusual variation in a season then it should be boiled to one fourth portion or one eighth portion.

While boiling the water if there is no ebullition, froth, if it remains clear and boiled down to one foruth of its quantity then that water becomes wholesome.

Water boiled down to quarter part should be used to pacify

vātadoṣa, boiled down to half to pacify *pittadoṣa*, and boiled down to three fourth to pacify *kaphadoṣa*. It is *laghu* and stimulates digestive capacity.

If boiled water is cooled down by pouring, it becomes constipating, if cooled down by fanning it becomes difficult to digest and if cooled down (by removal of vapour) by itself it pacifies all the three *doṣas*.

Water boiled in a day time becomes *guru* at the night and if boiled in night time beocmes *guru* on the (next) day.

Cool water is indicated in syncope, *pittadoṣa,* heat, burning sensation, poison, bleeding disorders, alcoholic intoxication, vertigo, exhaustion, feeling of darkness, vomiting, and haematemesis.

Cool water should not be given in the conditions like pain in the sides of the chest, coryza, diseases due to *vātadoṣa,* in disorders of throat, distension of abdomen, where there is no movement as peristalsis of abdomen, on whom purificatory processes have been carried out, in the initial stages of fever (toxic condition). hiccup, and during oleation therapy.

In the following conditions water should be used in less quantity: depressed digestive capacity, ascites, disorders of skin, fever, eye disorders, wounds and diabetes mellitus.

The water of the rivers which is clear and are swift in runing is *laghu* while water of those which are sluggish in their course and or covered with algae and is unclear due to mud etc. is *guru.*

Usually the water of the rivers, which run through *Marudeśa* is possessed of a bitter, saline, slightly *kaṣāya* and sweet taste. It is *laghu* in *vipāka* and is strength promoting.

वर्ज्यजलम् (Properties of unwholesome water)

तृणपर्णोत्करयुतं कलुषं विषसंयुतम् ॥३१८
योऽवगाहेत वर्षासु पिबेद्वाऽपि नवं जलम् ॥

स बाह्याभ्यन्तरान् रोगान् प्राप्नुयात्क्षिप्रमेव हि ॥३१९
अजीर्णे भेषजं वारि जीर्णे वारि बलप्रदम् ।

अमृतं भोजने वारि भुक्तस्योपरि तद्विषम् ॥३२०
तृषितो नैव भुञ्जीत क्षुधितो न जलं पिबेत् ।

तृषितस्य भवेद् गुल्मः क्षुधितस्य दकोदरम् ॥३२१
भुक्तस्याऽऽदौ जलं पीतमग्निसादं कृशाङ्गताम् ।

अन्ते करोति स्थूलत्वमूर्ध्वमामाशये कफम् ॥३२२
मध्ये मध्याङ्गतां साम्यधातूनां जरणं सुखम् ।

If a person takes bath in a water which is contaminated by withered grass, decomposed leaves, rubbish and poison or drinks early rain water he is immediately caught by external or internal diseases.

Water is just like a medicine who has indigestion, after digestion of food it is strength promoting, while taking food water is like a nectar but after completion of feeding it is just like a poison.

The one who is thirsty should not take food, and if one is hungry he should not drink water . Thirsty one (and taking food) gets tumour (diverticulosis) and hungry one (and drinking water) gets ascites.

Water taken before food causes depression of digestive capacity and causes emaciation, if the same taken after food causes obesity and accumulation of *kapha doṣa* in stomach. Water taken in the food keeps the body and its tissues in equilibrium, proper digestion and health.

पञ्चविधभौमजलम्
(Five types of soil and the properties of their water)

भूमिः पञ्चविधा ज्ञेया कृष्णा रक्ता सिता तथा ॥ ३२३
पीता नीला भवेच्चान्या गुणास्तासां प्रकीर्तिताः ॥

कृष्णा च मधुरा क्षारा कषाया पीतवर्णिनी ॥ ३२४
रक्ता सा च भवेत्तिक्ता मधुराम्ला सिता तथा ॥

नीला सकटुका ज्ञेया भूमिभागाज्जलं विदुः ॥ ३२५
सघनं मधुरं नीरं कृष्णभूमिप्रतिष्ठितम् ॥

पीताश्रितं कषायं स्यात् रक्तायाः पित्तलं स्मृतम् ॥ ३२६
सिताया मधुराम्लं स्यान्नीलाया कटुकं स्मृतम् ॥

जलं पञ्चविधम् एतत् भूमिभागेन लक्षयेत् ॥३२७

Soil is of five types 1) *kṛṣṇā* (black), 2) *raktā* (red), 3) *Sītā* (white), 4) *Pīta* (yellowish), and 5) *Nilā* (greenish). The taste of these soils are as follows:

Kṛṣṇā soil is sweet and salty; *Pītā* soil is *kaṣāya* (astringent);

Raktā soil is bitter; *Sitā* soil is sweet and sour; *Nīlā* soil is pungent. According to the taste of the soil, the taste of water should be understood.

Water in *kṛṣṇā* soil is viscid and sweet, water in *Pītā* soil is *kaṣāya,* water in *raktā* soil aggravates *pitta doṣa,* water in *sitā* soil is sweet and sour and water in *nīlā* soil is pungent. These five types of water are according to the types of soil.

नारिकेलोदकगुणाः Coconut water- properties & actions

वृष्यं पिपासादाहघ्नं नारिकेलोदकं लघु ।
तदेव जीर्णं विष्टम्भि गुरु पित्तकरं स्मृतम् ॥ ३२८

Cocoanut (shell) water is *vṛṣya,* alleviates thirst and burning sensation and is *laghu.* But the same when overmature it is constipating, *guru* and aggravates *pitta doṣa.*

(मांसवर्ग) मांसद्रव्याणि Māmsadravyāṇi

(Meat and other constituents of the body).

The topic is divided into three classes: (A) .The शरीरम् (Śarīram) The human body and its constituents mentioned in *Puruṣādi* class; (B) The constituents which are to be used i.e. *Dhatavaḥ* (tissues) and which are acted upon; (C) By animals having the same constituents.

"अस्मिन् शास्त्रे पञ्चमहाभूत शरीरि समवायः पुरुष इत्युच्यते । तस्मिन् क्रिया सोऽधिष्ठानं . . . .
तत्र पुरुषः प्रधानं, तस्योपकरणमन्यत; तस्मात् पुरुषोऽधिष्ठानम ।"
सु.सू. १. २२.

Here in this science, the *puruṣa* (the self or conscious organic individual) is described as the combination of the soul (the self) and the five primary material principles . It is he who is to be treated and the remaining all are the means of his treatment. (S. D. K.).

A) शरीर वर्ग Sarira vargaḥ

43 पुरुषः Puruṣaḥ

मानुषः पुरुषो वाऽथ शतायुर्नर एव च ।
कान्तो मर्त्यः पुमान् वक्ता दीर्घपेशी च मानवः ॥३२९

नरमांसमरवाद्यं स्यान्मूत्रमालेपनं मतम्
नेत्ररोगहरं वृष्यं पाण्डुशोफविनाशनम् ॥ ३३०

मानुषः (Mānuṣaḥ), पुरुषः (Puruṣaḥ), शतायुः ('Satāyuḥ), नरः (Naraḥ), कान्तः (Kāntaḥ), मर्त्यः (Martyaḥ), पुमान् (Pumān), वक्ता (Vaktā), दीर्घपेशी (Dīrghape'sī), मानवः (Mānavaḥ), are synonymous.

Human meat is unconsumable, human urine is useful in external application. It is beneficial in diseases of eye, *vṛṣya* and useful in anaemia and anasarca.

स्त्री Strī

स्त्री योषिद् वनिता योषा वासिता वामलोचना ।
प्रतीपदर्शिनी श्यामा कान्ता नार्यङ्गनाऽबला ॥३३१
रामा च कामिनी भीरुः सुन्दरी कामुका तथा ।
महिला ललना गौरी प्रोत्तग सीमन्तिनीति च ॥३३२
प्रमदा युवती चैव सैकवासा प्रकीर्तिता ॥

स्त्री (Strī), योषिद् (Yoṣid), वनिता (Vanitā), योषा (Yoṣā), वासिता (vāsitā), वामलोचना (Vāmalocanā), प्रतीपदर्शिनी (Pratīpadarsinī), श्यामा ('Syāmā), कान्ता (Kāntā), नारी (Nārī), अङ्गना (Aṅganā), अबला (Abalā), रामा (Rāmā), कामिनी (Kāminī), भीरुः (Bhīruḥ), सुन्दरी (Sundarī), कामुका (Kāmukā), महिला (Mahilā), ललना (Lalanā), गौरी (Gaurī), सीमन्तिनी (Sīmantinī) प्रमदा (Pramadā), युवती (Yuvatī), एकवासा (Ekvāsā) are synonymous.

शरीरम् 'Sarīram (Body)

शरीरं शकटं देहं पुरं कायं कलेवरम् ॥ ३३३
वपुश्चावयवस्थानमात्मा दशरथस्तथा ॥

शरीर ('Sarīram), शकटं ('Sakaṭam), देहं (Deham), पुरं (Puram), कायं (Kāyam), कलेवरं (Kalevaram), वपुः (Vapuḥ), अवयवस्थानं (Avayavasthānam), आत्मा (Ātmā), दशरथः (Da'sarathaḥ) are synonymous.

वाचा Vācā (Speech)

वाचा सरस्वती वाणी वाग्गौरी वचनी तथा ॥ ३३४
गिरा च भारती चैव ब्राह्मी भाषा च गीरसा ॥

---

१ 'कान्त्यः' क्वचित् पुस्तके पाठः ।

वाचा (Vācā), सरस्वती (Saraswatī), वाणी (Vāṇī), वाक् (Vāk), गौरी (Gaurī), वचनी (Vacanī), गिरा (Girā), भारती (Bhāratī), ब्राह्मी (Brāhmī), भाषा (Bhāṣā), गीः (Gīḥ), रसा (Rasā) are synonymous.

वायुः Vāyuḥ

वायुः प्रभञ्जनः कर्ता मारुतः श्वसनोऽनिलः ॥ ३३५
समीरणो मातरिश्वा पवनश्च सदागतिः ॥
प्राणोऽपान उदानश्च समानो व्यान एव च ॥ ३३६
कृकरो देवदत्तश्च नागः कूर्मो धनंजयः ॥
'तत्र रूक्षो लघुः शीतः खरः सूक्ष्मश्चलोऽनिलः' ॥३३७

(A.H.Su. 1.)

वायुः (Vāyuḥ), प्रभञ्जनः (Prabhañjanaḥ), कर्ता (Kartā), मारुतः (Mārutaḥ), श्वसनः (Śwasanaḥ), अनिलः (Anilaḥ), समीरणः (Samīraṇaḥ), मातरिश्वा (Mātariswā), पवनः (Pavanaḥ), सदागतिः (Sadāgatiḥ), etc. are synonymous.

Prāṇa, Apāna, Udāna, Samāna, Vyāna, Kṛkara, Devadatta, Nāga, Kūrma and *Dhanañjaya* are the types of *Vāyuḥ*.

Rūk'sa (rough or dry), *laghu* (light), *'sita* (cold), *khara* (Sharp), *sūk'sma* (penetrating) and *cala* (moving) are the qualtities of *vāyu*.

पित्तम् Pittam

पित्तं तेजोमयं तित्तं शिखी वैश्वानरोऽनलः ॥३३८
ज्वरः पक्ता तृषाकर्ता शोषं चैव प्रकीर्तितम् ॥
'पित्तं सस्नेहतीक्ष्णोष्णं लघु विस्रं सरं द्रवम्' । ½ (A.H.Su. 1.)

आग्नेयमुष्णं विशदं सतीक्ष्णं सरं द्रवं विस्रतरं विदाहि ॥
विनीलमम्लं कटुकं च पित्तं पक्वाशयामाशयमध्यवर्ति ॥ ३३९

पित्तम् (Pittam), तेजोमयं (Tejomayam), तित्तं (Tiktam), शिखी(Śikhī), वैश्वानरः (Vaisvānaraḥ), अनलः (Analaḥ), ज्वरः (Jwaraḥ), पक्ता (Paktā), तृषाकर्ता (Tṛṣākartā), शोषं (Sośam) are synonymous.

Pitta is slightly unctuous, sharp, hot (*uṣṇa*), light (*laghu*), having fishy smell (*visram*), laxative (*saram*) and fluid (*dravam*).

Pitta is having predominance of *Agni*, *uṣna* (hot), non slimy, irritant, laxative, fluid, having fishy smell, causing burning with hyperacidity, green in colour, sour, pungent and is predominantly in between *Āmāśaya* and *Pakvāśaya*.

श्लेष्मा Sleṣmā

श्लेष्मा बलासः सततो बलवान्समकृत्तथा ।
सोमयोनिरनिर्वाणो सुनिद्राजनकः कफः ॥३४०
"स्निग्धः शीतो गुरुर्मन्दः श्लक्ष्णो मृत्स्नः स्थिरः कफः ।"½
(A.H.Su. 1.)
स्निग्धो मृदुर्मधुर पिच्छिल शीतसान्द्रः ।
श्वेतो गुरुश्च लवणानुरसो विदाहात् ॥
श्लेष्मा वसत्युरसि मूर्धनि सर्वसन्धि
ष्वामाशयेषु वसति तत्र परं विशेषात् ॥ ३४०

श्लेष्मा (Śleṣmā), बलासः (Balāsaḥ), सततः (Satataḥ), बलवान् (Balawān), समकृत् (Samakṛt), सोमयोनिः (Somoyoniḥ), अनिर्वाणः(Anirwāṇaḥ), सुनिद्राजनकः (Sunidrājanakaḥ), कफः (Kaphaḥ) are synonymous.

Kapha is unctuous, *śīta* (cold), *guru* (heavy), *manda* (dull), *ślakṣṇa* (slippery though being hard), slimy and static.

Kapha is unctuous, soft, sweet, slimy, cold, viscid, white, *guru* (heavy), salty in subsidiary taste after partial digestion, remains predominantly in chest, head, all the joints and especially in *Āmaśaya.*

मोहः Mohah

त्रिदोषसंभवो मोहः संकरो मिश्र एव च ।
संनिपातो मतिभ्रंशः संन्यासो नष्टसंज्ञकः ॥३४२

त्रिदोषसंभवः (Tridoṣasambhavaḥ), मोहः (Mohaḥ), संकरः (Sankaraḥ), मिश्रः (Miśraḥ), संनिपातः (Sannipātaḥ), मतिभ्रंशः (Matibhramśaḥ), संन्यासः (Sannyāsaḥ), नष्टसंज्ञकः (Naṣṭasanjñakaḥ) are synonymous.

प्रकृतयः Prakṛtayaḥ - Body constitutions.

कृशो रूक्षोऽल्पकेशश्च चलचित्तोऽनवस्थितः ।
बहुवाग्व्योमगः स्वप्ने वातप्रकृतिकोऽधमः ॥ ३४३

अकालपलितो गौरः प्रस्वेदी कोपनो बुधः ।
स्वप्ने च दीप्तिमत्प्रेक्षी पित्तलो मध्यमो नरः ॥३४४

स्थिरचित्तः सुपुष्टाङ्गः सुप्रजः स्निग्धमूर्धजः ।
स्वप्ने जलाशयालोकी श्लेष्मप्रकृतिरुत्तमः ॥३४५

A person of *vātaprakṛti* : His body builtup is thin, rough, having less amount of hair, has unstable mind, is disordered, a chatterbox and in the dreams he flies in the sky. This type of *prakṛti* (body coustitution) is called as *Adhama prakṛti.*

A person of *pittaprakṛti* : His hair bcome grey at early age, has fair, complexion, sweats excessively, prompt to anger, intelligent and in the dreams he observes bright objects. This type of *prakṛti* (body constitution) is called as *Madhyama prakṛti.*

A person of *kapha prakṛti* : His mind is stable, has a well nourished body, has many children, his hair are unctuous and in the dreams he observes water reservoirs. This type of *prakṛti* (body constituation) is called as *Uttama prakṛti.*

44. (शरीर) धातवः (Śarīra) Dhātavaḥ - Body Tissues.

अस्थि Asthi

अस्थि हड्डं बलकरं संधानं देहधारणम् ।
सकलं मांसलिप्तं च सर्वमेदःसमुद्भवम् ॥ ३४६

अस्थि (Asthi), हड्डं (Haḍḍam), बलकरं (Balakaram), संधानं (Sandhānam), देहधारणं (Dehadhāraṇam), सकलं (Sakalam), मांसलिप्तं (Māmsaliptam), सर्वमेदः समुद्भवं (Sarvamedahsamudbhavam) are synonymous.

मांसम् (Māmsam).

आमिषं लोमनं मांसं रस्यं शोणितसंभवम् ।
अङ्गजं पिशितं कीरं क्रव्यं राक्षसभोजनम् ॥ ३४७

आमिषं (Āmiṣam), लोमनं (Lomanam), मांसं (Māmsam), रस्यं (Rasyam), शोणितसंभवम् (Śoṇitasambhavam), अङ्गजम् (Angajam), पिशितं (Piśitam), कीरं (Kīram), क्रव्यं (Kravyam), राक्षसभोजनम् (Rākṣasabhojanam) are synonymous.

वसा Vasa

वस्रा वसा पीतधरा मेदोमांससमुद्भवा ।
सर्वस्नेहप्रधाना च वसाऽस्थिजननी तथा ॥३४८

वस्रा (Vasrā), वसा (Vasā), पीतधरा (Pītadharā), मेदोमांससमुद्भवा (Medomāmsasamudbhawā), सर्वस्नेहप्रधाना (Sarvasnehapradhānā), वसा (Vasā), अस्थिजननी (Asṭhijananī) are synonymous.

रक्तम् (Raktam)

रक्तं तु शोणितं विस्रमसृग्लोहितमेव च ।
आग्नेयमामिषकरं प्राणदं रससंभवम् ॥३४९
अशुद्धं रुधिरं चैव रक्तनाम प्रकीर्तितम् ।

रक्तं (Raktam), शोणितं (Śonitam), विस्रं (Visram), असृक् (Asṛk), लोहितं (Lohitam), आग्नेयं (Āgneyam), आमिषकरं (Āmiṣakaram), प्राणदं (Prāṇadam), रससंभवम् (Rasasambhavam), अशुद्धं (Aśuddham), रुधिरं (Rudhiram) are synonymous.

शुक्रम् Śukram.

शुक्रं तेजो बलं पुंस्त्वं पौरुषं हर्षसंभवम् ।
रेतो वीर्यं वृद्धिकरं शिरःस्थं सप्तधातुजम् ॥३५०

शुक्रं (Śukram), तेजः (Tejaḥ), बलं (Balam), पुंस्त्वं (Pumstvam), पौरुषं (Pauruṣam), हर्षसंभवं (Harṣasambavam), रेतः (Retaḥ), वीर्यं (Vīryam), वृद्धिकरं (Vṛddhikaram), शिरःस्थं (Śirastham), सप्तधातुजम् (Saptadhātujam) are synonymous.

मज्जा Majjā

अस्थिसारस्तथा मज्जा बीजं तेजोऽस्थिसंभवम् ॥

अस्थिसारः (Asṭhisārah), मज्जा (Majjā), बीजं (Bījam), तेजः (Tejaḥ), अस्थिसंभवम् (Asthisambhavam) are synonymous.

रसः Rasaḥ

रसः प्राणप्रदः पथ्यः षड्रसो ह्यन्नसंभवः ॥ ३५१
रक्तस्य धातुकर्ता च स च रक्तपिता स्मृतः ॥

रसः (Rasaḥ), प्राणप्रदः (Prāṇapradaḥ), पथ्यः (Pathyaḥ), षड्रसः (Ṣaḍrasaḥ), अन्नसंभवः (Annasambhavaḥ), रक्तधातुकर्ता (Raktadhātukartā), रक्तपिता (Raktapitā) are synonymous.

सप्तधातुजनिक्रमः Genesis of saptadhātus

रसाद्रक्तं ततो मांसं मांसान्मेदोऽस्थि मेदसः ॥ ३५२
अस्थ्नो मज्जा ततः शुक्रमिति तेषां जनिक्रमः ॥

Rasadhātu produces *rakta*, from *raktadhātu* is formed *māmsadhātu,* from *māmsadhātu* orginates *medodhatu* which gives rise to *asthi dhātu*. From *asthi dhātu* originates *majjā* which in its turn produces *śukradhātu.*

C) प्राणीवर्गः

45 हस्ती Hastī (An elephant)

हस्ती द्विपो गजो नागः इभोऽथ द्विरदः करी ॥ ३५३
वारणः कुञ्जरो दन्ती मातङ्गः षष्टिहायनः ॥

कुम्भी स्तम्बेरमः पद्मी सिन्धुरश्च मतङ्गजः ॥ ३५४
करेणुः करिणी प्रोक्ता कलभः करिशावकः ॥

हस्तिनी धेनुका ज्ञेया गजस्त्री गजगामिनी ॥ ३५५
हस्ती कफानिलौ हन्यादुष्णः पित्तास्रकोपनः ।

हस्ती (Hastī), द्विपः (Dwipaḥ), गजः (Gajaḥ), नागः (Nāgaḥ), इभः (Ibhaḥ), द्विरदः (Dwiradaḥ), करी (Karī), वारणः (Wāraṇaḥ), कुञ्जरः (Kuñjaraḥ), दन्तीन् (Dantin), मातङ्गः (Mātaṅgaḥ), षष्टिहायनः (Ṣaṣṭihāyanaḥ), कुम्भी (Kumbhī), स्तम्बेरमः (Stamberamaḥ), पद्मी (Padmī), सिन्धुरः (Sindhuraḥ), मतङ्गजः (Mataṅgajaḥ) are synonymous and करेणुः (Karenuḥ), करिणी (Kariṇī) is she elephant हस्तिनी (Hastinī), धेनुका (Dhenukā), गजस्त्री (Gajastrī), and गजगामिनी (Gajagāminī) are synonyms for she elephant; and young one is called कलभः (Kalabhaḥ) of which synonym is करिशावक (Kariśavakā).

The flesh (or meat) of an elephant pacifies *kapha vāta doṣas, uṣṇavīrya* and aggravates *rakta* and *pittadoṣas.*

46 अश्वः Aśwah (a horse)

घोटोऽश्वस्तुरगो वाजी हरिहंसस्तुरंगमः ॥ ३५६
शालिहोत्रः जवी सप्तिस्तुरङ्गश्च ययुर्हयः ॥
घोटिका वडवा वामी प्रसूकाऽश्वा च वाजिनी ॥ ३५७
आश्वं सलवणं स्निग्धं बल्यं च गुरु बृंहणम् ॥

घोटकस्तु कटुः पाके दीपनः कफपित्तकृत् ॥ ३५८
वातहृद् बृंहणो बल्यश्चक्षुष्यो मधुरो लघुः ॥

घोटः (Ghoṭaḥ), अश्वः (Aśwaḥ), तुरगः (Turagaḥ), वाजी (Wājī), हरिः (Hariḥ), हंसः (Hansaḥ), तुरंगमः (Turangamaḥ), शालिहोत्रः (Śālihotraḥ), जवी (Javī), सप्तिः (Saptiḥ), तुरङ्गः (Turangaḥ), ययुः (Yayuḥ), हयः (Hayaḥ) are synonymous.

घोटिका (Ghoṭikā), वडवा (Vaḍawā), वामी (Vāmi), प्रसूका (Prasūkā) अश्वा (Aśwā), वाजिनी (Wājinī) are synonyms for mare.

The flesh of a horse is salty, unctuous, strength promoting, *guru* and increases the bulk of the body.

It is pungent in *vipāka*, stimulates digestive capacity, aggravates *kapha*, *pitta* and pacifies *vātadoṣa,* is beneficial to the eyes, is sweet in taste and *laghu.*

47 उष्ट्रः Uṣtraḥ (A Camel)

उष्ट्रः क्रमेलको धूम्रः करभो दीर्घमार्गगः ॥ ३५९
ग्रीवाङ्कुशः कुनासश्च दीर्घग्रीवोऽथ धूसरः ॥

वक्रग्रीवो दीर्घजङ्घो धूम्रो दासेरको मयः ॥ ३६०
उष्ट्रमांसं लघु स्वादु चक्षुष्यमनिलापहम् ॥

ऊष्णमर्शःप्रशमनं मेदःपित्तकफापहम्[१] ॥ ३६१

उष्ट्रः (Uṣtraḥ), क्रमेलकः (Kramelakaḥ), धूम्रः (Dhūmraḥ), करभः (Karabhaḥ), दीर्घमार्गगः (Dīrghamārgagaḥ), ग्रीवाङ्कुशः (Grīvān'kuśaḥ), कुनासः (Kunāsaḥ), दीर्घग्रीवः (Dīrghagrīvaḥ), धूसरः (Dhūsaraḥ), वक्रग्रीवः (Vakragrīvaḥ), दीर्घजङ्घः (Dīrghajanghaḥ), धूम्रः (Dhūmraḥ), दासेरकः (Dāserakaḥ), मयः (Mayaḥ) are synonymous .

The flesh of a camel is sweet in taste, *uṣṇavīrya* and pacifies *vātadoṣa.* It is *laghu,* beneficial to eyes, pacifies piles. It decreases *meda* (fatty tissue) and *kapha-pitta doṣas.*

48 गर्दभः Gardabhaḥ (An ass)

गर्दभः शङ्कुकर्णश्च बालेयो रासभः खरः ॥
भारवाहो भूमिगमो धूसरो रेणुभूषितः ॥ ३६२

गार्दभं वातनुद् बल्यं बृंहणं कफपित्तकृत् ॥
कटु पाके लघु श्रेष्टं तस्माद् वन्यखरोद्भवम् ॥ ३६३

---

१ 'कफावहम्' इति चौखम्बा मुद्रित पुस्तके पाठ। 'कफप्रदम्' इति क्वचित पुस्तके पाठः।

गर्दभः (Gardabhaḥ), शङ्कुकर्णः (Śaṅkukarṇaḥ), बालेयः (Bāleyaḥ), रासभः (Rāsabhaḥ), खरः (Kharaḥ), भारवाहः (Bhāravāhaḥ), भूमिगमः (Bhūmigamaḥ), धूसरः (Dhūsaraḥ), रेणुभूषितः (Reṇubhūṣitaḥ) are synonymous.

The flesh of an ass is pungent in taste, and *laghu* in *vipāka,* pacifies *vātadoṣa,* promotes strength and body and aggravates *kapha pitta doṣās*.

The flesh of a wild ass has better qualities than those of the domestic one.

अश्वतरः Aśwataraḥ (A mule) (66)

तज्जो द्युगाम्यश्वतरः शीघ्रगो वेगपूजितः ॥
बल्यमाश्वतरं मांसं बृंहणं कफपित्तलम् ॥ ३६४

अश्वतरः (Aśwataraḥ), द्युगामी (Dyugāmī), शीघ्रगः (Śīghragaḥ), and वेगपूजितः (Vegapūjitaḥ)are the synonyms for *Aśvatarah.*

The flesh of a mule promotes strength and is body promoting. It aggravates *kapha* and *pitta doṣas.*

49 अजः Ajaḥ (A goat)

छगलो बर्करश्छागस्तथा बस्तः पयस्वलः ।
अजो बूकडको मेध्यो लम्बकर्णः पशुस्तथा ॥३६५

छागमांसं गुरु स्निग्धं लघुपाकं त्रिदोषनुत् ॥३६६
अदाहि रुचिदं नाऽतिशीतं पीनसनाशनम् ॥
देहधातुसमानत्वादनभिष्यन्दि दीपनम् ॥३६७

छगलः (Chagalaḥ), बर्करः (Barkaraḥ), छागः (Chāgaḥ), बस्तः (Bastaḥ), पयस्वलः (Payaswalaḥ), अजः (Ajaḥ), बूकडकः (Būkaḍakaḥ), मेध्यः (Medhyaḥ), लम्बकर्णः (Lambakarṇaḥ), पशुः (Paśhuḥ), are synonymous.

The flesh of a goat is *guru,* unctuous, *laghu* after *vipāka* and pacifies the three *doṣas*, does not cause burning and regurgiration, appetizing, not too *śītavīrya,* and useful in chronic coryza. Being similar (in properties) to the human tissues it is *anabhiṣyandi* (does not cause secretion of *doṣas* in the channels of the body) and stimulates the digestive capacity.

50 अविः Aviḥ (A ram)

भेडो मेषो हुडो मेण्ढ्र उरभ्र उरणोऽविकः ।
अविः पशुस्तथैवेड एडकः पृष्ठशृंगकः ॥३६८

ऊर्णायु रोमशो वृष्णिर्मेदपुच्छस्तु बर्बुकः ।
मेषमांसं गुरुस्निग्धं बल्यं पित्तकफप्रदम् ॥३६९

*मेषपुच्छामिषं वृष्यं कफपित्तकरं गुरु ॥

भेडः (Bheḍaḥ), मेषः (Meṣaḥ), हुडः (Huḍaḥ), मेण्ढ्रः (Meṇḍhraḥ), उरभ्रः (Urabhraḥ), उरणः (Uraṇaḥ), अविकः (Avikaḥ), अविः (Aviḥ), पशुः (Paśuḥ), एडः (Eḍaḥ), एडकः (Eḍakaḥ), पृष्ठशृंगकः (Pṛṣṭhaśṛṅgakaḥ), ऊर्णायुः (Ūrṇāyuḥ), रोमशः (Romaśaḥ), वृष्णिः (Vṛṣṇiḥ), मेदपुच्छः (Medapucchaḥ), बर्बुकः (Barbukaḥ) are synonyms.

The flesh of a ram is *guru,* unctuous, strength promoting, aggravates *kaphapitta doṣas* and is *vṛṣya.*

51 वृकः Vṛkaḥ (A wolf)

ईहामृगस्तु कोकः स्याद् वृको वत्सादनोऽविभुक् ॥ ३७०

ईहामृगः (Ihāmṛgaḥ), कोकः (Kokaḥ), वृकः (Vṛkaḥ), वत्सादनः (Vatsādanaḥ), अविभुक् (Avibhuk) are synonymous.

52 व्याघ्रः Vyāghraḥ (A tiger)

व्याघ्रः पञ्चनखो द्वीपी शार्दूलोऽथ गुहाशयः ।
पुण्डरीकस्तीक्ष्णदंष्ट्रस्तपस्वी घोरदर्शनः ॥ ३७१
द्वीपी स्निग्धो भवेच्चोष्णो मधुरो लघुदीपनः ।
वातघ्नः पित्तशमनो बल्यो वृष्यो रुचिप्रदः ॥३७२

व्याघ्रः (Vyāghraḥ), पञ्चनखः (Pañcanakhaḥ), द्वीपी (Dwīpī), शार्दूलः (Śardūlaḥ), गुहाशयः (Guhāśayaḥ), पुण्डरीकः (Puṇḍarīkaḥ), तीक्ष्णदंष्ट्रः (Tīkṣṇadamṣtraḥ), तपस्वी (Tapasvī), घोरदर्शनः (Ghoradarśanaḥ) are synonymous.

The flesh of a tiger is sweet in taste, *uṣṇavīrya, laghu,* unctuous pacifies *vāta* and *pitta doṣās.* It stimulates digestive capacity, strength promoting, is *vṛṣya* and appetizing.

शरभः Śarabhaḥ (67) (A leoperd or panther)

शरभश्चित्रकायः स्यादुपव्याघ्रो मृगान्तकः ।
शूरश्च क्षुद्रशार्दूलश्चित्रव्याघ्र इतीरितः ॥३७३

* 'मेदः पुच्छामिषं' इति साधुपाठः भविष्यति ।

शरभः (Śarabhaḥ), चित्रकायः (Citrakāyaḥ), उपव्याघ्रः (Upavyāghraḥ), मृगान्तकः (Mṛgāntakaḥ), शूरः ('Suraḥ), क्षुद्रशार्दूलः (Kśudraśārdūlaḥ), चित्रव्याघ्रः (Citravyāghraḥ) are synonymous.

53 केसरी Kesarī (A lion) (सिंहः Simhaḥ)

सिंहः पञ्चमुखो दृप्तः क्रव्यात्पञ्चाननो हरिः ।
केशरी मृगराजश्च विक्रान्तः श्वेतपिङ्गलः ॥३७४

सिंहः (Simhaḥ), पञ्चमुखः (Pañcamukhaḥ), दृप्तः (Dṛptaḥ), क्रव्यात् (Kravyāt), पंचाननः (Pañcānanaḥ), हरिः (Hariḥ), केशरी (Ke'sarī), मृगराजः (Mṛgarājaḥ), विक्रान्तः (Vikrāntaḥ), श्वेतपिङ्गलः ('Svetapiṅgalaḥ), are synonymous.

54 सूकरः Sūkaraḥ (A pig) वराहः Varāhaḥ

सूकरो वज्रदंष्ट्रश्च वराहो रोमशः किरिः ।
दंष्ट्री दन्तायुधः क्रोडः पीनस्कन्धो बहुप्रजः ॥३७५

स्नेहनं बृंहणं वृष्यमामघ्नमनिलापहम् ।
वाराहं स्वेदनं बल्यं रोचनं श्रमनुद् गुरु ॥३७६

ग्रामसूकरजं विस्रं पित्तलं बलकृद् गुरु ।

सूकरः (Sūkaraḥ), वज्रदंष्ट्रः (Vajradamṣtraḥ), वराहः (Varāhaḥ), रोमशः (Romaśaḥ), किरिः (Kiriḥ), दंष्ट्री (Damṣtrī), दन्तायुधः (Dantāudhaḥ), क्रोडः (Kroḍaḥ), पीनस्कन्धः (Pīnaskandhaḥ), बहुप्रजः (Bahuprajaḥ),are synonymous.

The flesh of a pig is unctuous, bulk promoting, *vṛsya,* pacifies *āma* and *vātadoṣa*. It is sweat promoting, strength promoting, appetizing, fatigue decreasing and *guru.*

The flesh of a domestic pig is fishy smelling, aggravates *pitta doṣa* and is *guru.*

55 मृगः Mṛgaḥ (A deer) हरिणः Hariṇaḥ

मृगोऽथ हरिणो न्यङ्कुः सारङ्गः पृषतोरुरुः ॥ ३७७
एणः श्यामलपृष्ठश्च कुरङ्गश्चारुलोचनः ॥

एणमांसं हिमं रुच्यं ग्राहिदोषत्रयापहम् ॥३७८
षड्रसं बलदं पथ्यं लघु हृद्यं कफास्रजित् ॥

मृगः (Mṛgaḥ), हरिणः (Hariṇaḥ), न्यङ्कुः (Nyankuḥ), सारङ्गः (Sārangaḥ), पृषतः (Pṛṣataḥ), रुरुः (Ruruḥ) are the मृगजातयः (varieties or kinds). एणः (Eṇaḥ) is श्यामलपृष्ठः (Śyāmal pṛsthaḥ - Blackish skin coat) and कुरङ्गः (Kurangaḥ) and चारुलोचनः (Carulocanah) (having beautiful eyes), are synonymous.

These are various kinds of मृग (Mṛga) - Deer.

The meat of *eṇa* (a type of deer) is having all the six tastes. *śītavīrya,* appetizing, astringent (withholds elimination of faeces and urine) and pacifies all the three *doṣas.*

It is *laghu*, strength promoting, beneficial to health, *laghu,* cordial and pacifies *kapha* and *rakta doṣas.*

56 महिषः Mahiṣaḥ (A buffaelo)

महिषः कासरः शृङ्गी श्यामः कृष्णो लुलायकः ॥३७९
विषाणी कलुषो दंशी पीनस्कन्धो रजस्वलः ॥

महिषी मन्दगमना महाक्षीरा पयस्विनी ॥३८०
लुलायकान्ता कलुषा तुरङ्गद्वेषिणी च सा ॥

स्निग्धोष्णो महिषस्तित्तगे निद्राशुक्रबलप्रदः ॥ ३८१
मधुरस्तर्पणो वृष्यो गुरुमांसश्च दार्ढ्यकृत् ।
तद्वदरण्यजो ज्ञेयो विशेषाच्छोणिते हितः ।३८२

महिषः (Mahiṣaḥ), कासरः (Kāsaraḥ), शृङ्गी (Sṛngī), श्यामः (Śyāmaḥ), कृष्णः (Kṛṣṇaḥ), लुलायकः (Lulāyakaḥ), विषाणी (Viṣāṇī), कलुषः (Kaluṣaḥ), दंशी (Damśī), पीनस्कन्धः (Pīnaskandhaḥ), रजस्वलः (Rajaswalaḥ), are synonyms.

महिषी (Mahiṣī), मन्दगमना (Mandagamanā), महाक्षीरा (Mahāksīrā), पयस्विनी (Payaswinī), लुलायकान्ता (Lulāyakāntā), कलुषा (Kaluṣā), तुरङ्गद्वेषिणी (Turangadwesṇī) are synonyms of she buffalo.

The meat (or flesh) of a buffalo is bitter and sweet, *uṣṇavīrya.* It is unctuous and promotes sleep, *'sukradhātu,* strength, satiating, is *vṛṣya, guru* and provides firmness (of muscular tissue).

The flesh (meat) of a wild buffalo has similar properties but is more useful in blood disorders.

57 बलीवर्दः Balivardah (Ox- cow) (वृषभः – Vṛṣabhaḥ)

बलीवर्दो दान्त उग्रो गोरक्षो धूर्वहः स्थिरः ।
अनड्वान वृषभो दम्यः ककुद्मान वृषभो वृषः ॥३८३

गौः श्रृङ्गिणी सौरभेयी दोग्ध्री धेनुः पयस्विनी ।
गोमांसं वातहृद् बल्यं अपथ्यं पीनसप्रणुत् ॥३८४
कीर्तितं नात्यभिष्यन्दि मांसं प्रायस्तु जाङ्गलम् [1] ॥

बलीवर्दः (Balīvardaḥ), दान्तः (Dāntaḥ), उग्रः (Ugraḥ), गोरक्षः (Gorakśaḥ), धूर्वहः (Dhūrvaḥaḥ), स्थिरः (Sthiraḥ), दम्यः (Damyah), ककुद्मान् (Kakudamān) अनड्वान् (Anandwān), वृषभः (Vṛsabhaḥ), वृषः (Vṛsah) are synonymous.

गौः (Gauḥ), श्रृंगिणी (Śṛṅginị), सौरभेयी (Saurabheyī), दोग्ध्री (Daugdhrī), धेनुः (Dhenuḥ), पयस्विनी (Payaswinī) are synonyms.

The meat (or flesh) of an ox pacifies *vātadoṣa,* promotes strength, not beneficial to the human body, and alleviates rhinitis. Usually, the same of the wild ox is not much *abhisyandi.*

58 मत्स्यः Matsyaḥ (A fish) Matsya vargaḥ - मत्स्यवर्गः

मत्स्यो मीनोऽथ शकुनी कंण्ठी माङ्गल्यदर्शनः ॥३८५
रोहितः* कण्ठकालश्च पाठीनः शकुलस्तथा ॥

मत्स्यः (Matsyaḥ), मीनः (Mīnaḥ), शकुनी (Śakunī), कण्ठी (Kaṇṭhī), माङ्गल्यदर्शनः (Māṅgalyadarśanaḥ), रोहितः (Rohitaḥ), कण्ठकालः (Kaṇṭhakālaḥ), पाठीनः (Paṭhīnaḥ), शकुलः (Śakulaḥ) are synonymous.

कफपित्तकरा मत्स्या बल्याः शक्तिविवर्धनाः ॥३८६
व्यायामिनां च दीप्ताग्नेर्व्यवायीनां च पूजिताः ॥
कषायानुरसाः स्वादुवातघ्नाः नातिपित्तलाः ।३८७

A fish aggravates *kapha* and *pitta dosas* and promotes strength and is recommended to those who are having good digestive (and metabolic) capacity, engaged in exercise and copulation. It is sweet in taste and *kaṣāya* in subsidiary taste. It pacifies *vātadoṣa* and does not aggravate *pitta doṣa* much.

केषांचन विशिष्ट मत्स्यानां गुणकर्माणि

Properties & Actions of certain kinds of fishes.

रोहितः सर्वमत्स्यानां वरो वृष्योऽर्धवातजित्[2] ।
कषायो मधुरो रूक्षो विशदो रोचनो लघुः ॥३८८

---

१ ग्राम्या वन्याभेदेन च द्विविधा गोः अत्र वर्णिता दृश्यते ।
२ 'अर्धवात' इत्यनेन पक्षवधः गृह्यते ।
* Though here are mentioned as synonyms they are different kinds also. See below.

ग्राही तु नन्दिकावर्तस्तस्यानु शकलः स्मृतः ।
रणजित् शतशङ्खश्च गोमत्स्योऽलिस्त्रिकण्टकः ॥३८९
कण्टकैः स तु विज्ञेयो म्रक्ष्यमाणः सुनिर्विषः ।
श्रृङ्गी तु वातशमनी तथा श्लेष्मप्रकोपणी ॥ः३९०
विपाके मधुरो वृष्यो मुद्गरो वातहा गुरुः ।
अलिमत्स्यो गुरुः स्निग्धः कषायो रुक्ष एव च ॥ ३९१
मुखमत्स्यो गुरुः स्निग्धः श्लेष्मलो वातनाशनः ॥

इरसो मधुरः स्निग्धः पित्तश्लेष्मातिकोपनः ॥ ३९२
पुलङ्गः स्निग्धमधुरो गुरु विष्टम्भिशीतलः ॥

Rohita is said to be the best among fishes of all kinds. It is sweet and *kaṣāya* in taste, *vṛṣya,* useful in hemiplegia (or ? faciel palsy), roughening. nonslimy, delightful and *laghu* (light to digest).

Nandikāvarta is astringent, following this are *'Sakala, Raṇajit, 'Saia 'sankha*, *Gomatsya, Ali* and *Trikaṇṭaka* which has got thorns and becomes poisonless after repeated washings.

'Sṛṅgī pacifies *vātadoṣa* and aggravates *kaphadoṣa*. *Mudgara* is sweet in *vipāka, vṛṣya,* pacifies *vātadoṣa* and is *guru.*

Alimatsya is *kaṣāya* in taste, *guru* (heavy to digest), unctuous and roughening.

Mukhamatsya pacifies *vātadoṣa*, aggravates *kaphadoṣa*, is *guru* (heavy to digest) and unctuous.

Irasa is sweet in taste, unctuous, and aggravates *pitta* and *kapha doṣas.*

Pulaṅga is sweet in taste, *'sītavīrya,* unctuous, *guru* and constipating.

मत्स्यभेदाः Some other kinds of fish

राजीवः शकुली शृङ्गी वागूरः शल्यचुल्लकौ ॥३९३
पाठीनः कुलिशश्चैव नन्द्यावर्तश्च रोहितः ॥

मुद्गरस्तिमिराद्या तु ज्ञेयास्तद्भेदजातयः ॥३९४
तद्भेदो मकराख्योऽन्यो मातङ्गमकरोऽपरः ॥

चिरलुश्च तिमिंश्चैव तथाऽन्यश्च तिमिङ्गिलः॥ ३९५
तिमिङ्गिलगिलश्चेति महामत्स्या अमी मताः ॥

राजीवः (Rājīvaḥ), शकुली ('Sakulī), शृङ्गी (Śṛngī), वागूरः (Vāgūraḥ), शल्यः ('Salyaḥ), चुल्लकः (Cullakaḥ), पाठीनः (Pāthīnaḥ), कुलिशः (Kuli'saḥ), नन्द्यावर्तः (Nandyāvartaḥ), मुद्गरः (Mudgaraḥ) रोहितः (Rohitaḥ) and तिमिरः (Timiraḥ), etc. are their different types

The other kind of *Timīra i*s called as Makara (मकर), and another is मातङ्गमकर (Mātanga makara), चिरलुः (Ciraluh), तिमिः (Timiḥ), the other type तिमिङ्गिलः (Timinghilaḥ) and तिमिङ्गिलगिलः (Timingilagilaḥ) are called as महामत्स्याः (Mahāmatsyāḥ)

रोहितः Rohitaḥ

रक्तगोऽपरो रक्तमुखो रोहितो मत्स्यपुंगवः ॥३९६

The other type of *Rohita* is having red coloured mouth, is to be the best among all fishes.

पाठीनः Pāṭhīnaḥ

सहस्रदंष्ट्रः पाठीनः कृष्णवर्णो महाशिराः ।

Pāṭhīna is having many teeth, black colour and is having a big head.

शफरी, प्रोष्ठी चिलिचिमश्च Śapharī, Prosṭhī & Cilicimaḥ.

शफरी क्षुद्रमत्स्यः स्यात् प्रोष्ठी तु क्षुद्रमत्सिका ॥ ३९७
जलमीनश्चिलिचिमो मीनः ख्यातः समुद्रजः ॥

Śapaharī is a small fish and *Prosṭhī* is very small. *Cilicima* known also as *Jalamīna* is a (very small) fish from the sea.

मत्स्य सामान्य गुणकर्माणि
General properties & actions of fishes*

मत्स्या बलप्रदा वृष्या गुरवः कफपित्तलाः ॥ ३९८
ऊष्णाभिष्यन्दिनः स्निग्धा बृंहणा पवनापहाः ॥

The fish in general promotes strength, is *vṛsya, guru.*, aggravates *kapha pitta doṣas* and pacifies *vāta doṣa, usṇavīrya, abhiṣyandi* (causing

* These have been already mentioned or may be in relation to Rohita, Pāthina etc. only.

obstruction in the channels due to excessive secretion of *doṣas*), unctuous and body promoting.

नादेयादि मत्स्याः

Types of fishes according to habitat like rivers etc.& their properties

नादेया बृंहणा मत्स्या गुरवोऽनिलनाशनाः ॥ ३९९
कौपा वृष्या कफाष्ठीला मूत्रकृच्छ्रविबन्धदाः ।

ताडागा गुरवो वृष्याः शीतला बलमूत्रलाः ॥ ४००
ताडागवन्निर्झरजा बलायुर्मतिदृक्कराः ।

सरोजा मधुरा स्निग्धा बल्या वातनिबर्हणाः ॥४०१
सामुद्रा गुरवो नातिपित्तला पवनापहाः ॥

तत्रापि लवणाम्भोजाः ग्राहिणो दृष्टिनाशनाः ॥ ४०२
ह्रदोद्भवा बलकरा ये तु स्वच्छजलोद्भवाः ।

A fish from the rivers promotes body weight, is *guru* and pacifies *vātadoṣa.* Fish from a well is *vṛṣya,* aggravates *kapha doṣa,* causes aṣṭhīlā (prostatic enlargement), dysuria and constipation.

A fish from big lakes is *guru, vṛṣya, 'sītavīrya,* strength promoting and diuretic.

A fish from springs is similar in properties to that of a lake and promotes strength, longevity, intellect and vision.

A fish from the lakes is sweet in taste, unctuous, strength promoting and pacifeis *vātadoṣa.*

A fish from the sea is *guru.,* does not aggravate *pitta* much and pacifies *vāta doṣa,* those from very salty water are constipating and harmful to vision.

A fish from bigger lakes especially from clear water is strength promoting.

शिशुमारादीनां गुणकर्माणि Properties of 'si 'sumāra etc. (Popoise etc.)

शिशुमाराद्वते तुल्यो मकरस्तु त्रिदंष्ट्रकः ॥४०३
शिशुमारो गुरुर्वृष्यः कफकृत् वातनाशनः ॥

बृंहणो बलदः स्निग्धस्तद्वत मकरमादिशेत् ॥४०४

Except *'Si'sumāra*(शिशुमार), मकरः (Makaraḥ) and त्रिदंष्ट्रकः (Tridamṣṭrakaḥ) are similar in properties. *'Sisumāra* is *guru* (heavy) and *vṛsya,* aggravtes *kapha* and pacifies *vāta.* It is bulk promoting and gives strength.

59 कच्छपः Kacchapaḥ (A tortoise)

कच्छपः कमठः कूर्मो गूढाङ्गो धरणीधरः ।
कच्छेष्टः पल्वलावासो वृत्तः कठिनपृष्ठकः ॥४०५

कच्छपोऽन्यो महामत्स्यः कूर्मराजः प्रतिष्ठितः ।
गुप्ताङ्गश्चित्रपृष्ठश्च धरणीधरणक्षमः ॥४०६

कच्छपो बलदः स्निग्धो वातघ्नः पुंस्त्वकारकः ।

कच्छपः (Kacchapaḥ), कमठः (Kamaṭhaḥ), कूर्मः (Kūrmaḥ), गूढाङ्गः (Gūḍhāngaḥ), धरणीधरः (Dharaṇidharaḥ), कच्छेष्टः (Kaccheṣṭaḥ), पल्वलावासः (Palvalāvāsaḥ), वृत्तः (Vṛttaḥ), कठिनपृष्ठकः . (Kaṭhinaprsṭhkaḥ) are synonyms for *kacchapa.*

There is an other type of कच्छप (Kacchapa). Its synonyms are महामत्स्यः (Mahāmatsyaḥ), कूर्मराजः (Kūrmarājaḥ), गुप्ताङ्गः (Guptāngaḥ), चित्रपृष्ठः (Citraprṣṭhaḥ), धरणीधरणक्षमः (Dharaṇidharaṇaksamaḥ).

Kaccapaḥ is strength giving, unctuous, pacifier of *vāta* and is *vṛsya.*

60 आमूषिका Āmūṣikā (The musk rat)

दीर्घतुण्डी नखी ज्ञेयाऽऽ मूषिकाऽन्या छुछुन्दरी ।४०७

दीर्घतुण्डी (Dīrghatuṇḍī), नखी (Nakhī) are synonyms for आमूषिका (Āmūṣikā); there is an other type of आमूषिका (Āmūṣikā) called as छुछुन्दरी (Chuchundarī).

मूषकः Muṣakaḥ (68) (A mouse)

मूषकः खनकः पिङ्ग आखुरुन्दुरको नखी ॥
मूषको मधुरः स्निग्धो व्यवायी शुक्रवर्धनः ।४०८

मूषकः (Muṣakaḥ), खनकः (Khanakaḥ), पिङ्गः (Pingaḥ), आखुः Akhuḥ), उन्दुरकः (Undurakaḥ), नखी (Nakhī) are synonymous.

The meat of *muṣaka* is sweet in taste, unctuous, increases desire for copulation and increases *'sukra.*

महामूषकः Mahāmūṣakaḥ (69) (A rat)

अन्यो महाभूषकः स्यान्मोषी विघ्नेशवाहनः ॥
महाङ्गः सस्यमारी च भूफलो भित्तिपातनः ॥ ४०९

There is an another type of मूषक (Mūṣaka) called as महामूषकः (Mahāmūṣakaḥ) of which मोषी (Moṣī), विघ्नेशवाहनः (Vighne'savāhanaḥ), महाङ्गः(Mahāṅgaḥ), सस्यमारी (Sasyamārī), भूफलः (Bhūphalaḥ) and भित्तिपातनः (Bhittipātanaḥ) are synonymous.

61 बिडालः Biḍālaḥ (A cat)

बिडालो मूषकद्वेषी वृषदंशो बिडालकः ।*
शालावृकश्च मार्जारो मायावी दीप्तलोचनः ॥ ४१०

बिडालः (Biḍālaḥ), मूषक द्वेषी (Mūṣakadweṣī), वृषदंशः (Vṛṣadam'saḥ), बिडालकः (Biḍālakaḥ), शालावृकः ('Sālāvṛkaḥ), मार्जारः (Mārjāraḥ), मायावी (Māyāvī) and दीप्तलोचनः (Dīptalocanaḥ) are synonymous.

बिडाल विशेषाः** (70) (Civet cat etc.)
Certain other types of Biḍalḥ

लोमशोऽन्यो बिडालश्च पूतिकः पूतिकेशरः ॥
सुगन्धिमूत्रपतनो गन्धमार्जार संज्ञकः ॥४११

तृतीयः पिङ्गलश्चान्य उग्र उग्रबिडालकः ॥
सुगन्धिमूत्रवृषणः कस्तूरीति निगद्यते ॥४१२

There is an other type of *Biḍāla* (बिडाल) called by the synonyms लोमशः (Loma'saḥ), पूतिकः (Pūtikaḥ), पूतिकेशरः (Pūtikesaraḥ), सुगन्धिमूत्रपतनः (Sugandhi mūtrapatanaḥ), गन्धमार्जारः (Gandhamārjāraḥ). The third type of *Biḍāla* बिडाल is पिङ्गलः (Piṅgalaḥ), उग्रः (Ugraḥ), उग्रबिडालकः

---

* (अन्यच्च –
"बिडालो विषदन्तश्च मार्जारोऽथ बिडालकः ।
ओतुर्मूषकशत्रुश्च मायावी दीप्तलोचनः ॥") इत्यधिक पाठः आनन्दाश्रम मुद्रित पुस्तके दृश्यते ।

** The type Gandhamārjāraka गन्धमार्जारक seems to be *Viverra zibetha* Linn. commonly known as *Javādi* (जवादी) and the other type seems to be *Yūnanī* (युनानी) drug जुंदबेदस्तर (Jundabedastar) (castor fibre). (See Bha. Pr. Chunekar)

(Ugrabiḍālakaḥ), सुगन्धिमूत्रवृषणः (Sugandhimūtravṛṣaṇaḥ), कस्तूरी (Kastūrī) are its synonyms.

62 श्रृगालः Śṛgālaḥ (A Jackal)

श्रृगालो जम्बुकः फेरुर्गोमायुः क्रोष्टुकः शिवः ॥
भल्लूको मृगधूर्तश्च शालावृकश्च फेरवः ॥ ४१३

श्रृगालः (Śṛgālaḥ), जम्बुकः (Jambukaḥ), फेरुः (Pheruḥ), गोमायुः (Gomāyuḥ), क्रोष्टुकः (Kroṣṭukaḥ), शिवः (Śivaḥ), भल्लुकः (Bhallūkaḥ), मृगधूर्तः (Mṛgadhūrtaḥ), शालावृकः (Śālāvṛkaḥ) are synonymous.

तरक्षुः Tarakśuḥ (A heyna)

तरक्षुर्मृगभक्षश्च तरस्वी घोरदर्शनः ॥

तरक्षुः (Tarakśuḥ), मृगभक्षः (Mṛgabhaksaḥ), तरस्वी (Tarasvī), घोरदर्शनः (Ghoradarśanaḥ) are synonymous.

कुक्कुरः Kukkuraḥ (72) (सारमेयः - Sārameyaḥ) (A dog)

कुक्कुरः सारमेयश्च भषकः श्वानकः शुनः ॥ ४१४
भूस्तरो वक्रलाङ्गूलो भल्लूको रात्रिजागरः ॥

कुक्कुरः (Kukkuraḥ), सारमेयः (Sārameyaḥ), भषकः (Bhaṣakaḥ), श्वानकः (Śwānakaḥ), शुनः (Śunaḥ), भूस्तरः (Bhūstaraḥ), वक्रलाङ्गूलः (Vakralāṅg-ulaḥ), भल्लूकः (Bhallūkaḥ), रात्रिजागरः (Rātrijāgaraḥ) are synonymous.

63 मर्कटः Markaṭaḥ (A monkey)

मर्कटो वानरः कीशो हरिः शाखामृगः कपिः ॥ ४१५
प्लवङ्गमो वनौकश्च प्लवंगः प्लवगः प्लवः ॥

कषायो बद्धविण्मूत्र आमवातकफापहः ॥ ४१६
वानरः पवनश्वासमेदःपाण्डुकृमीञ्जयेत् ॥

मर्कटः (Markaṭaḥ), वानरः (Vānaraḥ), कीशः (Kīśaḥ), हरिः (Hariḥ), शाखामृगः (Śākhāmṛgaḥ), कपिः (Kapiḥ), प्लवंगमः (Plavaṅgamaḥ), वनौकः (Vanaukaḥ), प्लवंगः (Plavaṅgaḥ), प्लवगः (Plavagaḥ), प्लवः (Plavaḥ) are synonymous.

The meat of *Vānara* is astringent and causes binding of faeces and urine. It pacifies *āmavāta* and *kapha*. It is useful in *Vātadosa,* dyspnoea, vitiation of *meda*, anaemia and intestinal worms.

64 बर्हिः Barhiḥ (A peacock) (Mayūraḥ)

मयूरो नर्तको बर्हि नीलकण्ठः शिखी ध्वजी ॥ ४१७
मेघारावः कलापी च शिखण्डी चित्रपिच्छकः ॥

मयूरमांसं सुस्निग्धं वातघ्नं शुक्रवर्धनम् ॥ ४१८
बल्यं मेधाकरं प्रोक्तं चक्षूरोग विनाशनम् ॥

मयूरः (Mayūraḥ), नर्तकः (Nartakaḥ), बर्हि : (Barhiḥ), नीलकण्ठः (Nīlakaṇṭhaḥ), शिखी (Śikhī), ध्वजी (Dwajī), मेघारावः (Meghārāvaḥ), कलापी (Kalāpī), शिखण्डी (Śikhaṇḍī), चित्रपिच्छकः (Citrapicchakaḥ) are synonymous.

The meat of peacock is unctuous, pacifies *vāta,* and increases *śukra.* It is strength promoting, intelligence promoting and is beneficial for the diseases of eye.

65 शिलीमुखः (भ्रमरः) Śilīmukhaḥ (Bhramaraḥ)

भ्रमरः षट्पदो भृङ्गो भृङ्गराजः शिलीमुखः ॥ ४१९
द्विरेफोऽलिर्मधुकरो मधुपो मधुलिट् स्मृतः ॥

स च षट्चरणः प्रोक्तो झंकारी पुष्पलोलुपः ॥ ४२०
नीलो घुमुघुमारावो मधुकृन्मधुरस्वरः ॥

अपरः क्षुद्रभृङ्गारः पूतिभृङ्गः कुभृङ्गकः ॥४२१
भ्रमरो रूक्ष ऊष्णश्च तैलयोगेक्षणापहः ॥

कर्णरोगशिरोव्याधीन् मुखरोगान्निहन्ति च ॥ ४२२

भ्रमरः (Bhramaraḥ), षट्पदः (Ṣaṭpadaḥ), भृङ्गः (Bhṛṅgaḥ), भृङ्गराजः (Bhṛṅgarājaḥ), शिलीमुखः (Śilīmukhaḥ), द्विरेफः (Dvirephaḥ), अलिः (Aliḥ), मधुकरः (Madhukaraḥ), मधुपः (Madhupaḥ), मधुलिट् (Madhuliṭ), षट्चरणः (Ṣatcaraṇaḥ), झंकारी (Jhaṅkārī), पुष्पलोलुपः (Puspalolupaḥ), नीलः (Nīlaḥ), घुमुघुमारावः (Ghumughumārāvaḥ), मधुकृत (Madhukṛt), मधुरस्वरः (Madhuraswaraḥ) are synonymous.

There is an another type of भ्रमरः *Bhramarah* called by क्षुद्रभृङ्गारः

(Kśudrabhṛṅgārah), पूतिभृङ्गः (Pūtibhrngaḥ) and कुभृङ्गकः (Kubhṛngakaḥ). are it's synonyms.

Bhramara is *rūkśa, uṣṇavīrya* and useful in the processing of certain oils (? harmful to vision) and in the diseases of ear, head and mouth.

66 शुकः Śukaḥ (A parrot)

शुकः कीरो रक्तमुखो मेधावी प्रियदर्शनः ॥
अन्यो महान् राजशुकः शतपत्रो निगद्यते ॥ ४२३

शुको बल्योऽतिवृष्यश्च वीर्यवृद्धिकरः परः ॥
वातघ्नो बृंहणो ज्ञेयः तथा राजशुकः स्मृतः ॥ ४२४

शुकः (Śukaḥ), कीरः (Kīraḥ), रक्तमुखः (Raktamukhaḥ), मेधावी (Medhāvī), प्रियदर्शन (Priyadarśanaḥ) are synonymous.

There is an other type of शुकः (Śukkaḥ), of greater size called as राजशुकः (Rājaśukaḥ). It is called as शतपत्रः (Śatapatraḥ).

The meat of *śuka* is strength promoting, *vṛsya,* increases *śukra* pacifies *vātadoṣa,* and is bulk promoting. *Rājasuka* is having the similar properties.

67 सारिका Sārikā (A myna) *

गोराटिका गोकिरीटी गौरका कलहाकुला ।
मेधाविनी सारिकाऽन्या दूतिका प्रियवादिनी ॥४२५

सारिका च भवेत् स्निग्धा वातहा बृंहणी स्मृता ॥
वीर्यसंजननी वृष्या मेध्या चैव रसायनी ॥ ४२६

गोराटिका (Gorāṭikā), गोकिरीटी (Gokirīṭī), गौरका (Gaurakā), कलहाकुला (Kalahākulā), मेधाविनी (Medhāvinī) are synonyms of सारिका (Sārikā). There is an another *Sārikā* called by the synonyms दूतिका (Dūtikā) and प्रियवादिनी (Priyavādinī).

Sārikā is unctuous, pacifies *vāta doṣa* and is bulk promoting, increases *śukradhātu*, is *vṛsya*, intellect promoting and *rasāyana.*

68 चक्रवाकः Cakravākaḥ (The ruddy goose)

चक्रवाकस्तु चक्राह्वश्चक्री चक्ररथो रथी ॥
रथाङ्गनामा रथिकः कामी चक्रोऽथ चक्रवाक् ॥ ४२७

---

* *Acridotheris tristis* Linn.

चक्रवाको महास्निग्धः शुक्लो गुरुरेव च ।
बल्योऽथ रुचिकृद् वातहरो दोषविनाशनः ॥ ४२८

चक्रवाकः (Cakravākaḥ), चक्राह्वः (Cakrāhvaḥ), चक्री (Cakrī), चक्ररथः (Cakrarathaḥ), रथी (Rathī), रथाङ्गनामा (Rathāṅganāmā), रथिकः (Rathikaḥ), कामी (Kāmī), चक्रः (Cakraḥ), चक्रवाक् (Cakravāk) are synonymous.

Cakravāka is extremely unctuous, increases *śukra,* is *guru,* strength promoting, increases appetite and pacifies *vātadoṣa.*

69 हंसः Hamsaḥ (A swan)

हंसः श्वेतो धार्तराष्ट्रो राजहंसो मनोरमः ।
कलहंसोऽपरः प्रोक्तो जलपादोऽथ बंधुरः ॥४२९

हंसः स्निग्धो गुरुर्वृष्यो वीर्योष्णः स्वरवर्णकृत् ।
वातास्रपित्तशमनो बृंहणो बलवर्धकः ॥४३०

हंसः (Hamsaḥ), श्वेतः (Śwetaḥ), धार्तराष्ट्रः (Dhārtarāṣṭraḥ), राजहंसः (Rājahamsaḥ), मनोरमः (Manoramaḥ) are synonymous. There is an another type of हंसः (Hamsaḥ) called as कलहंसः (Kalahamsaḥ), जलपादः (Jalapādaḥ), and बंधुरः(Bandhuraḥ) are its synonyms.

Two Types are described A) *Hamsaḥ* and (B) *Rājahamsaḥ.*

Hamsa is unctuous, *guru, vṛṣya, uṣṇavīrya,* beneficial to voice and complexion, useful in *vātarakta* (gout), pacifies *pittadoṣa,* bulk promoting of the body and strength promoting.

70 कुक्कुटः Kukkuṭaḥ (A Cock)

कुक्कुटः ताम्रचूडश्च दक्षः शौण्डोऽथ विष्किरः ॥
कालज्ञः कृकवाकुश्च नियोद्धा चरणायुधः ॥ ४३१

कुक्कुटः स्वादुस्निग्धोष्णः स्वराग्नीन्द्रियदादर्यकृत् ॥
बृंहणो वातहा वृष्यो लघुर्बलकरः स्मृतः ॥ ४३२
अन्यस्तद्वद् गुणो ग्राम्यो* विशेषेण गुरुस्तथा ॥

कुक्कुटः (Kukkuṭaḥ), ताम्रचूडः (Tāmracūḍaḥ), दक्षः (Dakśaḥ), शौण्डः

---

१ अन्यच्च 'कारण्डवः प्लवो मञ्जुर्वरटा हंस योषिता' इति आनन्दाश्रम पुस्तके अधिकः पाठः ।
* निघण्टुकारेण ग्राम्यवन्य भेदेन द्विविधः कुक्कुटः निर्दिष्टः इति गुणकर्मवर्णनेन दृश्यते ।
The compiler has mentioned two types of कुक्कुटः (kukkuṭaḥ) (a) ग्राम्य Grâmyaḥ (b) वन्यः (Vanyaḥ)

(Śauṇḍaḥ), विष्किरः (Viṣkiraḥ), कालज्ञः (Kālajñaḥ), कृकवाकुः (Kṛkawākuḥ), नियोद्धा (Niyoddhā), चरणायुधः (Caraṇāyudhaḥ) are synonymous.

Kukkuṭa is sweet in taste, *uṣṇavīrya,* unctuous, pacifies *vātadoṣa,* is useful in the stability of voice, digestive capacity, and organs of perception. It is bulk promoting, *vṛsya, laghu* (easy to digest) and strength promoting. ग्राम्य कुक्कुट (Grāmya kukkuṭa). Domestic *kukkuṭa* (cock) is of the same properties but is especially *guru.*

71 लावः Lāvaḥ (quail)

लावस्तु लावको ज्ञेयश्चित्रदेहश्चतुर्विधः ॥ ४३३
पांसुलो गौरकोऽन्यश्च पौण्ड्रको दर्भरस्तथा ॥

लावो हृद्यो हिमः स्निग्धो ग्राही वह्निप्रदीपनः ॥ ४३४
गुरूष्णो मधुरः किञ्चित् सर्वदोषहरो मतः ॥

पांसुलः श्लेष्मलस्तेषां वीर्योष्णोऽनिलनाशनः ॥ ४३५
गौरको कफवातघ्नो रूक्षो वह्निप्रदीपनः ॥

पौण्ड्रकः. पित्तकृत् किञ्चिल्लघुः श्लेष्मानिलापहः ॥ ४३६
दर्भरो रक्तपित्तघ्नो हृदामयहरो हिमः ॥

लावः (Lāvaḥ), लावकः (Lāvakaḥ) and चित्रदेहः (Citradehaḥ) are synonymous. It is of four types (a) पांसुलः (Pāmsulaḥ), (b) गौरकः (Gaurakaḥ), (c) पौण्ड्रकः (Pauṇḍrakaḥ) and (d) दर्भरः (Darbharaḥ).

Lāva is cordial, *'sitavīrya*, unctuous, astringent and stimulates digestive capacity, is *guru, uṣṇa,* slightly sweet in taste and pacifies all the *doṣas.*

Out of these *Pāmsula* aggravates *kaphadoṣa, uṣṇavīrya* and pacifies *vātadoṣa.*

Gauraka pacifies *kapha vāta doṣas,* is roughning and stimulates digestive capacity.

Pauṇḍraka aggravates *pittadoṣa*, is slightly *laghu* and pacifies *kapha- vāta.*

Darbhara is useful in bleeding disorders, diseases of heart and is *'sitavīrya*.

72 कोकिल : Kokilaḥ (The Indian Cuckoo)

कोकिलः परपुष्टश्च कृष्णः परभृतोऽसितः ॥ ४३७
वसन्तदूतस्ताम्राक्षो गन्धर्वो वनभूषणः ॥

कोकिला परपुष्टा च धूर्ता परभृताऽसिता ॥ ४३८

कोकिलः (Kokilaḥ), परपुष्टः (Parapuṣṭaḥ), कृष्णः (Kṛṣṇaḥ), परभृतः (Parabhṛtaḥ), असितः (Asitaḥ), वसन्तदूतः (Vasantadūtaḥ), ताम्राक्षः (Tāmrākśaḥ), गन्धर्वः (Gandharvaḥ), वनभूषणः (Vanabhūṣaṇaḥ) are synonymous.

The synonyms for कोकिला (Kokilā) are परपुष्टा (Parapuṣṭā), धूर्ता (Dhūrtā), परभृता (Parabhṛtā), and असिता (Asitā).

काकः Kākaḥ (73) (A crow etc.)

Under this subheading the compiler has mentioned (a) काकः (Kākaḥ) (b) द्रोणकाकः (Droṇakākaḥ), (c) भल्लः (Bhallaḥ), (d) भासः (Bhāsaḥ) and (e) दात्यूहः (Dātyūhaḥ).

काकोऽथ वायसो ध्वाङ्क्षः काणोऽरिष्ट उलूकजित् ॥
बलिभुक्चिरजीवी च धूलिजङ्घो निमित्तकृत् ॥४३९
काकद्रोणो द्रोणकाकः स्यात्काणोऽपि च वायसः ।½
रूक्षो भल्लो भल्लको भल्लशल्यो
दुर्घोषः स्यात् भल्लको पृष्ठदृष्टिः ।
द्रागीश्चासौ दीर्घकेशश्चिरायु
र्ज्ञेयः सोऽयं दुःस्वरो दीर्घदर्शी ॥४४०
भासः शिवोऽनुभासेत गृध्राकारो रजःप्रभः ।
जलकाकस्तु दात्यूहः स च स्यात् कालकण्टकः ॥४४१
सर्वकाकभवं मांसं चक्षुष्यं दीपनं लघु ।
आयुष्यं बृंहणं बल्यं क्षतदोषक्षयापहम् ॥ ४४२

A) काकः (Kākaḥ), वायसः (Wāyasaḥ), ध्वाङ्क्षः (Dhwāṅkśaḥ), काणः (Kāṇaḥ), अरिष्टः (Ariṣṭaḥ), उलूकजित् (Ulūkajit), बलिभुक् (Balibhuk) चिरजीवी (Cirajīvī), धूलिजङ्घः (Dhiūlijaṇghaḥ), निमित्तकृत् (Nimittakṛt) are synonymous.

B) काकद्रोणः (Kākadroṇaḥ), द्रोणकाकः(Droṇakākaḥ), काणवायसः (Kāṇawāyasaḥ) are synonymous.

C) रूक्षः (Rūkśaḥ), भल्लः (Bhallaḥ), भल्लकः (Bhallakaḥ), भल्लशल्यः (Bhallaśalyaḥ), दुर्घोषः (Durghoṣaḥ), पृष्ठदृष्टिः (Pṛṣṭhadṛṣṭiḥ), द्रागीः (Drāgīḥ), दीर्घकेशः (Dīrghakesaḥ), चिरायुः (Cirāyuḥ), दुःस्वरः (Duḥswaraḥ), दीर्घदर्शी (Dīrghadarsī) are synonymous.

D) भासः (Bhāsaḥ) is also called by the synonym शिवः (Sivaḥ). It simulates *Gṛdhṛa* and is having the colour of dust.

E) दात्यूहः (Dātyūhaḥ) is called by the synonyms जलकाकः (Jalakākaḥ) and कालकण्टकः (Kālakaṇṭakaḥ).

The flesh of all types of *kāka* is beneficial to eyes, stimulates digestive capacity and *laghu*.It is useful for providing longevity, bulk promoting, strength promoting, and removes impurities of the wounds and useful in consumption.

73 उलूकः Ulūkaḥ

Under this heading two types are described by the compiler (A) उलूकः Ulūkaḥ and (B) क्षुद्रोलूकः (Kṡudrolūkaḥ).

उलूको नक्तञ्चारी च दिवान्धः कौशिकस्तथा ।
कौशी घर्घरको भीरुः काकशत्रुर्निशाचरः ॥४४३
क्षुद्रोलूकः शाकुनेयः पिङ्गलो डुडुलश्च सः ॥
वृक्षाश्रयी बृहद्रावः पिङ्गलाक्षो भयंकरः ॥४४४
औलूकं पित्तलं भ्रान्तिकरं वातप्रकोपणम् ।

A) उलूकः (Ulūkaḥ), नक्तञ्चारी (Naktacārī), दिवान्धः (Divāndhaḥ), कौशिकः (Kauṡikaḥ), कौशी (Kauṡī), घर्घरकः (Ghargharakaḥ), भीरुः (Bhīruḥ), काकशत्रुः (Kākaṡatruḥ) , निशाचरः (Niṡācaraḥ) are synonymous.

B) क्षुद्रोलूकः (Kṡūdrolūkaḥ), शाकुनेयः (Ṡākuneyaḥ), पिङ्गलः (Piṅgalaḥ), डुडुलः (Ḍuḍulaḥ), वृक्षाश्रयी (Vṛkṡāṡrayī), बृहत्रावः (Bṛhatrāvaḥ), पिंगलाक्षः (Piṅgalākṡaḥ), भयंकरः (Bhayaṅkaraḥ) are synonymous.

The flesh of an *ulūka* aggravates *pitta* and *vātadoṣa* and causes giddiness.

74 सर्पः Sarpaḥ

सर्पो दंष्ट्री भुजंगोऽहिर्भुजगोऽथ सरीसृपः ॥ ४४५
उरगः कञ्चुकी व्यालो द्विजिह्वोऽथ भुजंगमः ॥
स च नागो विषधरः कुण्डली पन्नगः फणी ॥४४६
चक्षुःश्रवा दन्दशूको भोगी चाऽऽशीविषः स्मृतः ॥

सर्पः (Sarpaḥ) , दंष्ट्री (Daṃṣṭrī), भुजंगः (Bhujaṅgaḥ), अहिः (Ahiḥ) , भुजगः (Bhujagaḥ) , सरीसृपः (Sarīsṛpaḥ), उरगः (Uragaḥ), कञ्चुकी (Kañcukī), व्यालः

(Vyālaḥ), द्विजिह्वः (Dwijivhaḥ), भुजंगमः (Bhujaṅgamaḥ), नागः (Nāgaḥ), विषधरः (Viṣadharaḥ), कुण्डली (Kuṇḍalī), पन्नगः (Pannagaḥ), फणी (Phaṇī), चक्षुःश्रवा (Cakṣuḥśravā), दन्दशूकः (Dandaśūkaḥ), भोगी (Bhogī), आशीविषः (Āśīviṣaḥ) are synonymous.

Out of these synonyms probabaly the synonyms नागः (Nāgaḥ) on wards are for poisonous species of serpents.

सर्पविशेषाः Sarpaviśeṣāḥ (Types of serpents)

राजिलो जलसर्पस्तु विरुलः स प्रकीर्तितः ॥४४७
श्वेतो नागोऽरुणः सर्पो व्यन्तरश्चित्रवर्णकः ॥
गोनसो मण्डलीपातः कुलङ्गः कृष्णडुण्डुभः ॥४४८
विविधाऽग्निकृताः सर्पा वातघ्ना स्वादुपाकिनः ।

दर्वीकरा मण्डलिनास्तेषूत्तगः कटुपाकिनः ॥४४९
स्वादवश्चातिचक्षुष्याः सृष्टविण्मूत्रमारुताः ।

राजीमदादयः स्वादे रसे पाके कफावहाः ॥ ४५०
स्निग्धाः शीताः स्तब्धवर्चः सशुक्रबलवर्धना ॥

कृष्णसर्पादयस्तेषां बल्याश्चोष्णानिलापहाः ॥ ४५१
शुक्रसंधानकृच्छ्रेष्ठा स्निग्धाः स्वापमलापहाः ॥

राजिल (Rājila) is जलसर्पः (Jalasarpaḥ) (aquatic in habitat), it is called as विरुलः (Virulaḥ); नाग (Nāga) is white coloured; सर्पः (Sarpaḥ) is pinkish coloured and व्यन्तर (Vyantara) is having various (variegated) colours. गोनस (Gonasa) अरुणः (Aruṇaḥ) मण्डलीपातः (Maṇḍalīpātaḥ) कुलङ्गः (Kulaṅgaḥ), कृष्णडुण्डुभः (Kṛṣṇaḍuṇḍubhaḥ) are some of the types of serpents.

The flesh of various types of serpents pacify *vātadoṣa* and are sweet in *vipāka.* Out of these *Darvīkara* and *Maṇḍalī* are sweet in taste and pungent in *vipāka*, extremely beneficial to the eyes and helpful to evacuation of faeces, urine and flatus etc.

Rājīmad are sweet in taste and in *vipāka* and aggravate *kapha doṣa.* These are unctuous, *śītavīrya,* check the process of evacuation and promote *śukra* and strength.

फणिनो धवलाङगा ये ते नागा इति कीर्तिताः ।
अन्ये स्तगादिवर्णाढ्या बोध्या सर्पादिनामभिः ॥ इति । Raj. ni. chapter 19.

Kṛṣṇasarpa etc. are strength promoting, *uṣṇavīrya* and pacify *vātadoṣa*. These are best in increasing *śukra,* and union promoting, unctuous and decrease (excessive) sleep and *malaṣ*.

75 मण्डूकः Maṇḍūkaḥ (A frog)

The compiler has mentioned two types under this heading (a) मण्डूकः (Maṇḍūkaḥ) and b) राजमण्डूकः (Rājamaṇḍūkaḥ.)

मण्डूको दर्दुरो मण्डो हरिर्भेकः कसूचकः । ४५२
महावित्तस्तु मण्डव्यो राजमण्डूक उच्यते ।।

मण्डूकः श्लेष्मलो नातिपित्तलो बलकारकः ।। ४५३

A) मण्डूकः (Maṇḍūkaḥ), दर्दुरः (Darduraḥ), मण्डः (Maṇḍaḥ), हरिः (Hariḥ), भेकः (Bhekaḥ), कसूचकः (Kasūcakaḥ) are synonymous.

B) महावित्तः (Mahāvittaḥ), मण्डव्यः (Maṇḍavyaḥ), राजमण्डूकः (Rājamaṇḍūkaḥ). Raj.Ni. has mentioned it by synonyms पीताङ्गः (Pītāṅgaḥ), पीतमण्डूकः (Pītamaṇḍūkaḥ).

Maṇḍūkaḥ aggravates *kaphadoṣa,* does not increase *pitta doṣa* much and is strength promoting.

कर्कटः Karkaṭaḥ (75) (A crab)

कर्कटः स्यात्कर्कटकः कुलीरश्च कुलीरकः ।
संदशकः पंकवासस्तिर्यग्गामी स चोर्ध्वदृक् ।।४५४
कर्कटो बृंहणो वृष्यः शीतलोऽसृग्गदापहः ।

कर्कटः (Karkaṭaḥ), कर्कटकः (Karkaṭakaḥ) , कुलीरः (Kulīraḥ), कुलीरकः (Kulīrakāḥ), संदशकः (Sandanśakaḥ), पंकवासः (Paṅkavāsaḥ), तिर्यग्गामी (Tiryaggāmī), ऊर्ध्वदृक् (Ūrdhwadṛk).

Karkaṭa is strength promoting, *vṛṣya, śītavīrya* and useful in blood disorders.

76 मलम् Malam (Faeces)

मलं विष्ठा पुरीषं च विट् किट्टं पूतिकं च तत् ।। ४५५

मलं (Malam), विष्ठा (Viṣṭhā), पुरीषं (Purīṣam), विट् (Viṭ), किट्टं (Kiṭṭam), पूतिकं (Pūtikam) are synonymous.

गोमयम् Gomayam (76)

गोमयं गोपुरीषं स्यात् गोविष्ठा गोमलं च तत् ॥

गोमयं (Gomayam), गोपुरीषं (Gopuriṣam), गोविष्ठा (Goviṣṭhā), गोमलं (Gomalam) are synonymous.

77 मूत्रम् Mūtram (Urine)

मूत्रं तु गुह्यनिष्यन्दः प्रस्रावः स्रवणः स्रवः ॥ ४५६

मूत्रं (Mūtram), गुह्यनिष्यन्दः (Guhyaniṣyandaḥ), प्रस्रावः (Prasrāvaḥ), स्रवणः (Sravaṇaḥ), स्रवः (Sravaḥ) are synonymous.

गोमूत्रं Gomūtram (Cow's Urine) (77)

गोमूत्रं गोजलं गोम्भो गोपानीयं च गोस्रवः ॥
गवापो गोकीलालं च गोनीरं सुरभीजलम् ॥ ४५७

गोमूत्रं कटु तिक्तोष्णं सक्षारं लेखनं सरम् ॥
लघ्वग्निदीपनं मेध्यं पित्तलं कफवातजित् ॥ ४५८
मूत्रप्रयोगसाध्येषु गव्यं मूत्रं प्रयोजयेत् ॥ S.S.Su. 45.221

गोमूत्रं (Gomūtram), गोजलं (Gojalam), गोम्भः (Gombhaḥ), गोपानीयं (Gopānīyam), गोस्रवः (Gosravaḥ), गवापः (Gavāpaḥ), गोकीलालं (Gokīlālam), गोनीरं (Gonīram), सुरभीजलम् (Surabhijalam) are synonymous.

Gomūtra is pungent, bitter and salty in taste. It pacifies *kapha* and *vāta doṣas* and aggravates *pitta doṣa.* It is salty, slimming, mild laxative, *laghu,* stimulates digestive capacity and promotes intellect. When urine is to be prescribed as a medicine *gomūtra* should be used.

अजामूत्रम् – Ajāmūtram (She goat's urine)

कासश्वासापहं शोफकामलापाण्डुरोगनुत् ॥ ४५९
कटुतिक्तान्वितं छागमीषन्मारुतकोपनम् ॥

S.S.Su. 45. 223.

Ajāmūtra (she goat's urine) is pungent and bitter in taste and slightly aggravates *vātadoṣa*. It is useful in cough, dyspnoea, oedema, jaundice and anaemia.

मेषीमूत्रम् - Meṣīmūtram (Ewe's urine) (79)

कासप्लीहोदरश्वासशोषवर्चोग्रहे हितम् ॥ ४६०
सक्षारं कटुकं तिक्तमुष्णं वातघ्नमाविकम् ॥ S.S.Su. 45. 224.

Meṣīmūtra is pungent, bitter and salty in taste, *uṣṇavīrya,* pacifies *vātadoṣa*. It is useful in cough, disorders of spleen, ascites, dyspnoea, consumption and constipation.

महिषीमूत्रम् - Mahiṣīmūtram (Urine of a she buffalo) (80)

दुर्नामोदरशूलेषु कुष्ठमेहादिव्याधिषु ॥ ४६१
आनाहशोफगुल्मेषु पाण्डुरोगे च माहिषम् ॥

S.S.Su. 45. 222.

Urine of a she buffalo is useful in piles, ascites, colics, skin disorders, polyuria (including diabetes melliuts), tympanites, anasarca, tumours (diverticulosis) and anaemia.

गजमूत्रम् Gajamūtram (Urine of an elephant) (81)

सतिक्तं लवणं भेदि वातघ्नं पित्तकोपनम् ॥ ४६२
तीक्ष्णं क्षारं किलासे च नागमूत्रं प्रयोजयेत् ॥

S.S.Su. 45. 226.

Gajamūtra is bitter and salty in taste, purgative, pacifies *vātadoṣa* and aggravates *pittadoṣa.* It is sharp and salty and used in white patches on the skin.

अश्वमूत्रं Aśwamūtram (Urine of a horse) (82)

दीपनं कटुतिक्तोष्णं वातचेतोविकारनुत ॥ ४६२
आश्वं कफहरं मूत्रं कृमिदद्रुषु शस्यते ॥

S.S.Su. 45. 225.

The urine of a horse is pungent and bitter in taste, *uṣṇavīrya,* pacify *vāta kapha doṣas,* psychological disorders, and is useful in worms and *dadru.* (a skin disorder with itching).

ऊष्ट्रमूत्रम् Uṣṭramūtram (Urine of a Camel) (83)

शोफकुष्ठोदरोन्मादमारुतकृमिनाशनम् ॥ ४६४
अर्शोघ्नं कारभं मूत्रं विजानीयाच्चिकित्सकः ॥

S.S.Su. 45. 228.

The urine of a camel is useful in oedema (anasarca), skin disorders, ascites, *unmāda* (psychological disorders), pacifies *vātadoṣa*, worms and piles.

गर्दभमूत्रम् Gardabhamūtram (Urine of an ass) (84)

गरचेतोविकारघ्नं तीक्ष्णं ग्रहणिरोगनुत् ॥ ४६५
दीपनं गार्दभं मूत्रं कृमिवातकफापहम् ॥

S.S.Su. 45. 227.

Urine of an *ass* pacifies *vāta* and *kapha doṣas,* is sharp, and useful in artificial poisoning, psycological disorders, diseases characterized by chronic diarrhoea (*Grahaṇī*), stimulates digestive capacity and is useful in worms.

मानुषमूत्रम् Mānuṣmūtram (Human Urine) (85)

पित्तरक्तकृमिहरं रोचनं कफवातजित् ॥ ४६६
तिक्तं मोहहरं मूत्रं मानुषं तु विषापहम् ॥

Human urine pacifies *kapha vāta doṣas,* bitter in taste, alleviates *pittarakta,* and worms; it is appetizing, useful in mental confusion and poisons.

78 मेदः Medaḥ (fats)

मेदस्तु मांससारः स्याच्छुभ्रं मांसजमीरितम् ॥ ४६७

मेदः (Medaḥ), मांससारः (Māmsasāraḥ), शुभ्रः (Śubhraḥ), मांसजम् (Māmsajam) are synonymous. (Though this has been mentioned earlier, here it is described in the sense of an animal fat.)

79 त्वक् Twak (Skin)

त्वक् चर्मासृग्धरा कृत्तिरजिनं देहचर्म च ॥
रक्तधारो रोमभूमिः शरीरावरणं तथा ॥ ४६८

त्वक् (Twak), चर्म (Carma), असृग्धरा (Asṛkdharā), कृत्तिः (Kṛttiḥ), अजिनं (Ajinam), देहचर्म (Dehacarma), रक्तधारः (Raktādhāraḥ), रोमभूमिः (Romabhūmiḥ), शरीरावरणं (Sarīrāvaraṇam) are synonymous.

80 रोम Roma (Hair of the body)

रोम लोम च त्वग्जं च चर्मजं च तनूरुहम् ॥
तच्च नेत्रस्थितं पक्ष्म मुखजं श्मश्रु उच्यते ॥ ४६९

रोम (Roma), लोम (Loma), त्वग्ज (Twakja), चर्मजं (Carmajam), तनूरुहं (Tanūruham) are synonymous. Those in relation to eylids are called as पक्ष्म *Paksma* while those in relation to face (beard) is called as *śmaśru*.

काञ्चनादिस्तु मत्स्यान्तो वर्गः षष्ठ उदाहृतः ।
धातुद्रव्यद्रवद्रव्यमांसद्रव्यसमाश्रयः ॥

Thus has been told the Suvarṇādi sixth chapter starting with metals like सुवर्ण Survaṇa and ending with मत्स्य Matsya etc. This group includes metalic substances, fluid substances and meat group.

इति सुवर्णादिः षष्ठो वर्गः ।

Thus ends the Suvarnādi Chapter Sixth.

अथ मिश्रकादिः सप्तमो वर्गः ।

MIŚRAKĀDIH CHAPTER VII

त्रिफला Triphalā.

हरीतकी चाऽऽमलकं बिभीतकमिति त्रयम् ।
त्रिफला च वरा श्रेष्ठतमं ज्ञेयं फलत्रिकम् ॥१॥

त्रिफला च त्रिदोषघ्नी दीपनी स्याद् रसायनी ।
वृष्या मेहहरा दिव्या नेत्ररोगहरा मता ॥ २॥

हरीतकी (Harītakī), आमलकम् (Āmalakam), and बिभीतकं (Bibhītakam). The fruits of these three together is called as (Triphalā), वरा (Varā), and श्रेष्ठतमं फलत्रिकं (Śreṣthatamam Phalatrikam) are its synonyms.

*Triphal*a pacifies the three *doṣas,* stimulates digestive capacity (*Agni*), is *rasāyana* and *vṛṣya*. It is useful in diseases characterized by polyuria, (including diabetes), is divine and beneficial in diseases of the eye.

स्वादुत्रिफला Swādu Triphalā

द्राक्षाखर्जूरकाश्मर्य फलानीति फलत्रयम् ।
सैव स्वादुर्द्वितीया तु त्रिफला त्रैफला स्मृता[१] ॥३॥
चक्षुष्या दीपनी रुच्या विषमज्वरनाशनी ॥

द्राक्षा (Drākśā), खर्जूर (Kharjūra), काश्मर्य (Kāśmarya); these three fruits together is called स्वादु त्रिफला (Swādu Triphalā) or स्वादु त्रैफला (Swādu Traiphalā)

It is beneficial to vision, appetizer, promotes desire for food, and useful in alleviating irregular fever. (*Viṣamajwara*).

सुगंधि त्रिफला Sugandhi Triphalā.

जातीफलं तथैला च लवङ्गफलमेव च ॥४॥

सुगन्धित्रिफला प्रोक्ता तृतीयं तु फलत्रिकम् ॥
संग्राहि मधुरा पाके कफवातविबन्धनुत् ॥५॥

---

१ आनन्दाश्रम मुद्रित पुस्तके द्राक्षा, दाडिम, खर्जूर फलानि मिलित्वा अन्या 'स्वादुत्रिफला' निर्दिष्टा ।

* द्रव्याणि मिश्रीकृत्य कथनात् पृथक् क्रमांकः न दत्तः । अस्मिन वर्गे १ विषाणि २ उपविषाणि ३ विषप्रशमननानि, इति त्रीण्येव शीर्षकानि ।

There is no seperate heading ģiven for Triphalā (त्रिफला) etc. only three heading names are mentioned in this chapter viz. 1) Viṣāṇi 2) Upviṣāṇī & 3) Viṣapraśamanani.
S.D.Kamat

जातीफलं (Jātīphalam), एला (Elā), लवङ्गं (Lavangam); these three constitute सुगन्धित्रिफला (Sugandhi Triphalā).

The third triphalā is astringent, sweet in *vipāka* and is useful in breaking constipation due to *kapha* and *vātadoṣas.*

त्रिकटुकम् *Trikaṭukam.*

पिप्पलीमरिचं शुण्ठी त्रयमेतद्विमिश्रितम् ।
त्रिकटु त्र्यूषणं व्योषं कटुत्रयमिहोच्यते ॥६॥
दीपनं रुचिदं वातश्लेष्ममन्दाग्निशूलनुत् ।

पिप्पली (Pippalī), मरिच (Marica) and शुण्ठी (Suṇṭhī), these three constitute त्रिकटु (Trikaṭu). त्र्यूषणं (Tryūṣaṇam), व्योषं (Vyoṣam) and कटुत्रयं (Kaṭutrayam) are it's synonyms.

It stimulates digestive capacity, promotes desire for food and alleviates decreased digestive capacity, and colics due to *kapha* and *vāta doṣas.*

त्रिकार्षिकं *Trikārṣikam;* चातुर्भद्रकम् *Cāturbhabhrakam*

नागराऽतिविषामुस्ता त्रयमेतत्त्रिकार्षिकम् ॥७॥
गुडूची संयुतं चैव चातुर्भद्रकमुच्यते ।॥
ज्वरघ्नं पाचनं प्रोक्तं त्रिदोषशमनं स्मृतम् ॥८॥
जीर्णज्वरारोचकघ्नं कण्ठामयविनाशनम् ॥

नागरम् (Nāgaram), अतिविषा (Ativiṣā), मुस्ता (Mustā); these three constitute त्रिकार्षिक (Trikārṣika); when गुडूची (Guḍūcī) is added to it then it is called as चातुर्भद्रक (Cāturbhadraka).

It is useful as antifebrile, digesṭant of *āma* and pacifies all the three *doṣas.* It is useful in chronic fevers, anorexia and diseases of the throat.

द्वितीयं चातुर्भद्रकम् *(2nd Cāturbhadrakam)*
कटुचातुर्भद्रकम् *(Kaṭucāturbhadrakam).*

एलात्वक्पत्रकैस्तुल्यैर्मरिचेन समन्वितैः॥९॥
कटुपूर्वमिदं चान्यच्चातुर्भद्रकमुच्यते ॥
चातुर्भद्रं रुचिकरं पित्तलं चाग्निदीपनम् ॥१०॥
रूक्षोष्णं च सुगंधि स्यात्तीक्ष्णं वर्ण्यं लघु स्मृतम् ।

एला (Elā), त्वक् (Twak), पत्रक (Patrak), मरिच(Marica) all together in equal parts constitute कटुचातुर्भद्र (Kaṭucāturbhadra).

It promotes appetite, aggravates *pitta,* stimulates digestive capacity, is *rūkśa* (roughening), *usnavirya,* aromatic, *tīkśṇa* (sharp), causes good complexion, and is *laghu* (light in digestion.).

तृतीयं चातुर्भद्रकम् (3rd cāturbhadrakam), त्रिजातक सहितं (with Trijātaka).

त्वगेलापत्रकैस्तुल्यैस्त्रिसुगंधि त्रिजातकम् ॥११॥
नागकेशरसंयुक्तं चातुर्भद्रकमुच्यते ॥
स्वरभेदश्वासकासमुखदोषविनाशनम् ॥१२॥
वृष्यं बल्यं च योगार्हं चातुर्जातं रसायनम् ॥

त्वक् (Twak), एला (Elā), पत्रक (Patraka), in equal parts is called as त्रिसुगंधि (Trisugandhi), or त्रिजातक (Trijātaka), with the addition of नागकेशर (Nāgakeśara) it is called as चातुर्भद्रक (Cāturbhadraka).

The third *cāturbhadraka* is useful in laryngitis, dyspnoea, cough, and disorders of the mouth. It is *vṛṣya,* promotes strength, acts synergistically with other medicines and is *rasāyana.*

पञ्चकोलकम् Pañcakolakam.

पिप्पली पिप्पलीमूलं चव्य चित्रकनागरम् ॥१३॥
एकत्र मिलितैरेभिः पञ्चकोलकमुच्यते ॥
पञ्चकोलं त्रिदोषघ्नं रुच्यं दीपनपाचनम् ॥१४॥
स्वरभेदहरं चैव शूलगुल्मार्तिनाशनम् ॥

पिप्पली (Pippalī), पिप्पलीमूलं (Pippalīmulam), चव्य (cavya), चित्रकः (citrakah), नागरम् (Nāgaram), all these together is called पञ्चकोलकम् (Pañcakolakam)

It pacifies three *doṣas,* promotes desire for food, is appetizer and digestant; and is useful in laryngitis, intestinal colics and pains due to tumors (or intestinal diverticulosis).

पञ्चवल्कलम् Pañcavalkalam.

न्यग्रोधोदुम्बराश्वत्थप्लक्षवेतस वल्कलैः ॥१५॥
सर्वैरेकत्र संयुक्तैः पञ्चवल्कलमुच्यते ।
रसे कषायं शीतं च वर्ण्यं दाहतृषापहम् ॥१६॥
योनिदोषं कफं शोफं हन्तीदं पञ्चवल्कलम् ।

न्यग्रोध (Nyagrodha), उदुम्बर (Udumbara), अश्वत्थ (Aśvattha), प्लक्ष (Plakśa), वेतस (Vetasa) (all belong to the 5th chapter), the stem barks of all these constitute पञ्चवल्कलम् (Pañcavalkalam).

It is *kaṣāya* (astringent) in taste, *śītavīrya,* pacifies *kaphadoṣa*, improves complexion, and is useful in buring sensation, thirst, alleviates disorders of female genital tract, and oedema (inflammation or swelling).

पञ्चभृङ्गम् Pañcabhṛṅgam.

देवदाली शमी भृङ्गा निर्गुण्डी शणकस्तथा ॥१७॥
रोगान्ते स्नानपानार्थं पञ्चभृङ्गमिति स्मृतम् ।

देवदाली (Devadālī), शमी (Śamī), भृङगा (Bhṛṅgā), निर्गुण्डी (Nirguṇḍī), and शण (Saṇa), all these constitute पञ्चभृङ्ग (Pañcabhṛṅga). It is used in convalecence for bathing and drinking purposes.

मध्यमपञ्चमूलम् Madhyamapañcamūlam.

बलापुनर्नवैरण्डशूर्पपर्णीद्वयेन तु ॥१८॥
मध्यमं कफवातघ्नं नातिपित्तकरं सरम् ॥

बला (Balā), पुनर्नवा (Punarnavā), एरण्ड (Eraṇḍa), शूर्पपर्णीद्वयम (Śūrpaparṇî dwayam). The roots of all these constitute मध्यमपञ्चमूलम् (Madhyama pañcamūlam). It pacifies *kapha* and *vāta doṣas*, is laxative and do not increase पित्त (Pitta) to a great extent.

लघुपञ्चमूलम् Laghupañcamūlam.

शालपर्णी पृश्निपर्णी बृहती कण्टकारिका ॥१९॥
तथा गोक्षुरकश्चैव पञ्चमूलं लघु स्मृतम् ।
पञ्चमूलं त्रिदोषघ्नं वातघ्नं लघुसंज्ञकम् ॥२०॥
ज्वरकासश्वासशूलमन्दाग्न्यरुचिनाशकम् ।

शालपर्णी (Śalaparṇī), पृश्निपर्णी (Pṛśniparṇī), बृहती (Bṛhatī), कण्टकारिका (Kaṇṭakārikā), and गोक्षुर (Gokśura), the roots of these five constitute लघुपञ्चमूलम् (Laghu Pañcamūlam).

Laghupañcamūlam pacifies all the three doṣās especially *vātadoṣa*.It is useful is fevers, cough, dyspnoea, colics, decreased digestive capacity and anorexia.

बृहत्पञ्चमूलम्-दशमूलम् *Bṛhatpancamūlam & Da'samūlam.*

बिल्वोऽग्निमंथः श्योनाकः काश्मर्यः पाटला तथा ॥२१॥
ज्ञेयं महापञ्चमूलं दशमूलमुभे स्मृतम् ।
उभयं पञ्चमूलं तु संनिपातज्वरापहम् ॥२२॥
कासे श्वासे च तन्द्रायां पार्श्वशूले च शस्यते ।

बिल्वः (Bilvaḥ), अग्निमंथः (Agnimanthaḥ), श्योनाकः (S'yonākaḥ), काश्मरी (Kās'marī), पाटला (Pāṭalā); the roots of these five constitute the महत्पञ्चमूलं (Mahatpañcamūlam) and both these two constitute दशमूलम् (Da'samūlam).

Da'samulam is useful in *sannipāta jwara* (fever caused by vitiation of three *doṣas*. It is useful in cough, dyspnoea, drowsiness, pain in the sides of the chest (eg. pleural pain).

जीवनीय पञ्चमूलम् *Jivanīya Pañcamūlam with properties*

अभीरुवीराजीवन्तीजीवकर्षभकैः स्मृतम् ॥२३॥
जीवनाख्यं तु चक्षुष्यं वृष्यं पित्तानिलापहम् ।

अभीरु (शतावरी) (S'atāvarī), वीरा (Vīrā), जीवन्ती (Jīvantī), जीवक `(Jīvaka) and ऋषभक(Ṛṣabhaka), the roots of these constitute the जीवनीय पञ्चमूलम् (Jīvanīya Pañcamūlam).

It pacifies *vāta* and *pitta doṣas* and is vision promoting and *vṛṣya.*

तृण पञ्चमूलम् *Tṛṇa pancamūlam*

तृणाख्यं पित्तजिद्दर्भशरकाशेक्षुशालयः ॥२४॥
एतैरेकीकृतं पञ्चमूलं तृणसंज्ञकम् ।
तृणादिपञ्चमूलं तु पित्तज्वरतृषापहम् ॥२५॥
हन्ति कृच्छ्राम्लपित्तं च स्त्रीरोगं रक्तपित्तकम् ।

दर्भः (Darbhaḥ), शरः (S'araḥ), काशः (Kās'aḥ), इक्षुः (Iks'uḥ), शालिः (S'ālih). The roots of all these five constitute तृण पञ्चमूलम् (Tṛṇa pañcamūlam).

Tṛṇa panchmūla pacifies *pittadoṣa* is useful in fevers due to *pittadoṣa,* thirst, dysuria, hyperacidity (*amlapitta*), bleeding disorders and disorders of female.

पञ्च-पञ्चमूलम् *Pañca Pañcamūlam*

बिल्वोऽग्निमंथः श्योनाकः काश्मर्यत्वक् च पाटला ॥२६॥
बलापुनर्नवैरण्डः शूर्पपर्णीद्वयं तथा ।

जीवकर्षभकौ मेदा जीवन्ती च शतावरी ॥२७॥
शरेक्षुदर्भकाशानां शालीनां मूलमेव च ।
गृध्रा[१] वरी श्वदंष्ट्रा च सैरेयं करमर्दिका ॥२८॥
इत्यौषधैः समुद्दिष्टं पञ्चमूलकपञ्चकम् ।

The roots mentioned in Bṛhat pañcamula (बृहतपञ्चमूल), Madhyama pañcamūla (मध्यमपञ्चमूल), Jīvanīya Pañcamula (जीवनीय पञ्चमूल), Tṛṇapañcamūla (तृण पञ्चमूल) together with the roots of गृध्रा (Gṛdhrā), वरी (Varī) (शतावरी), श्वदंष्ट्रा (Śvadanṣṭrā), सैरेय (Saireya), (सहचरः) and करमर्दिका (Karamardikā) is called as पञ्चपञ्चमूलक Pañcapañcamulam). The last five i.e *Gṛdhrā* to *Karamardikā* together called as कण्टक पञ्चमूलम् *Kaṇṭaka pañcamūlam*

जीवनीय गणः Jīvanīya Gaṇaḥ

जीवकर्षभकौ मेदे काकोल्यौ द्वे च योजिते ॥२९॥
द्वे शूर्पपर्ण्यौ जीवन्ती मधुकं चेत्ययं गणः ।
नाम्ना मधुर इत्युक्तो जीवनीयो रसायनः ॥३०॥
जीवनो जीवनीयश्च स्वादुर्मधुरकस्तथा ।
शुक्रदोषहरो बल्यो मूत्रदोषापहारकः ॥३१॥

जीवक (Jīvaka), ऋषभक (Ṛṣabhaka), मेदा (Medā), महामेदा (Mahāmedā), काकोली (Kākolī), क्षीरकाकोली (kśīrakākolī), माषपर्णी (Māṣaparṇī), मुद्गपर्णी (Mudgaparṇī), जीवन्ती (Jīvantī), and मधुकं (Madhukam), all these constitute जीवनीय गण (Jīvanīya group of drugs)

जीवनीय गण (Jīvanīya gaṇa), is also called as मधुरगण (Madhuragaṇa), रसायन गण (Rasāyana gaṇa), जीवन (Jīvana) and जीवनीय (Jīvanīya). It is sweet in taste and in *vipāka,* removes disorders from *śukradhātu* (substances for regeneration of tissues including progeny), strength promoting and eliminates disorders of urine.

वेशवारः Veśavāraḥ

शुण्ठीमरिचपिप्पल्या धान्यकाजाजिदाडिमम ।
पिप्पली मूलसंयुक्तं वेशवारमिति स्मृतम् ॥३२॥
वेशवारो भवेत्तीक्ष्णः सोऽग्नेर्वीर्यस्य वर्धकः ।

---

१ 'गृध्रा' is not mentioned in Dhn.Ni. However, in Suśruta Samhita (Sū. 38) *Grdghranakhī* is mentioned in its place which is identified as *capparis zeylanica* Linn. or *zizyphus jujuba* Lam. var. *fruiticosa* Hains (Balvantji p. 143) S. D. K.

शुण्ठी (Śuṇṭhī), मरिच (Marica), पिप्पली (Pippalī), धान्यकम् (Dhānyakam), अजाजी (Ajājī), दाडिमम् (Dāḍimam), पिप्पली मूलं (Pippalīmūlam), all these together is called as वेशवार (Veśavāraḥ).

Veśavāra is *tīkṣṇa* (sharp-irritant) and improves digestive capacity.

सम्भारः Sambhāraḥ.

कासमर्दकपत्राणां कृतं चूर्णमुलूखले ॥३३॥
वेशवारसमायुक्तं सप्ताहं भाजने स्थितम् ।

ततो हिंगुरसात्तेऽन्न मिश्रितास्तेन ते तथा ॥३४॥
दिवाकरकरैः शोष्या वटकाः कासमर्दकाः ।

शाकव्यञ्जनमांसानां संभार इति ते मताः ॥३५॥
अनेन संयुताः पाकाः वह्निवीर्यबलप्रदाः ।

Dried leaves of कासमर्द (Kāsamarda) are powdered to which is added the above mentioned वेशवार (Veśavāraḥ) and kept in a vessel for 1 week. Then the asafoetida water (हिंगुरस) is added to it and made into pills, and dried in sunlight. These are called as कासमर्द वटक (Kāsamarda vaṭaka). These are used as spices to prepare vegetables, curries, meat etc. while cooking them. These improve digestive capacity and promote virility and strength.

शिखरिणी Śikhariṇī

दध्नः पलानि द्वात्रिंशत्वगेलार्धपलं तथा ॥३६॥
मध्वाज्यस्य पलार्धार्धं मरिचस्य पलार्धकम् ।

पलान्यष्टौ च खण्डस्य पटे शुक्ले च गालयेत् ॥३७॥
कर्पूरवासिते भाण्डे छायायां स्थापयेदिह ।

एषा शिखरिणीत्युक्ता वृष्या दीप्तिविवर्धनी ॥३८॥
सदा पथ्या नियुद्धाध्वक्षीणदेहेषु पुष्टिदा ।

आयुष्यवर्धिनी चैव सर्वरोग प्रमर्दिनी ॥३९॥
सा स्याद्रुचिस्थैर्यकरी नराणां सर्वदा हिता ।

दधि (Curds)32 पलानि (palāni), त्वक् (Twak), एला (Elā), मधु (Madhu-Honey), आज्यं (Ājyam), मरिचम् (Maricam), each ½ पलम् (palam), शर्करा (Śarkarā)8 पलानि (palāni), all these should be well mixed, churned and strained through a white cloth and kept in a vessel already scented with a little कर्पूर (Karpūra-camphor). It is called as शिखरिणी (Śikhariṇī) which is *vṛṣya* and stimulates *Agni* i.e. stimulates digestive capacity.

It is always useful for those who are engaged in wrestling, and is nourishing to those who are weakened especially by walking long distance. It promotes longevity, appetite and is always wholesome.

सर्वौषधिकम् *Sarvauṣadhikam*

कुष्टं मांसी हरिद्रे द्वे मुराशैलेयचम्पकाः ॥ ४० ॥
वचाकर्पूरमुस्ता च सर्वौषधिकमुच्यते ।

सर्वौषधिस्त्रिदोषघ्नी मूत्रदाहापहा मता ॥ ४१॥
रसायन्यर्शःपित्तघ्नी मुखरोग विनाशिनी ।

कुष्टं (Kuṣṭham), मांसी (Māmsī), द्वे हरिद्रे (Dwe Haridre), मुरा (Murā), शैलेय (Śaileya), चम्पक (Campaka), वचा (Vacā), कर्पूर (Karpūra), मुस्ता (Mustā), all these together is called as सर्वौषधिकम् (Sarvauṣadhikam).

Survauṣadhika pacifies all the three *doṣas,* is useful in burning micturition, as a *rasāyan* (rejuvenation therapy), in piles, disorders due to *pitta doṣa,* and in the diseases of mouth.

सुगंधामलकम् *Sugandhāmalakam.*

सर्वौषधिकसंयुक्तः शुष्काश्चाऽऽमलकत्वचः ॥४२॥
सुगन्धामलकं ह्येतन्निर्दिशन्ति विचक्षणाः ।

सुगंधामलकं वृष्यं पवित्रं मूत्रदोषनुत् ॥४३॥
योनिदोषप्रशमनं हन्ति दोषत्रयं तथा ।

To the above mentioned सर्वौषधि (Sarvauṣadhi) drugs to which dried आमलकी (Āmalakī) fruits (powder) is added then it is called as सुगंधामलक (Sugandhāmalaka).

Sugandhāmalaka is *vṛṣya,* clean (*pavitra*), eliminates urinary disorders, pacifies all the three *doṣas* and alleviates the disorders of female genital tract.

पञ्चसुगन्धिकम् *Pañcasugandhikam.*

कंकोलकं पूगफलं लवङ्गकुसुमानि च ॥४४॥
जातीफलानि कर्पूरमेतत पञ्चसुगंधिकम् ।

पञ्चसुगंधिकं शीतं रक्तपित्तविनाशनम् ॥४५॥
हन्त्याशु मुखवैगन्ध्यं पीनसं च कफास्रजित् ।

कंकोलकम् (Kankolakam), पूगफलम् (Pūgaphalam), लवङ्गकुसुमम् (Lavanga Kusumam), जातीफलम् (Jātiphalam) and कर्पूरं (Karpūram). All these five together is called as पञ्चसुगंधिकम् (Pañcasugandhikam).

Pañcasugandhika is *śitavīrya*, and useful in haemorrhagic disorders (*Rakta pitta*), foul smell of the mouth, chronic cold and *kapharaktadoṣas*.

परार्ध, वाट्यपुष्पञ्च *Parārdham & Vāṭyapuṣpam.*

चन्दनं कुसुमं तुल्यं परार्धमभिधीयते ॥४६॥
त्रिभागकुसुमं यच्च तदुक्तं वाट्यपुष्पकम् ।

चन्दनं (Candanam) and कुसुमं (Kusumam - fragrant flowers) when they are mixed in equal parts it is called as परार्धम् (Parārdham). If the flowers are in 3 parts then it is called as वाट्यपुष्पकम् (Vāṭyapuṣpakm).

यक्षकर्दमः (महासुगन्धः) Yakśakardamaḥ (Mahāsugandhaḥ)

कुङ्कुमागरु कर्पूरो कस्तुरी चन्दनानि च ॥ ४७ ॥
महासुगन्ध इत्युक्तो नामतो यक्षकर्दमः ।

यक्षकर्दम एष स्याच्छीतस्त्वग्दोषहृत्तथा ॥ ४८ ॥
सुगंधिः कान्तिदश्चैव शिरोर्तिविषनाशनः ।

कुङ्कुम (Kunkuma), अगरु (Agaru), कर्पूर (Karpūra), कस्तूरी (Kastūri) and चन्दन (Candana) all these together is called as महासुगन्ध (Mahāsugandha) or यक्षकर्दमः (Yakśakardamaḥ).

This *yakśakardama* is *śitavīrya* and useful in disorders of skin. It is fragrant, improves complexion of the body and useful in headech and poisoning.

मन्थः *Manthaḥ.*

सत्तवः सर्पिषाभ्यक्तः शीतोदकपरिप्लुताः ॥४९॥
नातिद्रवा नातिसान्द्रा मन्थ इत्यभिधीयते ।
मन्थः पित्तहरो ज्ञेयो दाहारुचिविनाशनः ॥५०॥
शीतः श्रमापशमनो मूर्च्छादोषापहारकः ।

सक्तू (Saktū) i.e. powder of यव (yava - *Hordeum vualgare* Linn.) treated with some quantity of ghee (सर्पिषाभ्यक्तः) and then added the cold water so that the mixture is neither too fluid nor too semisolid, then it is called as मन्थ (Mantha).

Mantha pacifies *pittadoṣa* and is *śitavīrya* . It is useful in burning sensation, anorexia, and removes fatigue and fainting.

सन्तर्पणम् *Santarpaṇam.*

द्राक्षादाडिमखर्जूरैर्मर्दिताम्बु सशर्करम् ॥५१॥
लाजचूर्णं समध्वाज्यं संतर्पणमुदाहृतम् ।
तर्पणं शीतलं पाने नेत्ररोगविनाशनम् ॥५२॥
बल्यं रसायनं हृद्यं शुक्रवृद्धिकरं परम् ।

द्राक्षा (Drākṡa), दाडिम (Dāḍima), खर्जूर (kharjura), अम्बु सशर्करम् (Ambu sa śarkram = water added with sugar), लाजा (Lājā) in powder form with honey and ghee, all of these well mixed is called as संतर्पणम् (Santarpaṇam).

Santarpaṇa is refrigerating and useful in disorders of eyes. It gives strength, and is *rasāyana,* cordial and promotes semen (*śukradhātu).*

पञ्चामृतम् *Pañcāmṛtam.*

गव्यमाज्यं दधि क्षीरं माक्षिकं शर्करान्वितम् ॥५३॥
एकत्र मिलितं ज्ञेयं दिव्यं पञ्चामृतं परम् ।
अजीर्णभूतवातघ्नं ज्ञेयं पञ्चामृतं परम् ॥५४॥

Cow's Milk (क्षीरं), curds (दधि), ghee (आज्यं) along with honey and sugar mixed together is called as पञ्चामृतं *Pañcāmṛtam.*

Pañcāmṛta is useful in aggravated *vātadoṣa* due to indigestion.

पञ्चगव्यम् *Pañcagavyam.*

गोमूत्रं गोमयं क्षीरं दधिसर्पिस्तथैव च ।
समं योजितमेकत्र पञ्चगव्यमिति स्मृतम् ॥५५॥
पञ्चगव्यं देहशुद्धिकरं कफविनाशनम् ।

गोमूत्रम् (cow's urine), गोमयं (cow's faeces), गोक्षीरं (cow's milk), गोदधि (curds from cow's milk), गोसर्पि (ghee obtained by cow's milk) in equal quantity mixed together is called as पञ्चगव्यम (Pañcagavyam).

Pañcagavyam pacifies *kaphadoṣa* and has purificatory action on the body.

पञ्चाम्लकम् *Pañcāmlakam*

बीजपूरकजम्बीरं नारङ्गं साम्लवेतसम् ॥५६॥
फलपञ्चाम्लकं ख्यातं तिन्तिडीसहितं परम् ।

बीजपूरकं (Bījapūrakam), जम्बीरम् (Jambīram), नारङ्गम् (Nārangam), अम्लवेतसं (Amlāvetasam), तिन्तिडी (Tintiḍī), the sour fruits of all these five together is called as पञ्चाम्लकम् Pañcāmlakam.

द्वितीयं पञ्चाम्लकम् Second Pañcāmlakam.

कोलदाडिमवृक्षाम्लं चुक्रिका चाम्लवेतसः ॥५७॥
पञ्चाम्लकं समुद्दिष्टं विद्वद्भिश्च भिषग्वरैः ।

कोलम् (Kolam), दाडिमम् (Dāḍimam), वृक्षाम्लं (Vṛkṣāmlam), चुक्रिका (Cukrikā), अम्लवेतस (Amlavetasa), all these five together is called as (Second) पञ्चाम्लकम् (Pañcāmlakam).

पञ्चनिम्बकम् Pañcaṇimbakam.

निम्बस्य पत्रं त्वक्पुष्पफलमूलैः समन्वितम् ॥५८॥
पञ्चनिम्बमिति ख्यातं नामतः शास्त्रकोविदैः ।

Leaves, stembark, flowers, fruits and roots of the निम्ब (Nimba) together is called as पञ्चनिम्ब (Pañcanimba).

लवणपञ्चकम् Lavaṇa pañcakam.

सैंधवं रोमकं चैव सामुद्रलवणं तथा ॥५९॥
बिडं सौवर्चलाख्यं च युक्तं लवणपञ्चकम् ।

सैंधवं (Saindhavam), रोमकम् (Romakam), सामुद्रलवणं (Sāmudra lavaṇam), बिडं (Biḍam), and सौवर्चलम् (Sauvarcalam), these five together is called as लवणपञ्चकम् (Lavaṇa pañcakam).

पञ्चशैरीषम् Pañcaśairīsam.

शिरीषपत्रं त्वक्पुष्पफलमूलसमन्वितम् ॥६०॥
विषारिः सर्वतः ख्यातं पञ्चशैरीषमुच्यते ।

Leaves, stembark, flowers, fruits and roots of शिरीष (Śirīṣa) together is called as पञ्चशैरीष (Pañcaśairīṣa). It is antipoisonous.

पञ्चाङ्गम् Pañcāngam.

त्वक्पत्र फलमूलानि पुष्पं चैकस्य शाखिनः ॥६१॥
पञ्चाङ्गमिति बोद्धव्यं प्राज्ञैरेकत्र मिश्रितम् ।

Stembark, leaves, fruits, roots and flowers of the same plant together is called as पञ्चाङ्गम् (Pañcāṅgam).

पञ्चसार्पकम् *Pañcasārpakam*

शिरीषपञ्चपञ्चाङ्गमगदं पञ्चसार्पकम् ॥६२॥
सर्पदंष्ट्राविषध्वंसि विज्ञेयं शास्त्रकोविदैः ।

The roots, flowers, fruits, leaves, and strembark of शिरीष (śirīṣa) is called as पञ्चसार्पकम्. शिरीषपञ्चम् (Śirīṣapañcam), पञ्चाङ्गमगदं (Pañcāṅgamagadam) are its synonyms. *Pañcansārpakam agadam* is useful in snake poisoning.

पञ्चसूरणम् *Pañcasūraṇam.*

अत्यम्लपर्णी कांडीर मालाकन्द द्विसूरणैः ॥६३॥
प्रोक्तो भवति योगोऽयं पञ्चसूरण संज्ञकः ।

अत्यम्लपर्णी (Atyamlaparṇī), कांडीरः (Kāṇḍīrah), मालाकन्द (Mālākandaḥ), द्विसूरणैः (Two types of Sūraṇ), All these constitute पञ्चसूरणम् (Pañcasūraṇam).

पञ्चसिद्धौषधिः *Pañca Siddhauṣadhiḥ.*

[१]तैलकन्दः सुधाकन्दः क्रोडकन्दो रुदन्तिका ॥६४॥
सर्पनेत्रयुताः पञ्च सिद्धौषधिक संज्ञकाः ।

तैलकन्दः (Tail Kandaḥ), सुधाकन्दः (Suḍhākandaḥ), क्रोडकन्दः (Kroḍakandaḥ), रुदन्तिका (Radantikā) (and सर्पनेत्र i.e. सर्पाक्षी (Sarpākśī), all these are called as सिद्धौषधिः (Siddhauṣadhiḥ).

रक्तवर्गः *Raktavargah.*

दाडिमं किंशुकं लाक्षा बन्धूकं च निशाह्वयम् ॥६५॥
कुसुम्भपुष्पं मञ्जिष्ठा इत्येतैः रक्तवर्गकः ।

दाडिमं (Dāḍimam), किंशुकं (Kimśukam), लाक्षा (Lākśā), बन्धूकं (Bandhūkam), निशा (Niśā), कुसुम्भ पुष्पम (Kusumbḥapuṣpam), मञ्जिष्ठा (Mañjiṣṭhā). All these together is called as रक्तवर्गः (Raktavargaḥ).

---

१ All these drugs plants having tubers are not mentioned in Dhn. Ni. They should be understood from Raj. Nighaṇṭu.

शुक्लवर्गः Śuklavargaḥ.

खटिनी श्वेतसंयुक्तः शङ्खशुक्तिवराटिकाः ॥६६॥
भृष्टाश्मशर्करा चेति शुक्लवर्ग उदाहृतः ।

श्वेत खटिनी (Śwēta khaṭinī - white chalk), शङ्खः (Śaṅkhaḥ), शुक्तिः (Śuktiḥ), वराटिका (Varāṭikā), भृष्टाश्मशर्करा (Bhṛṣṭāṣmaśarkarā - Burnt white stone), all these together is called as शुक्लवर्ग Śuklavargaḥ.

पञ्चगणः Pañcagaṇaḥ.

विदारिगन्धा बृहती पृश्निपर्णी निदिग्धिका ॥६७॥
श्वदंष्ट्रा चेति संप्रोक्तो योगः पञ्चगणाभिधः ।

विदारिगन्धा (Vidārigandhā) बृहती (Bṛhatī), पृश्निपर्णी (Pṛśniparṇ ī), निदिग्धिका-कण्टकारी (Kanṭakārī), श्वदंष्ट्रा-गोक्षुरः (Gokśuraḥ), all these together is called as पञ्चगणः (Pañcagaṇāḥ).

मूत्राष्टकम् Mutrāṣṭakam.

मूत्रं गोजाविमहिषीगजाश्वोष्ट्रखरोद्भवम् ॥६८॥
सर्वमेकत्र संयुक्तं मूत्राष्टकमुदाहृतम् ।

The urine of गो (Go), अजा (Ajā), अवि (Avi), महिषी (Mahiṣī), गज (Gaja), अश्व (Aśwa), उष्ट्र (Uṣṭra), and खर (Khara) togetherly called as मूत्राष्टकम् (Mūtraṣṭakam).

क्षारत्रयम् Kśāratrayam.

सर्जिक्षारं यवक्षारं टंकणक्षारमेव च ॥६९॥
क्षारत्रयं समाख्यातं त्रिक्षारं च प्रकीर्तितम् ।

सर्जिक्षार (Sarjikśāra), यवक्षार (Yavakśāra), टंकणक्षार (Ṭaṅkaṇakśāra); all these together is called as क्षारत्रयम् (Kśāratrayam). or त्रिक्षार (Trikśāra)

क्षारपञ्चकम् Kśārapañcakam.

पलाशतिलमुष्काणां क्षाराः सर्जियवाग्रजैः॥७०॥
समांश मिलिताः पञ्च क्षारपञ्चकमादिशेत् ।

पलाश (क्षार) (Palāśa Kśāra), तिलक्षार (Tilakśāra), मुष्ककक्षार (Muṣkakakśāra), सर्जिक्षार (Sarjikśāra), यवक्षार (Yavakśāra), all these in equal quantity is called as क्षारपञ्चकम् (Kśārapañcakam).

क्षारषट्कम् *Kśāraṣaṭkam.*

कृष्णतिलजपालाशौ वचापामार्गजौ तथा ॥७१॥
कौटजो मुष्कजश्चैव क्षारषट्कं विनिर्दिशेत् ।

कृष्णतिलजक्षार (Kṛṣṇatilaja Kśāra), पालाशक्षार (Palāśa Kśāra), वचाक्षार (Vacā Kśāra), अपामार्गक्षार (Apāmārga Kśāra), कौटज (Kauṭaja Kśāra), मुष्ककज (Muṣkakaja Ksāra), all these together is called as (Ksāraṣaṭka).

क्षाराष्टकम् *Kśārāṣṭakam.*

अपामार्गपलाशार्कः तिलमुष्कयवाग्रजम् ॥७२॥
सर्जिकाटंकणयुतं क्षाराष्टकमुदाहृतम् ।

अपामार्गक्षार (Apāmārgakśāra), पलाशक्षार (Palāśakśāra), अर्कक्षार (Arkakśāra), तिलक्षार (Tilakśāra), मुष्ककक्षार (Muṣkaka Kśāra), यवक्षार (Yavakśāra), सर्जिकाक्षार (Sarjikākśāra), टंकण (Taṅkaṇa), all these together is called as (Kśārāṣṭakam).

त्रिलवणम् *Trilavaṇam.*

सैंधवं रुचकं चैव बिडं च लवणत्रयम् ॥७३॥
एतत्त्रिलवणं प्रोक्तं नामतत्त्वार्थकोविदैः ।

सैंधवम् (Saindhavam), रुचकम् (Rucakam), बिडम् (Biḍam), these three together is called as त्रिलवणं (Trilavaṇam).

लवणषट्कम् *Lavanasatkam*

सामुद्रसिंधुरुचकं बिडरोमकपांशुजम ॥७४॥
षडेते च समाख्याता लवणाः शास्त्रकोविदैः ।

सामुद्रलवणम् (Sāmudralavaṇam), सैंधवम् (Saindhavam), रुचकम् (Rucakam), बिडम् (Biḍam), रोमकम् (Romakam), पांशुजम् (Pāmśujam), all these six together is called as Lavaṇaṣaṭkam.

त्रिमधुरम् *Trimadhuram*

घृतं सिता माक्षिकञ्च विज्ञेयं मधुरत्रयम ॥७५॥
विद्यात्त्रिमधुरं चैव प्रोक्तं च मधुरत्रिकम् ।

घृतं (Ghṛtam= Ghee), सिता (Sitā=sugar), माक्षिकम् (Mākśikam =Honey), these three together is called as मधुरत्रयं (Madhuratrayam), त्रिमधुरम् (Trimadhuram) and मधुर त्रिकं(Madhuratrikam) are its synonyms.

षड्रसाः Ṣaḍrasāḥ

कटुतिक्तकषायाश्च लवणोऽम्लश्च पञ्चमः ॥७६॥
मधुरेण समायुक्ताः षड्रसाः समुदाहृताः ।

कटुः (Katuḥ- pungent), तिक्तः (Tiktaḥ- bitter), कषायः (Kaṣāyaḥ-astringent), लवणः (Lavanaḥ-salty), अम्लः (Amlaḥ-sour) and मधुरः (Madhuraḥ)-Sweet) These are six *Rasas*.

(*Rasa* - is the object of gustatory sense organ located in the tongue-mouth.) It is an indicator of the composition, properties and probable actions of the substance. Apart from this the word *Rasa* means *Pārada* पारद, mercury, expressed juice, and the first (fluid) *dhātu* from the diet produced in the body.

औषधम् *Auṣadham*

भैषज्यं भेषजं चैवमगदो जायुरौषधम् ॥७७॥
आयुर्योगो गदारातिरमृतं च तदुच्यते ।

तच्च पञ्चविधं प्रोक्तं स्वस्वयोग विशेषतः॥७८॥
रसश्चूर्णं कषायश्चावलेहः कल्क ईरितः ।

रसः पारदसंमिश्रो दिव्यद्रव्यसमन्वितः ॥७९॥
चूर्णं तु वस्तुभिः क्षुण्णैः कषायः क्वथितैस्तु तैः ।
अनेकैरवलेहः स्यात् कल्को मध्वादिमर्दितैः॥८०॥

औषधम् (Auṣadham), भैषज्यं (Bhaiṣajyam), भेषजं (Bheṣajam), अगदः (Agadaḥ), जायुः (Jāyuḥ), आयुर्योगः (Āyuryogaḥ), गदारातिः (Gadārātiḥ), and अमृतम् (Amṛtam) are synonymous.

पञ्चविध कल्प (Pañcavidha Kalpa-Processing for administration) : (1) रस Rasa (a) Expressed juice from the wet substances (b) The drug prepared with the help of mercury. (2) & (5) चूर्ण & कल्क - When plants or drugs are made into a (dry) powder form then it is called as चूर्ण (Cūrṇa); When in the wet state it is called as कल्क (Kalka -paste). (3) कषाय Kaṣāya or क्वाथ Kvātha. This is obtained by boiling of the drug materials (4) अवलेह (Avaleha) when various drug material in *Kalka* form with the addition of honey etc. is given then it is called as अवलेह (Avaleha -linctus).

(For precise definitions and procedures standard books on the subject should be referred. Here workable definitions are mentioned.)

पथ्यम् *Pathyam* (salutary)

आत्मनीनं तु पथ्यं स्यादायुष्यं च हितं च तत् ।

आत्मनीनम् (Ātmanīnam), पथ्यम् (Pathyam), आयुष्यम् (Āyuṣyam), हितम् (Hitam) are synonymous.

आरोग्यम् *Ārogyam* (Health)

पाटवं लाघवं वार्तमारोग्यं स्यादनामयम् ॥८१॥

पाटवं (Pāṭavam), लाघवं (Lāghavam), वार्तम् (Vārtam), आरोग्यं (Ārogyam), अनामयम् (Anāmayam) are synonymous.

नीरोगः *Nirogah* (Healthy, without disease)

अगदो नीरुजः स्यात्तु ह्यनार्तश्चैव कथ्यते ।

अगदः (Agadaḥ), नीरुजः (Nīrujaḥ), अनार्तः (Anartaḥ), are synonymous.

रोगी *Rogī* (A patient)

व्याधितो विकृतो ग्लास्नुर्ग्लानो मन्दस्तथाऽऽतुरः ॥८२॥
अभ्यान्तोऽभ्यमितो रुग्णश्चाऽऽमयावी च दुःसहः ॥

व्याधितः (Vyādhitaḥ), विकृतः (Vikṛtaḥ), ग्लास्नुः (Glāsnuḥ), ग्लानः (Glānaḥ), मन्दः (Mandaḥ), आतुरः (Āturaḥ),अभ्यान्तः (Abhyāntaḥ), अभ्यमितः (Abhyamitaḥ), रुग्णः (Rugṇaḥ), आमयावी (Āmayāvī), दुःसहः (Duḥsahaḥ), are synonymous.

वैद्यः *Vaidyah* (A Doctor)

वैद्यः श्रेष्ठोऽगदंकारी रोगहारी भिषग्विदः ॥८३॥
रोगज्ञो जीवनो विद्वानायुर्वेदश्चिकित्सकः ॥

वैद्यः (Vaidyaḥ), श्रेष्ठः (Śreṣṭhaḥ), अगदंकारी (Agadankārī), रोगहारी (Rogahārī), भिषग्विदः (Bhiṣagvidaḥ) , रोगज्ञः (Rogajñyaḥ), जीवनः (Jīvanaḥ), विद्वान् (Vidwān) आयुर्वेदः (Āyurvedaḥ), चिकित्सकः (Cikitsakaḥ) are synonymous.

आहारः *Āhārah*

अन्नं जीवनमाहारः कूरं कशिपुरोदनम् ॥८४॥
अन्धो भिस्साऽदनं भोज्यमन्नाद्यमशनं तथा ॥

अन्नं (Annam), जीवनम् (Jīvanam), आहारः (Āhāraḥ), कूरं (Kūram), कशिपुः (Kaśipuḥ), ओदनम् (Odanam), अन्धः (Andhaḥ), भिस्सा (Bhissā), अदनं (Adanam), भोज्यं (Bhojyam), अन्नाद्यं (Annadyam) and अशनं (Aśanam) are synonymous.

अष्टविधमन्नम् Aṣṭavidhamannam (Eight types of diet)

भोज्यं पेयं तथा चोष्यं लेह्यं खाद्यं च चर्व्यकम् ॥८५॥
निष्पेयं चैव भक्ष्यं स्यादन्नमष्टविधं स्मृतम् ।

भोज्यं (Bhojyam), पेयं (Peyam), चोष्यं (Choṣyam), लेह्यं (Lehyam), खाद्यं (Khādyam), चर्व्यकम् (Carvyakam), निष्पेयं (Niṣpeyam), and भक्ष्यं (Bhakṣyam). These are the eight types of food.

सप्तधातवः Saptadhātavāḥ (Seven metals)

सुवर्णरूप्य ताम्रं च रङ्गं यशदमेव च ॥८६॥
सीसं लोहं च सप्तैते धातवो गिरिसंभवाः ॥

सुवर्णम् (Suvarṇam), रूप्यम् (Rūpyam), ताम्रम् (Tāmram), रङ्गं (Ranga), यशदं (Yaśadam) सीसं (Sisam) and लोहं (Loham); these seven are धातु (Dhātus) (metals).

उपधातवः Upadhātvaḥ (Semimetals)

सप्तोपधातवः स्वर्णमाक्षिकं तारमाक्षिकम् ॥८७॥
तुत्थं कांस्यं च रीतिश्च सिन्दूरश्च शिलाजतुः ।

स्वर्णमाक्षिकं (Swarṇamākśikam), तारमाक्षिकम् (Tāramākśikam), तुत्थं (Tuttham), कांस्यं (Kāmsyam), रीतिः (Rītiḥ), सिन्दूरः (Sindūraḥ) and शिलाजतुः (Śilājatuḥ) are seven उपधातवः (Upadhātavaḥ).

नवरत्नानि Navaratnāni (Nine precious jewels)

मुक्ताफलं हीरकं च वैदूर्यं पद्मरागकम् ॥८८॥
पुष्परागं च गोमेदं नीलं गारुत्मतं तथा ॥

मुक्ता (Muktā), हीरकं(Hirakam),वैदूर्यम्(Vaidūryam),पद्मरागकम् (Padmarāgakam), पुष्परागं (Puṣparāgam), गोमेदम् (Gomedam), नीलं (Nīlam) and गारुत्मतं (Gārutmatam), these nine are called as महारत्नानि (Mahāratnāni)

पञ्चरत्नानि Pañcaratnāni. (five jewels)

पद्मनागेन्द्र नीलाख्यौ तथा मरकतः शुभः ॥८९॥
पुष्परागश्च वज्राख्यः पञ्च रत्नवराः स्मृताः ।

पद्मरागः (Padmarāgaḥ), इन्द्रनीलः (Indranīlaḥ), मरकतः (Marakataḥ), पुष्परागः (Puṣparāgaḥ), वज्रः (Vajraḥ), these five are called as पञ्चरत्नानि (Pañcaratnāni).

उपरत्नानि Uparatnāni. (Semi jewels)

उपरत्नानि काचश्च कर्पूराश्मा तथैव च ॥९०॥
मुक्ताशुक्तिस्तथा शङ्ख इत्यादीनि बहून्यपि ॥ ½ ॥

काच (Kāca), कर्पूराश्मा (Karpūrāśmā), मुक्ताशुक्तिः (Muktaśuktiḥ), शङ्खः (Śaṅkaḥ) etc. are उपरत्नानि (Uparatnāni).

उपरसाः Uparasāḥ

गंधो हिङ्गुलतालमभ्रतालकशिलाः स्त्रोतोंजनं टंकणम् ।
राजावर्तकचुम्बकौ स्फटिकया शङ्खः खटी गैरिकम् ॥९१॥

कासीसं रसकं कपर्दसिकता बोलाश्च कङ्कुष्ठकम् ।
सौराष्ट्री च मता अमी उपरसा सूतस्य किंचित् गुणैः ॥९२॥

गंधकः (Gandhakaḥ), हिङ्गुल (Hiṅgulaḥ), तालः (Tālaḥ), अभ्रकम (Abhrakam), स्त्रोतोंजनं (Srotoñjanam), टंकणम् (Ṭaṅkaṇam), राजावर्तः (Rajāvartaḥ), चुम्बकः (Cumbakaḥ), स्फटिका (Sphaṭikā), शङ्खः (Śaṅkhaḥ), खटी (Khaṭī), गैरिकम् (Gairikam), कासीसं (Kāsīsam), रसकं (Rasakam), कपर्दः (Kapardaḥ), सिकता (Sikatā), बोलः (Bolaḥ), कङ्कुष्ठकम् (Kaṅkuṣthakam), सौराष्ट्रीः (Saurāṣṭrī), these are called as उपरसाः (Uparasāḥ) which possess certain properties of mercury.

साधारणरसाः Sādhāraṇarasāḥ

कम्पिल्लः प्रथमो गौरीपाषाणो नवसागरः ।
कपर्दो वह्निजारश्च गिरिसिन्दूरहिङ्गुलौ ॥९३॥

बोदारश्रृङ्गमित्यष्टौ साधारणसाः स्मृताः । ½

कम्पिल्लः (Kampillaḥ), गौरीपाषाणः (Gaurīpāṣānaḥ), नवसागरः (Navasāgaraḥ), कपर्दः (Kapardaḥ), वह्निजारः (Vahnijāraḥ), गिरिसिन्दूरः (Girisindūraḥ), हिङ्गुलः (Hiṅgulaḥ), बोदारश्रृङ्गं (Bodārasṛṅgam) these eight are called as साधारणरसाः (Sādhāraṇa Rasāḥ).

धातवः Dhātavaḥ (in relation to planets)

तारं ताम्रं पित्तलं नागहेमं वङ्गं तीक्ष्णं कांस्यकं किट्टलोहम् ।
सूर्यादीनां नामभिः खेचराणां विज्ञातव्या धातवोऽनुक्रमेण ॥९४॥

तारं (Tāram), ताम्रं (Tāmram), पित्तलं (Pittalam), नागं (Nāgam), हेमं (Hemam), वङ्गम् (Vaṅgam), तीक्ष्णं (Tīkśnam), कांस्यम् (Kāmsyam), किट्टलोहम् (Kiṭṭaloham). These metals are related to the moving planets in the sky in their respective order beginning from the sun.

विषाणि - Viṣāṇi

विषं, विषभेदाश्च Viṣam & Viṣabhedāḥ ca.

स्थावरं जङ्गमं चैव द्विविधं विषमुच्यते ।
दशाधिष्ठानमाद्यं तु द्वितीयं षोडशाह्वयम् ॥९५॥

मूलं पत्रं फलं पुष्पं त्वक् क्षीरं सार एव च ।
निर्यासो धातवश्चैव कन्दश्च दशमः स्मृतः ॥९६॥

विष Viṣa (Poisonous substance) is of two types स्थावर Sthāvara (from immovable sources or substances and जंगम jaṅgama (from movable sources and substances). The sources of the first i.e. *sthāvara* are ten, while those of latter i.e. *Jaṅgama* are sixteen.

The roots, leaves, fruits, flowers, bark, latex, heartwood, exudates, metals and tubers. These ten are the sources of the immovables i.e. स्थावर and there are sixteen sources of the movable i.e. जंगम.

स्थावर विषाणि Sthāvara Viṣāṇi.

कालकूटं[1] वत्सनाभः श्रृङ्गकश्च प्रदीपनः ।
हालाहलो ब्रह्मपुत्रो हारिद्रः सक्तुकस्तथा ॥९७॥

सौराष्ट्रिक इति प्रोक्ता विषभेदा अमी नव ।

कालकूटं (Kālakūtam), वत्सनाभः (Vatṣanābhah), श्रृङ्गक (Śṛṅgakaḥ), प्रदीपनः (Pradipanaḥ) हालाहलः (Hālāhalaḥ), ब्रह्मपुत्रः (Brahmaputraḥ), हारिद्रः (Hāridraḥ), सक्तुकः (Saktukah) सौराष्ट्रिकः (Saurāṣtrikaḥ) these are the nine types (tubers?) of विष Viṣa.

वर्ज्यविषाणि Viṣāni - to be avoided.

कालकूटस्तथा मेषशृङ्गी दर्दुरकस्तथा ॥९८॥
हालाहलश्च कर्कोटी ग्रन्थिः हारिद्रकस्तथा ॥

1 These are mainly tuberous as it is clear from A.H. & A. Sang.
स्थिरमत्युल्बणं वीर्यं यत्कन्देषु प्रतिष्ठितम् ।
कालकूटेन्द्रवत्साख्यशृङ्गीहालाहलादिकम् । A.H. U. 35. 3.

रक्तशृङ्गी केशरश्च यमदंष्ट्रश्च पण्डितैः ॥९९॥
त्याज्यानीमानि योगेषु विषाणि दश तत्त्वतः ॥

कालकूट (Kālakūta), मेषशृङ्गी (Meṣaśṛṅgī), दर्दुरक (Darduraka), हालाहल (Halahāla), कर्कोटी (Karkoṭi), ग्रन्थिः (Granthih), हारिद्रक (Hāridraka), रक्तशृङ्गी (Raktasṛṅgi), केशर (Keśara), and यमदंष्ट्र (Yamadamṣṭra), these ten (tubers) विष Viṣa (Poisons) should not be used in medicinal preparations.

कालकूटः Kālakūṭaḥ

देवासुररणे देवैर्हतस्य पृथुमालिनः ॥१००॥
दैत्यस्य रुधिराज्जातः तरुरश्वत्थसंनिभः ॥
निर्यासः कालकूटोऽस्य मुनिभिः परिकीर्तितः ॥१०१॥
सोऽहिक्षेत्रे शृङ्गवेरे कोङ्कणे मलये भवेत् ॥

In the war which took place between Devas(देव) and Asuras(असुर) the daitya (दैत्य) by name Pṛthumālin was killed. From the blood of that (पृथुमालिन्) Pṛthumālina banyan like tree arose. The निर्यासः (gum resin) of this tree is called as कालकूट (Kālakūṭa). This tree occurs in अहिक्षेत्र (Ahikśetra), शृङ्गवेर (Śṛṅgavera), कोङ्कण (Konkaṇa) and मलय (Malaya).

*वत्सनाभः Vatsanābhaḥ**

सिन्दुवार सदृक्पत्रो वत्सनाभ्याकृतिस्तथा ॥ १०२ ॥
यत्पार्श्वे न तरोर्वृद्धिः वत्सनाभः स भाषितः ॥

The plant having leaves like सिन्दुवार (Chapter IV) and having characters like वत्सनाभी (Vatsanābhi)and in the viscinity of which there is no growth of plants is called as वत्सनाभ (Vatsanābha)

शृङ्गिकः Śṛṅgikaḥ

यस्मिन् गोशृङ्गके बद्धे दुग्धं भवति लोहितम् ॥१०३॥
स शृङ्गिक इति प्रोक्तो द्रव्यतत्त्वविशारदैः ॥

The plant of which tuberous root when tied to the cow's horn, the milk of which becomes red coloured is called as शृङ्गिक (Sṛṅgika).

---

* The compiler has mentioned वत्सनाभ Vatsanābha again on page 667. Therefore this may be different from the Amṛta Vatsanābha mentioned on page 667. S.D. Kamat

प्रदीपनः *Pradīpanaḥ*

वर्णतो लोहितो यः स्याद्दीप्तिमान् दहनप्रभः ॥१०४॥
महादाहकरः पूर्वैः कथितः स प्रदीपनः ॥

The plant which is red in colour and which has an illumination like fire, and which causes extreme burning is called as प्रदीपनः (Pradīpanaḥ).

हालाहलः *Hālāhalaḥ*

गोस्तनाभफलो गुच्छतालपत्रच्छदस्तथा ॥१०५॥
तेजसो यस्य दह्यन्ते समीपस्था द्रुमादयः ॥
असौ हालाहलो ज्ञेयः किष्किन्धायां हिमालये ॥१०६॥
दक्षिणाब्धितटे देशे कोकङ्णेऽपि च जायते ।

The plant having leaves like गुच्छताल (Gucchatāla) and fruits having resemblance to cow's teats and in the viscinity of which the other plants burn(i.e. do not grow) is called as हालाहल (Hālāhala). It occurs in Kiṣkindhā (किष्किन्धा), Himālaya (हिमालय), दक्षिणाब्धितटे (Southern part of the western ghat) and in Konkan.

ब्रह्मपुत्रः *Brahmputraḥ*

वर्णतो कपिलो यः स्यात्तथा भवति सारतः ॥१०७॥
ब्रह्मपुत्रः स विज्ञेयो जायते मलयाचले ॥

(The tubers) having grey coloured in appearance and internal substance of the same colour is called as ब्रह्मपुत्र (Brahmaputra). It occurs in मलयाचले (Malaya mountain).

हारिद्रः *Hāridraḥ*

हरिद्रातुल्यमूलो यो हारिद्रः स उदाहृतः ॥१०८॥

The tuberous roots of which resemble in appearance of हरिद्रा (*Curcuma longa*) is called as हारिद्र (Hāridra).

सक्तुकः *Saktukah*

यद्ग्रन्थिः सक्तुकेनेव पूर्णमध्यः स सक्तुकः ।

In the substance of the tubers of सक्तुक (Saktuka) there is a powder like substance or grains resembling the appearance of सक्तुक (Saktuka).

सौराष्ट्रिकः *Saurāstikah*

सुराष्ट्र विषये यः स्यात् स सौराँष्ट्रिकं उच्यते ॥१०९॥

The tuberous roots of सौराष्ट्रिक (Saurāṣṭrika) are found in the region of सौराष्ट्र (Saurașțra).

जंगमविषाश्रयाः *Sources of Vişa of immovables*

दृष्टिनिःश्वासदंष्ट्रा च नखमूत्र मलानि च ॥११०॥
शुक्रं लाला नखस्पर्शः संदंशं स्रावमर्दितम् ॥
गुदास्थिपित्तशुक्राणि दशषट् जङ्गमाश्रयाः ॥१११॥

Visualisation, exhalation (of expiratory air), teeth, nails, urine, faeces, semen, saliva, scratching by nails, bite, excretion, massaging, anus, bones, bile and semen these 16 are the sources of विष Vişa (poison) of immovables.

गुणकर्माणि Properties and actions of Vişa (Poison)

विषं प्राणहरं प्रोक्तं व्यवायि च विकासि च ।
आग्नेयं वातकफहृद् योगवाही मदावहम् ॥११२॥

स्थावरं जंगमं वाऽपि विषं जग्धं भिषग्वरैः ।
शीघ्रं दद्यात् व्यथां गुर्वीं प्रोक्तं च नरसत्तमैः ॥११३॥

तदेव युक्तियुक्तं तु प्राणदायि रसायनम् ।
योगवाही परं वातश्लेष्मजित् संनिपातहृत् ॥११४॥

The *visa* (poisonous substance) is rapidly devitalizing (प्राणहर), विकासि (*Vikāsi* -depressant) व्यवायी (*Vyavāyi*) readily absorbing and invading the tissues, *uṣṇavīrya,* pacifies *vāta* and *kapha doșas* is योगवाही (Yogavāhi) potentiating) and narcotic.

If any type of poison either *sthāvara* or *jaṅgam* is ingested by a person it gives an extreme distress.

But the same if taken by rational application, it is vitalizing, and *ras⁻ aya*na. It is potentiating (of other drugs), pacifies *vāta* and *kapha doșas* and is useful in conditions caused by vitiation of all the three *doșas* (Sannip⁻ ata).

हरितालम् *Haritalam*

हरितालं च गोदन्तं पीतकं नरमण्डनम् ।
आलं बिडालं गौरं च पिञ्जरं चित्रगन्धकम् ॥ ११५ ॥

हरितालं कटूष्णं च स्निग्धं कुष्ठोपघातकम् ।
विषकण्डुभूतहरं सुभगं केशहृत्परम् ॥११६॥

हरितालं (Haritālam), गोदन्तं (Godantam), पीतकं (Pītakam), नरमण्डनम् (Naramaṇḍanam), आलं (Ālam), बिडालम् (Biḍālam), गौरं (Gauram), पिञ्जरं (Piñjaram), चित्रगन्धकम् (Citragandhakam) are synonyms.

Haritāla is pungent in taste, *uṣṇavīrya,* unctuous, and useful in skin disorders, poison, pruritus, is antimicrobic, cosmetic and depilatory.

*अमृतम्-वत्सनाभः Amṛtam***

अमृतं स्यात् वत्सनाभो विषमुग्रं महौषधम् ।
गरलं मरणं नागं स्तोककं प्राणहारकम् ॥११७॥

गरलं स्थावराद्यं स्यात् प्रोक्तं चैकादशाह्वयम् । *
वत्सनाभोऽतिमधुरः सोष्णो वातकफापहः ॥११८॥

कण्ठरुक् संनिपातघ्नः पित्तसंशोधनोऽपि च ।

अमृतं (Amṛtam), वत्सनाभः (Vatsanābhaḥ), उग्रविषम् (Ugraviṣam), महौषधम् (Mahauṣadham), गरलं (Garalam), मरणं (Maraṇam), नागं(Nāgam), स्तोकं (Stokam), प्राणहारकम् (Prāṇahārakam), स्थावराद्यं (Sthavarādyam), गरलं (Garalam) are 11 synonyms of वत्सनाभ (Vastanābha).

Vatsanābha is sweet in taste, *uṣṇavīrya* and pacifies *vāta* and *kapha doṣas*. It is useful in disorders of throat, in *Sannipāta* (a condition with vitiation by three *doṣas*), and purifies *pitta* (or choleretic).

Aconitum ferox Wall ex ser.
(Fam. Ranunculaceae).

2 *उपविषाणि**** *Upaviṣāṇi*

अर्कक्षीरं स्नुहीक्षीरं लाङ्गली करवीरकः ॥११९॥
गुञ्जाऽहिफेनो धत्तूरः सप्तोपविषजातयः ॥ ½

(अन्यच्च

स्नुह्यर्क लाङ्गली गुञ्जा हयारिर्विषमुष्टिका ।
जेपालोन्मत्ताहिफेनं नवोपविषजातयः ॥)

---

* The Raj. Ni. has the same reading.

** there are many species of Aconite in India *Aconitum ferox* Wall. ex Ser. is usually accepted for Vatsanabha. वत्सनाभ S.D. Kamat

*** भल्लातकं चातिविषं चतुर्भागं च खाखसम् ।
करवीरं द्विधा प्रोक्तम् अहिफेनं द्विधा मतम् ॥
धत्तूरश्च चतुर्धा स्याद् द्विधा गुञ्जा च निर्विषा ।
विषमुष्टिलाङ्गली च गणश्चोपविषाह्वयः ॥
इत्यपि पाठः क्वचित् । चौखम्बा मुद्रित पुस्तके च संमतः । S.D. Kamat

The latex of अर्क (Arka - Chapter 4th), the latex of स्नुक् (Snuk-Chapter 1), लाङ्गली (Lāngalī- Chapter 4th) , करवीर (Karavīra) (Chapter 4th), गुञ्जा (Guñjā - Chapter 4th), अहिफेन (Ahiphena-Chapter VIth) , धत्तूरः (Dhattūraḥ - Chapter 4th) these seven are the types of उपविषाणि (Upaviṣāṇī - Subsidiary poisons). According to some others स्नुही (Snuhī), अर्क (Arka), लाङ्गली (Lāngalī), गुञ्जा (Guñjā), हयारिः (Hayāriḥ), विषमुष्टिः (Viṣamuṣatiḥ- Nux vomica- not mentioned in the Dhn. Ni)., जयपालः (Jayapālaḥ) (Chapter 1 st), उन्मत्त (Unmatta), अहिफेन (Ahiphena), are the nine types of उपविषाणि (Upaviśāṇi).

3 *विषप्रशमनानि*

पीतविषं नरं दृष्ट्वा सद्यो वमनमुत्तमम् ।
यावत्पीतातिविषं च तावत्तु वामयेत् सदा ॥१२०॥

सिञ्चेत् शीताम्भसा वक्त्रं मन्त्रपूतेन सत्वरम् ।
रजनी युग्मां[१]म्लकेन काञ्जिकेन तु पेषितम् ॥१२१॥

लेपेन च विषं हन्ति प्रलिप्तं नात्र संशयः ।
मातुलुङ्गरसेनापि धावनं काञ्जिकेन वा ॥१२२

अतिशीतेन तोयेन प्रलिप्तं नात्र संशयः ॥½

Here the methods are mentioned for the alleviation of the ingested poisons, (or with an external contact). If it is suspected that a person has (accidently) ingested poison, he should be vomitted immediately till the major portion of the poison goes out.

The cold water treated by मन्त्र (Mantras) should be sprinkled on the face immediately. The paste of हरिद्रा *Curcuma longa* and दारुहरिद्रा (*Berberis* sp.) made with sour काञ्जिकम् (Kāñjikam) should be applied locally. These can also be applied locally with the juice of मातुलुङ्ग (mātuluṅga) and washed with Kāñjī. Very cool water should be applied locally.

वर्गोऽयं मिश्रको नाम सप्तमः* परिकीर्तितः ।
द्रव्याण्युक्तानि गणशो मिश्रीकृत्य समासतः ॥१२३॥

---

१ रजनी युग्मकाम्लेन काञ्जिकेन तु पेषितम् । इति साधु भविष्यति ।
आनन्दाश्रम मुद्रित पुस्तके ग्रन्थान्तरादुद्धृतो पाठः ।

This reading is not found in Chaukhambā edition.

* One of the MṢṢ from Mumbai University shows 9 chapters instead of 7 chapters. The additional two chapters are mentioned separately.

'संध(ा)र्षिणी' पता गर्भा रक्षोघ्ना विडलांभसा । cont.....

Thus has been told the Mis'rakādi seventh chapter in which the drugs are mentioned by combinations and formulations.

गुडूच्यादिः शताह्वादिस्तथाऽन्यश्चन्दनादिकः ।
करवीरादिराम्रादिः सुवर्णादिर्विमिश्रकः ॥१२४॥

Thus in this Nighaṇṭu Guḍūcyādi, Satāhvādi, Candanādi, Karavīrādi, Āmrādi, Suvarṇādi and Miśrakādi chapters are described serially.

इति मिश्रकादिः सप्तमो वर्गः ।

Thus ends the Mis'rakādi Chapter Seventh.

(Contd.)मंदा मनोहरा कांता रत्नमाली धृतप्लवा ॥१२
शंखमूला कच्छविका पालना शास्यवर्जया ।
शूर्पपर्णी प्रहाकृष्णा सर्पाक्षी सूकरीति च ॥१३
एताश्चान्याऽपि बहवो याश्चान्या प्रथिता भुवि ।
विषघ्न्यः सर्व एवैताः संयोगेन विशेषतः ॥१४
विषहारि त्वयं वर्गो नवमः परिकीर्तितः ॥
गुडूच्यादिः शतपुष्पस्तथाऽन्यश्चन्दनादिकः ॥१५
करवीरादि आम्रादि सुवर्णादिर्विमिश्रितः ।
विषोपवविषवर्गश्च विषहारि तथैव च ॥१६
इत्येवमेते क्रमशो वर्गा नव प्रकीर्तिताः ॥
इति नवमो वर्गः ।
इत्यधिकः पाठः मुंबई विद्यापीठ संग्रहे हस्तलिखित पुस्तके दृश्यते ।
अशुद्धिप्रायोऽयं पाठः। अस्मिन् पुस्तके विषोपविषवर्गस्तथा विषप्रशमन वर्गश्च पृथक कृत्वा प्रदर्शितः दृश्यते ।

This reading is very corrupt; however certain plants like शूर्पपर्णी, etc. are mentioned as antidotal measures. S.D.Kamat.

Bibliography

A

A Ayur. -Adivasincha Ayurvdea, Marathi. MS. see Atmaram Awari.

Abhi.bu.dar. -Abhinava buti darpan, Edited by Shri Rupalalavaisya Hindi. Chaukhamba publication, Edit. 1940.

Abhi. Manj. -Abhidhan Manjari of Bhishagacharya-Nagari Sanskrit edited by Vaidyasarythi Press, 2nd Edition, 1952. See Krishnan.

Abhi. Raj. -Abhidhan Rajendra. prakrit and Ardhamagadhi Sanskrit (Nagari) Dictionary by Jaineshwar Swetambaracharya, Shree 1008 Shrimat Vijayarajendra Sureshwar 1918.(?)

Agharkar. -Dr. S. P. Agharkar. 'Medicinal Plants', Bombay State Gazetter, New series, Vol. 155, part Ist, 1953.

Agrawal. -Vasudeosharan Agrawal, 'Paninikaleen Bharat' (Hindi).

Ainslie. -Dr. Whitelow Ainslie- 'Materia Medica' Volume I, London, 1826.

Amar. -Amarakosha of Amarsimha, See Bhanuji; Kshiraswami; Maheswar.

A.P. Yoj. -'Amachi Panchawarshik Yojana' Forest Dept. M.S. Poona 1957.

Apte. -Apte's Sanskrit -English Dictionary, 1968.

Apte-Kali. -Dr. M.V. Apte, 'Kalidasachi Vanashree, Maharashtra Sahitya Patrika, Poona, Vols.81, 82, 83, 1921.(Mar.)

Apte. Gode. -Apte's Sanskrit-English Dictionary, Enlarged by Dr. Gode and Shri Karve (1st Edit).

Apte. Vana. -Dr. M.V. Apte, 'Vanashree Srishti' Vols . 1 & II, Maharashtra Rajya Sahitya Ani Sanskriti Mandal, Bombay . (Under publication; figures drawn by Dr. Apte and Prof. S.D. Mahajan [Marathi].

Aruna. -See Ashta. hr.

Asia Res. - Asiatic Researches Society of Bengal See Sir W.Jones.

---

* Appendix C-2 Index of Referred Books from the published Vol. I

* This is now published in 1986.

Ashubodha.	-Ashubodha Bhattacharya 'Raj Nighantu (with notes Hindi).
Ashta. hr.	-Ashtang hridaya of Vagbhat with Arunadatta and Hemadri teeka edited by Dr.Anna Moreswar Kunte, introductions of Shri P. K. Gode and Vaidya Harishastri Paradkar, Nirnayasagar Press,1939. See Kunte Arunadatta, Hemadri Shivadipika, Indu, Shivasen, Dasapandit.
Ashta. hr. Kosh	-Ashtangahridaya kosh compiled by K.M. Vaidya Malabara South. Valapada -Nagari Sanskrit and Vernacular names in Nagari Edn. 1936. See Vaidya.
Ashtra. Sang.	-Ashtang Sangraha. Indu Virachit 'Shashilekha, teeka on 3rd Part, Edn. 1924.
A.V.	-Atharva Veda, Shaunakeeya Samhita, with Sayana-chary's Bhashya, Edited by S. P. Pandit , 1895-96. See Ramachandra Sharma, Shende, Satavalekar, Karambelkar.
Atmaram. Awari	-'Aadivaseencha Ayurved' by Atmaram Awari, Peth -Barhe. Dist. Nasik, [MS. Marathi].
Athawale	-Ayurvediya Vyadhi Vinischaya Uttarardha by Vaidya A.D. Athavale Ayurved Parangat Poona, Shaka 1884 Marathi.
Ayangar	-P. M. Shrinivas Ayangar, 'Life in Ancient India' S. Varadachari and Co., 1952.
Ayur. Patr.	-Ayurveda Patrika 'Ayurved Seva sangh, Nasik, (Vols. from 1958, Marathi).
Ayur. Ausha.	-Ayurved Aushadhi Shastra by Shri Durgaprasad Sharma, 1965. Vaidyanath Ayurved Bhavan (Hindi).
Ayu. Jyo.	-Ayurjyoti Masik, Ayurved Mahavidyalaya, Baroda Vol. II-2nd year.
Ayur. Pra.	-Ayurved Prakash of Madhavopadhya translated into Marathi and edited by R. V. Patwardhan, 1925.
Ayur. Vis. Kosh	-Ayurvedeeya Vishwa Kosh compiled by Babu Ramaji Simha and Babu Dalajit Simha Vaidya Vols. 3, 1937
Ayur O. Ni.	- Ayurvedeeya Aushadhi Nighantu, compiled by Tayil-kumar Krishnan. Central Ayurvediya Gaveshana Samitee 1966. (Chapter -Gunadipika).

B

Balavantji Bihar	-'Biharki Vanaspatiya' Hindi with Botanical names by -Thakur Balwant Simhaji M SC

Balwantji,	-'Vanaushadhi Darshika, Hindi by Thakur Balwant Simhaji
Van.Dar.	-Simhaji M.SC.
Balwantji,	-Introduction to Bh. Pra. Ni. by Th. Balwant Simha Hindi
Bh. Pr.Ni.	-Vidyotini teeka.
B. Ramaji	-Baburamji See Ayur, V. Kosh.
Bapalalji.	-'A review on controversy in Ayurved and Some contrioversial Drugs' by Bapalal G. Vaidya in Sachitra Ayur. Monthly. 10-1961 and 1962.
B.F.D	-Bombay Forest Department Commercial Timbers of Bombay State; Poona. 1957.
Bha.Pr.Ni.	-Bhavaprakash Nighantu of Bhavamishra. See Ramtej Dattaram; Vidyotini; Ganga Vishnu; Dwivedi; Chunekar.
Bhagirath.	-Pandit Bhagirath Sharma ' Sandigdha Nirnaya Vanaushadhi Shastra', 1936; Farrukabada, Hindi.
Bhanuji.	-Bhanuji Dixit. 'Teeka' in Amarkosh.
Bhide.	-Abhinava Marathi Jnanakosh, Edited by G. R. Bḥide, Kolhapur, Vols I-IV, (1963-70).
Birdwood	-H. M. Birdwood, C.S.I. 'The flora of Mahabaleshwar and Matheran (Revised Edn.) J.B.N.H. Soc., 1887-97.
Blatter & McCann.	-Blatter E. & Mc Cann. C. 'The Bomaby Grasses', I.C.A.R. Scientific Mongoraph No. 5, Delhi. (illustrated by Shri Bhide).
Bodas.	-V.V. Bodas, A. Visharad.. 'Dravyaguna Shastra (Marathi) 1965.
Bom. Gaz.	-Bomaby Gazetteers (old series) Thana, xiii, Nasik xv Colaba, xi; Baruch II-i, p. 1st.
Bom. S. Gaz.	-Bomaby State Gazetter. See Agharkar.
B.S.I.	-Botanical Survery of India. Poona and Calcutta.
Borkar	-Vaidya Datto Balal Borkar, Marathi translation of 'Yoga Ratnakar', etc.
Br. Ni.	-M.M. S. D. Pade.'Brihannighantu' -Marathi with Botanical names, 1897.
Borwankar	-Raghuvamsha with commentary of Kalidas. Translated by A.G. Borwankar. Chitrashala Prees, Poona. 1933.
Botany II	-Technical terms in Hindi. Ministry of Education Govt. of India, 1959.

C

Ca. -Charaka Samhita of Charakacharya with 'Ayurved Deepika' teeka of Chakrapani. Edited by Acharya Yadavji Trikamji, N. S. Press, Bom 1941.

Ca. -Charaka Samhita with Chakrapani's Ayurved Dipika and Jejjata's Nirantarapada Vyakhya, Edited by Pdt. Harishastri.Bombay Sanskrit Press. 1st part 1940, and II nd part 1941.

Cakra Ca. -See Ca.

Chakra Su. "Bhanumati' teeka on Sushrut Sam. Sutrasthan, by Chakrapani. Introduction by M. M. Gananathsen Saraswati. Published by Agra Univ., 1939.

Charak Gangdhar. -See Gangadhar.

Chakradutta. -'Chakradatta, Composed by Chakrapani Dutta with Hindi Sandipani Teeka by Jagadiswara Prasad Tripathi A.M.S. Chaukhamba 1949. See Tripathi.

Chembers. -Chembers English Dictionary, Indian Edn., 1966.

Chopra, Handa. -I.C. Chopra and K.L. Handa. 'Review of Indian -Medicinal Plants.' Indian Council of Agri,. Res., New Delhi (1st Edn.)

Chopra. -R.N. Chopra & associates. 'Glossary of Indian Medicinal Plants.' New Delhi, 1953.

C.A.D. -Committee for standard and genuine Ayurvedic Drugs, Bom. Gov. 1955.

Com.Pro. -Sir G. Watt., 'Commercial Products of India, 1908.

Cooke Fl. -Dr.T. Cooke (Principal, Science College, Poona 'Flora of the Presidency of Bombay' Vols. I-III reprinted -B.S.I. Calcutta. 1958.

D

Das Gupta -Hist. of Indian Philosophy by Surendranath Dasagupta. Vol. II, edn. 1932 (?) 37.

Dasapandit. -'Hridayabodhika Vyakhya' on Astha. hr. Su. 16-30 by Dasapandit. Introduction by P.K. Narayan Pillai. Published by Anantashayanam Rajakiya Mudranalaya (Vernacular names of plants of Malyalam alphabet). Ed. 1950.

Dattaram. -Bha. Pr. Ni. with Pr. Abhinava Ni. Hindi teeka by Dattaram Chobe, N. S. Press, Bombay 1950.

De Candolle. - Origin of cultivated plants by De Candolle, America. Edn. 1959.

Desai. -'Vanausadhi Sangraha' written by Dr. Vaman Ganesh Desai B.SC., L.M.S. 1927.

Dhamankar. -'Ayurvediya Aushadhikaran' Marathi,by Vaidya P. V. Dhamankar and G. V. Puranik, B.SC., Panvel, Colaba District. 1964.

Dipika. -Dipika teeka on Sharangdhar Samhita, which see.

Dra. Ratn. -Drawayaratnakar, with Marathi names of plants incomplete, MS.

Dalhan. -'Nibandha Sangraha teeka' on Sushrut Samhita by Dalhan. N. S. Press, Bombay, 1938.

Datta Sharma. -'Dhatu Upadhatuka Sodhan, by Thakur Dattasharma Vaidya, 1930 Lahor.

Dutta Botany -A class book of Botany by A.C. Dutta - Ed.1953.

Dymock. -Phamacographia indica, by Dr. William Dymock & associates in parts. Vols.3 of 1890-93

Dwivedi. -Bhasha teeka on Bh. P. Ni. by Viswanath Dwiledi B.A; Edn. 1954. Hindi with Bot. names.

Dwivedi. Raj. Ni. -Rajanighantuki vishesata by V. Dwivedi. Ayurvedic Mahasammelan Patrika p. 133. March 1963.

G

Gajendra gadkar. -commentary by S. D. Gajendragadkar and English translation of Kumarasambhava of Kalidas by R.D. Karmarkar, Ed. 1923.

Gambel -Flora of the Presidency of Madras, reprinted, B. S. I. 1957.

Gangadhar. & Charak. -'Jalpa Kalpataru' Teeka of Gangadhar and Chakrapani on Charak.

Ganga V. -Ganga Vishnu. Tippani on Bh. Pr. Ni. Saka 1860.

Garde. -Dr. G. K. Garde 'Vagbhat', translated into Marathi 1935.

Gananath. Bhanumati. Sanskrit Introduction on Su. Su. Bhanumati teeka of Chakrapani by Gananathsen Saraswati see Cha. Su.

Gananath sharir. -'प्रत्यक्ष शारीरस्य उपोद्घात भागः' कवि. गणनाथसेन एल. एम्.एस. इत्यनेन विरचितः । कालिकता XI. नथूराम शर्मा (Year not mentioned).

Ghanekar. -Dr. B.G. Ghankekar , 'Sushrut Sam. Hinidi teeka on Sutrasthan' Samvat 2039.

Gode. -Studies in Indian Litrary History, Vol. I. by Dr. P. K. Gode, M.A. D. Litt. Published by Singhi Jain Shastra Shikshapith. Bharatiya Vidya Bhavan, Bombay. 1953 A.D. Printed in Veda-Vidya Mudranalaya, Poona 2.

Gosh. -Materia Medica, edited by Samir Kumar Biwas 1957.

Gu. Dipika. -Gudharath Dipika teeka. See Sharnagadhar Sam.

H

Halalayudh. - 'Halayudh Kosh' edited by Jayashankar Joshi 1st edn.

Harshe. 'Shivkosh of Shivadatta', edited by Dr. R.G. Harshe Deccan College, Poona, 1952.

Hast. Ayur. -Hastyaurved of Palakapya, Anandrashram, Poona. 1st Ed.

Hemadri -See Astangahriday

Hemaraj -See Kash. Saṁhita.

Hoernle. -Translation of Su. su, Adhayas, 1 to 5 by A.F. R. Hoernle. As. Res. Soc. Bengal, New series No. 94, 1897.

Hill. -Economic Botany by Mr. Albert F. Hill, Fellow, Hardward University, 2nd Edn. 1952.

Hist. of Med. - History of Medicine brturi Castiglioni Translated from Italic and edited by E.B. Krumbhaar. March 1959 (Canada).

Indu. Asta. Sang. -Astanga Sangraha 'Shashilekha' teeka on Uttarsthan. by Indu, 1924.

I

Indu. Su. Ast. br. -Astanghriday. Teeka on Su. by Indu, Vaidyasarathi Granthalaya, Kottayanagar, 1956.

J

Jangale. -Vaidya Hiramani Motiram Jangale, 'Sachitra Vanausadhi Gunadarsha' Parts 1-2 (1st Edn.)

Joshi. -See Nighantaprakash.

K

Kaji -Principals of General Geography by Prof. Diwan Bahadur H. L. Kaji, 1951.

Kannya Lall. -The Indigenous drugs of India by Kannya Lall Dey Rai Bahadur; C.I. E. etc. 2nd Edition, 1890, Thakar & Co. Calcutta.

Karambelkar -"The Atharvavedic civilization' by Dr. V. W. Karambelkar, M.A. Ph. D. 1959.

Kamsutram -(कामसूत्रम्) of Vatsayanamuni. With Jayamangalavyakhya teeka of Yashodhara and Hindi Vyakhya of Devadatta Shastri. Chaukhamba Sanskrit series. Varanasi edt. 1960.

Kas. Sam, -Kashyap Samhita, with Sankrit intorduction by Nepal Rajaguru Shri Hemaraja Sharma with its Hindi translation by Satytapal Bhishagacharya. Kashi Sanskrit Granthamala, 1953.

Kau. Artha Shastra. -Kautiliya Arthashastra, by Acharya Chanakya. Sanskrit translated into Hindi by Gangaprasadji Shastri,, Published by Chaukhamba Prakashan V. Sam. 2010.

Ketkar. -See Prachin Maharashtra.

Kirtikar -Indian Medicinal Plants by Dr. L. Col. K. R. Kirtikar and Major B.D. Basu Edit. 1918.

Krishnan. -C. V. Krishnan Chokhanathapuram Venkitaramner Krishnan. Krishan of Chokkanathapuram village (in Palaghata Dist. Kerala). The Gentleman who gave transliteration of Malyalam alphabets into Roman and Nagari alphabets. See Abhi. Manj. Supra.

Kshiraswami. -Teeka on Amarkosh by Kśihiraswami. with introduction of Oak, 1913. Law Printing Press, Poona.

Kudatarkar. -'Dravyaguna Shastra' Marathi with Botanical names of plants written by Vaidya M.N.Kudtarkar Shastri and associate Parts II First edn.

Ku. Sambhabva. -'Kumarasmbhava of Kalidas. See Gajendragadkar.

Kunte. -See Ashtanga hridaya.

L

L. Ni. -Laghu Nighantu by Vyasa Keshavaram, edited by A. S. Paranjpe and associates. published by Dr. G. S.Pendse. for I. D. R.A. Poona, 1962.

Laghu. S. kau. -Laghu Siddhant Kaumudi. Introduction by Ramachandra Jha Vyakaranacharya. Chaukhamba Sanskrit pustakalaya, Banares, 1952.

Law. -Vimalcharan. Law. India as Described in early texts Buddha & Jain. Ist Edit.

Lisboa -'Economical plants' Bombay Gazetteer, Vol. XXV (old series).

Lok. Tilak -Arctic Home in the Vedas' 1st Edn. poona. by B.G. Tilak.

M

Madan. Ni. -Madanapal Nighantu, Hindi translation by Ramprasad.

Maha. S. Gazet -Maharashtra State Gazetteer Vol. I. A. Botany, Economic Botany (1st Edn.)

Mantri. -Dr. P. G. Mantri 'Bharatiya Vanaushadhi Sangraha', 1886. Marathi.

Medi. Kosh. Mediiniya Kosh. Chaukhamba Sanskrit series, Sam. 1997.

Mahaskar & - Dr. K. G. Mhaskar and J. F. Caius. "सर्पदंशे प्रयुज्यमाना भारतवर्षीया वनस्पतयः" and "भारतवर्षे समुत्पन्ने वनस्पतीनां गुणावगुण चर्चापदानि" शकाब्दे 1852 म्हैसूरपत्तने वाचिता.

Moos. -Vayaskar N. S. Mooss - 'Ayurvedic Flora Indica. Keral Edit. 1953.

Mukerji. -'Indian pharamaceutical Codex Vol,. I, Lucknow, 1947.

Mukerjee. -'plant Groups' 1957.

Mule. -'Rasadhatu prakash', part II, by Pra. P.D. Mule. Vidarbha.

Mahajan. -Prof. S. D. Mahajan and V.V. Divan. 'Contribution to the Flora of Kolhapur Dist. part I, Vegetation & Forest resources of Radhanagari area', Shivaji Uni. Journal, Vol,. I. 1969.

Mahajan. -'कोल्हापूर जिल्ह्यातील वनस्पति व प्राणि' दर्शन. (श्री. लोहिया कोल्हापूर.गौरव ग्रंथ) International Book Service, Poona 1971. संपादकः पु.ल. देशपांडे व ग. रं. भिडे.

Mahajan & Vaidya. -Vegetation of Grasslands around Kolhapur' Shivaji Uni.J. Vol. II 1970.

N

Nadkarni. - 'Indian Materia Medica'. in 2 parts by A. K. Nadkarni. 3rd edition.

Namjoshi -A blue print in Ayurvedic Research by Prof. A.N.Namjoshi. (Now M. L. A.)

Namjoshi -Studies in Pharmacognosy of Ayurvedic Drugs. by A.N.

Namjoshi, M.SC .etc. Published by Maha. State. Board of Research in Ayur. Drugs. Bom. 1960.

Narke G. G. -Hand Book of Indian Geology, 1951.

Narayan Upa. -'Narayaniya Upanishad', N. S. Press, Bombay

Nelson, A. -Medical Botany, 1951.

Ni. Adarsha. -'Nighantu Adarsha' (Gujarathi) by Vaidya Bapalal Gadabaddas Shaha, Parts 2. 1927.

Ni. Prakash. -'Nighanta Prakash' with Marathi translation by Bapu Gangadhar Joshi, Ganapat Krishnaji Litho. P. 1839.

Ni. Ratna. - Nighanta Ratnakar with Marathi translation edited by Navare Shastri (2 parts) N. S. Press. Bombay, 1936.

Ni. Shiro. -Nighanta Shiromani edit. by Vaidya, S.D. Pade. 1898.

O

Oak -Introduction to Teeka of Kseeraswami on Amarakosh by Late K. G. Oak. Law Printing Press; Poona. Edit. 1913

P

Patanjali. Patanjali Kalin Bharata. Hindi, written by Dr. Prabhudayal, Agnihotri, Bihar Rashtrabhasha Parishad Patna, 1st Edit. 1963.

Patwardhan. -See Ayurved prakash.

Phadke. -Dravyaguna Shastram' Sanskrit. Compiled by Vaidya G.A. phadake, Ayurvedacharya. Edited by Late Vaidya N.H. Joshi, Bombay , Edit 1960.

Dr. Pendse. Glossary of Vegetable Drugs in Vagbhat, published by Dr. G. S. Pendse, Veda-Vidya Mudranalaya, poona 2. 1965.

Potters. Potters new 'Cyclopaedia of Botanical Drugs' by R. C.W. Ren. 1956.

Prayog Ratna - 'Prayoga Ratnakar' ,Narayanbhatti.

Pra. Maha. -Prachin Maharashtra, written by Dr. S.V. Ketkar edit. 1936.

Priyawrata. -'Drawvyaguna Vijnyan' Hindi. compiled by Acharya Priyawrat Sharma, part 2 first Edit.

Puri & Mahajan -Dr. G. S. Puri and prof. S. D. Mahajan. 'Study of The Evergreen Vegetation of Mahabaleshwar'. Bull Bot. Serv. India, Vol. II, 1960.

R

Raghuwamsh. -Raghuwamsha of Mahakavi Kalidas with commentary of Mallinath .See Borwankar.

Raghuwir -Dr.Raghuwir, Dictionary, Vol IV of Botanical terms. 1st Edit.

Rasa. P. -Rasapaddhati by Bindu. Edited by Yadavji, N.S. Press, 1925

Rajawade. -Rajawade's Lekhsangraha, part 3. Edited by Shankar Narayan Joshi, Chitrashala Press, Poona. 1st Edit.

Ram Sharma -See A.V.

Ramtej. -Tippani on Bh.pr.Ni. by Ramtej Pande, 1947

Roxb. -Flora Indica by Dr.W. Roxburgh. Carey's edition, Vols.3 of 1832 and C.B. Clark's Edit. 1874.

R.Y.S. -Rasayoga Sagar, parts2 compiled by Pandit Hariprapannaji Sharma, Bombay, 1925.

Ru.Sam -Rutusamhar of Kalidas.

Ramprasad -See Madan Pal, N.

R.S.V. -Riksukta Vaijayanti (ऋक्सूक्त वैजयंती) edited by Prof. H.D. Velankar and associate. Tilak Vidyapithnagar, Poona 9, Shaka 1887, Edit. 1965.

S

San. Sa. Iti -Sanskrit Sahitya Itihas, by Wachspati Gairola, Choukhamba Publication, Edit.1960.

Santapau. - 'Flora of Khandala' Bot.Serv. India, 1958.

Satwalekar. -Pandit Shripad Damodar, Subodh Atharva Veda, 1st Edit.

Satyapal -See Kas. Sam.

Shabda Kalpa -Sabda Kalpadrum, Kosha, parts 2 Hindi Choukhamba Prakashan

Sara. Ni. -Saraswati Ni. by Jayatilaka Colombia, Cylon, 1914 (M/s. Anandashram Press Poona.)

Satyaprakash -Prachin Bharat me rasayanka vikas-Hindi.(प्राचीन भारतमे रसायनका विकास) written by Satyaprakash, D.Sc.Prayag Viswavidyalaya 1960. Prakashan Shakha Suchná vibhag, Uttar Pradesh.

S.K.S. -Shraut Kosh Sanskrit edited by C.G. Kashikar, V.S. Mandal, Tilak Mandir Poona 2. March 1958, V.V. mudranalaya Press Poona 2.

S.K.E. -Shraut Kosh Vol. 1, parts 1 and 2 English Section of 1958 and 1962 edited by C.G. Kashikar. Published by N.S. Sontake, V.S. Mandal , Tilak Road Poona 2

Sharn. Sam. -Sharngadhar Samhita with Dipika and Gudharth Dipika Comentatories and with foot notes, introduction Edited by Pandit Parshuram Shastri Vidyasagar, N.S. press, Bombay 1931.

Shri Ram -do- Hindi translation by Shri Ram.

Shende -Religion and Philosophy of A.V. by Dr. N.J. Shende Ph.D.1952.

Shivadas. -Tika on 'Drawyaguna Sangrah' of Chakrapani, by Shivdas, N.S. Press Bombay 1922

Shivasen. -'Tatwabodh Vyakhya' by Shivdas Sen on Astang Hr.Uttaratantra. Introduction by Jyotishyachandra Saraswati, Agra University, 1942.

Siva Kosh -See Harshe.

Su. -Sushrut Samhita of Sushrutacharya with Nibandha Sangrah tika of Dulhan. N.S. Press Bombay. Edit. 1938. See Dulhan, Chakra Su.; Ghanekar, U.C.Dutta, Hoernle. Intro. by Yadavji.

Suredranath Gupta -History of Indian Philosophy, 1932.

T

Talbot. -Forest Flora of Bombay presi. and Sindha, Vol.2nd, by Talbot, 1909.

Tripathi -See Chakradutta.

U

U.C.Dutt -'Materia Medica of the Hindus' by Dr.U.C.Dutt with Glossary of Indian M. plants by George King. Edit 1932.

Uphof - Dictionary of economical plants by Th. Uphof Hamnea publishing Co. 1957.

V

Vaidya -See Asta. Hr. Kosh

Varma -Hale White Mat Med-Hindi trans.1957.

Vana -shatak -Vanaspati Shatak with coloured plates, Hindi. by Durga Prasad Sharma, Vaidyanath, Ayurved Bhavan Gopal Lane, Calcutta 1965.

Vishwa-Kosh -Vishwa Prakash Kosh. Compiled by Babu Ramji Simha and Babu Dalpatji Simha Parts 3. Hindi Sanskrit Choukhamba Publishers 1960.

Vadikand. -Rasaratnakarantargata Vadikanda, Copied by Jivaramsastri son of Kalidas. Gondala Rasashala Kathiawad on 11-5-1922

Vartaka - Dr. V.D. Vartak, 'Katraj Ghatatil Vanaspati' (Marathi), 1st Edn. Some Additions to Flora of Sinhagad Hill, Poona Dist. Poona Agri. Coll. Mag S7(4), 1957.

Vidyotini -Bh.pr.Ni. with Hindi tika by Brahma Shankar Mishra and Intro. by Tha. Balwant Sinhaji, 1960.

W

Waring. -Pharmacopeia of India, 1868.

W.Jones -President As.Res.Soc.of Bengal.

M.Williams - Sanskrit English Dictionary.

Watt Dict. -'Dictionary of Economic Products of India' Vols. 6. parts 9, India House, London. (1889-1897).

Y

Yadavji -'Dravyaguna Vijnyan' by Acha. Yadavji Tricumji Vol. II, 1950., and Intro. Su.Sam.

Yog. Taran. -Yogtarangini of Trimalbhatta. Intro. by Maheshwarji Vyas, 1953.

INDEX - A

INDEX OF BOTANICAL NAMES, SYNONYMS AND OTHER DRUGS.

Index of Botanical names, synonyms and other drugs. Page No.

Abies spectabilis (D. Don) Spach. 147
Abies webbiana Lindl. 147
Abroma augusta Linn. 84
Abrus precatorius Linn. 291
Absinthium vulgare Gaertn. 171
Abutilon asiaticum G. Don 111-112
Abutilon asiaticum W. & A. 111
Abutilon indicum G. Don 111
Abutilon indicum (Linn.) Sw. 111-112
Acacia catechu (Linn.f.) Willd. 10
Acacia catechu var. *sundra* Prain 10
Acacia catechu Willd. 10
Acacia concinna DC. 90
Acacia concinna DC. var. ***rugata*** 89
Acacia farnesiana Willd. 489
Acacia ferruginea DC. 10
Acacia leucophloea (Roxb.) Willd. 11-490
Acacia leucophloea Willd. 11
Acacia polycantha Willd. 11-433
Acacia rugata (Lamk.) Merr. 89
Acacia sirissa Ham. 463
Acacia suma Buch.- Ham. 443
Acacia suma Kurz. 11-444
Acampe papillosa (Lindl.) Lindl. 332
Achatina fulica 223
Achras sapota Linn. 440
Achyranthes aspera Linn. 101
Aconitum bisma (Buch.- Ham.) Rap. 4
Aconitum ferox Wall. ex Ser. 667
Aconitum heterophyllum Wall. 4
Aconitum heterophyllm Wall. ex Royle 4
Acorus calamus Linn. 125
Adenanthera pavonia Linn. 193
Adhatoda beddomei C.B. Clarke 9
Adhatoda vasica Nees 9
Adhatoda zeylanica Medik. 9

Adiantum capillus - veneris Linn. 348
Adiantum lunulatum Burm. 347
Adiantum lunulatum Linn. 348
Adiantum philippense Linn. 347
Adiantum venustum Don 348
Adiantum venustum G. Don 348
Adina cordfolia (Roxb.) Benth. & Hook. 452
Adina cordfolia (Roxb.) Benth. & Hook. f. 196
Adina cordifolia (Willd. ex Roxb.) Hook. f. ex Brandis 452
Aegle marmelos Corr. 39
Aegle marmelos (Linn.) Corr. 39
Ageratum conyzoides Linn.
Aframomum melegueta K. Schum. 142
Aglaia elaeagnoidea (Juss.) Benth. 202
Aglaia roxburghiana Miq. 202
Agrostis linearis Linn. 368
Ailanthus excelsa Roxb. 13
Alangium lamarckii Thwait. 100
Alangium salvifolium Wang 100
Alangium salvifolium(Linn.f.) Wang 100
Albizia amara Boivin 464
Albizia julibrissin Durazz. 464
Albizia lebbeck Benth. 463
Albizia lebbeck (Linn.) Willd. 463
Albizia odoratissima Benth. 463
Albizia odoratissima (Linn. f.) Benth. 463
Albizia procera (Roxb.) Benth. 464
Aleurites moluccana Willd. 415
Aleurites triloba Forst. 415
Alhagi camelorum Fisch. 8
Alhagi maurorum Baker 8
Alhagi pseudalhagi (Bieb.) Desv. 8
Allium ascalonicum Linn. 313
Allium cepa Linn. 316
Allium esculentum Linn. 295
Allium leptophyllum Wall. 314
Allium macleanii Baker 316
Allium sativum Linn. 312
Allium xiphopetallum Ait. & Baker 312
Alpinia cardamomum Roxb. 141
Alpinia galanga Willd. 105

Alstonia scholaris (Linn.) R. Br. 238
Alstonia scholaris R. Br. 238
Altingia excelsa Noronha 205
Amanita muscaria Linn. 381
Amaranthus blitum Linn. 355
Amaranthus caudatus Linn. 355
Amaranthus lividus Linn. 355
Amaranthus oleraceus Willd. 355
Amaranthus paniculutus Linn. 355
Amaranthus spinosus Linn. 355
Amaranthus tricolor Linn. var. *tristis* (Willd.) Meharotra, Aswal et Bist 355
Amaranthus tristis Willd. 355
Amomum aromaticum Roxb. 142
Amomum melegueta Rosc. 142
Amomum subulatum Roxb. 142
Amoora rohituka W. & A. 486
Amorphophallus campanulatus Blume ex Decn. 385
Amorphophallus sylvaticus (Roxb.) Kunth. 385
Amyrys kataf Forsk. 253
Andersonia rohituka Roxb. 486
Andrographis paniculata Nees 99
Andropogon citratus DC. 300
Andropogon laniger Desf. 301
Andropogon martini Roxb. 29,300
Andropogon muricatus Retz. 18-200
Andropogon schoenanthus Linn. 300-29
Andropogon schoenanthus Linn. Willd. 301
Andropogon schoenanthus Roxb. 301
Andropogon sorghum Brot. 558
Andropogon squarrosus Hook f. non Linn. 18
Andropogon squarrousus Linn. 198
Anethum foeniculum Linn. 123
Anethum panmorium DC. (Roxb.) 123
Anethum sova Kurz 121
Angelica glauca Edg. 232,234
Anisomelis malabarica (?. R. Br.) 225
Anneslea spinosa Roxb. 375
Anogeissus latifolia Wall. ex. Bedd. 522
Anthemis nobilis Linn. 508
Anthocephalus cadamba Benth. & Hook. f. 452
Anthocephalus cadamba Miq. 452

Anthocephalus chinensis (Lamk.) A. Rich. ex Walp. 452
Anthocephalus indicus A. Rich. 452
Aphanamixis polystachya (Wall.) Parker 486
Apium graveolens Linn. 184
Apium involucratum Roxb. 183
Aplotaxis auriculata DC. 219
Aquilaria agallocha Roxb. 206
Aquilaria ovata Willd. 206
Areca catechu Linn. 214
Argemone mexicana Linn. 91
Argyreia nervosa (Burm. f.) Boj. 343
Argyreia speciosa Sweet 343
Aristolochia indica Linn. 341
Aristolochia serpentaria Linn. 200
Armoracia lepathifolia Gilib. 297
Arsenicum rubrum 245
Artemisia absinthium Linn. 171
Artemisia dubia 171
Artemisia indica Willd. 171
Artemisia maritima Linn. 171
Artemisia myriantha 171
Artemisia officinale Lam. 171
Artemisia pallens Wall. 228
Artemisia pallens Wall. ex DC. 228
Artemisia paniculata Roxb. 171,228
Artemisia vulgaris Linn. 170,171, 508,380
Arundo bambos Linn. 364
Arundo bengalensis Retz. 367
Arundo donax Linn. 367
Arundo karka Linn. et Willd. 366
Asclepias curassavica Linn. 289
Asparagus officinalis Linn. 115
Asparagus racemosus Willd. 115
Asparagus sarmentosus Linn. 116
Astercantha longifolia Nees 358
Auclandia lappa Falkoner 219
Azadirachata indica A. Juss. 12
Bacopa monnieri ((L.) Pennell 338
Baliospermum montanum Muell.- Arg. 84
Baliospermum montanum (Willd.)Muell.- Arg. 84
Balsamea erythrea Angler 253

Balsamea erythrea Erhenbung 253
Balsamodendron berryi Arnott 253
Balsamodendron kataf Kunth. 253
Balsamodendron mukul Hook. ex Stocks 252
Balsamodendron myrrha Nees 226,254
Balsamodendron opobalsamum Kunth. 253
Balsamodendron pubescense Stocks 253
Balsamondendron roxburghii Arn. 253
Bambusa arundinacea Aiton. 364
Bambusa arundinacea Retz. 364
Bambusa arundinacea (Retz.) Roxb. 364
Bambusa arundinacea Willd. 151
Bambusa stricta 364
Bambusa tulda (Roxb.) 365
Bambusa vulgaris Wendle 364
Barleria cristata Linn. 109
Barleria involucrata Nees 109
Barleria prionitis Linn. 109
Barringtonia acutangula (Linn.) Gaertn. 469
Basella alba Linn. 382
Basella rubra Linn. 382
Bassia butyracea Roxb. 407
Bassia latifolia (Roxb.) 407
Bassia longifolia Willd. 408
Bassia malabarica Bedd. 409
Bassia nerrifolia Moon 409
Bauhinia candida Willd. 73
Bauhinia malabarica Roxb. 72
Bauhinia purpurea Willd. 73
Bauhinia racemosa Lam. 72
Bauhinia tomentosa Willd. 73
Bauhinia vahlli W. & A. 6
Benincasa cerifera Savi 68
Benincasa hispida Cogn. 68
Benincasa hispida (Thunb.) Cogn. 68
Berberis aristata DC. 21
Beta cyclea 295
Beta cyclea var. *cyclea* 295
Bezoar 203
Bignonia chelonoides Wall. (Roxb.) 44
Bignonia glauca Dcne. 487

Bignonia indica Willd. (Roxb.) 42
Bignonia suaveolens Roxb. 43
Bignonia undulata Smith. 487
Biophytum sensitivum (Linn.) DC. 345
Blumea aromatica DC. 230
Blumea balsamifera DC. 231
Blumea balsamifera (Linn.) DC. 210
Blumea densiflora DC. 231
Blumea lacera (Burm. f.) DC. 230
Blumea lacera DC. 230
Boehmeria nivea Gaud. 565
Boerhaavia diffusa Linn. 107
*Boerhaavia procumbens (*Roxb.) 107
Boerhaavia repanda Willd. 107
Bombax ceiba Linn. 482
Bombax malabaricum DC. 482
Bombax orientle Spreng. 487
Bombax pentandrum Linn. 487
Borassus flabellifer Linn. 421
Borassus flabelliformis Roxb. 421
Boswellia glabra Roxb. 256
Boswellia serrata Roxb. 256
Boswellia serrata Roxb.ex Coleb. 256
Boswellia thurifera Roxb.ex. Flem. 256
Brassica alba 308
Brassica campestris Linn. *var.* ***dichotoma*** ssp. Roxb. 299
Brassica campestris Linn. var. *dichotomos* Roxb. 308
Brassica campestris Linn. var. ***glauca*** ssp. Roxb. 298
Brassica campestris Linn .var. ***toria*** Duthie & Fuller 298
Brassica juncea (Linn.) Czern. & Coss. 299
Brassica juncea Roxb. 299
Brassica niger Koch 308
Brassica nigra Koch 307
Brassica nigra (Linn.) Koch 306
Bryonia callosa Rottle. 64
Bryonia scabrella Linn. 99
Buchanania lanzan Spreng. 423
Buchanania latifolia Roxb. 423
Butea frondosa Koen. ex Roxb. 518
Butea frondosa Roxb. 518
Butea monosperma (Lam.) Kuntze 518

Butea monosperma (Lam.) Taub. 518
Butea parviflora Roxb. 518
Butea superba Roxb. 520
Caesalpinia bonducella Fleming 459,461
Caesalpinia crista Linn. 458
Caesalpinia digyna Rottl. 456,459
Caesalpinia oliosperma Roxb. 460
Caesalpinia sappan Linn. 194
Caesulia axillaris Willd. 281
Cajanus cajan (Linn.) Millsp. 549
Cajanus indicus Spreng. 549
Cajanus indicus var. *bicolor* 549
Cajanus indicus var. *flavus* 549
Callicarpa macrophylla Vahl 202-547
Calonyction aculeatum House 98
Calophyllum inophyllum Linn. 144-512
Calophyllum longifolium Wall. 512
Calotropis gigantea (Linn.) Dryand 284
Calotropis gigantea (Linn.) R. Br. ex Ait. 284
Calotropis gigantea R. Br. 284
Calotropis procera (Ait.) R. Br. 283
Calotropis procera R. Br. 283
Cannabis indica Lam. (Roxb.) 46
Cannabis sativa Linn. 46
Canscora decussata Roxb. 350
Canscora decussata (Roxb.) J.A. Schult. & J.H. Schult. 349
Canscora decussata R.& Seb. 349
Canscora diffusa R.Br. 350
Capparis aphylla Roth. 448
Capparis decidua Edgew. 448
Capparis decidua (Forsk.) Edgew. 448
Capparis trifoliata Roxb. 473
Cardiospermum halicacabum Linn. 291
Carissa carandas auct. non Linn. 449
Carissa carandas Linn. 449
Carissa carandas var. *hirsuta* 451
Carissa congesta Wight 449,450
Carissa diffusa Roxb. 450
Carissa lanceolata Dalz. 450
Carissa macrophylla Wall. 450
Carissa spinarum A.DC. 450
Carissa spinarum Linn. 450-207
Carissa villosa Roxb. 451
Carpopogon capitatum Roxb. 56
Carthamus oxycantha Bieb. 566

Carthamus tinctorius Linn. 566
Carum bulbocastanum Koch 158
Carum carvi Linn. 158
Carum copticum Benth. & Hook. f. 170
Carum nigrum Royle 154
Carum roxburghianum Benth. & Hook. f. 183
Caryophyllus aromaticus Linn. 215
Caryota urens Linn. 422
Casearia esculenta Roxb. 129
Casearia tomentosa Roxb. 128-129
Cassia absus Linn. 264
Cassia fistula Linn. & Willd. 81-82
Cassia obtusifolia Linn. 277
Cassia occidentalis Linn. 357
Cassia rhombifolia Roxb. 81- 82
Cassia sophera Linn. 357
Cassia tora Linn. & Willd. 277
Cassine glauca (Rottb.) Kuntz. 483
Cedrela toona Roxb. 203
Cedrus deodara Roxb. ex. D. Don 28
Cedrus deodara (Roxb.) Loud. 28
Cedrus libani Barrel var. *deodara* Hook. f. 28
Ceiba pentandra (L.) Gaertn. 482
Ceiba pentandra (Linn.) Gaertn. 486
Celastrus alnifolia Don. 103
Celastrus dependens Wall. 103
Celastrus multiflora Roxb. 103
Celastrus nutans Roxb. 103
Celastrus paniculatus Willd. 102
Celosia argentea Linn. 57
Centella asiatica Linn. 334-336
Centella asiatica (Linn.) Urban 336
Centratherum anthelminticum (Linn.) Kuntz 159
Centratherum anthelminticum (Willd.) Kuntz 159
Cephalandra indica Naud. 76
Cephalanthus pilulifer Lam. 454
Cerbera thevetia Linn. 277
Cetraria islandica (Linn.) Ach. 235
Chalacas paniculata Linn. 220
Chloroxylon swietenia DC. 488
Chrysanthemum coronarium Linn. 507

Chrysanthemum indicum Linn. 07
Cicer arietinum Linn. 553
Cinnamomum camphora F. Nees 209
Cinnamomum camphora (Linn.) Nees & Eberm. 209
Cinnamomum camphora (Linn.) Sieb. 209
Cinnamomum camphora Nees 209
Cinnamomum tamala (Ham.) Nees & Eberm. 146
Cinnamomum tamala Nees & Eberm. 146
Cinnamomum verum J.S. Preisl. 145
Cinnamomum zeylanicum Blume 145
Cissampelos hernandifolia Wall. 26
Cissampelos hexandra Roxb. 26
Cissampelos pareira Linn. 26
Citrullus colocynthis (Linn.) Schrad. 95
Citrullus colocynthis Schrad. 95
Citrus aurantium Linn. 393
Citrus aurantium Linn. ssp. *amara* Eng. 394
Citrus aurantium Linn. & Willd. 392
Citrus aurantium var. *aurantium* proper (in part) 392
Citrus buxifolia Poir. 393
Citrus limetta Risso. 390
Citrus limettioides Tanaka 390
Citrus limon (Linn.) Burm. f. 389
Citrus medica Linn. 396
Citrus medica var. ***limetta*** W. & A. 390
Citrus medica var. ***limonum*** sp. Risso. 389
Citrus medica var. *medica proper.* 396
Citrus reticulata Blanco. 392
Citrus sinensis (Linn.) Osbeck 392
Citrus vulgaris Risso 393
Civet cat 208
Clay 247
Clematis gouriana Roxb. 6
Clematis gouriana Roxb. ex DC. 6
Clematis triloba Linn. f. 6
Cleome felina 92
Cleome gynandra Linn. 185
Cleome icosandra Linn. 185,186
Cleome pentaphylla DC. 186
Cleome viscosa Linn. 185,186,234,334
Clerodendron indicum (L.) Kuntze 24

Clerodendron inerme *(*L.) Gaertn. 40
Clerodendron phlomidis Linn. f. 40
Clerodendron serratum (L.) Moon 24
Clerodendron serratum Spreng. 24
*Clerodendron siphonanthus (*R. Br.) C.B. Clarke 24
Clerodendrum inerme (Linn. f.) Gaertn. 40
Clerodendrum multiflorum (Burm. f.) O.Ktze. 40
Clitoria ternatea Linn. 324
Coccinia grandis (Linn.) Voiget 76
Coccinia indica W. & A. 76
Cocculus cordifolia DC. 2
Cocculus crispus DC. 3
Cocculus palmata DC. 3
Cocculus verrucosus Wall. 3
Coccus lacca 239
Cocos nucifera Linn. 425
Colchicum autamnale Linn. 326
Colchicum luteum Baker 325
Coleus amboinicus Lour. 232
Coleus aromaticus Benth. 232,234
Commelina longifolia Lamk. 310
Commelina siliciflora 311
Commelina silicifolia Roxb. 310
Commiphora africana 253
Commiphora mukul Engl. 252
Commiphora myrrha (Nees) Engl. 226
Commiphora opobalsamum (Linn.) Eng. 253
Commiphora roxburghii Engl. 252
*Commiphora wightii (*Arnott.) Bhandari 252
Communium sinense Rump. 220
Conch 271
Convolvulus arvensis Linn. 115
Convolvulus bilobatus Roxb. 93
Convolvulus hirsutus Willd. 354
Convolvulus microphyllus Sieb. ex Spreng. 351,353
Convolvulus nil Linn. (Roxb.) 98
Convolvulus pescaprea Linn. 93
Convolvulus pluricaulis Choisy 350-353
Copper pyrite 261
Copper sulphate 260
Cordia dichotoma Forst. f. 441

Cordia latifolia Roxb. 441
Cordia myxa Linn. 441
Cordia obliqua Willd. var. *tomentosa* (Willd.) Kazmi 441
Cordia obliqua Willd. var. *wallichi.* 441
Cordia rothii Roem. & Schult. 442
Cordia wallichi G. Don 441
Coriandrum sativum Linn. 156
Corydalis govaniana Wall. 218-219
Coscinium fenestratum 21
Coscinium fenestratum (Gaertn.) Colebr. 196
Crataeva nurvala Ham. 473
Crataeva nurvala Buch.- Ham. 473
Crataeva religiosa Forst. 473
Crinum asiaticum Linn. 380
Crocus sativus Linn. 197
Crossandra axillaris Nees 501
Crossandra infundibuliformis (Linn.) Nees 501
Crossandra undulaefolia Salisb. 501
Crotalaria retusa Linn. 75
Croton axilare Bl. 85
Croton polyandrum Wight. 85
Croton polyandrus Roxb. 84
Croton tiglium Linn. 86
Crozophora plicata A. Juss. 334
Cryptolepis buchanani Roem. & Schult. 60
Cucumis callosus (Rottl.) Cogn. 64
Cucumis melo Linn. ***proper*** 66
Cucumis melo Linn. var. *culta* 65
Cucumis melo Linn. var. *momordica* Duthie & Fuller 67
Cucumis melo var. ***momordica*** Duthie & Fuller 65
Cucumis momordica Roxb. 65
Cucumis psudocolocynthis Royle 64
Cucumis trigonus Roxb. 64
Cucumis trigonus Roxb. var. ***pubescens*** 64,67
Cucurbita pepo Willd. (non Linn.) 68
Cuminum cyminum Linn. 157
Curcuma angustifolia Roxb. 152
Curcuma caesia Roxb. 20
Curcuma longa Linn. (proper) 20
Curcuma zedoaria (Berg.) Rosc. 245
Curcuma zedoaria Rosc. 22, 245

Curcuma zedoaria Roxb. 245
Curcuma zerumbet Roxb. 22
Cyclea peltata Hook. 26
Cydonia oblonga Mill. 400
Cymbopogon jwarankusa (Jones) Schult. 241
Cymbopogon jwarankusa Schult. 240
Cymbopogon martini Stapf 29
Cymbopogon schoenanthus (Linn.) Spreng. 299
Cymbopogon schoenanthus (L.) Spreng. 28
Cynodon dactylon (L.) Pers. 368
Cyperus jeminious 16
Cyperus juncifolius Klein. 218
Cyperus pertenuis Roxb. 16
Cyperus rotundus Linn. 16
Cyperus scariosus Linn. 16
Cyperus stoloniferus Retz. 218
Daemia extensa R. Br. 31
Dalbergia arborea Willd. 460
Dalbergia emarginata Roxb. 474
Dalbergia latifolia Roxb. 474
Dalbergia latifolia Willd. 474
Dalbergia sissoo Roxb. 474
Dalbergia sissoo Roxb. ex DC. 474
Datura fastuosa Linn. 278
Datura fastuosa Linn. var. ***alba*** C.B. Clarke 278
Datura fastuosa Willd.
Datura metal Linn. 278
Datura metal Mukerji 278
Datura rubra Rumph. 278
Datura stramonium Linn. 278
Daucus carota Linn.var. ***sativa*** DC. 314
Delphinium semibarbatum Blenert ex Boiss. 97
Delphinium zalil Aitch. & Hemsl. 97
Dendrobium macraei Lindle 51-332
Dendrocalamus strictus Nees 365
Derris indica (Lam.) Bennet. 456
Desmodium gangeticumDC. 32
Desmodium gangeticum (Linn.) DC. 32
Desmodium laxiflorum DC. 32
Desmodium triquetrum DC. 34
Desmostachya bipinnata (Linn.) Stapf 362

Desmostachya bipinnata Stapf 362
Desmotrichum fimbriatum Blume 51
Dillenia indica **Linn.** 401
Dillenia pentagyna Roxb. 401
Dioscorea bulbifera Linn. 327
Dioscorea crispata Roxb. 329
Dioscorea jacquemontii Hook f. 328
Dioscorea pentaphylla Linn. 327
Dioscorea pulchella Roxb. 329
Dioscorea sativa. 327
Dioscorea sativa Thunb., non Linn. 329
Dioscorea triphylla Linn. 328
Dioscorea versicolor Buch.- Ham. ex Wall. 329
Diospyros embryopteris Pers. 402,404
Diospyros exculpta Buch.- Ham. 402
Diospyros glutinefera Roxb. 402
Diospyros glutinosa Koen. 402
Diospyros malabarica Desr. 402
Diospyros malabarica (Desr.) Kostel. 402
Diospyros melanoxylon Roxb. 402
Diospyros montana Roxb. 403
Diospyros peregrina Gurke 402,404
Diospyros tomentosa Roxb. 402,404
Dipterocarpus alatus Roxb. 478
Dipterocarpus turbinatus Gaertn. 477
Dolichos biflorus auct. non Linn. 557
Dolichos biflorus Linn. 557
Dolichos lablab Linn. 562
Dolichos lablab var. *lignosus* Prain 561
Dolichos lablab var. *typicus* Prain 561
Dolichos uniflorus Lamk. 557
Donax 'arundinaceus Beauv. 367
Doodia picta Roxb. 34
Dregia viridiflora Benth. ex. Hook f. 51
Dryobalanops aromatica Gaertn. f. 209
Dryobalanops camphora Colebr. 210
Echinocloa cruss-galli (Linn.) Beauv. var. *frumentacea* Wight 545
Echinocloa frumentacea Link 545
Echites frutescens Roxb. 59
Eclipta alba Hassk. 281
*Eclipta alba (*Linn.) Hassk. 281

Eclipta erecta 281
Eclipta prostrata Linn. 281
Elaeodendron glaucum Pers. 483
Elaeodendron paniculatum W. A. 484
Elettaria cardamomum (Linn.) Maton 141
Elettaria cardamomum Maton 141
Embelia ribes Burm. 130
Embelia robusta C. B.C. 131
Embelia tsjeriam - cottam A.DC. 131
Emblica officinalis Gaertn. 79
Ephedra gerardiana Wall. 381
Ephedra major Host 381
Ephedra nebrodensis Tineo 381
Ephedra vulgaris Hook. f. non A. Rich. 381
Eragrostis cynosuroides Beauv. 362
Erianthus munja Jesw. 363
Eriodendron anfractuosum DC. 482-486
Ervatamia coronaria Stapf 222
Ervum lens Linn. 550
Erythrina indica Lam. 520
Erythrina species 83
Eugenia aromatica Kuntz., Thunb. 215
Eugenia cerasoides Roxb. 433
Eugenia heyneana Wall. 434
Eugenia jambolana Lam. 433,435
Eugenia operculata Roxb. 433,435
Eugenia operculata var. *obovata* Kurz 435
Euphorbia antiquorum Linn. 89
Euphorbia ligularia Roxb. 88
Euphorbia neriifolia Linn. 88
Euphorbia nivulia Buch.- Ham. 88
Euphorbia thomsoniana Boiss. 90
Euphorbia tirucalli Linn. 89
Eurale ferox Salisb. 375
Eurale indica Planch. 375
Evolvulus alsinoides Linn. 352
Evolvulus alsinoides (Linn.) Linn. 352
Evolvulus angustifolius Roxb. 354
Evolvulus erecta 353
Evolvulus hirsutus Lam. 354
Evolvulus hirsutus Lam. et. Willd. 352

Extractum fellis bovini 203
Extractum berberis 265
Fagonia arabica Linn. 8
Fagonia cretica Linn. 8
Feronia elephantum Correa 188
Feronia limonia (Linn.) Swingle 188
Ferrous sulphate 251
Ferula assafoetida Boiss. 137
Ferula assafoetida Linn. 137
Ferula foetida Regel 137
Ferula narthex Boiss. 137
Ficus arnottiana Miq. 430
Ficus benghalensis Linn. 426
Ficus benjamina Willd. (non Linn.) 429
Ficus cunia Ham. ex Roxb. 438
Ficus glomerata Roxb. 436
Ficus gulereea Roxb. 437
Ficus heterophylla Linn. 437
Ficus heterophylla Linn var. *aquatiloba* Mic 436
Ficus heterophylla Linn. var. ***repens*** Willd. 436
Ficus heterophylla *Linn* var. ***scabrella*** Roxb. 436
Ficus hispida Linn. f. 438
Ficus indica Linn. 427
Ficus indicus Linn. 426
Ficus infectoria Roxb. 430
Ficus infectoria Willd. 429
Ficus lacor Buch.- Ham. 430
Ficus microcarpa Linn. f. 429
Ficus oppositifolia (Roxb.) Corum. 438
Ficus oppositifolia Willd. 437
Ficus racemosa Linn. 436
Ficus racemosa Wall. (non Roxb.) 437
Ficus religiosa Linn. 429
Ficus retusa Linn. 429
Ficus rumphii Blume 430
Ficus talboti G. King 430
Ficus tsiela 429
Ficus tsiela Roxb. 431
Ficus tsjakela Burm.f. 430
Ficus virens Aiton. 429
Flacourtia catafracta Roxb. 148

Flacourtia catafracta (Willd.) Roxb. 80
Flacourtia indica (Burm. f.) Merr. 405
Flacourtia indica Merr. 405
Flacourtia jangomas (Lour.) Raeusch. 80-148
Flacourtia ramontchi L' Herit. 405,406
Flacourtia sapida Roxb. 406
Foeniculum capillaceum Gilib. 123
Foeniculum vulgare Mill. 124
Fumaria officinalis Linn. 17
Fumaria parviflora Linn. 17
Gaertnera pangati Retz. 310
Galedupa arborea Roxb. 460
Galedupa indica Lam. 460
Galena 261
Gall stone 203
Garcinia indica Chois. 173
Garcinia indica (Dupetit -Thouras) Chois. 173
Garcinia pedunculata Roxb. 179
Garcinia purpurea Roxb. 173
Gardenia floribunda Roxb. 62
Gardenia gummifera Linn f. 139
Gardenia lucida Roxb. 139
Gardenia resinifera Roth. 139
Gentiana diffusa Vahl 351
Gentiana kurroo Royle 97
Gisekia pharnaceoides Linn. 236
Gloriosa superba Linn. 280
Glycine debilis Willd. 48
Glycine labialis Linn. 48
Glycyrrhiza glabra Linn. 52
Gmelina arborea Linn. 43
Gmelina arborea Roxb. 43
Grewia asiatica Linn. 416
Grewia populifolia Vahl 112
Grewia subinaequalis DC. 416
Guilandiana moringa Linn. 296
Gymnema aurantiacum Wall. ex Hook f. 50
Gymnema auriculatum Wall. ex Hook f. 50
Gymnema sylvestre R. Br. 31-289
Gymnosporia spinosa (Forsk.) Fiori 405-06
Gynandropsis gynandra (Linn.) Briquet 185

Gynandropsis pentaphylla DC. 185
Habenaria commelinifolia Wall. ex Lindl. 326
Habenaria intermedia D. Don 53
Harmonitis cordifolia 34
Hedychium coronarium Linn. 152
Hedychium spicatum Ham. 22
Hedychium spicatum Ham. ex Smith 22-245-152
Hedysarum alatum Roxb. 34
Hedysarum alhagi Linn. 8
Hedysarum gangeticum Linn. 32
Hedysarum gangeticum Willd. 32
Hedysarum tuberosum Roxb. 54
Helianthus annuus Linn. 187,334
Helicteres isora **Linn. & Willd.** 75
Helix aspera 223
Hellebore niger Linn. 15
Hemidesmus indicus (Linn.) R. Br. 60
Hemidesmus indicus R. Br. 60
Hemprichia erythrea Erhenbung 253
Hibiscus cannabinus Linn. 249
Hiptage benghalensis Kurz 509
Hiptage benghalensis (Linn.) Kurz 510
Hiptage madablota Gaertn. 510
Holarrhena antidysenterica (Roth.) DC. 132
Holarrhena antidysenterica Wall. 132
Holoptelea integrifolia Planch. 456
Holoptelea integrifolia (Roxb.) Planch. 456
Homonoia riparia Lour. 128
Hopea eglandulsoa Roxb. 255
Hopea odorata 479
Hopea odorata Roxb. 255
Hordeum sativum Pers. 539
Hordeum vulgare Linn. 539
Hoya viridiflora R.Br. 51
Hycinthoides alestris 6
Hydrocotyle asiatica Willd. 338
Hydrocotyle asiatica Willd. (Roxb.) 334
Hydrocotyle rotundifolia Roxb. 333
Hydrocotyle sibthorpioides Lam. 333
Hygrophila spinosa T. Anders. 358
Hygroryza aristata Nees 544

Hygroryza aristata(Retz.) Nees ex Wight & Arn. 544
Hyoscyamus niger Linn. 172
Hyoscyamus reticulatus Linn. 172
Hyperanthera concanensis (Vah.) Nimmo 297
Hyptis suaveolens Poit. 241
Ichnocarpus frutescens (Linn.) R. Br. 59
Ichnocarpus frutescens R. Br. 59
Imperata arundinacea Cyrill. 362
Imperata cylindrica Beauv. 362
Indigofera oblongifolia Forsk. 88
Indigofera paucifolia Del. 88
Inula helenium Linn. 104
Inula racemosa 23-105
Inula racemosa Hook. f. 105
Ipomoea biloba Forsk. 93
Ipomoea biloba Forsk. 343
Ipomoea bona- nox Boj. var. *grandiflora* 98
Ipomoea bonanox (Jack.) (Roxb.fl.) 98
Ipomoea bona-nox Linn. 98
Ipomoea caerulea Koen. 98
Ipomoea caerulea Roxb. 98
Ipomoea digitata auct. non Linn.. 55
Ipomoea digitata Linn. 55
Ipomoea grandiflora Roxb. 98
Ipomoea hederacea Jacq. 98
Ipomoea nil (Linn.) Roth. 98
Ipomoea obscura Ker- Gaul. 118
Ipomoea paniculata (Linn.) R. Br. 55
Ipomoea paniculata R. Br. 55
Ipomoea pes-caprea (Linn.) Sweet 93
Ipomoea pes-caprea Sweet 93,343
Ipomoea petaloidea Chois. 344
Ipomoea vitifolia Sweet 339
Iris decora Wall. 127
Iris germanica Linn. 23,127
Iris germanica Linn. var. *florentina* 25
Iris kumaonensis Wall. 127
Iris kumaonensis Wall. ex G. Don 127
Iris nepalensis D. Don 127
Iris soongariea Schrenk. 127
Iris versicolor Linn. 127

Jasminum angustifolium Vahl 493
Jasminum arborescens Roxb. 495,499
Jasminum arborescens Wooder. 499
Jasminum aureum Don 497
Jasminum auriculatum Linn. 505
Jasminum auriculutum Vahl 505
Jasminum bignoniaceum Wall. 505
Jasminum chrysanthemum Roxb. 505
Jasminum grandiflorum Linn. 496
Jasminum humile Linn. 505
Jasminum latifolium Grah. 499
Jasminum malabaricum Wight 499
Jasminum multiflorum Andr. 506
Jasminum multiflorum (Burm. f.) Andr. 506
Jasminum pubescens Linn. Willd. 506
Jasminum pubescens Watt (not of Willd.) 493
Jasminum pubescens Willd. 506
Jasminum roxburghianum Wall. 499
Jasminum sambac Ait. 493
Jasminum sambac (Linn.) Ait. 493-494
Jasminum undulatum Willd. 493
Jasminum zambac Roxb. 493
Jasminum zambac Willd. 495
Jateorhiza calumba Miers 3
Jateorhiza palmata Miers 3
Jatropha curcus Linn. 87
Jatropha glandulifera Roxb. 87
Jatropha montana 85
Jatropha multifida Linn. 85
Jonesia asoka Roxb. 516
Juglans regia Linn. 415
Juglans regia var. *kumaonica* DC. 415
Juniperus communis Linn. 128
Juniperus communis Linn. var. **saxatilils** Pallas 128
Justicia procumbens Linn. 17
Kaempferia galanga Linn. 22, 245
Lablab purpureus (Linn.) Sweet 561
Lagenaria siceraria (Molina) Standle. 63
Lagenaria siceraria Standle. 63
Lagenaria vulgaris Seringe 63
Land snail 223

Lannea coromandelica (Houtt.) Merr. 272
Lannea grandis(Dennst.) Engl. 272
Lathyrus sativus Linn. 560
Laurus cassia Roxb. 146
Leea aequata Roxb. 288
Leea hirta Roxb. 288
Lens culinaris Medik. (Medic.) 550
Lens esculenta Moench 550
Leptadenia reticulata Benth. 289
Leptadenia reticulata (Retz.) W. & Arn. 50
Leptadenia reticulata W. & A. 50
Lettsomia atropurpuria 93
Lettsomia nervosa Roxb. 343
Ligusticum ajoun Roxb. 170
Linum usitatissimum Linn. 565
Lippia nodiflora Mich. 311
Lippia nodiflora Rich. 311
Liqidamber orientalis Miller 204
Loranthus bicolor Roxb. var. *amplexifolia* Thunb. 332
Loranthus bicolor Roxb. var. *falcata* Kurz 332
Loranthus bicolor Roxb. var. *pubescens* 332
Loranthus longiflorus Desr. 332
*Luffa acutangula (*Linn.) Roxb. var. *amara* Clarke 71
Luffa acutangula Roxb. 71
Luffa acutangula Roxb. *var* ***amara*** Clarke 71
Luffa cylindrica (L.) M. Roem. 70
Luffa echinata Roxb. 64
Luffa pentandra Roxb. 70
Maba nigrescens Dalz. 488
Madhuca indica J.F. Gmel. 407
Madhuca latifolia (Roxb.) Macbride 407
Madhuca longifolia (Koen.) Macbride 407-408
Madhuca longifolia (L) Macbride 408
Maerua arenaria Hook. f. 5,6
Maerua oblongifolia (Forsk.) A. Rich. 5
Maerua ovalifolia Canw. 5
Majorana hortensis Moench. 302
Mallotus philippinensis (Lam.) Muel.- Arg. 257
Mallotus philippinensis Muel. - Arg. 257
Malus sylvestris Mill. 400
Malva rotundifolia Linn. 334

Mammea suriga (Ham. ex Roxb.) Kosterm. 144-512
Mangifera domestica Gaertn. 387
Mangifera indica Linn. 386
Mangifera sylvatica Roxb. 388
Mangle wurzil 295
Manilkara hexandra (Roxb.) Dubard. 439
Manilkara kauki (Linn.) Dub. 440
Maranta arundinacea Linn. 152
Marcilecia budrifolia 226
Marsdenia volubilis T. Cooke 50,51
Marsilea minuta Linn. 57
Marsilea quadrifolia Linn. 57
Matricaria bauna 507
Matricaria chamomilla Linn. 508
Medicago sativa Linn. 563
Melia azedarach Linn. 12
Melia composita Willd. 13
Melia dubia Cav.. 13
Melilotus alba Lam. 225
Melilotus altisima Thuill. not of Wall. 224
Melilotus hamosa Link. 225
Melilotus indica (Linn.) All. 225-562
Melilotus macrorhiza Pers. 225
Melilotus minima Roth. 225
Meliotus officinalis Billad. 226
Melilotus officinalis Lam. 224
Melilotus officinalis (Linn.) Medik. 224
Melilotus officinalis Willd. 225
Melilotus parviflora Desf. 225-563
Menispermum calumba Roxb. 3
Menispermum crispum Linn. 3
Menispermum fenastratum Gaertn. 4
Menispermum tomentosum Roxb. 3
Menispermum verrucosum Roxb. 3
Merremia turpethum (Linn.) Shah & Bhatt 94
Merremia vitifolia (Burm. f.) Hallier 339
Merremia vitifolia Hallier 339
Mesua coromondeliana Roxb. 143
Mesua ferrea Linn. 143
Metroxylon sagu Rottb. 153
Meyna laxiflora Robyns 244

Michelia champaca Linn. 500
Michelia excelsa Blume 500
Michelia nilagirica Zenk. 500
Microstylis musifera Ridley 45
Microstylis wallichi Lindle. 45
Mimosa catechu Linn. 10
Mimosa farnesiana Linn. 489
Mimosa ferruginea Roxb. 10
Mimosa mutabilis 477
Mimosa pudica Linn. 345
Mimosa rubricaulis 477
Mimosa sirissa Ham. 463
Mimosa suma Roxb. 11,443
Mimusops elengi Linn. 511
Mimusops hexandra Roxb. 439
Mimusops indica A.DC. 440
Mimusops kauki Linn. 440
Mimusops kauki Wall. 440
Mimusops manilkara Don 440
Mitragyna parvifolia Korth. 452
Mitragyna parvifolia (Roxb.) Korth. 452
Mogorium sambuc Lamk. 493
Momordica dioica Roxb. 69
Momordica dioica Roxb.ex Willd. 69
Momordica monadelpha Roxb. 76
Moniera cuneifolia Mich. 338
Moringa concanensis Nimmo 296
Moringa oleifera Lam. 296
Moringa oleifera Linn. 297
Moringa polygona DC. 296
Moringa pterygosperma Gaertn. 297
Morus acidosa Griff. 417
Morus alba var. *cuspidata* Bureau 417
Morus alba var. *indica* Bureau 417
Morus australis Poir. 417
Morus cuspidata Wall. 417
Morus indica Griff. 418
Morus indica Linn. 417
Morus nigra Linn. 418
Morus parvifolia Royle 417
*Mucuna pruriens (*Linn.) DC. 55

Mucuna prurita Hook. 55
Mukia scabrella Arn. 99
Mungorium sambac Lam. 495
Murraya exotica Linn. 220, 221
Murraya paniculata (L.) Jack. 220, 221
Murraya sumatrana Roxb. 220
Musa paradisiaca Linn. 318
Musa paradisiaca Linn. var. ***sapientum*** Kuntz. 316
Musa sapientum Linn. 316
Musk 208
Myrica malabarica 27
Myrica nagi Thunb. 27
Myrica sapida Wall. 27
Myristica fragrans Houtt. 211
Myristica malabarica Lam. 212
Myristica moschata (Willd.) Roxb. 212
Myristica officinalis Linn. 212
Nardostachys grandiflora DC. 217
Nardostachys jatamansi DC. 217
Nardus indicus 218
Nauclea cadamba Roxb. 452
Nauclea cordifolia Roxb. 455
Nauclea parvifolia Pers. 454
Nauclea parvifolia Willd. 452
Neerija paniculata Roxb. 484
Nelumbium speciosum Willd. 370-375
Nelumbo nucifera Gaertn. 370
Neptunea oleracea Lour. 347
Nerium coccineum Roxb. 276
Nerium indicum Mill. 275
Nerium odorum Soland. 275
Nerium oleander Linn. 277
Nerium pisidium Roxb. 276
Nigella indica Roxb. 154
Nigella sativa Linn. 154
Nymphaea cynea Roxb. 372
Nymphaea lotus Linn. 373
Nymphaea lotus Willd. 372
Nymphaea nouchali Burm. f. 371
Nymphaea parviflora 372
Nymphaea rubra Roxb. 372

Nymphaea stellata Willd. 371
Nymphaea versicolor Roxb. 372
Nymphaea rubra Roxb. ex Salisb. 373
Ochre 262
Ochrocarpus longifolius Benth. & Hook. f. 144-512
Ocimum basilicum Linn. 186,303
Ocimum gratissimum Linn. 305
Ocimum sanctum Linn. 508
Ocimum sanctum Linn. 302
Ocimum sanctum Willd. 302
Odina wodier Roxb. 272
Olea fragrans Linn. 285
Olea fragrans Thunb. 285
Onosma echioides (Linn.) 216
Onosma hispidum Wall. ex . Don 216
Operculina turpethum Silva Manso 94
Ophiorrhiza mungos Linn. 342
Opopanax bdellium 253
Origanum majorana Linn. 302
Oroxylum indicum (Linn.) Vent. 42
Oroxylum indicum Vent. 42
Orthosiphon pallidus Royle 304
Oryza abuensis 537
Oryza rufipogon Griff. 537
Oryza sativa Linn. 535
Os sepiae 263
Osmanthus acuminata Wall. 285
Osmanthus fragrans Lour. 284
Ougeinia dalbergioides Benth. 520
Oxalis corniculata Linn. 399
Paederia foetida Linn. 115
Paederia foetida Willd. 115
Paederia scandens (Lour.) Merr. 115
Pandanus fasicularis Lam. 521
Pandanus odoratissimus Roxb. 521
Pandanus odoratissimus (Willd.) Roxb. 521
Pandanus tectorius Soland. ex. Park. 521
Panicum colonum Linn. 546
Panicum crusgalli Linn. 546
Panicum dactylon Linn. 368
Panicum frumentaceum Roxb. 545

Panicum miliaceum Linn. 547
Panicum paludosum Roxb. 198
Papaver somniferum Linn. 568
Parmelia perlata Huds. Ach. 236
Parmelia perforata 236
Paspalum commersonii Lam. 543
Paspalum scrobiculatum Linn. 543
Paspalum scrobiculatum var. *commersonii* Stapf 543
Paspalum scrobiculatum var. *frumentaceum* Stapf 543
Patrinia jatamansi Don. 217
Pavetta indica Linn. 83-521
Pavonia odorata Linn. 200
Pedalium murex Linn. 38
Pentaptera arjuna Roxb. 465
Pentaptera tomentosa Roxb. 465
Pentatropis cynanchoides R. Br. 289
Pentatropis microphylla W. & A. 289
Pergularia daemia (Forsk.) Chiov. 31
Pergularia extensa N.E. Br. 31
Peristrophe bicalyculata Nees 288
Peristrophe bicalyculata (Retz.) Nees 288
Peucedanum graveolens Linn. 121
Peucedanum graveolens (Linn.) Hiern. 121
Peucedanum graveolens Linn.(in part.) 121
Pharbitis choisy 98
Phaseolus aconitifolius Jacq. 548
Phaseolus mungo Linn. 552
Phaseolus mungo Linn. non Roxb. & auct. 552
Phaseolus radiatus Linn. 541
Phaseolus radiatus Roxb. non Linn. 552
Phaseolus trilobus Ait. 49
Phaseolus trilobus Willd. 49
Phoenix acualis Buch. - Ham. 413
Phoenix dactylifera Linn. 412
Phoenix farinifera Roxb. 419
Phoenix farinifera Willd. 420
Phoenix pusilla Gaertn. 419,420
Phoenix sylvestris (Linn.) Roxb. 411
Phoenix sylvesris Roxb. 411
Phragmites karka Trim. 366
Phragmites karka Trim. ex Steud. 366
Phragmites maxmia Blatter & Mc Cann 367

Phragmites roxburghii Kunth. 366
Phyla nodiflora (Linn.) Greene 311
Phyllanthus fraternus Webster 240
Phyllanthus niruri auct. (non Linn). 240
Phyllanthus niruri Linn. 240
Phyllanthus urinaria Linn. 241
Physalis flexuosa Linn. 106
Picrorhiza kurroa Royle ex Benth. 15
Pimpinella anisum Linn. 124
Pimpinella involucratum W. & A. 183
Pinus damar 251
Pinus longifolia Roxb. 237
Pinus roxburghii Sargent 237
Pinus webbiana Wall. 147
Piper betle Linn. 272
Piper chaba W. Hunter 162
Piper cubeba Linn. 213
Piper glabrum Roxb. 162
Piper longum Linn. 160
Piper longum Rumph. 162
Piper nigrum Linn. 168
Piper officinarum DC. 163
Piper retrofractum 161
Piper retrofractum Vahl 162
Pistacia integerrima Stew.ex. Brandis 30
Pisum arvense Linn. 555
Pisum sativum Linn. 555
Pladera decussata Roxb. 349-350
Pladera sessiliflora Roxb. 350
Pladera virgata Roxb. 350
Plasmonium margaratiferum (Roxb.) Schott. 384
Plectranthus aromaticus Roxb. 232,234
Pluchea lanceolata Oliver 105
Plumbago auriculata Lam. 165
Plumbago capensis Thunb. 165
Plumbago coccinia Boiss. 165
Plumbago indica Linn. 165
Plumbago rosea Linn. 165
Plumbago zeylanica Linn. 165
Plumbi oxidum rubrum 246
Plumeria acutifolia Poir. 145-507

Plumeria rubra Linn. forma *acuminata* Sant, Irani & Shah. 145
Poa cynosuroides (Linn.) Willd. 362
Poa cynosuroides Retz. 362
Pogostemon parviflorus Benth. 302
Polanisia felina 92
Polanisia icosandra (Linn.) W. & A. 185
Polyalthia longifolia Benth. & Hook f. 517
Polyalthia longifolia (Sonn.) Thw. 517
Polygonatum cirrhifolium Royle 46
Polygonatum verticillatum All. 46
Pongamia glabra Vent. 456
Pongamia pinnata Merr. 456
Premna coriacea Clarke 41
Premna corymbosa Rottle. 40
Premna herbacea Roxb. 25
Premna integrifolia Linn. 40
Premna integrifolia Linn. 25
Premna spinosa Roxb. 40
Prosopis cineraria Druce. 443
Prosopis spicigera Linn. & Willd. 443
Prunus armeniaca Linn. 400
Prunus avium Linn. 400
Prunus cerasoides D. Don 242
Prunus cerasus Linn. 236-400
Prunus domestica Linn. 400
Prunus domestica L. var. ***communis*** Huds. 400
Prunus gilab. 236
Prunus mahaleb Linn. 201
Prunus persica Batsch. 400
Prunus puddum Roxb. ex Brandis non Miq. 242
Prunus puddum Roxb. ex Wall. 242
Psidium guajava Linn. 420
Psoralea corylifolia Linn. 61
Psoralea plicata Del. 61
Pterocarpus marsupium Roxb. 479
Pterocarpus santalinus Linn. f. 193
Pterospermum acerifolium Linn. 83
Ptychotis ajowan DC. 170
Ptychotis roxburghiana DC. 183
Pueraria tuberosa DC. 54
Pueraria tuberosa Roxb. ex Willd. 54

Punica granatum Linn. 155
Pupalia lappacea Moq. 380
Pyrus communis Linn. 400
Pyrus malus Linn. 400
Randia brandisi Gamble 62
Randia dumetorum Linn. 62
Ranunculus indicus Roxb. 309
Ranunculus sceleratus Linn. 309
Raphanus sativus Linn. 293
Rauwolfia serpentina 340
Rauvolfia serpentina Benth. ex Kurz 341
Realgar 245
Red oxide of Mercury. 246
Rhamnus jujuba Linn. 445
Rhamnus wightii W. & A. 488
Rheum emodi Wall. 180
Rheum emodi Wall. ex Meissn. 180
Rhus chinensis Mill. 175
Rhus coriaria Linn. 175
Rhus integerrima Wall. 30
Rhus javanica Linn. 175
Rhus parviflora Roxb. 173
Rhus parviflora Roxb. ex DC. 173
Rhus semialata Murray 175
Ricinus communis Linn. 117
Rondeletia exserta Roxb. 515
Rondeletia sinerea Wall. 515
Rosa brunonii Lindle 503
Rosa centifolia Linn. 502-509
Rosa damascena Mill. 509
Rosa gallica Linn. 508-509
Rosa gigantea Collet 502
Rosa indica Hook. f. in part, non Linn. 503-509
Rosa involucrata Roxb. 504
Rosa macrophylla Lindl. 509
Rosa moschata Herrm. 503
Rosa moschata Mill. 503
Rosa recurva Roxb. (C.B.C.) 503
Roscoea alpina Royle 47
Roscoea procera Wall . 47
Rubia cordifolia Linn. 7

Ruellia infundibuliformis Roxb. var. *aboli* 501
Ruellia longifolia Roxb. 358
Rumex acitosa Linn. 180
Rumex crispus Linn. 180
Rumex vesicarius Linn. 180
Rungia repens Nees 17
Saccharum arundinaceum Retz. 360
Saccharum bengalense Retz. 360
Saccharum ciliare Anders. 360
Saccharum cylindrica Linn. 362
Saccharum cylindricum Lam. 359
Saccharum exaltum Roxb. 363
Saccharum munja Roxb. 360
Saccharum officinarum Linn. 358
Saccharum sara Roxb. 360, 363
Saccharum semidecumbens Roxb. 359
Saccharum spontaneum Linn. 359
Saccolabium papillosum Lindl. 332
Salix alba Linn. 470
Salix caprea Linn. 468
Salix tetrasperma Roxb. 179-468
*Salix tetrasperma*Willd. 179
Salix tetrasperma Willd. (Roxb.) 177
Salmalia malabarica Schott. & Engl. 481
Salvadora oleoides Decne 410
Salvadora persica Linn. 410,411
Salvadora persica Linn.var. *wightiana* (Planch. ex Thw.) Verdc. 410
Sansevieria zeylanica Willd. 5
Santalum album Linn. 191
Santalum myrtifolium Roxb. 192
Santalum verum Linn. 191
Saraca asoca (Roxb.) De Wilde 516
Saraca indica auct., non Linn. 516
Saraca indica Linn. 516
Sarcostemma brevistigma W. & A.. 382
Saussurea lappa C. B. Clarke 219
Saussurea lappa (Decne.) Sch. Bip. 219
Saxifraga ligulata Wall. 58
Schleichera oleosa (Lour.) Merr. 387
Schleichera oleosa (Lour.) Oken 387
Schleichera trijuga Willd. 387

Schrebera swietenioides Roxb. 483
Schweinfurthia papilionacea (Burm. f.) Boiss 14
Schweinfurthia sphaerocarpa A. Br. 14
Scindapsus officinalis (Roxb.) Schott 164
Scindapsus offcinalis Schott 164
Selinum tenuifolium Wall. 229
Selinum vaginatum C. B. Clarke 229
Semecarpus anacardium Linn. 260
Semecarpus anacardium Linn.f. 260
Sena tora Roxb. 277
Serpent stone 203
Serratula anthelmintica Roxb. 159
Sesamum indicum Linn. 569
Sesbania aculeata Pers. 379
Sesbania aculeata Pers. var. *cannabina* Baker 379
Sesbania aegyptiaca Pers. 379
Sesbania cannabina (Retz.) Pers. 379
Sesbania sesban Merill. 379
Setaria italica Beauv. 547
Shorea robusta Gaertn. 250,477
Shorea robusta Gaertn.f. 250
Sida alba Linn. 113
Sida asiatica Linn. 111
*Sida asiatica*Willd. 111
Sida cordifolia Linn. 110
Sida humilis Linn. 379
Sida indica Linn. 111
Sida populifolia Lam. 111
Sida spinosa Linn. 113
Sinapis cuneifolia Roxb. 299
Sinapis dichotoma Roxb. 299
Sinapis dischotomos Roxb. 308
Sinapis glauca Roxb. 298
Sinapis glauca Royle. 298
Sinapis juncea Linn. 299
Sinapis ramosa Roxb. 299
Sinapis rugosa Roxb. 299
Sirium myrtifolium Roxb. 192
Solanum dulcamara Linn. 286
Solanum hirsutum Roxb. 36
Solanum indicum Linn. 35

Solanum melongena Linn. 37
Solanum nigrum Linn. 286
Solanum surattense Burm. f. 36
Solanum xanthocarpum Schrad. & Wendle. 36
Sorghum bicolor (Linn.) Moench
Sorghum bicolor (Linn.) Pers. 558
Sorghum vulgare (Linn.) Pers. 558
Soymida febrifuga A. Juss. 331
Spatholobus roxburghii Benth. 519
Sphaeranthus africanus Linn. 58
Sphaeranthus hirtus Willd. 59
Sphaeranthus indicus Linn. 59,452
Sphaeranthus mollis Roxb. 59
Sphenoclea pongatium Lam. 310
Sphenoclea zeylanica Gaertn. 310
Sphenoclea zeylanica Willd. 310
Spondias amara Lamk. 389
Spondias mangifera Willd. 389
Spondias pinnata (Linn. f.) Kurz 389
Stephania glabra Miers. 26
Stephania hernandifolia Walp. 26
Stephegyne parvifolia Korth. 452,454
Stereospermum chelonoides (Willd.) Roxb. 43
Stereospermum personatum (Hassk.) Chatterjee 44
Stereospermum suaveolens DC. Proder. 43
Stereospermum tetragonum DC. 44
Stramonia indica 278
Strychnos nux-vomica Linn. 403
Strychnos potatorum Linn. f. 267
Styrax officinalis Linn. 204
Sulphur 248
Swertia chirata Buch. - Ham. 14
Swietenia febrifuga Willd. 331
Symplocos beddomei C.B. Clarke 269
Symplocos chinensis (Lour.) Druce 270
Symplocos crataegoides Buch.- Ham. 270
Symplocos hamiltonia Wall. 268
Symplocos nervosa A.DC. 268,269
Symplocos paniculata Wall. 270
Symplocos racemosa Roxb. 268,269
Symplocos stocksii 268

Synantherias sylvatica Schott 384
Syzygium aromaticum (Linn.) Merr. & L. M. Perry 215
Syzygium aromaticum Merr. & Perry 215
Syzygium cumini (Linn.) Skeels 433
Syzygium heyneana Wall. 434
Syzygium heyneanum Wall. ex Gamble 434
Syzygium jambolanum DC. 433
Syzygium operculatum (Roxb.) Gamble 433
Syzygium zeylanica Wight 434,435
Syzygium zeylanicum (Linn.) DC. 434
Tacca aspera Roxb. 327
Tacca integrifolia Ker-Gawl. 327
Tacca leontopetaloides (Linn.) O. Kuntz. 327
Tacca pinnatifida Willd. ex Forst. 327
Tacca pinnatifolia Gaertn. 328
Tacca pinnatifolia Roxb. 327
Tamarindus indica Linn. 398
Taverniera nummularia Baker 53
Taverniera nummularia (Roth.) Arn. 53
Taxus baccata auct. (non Linn.) 147
Taxus baccata Linn. 147
Taxus baccata Linn. 231
Taxus wallichiana Zucc. 147
Tecoma glabra DC. 487
Tecoma undulata (G.Don) Seem. 487
Tecomella undulata (G. Don) Seem. 485
Tecomella undulata Seem. 488
Tecomella undulata (Sm.) Seem. 485
Tectona grandis Linn. 522
Teramnus labialis (Linn. f.) Spreng. 48
Teramnus labialis Spreng. 48
Terminalia angustifolia Willd. 78
Terminalia arjuna Bedd. 465
Terminalia arjuna (Roxb.) Wight & Arn. 465
Terminalia bellirica (Gaertn.) Roxb. 78
Terminalia bellirica Roxb. 78
Terminalia chebula (Gaertn.) Retz. 77
Terminalia chebula Retz. & Willd. 77
Terminalia citrina Roxb. var. ***malayana*** Kurz 77
Terminalia gangetica Roxb. 78
Terminalia glabra var. *tomentosa* Dalz. & Gibs. 465

Terminalia moluccana (Willd.) Roxb. 78
Terminalia tomentosa W. & A. 465
Thalictrum foliolosum DC. 97
Thesepsia populnea Soland. ex Correa 429
Thevetia nerifolia Juss. 129
Thevetia nerifolia Juss. ex Steud. 277
Thevetia peruviana Schum. 277
Tinospora cordifolia (Willd.) Hook. f. & Thoms. 2
Tinospora cordifolia (Willd.) Miers 2
Tinospora crispa (Linn.) Hook. f. & Thoms. 3
Tinsopora crispum Miers. 3
Tinospora malabarica (Lam.) Miers 3
Tinospora sinensis (Lour.) Merr. 3
Tinospora tomentosa Miers 3
Toona ciliata Roem. 203
Trachardis lacca 239
Trachyspermum ammi Sprague 170
Trachyspermum roxburghianum (DC.) Sprague 183
Trachyspermum roxburghianum (DC.) Wolff 183
Trianthema monogyna Linn. 108
Trianthema portulacastrum Linn. 108
Tribulus lanuginosus Willd. 38
Tribulus terrestris Linn. 38
Trichosanthes anguina Linn. 19
Trichosanthes bracteata (Lam.) Vogt. 96
Trichosanthes cucumerina Linn. 19
Trichosanthes cucumerina Linn. var. *anguina* (Linn.) Hains 19
Trichosanthes dioica Roxb. 19
Trichosanthes palmata Roxb. 96
Trifolium indicum Linn. 225,563
Trifolium officinale Willd. 225
Trifolium officinalis 225
Trigonella corniculata 225
Trigonella corniculata Linn. 226
Trigonella foenum-graecum Linn. 562
Trigonella uncata Boiss. 226
Triticum sativum Linn. 551
Typha elephantina Roxb. 30
Ulmus integrifolia Roxb. 456,560
Uniloa bipinnata Linn. 362
Uraria picta Desv. 34

Uraria picta (Jacq.) Desv. ex DC. 34
Valeriana dubia Bunge 222
Valeriana jatamansi Jones 222
Valeriana jatamansi Wall. 217
Valeriana officinalis Linn. 222
Valeriana wallichii DC. 222
Vanda roxburghii R. Br. 332
Vanda roxburghii. (R. Br.) 105
Vangueria spinosa Roxb. 244
Vateria indica 251
Vateria indica Linn. 255, 476
Vateria malabarica. 251
Vateria malabarica Blume 255,476
Vepris bilocularis Engler 207
Vepris bilocularis (W. & A.) Engler 207
Vernonia anthelmintica Willd. 159
Vernonia cineria Less. 111
Vernonia cineria (Linn.) Less. 111
Vetiveria zizanioides (Linn.) Nash 18
Vetiveria zizanioides Nash 18,198
Viburnum foetidum Wall. 41
Viburnum prunifolium Linn. 514
Vigna aconitifolia (Jacq.) Marechal 548
Vigna catjang Walp. 542
Vigna cylindrica Skeels 542
Vigna mungo (Linn.) Hepper. 552
Vigna radiata (Linn.) Wilczek.var. ***radiata*** Verdcourt 541
Vigna trilobata (Linn.) Verdocourt 48
Vigna unguiculata (Linn.) Walp. ssp. ***cylindrica*** (Linn.) Van Esettine 542
Viscum album Linn. 332
Vitex altissima Linn. f. 319
Vitex arborea Roxb. 320
Vitex leucoxylon Willd. 319
Vitex negundo Linn. 320
Vitex trifolia Willd. 320
Vitis pedata Vahl ex Wall. 348
Vitis vinifera Linn. 413
Viverra zibetha Linn. 208
Vogelia arabica Boiss. 165
Vogelia indica Gibs. 165
Wattakaka volubilis (L.) Stapf 51

Wedelia calandulacea Less. J. Murray 281
Wedelia calendulacea Less., non Rich. 281
Wedelia chinensis Merrill 281
Wendlandia exserta DC. 514
Wendlandia tinctoria DC. 515
Withania ashwagandha Kaul 106
Withania somnifera Dunal 106
Withania somnifera (Linn.) Dunal 106
Woodfordia floribunda Salisb. 243
Woodfordia fruiticosa Kurz 243
Woodfordia fruiticosa (Linn.) Kurz 243
Wrightia antidysenterica J. Graham 132
Wrightia tinctoria R. Br. 132
Wrightia tomentosa Roem. & Schult. 196
Xeromphis spinosa (Thunb.) Keay 62
Zanthoxylum alatum 103
Zanthoxylum alatum Roxb. 102,140
Zanthoxylum armatum DC. 140
Zanthoxylum budrunga Wall. 103
Zanthoxylum budrunga Wall. ex DC. 140
Zanthoxylum hostil 102
Zanthoxylum limonella (Dennst.) Alston 140
Zanthoxylum rhesta DC. 103,140
Zinc oxide 265
Zingiber officinale Rosc. 167
Zingiber zerumbet Rosc. ex Smith 126
Zizyphus jujuba Lam. 445
Zizyphus jujuba Mill. 446
Zizyphus mauritiana Lam. 445
Zizyphus microphylla Roxb. 446
Zizyphus nitida Roxb. 446
Ziziphus nummularia (Burm. f.) W. & A. 445
Zizphus nummularia W. & A. 445
Zizyphus sativa Gaertn. 446
Zizyphus vulgaris Lam. 446
(Zizyphus = Ziziphus)

INDEX - B

INDEX OF SANSKRTA NAMES, SYNONYMS ETC.

Here those names, synonyms etc. occuring in the text of Dhn. ni. and those occuring in clause II - a of the comments (from Raj. ni. which are useful for morphological identification) are only mentioned.

Abalā - Strī	अबला - स्त्री	615
Abdaḥ - Mustā	अब्दः - मुस्ता	15
Abdhibhūmijam-Hīrakam	अब्धिभूमिजम् - हीरकम्	532
Abhayā - Harītakī	अभया - हरीतकी	77
Abhayam - Uśīram	अभयम् - उशीरम्	198
Abhedyam - Hīrakam	अभेद्यं - हीरकम्	532
Abhidhāraḥ - Ghṛtam	अभिधारः - घृतम्	574
Abhīruḥ - Mahāśatāvarī	अभीरुः - महाशतावरी	116
Abhiṣavakrāntam-Mārdwīkam	अभिषवक्रान्तम् - मार्द्वीकम्	599
Abhiṣṭaḥ -Tilakaḥ (Raj. ni.)	अभीष्टः - तिलकः (रा.नि.)	514
Abhyañjanam - Tailam	अभ्यञ्जनम् - तैलम्	570
Abjam - Kumudam	अब्जम् - कुमुदम्	373
Ācamanam - Vālakam	आचमनम् - वालकम्	17
Adhaḥśalyaḥ - Apāmārgaḥ	अधःशल्यः -अपामार्गः	100
Āḍhakī - Saurāṣṭrī	आढकी - सौराष्ट्री	247
Āḍhakī (p. 549)	आढकी (p. 549)	
Adhikaṇṭakah - Yāsaḥ	अधिकण्टक :- यासः	8
Ādityakāntā - Suvarcalā	आदित्यकान्ता - सुवर्चला	333
Ādityavallī - Suvarcalā	आदित्यवल्ली- सुवर्चला	333
Afūkam (p. 567)	अफूकम् (p. 567)	
Agadaḥ - Kuṣṭham	अगदः - कुष्ठम्	219
Āgahaṭṭakaḥ-Rakt. Apāmārgaḥ	आघट्टकः - र. अपामार्गः (रा.नि.)	101
Agaru (p.206)	अगरु (p.206)	
Agaruḥ - Śiṁśapā	अगरुः - शिंशपा	473
Āgneyam - Raktam	आग्नेयम् - रक्तम्	619
Agnibhāsā - Jyotiṣmatī	अग्निभासा - ज्योतिष्मती	103
Agnijihvā-Kalikārī (Raj.ni.)	अग्निजिह्वा- कलिकारी (रा. नि.)	281
Agnikaḥ - Bhallātakaḥ	अग्निकः - भल्लातकः	259
Agnikaḥ - Citrakaḥ	अग्निकः - चित्रकः	165
Agnikaḥ - Tumbaruḥ	अग्निकः - तुम्बरुः	140
Agnimanthaḥ (p. 40)	अग्निमन्थः (p. 40)	
Agnimathanaḥ-Agnimanthaḥ	अग्निमथनः - अग्निमंथः	40
Agnimukhaḥ - Bhallātakaḥ	अग्निमुखः - भल्लातकः	259

Agnimukhī - Kalikārī	अग्निमुखी - कलिकारी	280
Agnivallabhaḥ - Rālaḥ	अग्निवल्लभः - रालः	250
Agryā - Rocanā	अग्र्या - रोचना	203
Agūḍhagandham - Hingu	अगूढगन्धम् - हिंगु	137
Āhāraḥ	आहारः	
660,661	Ahicchatrā - Śarkarā	
अहिच्छत्रा -शर्करा	188	
Ahifenam - Afūkam	अहिफेनम् - अफूकम्	568
Ahiḥ - Sarpaḥ	अहिः - सर्पः	638
Ahimāraḥ - Irimedaḥ	अहिमारः - इरिमेदः	489
Ahimārakaḥ - Irimedaḥ	अहिमारकः - इरिमेदः	489
Ahimedaḥ - Irimedaḥ	अहिमेदः - इरिमेदः	489
Aindrī - Indravāruṇī	ऐन्द्री - इन्द्रवारुणी	95
Airāvatikaḥ - Nārangaḥ	ऐरावतिकः- नारङ्गः	391
Ajādadhi	अजादधि	583
Ajagandhā (p. 184)	अजगन्धा (p. 184)	
Ajāghṛtam	अजाघृतम्	575
Ajaḥ - Chāgaḥ	अजः - छागः	622
Ajājī - Jīrakam	अजाजी - जीरकम्	156
Ajakarṇaḥ-Sarjakaḥ (Raj. ni.)	अजकर्णः - सर्जकः (रा. नि.)	477
Ajamodā (p. 183)	अजमोदा (p. 183)	
Ajāmūtram	अजामूत्रम्	641
Ajāntrī - Vṛddhadārukaḥ	अजान्त्री - वृद्धदारुकः	343
Ajāpayaḥ	अजापयः	578
Ajarā - Vṛddhadārukaḥ (Raj. ni.)	अजरा - वृद्धदारुकः (रा. नि.)	343
Ajaśṛngī (p. 31)	अजश्रृ गी (p. 31)	
Ajaṭā - Tāmalakī	अजटा -तामलकी	240
Ajinam - Twak	अजिनम् - त्वक्	644
Ajitā - Saurāṣṭrī	अजिता - सौराष्ट्री	247
Ājyam - Ghṛtam	आज्यम् - घृतम्	574
Ākhuḥ - Mūṣakaḥ	आखुः - मूषकः	630
Ākhuparṇikā - Dravantī	आखुपर्णिका - द्रवन्ती	87
Ākhuviṣahā - Jīmūtakaḥ	आखुविषहा - जीमूतकः	64
Akśaḥ - Bibhītakaḥ	अक्षः - बिभीतकः	78
Akśam - Sauvarcalam	अक्षम् - सौवर्चलम्	136
Akśapīḍā - Yavatiktā	अक्षपीडा - यवतिक्ता	98
Akśasasyaḥ - Kapitthaḥ	अक्षसस्यः - कपित्थः	187
Akśataḥ - Yavaḥ	अक्षतः - यवः	538
Akśatailam	अक्षतैलम्	572
Ākśika sīdhuḥ	आक्षिकसीधुः	601

Akśoḍaḥ (p. 414)	अक्षोडः (p. 414)	
Ālakam - Śāliparṇī viśeṣaḥ	आलकम् - शालिपर्णी विशेषः	32
Alaktakaḥ -Lākśā	अलक्तकः - लाक्षा	239
Alaktam - Kusumbham	अलक्तम् - कुसुम्भम्	566
Ālam- Haritālam	आलं -हरितालम्	667
Alarkaḥ - Rājārkaḥ	अलर्कः - राजार्कः	282
Aliḥ - Matsyaviśeṣaḥ	अलिः - मत्स्यविशेषः	627
Aliḥ - Bhramaraḥ	अलिः - भ्रमरः	633
Alimatsyaḥ-Matsyaviśeṣaḥ	अलिमत्स्यः - मत्स्यविशेषः	627
Aliskandhaḥ - Kulatthaḥ	अलिस्कन्धः - कुलत्थः	557
Allakā - Dhānyakam	अल्लका - धान्यकम्	156
Ālocakam -Kānta Loham	आलोचकम् - कान्तलोहम्	528
Alpakśupaḥ-Vaiparītyā Lajjāluḥ	अल्पक्षुपः - वैपरीत्या लज्जालुः	345
Ālūkam - Elavālukam	आलूकम् - एलवालुकम्	236
Āmaghnī - Kaṭukā	आमघ्नी - कटुका	15
Amalā - Sātalā	अमला - सातला	89
Āmalakī (p.79)	आमलकी (p.79)	
Āmalakīpatram - Tālīsam	आमलकीपत्रम् - तालीसम्	147
Āmaṇḍaḥ - Eraṇḍaḥ	आमण्डः - एरण्डः	117
Amaradāruḥ - Devadāruḥ	अमरदारुः - देवदारुः	27
Ambā - Ambaṣṭhā	अम्बा - अम्बष्ठा	249
Ambālikā - Ambaṣṭhā	अम्बालिका - अम्बष्ठा	249
Ambaṣṭhā - Pāthā	अम्बष्ठा - पाठा	26
Ambaṣṭhā (p. 248)	अम्बष्ठा (p. 248)	
Ambaṣṭhā - Karañjaḥ	अम्बष्ठा - करञ्जः	462
Ambaṣṭhakā - Ambaṣṭhā	अम्बष्ठका - अम्बष्ठा	249
Ambaṣṭhakī -Pāthā	अम्बष्ठकी - पाठा	26
Ambhaḥ - Jalam	अम्भः - जलम्	605
Ambhojam - Kumudam	अम्भोजम् - कुमुदम्	373
Ambikā - Ambaṣṭhā	अम्बिका - अम्बष्ठा	249
Ambu - Jalam	अम्बु - जलम्	605
Ambu - Vālakam	अम्बु - वालकम्	17
Ambudharaḥ - Mustā	अम्बुधरः - मुस्ता	15
Ambujam - Kumudam	अम्बुजम् - कुमुदम्	373
Ambuprasādanaphalam-Katakam	अम्बुप्रसादनफलम् - कतकम्	267
Amburuhā-Padmacāriṇī (Raj. ni.)	अम्बुरुहा - पद्मचारिणी (रा.नि.)	325
Ambuvāsinī - Pāṭalā	अम्बुवासिनी - पाटला	43
Āmiṣakaram - Raktam	आमिषकरम् - रक्तम्	619
Āmiṣam - Māmsam	आमिषम् - मांसम्	618

Amlaḥ - Amlavetasaḥ	अम्लः - अम्लवेतसः	177
Amlaloṇikā-Kśudrāmlikā	अम्ललोणिका - क्षुद्राम्लिका	399
Amlamahiruhaḥ-Vṛkśāmlam	अम्लमहीरुहः - वृक्षाम्लम्	173
Amlānaḥ-Taruṇī (Raj. ni.)	अम्लानः - तरुणी (रा. नि.)	501
Amlanāyakaḥ-Amlavetasaḥ (Raj. ni.)	अम्लनायकः - अम्लवेतसः (रा.नि.)	177
Amlapatrakaḥ-Aśmantakaḥ	अम्लपत्रकः - अश्मन्तकः	72
Amlaśākhaḥ - Vrkśāmlam	अम्लशाखः - वृक्षाम्लम्	173
Amlavāṭakaḥ - Āmrātakaḥ	अम्लवाटकः - आम्रातकः	388
Amlavetasaḥ (p. 177)	अम्लवेतसः (p. 177)	
Amlavṛkśaḥ - Vṛksāmlam	अम्लवृक्षः - वृक्षाम्लम्	173
Amlīkā - Amlikā	अम्लीका - अम्लिका	398
Amlikā (p. 398)	अम्लिका (p. 398)	
Āmodajananī- Tāmbūlī	आमोदजननी - ताम्बूली	273
Amoghā - Pāṭalā	अमोघा - पाटला	43
Amoghā - Viḍaṅgam	अमोघा - विडङ्गम्	130
Āmraḥ (p. 385)	आम्रः (p. 385)	
Āmrāntaḥ - Rājāmraḥ	आम्रान्तः - राजाम्रः	388
Āmrātakaḥ (p. 388)	आम्रातकः (p. 388)	
Amṛṇālam - Lāmajjakam	अमृणालम् - लामज्जकम्	241
Amṛtā - Guḍūcī	अमृता - गुडूची	2
Amṛtā - Saurāṣṭrī	अमृता - सौराष्ट्री	247
Amṛtā - Tāmbūlī	अमृता - ताम्बूली	273
Amṛtā - Harītakī	अमृता - हरीतकी	77
Amṛtakaṇḍā gūḍūcikā-Kandaguḍūcī	अमृतकन्दागुडूचिका- कंदगुडूची	2
Amṛtalatā - Guḍūcī	अमृतलता - गुडूची	2
Amṛtam - Ghṛtam	अमृतम् - घृतम्	574
Amṛtam - Jalam	अमृतम् - जलम्	605
Amṛtam - Vatsanābhaḥ	अमृतम् - वत्सनाभः	667
Amṛtāphalaḥ - Paṭolaḥ	अमृताफलः - पटोलः	18
Amṛtāphalākhyam-Pālevatam (Raj. ni.)	अमृतफलाख्यम् -पालेवतम् (रा.नि.)	419
Amṛtaphalam - Āmalakī	अमृतफलम् - आमलकी	79
Amṛtasambhavā - Guḍūcī	अमृतसंभवा - गुडूची	2
Amṛtāsaṅgā - Saurāṣṭrī	अमृतासङ्गा - सौराष्ट्री	247
Amṛtāsaṅgam - Tuttham	अमृतासङ्गम् - तुत्थम्	260
Amṛtavallī - Guḍūcī	अमृतवल्ली - गुडूची	2
Amṛtodbhavā - Tāmbūlī	अमृतोद्भवा - ताम्बूली	273
Amśūdakam	अंशूदकम्	607
Amśukam - Tamālapatram	अंशुकम् - तमालपत्रम्	146

Āmūṣikā (p. 630) आमूषिका (p. 630)
Anaḍvān - Vṛṣabhaḥ अनड्वान् - वृषभः 626
Analaḥ - Citrakaḥ अनलः - चित्रकः 165
Analaḥ - Pittam अनलः - पित्तम् 616
Anantā - Dūrvā अनन्ता - दूर्वा 368
Anantā - Tāmbūlī अनन्ता - ताम्बूली 273
Anantaḥ - Yāsaḥ अनन्त : -यासः 8
Anāryakam - Agaru अनार्यकम् - अगरु 206
Anāryatiktakaḥ-Kirātatiktakaḥ अनार्यतिक्तकः - किराततिक्तकः 13
Aṇḍagajaḥ - Cakramardaḥ अण्डगजः - चक्रमर्दः 277
Aṅgajam - Māmsam अङ्गजम् - मांसम् 618
Aṅganā -Strī अङ्गना - स्त्री 615
Aṅgāravallī - Bhārngī अङ्गारवल्ली - भार्ङ्गी 24
Aṅgāravallikā - Karañjaḥ अंगारवल्लिका - करञ्जः 462
Aṅghribalā - Pṛśniparṇī अङ्घ्रिबला - पृश्निपर्णी 33
Anilaḥ - Vāyuḥ अनिलः - वायुः 616
Ānīlam - Vaṅgaṃ आनीलम् - वङ्गम् 525
Anilāpahaḥ - Kulatthaḥ अनिलापहः - कुलत्थः
Anirvāṇaḥ - Sleṣmā अनिर्वाणः - श्लेष्मा 617
Añjalikārikā - Raktapādī अञ्जलिकारिका - रक्तपादी 344
Añjanam (p. 261) अञ्जनम् (p. 261)
Aṅkavṛkśaḥ - Kadambaḥ अंकवृक्षः - कदम्बः 451
Aṅkolakaḥ - Aṅkoṭakaḥ अङ्कोलकः - अङ्कोटकः 99
Aṅkoṭakaḥ (p.99) अङ्कोटकः (p.99)
Annasambhavaḥ - Rasaḥ अन्नसंभवः - रसः 619
Anṛju - Tagaram अनृजु - तगरम् 221
Anujam - Prapauṇḍarīkam अनुजम् - प्रपौण्डरीकम् 243
Anyā Indravāruṇī - Viśālā अन्या इन्द्रवारुणी- विशाला 95
Anyāmṛt - Saurāṣṭrī अन्यामृत् - सौराष्ट्री 247
Āpaḥ - Jalam आपः - जलम् 605
Apāmāragaḥ (p.100) अपामार्ग : (p.100)
Apāmārgaḥ - Raktapuṣpaḥ (p.101) अपामार्गः - रक्तपुष्पः (p.101)
Aparā Hapuṣā (p.128) अपरा हपुषा (p.128)
Aparā Raktapādī-Viśvagranthiḥ अपरा रक्तपादी - विश्वग्रंथिः 347
Aparājitā -Viṣṇukrāntā (Raj.ni.) अपराजिता - विष्णुक्रान्ता (रा.नि.) 353
Aparājitā - Śamī (Raj. ni.) अपराजिता - शमी (रा.नि.) 443
Aparājitā - Aśvakśurakaḥ अपराजिता - अश्वक्षुरकः 323
Aparājitā - Balāmoṭā अपराजिता - बलामोटा 378
Apetarākśasī - Surasā अपेतराक्षसी - सुरसा 301
Aphenakam - Afūkam अफेनकम् - अफूकम् 568

Āpītaḥ - Tūṇiḥ आपीतः - तूणिः 202
Āpitam - Padmakesaram आपीतम् - पद्मकेसरम् 377
Apuṣpaphalasambandhaḥ - Udumbaraḥ अपुष्पफलसम्बन्धः - उदुम्बरः 436
Āragvadhaḥ (p.80) आरग्वधः (p.80)
Aralukaḥ - Śyonākaḥ अरलुकः - श्योनाकः 41
Āram - Pittalam आरम् - पित्तलम् 526
Āranālam - Kāñjikam आरनालम् - काञ्जिकम् 595
Araṇī - Agnimanthaḥ अरणी -अग्निमंथः 40
Araṇī (Varaṇī) (p.85) अरणी (वरणी) (p.85)
Araṇikaḥ - Agnimanthaḥ अरणिकः -अग्निमंथः 40
Araṇyadhānyanāmā - Śāliḥ अरण्यधान्यनामा - शालिः 535
Āraṇyadhānyanāmā - Nīvāraḥ अरण्यधान्यनामा - नीवारः 543
Araṇyakadalī -Girikadalī (Raj. ni.) अरण्यकदली-गिरिकदली (रा. नि.) 317
Araṇyakadalī -Kāṣṭhakadalī अरण्यकदली - काष्ठकदली 317
Aravindam - Kumudam अरविन्दम् - कुमुदम् 373
Ardhacandrā - Trivṛt अर्धचन्द्रा - त्रिवृत् 93
Ārdrā - Ativiṣā आर्द्रा - अतिविषा 4
Ārdrakam - Śuṇṭhī (viśeṣaḥ) आर्द्रकम् - शुण्ठी (विशेषः) 167
Ārdramāṣā - Māṣaparṇī आर्द्रमाषा -माषपर्णी 48
Ārevataḥ - Āragvadhaḥ आरेवतः - आरग्वधः 80
Ārevatam - Pālevatam आरेवतम् - पालेवतम् 418
Arimardaḥ - Kāsamardaḥ अरिमर्दः - कासमर्दः 356
Arimedaḥ - Bilvaḥ अरिमेदः - बिल्वः 39
Arimedaḥ - Irimedaḥ अरिमेदः - इरिमेदः 489
Arimedakaḥ - Irimedaḥ अरिमेदकः - इरिमेदः 489
Ariṣṭā - Gāṅgerukī अरिष्टा - गांगेरुकी 112
Ariṣṭā - Kaṭukā अरिष्टा -कटुका 15
Ariṣṭaḥ अरिष्टः 602
Ariṣṭaḥ - Laśunaḥ अरिष्टः - लशुनः 312
Ariṣṭaḥ - Kākaḥ अरिष्टः - काकः 637
Ariṣṭaḥ - Nimbaḥ अरिष्टः - निम्बः 12
Arjakaḥ - Kuṭherakaḥ अर्जकः - कुठेरकः 304
Arjunaḥ (p. 464) अर्जुनः (p. 464)
Arkacandanam -Raktacandanam (Raj. ni.)
अर्कचन्दनम् - रक्तचंदनम् (रा.नि.) 193
Arkaḥ (p. 281) अर्कः (p. 281)
Arkavedham - Tālīsam (Raj. ni.) अर्कवेधम् - तालीसम् (रा. नि.) 148
Ārogyam आरोग्यम 660
Ārogyaśimbī - Karṇikāraḥ आरोग्यशिम्बी - कर्णिकारः 81
Arśoghnaḥ - Sūraṇaḥ अर्शोघ्नः - सूरणः 383

Ārtagalā -Saireyakaḥ (Raj. ni.)	आर्तगला - सैरेयकः (रा.नि.)	110
Arthasiddhakaḥ-Sinduvāraḥ (Raj. ni.)	अर्थसिद्धकः - सिन्दुवारः (रा.नि.)	319
Ārukam (p. 399)	आरुकम् (p. 399)	
Aruṇā - Mañjiṣṭhā	अरुणा -मञ्जिष्ठा	7
Aruṇaḥ - Citrakaḥ	अरुणः - चित्रकः	165
Aruṣkaḥ - Bhallātakaḥ	अरुष्कः - भल्लातकः	259
Aśanaḥ (p. 479)	अशनः (p. 479)	
Aśaniḥ - Hīrakam	अशनिः - हीरकम्	532
Āsavadruḥ-Tālaḥ (Raj. ni.)	आसवद्रुः - तालः (रा. नि.)	421
Āsavam	आसवम्	600
Aśiram - Hīrakam	अशिरं - हीरकम्	532
Aśirī - (type of) Kāśaḥ	अशिरी - (अन्यः) काशः	359
Asitā - Kokilā	असिता - कोकिला	637
Asitā Āḍhakī - Āḍhakī	असिता आढकी - आढकी	549
Asitaḥ - Kokilaḥ	असितः - कोकिलः	637
Asitānanaḥ - Bilvaḥ	असिताननः - बिल्वः	39
Āśīviṣaḥ - Sarpaḥ	आशीविषः - सर्पः	639
Aśmabhedakaḥ-Pāṣāṇabhedaḥ	अश्मभेदकः - पाषाणभेदः	57
Aśmagarbhajam-Gārutmatam	अश्मगर्भजम् - गारुत्मतम्	531
Aśmaghnaḥ-Pāṣāṇabhedaḥ	अश्मघ्नः - पाषाणभेदः	57
Aśmajatuḥ - Śilājatuḥ	अश्मजतुः - शिलाजतुः	266
Aśmantakaḥ (p.72)	अश्मन्तकः (p.72)	
Aśokaḥ (p. 516)	अशोकः (p. 516)	
Aśokarohiṇī - Kaṭukā	अशोकरोहिणी -कटुका	15
Āsphotā - Sārivā	आस्फोता - सारिवा	59
Āsphoṭaḥ - Arkaḥ	आस्फोटः - अर्कः	282
Asram - Kumkumam	अस्रम् - कुंकुमम्	197
Asṛg - Spṛkkā	असृग् - स्पृक्का	224
Asṛgdharā - Twak	असृग्धरा - त्वक्	644
Asṛk - Kumkumam	असृक् - कुंकुमम्	197
Asṛk - Raktam	असृक् - रक्तम्	619
Aṣṭapadī - Mallikā	अष्टपदी - मल्लिका	493
Aṣṭavidhamannam	अष्टविधमन्नम्	661
Asthi (p.618)	अस्थि (p. 618)	
Asthijananī - Vasā	अस्थिजननी -वसा	619
Asthisambandhanaḥ-Kaṅguḥ	अस्थिसम्बन्धनः - कङ्गुः	547
Asthisambhavam - Majjā	अस्थिसंभवम् - मज्जा	619
Asthisāraḥ - Majjā	अस्थिसारः - मज्जा	619
Astram - Vyāghranakham	अस्त्रम् - व्याघ्रनखम्	223

Aśuddham - Raktam	अशुद्धम - रक्तम्	619
Āsuram - Biḍam	आसुरम - बिडम्	135
Āsurī (p 305)	आसुरी (p 305)	
Aśvā dadhi	अश्वा दधि	584
Aśvagandhā (p.105)	अश्वगन्धा (p.105)	
Aśvaghnī - Tejasvinī	अश्वघ्नी - तेजस्विनी	102
Aśvāghṛtam	अश्वाघृतम्	575
Aśvaḥ (p. 620)	अश्वः (p. 620)	
Aśvahā - Karavīraḥ	अश्वहा - करवीरः	275
Aśvakśurā - Aśvakśurakaḥ	अश्वक्षुरा -अश्वक्षुरकः	323
Aśvakśurakaḥ (p. 323)	अश्वक्षुरकः (p. 323)	
Aśvamārakaḥ - Karavīraḥ	अश्वमारकः - करवीरः	275
Aśvamohakaḥ - Karavīraḥ	अश्वमोहकः - करवीरः	275
Aśvamūtram	अश्वमूत्रम	642
Aśvamūtrī - Śallakī	अश्वमूत्री - शल्लकी	256
Aśvāpayaḥ	अश्वापयः	579
Aśvapucchikā - Māṣaparṇī	अश्वपुच्छिका - माषपर्णी	48
Aśvataraḥ (p. 622)	अश्वतरः (p. 622)	
Aśvatthaḥ - Pippalaḥ	अश्वत्थः - पिप्पलः	427
Aśvatthaphalā-Aparā Hapuṣā	अश्वत्थफला - अपरा हपुषा	128
Aśvatthasannibhā-Aśvatthī	अश्वत्थसंनिभा - अश्वत्थी	428
Aśvāvarohakaḥ-Aśvagandhā	अश्वावरोहकः - अश्वगन्धा	105
Aśvghnaḥ - Karavīraḥ	अश्वघ्नः - करवीरः	275
Āṭarūṣaḥ - Vāsakaḥ	आटरूषः - वासकः	9
Aṭarūṣakaḥ - Vāsakaḥ	आटरूषकः - वासकः	9
Atasī (p. 564)	अतसी (p. 564)	
Atasītailam	अतसीतैलम्	570
Aṭavīmūlakam - Gṛñjanam	अटवीमूलकम् - गृञ्जनम्	294
Āṭavyā - Kāsaghnī	आटव्या - कासघ्नी	37
Atibalā (p.113)	अतिबला (p.113)	
Aticarā - Padmacāriṇī	अतिचरा -पद्मचारिणी	325
Aticchatrā - Śatapuspā	अतिच्छत्रा - शतपुष्पा	121
Aticchatrakaḥ - Bhūṣṭṛṇaḥ	अतिच्छत्रकः - भूस्तृणः	300
Atigandhikā - Hapuṣā	अतिगन्धिका - हपुषा	128
Atiguhā - Śaliparṇī	अतिगुहा - शालिपर्णी	32
Atiguhā - Pṛṣni. viśeṣaḥ	अतिगुहा - पृश्नि. विशेषः	33
Atikesarā - Kubjakaḥ	अतिकेसरा - कुब्जकः	503
Atimuktakaḥ - Tindukaḥ	अतिमुक्तकः - तिन्दुकः	402
Atimuktakaḥ (p. 509)	अतिमुक्तकः (p. 509)	

Atirasā - Rāsnā अतिरसा - रास्ना 104
Atiruhā - Māmsarohiṇī अतिरुहा - मांसरोहिणी 330
Atithiḥ - Śilājatuḥ अतिथिः - शिलाजतुः 266
Atitikṣṇā - Āsurī अतितीक्ष्णा - आसुरी 306
Ativiṣā (p.4) अतिविषा (p.4)
Ātmā - Śarīram आत्मा - शरीरम् 615
Ātmaguptā - Kapikacchuḥ आत्मगुप्ता - कपिकच्छुः 55
Ātmaguptātailam आत्मगुप्तातैलम् 572
Ātmarakṣā - Viśālā आत्मरक्षा - विशाला 95
Aṭṭahāsaḥ - Kundaḥ अट्टहासः - कुन्दः 506
Atyarkaḥ - Rājārkaḥ अत्यर्कः - राजार्कः 282
Atyarkaḥ - Śuklārkaḥ अत्यर्कः - शुक्लार्कः 283
Atyugragandhā - Aśvakṣurakaḥ अत्युग्रगन्धा -अश्वक्षुरकः 323
Atyugram - Hiṅgu अत्युग्रम् - हिंगु 137
Audbhidam (p. 136) औद्भिदम् (p. 136)
Aurabhrapayaḥ औरभ्रपयः 579
Aurvam - Audbhidam और्वम् - औद्भिदम् 136
Auṣadham औषधम् 659
Avadamśakṣamaḥ - Śigruḥ अवदंशक्षमः - शिग्रुः 295
Avākpuṣpī - Śatapuṣpā अवाक्पुष्पी - शतपुष्पा 121
Avalgujā- Bākucī अवल्गुजा - बाकुची 61
Avandhyā - Karkoṭakī अवन्ध्या - कर्कोटकी 69
Avantisomam - Kāñjikam अवन्तिसोमम् - काञ्जिकम् 595
Āvartakī - Araṇī आवर्तकी - अरणी 85
Āvartakī - Viṣāṇikā (p. 74) आवर्तकी - विषाणिका (p.74)
Āvartam - Hemamākṣikam आवर्तम् - हेममाक्षिकम् 261
Avayavasthānam - Śarīram अवयवस्थानम् - शरीरम् 615
Āvegī -Vṛddhadārukaḥ आवेगी - वृद्धदारुकः 343
Avibhuk - Vṛkaḥ अविभुक् - वृकः 623
Āvignam - Karamardakam आविग्नम् - करमर्दकम् 448
Aviḥ (p. 622) अविः (p. 622)
Āvikaghṛtam आविकघृतम् 575
Avikaḥ - Aviḥ अविकः - अविः 623
Āvikam dadhi आविकं दधि 584
Avimuktaḥ - Atimuktakaḥ अविमुक्तः - अतिमुक्तकः 509
Avyathā - Harītakī अव्यथा - हरीतकी 77
Ayaḥ - Loham अयः - लोहम् 528
Ayaḥśiṣṭam - Maṇḍūram अयः शिष्टम् - मण्डूरम् 529
Bākucī (p.61) बाकुची (p.61)

Badaram (p. 445)	बदरम् (p. 445)	
Baheḍakaḥ - Bibhītakaḥ	बहेडकः - बिभीतकः	78
Bahubījā - Girikadalī (Raj. ni.)	बहुबीजा- गिरिकदली (रा. नि.)	317
Bahucchinnā - Kandaguḍūcī	बहुच्छिन्ना - कंदगुडूची	2
Bahudhāram - Hīrakam	बहुधारम् - हीरकम्	532
Bahugandhaḥ -Kunduruḥ(Raj.ni.)	बहुगन्धः - कुन्दुरुः (रा. नि.)	254
Bahulā - Elā	बहुला - एला	141
Bahulā - Tāmbūlī	बहुला - ताम्बूली	273
Bahulacchadaḥ - Śigruḥ (Raj. ni.)	बहुलच्छदः - शिग्रुः (रा. नि.)	296
Bahulacchadaḥ -Madhuśigrukaḥ (Raj. ni)	बहुलच्छदः -मधुशिग्रुकः (रा. नि.)	296
Bahumañjarī - Surasā	बहुमञ्जरी - सुरसा	301
Bahupādaḥ - Vaṭaḥ	बहुपादः - वटः	426
Bahupatrā - Taruṇī (Raj. ni.)	बहुपत्रा - तरुणी (रा. नि.)	501
Bahupatrikā - Methikā	बहुपत्रिका - मेथिका	562
Bahuphenā - Sātalā	बहुफेना - सातला	89
Bahuprajaḥ - Sūkaraḥ	बहुप्रजः - सूकरः	624
Bahuputrikā - Mahāśatāvarī	बहुपुत्रिका - महाशतावरी	116
Bahutiktā - Kākamācī (Raj. ni.)	बहुतिक्ता - काकमाची (रा. नि.)	286
Bahuvādinī - Vijayā	बहुवादिनी - विजया	46
Bahuvāraḥ - Śleṣmātakaḥ	बहुवारः - श्लेष्मातकः	441
Bahvī - Dūrvā	बह्वी - दूर्वा	368
Bakkasaḥ	बक्कसः	599
Bakulaḥ (p. 510)	बकुलः (p. 510)	
Balā - Tāmbūlī	बला - ताम्बूली	273
Balā (p.110)	बला (p.110)	
Balā pañcakam (p.113-14)	बलापञ्चकम् (p.113-14)	
Balabhadrā - Trāyamāṇā	बलभद्रा - त्रायमाणा	97
Baladevā - Trāyamāṇā	बलदेवा - त्रायमाणा	97
Balāḍhyaḥ - Māṣaḥ	बलाढ्यः - माषः	552
Balāhakaḥ - Mustā	बलाहकः - मुस्ता	15
Balakaram - Asthi	बलकरम् - अस्थि	618
Balam - Kāṃsyam	बलम् - कांस्यम्	527
Balam - Śukram	बलम् - शुक्रम्	619
Balāmoṭā (p. 378)	बलामोटा (p. 378)	
Bālapatraḥ - Khadiraḥ	बालपत्रः - खदिरः	10
Bālapatraḥ - Yāsaḥ	बालपत्रः - यासः	8
Bālapuṣpā - Yūthikā	बालपुष्पा - यूथिका	504
Bālaroganāśinī - Ativiṣā	बालरोगनाशिनी - अतिविषा	4

Balāsaḥ - Śleṣmā	बलासः - श्लेष्मा	617
Bālasātmyam- Dugdham	बालसात्म्यम् - दुग्धम्	577
Balātrayam (113)	बलात्रयम् (p. 113)	
Balavān - Śleṣmā	बलवान् - श्लेष्मा	617
Bāleṣṭam - Badaram	बालेष्टं - बदरम्	445
Bāleyaḥ - Gardabhaḥ	बालेयः - गर्दभः	622
Bālhīkam - Hiṅgu	बाल्हीकम् - हिंगु	137
Bālhīkam - Kumkumam	बाल्हीकम् - कुंकुमम्	197
Balī - Gandhakaḥ	बली - गन्धकः	248
Balī - Kunduruḥ	बली- कुन्दुरुः	254
Balibhuk - Kākaḥ	बलिभुक् - काकः	637
Balikā - Atibalā	बलिका - अतिबला	113
Balīvardaḥ - Vṛṣabhaḥ	बलीवर्दः - वृषभः	625
Balivasā - Gandhakaḥ	बलिवसा - गन्धकः	248
Balyā - Aśvagandhā	बल्या - अश्वगन्धा	106
Bāṇaḥ - Śaraḥ	बाणः - शरः	363
Bāṇāhvaḥ - Muñjaḥ	बाणाह्वः - मुञ्जः	360
Bandhūka puṣpakaḥ - Aśanaḥ	बन्धूकपुष्पकः - अशनः	479
Bandhuraḥ - Hamsaviśeṣaḥ	बंधुरः - हंसविशेषः	635
Bandhuraḥ - Ṛṣabhaḥ	बन्धुरः - ऋषभः	45
Barbarā - Ajagandhā	बर्बरा - अजगन्धा	184
Barbaram - Bolam	बर्बरम् - बोलम्	226
Barbarikam (p. 195)	बर्बरिकम् (p. 195)	
Barbarodbhavam - Barbarikam	बर्बरोद्भवम् - बर्बरिकम्	195
Barbukaḥ - Aviḥ	बर्बुकः - अविः	623
Barhicūḍam - Sthauṇeyakam	बर्हिचूडम् - स्थौणेयकम्	230
Barhiḥ - Kuśaḥ	बर्हिः - कुशः	361
Barhiḥ - Mayūraḥ	बर्हिः - मयूरः	633
Barkaraḥ - Chāgaḥ	बर्करः - छागः	622
Bāṣpikā - Hiṅgupatrī	बाष्पिका - हिंगुपत्री	138
Bastagandhā - Ajagandhā	बस्तगन्धा - अजगन्धा	184
Bastaḥ - Chāgaḥ	बस्तः - छागः	622
Bastakarṇaḥ - Sarjakaḥ (Raj. ni.)	बस्तकर्णः - सर्जकः (रा. नि.)	477
Bastamodā - Ajamodā	बस्तमोदा - अजमोदा	183
Bastāntrī - Vṛṣamedhā	बस्तान्त्री -वृषमेधा	118
Baṭṭaloham - Bartaloham	बट्टलोहम् - बर्तलोहम्	528
Bahurecanī - Śuklabhaṇḍī (Raj. ni.)	बहुरेचनी - शुक्लभण्डी (रा. नि.)	94
Bahudugdhaḥ -Godhūmaḥ (Raj. ni.)	बहुदुग्धः - गोधूमः (रा नि.)	551
Bhadrā - Samī (Raj. ni.)	भद्रा - शमी (रा.नि.)	443

Bhadrā - Tāmbūlī	भद्रा - ताम्बूली	273
Bhadrā - Kaṭphalaḥ	भद्रा - कट्फलः	27
Bhadrā - Kṛ. Sārivā	भद्रा - कृ. सारिवा	60
Bhadradāruḥ - Devadāruḥ	भद्रदारुः - देवदारुः	27
Bhadrailā (p. 142)	भद्रैला (p. 142)	
Bhadrakāṣṭham - Devadāruḥ	भद्रकाष्ठम् - देवदारुः	27
Bhadralatā - Haridrā	भद्रलता - हरिद्रा	20
Bhadram - Saugandhikam	भद्रम् - सौगन्धिकम्	371
Bhadramustaḥ - Mustā	भद्रमुस्तः - मुस्ता	15
Bhadraparṇī - Prasāraṇī	भद्रपर्णी - प्रसारणी	114
Bhadraśrīḥ - Candanam	भद्रश्रीः–चन्दनम्	191
Bhadrataruṇī - Kubjakaḥ	भद्रतरुणी -कुब्जकः	503
Bhadraudanī - Balā	भद्रौदनी - बला	110
Bhadravatī - Kaṭphalaḥ	भद्रवती - कट्फलः	27
Bhadravallī - Mallikā (Raj. ni.)	भद्रवल्ली - मल्लिका (रा. नि.)	494
Bhadrayavaḥ - Indrayavaḥ	भद्रयवः - इन्द्रयवः	131
Bhakśakaḥ - Gokśuraḥ	भक्षकः - गोक्षुरः	38
Bhakśaṭakaḥ - Gokśuraḥ	भक्षटकः - गोक्षुरः	38
Bhallaḥ (Kākaḥ) (p.637)	भल्लः (काकः) (p.637)	
Bhallakaḥ - Bhallaḥ	भल्लकः - भल्लः	637
Bhallaśalyaḥ - Bhallaḥ	भल्लशल्यः - भल्लः	637
Bhallātaḥ - Bhallātakaḥ	भल्लातः - भल्लातकः	259
Bhallātakaḥ (p. 259)	भल्लातकः (p. 259)	
Bhallūkaḥ - Sārameyaḥ	भल्लूकः - सारमेयः	632
Bhallūkaḥ - Śṛgālaḥ	भल्लूकः - शृगालः	632
Bhallūkaḥ - Śyonākaḥ	भल्लूकः - श्योनाकः	41
Bhāṇḍī - Mañjiṣṭhā	भाण्डी - मञ्जिष्ठा	7
Bhaṇḍī - Mañjiṣṭhā	भण्डी - मञ्जिष्ठा	7
Bhaṇḍikaḥ - Śirīṣaḥ	भंडिकः- शिरीषः	463
Bhaṇḍīraḥ - Taṇḍulīyakaḥ	भण्डीरः - तण्डुलीयकः	355
Bhaṅgurā - Priyaṅguḥ (Raj. ni.)	भङ्गुरा - प्रियङ्गुः (रा.नि.)	201
Bhaṅgurā - Ativiṣā	भङ्गुरा- अतिविषा	4
Bhaṇṭākī - Vṛntākī	भण्टाकी - वृन्ताकी	37
Bhaṇṭikā - Vṛntākī	भण्टिका - वृन्ताकी	37
Bhayaṅkaraḥ - Kśudrolūkaḥ	भयंकरः - क्षुद्रोलूकः	638
Bhāratī - Brāhmī (Raj. ni.)	भारती - ब्राह्मी (रा.नि.)	336
Bhāratī - Vācā	भारती - वाचा	616
Bhāravāhaḥ - Gardabhaḥ	भारवाहः - गर्दभः	622
Bhāravāhī - Nīlinī	भारवाही - नीलिनी	87

Bhārgavā - Bhārṅgī	भार्गवा - भाङ्गी	24
Bhārgavakam - Hīrakam	भार्गवकम् - हीरकम्	532
Bhārgavam - Hīrakam	भार्गवम् - हीरकम्	532
Bhārgavī - Dūrvā	भार्गवी - दूर्वा	368
Bhārṅgī (p.24)	भाङ्गी (p.24)	
Bhāṣā - Vācā	भाषा - वाचा	616
Bhāsaḥ - Kākaḥ (p.637)	भासः - काकः (p.637)	
Bhaṣakaḥ - Sārameyaḥ	भषकः - सारमेयः	632
Bhāskaraḥ - Arkaḥ	भास्करः - अर्कः	282
Bhasmagarbhā - Śiṃśapā	भस्मगर्भा - शिंशपा	473
Bahulavalkalaḥ - Priyālaḥ	बहुलवल्कलः-प्रियालः	423
Bhautikam - Mauktikam	भौतिकम् - मौक्तिकम्	533
Bhavam (p. 401)	भवम् (p. 401)	
Bhāvanam - Bhavam	भावनम् - भवम्	401
Bhaviṣyam - Bhavam	भविष्यम् - भवम्	401
Bhavyam - Bhavam	भव्यम् - भवम्	401
Bheḍaḥ - Aviḥ	भेडः - अविः	623
Bhedaḥ - Padmabījam	भेडः - पद्मबीजम्	375
Bhedakaḥ - Amlavetasaḥ	भेदकः - अम्लवेतसः	177
Bhekaḥ - Maṇḍūkaḥ	भेकः - मण्डूकः	640
Bhiduram - Hīrakam	भिदुरम् - हीरकम्	531
Bhikṣuśīrṣikā - Śrāvaṇī	भिक्षुशीर्षिका - श्रावणी	58
Bhillī - Lodhraḥ	भिल्ली - लोध्रः	268
Bhīmaḥ - Amlavetasaḥ	भीमः - अम्लवेतसः	177
Bhiraṭikā - Śvetakāmbhojī	भिराटिका -श्वेतकाम्भोजी	292
Bhīruḥ - Strī	भीरुः - स्त्री	615
Bhīruḥ - Ulūkaḥ	भीरुः - उलूकः	638
Bhiṣagjitā - Guḍūcī	भिषग्जिता - गुडूची	2
Bhīṣaṇaḥ - Kunduruḥ	भीषणः - कुन्दुरुः	254
Bhiṣaṅmātā - Vāsakaḥ	भिषङ्माता - वासकः	9
Bhittipātanaḥ - Mahāmūṣakaḥ	भित्तिपातनः - महामूषकः	631
Bhogī - Sarpaḥ	भोगी - सर्पः	639
Bhogigandhikā - Nākulī	भोगिगन्धिका - नाकुली	339
Bhramarabāndhavā - Vāsantī	भ्रमरबान्धवा - वासन्ती	498
Bhramaraḥ (p. 633)	भ्रमरः (p. 633)	
Bhramaram - Loham	भ्रमरम् - लोहम्	528
Bhrāmaram -Kānta Loham	भ्रामरम् -कान्तलोहम्	528
Bhramareṣṭā - Jambūḥ	भ्रमरेष्टा - जम्बूः	433
Bhramarotsavaḥ -Atimuktakaḥ	भ्रमरोत्सवः - अतिमुक्तकः	509

Bhrāntaḥ - Dhattūraḥ (Raj. ni.)	भ्रान्तः - धत्तूरः (रा. नि.)	279
Bhṛṅgaḥ - Bhṛamaraḥ	भृङ्गः - भ्रमरः	633
Bhṛṅgaḥ - Bhṛṅgarājaḥ	भृङ्गः -भृङ्गराजः	281
Bhṛṅgajā - Bhārṅgī	भृङ्गजा - भार्ङ्गी	24
Bhṛṅgam - Twak	भृङ्गम -त्वक्	145
Bhṛṅgamohī - Campakaḥ (Raj.ni.)	भृङ्गमोही - चम्पकः (रा. नि.)	500
Bhṛṅgānandā - Yūthikā (Raj. ni.)	भृङ्गानन्दा - यूथिका (रा.नि.)	504
Bhṛṅgāraḥ - Bhṛṅgarājaḥ	भृङ्गारः -भृङ्गराजः	281
Bhṛṅgarājaḥ - Bhṛamaraḥ	भृङ्गराजः - भ्रमरः	633
Bhṛṅgarajaḥ - Bhṛṅgarājaḥ	भृङ्गरजः - भृङ्गराजः	281
Bhṛṅgarājaḥ (p. 280)	भृङ्गराजः (p. 280)	
Bhṛṅgārakaḥ - Bhṛṅgarājaḥ	भृङ्गारकः - भृङ्गराजः	281
Bhṛṅgāram - Lavaṅgam	भृङ्गारम् - लवङ्गम्	214
Bhṛṅgareṇuḥ - Bhṛṅgarājaḥ	भृङ्गरेणुः - भृङ्गराजः	281
Bhṛṅgasuhṛt - Kundaḥ	भृङ्गसुहृत् - कुन्दः	506
Bhṛṅgeṣṭā - Taruṇī (Raj. ni.)	भृङ्गेष्टा - तरुणी (रा. नि.)	501
Bhūdhātrī - Tāmalakī	भूधात्री -तामलकी	240
Bhujagaḥ - Sarpaḥ	भुजगः - सर्पः	638
Bhujaṅgaḥ - Sarpaḥ	भुजंगः - सर्पः	638
Bhujaṅgamaḥ - Sarpaḥ	भुजंगमः - सर्पः	639
Bhujangamam - Sīsakam	भुजंगमम्- सीसकम्	526
Bhūkadambakaḥ - Yawānī (Raj. ni.)	भूकदम्बकः - यवानी (रा. नि.)	170
Bhūlagnā - Śaṅkhapuṣpī (Raj. ni.)	भूलग्ना - शंखपुष्पी (रा.नि.)	349
Bhūmigamaḥ - Gardabhaḥ	भूमिगमः - गर्दभः	622
Bhūmigandhikam - Śāliparṇī viśeṣaḥ	भूमिगंधिकम् - शालिपर्णी विशेषः	32
Bhūmijaḥ - Kadambaḥ (Raj. ni.)	भूमिजः- कदम्बः (रा.नि.)	453
Bhūmijambuḥ - Jambūḥ (Raj. ni.)	भूमिजम्बूः - जम्बूः (रा. नि.)	434
Bhūmikadmbaḥ - Kadambaḥ (Raj. ni.)	भूमिकदम्बः - कदम्बः (रा. नि.)	452
Bhūmilagnā - Viṣṇukrāntā	भूमिलग्ना - विष्णुक्रान्ता	352
Bhūmirajaḥ - Vaikrāntam	भूमिरजः - वैक्रान्तम्	531
Bhūmisahaḥ - Sāgaḥ	भूमिसहः - सागः	522
Bhūnimbaḥ - Kadambaḥ (Raj. ni.)	भूनिम्बः - कदम्बः (रा. नि)	453
Bhūnimbaḥ - Kirātatiktakaḥ	भूनिम्बः - किराततित्तक्कः	13
Bhūpadī - Mallikā	भूपदी - मल्लिका	493
Bhūphalaḥ - Mahāmūṣakaḥ	भूफलः - महामूषकः	631
Bhūribalā - Atibalā	भूरिबला - अतिबला	113
Bhūrigandhā - Murā	भूरिगन्धा - मुरा	229
Bhūṣaṇārham - Suvarṇam	भूषणार्हम् - सुवर्णम्	523
Bhūṣaṇārham- Pravālam	भूषणार्हम्- प्रवालम्	534

Bhūṣaṇārhatamam - Mauktikam	भूषणार्हतमम् - मौक्तिकम्	533
Bhūstaraḥ - Sārameyaḥ	भूस्तरः - सारमेयः	632
Bhūstṛṇaḥ (p. 299)	भूस्तृणः (p. 299)	
Bhūtadrumaḥ - Śleṣmātakaḥ (Raj. ni.)	भूतद्रुमः - श्लेष्मातकः (रा. नि.)	441
Bhūtaghnī - Surasā	भूतघ्नी - सुरसा	301
Bhūtajaṭā - Māmsī (Raj.ni.)	भूतजटा - मांसी (रा.नि.)	217
Bhūtajaṭā - Gandhamāmsī	भूतजटा - गन्धमांसी	217
Bhūtakeśī - Śephālikā	भूतकेशी - शेफालिका	321
Bhūtakeśī - Gandhamāmsī	भूतकेशी - गन्धमांसी	217
Bhūtalikā - Spṛkkā (Raj.ni.)	भूतलिका - स्पृक्का (रा. नि.)	224
Bhūtanāśanaḥ - Sarṣapaḥ	भूतनाशनः - सर्षपः	297
Bhūtanāśanam - Hiṅgu	भूतनाशनम् - हिंगु	137
Bhūtavāsaḥ - Bibhītakaḥ	भूतवासः - बिभीतकः	78
Bhūtavidrāvaṇī - Jīvantī (Raj. ni.)	भूतविद्रावणी - जीवन्ती (रा.नि.)	50
Bhūtidam - Kattṛṇam	भूतिदम् - कत्तृणम्	28
Bhūtiḥ - Bhūstṛṇaḥ	भूतिः - भूस्तृणः	300
Bhūtiḥ - Kattṛṇam	भूतिः - कत्तृणम्	28
Bhūtikaḥ - Bhūstṛṇaḥ	भूतिकः - भूस्तृणः	300
Bhvāmalakī - Tāmalakī	भ्वामलकी - तामलकी	240
Bibhīṣaṇaḥ - Nalaḥ	बिभीषणः - नलः	366
Bibhītakaḥ (p.78)	बिभीतकः (p.78)	
Biḍālaḥ (p. 631)	बिडालः (p. 631)	
Biḍālakaḥ - Bidālaḥ	बिडालकः - बिडालः	631
Biḍālam- Haritālam	बिडालं-हरितालम्	667
Biḍālikā - Vidārī	बिडालिका -विदारी	54
Biḍam (p. 135)	बिडम् (p. 135)	
Bījakaḥ - Aśanaḥ	बीजकः - अशनः	479
Bījakaḥ - Bījapūraḥ	बीजकः- बीजपूरः	396
Bījam - Majjā	बीजम् - मज्जा	619
Bījapūraḥ (p. 395)	बीजपूरः (p. 395)	
Bījapūrṇaḥ - Bījapūraḥ	बीजपूर्णः - बीजपूरः	396
Bījarecakaḥ - Jayapālaḥ	बीजरेचकः - जयपालः	86
Bījasnehaḥ - Kimśukaḥ	बीजस्नेहः - किंशुकः	518
Bījavaraḥ - Rājamāṣaḥ	बीजवरः - राजमाषः	542
Bilvagandhakaḥ - Kuṭherakaḥ	बिल्वगंधकः - कुठेरकः	304
Bilvaḥ (p.39)	बिल्वः (p.39)	
Bilvikā - Hiṅgupatrī	बिल्विका - हिंगुपत्री	138
Bimbī (p.76)	बिम्बी (p.76)	
Bindukinī - Āvartakī	बिन्दुकिनी - आवर्तकी	74

Bisam (p. 376)	बिसम् (p. 376)	
Bisinī - Bisam	बिसिनी - बिसम्	376
Bodhivṛkṣaḥ - Pippalaḥ	बोधिवृक्षः - पिप्पलः	427
Bolam (p.226)	बोलम् (p.226)	
Boṭam - Śāliparṇī viśeṣaḥ	बोटम् - शालिपर्णी विशेषः	32
Brahamaputraḥ	ब्रह्मपुत्रः	665
Bṛahatpālī (p.159)(Jī.viśeṣaḥ)	बृहत्पाली (जीरक विशेषः) (159)	
Bṛahatpuṣpī - Śaṇapuṣpī	बृहत्पुष्पी - शणपुष्पी	75
Brahmabhūmijā-a type of Śreyasī (Raj.ni.)	ब्रह्मभूमिजा-श्रेयसी विशेषः(रा.नि.)	163
Brahmacāriṇam - Tūdam	ब्रह्मचारिणम् - तूदम्	417
Brahmadāru - Tūdam	ब्रह्मदारु - तूदम्	417
Brahmajaṭaḥ - Damanaḥ	ब्रह्मजटः - दमनः	228
Brāhmakandaḥ - Vārāhī (Raj. ni.)	ब्राह्मकन्दः - वाराही (रा. नि.)	327
Brahmakāṣṭhakam - Tūdam	ब्रह्मकाष्ठकम् - तूदम्	417
Brahmamekhalaḥ - Muñjaḥ	ब्रह्ममेखलः - मुञ्जः	360
Brāhmaṇayaṣṭikā - Bhārṅgī	ब्राह्मणयष्टिका - भाङ्र्गी	24
Brāhmaṇeṣṭam - Tūdam	ब्राह्मणेष्टम् - तूदम्	417
Brāhmaṇī - Spṛkka	ब्राह्मणी - स्पृक्का	224
Brahmāṇī - Pittalam	ब्रह्माणी - पित्तलम्	526
Brahmaṇyam - Tūdam	ब्रह्मण्यम् - तूदम्	417
Brahmapādapaḥ - Vikaṅkataḥ (Raj. ni.)	ब्रह्मपादपः -विकंकतः (रा.नि.)	405
Brahmapavitraḥ -Kuśaḥ (Raj. ni.)	ब्रह्मपवित्रः - कुशः (रा.नि.)	362
Brahmaputrī - Vārāhī (Raj. ni.)	ब्रह्मपुत्री - वाराही (रा. नि.)	327
Brahmarītiḥ - Pittalam	ब्रह्मरीतिः - पित्तलम्	526
Brahmasuvarcalā - Bhārṅgī	ब्रह्मसुवर्चला - भाङ्र्गी	24
Brahmasuvarcalā - Brāhmī	ब्रह्मसुवर्चला - ब्राह्मी	336
Brahmavṛkṣaḥ - Kiṃśukaḥ	ब्रह्मवृक्षः - किंशुकः	518
Brahmavṛkṣakaḥ - Kiṃśukaḥ	ब्रह्मवृक्षकः - किंशुकः	518
Brāhmī - Vācā	ब्राह्मी - वाचा	616
Brāhmī (p. 336)	ब्राह्मी (p. 336)	
Bṛhaddalā - Vaiparītyā Lajjāluḥ	बृहद्दला -वैपरीत्या लज्जालुः	345
Bṛhadelā - Bhadrailā	बृहदेला -भद्रैला	142
Bṛhadrāvaḥ - Kṣudrolūkaḥ	बृहद्रावः - क्षुद्रोलूकः	638
Bṛhatī (p.34)	बृहती (p.34)	
Bṛhatpañcamūlam	बृहत्पञ्चमूलम्	649
Bṛhatpārevatam -Pālevatam (Raj. ni.)	बृहत्पारेवतम् -पालेवतम् (रा.नि.)	418
Bṛhatparṇaḥ - Paṭṭikārodhraḥ	बृहत्पर्णः -पट्टिकारोध्रः	270
Bṛhatphalā - Mahābalā	बृहत्फला - महाबला	111

Bṛhatphalā - Kūṣmāṇḍikā	बृहत्फला - कूष्माण्डिका	68
Bṛhatpīluḥ (Raj. ni.) (p.410)	बृहत्पीलुः (रा.नि.) (p.410)	
Bṛhatpuṣpā - Kubjakaḥ	बृहत्पुष्पा - कुब्जकः	503
Bṛhattiktā - Pāṭhā	बृहत्तिक्ता - पाठा	26
Bahuvāhā - Kāsaghnī	बहुवाहा - कासघ्नी	37
Budharatnam - Gārutmatam	बुधरत्नम् - गारुत्मतम्	531
Būkaḍakaḥ - Chāgaḥ	बूकडकः - छागः	622
Bukaḥ (p. 284)	बुकः (p. 284)	
Chacchikā - Takram	छच्छिका - तक्रम्	587
Caityadrumaḥ - Pippalaḥ	चैत्यद्रुमः -पिप्पलः	427
Cakraḥ - Cakravākaḥ	चक्रः - चक्रवाकः	635
Cakrāhvaḥ - Cakramardaḥ	चक्राह्वः - चक्रमर्दः	277
Cakrāhvaḥ - Cakravākaḥ	चक्राह्वः - चक्रवाकः	635
Cakralakṣaṇā- Guḍūcī	चक्रलक्षणा - गुडूची	2
Cakramardaḥ (p. 277)	चक्रमर्दः (p. 277)	
Cakrāṅgī - Kaṭukā	चक्राङ्गी -कटुका	15
Cakrarathaḥ - Cakravākaḥ	चक्ररथः - चक्रवाकः	635
Cakravāk - Cakravākaḥ	चक्रवाक्- चक्रवाकः	635
Cakravākaḥ (p. 634)	चक्रवाकः (p. 634)	
Cakravartinī - Māṃsī (Raj.ni.)	चक्रवर्तिनी - मांसी (रा.नि.)	217
Cakravartinī -Jantukārī	चक्रवर्तिनी - जन्तुकारी	324
Cakrī - Cakramardaḥ	चक्री - चक्रमर्दः	277
Cakrī - Cakravākaḥ	चक्री- चक्रवाकः	635
Cakrikaḥ - Cakramardaḥ	चक्रिकः - चक्रमर्द	277
Cakṣuḥśravā - Sarpaḥ	चक्षुःश्रवा - सर्पः	639
Cakṣuṣyā (p. 263)	चक्षुष्या (p. 263)	
Calaḥ - Nakham	चलः - नखम्	223
Calapatraḥ - Pippalaḥ	चलपत्रः -पिप्पलः	427
Camarikaḥ - Kovidāraḥ	चमरिकः - कोविदारः	73
Cāmīkaram - Suvarṇam	चामीकरम् - सुवर्णम्	523
Campakarambhā - Suvarṇakadalī	चम्पकरम्भा- सुवर्णकदली	318
Cāmpeyaḥ - Campakaḥ	चाम्पेयः - चम्पकः	500
Cāmpeyam - Nāgakesaram	चाम्पेयम् - नागकेसरम्	143
Caṇakaḥ (p. 553)	चणकः (p. 553)	
Cāṇākhyamūlkam (p. 293)	चाणाख्यमूलकम् (p. 293)	
Cañcuḥ - Raktairaṇḍaḥ	चञ्चुः - रक्तैरण्डः	117
Caṇḍā - Dravantī	चण्डा - द्रवन्ती	87
Caṇḍā - Corakaḥ	चण्डा - चोरकः	232
Caṇḍā - Kapikacchuḥ	चण्डा - कपिकच्छुः	55

Caṇḍakaḥ - Karavīraḥ चण्डकः - करवीरः 275
Candanā - Kr. Sārivā चन्दना - कृ. सारिवा 60
Candana Sārivā - Kr. Sārivā चन्दनसारिवा - कृ. सारिवा 60
Candanagopā - Kr. Sārivā चन्दनगोपा - कृ. सारिवा 60
Candanam (p. 191) चन्दनम् (p. 191)
Candanapuspam - Lavangam चन्दनपुष्पम् - लवङ्गम् 214
Caṇḍātakaḥ - Karavīraḥ चण्डातकः - करवीरः 275
Caṇḍīkusumaḥ - Karavīraḥ (Raj. ni.)चण्डीकुसुमः - करवीरः (रा. नि.) 276
Candrabhūtiḥ - Raupyam चन्द्रभूतिः - रौप्यम् 524
Candracandanam - Haricandanamचन्द्रचन्दनम् - हरिचन्दनम् 196
Candragandhā- Śaṭhī चन्द्रगन्धा - शठी 22
Candraḥ - Karpūraḥ चन्द्रः -कर्पूरः 209
Candrahāsā - Guḍūcī चन्द्रहासा- गुडूची 2
Candrahāsam - Raupyam चन्द्रहासम् - रौप्यम् 524
Candrakaḥ - Aśmantakaḥ चन्द्रकः - अश्मन्तकः 72
Candrakānta Jalam चन्द्रकान्तजलम् 607
Candralekhā - Bākucī चन्द्रलेखा - बाकुची 61
Candrāṇī - Śaṭhī चन्द्राणी - शठी 22
Candrapuṣpā - Kāsaghnī चन्द्रपुष्पा - कासघ्नी 37
Candrapuṣpā - Lakśmaṇā चन्द्रपुष्पा - लक्ष्मणा 37
Candrāspadā - Karkaṭaśṛṅgī चन्द्रास्पदा - कर्कटश्रृंगी 30
Candravallī - Prasāraṇī (Raj. ni.) चन्द्रवल्ली - प्रसारणी (रा.नि.) 115
Candravapuḥ - Raupyam चन्द्रवपुः - रौप्यम् 524
Cāngerī - Kśudrāmlikā चांगेरी - क्षुद्राम्लिका 399
Capalā - Pippalī चपला - पिप्पली 160
Capalaḥ - Pāradaḥ चपलः - पारदः 529
Cāpavaṭaḥ - Priyālaḥ चापवटः -प्रियालः 423
Cāraḥ- Priyālaḥ चारः -प्रियालः 424
Caraṇāyudhaḥ - Kukkuṭaḥ चरणायुधः - कुक्कुटः 636
Cāraṭī - Padmacāriṇī चारटी- पद्मचारिणी 325
Carma - Twak चर्म - त्वक् 644
Carmajam - Roma चर्मजम् - रोम 644
Carmakaṣā - Sātalā चर्मकषा - सातला 89
Carmakasā - Māmsarohiṇī चर्मकसा - मांसरोहिणी 330
Carmānurañjanam - Hiṅgulam चर्मानुरञ्जनम् - हिंगुलम् 530
Carmaraṅgā - Āvartakī चर्मरङ्गा - आवर्तकी 74
Cāru - Kumkumam चारु - कुंकुमम् 197
Cārudarśanaḥ - Plakśaḥ चारुदर्शनः -प्लक्षः 429
Cāruḥ - Padmakaḥ चारुः - पद्मकः 242

Cārukesarā - Taruṇī चारुकेसरा - तरुणी 501
Cārulocanaḥ - Hariṇaḥ चारुलोचनः - हरिणः 625
Cārumodā - Yūthikā चारुमोदा - यूथिका 504
Cāruparṇī - Prasāraṇī चारुपर्णी - प्रसारणी 114
Cāruphalā - Drākṡā चारुफला - द्राक्षा 413
Cāruratnam - Suvarṇam चारुरत्नम् - सुवर्णम् 523
Cārurūpam - Suvarṇam चारुरूपम् - सुवर्णम् 523
Caṭakī- Cūḍāmaṇiḥ चटकी - चूडामणिः 291
Caturaṅgulaḥ - Āragvadhaḥ चतुरङ्गुलः - आरग्वधः 80
Cāturbhadrakam चातुर्भद्रकम् 646
Cāturjātakasangatā - Marjikā चातुर्जातकसंगता - मर्जिका 605
Catuṣparṇī - Kṡudrāmlikā चतुष्पर्णी - क्षुद्राम्लिका 399
Catuṣphalā -Gāngerukī (Raj. ni.) चतुष्फला - गांगेरुकी (रा.नि.) 112
Cauhāraḥ - Yawānikā चौहारः - यवानिका 171
Cavalaḥ - Rājamāṣaḥ चवलः - राजमाषः 542
Cāvalikā - Dhānyakam चावलिका - धान्यकम् (रा. नि.) 156
Cavikā (p.161) चविका (p.161)
Cavikam - Cavikā चविकम् - चविका 162
Cavikāṡiraḥ - Pippalīmūlam चविकाशिरः - पिप्पलीमूलम् 161
Cavyam - Cavikā चव्यम् - चविका 162
Cavyaphalā - Ṡreyasī (Raj. ni.) चव्यफला - श्रेयसी (रा.नि.) 163
Cetakī - Harītakī चेतकी - हरीतकी 77
Cetikā - Jātī चेतिका - जाती 496
Chadanam - Tamālapatram छदनम् - तमालपत्रम् 146
Chāgaḥ (p. 622) छागः (p. 622)
Chagalaḥ - Chāgaḥ छगलः - छागः 622
Chagalāntrī - Vṛddhadārukaḥ छगलान्त्री - वृद्धदारुकः 343
Chagalāntrikā - Vṛṣamedhā छगलान्त्रिका -वृषमेधा 118
Chakṡuṣyam - Prapauṇḍarīkam चक्षुष्यम् -प्रपौण्डरीकम् 243
Campakaḥ (p. 499) चम्पकः (p. 499)
Chandrabālā - Elā चन्द्रबाला - एला 141
Chardanaḥ - Madanaḥ छर्दनः - मदनः 62
Chardikā - Viṡṇukrāntā (Raj. ni.) छर्दिका -विष्णुक्रान्ता (रा.नि.) 353
Chatrā - Miṡreyā (Raj. ni.) छत्रा - मिश्रेया (रा. नि.) 123
Chatradhānyam - Dhānyakam छत्रधान्यम् - धान्यकम् 156
Chatraḥ - Bhūstṛnaḥ छत्रः - भूस्तृणः 300
Chatrākī- Gandhanākulī छत्राकी - गन्धनाकुली 342
Chatraparṇaḥ - Saptaparṇaḥ छत्रपर्णः - सप्तपर्णः 238
Chatrapuṣpakaḥ - Tilakaḥ छत्रपुष्पकः - तिलकः 513

Chedanīyam - Katakam	छेदनीयम् - कतकम्	267
Chinnā - Guḍūcī	छिन्ना - गुडूची	2
Chinnagranthinikā-Mahāśravaṇī	छिन्नग्रन्थिनिका - महाश्रावणी	58
Chinnāṅgī - Guḍūcī	छिन्नांगी - गुडूची	2
Chinnapatrā -Ambaṣṭhā (Raj. ni.)	छिन्नपत्रा - अम्बष्ठा (रा.नि.)	249
Chinnaruhā - Guḍūcī	छिन्नरुहा - गुडूची	2
Chinnaruhaḥ - Tilakaḥ (Raj. ni.)	छिन्नरुहः - तिलकः (रा.नि.)	514
Chinnodbhavā - Guḍūcī	छिन्नोद्भवा -गुडूची	2
Chuchundarī - Anyā Āmūṣikā	छुछुन्दरी -अन्या आमूषिका	630
Ciḍā - Saralaḥ	चिडा - सरलः	237
Ciḍā - Kapaṭam	चिडा - कपटम्	29
Cikkā - Pūgaphalam	चिक्का - पूगफलम्	213
Cikkaṇā - Pūgaphalam	चिक्कणा- पूगफलम्	213
Cikkaṇam - Pūgaphalam	चिक्कणम् - पूगफलम्	213
Cilicimaḥ - Matsyaviśeṣaḥ	चिलिचिमः -मत्स्य विशेषः	628
Cīnakaḥ - Kanguḥ	चीनकः - कङ्गुः	546
Ciñcā - Amlikā	चिञ्चा - अम्लिका	398
Ciñcikā - Amlikā	चिञ्चिका - अम्लिका	398
Cirabilvakaḥ - Karañjaḥ	चिरबिल्वकः - करञ्जः	456
Cirajīvī - Jīvakaḥ	चिरजीवी - जीवकः	44
Cirajīvī - Kākaḥ	चिरजीवी - काकः	637
Cirajīvikā - Śālmalī	चिरजीविका - शाल्मली	481
Ciraluḥ - Mahāmatsyaviśeṣaḥ	चिरलुः - महामत्स्य विशेषः	628
Cirapatrakaḥ - Sarjakaḥ	चिरपत्रकः - सर्जकः	476
Cīrapiṣṭakam - Sīsakam	चीरपिष्टकम् - सीसकम्	526
Cirāyuḥ - Bhallaḥ	चिरायुः - भल्लः	637
Cirbhaṭam (p.66)	चिर्भटम् (p. 66)	
Cīritapatrakā - Nākulī	चीरितपत्रका - नाकुली	339
Cirapākī - Kapitthaḥ	चिरपाकी - कपित्थः	187
Citrā - Dravantī	चित्रा - द्रवन्ती	86
Citrabhānuḥ -Citrakaḥ	चित्रभानुः - चित्रकः	165
Citrabheṣajā - Kākodumbarikā	चित्रभेषजा - काकोदुम्बरिका	438
Citradehaḥ - Lāvaḥ	चित्रदेहः - लावः	636
Citragandhakam - Haritālam	चित्रगन्धकं- हरितालं	667
Citraghanā - Sātāla (Raj. ni.)	चित्रघना - सातला (रा.नि.)	89
Citraḥ - Aśokaḥ	चित्रः - अशोकः	516
Citraḥ - Tilakaḥ	चित्रः - तिलकः	513
Citraḥ - Eraṇḍaḥ	चित्रः - एरण्डः	117
Citrakaḥ (p. 164)	चित्रकः (p. 164)	

Citrakāyaḥ - Śarabhaḥ	चित्रकायः - शरभः	624
Citraphalā - Viśala	चित्रफला - विशाला	95
Citraphalā - Vṛntākī (Raj. ni.)	चित्रफला - वृन्ताकी (रा. नि.)	37
Citraphalam - Śīrṇavṛntam	चित्रफलं - शीर्णवृन्तम्	66
Citrapicchakaḥ - Mayūraḥ	चित्रपिच्छकः - मयूरः	633
Citrapṛṣṭhaḥ - Anyaḥ Kacchapaḥ	चित्रपृष्ठः -अन्यः कच्छपः	630
Citrapuṣpī - Ambaṣṭhā (Raj. ni.)	चित्रपुष्पी - अम्बष्ठा (रा. नि.)	249
Citrataṇḍulā - Viḍaṅgam	चित्रतण्डुला - विडङ्गम्	130
Citravarṇakaḥ-(Sarpaḥ)-Vyantaraḥ	चित्रवर्णकः (सर्पः) - व्यन्तरः	639
Citravyāghraḥ - Śarabhaḥ	चित्रव्याघ्रः - शरभः	624
Citrayodhī - Arjunaḥ	चित्रयोधी -अर्जुनः	464
Cocam -Twak	चोचम् - त्वक्	145
Corakaḥ (p. 232)	चोरकः (p. 232)	
Cūḍāmaṇiḥ (p.291)	चूडामणिः (p.291)	
Cūḍāmlabījam-Vṛkśāmlam (Raj.ni.)	चूडाम्लबीजम्-वृक्षाम्लम् (रा.नि.)	173
Cukrā - Amlikā	चुक्रा- अम्लिका	398
Cukram - Śūktam	चुक्रम् - शुक्तम्	594
Cukrikā - Amlikā	चुक्रिका - अम्लिका	398
Cūlinī - Śālmalī	चूलिनी - शाल्मली	481
Cullakaḥ - Matsyabhedaḥ	चुल्लकः - मत्स्यभेदः	628
Cumbakam -Kānta Loham	चुम्बकम् -कान्तलोहम्	528
Curṇam - Kamkolam	चूर्णम् - कंक्कोलम्	213
Curṇapāradam - Hiṅgulam	चूर्णपारदम् - हिंगुलम्	530
Cūtaḥ - Āmraḥ	चूतः - आम्रः	385
Dadhi - Śriveṣṭakaḥ	दधि - श्रीवेष्टकः	255
Dadhi (582)	दधि (582)	
Dadhibhavam - Navanītam	दधिभवम् - नवनीतम्	591
Dadhimaṇḍodbhavam - Navanītam	दधिमण्डोद्भवम् - नवनीतम्	591
Dadhiphalaḥ - Kapitthaḥ	दधिफलः - कपित्थः	187
Dadhipuṣpī (p.55)	दधिपुष्पी (p.55)	
Dadhitthaḥ - Kapitthaḥ	दधित्थः - कपित्थः	187
Dadhyamlam - Mathita dadhi	दध्यम्लम् - मथित दधि	583
Dāḍimaḥ (p. 155)	दाडिमः (p. 155)	
Dāḍimapuṣpakaḥ - Rohitakaḥ	दाडिमपुष्पकः - रोहितकः	485
Dāḍimīsāraḥ - Daḍimaḥ	दाडिमीसारः -दाडिमः	155
Dadrughnaḥ-Cakramardaḥ (Raj.ni.)	दद्रुघ्नः - चक्रमर्दः (रा.नि.)	277
Dagdham - Śāliparṇī viśeṣaḥ	दग्धम् - शालिपर्णी विशेषः	32
Dagdharuhaḥ - Tilakaḥ (Raj. ni.)	दग्धरुहः - तिलकः (रा.नि.)	514
Dāhadā - Tāmbūlī	दाहदा - ताम्बूली	273
Dahanaḥ - Bhallātakaḥ	दहनः - भल्लातकः	259

Dahanaḥ - Citrakaḥ दहनः – चित्रकः 165
Dahanam - Śuktam दहनम् – शुक्तम् 594
Daityā - Murā दैत्या – मुरा 229
Dakśaḥ - Kukkuṭaḥ दक्षः – कुक्कुटः 636
Dākśiṇātyakaḥ - Nārikelaḥ दाक्षिणात्यकः – नारिकेलः 425
Dalam - Tamālapatram दलम् – तमालपत्रम् 146
Dalapuṣpā - Ketakī (Raj. ni.) दलपुष्पा – केतकी (रा.नि.) 521
Damaḥ (p. 229) दमः (p. 229)
Damanaḥ (p. 228) दमनः (p. 228)
Damavaśānvitaḥ - Damaḥ दमवशान्वितः – दमः 229
Daṁśaḥ - Śigruḥ दंशः – शिग्रुः 295
Daṁśī - Mahiṣaḥ दंशी– महिषः 625
Daṁṣṭrī - Sūkaraḥ दंष्ट्री – सूकरः 624
Daṁṣṭrī - Sarpaḥ दंष्ट्री – सर्पः 638
Damyaḥ - Vṛṣabhaḥ दम्यः – वृषभः 626
Dānavapriyā - Tāmbūlī दानवप्रिया – ताम्बूली 273
Daṇḍāhatam - Mathita dadhi दण्डाहतं – मथित दधि 583
Dandaśūkaḥ - Sarpaḥ दन्दशूकः – सर्पः 639
Ḍāṅgarī - Ḍaṅgarī डाङ्गरी – डङ्गरी 67
Ḍāṅgārī - Ḍaṅgarī डाङ्गारी – डङ्गरी 67
Ḍaṅgarī (p.67) डङ्गरी (p.67)
Ḍaṅgariḥ - Ḍaṅgarī डङ्गरिः – डङ्गरी 67
Dantadhāvanaḥ - Khadiraḥ दन्तधावनः – खदिरः 9
Dāntaḥ - Damanaḥ दान्तः – दमनः 228
Dāntaḥ - Vṛṣabhaḥ दान्तः – वृषभः 626
Dantaharṣaṇaḥ - Jambīraḥ दन्तहर्षणः – जम्बीरः 389
Dantaśaṭhā - Kśudrāmlikā दन्तशठा – क्षुद्राम्लिका 399
Dantaśaṭhaḥ - Jambīraḥ दन्तशठः– जम्बीरः 389
Dantāyudhaḥ - Sūkaraḥ दन्तायुधः – सूकरः 624
Dantī - Hasti दन्ती – हस्ति 620
Dantī (p.84) दन्ती (p.84)
Dantībījam - Jayapālaḥ दन्तीबीजम् – जयपालः 86
Daradam - Hiṅgulam दरदम् – हिंगुलम् 530
Darbha patraḥ - Kāśaḥ (Raj. ni.) दर्भपत्रः – काशः (रा.नि.) 359
Darbharaḥ - Lāvaḥ दर्भरः – लावः 636
Darduraḥ - Maṇḍūkaḥ दर्दुरः – मण्डूकः 640
Dāru - Devadāruḥ दारु – देवदारुः 27
Dāruharidrā (p.21) दारुहरिद्रा (p.21)
Dārukaṇṭakaḥ - Pittalam दारुकण्टकः – पित्तलम् 526

Dāruṇaḥ - Citrakaḥ	दारुणः - चित्रकः	165
Dāruniśā - Dāruharidrā	दारुनिशा - दारुहरिद्रा	21
Dārupatrikā - Hiṅgupatrī	दारुपत्रिका - हिंगुपत्री	138
Dārvīkwāthasamudbhavam - Rasāñjanam	दार्वीक्वाथसमुद्भवम् - रसाञ्जनम्	265
Daśamūlam	दशमूलम्	649
Dāsapuram - Paripellavam	दासपुरम् - परिपेल्लवम्	222
Dāśapuram - Jalamustam	दाशपुरम् - जलमुस्तम्	16
Daśarathaḥ - Śarīram	दशरथः - शरीरम्	615
Dāserakaḥ - Uṣṭraḥ	दासेरकः - उष्ट्रः	621
Dāsī - Kākajaṅghā	दासी - काकजङ्घा	287
Dāsī -Saireyakaḥ (Raj. ni.)	दासी - सैरेयकः (रा.नि.)	110
Dātyūhaḥ - Kākaḥ (p.637)	दात्यूहः -काकः (p.638)	
Daugdhrī - Goḥ	दौग्ध्री - गोः	626
Dehacarma - Twak	देहचर्म - त्वक्	644
Dehadhāraṇam - Asthi	देहधारणम् - अस्थि	618
Dehaḥ - Śarīram	देहः - शरीरम्	615
Devadālī - Jīmūtakaḥ	देवदाली - जीमूतकः	64
Devadāruḥ (p.27)	देवदारुः (p.27)	
Devadaṁśakam - Kattṛṇam	देवदंशकम् - कत्तृणम्	28
Devadundubhiḥ - Surasā	देवदुन्दुभिः - सुरसा	301
Devakāṣṭham - Devadāruḥ	देवकाष्ठम् - देवदारुः	27
Devakusumam - Lavaṅgam	देवकुसुमम् - लवङ्गम्	214
Devamaṇiḥ - Mahāmdeā	देवमणिः - महामेदा	46
Devanālaḥ - Mahānalaḥ	देवनालः - महानलः	367
Devānāmpriyā - Tāmbūlī	देवानांप्रिया - ताम्बूली	273
Devanirmitā - Guḍūcī	देवनिर्मिता - गुडूची	2
Devapriyaḥ-Bhṛṅgarājaḥ (Raj.ni.)	देवप्रियः - भृङ्गराजः (रा. नि.)	281
Devaputrī - Spṛkkā	देवपुत्री - स्पृक्का	224
Devārhā - Mahābalā (Raj. ni.)	देवार्हा - महाबला (रा.नि.)	111
Devasahā - Mahābalā	देवसहा - महाबला	111
Devaśekharaḥ-Damanaḥ (Raj.ni.)	देवशेखरः - दमनः (रा. नि.)	228
Devaśreṇī -Mūrvā	देवश्रेणी - मूर्वा	5
Devatā - Dhattūraḥ	देवता - धत्तूरः	278
Devatāḍaḥ - Jīmūtakaḥ	देवताडः - जीमूतकः	64
Devī - Spṛkkā	देवी - स्पृक्का	224
Devī - Murvā	देवी-मूर्वा	5
Devī - Pāṭhā	देवी - पाठा	26
Devī - Vandhyakarkoṭakī	देवी - वन्ध्यकर्कोटकी	68

Devī -Karkoṭakī देवी - कर्कोटकी 69
Dhamanaḥ - Nalaḥ धमनः - नलः 366
Dhamanī - Nalikā धमनी - नलिका 216
Dhāmārgavaḥ (p.69) धामार्गवः (p.69)
Dhanañjayaḥ - Arjunaḥ धनंजयः -अर्जुनः 464
Dhāneyakam - Dhānyakam धानेयकम् - धान्यकम् 156
Dhānī - Dhānyakam धानी - धान्यकम् 156
Dhānī - Pīluḥ धानी - पीलुः 409
Dhanuḥ - Bhallātakaḥ धनुः - भल्लातकः 259
Dhanurdrumaḥ -Vamsaḥ (Raj.ni.) धनुर्द्रुमः - वंशः (रा.नि.) 365
Dhanvayāsaḥ (p. 7) धन्वयासः (p. 7)
Dhanvayavāsakaḥ - Dhanvayāsaḥ धन्वयवासकः - धन्वयासः 7
Dhānyā - Dhānyakam धान्या - धान्यकम् 156
Dhānyakā - Dhānyakam धान्यका - धान्यकम् 156
Dhānyakam (p. 155) धान्यकम् (p. 155)
Dhānyamāṣaḥ - Māṣaḥ धान्यमाषः - माषः 552
Dhānyāmlam - Kāñjikam धान्याम्लम् - काञ्जिकम् 595
Dhārā - Guḍūcī धारा - गुडूची 2
Dharā - Medā धरा - मेदा 46
Dhārākadambaḥ - Kadambaḥ धाराकदम्बः - कदम्बः 451
Dharaṇī dharaṇakṡamaḥ - Anyaḥ kacchapaḥ
धरणीधरणक्षमः -अन्यः कच्छपः 630
Dharaṇīdharaḥ - Kacchapaḥ धरणीधरः - कच्छपः 630
Dhārāphalā - Kośātakī धाराफला - कोशातकी (रा.नि.) 72
Dharmapattanam - Maricam धर्मपत्तनम् - मरिचम् 168
Dharmavṛkṡaḥ - Pippalaḥ धर्मवृक्षः -पिप्पलः 427
Dhārtarāṣṭraḥ - Hamsaḥ धार्तराष्ट्रः - हंसः 635
Dhārtarāṣṭrapadī -Viśvagranthiḥ (Raj. ni.)
धार्तराष्ट्रपदी -विश्वगंथिः (रा.नि.) 348
Dhātakī - Dhātukī धातकी - धातुकी 242
Dhātavaḥ धातवः 663
Dhātrīphalam - Āmalakī धात्रीफलम् - आमलकी 79
Dhattūraḥ (p. 278) धत्तूरः (p. 278)
Dhātuhā - Gandhakaḥ धातुहा - गन्धकः 248
Dhātujamadrijam - Śilājatuḥ धातुजमद्रिजम् - शिलाजतुः 266
Dhātukāsīsam - Kāsīsam धातुकासीसम् - कासीसम् 251
Dhātukī (p. 242) धातुकी (p. 242)
Dhātumākṡikam - Hemamākṡikam धातुमाक्षिकम् - हेममाक्षिकम् 261
Dhavaḥ (p. 522) धवः (p. 522)

Dhavalaḥ - Śaṅkhaḥ	धवलः - शंखः	271
Dhavalaḥ - Dhavaḥ (Raj.ni.)	धवलः - धवः (रा.नि.)	522
Dhāvanī - Kaṇṭakārī	धावनी - कण्टकारी	35
Dhāvanī - Pṛśniparṇī	धावनी - पृश्निपर्णी	33
Dhenudugdham - Cirbhaṭam	धेनुदुग्धम् -चिर्भटम्	67
Dhenuḥ - Goḥ	धेनुः - गोः	626
Dhenukā - Hastinī	धेनुका - हस्तिनी	620
Dhīraḥ - Ṛṣabhaḥ	धीरः - ऋषभः	45
Dhīram - Puṣkaramūlam	धीरम् - पुष्करमूलम्	23
Dhruvā - Śāliparṇī	ध्रुवा - शालिपर्णी	32
Dhruvaḥ - Vaṭaḥ	ध्रुवः- वटः	426
Dhūlijaṅghaḥ - Kākaḥ	धूलिजङ्घः - काकः	637
Dhūlikadambaḥ - Kadambaḥ	धूलिकदम्बः - कदम्बः	452
Dhūmraḥ - Uṣṭraḥ	धूम्रः - उष्ट्रः	621
Dhūmraḥ - Turuṣkaḥ	धूम्रः - तुरुष्कः	204
Dhūhmravarṇaḥ - Turuṣkaḥ	धूम्रवर्णः- तुरुष्कः	204
Dhūpavṛkśaḥ - Śrīveṣṭakaḥ	धूपवृक्षः - श्रीवेष्टकः	255
Dhurandhurī - Dhavaḥ	धुरन्धुरी - धवः	522
Dhūrtā - Kokilā	धूर्ता - कोकिला	637
Dhūrtaḥ - Dhattūraḥ	धूर्तः - धत्तूरः	278
Dhūrtam - Biḍam	धूर्तम् - बिडम्	135
Dhūrvahaḥ - Vṛṣabhaḥ	धूर्वहः - वृषभः	626
Dhūsaraḥ - Uṣṭraḥ	धूसरः - उष्ट्रः	621
Dhūsaraḥ - Gardabhaḥ	धूसरः - गर्दभः	622
Dhvāṅkśajaṅghā - Kākajaṅghā	ध्वाङ्क्षजङ्घा - काकजङ्घा	287
Dhvāṅkśanakhī - Kākādanī	ध्वाङ्क्षनखी - काकादनी	290
Dhwajadrumaḥ - Tālaḥ	ध्वजद्रुमः - तालः	419
Dhwajavṛkśaḥ - Māḍaḥ	ध्वजवृक्षः - माडः	422
Dhwāṅkśaḥ - Kākaḥ	ध्वाङ्क्षः - काकः	637
Dhwāṅkśamācī - Kākamācī	ध्वाङ्क्षमाची - काकमाची	285
Dhwāṅkśanāsā - Kākanāsā	ध्वाङ्क्षनासा - काकनासा	289
Dhwāṅkśanāśinī - Aparā Hapuṣā	ध्वाङ्क्षनाशिनी - अपरा हपुषा	128
Dhwāṅkśatuṇḍaphalā - Kākanāsā	ध्वाङ्क्षतुण्डफला - काकनासा	289
Dhwāṅkśolikā - Kākolī	ध्वांक्षोलिका - काकोली	47
Dhyāmakam - Kattṛṇam	ध्यामकम् - कत्तृणम्	28
Dīnam - Tagaram	दीनम् - तगरम्	221
Dīpanī - Yawānī	दीपनी - यवानी	169
Dīpanī - Methikā	दीपनी - मेथिका	562
Dīpanīyā - Yawānī	दीपनीया - यवानी	169

Dīpavṛkśaḥ - Saralaḥ	दीपवृक्षः - सरलः	237
Dīptā - Kalikārī	दीप्ता - कलिकारी	280
Dīptā - Sātalā	दीप्ता - सातला	89
Dīptalocanaḥ - Biḍālaḥ	दीप्तलोचनः - बिडालः	631
Dīptiḥ - Lākśā	दीप्तिः - लाक्षा	239
Dīpyā (p. 412)	दीप्या (p. 412)	
Dīpyaḥ - Yawānī	दीप्यः - यवानी	169
Dīpyakaḥ - Ajamodā	दीप्यकः - अजमोदा	183
Dīpyakaḥ - Yawānī	दीप्यकः- यवानी	169
Dīpyam - Jīrakam	दीप्यम् - जीरकम्	157
Dīrghadaṇḍakaḥ - Eraṇḍaḥ	दीर्घदण्डकः - एरण्डः	117
Dīrghadarśī - Bhallaḥ	दीर्घदर्शी - भल्लः	637
Dīrghagrīvaḥ - Uṣṭraḥ	दीर्घग्रीवः - उष्ट्रः	621
Dīrghaḥ - Māḍaḥ	दीर्घः - माडः	422
Dīrghajaṅghaḥ - Uṣṭraḥ	दीर्घजङ्घः - उष्ट्रः	621
Dīrghajīrakaḥ - Śuklajīrakaḥ	दीर्घजीरकः - शुक्लजीरकः	157
Dīrghakaḥ - Śuklajīrakaḥ	दीर्घकः - शुक्लजीरकः	157
Dīrghakaḥ - Śigruḥ	दीर्घकः - शिग्रुः	295
Dīrghakam - Jīrakam	दीर्घकम् - जीरकम्	156
Dīrghakaṇā - Śuklajīrakaḥ	दीर्घकणा - शुक्लजीरकः	157
Dīrghakeśaḥ - Bhallaḥ	दीर्घकेशः - भल्लः	637
Dīrghakīlakaḥ - Aṅkoṭakaḥ	दीर्घकीलकः - अङ्कोटकः	99
Dīrgham - Kattṛṇam (Raj. ni.)	दीर्घम् - कत्तृणम् (रा.नि)	28
Dīrghamārgagaḥ - Uṣṭraḥ	दीर्घमार्गगः - उष्ट्रः	621
Dīrghamūlaḥ - Moraṭaḥ	दीर्घमूलः - मोरटः	6
Dīrghamūlam - Lāmajjakam	दीर्घमूलम् - लामज्जकम्	241
Dīrghanisvanaḥ - Śaṅkhaḥ	दीर्घनिस्वनः - शंखः	271
Dīrghapādapaḥ - Pūgīvṛkśaḥ	दीर्घपादपः -पूगीवृक्षः	214
Dīrghaparṇī - Pṛśni. viśesaḥ	दीर्घपर्णी - पृश्नि. विशेषः	33
Dīrghaparṇī - Trapusam	दीर्घपर्णी - त्रपुसम्	65
Dīrghapatrā - Kadalī	दीर्घपत्रा - कदली	316
Dīrghapatraḥ - Jaladaḥ	दीर्घपत्रः -जलदः	408
Dīrghapatraḥ - Sāgaḥ (Raj. ni.)	दीर्घपत्रः - सागः (रा.नि.)	522
Dīrghapatraḥ - Punarnavā	दीर्घपत्रः - पुनर्नवा	107
Dīrghapatraḥ - Tālaḥ (Raj. ni.)	दीर्घपत्रः -तालः (रा.नि.)	421
Dīrghapatrakaḥ - Laśunaḥ	दीर्घपत्रकः - लशुनः	312
Dīrghapatrakaḥ - Vetasaḥ	दीर्घपत्रकः - वेतसः	467
Dīrghapatrikā - Śvetavacā	दीर्घपत्रिका - श्वेतवचा	126
Dīrghapatrakaḥ - Jaladaḥ	दीर्घपत्रकः -जलदः	408

Dīrghapeśī - Puruṣaḥ दीर्घपेशी - पुरुषः 615
Dīrghaphalā -Jantukārī (Raj. ni.) दीर्घफला - जन्तुकारी (रा. नि.) 325
Dīrghaphalaḥ-Kapitthaḥ (Raj. ni.) दीर्घफलः - कपित्थः (रा.नि.) 188
Dīrghaphalaḥ - Āragvadhaḥ दीर्घफलः - आरग्वधः 80
Dīrghapuṣpaḥ - Śwetamandāraḥ दीर्घपुष्पः - श्वेतमन्दारः 283
Dīrgharaṅgā - Haridrā दीर्घरङ्गा - हरिद्रा 20
Dīrghaskandhaḥ - Tālaḥ दीर्घस्कन्धः - तालः 421
Dīrghataruḥ - Tālaḥ दीर्घतरुः - तालः 421
Dīrghatuṇḍī - Āmūṣikā दीर्घतुण्डी - आमूषिका 630
Dīrghātyarkaḥ - Śwetamandāraḥ दीर्घात्यर्कः - श्वेतमन्दारः 283
Dīrghavālukaḥ - Vṛddhadārukaḥ दीर्घवालुकः - वृद्धदारुकः 343
Dīrghavṛntakaḥ - Śyonākaḥ दीर्घवृन्तकः - श्योनाकः 41
Dīrghāyuḥ - Jīvakaḥ दीर्घायुः - जीवकः 44
Dīrghikā - Hiṅgupatrī दीर्घिका - हिंगुपत्री 138
Dīrghorvāruḥ - Ḍaṅgarī दीर्घोर्वारुः - डङ्गरी 67
Dirghamūlaḥ- Yāsaḥ दीर्घमूलः - यासः 8
Dīvāndhaḥ - Ulūkaḥ दिवान्धः- उलूकः 638
Divijam - Haricandanam दिविजम् - हरिचन्दनम् 196
Divyam - Lavaṅgam दिव्यम् - लवङ्गम् 214
Divyam - Haricandanam दिव्यम्- हरिचन्दनम् 196
Divyatejā - Brāhmī दिव्यतेजा -ब्राह्मी 336
Dolā (Tūṇī) - Nīlinī दोला (तृणी) - नीलिनी 87
Doṣotkleśī - Sumukhaḥ दोषोत्क्लेशी - सुमुखः 305
Drāgīḥ - Bhallaḥ द्रागीः - भल्लः 637
Drākṣā (p. 413) द्राक्षा (p. 413)
Dravadravyāṇi (p. 569) द्रवद्रव्याणि (p. 569)
Dravamamlam - Mathita dadhi द्रवमम्लम् - मथित दधि 583
Drāvaṇakaḥ - Ṭaṅkaṇaḥ द्रावणकः - टंकणः 134
Dravantī (p.86) द्रवन्ती (p.86)
Drāvī - Ṭaṅkaṇaḥ द्रावी - टंकणः 134
Drāviḍaḥ - Karcūraḥ द्राविडः - कर्चूरः 244
Draviḍam - Biḍam द्रविडम् - बिडम् 135
Drāviḍī - Elā द्राविडी - एला 141
Dṛḍham - Elavālukam दृढम् - एलवालुकम् 236
Dṛḍham - Hīrakam दृढम् - हीरकम् 532
Dṛḍhapādā - Yavatiktā दृढपादा - यवतिक्ता 98
Dṛḍhaphalaḥ - Nārikelaḥ दृढफलः - नारिकेलः 425
Dṛḍhaprarohaḥ - Plakṣaḥ दृढप्ररोहः - प्लक्षः 429
Dṛḍhaskandhaḥ - Rājādanaḥ दृढस्कन्धः - राजादनः 439

Dṛḍhavalkā -Ambaṣṭhā (Raj. ni.)	दृढवल्का - अम्बष्ठा (रा.नि.)	249
Dṛḍhavalkaḥ - Pūgīvṛkṡaḥ	दृढवल्कः -पूगीवृक्षः	214
Drekī - Mahānimbaḥ	द्रेकी - महानिम्बः	12
Dṛkprasādā - Cakṡuṣyā	दृक्प्रसादा - चक्षुष्या	264
Droṇakākaḥ (p. 637)	द्रोणकाकः (p. 637)	
Dṛptaḥ - Simhaḥ	दृप्तः - सिंहः	624
Dṛṣadaṡmajit - Pāṣāṇabhedaḥ	दृषदश्मजित् - पाषाणभेदः	57
Drumavyādhiḥ - Lākṡā	द्रुमव्याधिः - लाक्षा	239
Drumeṡvaraḥ - Tālaḥ	द्रुमेश्वरः - तालः	421
Ḍuḍulaḥ - Kṡudrolūkaḥ	डुडुलः - क्षुद्रोलूकः	638
Dyugāmī - Aṡwataraḥ	द्युगामी - अश्वतरः	622
Dugdham (p. 577)	दुग्धम् (p. 577)	
Duḥsparṡā - Dhanvayāsaḥ	दुःस्पर्शा - धन्वयासः	7
Duḥsparṡā - Kaṇṭakārī	दुःस्पर्शा - कण्टकारी	35
Durabhigrahā — Kapikacchuḥ	दुरभिग्रहा - कपिकच्छुः	55
Durabhigrahaḥ - Apāmārgaḥ	दुरभिग्रहः -अपामार्गः	100
Durālabhā - Dhanvayāsaḥ	दुरालभा - धन्वयासः	7
Dūralambhā - Dhanvayāsaḥ	दुरालम्भा -धन्वयासः	7
Dūramūlaḥ - Muñjaḥ (Raj. ni.)	दूरमूलः - मुञ्जः (रा.नि.)	360
Dūramūlaḥ - Yāsaḥ	दूरमूलः - यासः	8
Durārohā - Kharjurī	दुरारोहा - खर्जूरी	411
Durāruhaḥ - Bilvaḥ	दुरारुहः - बिल्वः	39
Durāruhaḥ - Tālaḥ	दुरारुहः -तालः	421
Durdharaḥ - Ṛṣabhaḥ	दुर्धरः - ऋषभः	45
Durdrumaḥ - Palāṇḍuḥ	दुर्द्रुमः - पलाण्डुः	315
Durgaḥ - Gugguluḥ	दुर्गः - गुग्गुलुः	252
Durgandhā - Bākucī	दुर्गन्धा - बाकुची	61
Durghoṣaḥ - Bhallaḥ	दुर्घोषः - भल्लः	637
Durgrahā - Apāmārgaḥ	दुर्ग्रहा -अपामार्गः	100
Duḥsvaraḥ - Bhallaḥ	दुःस्वरः - भल्लः	637
Durjarā - Jyotiṣmatī	दुर्जरा - ज्योतिष्मती	103
Durlabhā - Lakṡmaṇā	दुर्लभा - लक्ष्मणा	36
Durlabhaḥ - Karcūraḥ	दुर्लभः - कर्चूरः	244
Durmarā - Dūrvā	दुर्मरा - दूर्वा	368
Durmohā - Kākādanī	दुर्मोहा - काकादनी	290
Durnāmāriḥ - Sūraṇaḥ	दुर्नामारिः - सूरणः	383
Dūrvā (p. 367)	दूर्वा (p. 367)	367
Durvarṇam - Elavālukam	दुर्वर्णम् - एलवालुकम्	236
Durvidheyā - Ṡaṭhī	दुर्विधेया - शठी	22

Duṣpatraḥ - Corakaḥ	दुष्पत्रः - चोरकः	232
Duṣpradharṣā - Kharjūrī	दुष्प्रधर्षा - खर्जूरी	411
Duṣpradharṣiṇī - Kaṇṭakārī	दुष्प्रधर्षिणी - कण्टकारी	35
Dūtikā - Sārikā	दूतिका - सारिका	634
Dhwajī - Mayūraḥ	ध्वजी - मयूरः	633
Dwijā - Reṇukā	द्विजा -रेणुका	220
Dwijaḥ - Tumbaruḥ (Raj. ni.)	द्विजः - तुम्बरुः (रा. नि.)	140
Dwijapriyā - Somavallī	द्विजप्रिया - सोमवल्ली	380
Dwijihvaḥ - Sarpaḥ	द्विजिह्वः - सर्पः	639
Dwijkutsitaḥ - Ślseṣmātakaḥ	द्विजकुत्सितः - श्लेष्मातकः	441
Dwipaḥ - Hasti	द्विपः - हस्ति	620
Dwīpajam pārevatam - Pālevatam (Raj. ni.)	द्वीपजंपारेवतं - पालेवतं (रा.नि.)	418
Dwīpakharjūrī - Pālevatam (Raj. ni.)	द्वीपखर्जूरी - पालेवतम् (रा.नि.)	418
Dwīpamaricam - Kamkolam	द्वीपमरिचम् - कंकोलम्	213
Dwipapippalī - Śreyasī	द्विपपिप्पली - श्रेयसी	163
Dwīpī - Citrakaḥ	द्वीपी - चित्रकः	165
Dwīpī - Vyāghṛaḥ	द्वीपी - व्याघ्रः	623
Dwīpiśatruḥ - Śatāvarī	द्वीपिशत्रुः - शतावरी	115
Dwīpijam Nakham - Vyāghranakham	द्वीपिजंनखम् - व्याघ्रनखम्	224
Dwīpikā - Śatāvarī	द्वीपिका - शतावरी	115
Dwiradaḥ - Hasti	द्विरदः - हस्ति	620
Dwirephagaṇasammatā - Taruṇī	द्विरेफगणसंमता - तरुणी	501
Dwirephaḥ - Bhramaraḥ	द्विरेफः - भ्रमरः	633
Dwitīyam Cāturbhadrakam	द्वितीयं चातुर्भद्रकम्	646
Dwitīyam Pañcāmlakam	द्वितीयं पञ्चाम्लकम्	655
Eḍaḥ - Aviḥ	एडः - अविः	623
Eḍakaḥ - Aviḥ	एडकः - अविः	623
Eḍgajaḥ - Cakramardaḥ	एडगजः - चक्रमर्दः	277
Ekāṣṭhīlaḥ - Rājārkaḥ	एकाष्ठीलः - राजार्कः	282
Ekavāsā - Strī	एकवासा - स्त्री	615
Elā. (p.141)	एला (p.141)	
Elāgandhikam-Elavālukam (Raj. ni.)	एलागन्धिकम्-एलवालुकम् (रा.नि.)	236
Elavālukam (p. 236)	एलवालुकम् (p. 236)	
Elvālukam - Elavālukam	एल्वालुकम् - एलवालुकम्	236
Eṇaḥ - Hariṇaḥ	एणः - हरिणः	625
Eranḍaḥ (p.117)	एरण्डः (p.117)	
Eranḍatailam	एरण्डतैलम्	571
Falgū - Kākodumbarikā	फल्गू - काकोदुम्बरिका	437
Fālgunī - Kākodumbarikā	फाल्गुनी - काकोदुम्बरिका	437

Falguvṛntākaḥ - Śyonākaḥ	फल्गुवृन्ताकः - श्योनाकः	41
Feruḥ - Śṛgālaḥ	फेरुः - शृगालः	632
Gaganāmbu	गगनाम्बु	606
Gairikam (p. 262)	गैरिकम् (p. 262)	
Gajabhakśyā- Śallakī	गजभक्ष्या - शल्लकी	256
Gajacirbhaṭā - Sve. indravāruṇī	गजचिर्भटा - इन्द्रवारुणी (श्वे.)	96
Gajadantaphalā - Ḍaṅgarī	गजदन्तफला - डङ्गरी	67
Gajagāmini - Hastinī	गजगामिनी - हस्तिनी	620
Gajaḥ - Hasti	गजः - हस्ति	620
Gajakṛṣṇā - Śreyasī	गजकृष्णा - श्रेयसी	163
Gajamūtram	गजमूत्रम्	642
Gajāṇḍam -Piṇḍamūlam (Raj. ni.)	गजाण्डम् - पिण्डमूलम् (रा.नि)	294
Gajapippalī - Śreyasī	गजपिप्पली - श्रेयसी	163
Gajastrī - Hastinī	गजस्त्री - हस्तिनी	620
Gajavallabhā-Girikadalī (Raj. ni.)	गजवल्लभा - गिरिकदली (रा. नि.)	317
Gālavaḥ - Madanaḥ	गालवः - मदनः	62
Gāloḍyam - Padmabījam	गालोड्यम् - पद्मबीजम्	375
Gambhārī - Kāśmarī	गम्भारी - काश्मरी	42
Gambhīraḥ - Jambīraḥ	गम्भीरः - जम्बीरः	389
Gaṇahāsaḥ - Corakaḥ	गणहासः - चोरकः	232
Gaṇarūpakaḥ - Rājārkaḥ	गणरूपकः - राजार्कः	282
Gaṇḍadūrvā - Dūrvā	गण्डदूर्वा - दूर्वा	368
Gaṇḍālī - Dūrvā	गण्डाली - दूर्वा	368
Gaṇḍālī - Mañjiṣṭhā	गण्डाली - मञ्जिष्ठा	7
Gaṇḍamālikā - Raktapādī (Raj. ni.)	गण्डमालिका - रक्तपादी (रा. नि.)	345
Gandhā - Ajagandhā	गन्धा - अजगन्धा	184
Gandhacelikā - Kastūrikā	गन्धचेलिका - कस्तूरिका	208
Gandhadalā - Ajamodā (Raj.ni.)	गन्धदला - अजमोदा (रा. नि.)	183
Gandhāḍhyā - Taruṇī	गन्धाढ्या - तरुणी	501
Gandhāḍhyā - Murā	गन्धाढ्या - मुरा	229
Gandhagarbhaḥ - Bilvaḥ	गन्धगर्भः - बिल्वः	39
Gandhaḥ - Vaṭasaugandhikaḥ	गन्धः - वटसौगन्धिकः	248
Gandhakaḥ - Vaṭasaugandhikaḥ	गन्धकः - वटसौगन्धिकः	248
Gandhakaḥ (p. 247)	गन्धकः (p. 247)	
Gandhakārī - Raktapādī	गन्धकारी - रक्तपादी	344
Gandhakusumaḥ - Bījapūraḥ	गन्धकुसुमः- बीजपूरः	396
Gandhakuṭī - Murā	गन्धकुटी - मुरा	229
Gandhālī -Śaṭhī	गंधाली - शटी	22
Gandham - Śāliparṇī viśeṣaḥ	गन्धम् - शालिपर्णी विशेषः	32

Gandhamādanaḥ - Gandhakaḥ गन्धमादनः - गन्धकः 248
Gandhamādanaḥ - Vaṭasaugandhikaḥ गन्धमादनः - वटसौगन्धिकः 248
Gandhamālinī - Murā गन्धमालिनी - मुरा 229
Gandhamāmsī (p. 217) गन्धमांसी (p. 217)
Gandhamārjāraḥ - Biḍālaḥ गन्धमार्जारः - बिडाल 631
Gandhamūlā - Padmacāriṇī गन्धमूला - पद्मचारिणी 325
Gandhamūlaḥ - Karcūraḥ गन्धमूलः - कर्चूरः 244
Gandhanākulī (p. 342) गन्धनाकुली (p. 342)
Gandhaphalaḥ - Kapitthaḥ गन्धफलः - कपित्थः 187
Gandhapalāśī (p.22) गन्धपलाशी (p.22)
Gandhapāṣāṇaḥ - Vaṭasaugandhikaḥ गन्धपाषाणः - वटसौगन्धिकः 248
Gandhapāṣāṇaḥ - Gandhakaḥ गन्धपाषाणः - गन्धकः 248
Gandhapuṣpaḥ - Aṅkoṭakaḥ गन्धपुष्पः - अङ्कोटकः 99
Gandhapuṣpaḥ-Śleṣmātakaḥ (Raj. ni.) गन्धपुष्पः-श्लेष्मातकः(रा. नि.) 441
Gandhapuṣpakaḥ - Vetasaḥ गन्धपुष्पकः - वेतसः 467
Gandharasam - Bolam गन्धरसम् - बोलम् 226
Gandharvaḥ - Kokilaḥ गन्धर्वः - कोकिलः 637
Gandharvahastakaḥ - Eraṇḍaḥ गन्धर्वहस्तकः - एरण्डः 117
Gandhasāram - Candanam गन्धसारम् - चन्दनम 191
Gandhāśmā - Gandnakaḥ गन्धाश्मा - गन्धकः 248
Gandhatṛṇaḥ -(Sugandha) Bhūstṛṇaḥ (Raj. ni.) गन्धतृणः - (सुगंध) भूस्तृणः (रा. नि.) 300
Gandhavadhūḥ - Kapaṭam गन्धवधूः - कपटम् 29
Gandhavalkam - Twak (Raj. ni.) गन्धवल्कम् - त्वक् (रा. नि.) 146
Gandhavṛkṣaḥ-Sarjakaḥ (Raj.ni.) गन्धवृक्षः - सर्जकः (रा. नि.) 477
Gandhavṛkṣaḥ - Varuṇaḥ गन्धवृक्षः - वरुणः 472
Gandhavatī - Murā गन्धवती - मुरा 229
Gandhotkaṭaḥ - Damanaḥ गन्धोत्कटः - दमनः 228
Gaṇḍīrah - Snuhī गण्डीरः - स्नुही 88
Gaṇerukā (P. 521) गणेरुका (P. 521)
Gaṇeśakuśumaḥ-Karavīraḥ (Raj.ni.) गणेश कुसुमः - करवीरः (रा. नि.)276
Gāngerukī (p.112) गांगेरुकी (p.112)
Gāngeyaḥ - Mustā गांगेयः - मुस्ता 15
Gaṇikā - Yūthikā गणिका - यूथिका 504
Gaṇikārikā -Gaṇerukā गणिकारिका - गणेरुका 521
Gañjākinī - Vijayā गञ्जाकिनी - विजया 46
Garāgarī - Jīmūtakaḥ गरागरी - जीमूतकः 64
Garaghnaḥ - Sumukhaḥ गरघ्नः -सुमुखः 305
Garalam - Vatasanābhaḥ गरलम् - वत्सनाभः 667
Garalāriḥ - Gārutmatam गरलारिः - गारुत्मतम 531

Garbhapātinī - Kalikārī	गर्भपातिनी - कलिकारी	280
Garbhāriḥ - Elā (Raj. ni.)	गर्भारिः - एला (रा. नि.)	141
Gardabhaḥ (p. 621)	गर्दभः (p. 621)	
Gardabhamūtram	गर्दभमूत्रम्	643
Gardabhāṇḍaḥ - Plakśaḥ	गर्दभाण्डः -प्लक्षः	429
Gardabhaśākam - Bhārngī	गर्दभशाकम् - भाङ्गी	24
Gardabhī - Kāsaghnī	गर्दभी - कासघ्नी	37
Gardabhī dadhi	गर्दभीदधि	585
Gardabhīghṛtam	गर्दभी घृतम्	576
Gardabhīpayaḥ	गर्दभीपयः	580
Gāruḍam - Gārutmatam	गारुडम् - गारुत्मतम्	531
Garuḍodgīrṇam - Gārutmatam	गरुडोद्गीर्णम् - गारुत्मतम्	531
Gauḍa sīdhuḥ	गौडसीधुः	600
Gauḍikaḥ - Jaladaḥ	गौडिकः -जलदः	408
Gaulyaḥ - Kāśaḥ (Raj. ni.)	गौल्यः - काशः (रा. नि.)	359
Gaurā- Suvarṇakadalī	गौरा- सुवर्णकदली	318
Gaurah - Karañjah	गौरः - करञ्जः	456
Gaurah - Śāliḥ	गौरः -शालिः	535
Gaurajīrakaḥ - Śuklajīrakaḥ	गौरजीरकः - शुक्लजीरकः	157
Gaurakā - Sārikā	गौरका - सारिका	634
Gaurakaḥ - Lāvaḥ	गौरकः - लावः	636
Gauram- Haritālam	गौरम् -हरिताल	667
Gauram -Padmakesaram	गौरम् - पद्मकेसरम्	377
Gaurarambhā - Suvarṇakadalī	गौररम्भा- सुवर्णकदली	318
Gaurī - Haridrā	गौरी - हरिद्रा	20
Gaurī - Rocanā	गौरी - रोचना	203
Gaurī - Surasā	गौरी - सुरसा	301
Gaurī - Strī	गौरी - स्त्री	615
Gaurī - Vācā	गौरी - वाचा	616
Gauri - Dhavaḥ	गौरी - धवः	522
Gārutmatam (p. 531)	गारुत्मतम् (p. 531)	
Gavādanī - Aśvakśurakaḥ	गवादनी -अश्वक्षुरकः	323
Gavādanī - Indravāruṇī	गवादनी - इन्द्रवारुणी	95
Gavākśī - Mallikā	गवाक्षी - मल्लिका	493
Gavākśī - Indravāruṇī	गवाक्षी - इन्द्रवारुणी	95
Gavāmpriyaḥ - Śyāmākaḥ	गवांप्रियः - श्यामाकः	545
Gavāpaḥ - Gomūtram	गवापः - गोमूत्रम्	641
Gavedhukam - Gairikam	गवेधुकम् - गैरिकम्	262
Gāyatrī - Khadiraḥ	गायत्री - खदिरः	9

Ghanacchadam-Tālīsam (Raj.ni.) घनच्छदम् - तालीसम् (रा.नि.) 148
Ghanaḥ - Mustā घनः - मुस्ता 15
Ghanam - Loham घनम् - लोहम् 528
Ghanam - Vaṅgam घनम् - वङ्गम् 525
Ghanaskandhaḥ - Kṣudrāmraḥ घनस्कन्धः - क्षुद्राम्रः 387
Ghanasvanaḥ - Taṇḍulīyakaḥ घनस्वनः - तण्डुलीयकः 355
Ghaṇṭālī - Kośātakī घण्टाली - कोशातकी 71
Ghargharakaḥ - Ulūkaḥ घर्घरकः - उलूकः 638
Ghārīḥ - Rājamāṣaḥ घारीः - राजमाषः 542
Gholam - Mathita dadhi घोलम् - मथित दधि 583
Ghoṇṭāphalam - Pūgaphalam घोण्टाफलम् - पूगफलम् 213
Ghoradarśanaḥ- Tarakṣuḥ घोरदर्शनः - तरक्षुः 632
Ghoradarśanaḥ - Vyāghraḥ घोरदर्शनः - व्याघ्रः 623
Ghoṣā - Śatapuṣpā घोषा - शतपुष्पा 121
Ghoṣam - Kāmsyam घोषम् - कांस्यम् 527
Ghoṣapuṣpam - Kāmsyam घोषपुष्पम् - कांस्यम् 527
Ghoṭaḥ - Aśvaḥ घोटः - अश्वः 621
Ghotikā - Aśvā घोटिका - अश्वा 621
Ghṛtahetuḥ - Navanītam घृतहेतुः - नवनीतम् 591
Ghṛtam (p. 574) घृतम् (p. 574)
Ghṛtamaṇḍalikā - Viśvagranthiḥ घृतमण्डलिका -विश्वग्रंथिः 347
Ghṛtaparṇaḥ - Karañjaḥ घृतपर्णः - करञ्जः 456
Ghumgumārāvaḥ - Bhramaraḥ घुमघुमारावः - भ्रमरः 633
Ghuṇapriyā - Dantī घुणप्रिया - दन्ती 84
Ghuṇapriyā- Ativiṣā घुणप्रिया - अतिविषा 4
Guhyaniṣyandaḥ - Mūtram गुह्यनिष्यन्दः - मूत्रम् 641
Giḥ - Vācā गीः - वाचा 616
Girā - Vācā गिरा - वाचा 616
Girijā - Girikadalī (Raj. ni.) गिरिजा - गिरिकदली (रा. नि.) 317
Girijā - Mallikā (Raj. ni.) गिरिजा - मल्लिका (रा. नि.) 494
Girijaḥ - Godhūmaḥ गिरिजः :- गोधूमः 551
Girijāśmajam - Śilājatuḥ गिरिजाश्मजम् - शिलाजतुः 266
Girikadalī (p. 317) गिरिकदली (p. 317)
Girikarṇī - Aśvakṣurakaḥ गिरिकर्णी -अश्वक्षुरकः 323
Girikarṇikā - Aśvakṣurakaḥ गिरिकर्णिका -अश्वक्षुरकः 323
Girimallikā - Kuṭajaḥ गिरिमल्लिका - कुटजः 131
Giripīluḥ - Paruṣakaḥ गिरिपीलुः -परुषकः 416
Girirambhā - Girikadalī (Raj. ni.) गिरिरम्भा - गिरिकदली (रा. नि.) 317
Girisānujā - Trāyamāṇā गिरिसानुजा - त्रायमाणा 97

Girisindukaḥ - Śephālikā गिरिसिन्दुकः - शेफालिका 321
Girisindūram (p. 246) गिरिसिन्दूरम् (p.246)
Godadhi गोदधि 583
Godantam - Haritālam गोदन्तम्- हरितालम् 667
Godhāpadī-Viśvagranthiḥ (Raj. ni.) गोधापदी -विश्वग्रंथिः (रा. नि.) 348
Godhāskandhaḥ - Irimedaḥ गोधास्कन्धः - इरिमेदः 489
Godhūmaḥ (p. 551) गोधूमः (p. 551)
Godhūmsambhavā -Vamśarocanā (Type)
गोधूमसंभवा - वंशरोचना (विशेषः) 150
Godugdham गोदुग्धम् 578
Goghṛtam गोघृतम् 574
Goḥ (p. 626) गोः (p. 626)
Gojalam - Gomūtram गोजलम् - गोमूत्रम् 641
Gokaṇṭakaḥ - Gokśuraḥ गोकण्टकः - गोक्षुरः 38
Gokīlālam - Gomūtram गोकीलालम् - गोमूत्रम् 641
Gokiriṭī - Sārikā गोकिरीटी - सारिका 634
Gokśuraḥ (p.38) गोक्षुरः (p.38)
Gokśurakaḥ - Gokśuraḥ गोक्षुरकः - गोक्षुरः 38
Golā - Manaḥśilā गोला - मनःशिला 246
Golakaḥ - Muṣkakah गोलकः - मुष्ककः 483
Golhā - Bimbī गोल्हा - बिम्बी 76
Golīdhaḥ - Muṣkakaḥ (Raj. ni.) गोलीढः - मुष्ककः (रा. नि.) 483
Golomī - Dūrvā गोलोमी दूर्वा 368
Golomī - Vacā गोलोमी - वचा 125
Gomalam - Gomayam गोमलम् - गोमयम् 641
Gomatī - Rocanā गोमती - रोचना 203
Gomatsyaḥ - Matsyaviśeṣaḥ गोमत्स्यः - मत्स्यविशेषः 627
Gomayam - Gomalam गोमयम् -गोमलम् 641
Gomāyuḥ - Sṛgālaḥ गोमायुः - श्रृगालः 632
Gombhaḥ - Gomūtram गोम्भः - गोमूत्रम् 641
Gomūtram (p. 641) गोमूत्रम् (p. 641)
Gonardam - Paripellavam गोनर्दम् - परिपेल्लवम् 222
Gonasaḥ - Sarpa viśeṣaḥ गोनसः - सर्पविशेषः 639
Gonasam - Vaikrāntam गोनसम् - वैक्रान्तम् 530
Gonīram - Gomūtram गोनीरम् - गोमूत्रम् 641
Gopā - Sārivā गोपा - सारिवा 59
Gopakam - Bolam गोपकम् - बोलम् 226
Gopakaṇṭaḥ - Vikaṅkataḥ गोपकण्टः - विकंकतः 405
Gopakanyā - Sārivā गोपकन्या - सारिवा 59
Gopanam - Tamālapatram गोपनम - तमालपत्रम् 146

Gopānīyam - Gomūtram गोपानीयम् - गोमूत्रम् 641
Gopatiḥ - Ṛṣabhaḥ गोपतिः - ऋषभः 45
Gopavallī - Sārivā गोपवल्ली - सारिवा 59
Gopuraḥ - Kunduruḥ गोपुरः - कुन्दुरुः 254
Gopurakaḥ - Kunduruḥ(Raj. ni.) गोपुरकः - कुन्दुरुः : (रा. नि.) 254
Gopurīṣam - Gomayam गोपुरीषम् - गोमयम् 641
Goputam - Paripellavam गोपुटम् - परिपेल्लवम् 222
Gorakšaḥ - Vṛṣabhaḥ गोरक्षः - वृषभः 626
Gorakšakarkaṭī - Cirbhaṭam गोरक्षकर्कटी - चिर्भटम् 67
Goraṅkaḥ - Jaladaḥ गोरङ्कः -जलदः 408
Gorasam - Mathita dadhi गोरसम् - मथित दधि 583
Gorāṭikā - Sārikā गोराटिका - सारिका 634
Gošīrṣam - Candanam गोशीर्षम् - चन्दनम् 191
Gosravaḥ - Gomūtram गोस्रवः - गोमूत्रम् 641
Gostanī - Uttarāpathikā गोस्तनी -उत्तरापथिका 414
Govandanī - Priyaṅguḥ गोवन्दनी - प्रियङ्गुः 201
Goviṣṭhā - Gomayam गोविष्ठा - गोमयम् 641
Grahabhūtopašamanam- Vyāghranakham ग्रहभूतोपशमनम्-व्याघ्रनखम् 224
Grahaghnaḥ - Sarṣapaḥ ग्रहघ्नः - सर्षपः 297
Grāhī - Kapitthaḥ ग्राही - कपित्थः 187
Graiṣmī - Vāsantī (Raj. ni.) ग्रैष्मी - वासन्ती (रा. नि) 499
Graiṣmī (p. 498) ग्रैष्मी (p. 498)
Grāmasūkaraḥ - Sūkaraḥ (type of) ग्रामसूकरः - सूकरविशेषः 624
Grāmyā - Surasā ग्राम्या - सुरसा 301
Grāmyā - Nīlinī ग्राम्या - नीलिनी 87
Grāmyakukkuṭaḥ-Kukkuṭavišesaḥ ग्राम्यकुक्कुटः - कुक्कुट विशेषः 636
Granthidalaḥ - Corakaḥ (Raj. ni.) ग्रन्थिदलः - चोरकः (रा. नि.) 232
Granthikam - Pippalīmūlam ग्रन्थिकम् - पिप्पलीमूलम् 161
Granthilaḥ-Taṇḍulīyakaḥ(Raj.ni.) ग्रन्थिलः - तण्डुलीयकः (रा.नि.) 356
Granthilaḥ - Karīraḥ ग्रन्थिलः - करीरः 448
Granthilaḥ - Corakaḥ (Raj. ni.) ग्रन्थिलः - चोरकः (रा. नि.) 232
Granthilaḥ - Vikankataḥ ग्रन्थिलः - विकंकतः 405
Granthiparṇaḥ-Corakaḥ (Raj.ni.) ग्रन्थिपर्णः - चोरकः (रा. नि.) 232
Gṛdhrā गृध्रा 650
Gṛhadrumaḥ - Sāgaḥ (Raj. ni.) गृहद्रुमः - सागः (रा.नि.) 522
Grīṣmodbhavā -Graiṣmī (Raj.ni.) ग्रीष्मोद्भवा - ग्रैष्मी (रा. नि.) 499
Grīvāṅkušaḥ - Uṣṭraḥ ग्रीवाङ्कुशः - उष्ट्रः 621
Gṛñjanaḥ - Lašunaḥ गृञ्जनः - लशुनः 312
Gṛñjanam (p. 294) गृञ्जनम् (p. 294)
Gṛñjaram (Garjaram) (p. 314) गृञ्जरम् (गर्जरम्) (p. 314)

Gṛṣṭiḥ - Vārāhī	गृष्टिः - वाराही	326
Gṛṣṭikā - Vārāhī	गृष्टिका - वाराही	326
Guḍā - Snuhī	गुडा - स्नुही	88
Guḍaḥ (p. 357)	गुडः (p. 357)	
Guḍamañjarī - Jinginī	गुडमञ्जरी - जिंगिणी	272
Guḍaphalaḥ - Pīluḥ	गुडफलः - पीलुः	409
Guḍaphalam - Badaram	गुडफलम् - बदरम्	445
Guḍapuṣpaḥ - Madhūkaḥ	गुडपुष्पः -मधूकः	406
Guḍāśrayaḥ - Akṣoḍaḥ	गुडाश्रयः - अक्षोडः	414
Gūḍhamallikā-Aṅkoṭakaḥ (Raj. ni.)	गूढमल्लिका - अङ्कोटकः (रा.नि.)	100
Gūḍhāṅgaḥ - Kacchapaḥ	गूढाङ्गः - कच्छपः	630
Gūḍhapatraḥ - Karīraḥ	गूढपत्रः - करीरः	448
Gūḍhapuṣpaḥ - Bakulaḥ	गूढपुष्पः - बकुलः	511
Gūḍhapuṣpaḥ - Saptaparṇaḥ	गूढपुष्पः - सप्तपर्णः	238
Guḍūcī (p. 1)	गुडूची (p. 1)	
Gugguluḥ (p. 252)	गुग्गुलुः (p. 252)	
Guhā - Pṛśniparṇī	गुहा - पृश्निपर्णी	32
Guhāśayaḥ - Vyāghraḥ	गुहाशयः - व्याघ्रः	623
Guhyapatraḥ - Pippalaḥ	गुह्यपत्रः -पिप्पलः	427
Gulmakaḥ - Karavīraḥ	गुल्मकः - करवीरः	275
Gundrā - Kuśaḥ	गुन्द्रा - कुशः	362
Guñjā - Cūḍāmaniḥ	गुञ्जा - चूडामणिः	291
Guṇojjvalā- Yūthikā	गुणोज्ज्वला - यूथिका	504
Gunṭhaḥ (p.29)	गुण्ठः (p.29)	29
Guptāṅgaḥ - Anyaḥ Kacchapaḥ	गुप्ताङ्गः -अन्यः कच्छपः	630
Guruśreṣṭham - Vaṅgam	गुरुश्रेष्ठम् - वङ्गम्	525
Guvākaḥ - Pūgaphalam	गुवाकः - पूगफलम्	213
Haḍḍam - Asthi	हड्डम् - अस्थि	618
Haimaḥ - Kirātatiktakaḥ	हैमः -किराततिक्तकः	13
Haimavatī - Harītakī	हैमवती - हरीतकी	77
Haimavatī - Kṣīriṇī	हैमवती - क्षीरिणी	90
Haimavatī - Reṇukā (Raj. ni.)	हैमवती -रेणुका (रा.नि.)	221
Haimavatī - Śvetavacā (Dhn.ni.)	हैमवती - श्वेतवचा (ध.नि.)	125,126
Hālā - Surā	हाला - सुरा	596
Haladīkā - Haridrā	हलदीका - हरिद्रा	20
Hālāhalaḥ	हालाहलः	665
Halinī - Kalikārī	हलिनी - कलिकारी	280
Haṃsaḥ - Aśvaḥ	हंसः - अश्वः	621
Haṃsaḥ (p. 635)	हंसः (p. 635)	

Hamsapādī - Viśvagranthiḥ	हंसपादी - विश्वग्रंथिः	347
Hamsapadī - Viśvagranthiḥ	हंसपदी -विश्वग्रंथिः	347
Hanuḥ - Nakham	हनुः - नखम्	223
Hapuṣā (p.127)	हपुषा (p.127)	
Hārahūrā-Uttarāpathikā (Raj. ni.)	हारहूरा -उत्तरापथिका (रा. नि.)	414
Haravallabhaḥ - Dhattūraḥ	हरवल्लभः - धत्तूरः	278
Hareṇuḥ - Kalāyaḥ	हरेणुः - कलायः	554
Hareṇukā - Reṇukā	हरेणुका -रेणुका	220
Haricandanam - Raktacandanam	हरिचन्दनम् - रक्तचंदनम्	193
Haricandanam - Kālīyakam	हरिचन्दनम् - कालीयकम्	194
Haricandanam (Raj. ni.) (p.195)	हरिचन्दनम् (रा.नि.) (p.195)	
Haridarbhaḥ - Kuśaḥ (Raj. ni.)	हरिदर्भः - कुशः (रा.नि.)	362
Haridrā (p.20)	हरिद्रा (p.20)	
Haridrā patrakandakā-Gandhapalāśī	हरिद्रापत्रकन्दका - गन्धपलाशी	22
Hāridraḥ	हारिद्रः	665
Harigandham - Haricandanam	हरिगन्धम् - हरिचन्दनम्	196
Hariḥ - Maṇḍukaḥ	हरिः - मण्डूकः	640
Hariḥ - Aśvaḥ	हरिः - अश्वः	621
Hariḥ - Markaṭaḥ	हरिः - मर्कटः	632
Hariḥ - Simhaḥ	हरिः - सिंहः	624
Harimanthaḥ - Caṇakaḥ	हरिमन्थः - चणकः	553
Hariṇaḥ (p.624)	हरिणः (p.624)	
Harinetram - Puṇḍarīkam	हरिनेत्रम् -पुण्डरीकम्	370
Hariṇī - Yūthikā	हरिणी - यूथिका	504
Harinmaṇiḥ - Gārutmatam	हरिन्मणिः - गारुत्मतम्	531
Hariparṇam - Mūlakam	हरिपर्णम् -मूलकम्	293
Haripriyā - Surasā (Raj. ni.)	हरिप्रिया - सुरसा (रा. नि.)	301
Hari(li)priyaḥ - Kadambaḥ	हरि(लि) प्रियः - कदम्बः	452
Haritā - Uttarāpathikā (Raj. ni.)	हरिता - उत्तरापथिका(रा. नि.)	414
Haritā - Balāmoṭā	हरिता - बलामोटा	378
Haritaḥ - Mudgaḥ	हरितः -मुद्गः	540
Haritaḥ Palāṇḍuḥ - Palāṇḍuḥ	हरितः पलाण्डुः - पलाण्डुः	315
Harītakī (p.76)	हरीतकी (p.76)	
Haritālam (p.667)	हरितालम् (p.667)	667
Haritam - Dūrvā	हरितम् - दूर्वा	368
Haritam - Sthauṇeyakam	हरितम् - स्थौणेयकम्	230
Haritamagadhā - Śreyasī	हरितमगधा - श्रेयसी	163
Haritaśākaḥ - Śigruḥ	हरितशाकः - शिग्रुः	295
Harivālukam - Elavālukam	हरिवालुकम् - एलवालुकम्	236
Harṣasambhavam - Śukram	हर्षसंभवम् - शुक्रम्	619

Hartalam -Tīkśṇa Loham	हर्तालम् -तीक्ष्णलोहम्	528
Hāsaḥ - Śāliḥ	हासः -शालिः	535
Hastaparṇaḥ - Raktairaṇḍaḥ	हस्तपर्णः - रक्तैरण्डः	117
Hastī (p. 619)	हस्ती (p. 619)	
Hasticāriṇī - Karañjaḥ	हस्तिचारिणी - करञ्जः	461
Hastidantī - (Śve.) indravāruṇī	हस्तिदन्ती - इन्द्रवारुणी (श्वे.)	96
Hastighoṣā - Kośātakī	हस्तिघोषा- कोशातकी	71
Hastikandakam-Mūlakam (Raj.ni.)	हस्तिकन्दकम् -मूलकम् (रा. नि.)	293
Hastikarṇī - Raktairaṇḍaḥ	हस्तिकर्णी - रक्तैरण्डः	117
Hastimagadhā - Śreyasī	हस्तिमगधा - श्रेयसी	163
Hastimayūrakaḥ - Ajamodā	हस्तिमयूरकः - अजमोदा	183
Hastidantaphalā - Urvāruḥ	हस्तिदन्तफला -उर्वारुः	65
Hastinī dadhi	हस्तिनी दधि	585
Hastinīghṛtam	हस्तिनीघृतम्	576
Hastinīpayaḥ	हस्तिनीपयः	580
Hastiparṇinī - Trapusam	हस्तिपर्णिनी - त्रपुसम्	65
Hastirohaṇakaḥ - Karañjaḥ	हस्तिरोहणकः - करञ्जः	461
Hastiviṣāṇikā - Kadalī	हस्तिविषाणिका - कदली	316
Hāṭakam - Suvarṇam	हाटकम् - सुवर्णम्	523
Haviḥ - Ghṛtam	हविः - घृतम्	574
Hayabhakśā - Dīpyā	हयभक्षा - दीप्या	412
Hayaḥ - Aśvaḥ	हयः - अश्वः	621
Hayamāraḥ - Karavīraḥ	हयमारः - करवीरः	275
Hema - Suvarṇam	हेम- सुवर्णम्	523
Hemadugdhaḥ- Udumbaraḥ	हेमदुग्धः - उदुम्बरः	436
Hemagauraḥ - Kinkirātaḥ	हेमगौरः - किंकिरातः	511
Hemāhvā - Sarvakśīrī	हेमाह्वा -सर्वक्षीरी	91
Hemakāñcanam - Nāgakesaram	हेमकाञ्चनम् - नागकेसरम्	143
Hemakāntā - Dāruharidrā	हेमकान्ता - दारुहरिद्रा	21
Hemakśīrī - Sarvakśīrī	हेमक्षीरी -सर्वक्षीरी	91
Hemamākśikam (p. 261)	हेममाक्षिकम् (p. 261)	
Hemaphalā - Suvarṇakadalī	हेमफला- सुवर्णकदली	318
Hemapuṣpaḥ - Campakaḥ	हेमपुष्पः - चम्पकः	500
Hemavarṇavatī - Dāruharidrā	हेमवर्णवती - दारुहरिद्रा	21
Hemayūthikā - Yūthikā (Raj. ni.)	हेमयूथिका - यूथिका (रा. नि.)	504
Hemdugdhā - Kśīriṇī	हेमदुग्धा - क्षीरिणी	90
Himaḥ - Karpūraḥ	हिमः -कर्पूरः	209
Himam - Lāmajjakam	हिमम् - लामज्जकम्	241
Himavālukaḥ - Karpūraḥ	हिमवालुकः-कर्पूरः	209

Himāvatī - Kṡiriṇī	हिमावती - क्षीरिणी	90
Himsrā - Māmsī	हिंस्रा- मांसी	217
Hingusivāṭikā- Nāḍīhingu	हिङगुशिवाटिका - नाडीहिंगु	139
Hingu (p. 37)	हिङ्गु (p. 37)	
Hingūlam - Hingulam	हिङ्गूलम् - हिंगुलम्	530
Hingulam (p. 530)	हिङ्गुलम् (p. 530)	
Hingupatrī (p.138)	हिंगुपत्री (p.138)	
Hīrā - Kāṡmarī	हीरा - काश्मरी	42
Hīrakam (p. 532)	हीरकम् (p. 532)	
Hiraṇyam - Suvarṇam	हिरण्यम् - सुवर्णम्	523
Hispitthaḥ - Vanamethikā	हिस्पित्थः - वनमेथिका	563
Hlādā - Ṡallakī	ह्लादा- शल्लकी	256
Homadhānyam - Tilaḥ	होमधान्यम् - तिलः	568
Hṛdyā - Tāmbūli	हृद्या - ताम्बूली	273
Hṛdyagandhā - Jātī	हृद्यगन्धा - जाती	496
Hṛdyagandhaḥ - Bilvaḥ	हृद्यगन्धः - बिल्वः	39
Hṛdyagandhakam - Sauvarcalam	हृद्यगन्धकम् - सौवर्चलम्	136
Hṛdyam - Jīrakam	हृद्यम् - जीरकम्	156
Hṛdyam - Mārdwīkam	हृद्यम्- मार्द्वीकम्	599
Huḍah - Aviḥ	हुडः - अविः	623
Huḍumbaḥ - Godhūmaḥ	हुडुम्बः :- गोधूमः	551
Ibhāḥ - Hasti	इभः - हस्ति	620
Ibhakaṇā - Ṡreyasī	इभकणा - श्रेयसी	163
Ibhamūlakaḥ - Guṇṭhaḥ	इभमूलकः - गुण्ठः	29
Īhāmṛgaḥ - Vṛkaḥ	ईहामृगः - वृकः	623
Ikṡugandhā - Kṡiravidārī	इक्षुगन्धा - क्षीरविदारी	54
Ikṡugandhaḥ - Ikṡuḥ	इक्षुगन्धः - इक्षुः	358
Ikṡuḥ (p. 357)	इक्षुः (p. 357)	
Ikṡukaḥ -(Sthūla) Ṡaraḥ	इक्षुकः - (स्थूल) शरः	363
Ikṡukāṇḍaḥ - Kāṡaḥ	इक्षुकाण्डः - काशः	359
Ikṡukusumaḥ - Kāṡaḥ	इक्षुकुसुमः - काशः	359
Ikṡuraḥ - Ikṡuḥ	इक्षुरः - इक्षुः	358
Iksuraḥ -(Sthūla) Ṡaraḥ	इक्षुरः - (स्थूल) शरः	363
Ikṡusāraḥ - Guḍaḥ	इक्षुसारः - गुडः	358
Ikṡuvālikā - Ikṡuḥ	इक्षुवालिका - इक्षुः	358
Ikṡuvallī - Kṡiravidārī	इक्षुवल्ली - क्षीरविदारी	54
Ikṡuyonī - Ikṡuḥ	इक्षुयोनी - इक्षुः	358
Ikṡvākuḥ - Kaṭukālāmbunī	इक्ष्वाकुः - कटुकालाम्बुनी	63
Ikṡvārikā- Kāṡaḥ	इक्ष्वारिका - काशः	359

Indīvaram - Saugandhikam	इन्दीवरम् - सौगन्धिकम्	371
Indīvarī - Śatāvarī	इन्दीवरी - शतावरी	115
Indradāruḥ - Devadāruḥ	इन्द्रदारुः - देवदारुः	27
Indrāhvā - Indravāruṇī	इन्द्राह्वा- इन्द्रवारुणी	95
Indrākśaḥ - Ṛṣabhaḥ	इन्द्राक्षः - ऋषभः	45
Indrāṇī - Śephālikā (Raj. ni.)	इन्द्राणी - शेफालिका (रा. नि.)	321
Indravāruḥ - Indravāruṇī	इन्द्रवारुः - इन्द्रवारुणी	95
Indravāruṇī (p.94)	इन्द्रवारुणी (p.94)	
Indravṛkśaḥ - Kuṭajaḥ	इन्द्रवृक्षः - कुटजः	131
Indravṛkśaḥ - Devadāruḥ	इन्द्रवृक्षः - देवदारुः	27
Indrayavaḥ (p.131)	इन्द्रयवः (p.131)	
Induḥ - Karpūraḥ	इन्दुः -कर्पूरः	209
Indukalikā - Ketakī (Raj. ni.)	इन्दुकलिका - केतकी (रा.नि.)	521
Indulekhā - Bākucī	इन्दुलेखा - बाकुची	61
Irā - Surā	इरा - सुरा	596
Irasaḥ - Matsyaviśeṣaḥ	इरसः - मत्स्यविशेषः	627
Irimedaḥ (p. 489)	इरिमेदः (p. 489)	
Īṣadraktam- Kśudramutpalam	ईषद्रक्तम् - क्षुद्रमुत्पलम्	374
Īśānī - Śamī	ईशानी - शमी	442
Īṣannīlam - Kśudramutpalam	ईषन्नीलम् - क्षुद्रमुत्पलम्	374
Īṣatśvetam - Kśudramutpalam	ईषतश्वेतम् - क्षुद्रमुत्पलम्	
Iṣṭakāpathakam - Lāmajjakam	इष्टकापथकम् - लामज्जकम्	241
Iṣuḥ - Śaraḥ	इषुः - शरः	363
Īśvarī - Nākulī (Raj. ni.)	ईश्वरी - नाकुली (रा. नि.)	340
Jagalaḥ	जगलः	599
Jagalaḥ - Surā	जगलः - सुरा	596
Jaladaḥ - Śaṅkhaḥ	जलदः - शङ्खः	271
Jaladaḥ - Mustā	जलदः - मुस्ता	15
Jaladaḥ (p. 408)	जलदः (p. 408)	
Jalajaḥ - Śaliḥ	जलजः - शालिः	535
Jalakākaḥ - Dātyūhaḥ	जलकाकः - दात्यूहः	638
Jalakāmaḥ - Vetasaḥ	जलकामः - वेतसः	467
Jalākhyakaḥ - Jaladaḥ	जलाख्यकः -जलदः	408
Jalālūkam - Padmamūlam	जलालूकम् - पद्ममूलम्	377
Jalam - Vālakam	जलम् - - वालकम्	17
Jalam (p. 605)	जलम् (p. 605)	
Jalamadhūkaḥ - Jaladaḥ	जलमधूकः - जलदः	408
Jalamustam. (p.16)	जलमुस्तम् (p.16)	
Jalapādaḥ - Hamsaviśeṣaḥ	जलपादः - हंसविशेषः	635
Jalapippalī (p. 310)	जलपिप्पली (p. 310)	

Jalasarpaḥ (p. 638)	जलसर्पः (p.639)	
Jalāśrayam - Lāmajjakam	जलाश्रयम् - लामज्जकम्	241
Jalaukaḥsamvṛtaḥ - Vetasaḥ	जलौकःसंवृतः - वेतसः	467
Jalavāsam - Uśīram (Raj, ni.)	जलवासम् - उशीरम् (रा.नि.)	199
Jalavetasaḥ- Vetasaḥ	जलवेतसः - वेतसः	467
Jālinī - Kośātakī	जालिनी - कोशातकी	71
Jalodbhavā -Laghubrāhmī (Raj. ni.)	जलोद्भवा - लघुब्राह्मी (रा.नि.)	336
Jāmbava sīdhuḥ	जाम्बव सीधुः	601
Jambhaḥ - Jambīraḥ	जम्भः - जम्बीरः	389
Jambhalaḥ - Arkaḥ	जम्भलः - अर्कः	282
Jambhalaḥ - Jambīrah	जम्भलः - जम्बीरः	389
Jambīraḥ (p. 302)	जम्बीरः (p. 302)	
Jambīraḥ (p. 389)	जम्बीरः (p. 389)	
Jambūḥ (p. 433)	जम्बूः (p. 433)	
Jambūkaḥ - Ketakī	जम्बूकः - केतकी	520
Jambukaḥ - Śṛgālaḥ	जम्बुकः - श्रृगालः	632
Jambukaḥ - Śyonākaḥ	जम्बुकः - श्योनाकः	41
Jāmbūnadam- Suvarṇam	जाम्बूनदम् - सुवर्णम्	523
Janā - Kaṭukā	जना - कटुका	15
Jananī - Jantukārī	जननी - जन्तुकारी	324
Jananī - Kaṭukā	जननी - कटुका	15
Janapriyaḥ - Śigruḥ (Raj. ni.)	जनप्रियः - शिग्रुः (रा. नि.)	296
Jantughnam - Hiṅgu	जन्तुघ्नम् - हिंगु	137
Jantuhantrī - Viḍaṅgam	जन्तुहन्त्री - विडङ्गम्	130
Jantukā - Nāḍihiṅguh	जन्तुका - नाडीहिंगुः	139
Jantukā -Jantukārī	जन्तुका - जन्तुकारी	324
Jantukārī (p. 324)	जन्तुकारी (p. 324)	
Jantukṛṣṇā - Jantukārī	जन्तुकृष्णा - जन्तुकारी	324
Jantunāśanaḥ - Yawānikā	जन्तुनाशनः - यवानिका	171
Jaraṇā - Kṛṣṇajīrakaḥ	जरणा - कृष्णजीरकः	158
Jaranaḥ - Kāsamardaḥ	जरणः - कासमर्दः	357
Jaraṇam - Hiṅgu	जरणम् - हिंगु	137
Jartilaḥ - Tilaḥ (Vanodbhavaḥ)	जर्तिलः - तिलः (वनोद्भवः)	569
Jaṭā - Māmsī	जटा - मांसी	217
Jaṭālaḥ -Muṣkakaḥ (Raj. ni.)	जटालः - मुष्ककः (रा. नि.)	483
Jātarūpam - Suvarṇam	जातरूपम् - सुवर्णम्	523
Jaṭāyuḥ - Gugguluḥ	जटायुः - गुग्गुलुः	252
Jātī (p. 496)	जाती (p. 496)	
Jātikośā - Jātipatrī	जातिकोशा - जातिपत्री	211

Jaṭilā - Māmsī	जटिला - मांसी	217
Jaṭilā - Vacā	जटिला - वचा	125
Jātīpatrī (p. 211)	जातिपत्री (p. 211)	
Jātīphalam (p. 211)	जातीफलम् (p. 211)	
Jatīphalarasam - Āmalakī	जातीफलरसम् - आमलकी	79
Jātīsasyam - Jātīphalam	जातीसस्यम् - जातीफलम्	211
Jatiśṛṅgam - Jātīphalam	जातिशृङ्गम् - जातीफलम्	211
Jatudrumaḥ - Kśudrāmraḥ	जतुद्रुमः - क्षुद्राम्रः	387
Jatuḥ - Lākśā	जतुः - लाक्षा	239
Jatukā - Jantukārī	जतुका - जन्तुकारी	324
Jatvaśmajam - Śilājatuḥ	जत्वश्मजम् - शिलाजतुः	266
Javī - Aśvaḥ	जवी - अश्वः	621
Jayā - Agnimanthaḥ	जया -अग्निमंथः	40
Jayā - Harītakī	जया - हरीतकी	77
Jayantī - Balāmoṭā	जयन्ती - बलामोटा	378
Jayantī - Haridrā	जयन्ती - हरिद्रा	20
Jayantikā - Haridrā (Raj. ni.)	जयन्तिका - हरिद्रा (रा.नि.)	20
Jayapālaḥ (p.85)	जयपालः (p.85)	
Jayāvahā - Araṇī	जयावहा - अरणी	85
Jayāvahā - Balāmoṭā	जयावहा - बलामोटा	378
Jhaṅkārī - Bhramaraḥ	झंकारी - भ्रमरः	633
Jhaṣā - Gāṅgerukī	झषा - गांगेरुकी	112
Jhiñziṇī - Jiṅgiṇī	झिञ्झिणी - जिंगिणी	272
Jihmaśalyaḥ - Khadiraḥ	जिह्मशल्यः - खदिरः	10
Jihmam - Tagaram	जिह्मम् - तगरम्	221
Jīmūtaḥ - Mustā	जीमूतः - मुस्ता	15
Jīmūtakaḥ (p.63)	जीमूतकः (p.63)	
Jiṅgī - Mañjiṣṭhā	जिङ्गी - मञ्जिष्ठा	7
Jiṅgiṇī (p. 272)	जिं गिणी (p. 272)	
Jīrakam (p.156)	जीरकम् (p.156)	
Jīrṇam - Śaileyam	जीर्णम् - शैलेयम्	235
Jīrṇaparṇaḥ - Paṭṭikārodhraḥ	जीर्णपर्णः -पट्टिकारोध्रः	270
Jīrṇāphañjī-Vṛddhadārukaḥ (Raj.ni.)	जीर्णाफञ्जी - वृद्धदारुकः (रा. नि.)	343
Jīrṇapuṣpakam - Paripellavam	जीर्णपुष्पकम् - परिपेल्लवम्	222
Jirṇavajram - Vaikrāntam	जीर्णवज्रम् - वैक्रान्तम्	531
Jīvakaḥ (p.44)	जीवकः (p.44)	
Jīvanī - Guḍūcī	जीवनी - गुडूची	2
Jīvanī - Jīvantī	जीवनी - जीवन्ती	49
Jīvanīyā - Jīvantī	जीवनीया - जीवन्ती	49

Jīvanīya Gaṇaḥ	जीवनीयगणः	650
Jīvanīya pañcamūlam	जीवनीय पञ्चमूलम्	649
Jīvaniyam - Ghṛtam	जीवनीयम् - घृतम्	574
Jīvantī - Tāmbūlī	जीवन्ती - ताम्बूली	273
Jīvantī (p.49)	जीवन्ती (p.49)	
Jīvavardhinī - Jīvantī	जीववर्धनी - जीवन्ती	49
Jīvitam- Dugdham	जीवितम् - दुग्धम्	577
Juṅgakaḥ - Vṛddhadārukaḥ	जुङ्गकः - वृद्धदारुकः	343
Jūrṇā (p. 558)	जूर्णा (p. 558)	
Jūrṇāhvaḥ - Jurnā	जूर्णाह्वः - जूर्णा	557
Jwalanābham - Śāliparṇī viśeṣaḥ	ज्वलनाभम् - शालिपर्णी विशेषः	32
Jwalanī - Gandhapalāśī	ज्वलनी - गन्धपलाशी	22
Jwaraḥ - Pittam	ज्वरः - पित्तम्	616
Jwaranāśinī - Guḍūcī	ज्वरनाशिनी - गुडूची	2
Jwarāntakaḥ - Kirātatiktaḥ	ज्वरान्तकः - किराततिक्तः	14
Jyotiṣmatī (p.103)	ज्योतिष्मती (p.103)	
Jyotiṣkā - Methikā	ज्योतिष्का - मेथिका	562
Jyotiṣkaḥ - Citrakaḥ	ज्योतिष्कः - चित्रकः	165
Jyotiṣkāyā - Jyotiṣmatī	ज्योतिष्काया - ज्योतिष्मती	103
Kabarī - Hiṅgupatrī	कबरी - हिंगुपत्री	138
Kacam - Vālakam	कचम् - वालकम्	17
Kacchapaḥ (p. 630)	कच्छपः (p. 630)	
Kaccheṣṭaḥ - Kacchapaḥ	कच्छेष्टः - कच्छपः	630
Kacchūghnī - Aparā Hapuṣā	कच्छूघ्नी- अपरा हपुषा	128
Kacchurā - Dhanvayāsaḥ	कच्छुरा - धन्वयासः	7
Kadalī (p.316)	कदली (p.316)	
Kadambaḥ (p. 451)	कदम्बः (p. 451)	
Kadambapuṣpikā - Mahāśrāvaṇī	कदम्बपुष्पिका - महाश्रावणी	58
Kādambaryaḥ - Kadambaḥ	कादम्बर्यः - कदम्बः	451
Kādambarī - Surā	कादम्बरी - सुरा	596
Kādambaryaḥ - Kadambaḥ	कादम्बर्यः - कदम्बः	452
Kaḍāram - Muṇḍaloham	कडारम् -मुण्डलोहम्	528
Kairalā - Viḍaṅgam	कैरला - विडङ्गम्	130
Kaivartamustam - Jalamustam	कैवर्तमुस्तम् - जलमुस्तम्	16
Kākabhāṇḍikā - Karañjaḥ	काकभाण्डिका - करञ्जः	462
Kākādanī - Śvetakāmbhojī	काकादनी -श्वेतकाम्भोजी	292
Kākādanī (p. 290)	काकादनी(p. 290)	
Kākadroṇaḥ - Droṇakākaḥ	काकद्रोणः -द्रोणकाकः	637
Kākaghnī - Karañjaḥ	काकघ्नी - करञ्जः	462

Kākaḥ - Śāliḥ	काकः - शालिः	535
Kākaḥ (p.637)	काकः (p.637)	
Kākāhvā - Kākamācī	काकाह्वा - काकमाची	285
Kākajambūḥ - Jambūḥ	काकजम्बूः - जम्बूः	433
Kakajaṅghā (p. 287)	काकजङ्घा (p. 287)	
Kākākṣī - Śuklabhāṇḍī	काकाक्षी - शुक्लभण्डी	94
Kākalī-Nirbījā-Uttarāpathikā (Raj.ni.)	काकली निर्बीजा-उत्तरापथिका (रा. नि.)	414
Kākamācī (p. 285)	काकमाची (p. 285)	
Kākamātā - Kākamācī (Raj. ni.)	काकमाता - काकमाची (रा.नि.)	286
Kākaṇantī - Kākādanī	काकणन्ती - काकादनी	290
Kākaṇantikā - Kākādanī	काकणन्तिका - काकादनी	290
Kākanāsā (p.288)	काकनासा (p.288)	
Kākāṇḍī - Dadhipuṣpī	काकाण्डी - दधिपुष्पी	56
Kākapādā - Kākajaṅghā	काकपादा - काकजङ्घा	287
Kākapādaḥ - Vikaṅkataḥ	काकपादः - विकंकतः	405
Kākaphalā - Jambūḥ (Raj. ni.)	काकफला - जम्बूः (रा. नि.)	434
Kākapīluḥ - Śvetakāmbhojī	काकपीलुः -श्वेतकाम्भोजी	292
Kākapīluḥ - Kākādanī	काकपीलुः - काकादनी	290
Kākasāhvayā - Cūḍāmaṇiḥ	काकसाह्वया - चूडामणिः	291
Kākaśatruḥ - Ulūkaḥ	काकशत्रुः - उलूकः	638
Kākatindukaḥ - Tindukaḥ	काकतिन्दुकः - तिन्दुकः	402
Kākatuṇḍaphalā - Kākanāsā	काकतुण्डफला - काकनासा	289
Kākatuṇḍī - Pittalam	काकतुण्डी - पित्तलम्	526
Kākavallī - Karañjaḥ	काकवल्ली - करञ्जः	462
Kakendukaḥ - Kākatindukaḥ	काकेन्दुकः - काकतिन्दुकः	402
Kākekṣuḥ - Kāśaḥ	काकेक्षुः - काशः	359
Kākodumbarikā (p. 437)	काकोदुम्बरिका (p. 437)	
Kākolī (p.47)	काकोली (p.47)	
Kākṣī - Saurāṣṭrī	काक्षी - सौराष्ट्री	247
Kakubhaḥ - Arjunaḥ	ककुभः -अर्जुनः	464
Kakud - Ṛṣabhaḥ	ककुद् - ऋषभः	45
Kakudmān - Vṛṣabhaḥ	ककुद्मान् - वृषभः	626
Kālaḥ - Kāsamardaḥ	कालः - कासमर्दः	356
Kalā - Manaḥśilā	कला - मनःशिला	246
Kālā - Mañjiṣṭhā	काला - मञ्जिष्ठा	7
Kālā - Nīlinī	काला - नीलिनी	87
Kālā - Trivṛt	काला -त्रिवृत्	93
Kalabhaḥ- Hastiśāvakaḥ	कलभः - हस्तिशावकः	620

Kalahākulā - Sārikā	कलहाकुला - सारिका	634
Kalahamsaḥ - Hamsaviśeṣaḥ	कलहंसः - हंसविशेषः	635
Kālajñaḥ - Kukkuṭaḥ	कालज्ञः - कुक्कुटः	636
Kalakalodbhavaḥ - Rālaḥ	कलकलोद्भवः - रालः	250
Kālakaṇṭakaḥ - Datyūhaḥ	कालकण्टकः - दात्यूहः	638
Kālakuṣṭham - Kamkuṣṭham	कालकुष्ठम् - कंकुष्ठम्	259
Kālakūṭaḥ	कालकूटः	664
Kālalavaṇam - Sauvarcalam	काललवणम् - सौवर्चलम्	136
Kālaloham -Tikṣna Loham	काललोहम् -तीक्ष्णलोहम्	528
Kālamālah - Śalukaḥ	कालमालः - शालुकः	304
Kālameṣī - Trivṛt	कालमेषी -त्रिवृत	93
Kālameṣī - Bākucī	कालमेषी - बाकुची	61
Kālameṣī - Mañjiṣṭhā	कालमेषी - मञ्जिष्ठा	7
Kālameṣikā - Mañjiṣṭhā	कालमेषिका - मञ्जिष्ठा	7
Kalanaḥ - Vetasaḥ	कलनः - वेतसः	467
Kālaniryāsaḥ - Gugguluḥ	कालनिर्यासः - गुग्गुलः	252
Kālānusāryakam - Śaileyam	कालानुसार्यकम् - शैलेयम्	235
Kālānusāryam - Tagaram	कालानुसार्यम् - तगरम्	221
Kālapālakam - Kamkuṣṭham	कालपालकम् - कंकुष्ठम्	259
Kālapeśikā - Kṛṣṇajīrakaḥ	कालपेशिका - कृष्णजीरकः	158
Kalāpī -Mayūraḥ	कलापी - मयूरः	633
Kālapuṣpaḥ-Dhattūraḥ (Raj. ni.)	कालपुष्पः - धत्तूरः (रा. नि.)	278
Kalaśī - Pṛsniparnī	कलशी - पृश्निपर्णी	33
Kālaskandhaḥ - Tindukaḥ	कालस्कन्धः - तिन्दुकः	402
Kalavṛntikā - Pāṭalā	कालवृन्तिका - पाटला	43
Kalāvṛttaḥ - Kulatthaḥ	कलावृत्तः - कुलत्थः	557
Kalāyaḥ (Vartulaḥ) (p. 554)	कलायः (वर्तुलः) (p. 554)	
Kalevaram - Śarīram	कलेवरम् - शरीरम्	615
Kāleyakam (p. 207)	कालेयकम् (अगरु) (p. 207)	
Kāleyakā - Dāruharidrā	कालेयका - दारुहरिद्रा	21
Kalhāram- Kumudam	कल्हारम् - कुमुदम्	373
Kālī - Potakī	काली - पोतकी	382
Kalidrumaḥ - Bibhītakaḥ	कलिद्रुमः - बिभीतकः	78
Kāliḥ - Kṛṣṇajīrakaḥ	कालिः - कृष्णजीरकः	158
Kāliḥ - Dhattūraḥ	कालिः - धत्तूरः	278
Kālikā - Upakuñcī	कालिका - उपकुञ्ची	154
Kalikārī (p. 280)	कलिकारी (p. 280)	
Kālindī - Trivṛt	कालिन्दी - त्रिवृत	93
Kalingaḥ - Kuṭajaḥ	कलिङ्गः - कुटजः	131

Kaliṅgakāḥ - Indrayavāḥ	कलिङ्गकाः - इन्द्रयवाः	131
Kālīyakam (p. 194)	कालीयकम् (p. 194)	
Kalkaḥ - Turuṣkaḥ	कल्कः - तुरुष्कः	204
Kalkidharmaghnaḥ-Bibhītakaḥ (Raj.ni.)	कल्किधर्मघ्नः-बिभीतकः(रा.नि.)	78
Kalkihāryaḥ - Bibhītakaḥ	कल्किहार्यः - बिभीतकः	78
Kālmikābhedā - Karañjaḥ	काल्मिकाभेदा - करञ्जः	462
Kaluṣā - Mahiṣī	कलुषा - महिषी	625
Kaluṣaḥ - Mahiṣaḥ	कलुषः - महिषः	625
Kam - Jalam	कम् - जलम्	605
Kāmadā - Tāmbūlī	कामदा - ताम्बूली	273
Kāmajananī - Tāmbūlī	कामजननी - ताम्बूली	273
Kamalam - Raktapadmam	कमलम् - रक्तपद्मम्	372
Kamaṇḍaluḥ - Plakśaḥ	कमण्डलुः -प्लक्षः	429
Kamāṅgaḥ - Āmraḥ	कामाङ्गः - आम्रः	385
Kāmarūpakā - Vandakā	कामरूपका - वन्दका	331
Kāmaśaraḥ - Āmraḥ	कामशरः - आम्रः	386
Kamaṭhaḥ - Kacchapaḥ	कमठः - कच्छपः	630
Kāmbojī - Māṣaparṇī	काम्बोजी - माषपर्णी	48
Kambuḥ - Śaṅkhaḥ	कम्बुः -शङ्खः	271
Kambumālinī - Śaṅkhapuṣpī	कम्बुमालिनी - शंखपुष्पी	349
Kambupuṣpī - Śaṅkhapuṣpī	कम्बुपुष्पी - शंखपुष्पी	348
Kāmī - Cakravākaḥ	कामी - चक्रवाकः	635
Kāmikāntam - Mārdwīkam	कामिकान्तम् - मार्द्वीकम्	599
Kāminī - Vandakā	कामिनी - वन्दका	331
Kāminī -Strī	कामिनी - स्त्री	615
Kamkolam (p.213)	कंकोलम् (p.213)	
Kamkuṣṭham (p. 258)	कंकुष्ठम् (p. 258)	
Kampillaḥ - Kampillakaḥ	कम्पिल्लः - कम्पिल्लकः	257
Kampillakaḥ (p. 257)	कम्पिल्लकः (p. 257)	
Kāmsyakam - Kāmsyam	कांस्यकम् - कांस्यम्	527
Kāmsyam (p. 526)	कांस्यम् (p. 526)	
Kāmukā -Srtī	कामुका - स्त्री	615
Kaṇā - Bṛhatpālī	कणा - बृहत्पाली	159
Kaṇā - Pippalī	कणा - पिप्पली	160
Kaṇā - Śuklajīrakaḥ	कणा - शुक्लजीरकः	157
Kāṇaḥ - Kākaḥ	काणः - काकः	637
Kaṇajīrakaḥ - Kṛṣṇajīrakaḥ	कणजीरकः - कृष्णजीरकः	158
Kaṇajīrakaḥ - Śuklajīrakaḥ	कणजीरकः - शुक्लजीरकः	157
Kanakaḥ - Kāsamardaḥ	कनकः - कासमर्दः	356
Kanakaḥ - Dhattūraḥ	कनकः - धत्तूरः	278

Kanakaḥ - Tūniḥ	कनकः - तूणिः	202
Kanakam - Nāgakesaram	कनकम् - नागकेसरम्	143
Kanakam - Suvarṇam	कनकम् - सुवर्णम्	523
Kanakaprasavā-Ketakī (Raj. ni.)	कनकप्रसवा - केतकी (रा.नि.)	521
Kanakarambhā - Suvarṇakadalī	कनकरम्भा - सुवर्णकदली	318
Kanakakṡirī - Sarvakṡirī	कनकक्षीरी -सर्वक्षीरी	91
Kanakastambhā - Suvarṇakadalī	कनकस्तम्भा - सुवर्णकदली	318
Kāṇavāyasaḥ - Droṇakākaḥ	काणवायसः -द्रोणकाकः	637
Kāñcanaḥ - Campakaḥ	काञ्चनः - चम्पकः	500
Kāncanakadalī - Suvarṇakadalī	काञ्चनकदली - सुवर्णकदली	318
Kāñcanakam- Padmakesaram	काञ्चनकम् - पद्मकेसरम्	377
Kāñcanakṡirī - Kṡiriṇī	काञ्चनक्षीरी - क्षीरिणी	90
Kāñcanam - Suvarṇam	काञ्चनम् - सुवर्णम्	523
Kāñcanī - Sarvakṡirī	काञ्चनी -सर्वक्षीरी	91
Kañcukā - Aṡvagandhā	कञ्चुका - अश्वगन्धा	105
Kañcukī - Yavaḥ (Raj. ni.)	कञ्चुकी - यवः (रा. नि.)	539
Kañcukī - Sarpaḥ	कञ्चुकी - सर्पः	638
Kandā- Kandaguḍūcī	कन्दा - कंदगुडूची	2
Kaṇḍaḥ - Sūraṇaḥ	कन्दः - सूरणः	383
Kāṇḍaḥ - Ṡaraḥ	काण्डः - शरः	363
Kāṇḍahīnaḥ - Lodhraḥ	काण्डहीनः - लोध्रः	267
Kāṇḍakam - Vālukam	काण्डकम् - वालुकम्	66
Kāṇḍakāṇḍakaḥ - Kāṡaḥ(Raj. ni.)	काण्डकाण्डकः - काशः (रा.नि.)	359
Kāṇḍakaṭukaḥ - Kāṇḍīraḥ	काण्डकटुकः -काण्डीरः	309
Kandalī - Padmabījam (Raj. ni.)	कन्दली - पद्मबीजम् (रा. नि.)	375
Kandaphalam - Kamkolam	कन्दफलम् - कंकोलम्	213
Kandārhaḥ - Sūraṇaḥ	कन्दार्हः - सूरणः	383
Kandarohiṇī - Kandaguḍūcī	कन्दरोहिणी - कंदगुडूची	2
Kāṇḍaruhā - Kaṭukā	काण्डरुहा -कटुका	15
Kandasūraṇaḥ - Sūraṇaḥ	कन्दसूरणः - सूरणः	383
Kāṇḍatiktaḥ - Kirātatiktakaḥ	काण्डतिक्तः - किराततिक्तकः	13
Kandavardhanaḥ - Sūraṇaḥ	कन्दवर्धनः - सूरणः	383
Kāṇḍekṡuḥ - Kāṡaḥ	काण्डेक्षुः - काशः	359
Kāṇḍīraḥ (p.308)	काण्डीरः (p.308)	
Kandodbhavā - Kandaguḍūcī	कन्दोद्भवा - कंदगुडूची	2
Kaṇḍulā - Kapikacchuḥ	कण्डुला - कपिकच्छुः	55
Kaṅguḥ (p. 546)	कङ्गुः (p. 546)	
Kaṅgukaḥ - Kaṅguḥ	कङ्गुकः - कङ्गुः	546
Kaṅgunī - Kaṅguḥ	कङ्गुनी - कङ्गुः	547
Kaṅgunī - Priyaṅguḥ	कङ्गुनी - प्रियङ्गुः	201
Kāñjikam (p. 595)	काञ्जिकम् (p. 595)	

Kaṅkatā - Atibalā	कङ्कता - अतिबला	113
Kaṅkeliḥ - Aśokaḥ (Raj. ni.)	कंकेलिः - अशोकः (रा.नि.)	516
Kākśi - Saurāṣṭrī	काक्षी - सौराष्ट्री	247
Kāṅkśī - Saurāṣṭrī	कांक्षी - सौराष्ट्री	247
Kāntā - Srtī	कान्ता - स्त्री	615
Kāntā - Vārāhī	कान्ता - वाराही	326
Kāntā - Bṛhatī	कान्ता - बृहती	35
Kāntā - Graiṣmī	कान्ता - ग्रैष्मी	498
Kaṇṭadalā - Ketakī (Raj. ni.)	कण्टदला - केतकी (रा.नि.)	521
Kāntaḥ - Puruṣaḥ	कान्तः - पुरुषः	615
Kaṇṭakāḍhyā - Kubjakaḥ	कण्टकाढ्या - कुब्जकः	503
Kaṇṭakādhyā - Śālmalī	कण्टकाढ्या - शाल्मली	481
Kaṇṭakādhyaḥ - Bilvaḥ	कण्टकाढ्यः - बिल्वः	39
Kaṇṭakaphalaḥ-Dhattūraḥ (Raj.ni.)	कण्टकफलः - धत्तूरः (रा.नि.)	278
Kaṇṭakārī - Lakśmaṇā	कण्टकारी - लक्ष्मणा	36
Kaṇṭakārī (p.35)	कण्टकारी (p.35)	
Kaṇṭakatrikaḥ - Gokśuraḥ	कण्टकत्रिकः - गोक्षुर	38
Kaṇṭakī - Vamśaḥ (Raj. ni.)	कण्टकी - वंशः (रा.नि.)	364
Kaṇṭakī - Khadiraḥ	कण्टकी - खदिरः	10
Kaṇṭakinī - Kaṇṭakārī	कण्टकिनी - कण्टकारी	35
Kāntalakaḥ - Tūṇiḥ	कान्तलकः - तूणिः	202
Kaṇṭālikā - Kaṇṭakāri	कण्टालिका - कण्टकारी	35
Kāntam - Loham	कान्तम् - लोहम्	528
Kāntam - Kāntaloham	कान्तम् - कान्तलोहम्	528
Kaṇṭam -Muṇḍaloham	कण्टम् - मुण्डलोहम्	528
Kāntāraḥ - Ikśuḥ	कान्तारः - इक्षुः	357
Kaṇṭhakālaḥ - Matsayḥ	कण्ठकालः - मत्स्यः	626
Kaṇṭhī - Kalāyaḥ	कण्ठी - कलायः	554
Kaṇṭhī - Matsayḥ	कण्ठी - मत्स्यः	626
Kaṇṭī - Apāmārgaḥ	कण्टी -अपामार्गः	100
Kāntiḥ - Vārāhī	कान्तिः - वाराही	326
Kanyakā - Bhadrailā	कन्यका -भद्रैला	142
Kaphaḥ - Śleṣmā	कफः - श्लेष्मा	617
Kapaṭā -Kāsaghnī	कपटा - कासघ्नी	37
Kapaṭam (p.29)	कपटम् (p.29)	
Kapaṭeśvarī - Kāsaghnī	कपटेश्वरी - कासघ्नी	37
Kapī - Āmrātakaḥ	कपी - आम्रातकः	388
Kapicūtaḥ - Āmrātakaḥ	कपिचूतः - आम्रातकः	388
Kapiḥ - Markaṭaḥ	कपिः - मर्कटः	632
Kapiḥ - Turuṣkaḥ	कपिः - तुरुष्कः	204

Kapijaḥ - Turuṣkaḥ	कपिजः - तुरुष्कः	204
Kapikacchuḥ (p.55)	कपिकच्छुः (p.55)	
Kapilā - Śimśapā	कपिला - शिंशपा	473
Kapilā - Pittalam	कपिला - पित्तलम्	526
Kapilā - Reṇukā	कपिला -रेणुका	220
Kapilā - Uttarāpathikā	कपिला -उत्तरापथिका	413
Kapiloham - Pittalam	कपिलोहम् - पित्तलम्	526
Kapilolā - Reṇukā	कपिलोला -रेणुका	220
Kapīluḥ - Kākatindukaḥ	कपीलुः - काकतिन्दुकः	402
Kapipippalī - Rakt. Apāmārgaḥ	कपिपिप्पली -र. अपामार्गः	101
Kapipriyaḥ - Kapitthaḥ	कपिप्रियः - कपित्थः	187
Kapipriyaḥ - Āmrātakaḥ	कपिप्रियः - आम्रातकः	389
Kapīṣṭaḥ - Rājādanaḥ	कपीष्टः - राजादनः	439
Kapītailam - Turuṣkaḥ	कपितैलम् - तुरुष्कः	204
Kapītanaḥ - Śirīṣaḥ	कपीतनः शिरीषः	463
Kapītanaḥ - Plakṣaḥ	कपीतनः -प्लक्षः	428
Kapitthaḥ (p. 187)	कपित्थः (p. 187)	
Kapittham - Elavālukam	कपित्थम् - एलवालुकम्	236
Kapotacaraṇā - Nalikā	कपोतचरणा - नलिका	216
Kapotam - Añjanam	कपोतम् - अञ्जनम्	262
Kapotavarṇā - Elā	कपोतवर्णा - एला	141
Kapotavegā - Brāhmī	कपोतवेगा - ब्राह्मी	336
Karabhaḥ - Uṣṭraḥ	करभः - उष्ट्रः	621
Karabhavallabhaḥ - Pīluḥ	करभवल्लभः - पीलुः	409
Karacchadaḥ - Sāgaḥ	करच्छदः - सागः	522
Karahāṭaḥ - Madanaḥ	करहाटः - मदनः	62
Karahāṭakam - Padmamūlam	करहाटकम् - पद्ममूलम्	377
Karajaḥ - Nakham	करजः - नखम्	223
Karakaḥ - Dāḍimaḥ	करकः -दाडिमः	155
Karālaḥ - Tripuṭaḥ	करालः - त्रिपुटः	560
Karālaḥ - Śālukaḥ	करालः - शालुकः	304
Karamardakam (p. 449)	करमर्दकम् (p. 449)	
Karamardam - Karamardakam	करमर्दम् - करमर्दकम्	449
Karamardikā - Drākṣā	करमर्दिका - द्राक्षा	413
Karambhā - Priyaṅguḥ	करम्भा - प्रियङ्गुः	201
Karāmlam - Karamardakam	कराम्लम् - करमर्दकम्	449
Karaṅgekṣuḥ - Ikṣuḥ (Raj. ni.)	करङ्गेक्षुः - इक्षुः (रा.नि.)	358
Karañjaḥ (p. 455)	करञ्जः (p. 455)	
Kararuhaḥ - Nakham	कररुहः - नखम्	223
Karaṭaḥ - Tripuṭaḥ	करटः - त्रिपुटः	560
Kāravallī - Kāṇḍiraḥ	कारवल्ली -काण्डीरः	309
Kāravī - Śatapuṣpā	कारवी - शतपुष्पा	121

Kāravī - Ajagandhā	कारवी - अजगन्धा	184
Kāravī - Ajamodā	कारवी- अजमोदा	183
Karavīraḥ (p. 275)	करवीरः (p. 275)	
Karbudāraḥ - Śleṣmātakaḥ	कर्बुदारः - श्लेष्मातकः	441
Karcūraḥ (p. 244)	कर्चूरः (p. 244)	
Kareṇuḥ - Hastinī	करेणुः - हस्तिनी	620
Karī - Hasti	करी - हस्ति	620
Karikaṇā - Cavikā (Raj. ni.)	करिकणा - चविका (रा.नि.)	162
Karikaṇā - Śreyasī	करिकणा - श्रेयसी	163
Kariṇī - Hastinī	करिणी - हस्तिनी	620
Karīraḥ - Vamśāgram	करीरः - वंशाग्रम्	
Karīraḥ (p.448)	करीरः (p.448)	
Kariśāvakaḥ - Hastiśāvakaḥ	करिशावकः - हस्तिशावकः	620
Karkandhukam - Badaram	कर्कन्धुकम् - बदरम्	445
Karkaśacchadaḥ - Paṭolaḥ	कर्कशच्छदः - पटोलः	18
Karkaśaḥ - Kāsamardaḥ	कर्कशः - कासमर्दः	356
Karkaṭaḥ - Bilvaḥ	कर्कटः - बिल्वः	39
Karkaṭaḥ (p.640)	कर्कटः (p.640)	
Karkaṭakaḥ - Karkaṭaḥ	कर्कटकः - कर्कटः	640
Karkaṭaśṛṅgī - Śṛṅgī	कर्कटशृंगी - शृंगी	30
Karkaṭāvhayā - Karkaṭaśṛṅgī	कर्कटाह्वया - कर्कटशृंगी	30
Karkaṭī - Urvāruḥ	कर्कटी -उर्वारुः	65
Karkoṭakaḥ - Ikśuḥ	कर्कोटकः - इक्षुः	357
Karkoṭakī - Dhāmārgavaḥ	कर्कोटकी - धामार्गवः	70
Karkoṭakī (p.69)	कर्कोटकी (p.69)	
Kārmukaḥ - Vamśaḥ	कार्मुकः - वंशः	364
Kārmukaḥ - Mahānimbaḥ	कार्मुकः - महानिम्बः	12
Kārmukaḥ - Somavalkaḥ	कार्मुकः- सोमवल्कः	10
Kārmukaḥ -Atimuktakaḥ	कार्मुकः - अतिमुक्तकः	509
Karṇābharaṇakaḥ - Karṇikāraḥ	कर्णाभरणकः -कर्णिकारः	81
Karṇapūrakaḥ - Aśokaḥ	कर्णपूरकः - अशोकः	516
Karṇapūrakaḥ-Kadambaḥ (Raj.ni.)	कर्णपूरकः - कदम्बः (रा. नि.)	453
Karṇapūrakaḥ - Kadambaḥ	कर्णपूरकः - कदम्बः	451
Karṇī - Āragvadhaḥ	कर्णी - आरग्वधः	80
Karṇiḥ - Gaṇerukā	कर्णिः - गणेरुका	521
Karṇikā - Agnimanthaḥ	कर्णिका -अग्निमंथः	40
Karṇikā - Taruṇī	कर्णिका - तरुणी	501
Karṇikā -Kākolī	कर्णिका - काकोली	47
Karṇikāraḥ - Āragvadhaḥ	कर्णिकारः - आरग्वधः	80
Karṇikāraḥ - Gaṇerukā	कर्णिकारः -गणेरुका	521
Karṇikāraḥ (p.81)	कर्णिकारः (p.81)	
Karparālaḥ - Akśoḍaḥ	कर्परालः - अक्षोडः	414

Karparikātuttham - Tuttham कर्परिकातुत्थम् - तुत्थम् 260
Karparītuttham - Tuttham कर्परीतुत्थम् - तुत्थम् 260
Karparītutthakam - Tuttham कर्परीतुत्थकम् - तुत्थम् 260
Karpūraḥ (p. 208) कर्पूरः (p. 208)
Kārśaḥ - Karcūraḥ कार्शः - कर्चूरः 244
Karṣaṇaḥ - Kulatthaḥ कर्षणः- कुलत्थः 557
Karṣaṇī - Kṣīriṇī कर्षणी - क्षीरिणी 90
Karṣaphalaḥ - Bibhītakaḥ कर्षफलः - बिभीतकः 78
Kartā - Vāyuḥ कर्ता - वायुः 616
Karvīrabhujā - Āḍhakī करवीरभुजा - आढकी 548
Karvīrakaḥ - Karavīraḥ करवीरकः - करवीरः 275
Kāsaghnī (p.37) कासघ्नी (p.37)
Kāsaghnī - Bhaṛngī कासघ्नी - भार्ङ्गी 24
Kāśaḥ (p. 359) काशः (p. 359)
Kāsamaradakaḥ - Kāsamardaḥ कासमर्दकः - कासमर्दः 356
Kāsamardaḥ (p. 356) कासमर्दः (p. 356)
Kāsamuktidaḥ - Paṭolaḥ कासमुक्तिदः - पटोलः 18
Kāsaraḥ - Mahiṣaḥ कासरः - महिषः 625
Kāsāriḥ - Kāsamardaḥ कासारिः - कासमर्दः 356
Kaṣāyā - Kharjūrī कषाया - खर्जूरी 411
Kaṣāyā - Ambaṣṭhā कषाया - अम्बष्टा 249
Kaṣāyaḥ - Sarjakaḥ कषायः - सर्जकः 477
Kāsīsam (p.251) कासीसम् (p.251)
Kāśmarī (p.42) काश्मरी (p.42)
Kāśmaryā - Kāśmarī काश्मर्या - काश्मरी 42
Kāṣmaryaḥ - Kāśmarī काश्मर्यः - काश्मरी 42
Kaśmīrajīrakā - Kṛṣṇajīrakaḥ कश्मीरजीरका - कृष्णजीरकः 158
Kāśmīram - Kumkumam काश्मीरम् - कुंकुमम् 197
Kāśmīram - Puskaramūlam काश्मीरम् - पुष्करमूलम् 23
Kāśmīrikā - Drākśā काश्मीरिका - द्राक्षा 413
Kāṣṭhajambuḥ - Jambūḥ (Raj. ni.) काष्ठजम्बूः - जम्बूः (रा. नि.) 434
Kāṣṭhakadalī (p. 317) काष्टकदली (p. 317)
Kāṣṭhapāṭalā (p.44) काष्ठपाटला (p.44)
Kāṣṭharajanī - Dāruharidrā काष्ठरजनी - दारुहरिद्रा 21
Kāṣṭhasārivā - Sārivā काष्ठसारिवा - सारिवा 59
Kastūrī (biḍālaḥ) - Ugrabiḍālakaḥ कस्तूरी (बिडालः) - उग्रबिडालकः 631
Kastūrikā (p. 208) कस्तूरिका (p. 208)
Kasūcakaḥ - Manḍūkaḥ कसूचकः - मण्डूकः 640
Kaṭabhī - Aśvakśurakaḥ कटभी-अश्वक्षुरकः 323
Kaṭabhī - Jyotiṣmatī कटभी - ज्योतिष्मती 103
Katakam (p. 266) कतकम् (p. 266)
Katam - Katakaṃ कतम - कतकम 267

Kaṭambharaḥ - Śyonākaḥ कटंभरः - श्योनाकः 41
Kaṭankaṭerī - Dāruharidrā कटंकटेरी - दारुहरिद्रा 21
Kataphalam - Katakam कतफलम् - कतकम् 267
Kaṭhillaḥ - Punarnavā कठिल्लः - पुनर्नवा 107
Kathillakaḥ - Punarnavā कठिल्लकः - पुनर्नवा 107
Kaṭhinā-Kākodumbarikā (Raj.ni.) कठिना - काकोदुम्बरिका (रा.नि.)438
Kaṭhinapṛṣṭhakaḥ - Kacchapaḥ कठिनपृष्ठकः - कच्छपः 630
Kaṭphalaḥ (p. 26) कट्फलः (p.26)
Kattṛṇam (p.28) कत्तृणम् (p.28)
Kaṭu - Cāturbhadrakam कटु चातुर्भद्रकम् 646
Kaṭuvārtākinī - Lakṣmaṇā कटुवार्ताकिनी - लक्ष्मणा 37
Kaṭubhadram - Śuṇṭhī कटुभद्रम् - शुण्ठी 167
Kaṭugranthiḥ - Pippalīmūlam कटुग्रन्थिः -पिप्पलीमूलम् 161
Kaṭuḥ - Sarṣapaḥ (Raj. ni.) कटुः - सर्षपः (रा. नि.) 298
Kaṭuh - Citrakaḥ कटुः - चित्रकः 165
Kaṭukā (p.14) कटुका (p.14)
Kaṭukaḥ - Sarṣapaḥ कटुकः - सर्षपः 297
Kaṭukālāmbunī (p.62) कटुकालाम्बुनी (p.62)
Kaṭukam - Kamkolam कटुकं (फलम्) - कंकोलम् 213
Kaṭukam - Trapusam कटुकम् - त्रपुसम् 65
Kaṭukarohiṇī - Kaṭukā कटुकरोहिणी -कटुका 15
Kaṭuniṣpāvaḥ-Niṣpāvaḥ (Raj.ni.) कटुनिष्पावः - निष्पावः (रा. नि.) 560
Kaṭuparṇī - Kṣīriṇī कटुपर्णी - क्षीरिणी 90
Kaṭupatrakaḥ - Sumukhaḥ कटुपत्रकः - सुमुखः : 305
Kaṭuphalā - Kākamācī कटुफला - काकमाची 285
Kaṭurohiṇī - Kaṭukā कटुरोहिणी -कटुका 15
Kaṭusnehaḥ - Sarṣapaḥ कटुस्नेहः - सर्षपः 297
Kaṭutiktakā - Śaṇapuṣpī कटुतिक्तका - शणपुष्पी 75
Kaṭutrayam -Trikaṭukam कटुत्रयम् - त्रिकटुकम् 646
Kaṭuvārtākinī - Kāsaghnī कटुवार्ताकिनी - कासघ्नी 37
Kaṭvangaḥ - Śyonākaḥ कट्वङ्गः - श्योनाकः 41
Kaṭvī - Kākamācī कट्वी - काकमाची 285
Kauberam - Kuṣṭham कौबेरम् - कुष्ठम् 219
Kauntī - Reṇukā कौन्ती -रेणुका 220
Kauśī - Ulūkaḥ कौशी - उलूकः 638
Kauśikaḥ - Gugguluḥ कौशिकः - गुग्गुलुः 252
Kauśikaḥ - Ulūkaḥ कौशिकः - उलूकः 638
Kausumam - Puspāñjanam कौसुमम् - पुष्पाञ्जनम् 266
Kausumāñjanam - Puṣpāñjanam कौसुमाञ्जनम् - पुष्पाञ्जनम् 266
Kausumbham - Kusumbham कौसुम्भम् - कुसुम्भम् 566
Kauṭaḥ - Kuṭajaḥ कौटः - कुटजः 131
Kauṭajah - Kuṭajaḥ कौटजः - कुटजः 131

Kauṭilyam - Cāṇākhyamūlakam (Raj. ni.)	कौटिल्यम्-चाणाख्यमूलकम् (रा. नि.)	294
Kavacaḥ - Parpaṭaḥ	कवचः - पर्पटः	17
Kāyaḥ - Śarīram	कायः - शरीरम्	615
Kāyasthā - Elā (Raj. ni.)	कायस्था - एला (रा.नि.)	141
Keśahantrī - Śamī	केशहन्त्री - शमी	442
Keśamuṣṭiḥ - Mahānimbaḥ	केशमुष्टिः - महानिम्बः	12
Keśaraḥ - Bījapūraḥ	केशरः - बीजपूरः	396
Kesaram - Kāsīsam	केसरम् - कासीसम्	251
Kesaram - Nāgakesaram	केसरम् - नागकेसरम्	143
Keśarāmlaḥ - Bījapūraḥ	केशराम्लः - बीजपूरः	396
Keśarañjanaḥ - Bhṛṅgarājaḥ	केशरञ्जनः -भृङ्गराजः	281
Keśarī - Bījapūraḥ	केशरी - बीजपूरः	396
Keśarī - Simhaḥ	केशरी - सिंहः	624
Keśarūhā - Araṇī	केशरुहा - अरणी	85
Keśarūhā - Balāmoṭā	केशरुहा - बलामोटा	378
Keśarūpā - Vandakā (Raj. ni.)	केशरूपा - वन्दका (रा. नि.)	331
Keśavāvāsaḥ - Pippalaḥ	केशवावासः -पिप्पलः	427
Keśī - Gandhamāmsī	केशी - गन्धमांसी	217
Keśyaḥ - Bhṛṅgarājaḥ (Raj. ni.)	केश्यः - भृङ्गराजः (रा. नि.)	281
Keśyam - Vālakam	केश्यम् - वालकम्	17
Ketakī (p. 520)	केतकी (p. 520)	
Ketuḥ - Agnimanthaḥ	केतुः -अग्निमंथः	40
Khadiraḥ (P. 9)	खदिरः (P. 9)	
Khanakaḥ - Mūṣakaḥ	खनकः - मूषकः	630
Khaṇḍā - Gāṅgerukī	खण्डा - गांगेरुकी	112
Khaṇḍakaḥ - Rājamudgaḥ	खण्डकः - राजमुद्गः	541
Khaṇḍalavaṇam - Biḍam	खण्डलवणम् - बिडम्	135
Khaṇḍikaḥ - Tripuṭaḥ	खण्डिकः - त्रिपुटः	560
Khāṇḍavarasā - Marjikā	खाण्डवरसा - मर्जिका	605
Khapuram - Pūgaphalam	खपुरम् - पूगफलम्	213
Kharadrumaḥ - Śrīveṣṭakaḥ	खरद्रुमः - श्रीवेष्टकः	255
Kharagandhinikā - Gāṅgerukī	खरगन्धिनिका - गांगेरुकी	112
Kharaḥ - Gardabhaḥ	खरः - गर्दभः	622
Kharaḥ - Kuśaḥ	खरः - कुशः	361
Kharāhvā - Ajamodā	खराह्वा - अजमोदा	183
Kharakaśālī - Ikśuḥ	खरकशाली - इक्षुः	358
Kharamañjarī - Apāmārgaḥ	खरमञ्जरी -अपामार्गः	100
Kharaparṇaḥ - Kimśukaḥ	खरपर्णः - किंशुकः	518
Kharapatraḥ - Jambīraḥ	खरपत्रः - जम्बीरः	302
Kharapuṣpā - Ajagandhā	खरपुष्पा - अजगन्धा	184
Kharasāram - Tikṣṇa Loham	खरसारम् -तीक्ष्णलोहम्	528

Kharaskandhā - Kharjūrī	खरस्कन्धा - खर्जूरी	411
Kharaskandhaḥ - Priyālaḥ	खरस्कन्धः - प्रियालः	424
Kharaśūkaḥ - Śāliḥ	खरशूकः - शालिः	535
Kharayaṣṭikā - Balā	खरयष्टिका - बला	110
Khārjūram	खार्जूरम्	600
Kharjūrī (P. 411)	खर्जूरी (P. 411)	
Khastilaḥ (p. 567)	खस्तिलः (p. 567)	
Khastilavalkalaḥ (p. 567)	खस्तिलवल्कलः (p. 567)	
Khaṭvā - Dadhipuṣpī	खट्वा - दधिपुष्पी	56
Khaṭvāṅgī - Dadhipuṣpī	खट्वाङ्गी - दधिपुष्पी	56
Khuraḥ - Nakham	खुरः - नखम्	223
Kīcakaḥ - Vaṁśaḥ	कीचकः - वंशः	364
Kīlālam - Jalam	कीलालम् - जलम्	605
Kīlapādikā-Viśvagranthiḥ (Raj.ni.)	कीलपादिका-विश्वग्रंथिः (रा.नि.)	347
Kilāṭaḥ - Mudgaḥ	किलाटः -मुद्गः	540
Kilimam - Devadāruḥ	किलिमम् - देवदारुः	27
Klītanam - Klītanakam	क्लीतनम् - क्लीतनकम्	52
Kiṁśukaḥ (p. 517)	किंशुकः (p. 517)	
Kiṇihī - Apāmārgaḥ	किणिही -अपामार्गः	100
Kiñjalkam - Padmakesaram	किञ्जल्कम् - पद्मकेसरम्	377
Kiñjam -Padmakesaram	किञ्जम् - पद्मकेसरम्	377
Kiṅkiṇī - Vikaṅkataḥ	किंकिणी - विकंकतः	405
Kiṅkirāṭaḥ - Kiṅkirātaḥ	किंकिराटः - किंकिरातः	511
Kiṁkirātaḥ (p. 511)	किं किरातः (p. 511)	
Kīraḥ - Śukaḥ	कीरः - शुकः	634
Kīram - Māṁsam	कीरम् - मांसम्	618
Kirātaḥ - Kirātatiktkaḥ	किरातः - किराततिक्तकः	14
Kirātakaḥ - Kirātatiktakaḥ	किरातकः- किराततिक्तकः	13
Kirātatiktakaḥ (p.13)	किराततिक्तकः (p.13)	
Kīreṣṭaḥ - Āmraḥ	कीरेष्टः - आम्रः	385
Kīreṣṭaḥ - Akṣoḍaḥ	कीरेष्टः - अक्षोडः	414
Kiriḥ - Sūkaraḥ	किरिः - सूकरः	624
Kirīṭī - Arjunaḥ	किरीटी -अर्जुनः	464
Kīrṇapuṣpaḥ - Moraṭaḥ	कीर्णपुष्पः - मोरटः	6
Kīśaḥ - Markaṭaḥ	कीशः - मर्कटः	632
Kitavaḥ - Dhattūraḥ	कितवः - धत्तूरः	278
Kitavaḥ - Corakaḥ	कितवः - चोरकः	232
Kiṭṭaloham - Maṇḍūram	किट्टलोहम् - मण्डूरम्	529
Kiṭṭam - Malam	किट्टम् - मलम्	640
Klītanakam (p.52)	क्लीतनकम् (p.52)	
Klītanī - Nīlinī (Raj. ni.)	क्लीतनी - नीलिनी (रा.नि.)	88
Klītikā - Klītanakam	क्लीतिका - क्लीतनकम्	52

Kodravaḥ (p. 543)	कोद्रवः (p. 543)	
Kohalaḥ	कोहलः	599
Kokaḥ - Vṛkaḥ	कोकः - वृकः	623
Kokanadam - Raktapadmam	कोकनदम् - रक्तपद्मम्	372
Kokilā (p.637)	कोकिला (p.637)	
Kokilaḥ (p. 636)	कोकिलः (p. 636)	
Kokilākṡakaḥ - Ikṡuḥ	कोकिलाक्षकः - इक्षुः	358
Kokilotsavaḥ - Āmraḥ	कोकिलोत्सवः -आम्रः	386
Kolā - Pippalī	कोला - पिप्पली	160
Kolakam - Kamkolam	कोलकम् - कंकोलम्	213
Kolakam - Maricam	कोलकम् - मरिचम्	168
Kolakam - Badaram	कोलकम् - बदरम्	445
Kolam - Badaram	कोलम् - बदरम्	445
Kolamūlam - Pippalīmūlam	कोलमूलम् - पिप्पलीमूलम्	161
Kolavallī - Cavikā	कोलवल्ली - चविका	162
Kopanakaḥ - Corakaḥ	कोपनकः - चोरकः	232
Koradūṣaḥ -Kodravaḥ	कोरदूषः - कोद्रवः	542
Korangī - Pippalī (Raj. ni.)	कोरङ्गी - पिप्पली (रा.नि.)	160
Korangī - Elā	कोरङ्गी - एला	141
Koṡāmraḥ - Kṡudrāmraḥ	कोशाम्रः - क्षुद्राम्रः	387
Koṡāmratailam	कोशाम्रतैलम्	572
Koṡaphalā - Dhāmārgavaḥ	कोशफला -धामार्गवः	70
Koṡātakī (p.70)	कोशातकी (p.70)	
Koṡī- Nakham	कोशी - नखम्	223
Koṭarapuṣpī - Vṛddhadārukaḥ	कोटरपुष्पी - वृद्धदारुकः	343
Koṭikā - Spṛkkā	कोटिका - स्पृक्का	224
Kovidāraḥ (p.73)	कोविदारः (p.73)	
Krakacacchadaḥ - Ketakī	क्रकचच्छदः - केतकी	520
Krakacaḥ - Karīraḥ	क्रकचः - करीरः	448
Krakacapatraḥ - Sāgaḥ (Raj.ni.)	क्रकचपत्रः - सागः (रा.नि.)	522
Kramelakaḥ - Uṣṭraḥ	क्रमेलकः - उष्ट्रः	621
Kramukaḥ - Paṭṭikārodhraḥ	क्रमुकः -पट्टिकारोध्रः	270
Kramukaḥ - Pūgīvṛkṡaḥ	क्रमुकः -पूगीवृक्षः	214
Kramukam - Tūdam	क्रमुकम् - तूदम्	417
Kramukaprasūnaḥ - Kadambaḥ (Raj. ni.)	क्रमुकप्रसूनः - कदम्बः (रा. नि.)	452
Krāntasamjñam - Vaikrāntam	कान्तसंज्ञम् - वैक्रान्तम्	531
Krauñcādanaḥ - Padmabījam	क्रौञ्चादनः - पद्मबीजम्	375
Krauñcaḥ - Padmabījam	क्रौञ्चः - पद्मबीजम्	375
Kravyādī - Māmsī	क्रव्यादी - मांसी	217
Kravyam - Māmsam	क्रव्यम् - मांसम्	618
Kravyāt- Simhaḥ	क्रव्यात् - सिंहः	624

Kṛkavākuḥ - Kukkuṭaḥ	कृकवाकुः - कुक्कुटः	636
Kṛmighnaḥ - Bījapūraḥ	कृमिघ्नः - बीजपूरः	396
Kṛmighnī - Viḍaṅgam	कृमिघ्नी - विडङ्गम्	130
Kṛmihā - Viḍaṅgam	कृमिहा - विडङ्गम्	130
Kṛmijā - Lākṡā	कृमिजा - लाक्षा	239
Kṛmijagdham - Agaru	कृमिजग्धम् - अगरु	206
Kṛmīlakaḥ - Makuṣṭhakaḥ	कृमीलकः - मकुष्ठकः	548
Kṛmitaruḥ - Kṡudrāmraḥ	कृमितरुः - क्षुद्राम्रः	387
Kroḍaḥ - Sūkaraḥ	क्रोडः - सूकरः	624
Kroḍakanyā - Vārāhī (Raj. ni.)	क्रोडकन्या - वाराही (रा. नि.)	327
Kroṣṭukaḥ - Sṛgālaḥ	क्रोष्टुकः - श्रृगालः	632
Kroṣṭukapuchhikā - Pṛṣniparṇī	क्रोष्टुकपुच्छिका - पृश्निपर्णी	33
Kṛṣṇā - Drākṡā	कृष्णा - द्राक्षा	413
Kṛṣṇā - Pippalī	कृष्णा - पिप्पली	160
Kṛṣṇabhedā - Kaṭukā	कृष्णभेदा -कटुका	15
Kṛṣṇacūḍikā-Cūḍāmaniḥ(Raj.ni.)	कृष्णचूडिका - चूडामणिः (रा. नि.)	291
Kṛṣṇadhattūrakaḥ-Dhattūraḥ (Raj.ni.)	कृष्णधत्तूरकः - धत्तूरः (रा.नि.)	279
Kṛṣṇaḍunḍubhaḥ-Sarpaviṡeṣaḥ	कृष्णडुण्डुभः - सर्पविशेषः	639
Kṛṣṇāgaru - Agaru	कृष्णागरु - अगरु	206
Kṛṣṇaḥ - Citrakaḥ	कृष्णः - चित्रकः	165
Kṛṣṇaḥ - Ikṡuḥ (Raj. ni.)	कृष्णः - इक्षुः (रा.नि.)	358
Kṛṣṇaḥ - Kokilaḥ	कृष्णः - कोकिलः	637
Kṛṣṇaḥ - Mahiṣaḥ	कृष्णः - महिषः	625
Kṛṣṇājājī - Kṛṣṇajīrakaḥ	कृष्णाजाजी - कृष्णजीरकः	158
Kṛṣṇajaṭā - Māmsī	कृष्णजटा - मांसी	217
Kṛṣṇajīrakaḥ (p. 158)	कृष्णजीरकः (p. 158)	
Kṛṣṇakā - Āsurī	कृष्णका - आसुरी	306
Kṛṣṇakañcukaḥ - Caṇakaḥ	कृष्णकञ्चुकः - चणकः	553
Kṛṣṇalā - Cūḍāmaniḥ	कृष्णला - चूडामणिः	291
Kṛṣṇalavaṇam - Sauvarcalam	कृष्णलवणम् - सौवर्चलम्	136
Kṛṣṇalohakam - Loham	कृष्णलोहकम् - लोहम्	528
Kṛṣṇam - Añjanam	कृष्णम् - अञ्जनम्	262
Kṛṣṇam - Maricam	कृष्णम् - मरिचम्	168
Kṛṣṇamallikā - Ṡālukaḥ	कृष्णमल्लिका - शालुकः	304
Kṛṣṇamudgaḥ - Mudgaḥ	कृष्णमुद्गः -मुद्गः	540
Kṛṣṇamūlī Sārivā (p.60)	कृष्णमूली सारिवा (p.60)	
Kṛṣṇamūṣaṇam - Maricam	कृष्णमूषणम् - मरिचम्	168
Kṛṣṇamuṣkakaḥ-Muṣkakaḥ (Raj.ni.)	कृष्णमुष्ककः - मुष्ककः (रा. नि.)	483
Kṛṣṇapākaphalam-Karamardakam	कृष्णपाकफलम् - करमर्दकम्	449
Kṛṣṇaphalā - Bākucī	कृष्णफला - बाकुची	61
Kṛṣṇārjakaḥ - Sālukaḥ	कृष्णार्जकः - शालुकः	304
Kṛṣṇaṡālih - Ṡālih	कृष्णशालिः-शालिः	535

Kṛṣṇaśālukaḥ - Śālukaḥ	कृष्णशालुकः - शालुकः	304
Kṛṣṇaśamjñaḥ - Śephālikā	कृष्णसंज्ञः - शेफालिका	321
Kṛṣṇasārā - Śimśapā	कृष्णसारा - शिंशपा	473
Kṛṣṇasarṣapaḥ - Rājakśavakaḥ	कृष्णसर्षपः - राजक्षवकः	299
Kṛṣṇaśigruḥ - Śigruḥ (Raj. ni.)	कृष्णशिग्रुः - शिग्रुः (रा. नि.)	296
Kṛṣṇavallī - Kr. Sārivā	कृष्णवल्ली - कृ. सारिवा	60
Kṛṣṇavrīhiḥ - Vrīhiḥ	कृष्णव्रीहिः - व्रीहिः	538
Kṛṣṇavṛntakā - Kāśmarī	कृष्णवृन्तका - काश्मरी	42
Kṛṣṇavṛntā - Māṣaparṇī	कृष्णवृन्ता -माषपर्णी	48
Kṛṣṇāyasam - Loham	कृष्णायसम् - लोहम्	528
Kṛṣṇodumbarikā - Kakodumbarikā (Raj. ni.)	कृष्णोदुम्बरिका-काकोदुम्बरिका (रा.नि.)	438
Kṛṣṇoragaḥ - Sīsakam	कृष्णोरगः - सीसकम्	526
Kṛtacchidrā - Kośātaki	कृतच्छिद्रा - कोशातकी	71
Kṛtakaḥ - Turuṣkaḥ	कृतकः - तुरुष्कः	204
Kṛtakam - Biḍam	कृतकम् - बिडम्	135
Kṛtamālakaḥ - Karṇikāraḥ	कृतमालकः - कर्णिकारः	81
Kṛtaphalam - Kamkolam	कृतफलम् - कंकोलम्	213
Kṛtatrāṇā - Trāyamāṇā	कृतत्राणा - त्रायमाणा	97
Kṛtavedhanam - Kośātakī	कृतवेधनम् - कोशातकी	70
Kṛtavedhanī - Kośātakī	कृतवेधनी - कोशातकी	71
Kṛtrimaḥ - Turuṣkaḥ	कृत्रिमः - तुरुष्कः	204
Kṛtrimakam - Biḍam	कृत्रिमकम् - बिडम्	135
Kṛttiḥ - Twak	कृत्तिः - त्वक्	644
Krūraḥ (p.108)	क्रूरः (p.108)	
Kśamāśāntiparaḥ - Damaḥ	क्षमाशान्तिपरः - दमः	229
Kśaṇaḥ - Rālaḥ	क्षणः - रालः	250
Kśāram - Biḍam	क्षारम् - बिडम्	135
Kśāram - Sāmudram	क्षारम् - सामुद्रम्	136
Kśārapañcakam	क्षारपञ्चकम्	657
Kśāraṣaṭkam	क्षारषट्कम्	658
Kśāraśreṣṭhaḥ -Muṣkakaḥ	क्षारश्रेष्ठः - मुष्ककः	483
Kśāraśreṣṭhaḥ - Kimśukaḥ	क्षारश्रेष्ठः - किंशुकः	518
Kśārāṣṭakam	क्षाराष्टकम्	658
Kśāratrayam	क्षारत्रयम्	657
Kśataghnī - Lākśā	क्षतघ्नी - लाक्षा	239
Kśatakśamaḥ - Khadiraḥ	क्षतक्षमः - खदिरः	10
Kśatriyavarā - Kaṭukālāmbunī	क्षत्रियवरा - कटुकालाम्बुनी	63
Kśaudrajā - Mādhvīsitā	क्षौद्रजा - माध्वी सिता	594
Kśaudram - Madhu	क्षौद्रम् - मधु	591
Kśaudraśarkarā - Madhvīsita	क्षौद्रशर्करा - माध्वी सिता	594
Kśavaḥ - Āsurī	क्षवः - आसुरी	306

Kśemakaḥ - Corakaḥ	क्षेमकः - चोरकः	232
Kśetradūtī - Lakśmaṇā	क्षेत्रदूती - लक्ष्मणा	36
Kśetraruhā - Vālukam (Raj. ni.)	क्षेत्ररुहा - वालुकम् (रा.नि.)	66
Kśetriṇī - Mañjiṣṭhā	क्षेत्रिणी - मञ्जिष्ठा	7
Kśīrā - Kākolī	क्षीरा - काकोली	47
Kśīradrumaḥ - Pippalaḥ	क्षीरद्रुमः -पिप्पलः	427
Kśīrakākolī (p.47)	क्षीरकाकोली (p.47)	47
Kśīrakandā - Kśīravidārī	क्षीरकन्दा - क्षीरविदारी	54
Kśīrakāṇḍakaḥ - Arkaḥ (Raj.ni.)	क्षीरकाण्डकः - अर्कः (रा नि.)	283
Kśīram - Dugdham	क्षीरम् - दुग्धम्	577
Kśīramadhurā - Kśīrakākolī	क्षीरमधुरा - क्षीरकाकोली	47
Kśīramoraṭaḥ - Moraṭaḥ	क्षीरमोरटः - मोरटः	6
Kśīrapalāṇḍuḥ - Palāṇḍuḥ	क्षीरपलाण्डुः - पलाण्डुः	315
Kśīraparṇī - Arkaḥ	क्षीरपर्णी - अर्कः	282
Kśīrasrāvaḥ - Śrīveṣṭakaḥ	क्षीरस्रावः - श्रीवेष्टकः	255
Kśīraśīrṣaḥ - Śrīveṣṭakaḥ	क्षीरशीर्षः - श्रीवेष्टकः	255
Kśīraśuklā - Kśīrakākolī	क्षीरशुक्ला - क्षीरकाकोली	47
Kśīraśuklā - Kśīravidārī	क्षीरशुक्ला - क्षीरविदारी	54
Kśīravallī - Kśīravidārī	क्षीरवल्ली - क्षीरविदारी	54
Kśīravidārī (p.54)	क्षीरविदारी (p.54)	
Kśīraviṣāṇikā - Kśīrakākolī	क्षीरविषाणिका - क्षीरकाकोली	47
Kśīravṛkśaḥ-Rajādanaḥ (Raj.ni.)	क्षीरवृक्षः - राजादनः (रा.नि.)	439
Kśīravṛkśaḥ - Udumbaraḥ	क्षीरवृक्षः - उदुम्बरः	436
Kśīrī - Rājādanaḥ	क्षीरी - राजादनः	439
Kśīrī - Vaṭaḥ	क्षीरी - वटः	426
Kśīriṇī (p. 90)	क्षीरिणी (p. 90)	
Kśuvakaḥ - Āsurī	क्षुवकः - आसुरी	306
Kśudhābhijanakaḥ-Rājakśavakaḥ	क्षुधाभिजनकः - राजक्षवकः	299
Kśudrā - Kaṇṭakārī	क्षुद्रा - कण्टकारी	35
Kśudrabhṛṅgāraḥ - Bhramaraḥ	क्षुद्रभृङ्गारः - भ्रमरः	634
Kśudracandanam-Raktacandanam	क्षुद्रचन्दनम् - रक्तचन्दनम्	193
Kśudrakuliśam -Vaikrāntam	क्षुद्रकुलिशम् - वैकान्तम्	531
Kśudramātā - Kāsaghnī	क्षुद्रमाता - कासघ्नी	37
Kśudrāmlikā (p. 399)	क्षुद्राम्लिका (p. 399)	
Kśudrāmraḥ (p. 387)	क्षुद्राम्रः (p. 387)	
Kśudramutpalam (p. 374)	क्षुद्रमुत्पलम् (p. 374)	373
Kśudrāpāmargaḥ-Rakt.Apāmārgaḥ	क्षुद्रअपामार्गः- र. अपामार्गः	101
Kśudraparṇaḥ - Kuṭherakaḥ	क्षुद्रपर्णः - कुठेरकः	304
Kśudrapatrā-Laghubrāhmī (Raj.ni.)	क्षुद्रपत्रा- लघुब्राह्मी (रा.नि.)	336
Kśudraphalā - Indravāruṇī	क्षुद्रफला - इन्द्रवारुणी	95
Kśudrasahā - Mudgaparṇī	क्षुद्रसहा -मुद्गपर्णी	49
Kśudraśārdūlaḥ - Śarabhaḥ	क्षुद्रशार्दूलः - शरभः	624

Kśudravarṣābhūḥ - Punarnavā	क्षुद्रवर्षाभूः - पुनर्नवा	107
Kśudrolūkaḥ - Ulūkaḥ (p. 638)	क्षुद्रोलूकः - उलूकः (p. 638)	
Kśumā - Atasī	क्षुमा - अतसी	565
Kśuraḥ - Muñjaḥ	क्षुरः - मुञ्जः	360
Kśuraḥ - Śaraḥ	क्षुरः - शरः	363
Kśurakaḥ - Tilakaḥ	क्षुरकः - तिलकः	513
Kśurapatraḥ - Śaraḥ (Raj. ni.)	क्षुरपत्रः - शरः (रा.निः)	364
Kśveḍā - Kośātakī	क्ष्वेडा - कोशातकी	71
Kśveḍaḥ - Jīvakaḥ	क्ष्वेडः - जीवकः	44
Kuberākśī -Kaṣṭhapāṭalā	कुबेराक्षी - काष्ठपाटला	44
Kubhṛṅgakaḥ - Bhramaraḥ	कुभृङ्गकः - भ्रमरः	634
Kubjakaḥ (p. 502)	कुब्जकः (p. 502)	
Kubjakaṇṭakaḥ- Somavalkaḥ	कुब्जकण्टकः - सोमवल्कः	10
Kucandanam - Pataṅgam	कुचन्दनम् - पतङ्गम्	194
Kucaphalaḥ-Dāḍimaḥ (Raj.ni.)	कुचफलः -दाडिमः (रा.नि.)	155
Kuddālaḥ - Kovidāraḥ	कुद्दालः - कोविदारः	73
Kuddālī - Aśmantakaḥ	कुद्दाली - अश्मन्तकः	72
Kuḍmalam - Saugandhikam	कुड्मलम् - सौगन्धिकम्	371
Kuham - Badaram	कुहम् - बदरम्	445
Kujam - Saugandhikam	कुजम् - सौगन्धिकम्	371
Kukkuraḥ - Sārameyaḥ	कुक्कुरः - सारमेयः	632
Kukkuṭaḥ - Śitivāraḥ	कुक्कुटः -शितिवारः	56
Kukkuṭaḥ (p. 635)	कुक्कुटः (p. 635)	
Kukkuṭī - Śālmalī	कुक्कुटी - शाल्मली	481
Kulakaḥ - Paṭolaḥ	कुलकः - पटोलः	18
Kulālī - Cakśuṣyā	कुलाली - चक्षुष्या	264
Kulaṅgaḥ - Sarpaviśeṣaḥ	कुलङ्गः - सर्पविशेषः	639
Kulatthaḥ (p. 556)	कुलत्थः (p. 556)	
Kulatthikā - Cakśuṣyā	कुलत्थिका - चक्षुष्या	264
Kulī - Bṛhatī	कुली - बृहती	35
Kulī - Kovidāraḥ	कुली - कोविदारः	73
Kulīrā - Karkaṭaśṛṅgī	कुलीरा - कर्कटशृंगी	30
Kulīraḥ - Karkaṭaḥ	कुलीरः - कर्कटः	640
Kulīrakaḥ - Karkaṭaḥ	कुलीरकः - कर्कटः	640
Kulīraśṛṅgī - Karkaṭaśṛṅgī	कुलीरशृङ्गी - कर्कटशृङ्गी	30
Kuliśaḥ - Matsyabhedaḥ	कुलिशः - मत्स्यभेदः	628
Kuliśam - Hīrakam	कुलिशम् - हीरकम्	532
Kulmāṣābhiṣutam - Kāñjikam	कुल्माषाभिषुतम् - काञ्जिकम्	595
Kumārakaḥ - Varuṇaḥ	कुमारकः - वरुणः	472
Kumarī - Taruṇī	कुमारी - तरुणी	501
Kumārikā - Karkoṭakī	कुमारिका - कर्कोटकी	69
Kumārikā - Mallikā (Raj. ni.)	कुमारिका - मल्लिका (रा. नि.)	494

Kumārikā - Vandhyakarkoṭakī	कुमारिका - वन्ध्यकर्कोटकी	68
Kumbhakārī - Cakṡuṣyā	कुम्भकारी - चक्षुष्या	264
Kumbhaphalā - Kūṣmāṇḍikā	कुम्भफला - कूष्माण्डिका	68
Kumbhāraḥ - Kovidāraḥ	कुम्भारः - कोविदारः	73
Kumbhī - Hasti	कुम्भी - हस्ति	620
Kumbhībījam - Jayapālaḥ	कुम्भीबीजम् - जयपालः	86
Kumbhīkā - Kaṭphalaḥ	कुम्भीका - कट्फलः	27
Kumbhīkā - Pāṭalā	कुम्भीका - पाटला	43
Kumbhinīphalam -Jayapālaḥ	कुम्भिनीफलम् - जयपालः	86
Kumkumam (p. 197)	कुंकुमम् (p. 197)	
Kumudā - Kaṭphalaḥ	कुमुदा - कट्फलः	27
Kumudā - (Pṛṡni.) viṡeṣaḥ	कुमुदा - (पृश्नि.) विशेषः	33
Kumudagandhinī - Ṡuklabhaṇḍī	कुमुदगन्धिनी - शुक्लभण्डी	94
Kumudam (p. 373)	कुमुदम् (p. 373)	
Kumudvatī- Padminī	कुमुद्वती - पद्मिनी	374
Kunāsaḥ - Uṣṭraḥ	कुनासः - उष्ट्रः	621
Kunaṭī - Manaḥṡilā	कुनटी - मनःशिला	246
Kuñcī - Upakuñcī	कुञ्ची - उपकुञ्ची	154
Kuñcikā - Upakuñcī	कुञ्चिका -उपकुञ्ची	154
Kuñcikā - Methikā	कुञ्चिका - मेथिका	562
Kuñcitam - Tagaram	कुञ्चितम् - तगरम्	221
Kundaḥ (p. 506)	कुन्दः (p. 506)	
Kuṇḍalī - Kovidāraḥ	कुण्डली - कोविदारः	73
Kuṇḍalī - Sarpaḥ	कुण्डली - सर्पः	639
Kuṇḍalī- Guḍūcī	कुण्डली - गुडूची	2
Kundraḥ - Kunduruḥ	कुन्द्रः - कुन्दुरुः	254
Kunduruḥ (p. 254)	कुन्दुरुः (p. 254)	
Kundurukaḥ - Kunduruḥ	कुन्दुरुकः - कुन्दुरुः	254
Kundurukī - Ṡallakī	कुन्दुरुकी - शल्लकी	256
Kuñjarā - Dhātukī	कुञ्जरा - धातुकी	242
Kuñjaraḥ - Hasti	कुञ्जरः - हस्ति	620
Kuntalavardhanaḥ - Bhṛṅgarājaḥ (Raj. ni.)	कुन्तलवर्धनः - भृङ्गराजः (रा.नि.)	281
Kuṇṭham - Guṇṭhaḥ	कुण्ठम् - गुण्ठः	29
Kūpyam - Raupyam	कूप्यम् - रौप्यम्	524
Kurabakaḥ - Ṡwetamandāraḥ	कुरबकः - श्वेतमन्दारः	283
Kurabakaḥ - Saireyakaḥ	कुरबकः - सैरेयकः	109
Kuraṅgaḥ - Hariṇaḥ	कुरङ्गः - हरिणः	625
Kuraṇṭakaḥ -Saireyakaḥ	कुरण्टकः - सैरेयकः	109
Kūrcaṡekharaḥ - Nārikelaḥ	कूर्चशेखरः - नारिकेलः	425
Kūrcaṡīrṣakaḥ - Jīvakaḥ	कूर्चशीर्षकः - जीवकः	44
Kūrmaḥ - Kacchapaḥ	कूर्मः - कच्छपः	630

Kūrmarājaḥ-Anyaḥ Kacchapaḥ कूर्मराजः -अन्यः कच्छपः 630
Kuruṭaḥ - Sitivāraḥ (Raj. ni.) कुरुटः - शितिवारः (रा. नि.) 57
Kuruvindaḥ - Māṣaḥ कुरुविन्दः - माषः 552
Kuruvindakaḥ - Mustā कुरुविन्दकः - मुस्ता 15
Kuśah (p. 361) कुशः (p. 361)
Kuśaḥ alpaḥ - Kuśaḥ (Raj. ni.) कुशः अल्पः - कुशः (रा.नि.) 362
Kuśālmaliḥ - Rohitakaḥ कुशाल्मलिः - रोहितकः 485
Kuśeśayam - Kumudam कुशेशयम् - कुमुदम् 373
Kuśimśapā - Śimśapā कुशिंशपा - शिंशपा 473
Kūṣmāṇḍī - Kūṣmāṇḍikā कूष्माण्डी - कूष्माण्डिका 68
Kūṣmāṇḍikā (p.68) कूष्माण्डिका (p.68)
Kusumbhakam-Śāliparṇī viśeṣaḥ कुसुम्भकम् - शालिपर्णी विशेषः 32
Kuṣṭhahā - Paṭolaḥ कुष्ठहा - पटोलः 18
Kuṣṭham (p.218) कुष्ठम् (p.218)
Kuṣṭhanāśanaḥ-Sarṣapaḥ (Raj.ni.) कुष्ठनाशनः - सर्षपः (रा. नि.) 298
Kuṣṭhanāśinī - Bākucī कुष्ठनाशिनी - बाकुची 61
Kuṣṭhghnī-Kākodumbarikā (Raj.ni.) कुष्ठघ्नी-काकोदुम्बरिका (रा.नि.) 438
Kustumbaruḥ - Dhānyakam कुस्तुम्बरुः - धान्यकम् 156
Kusumāsavam - Madhu कुसुमासवम् - मधु 592
Kusumbhakā - Dāruharidrā कुसुम्भका - दारुहरिद्रा 21
Kusumbham (p. 566) कुसुम्भम् (p. 566)
Kusumbhatailam कुसुम्भतैलम् 571
Kuṭajaḥ (p.131) कुटजः (p.131)
Kuṭannaṭaḥ - Śyonākaḥ कुटंनटः - श्योनाकः 41
Kuṭannaṭam - Paripellavam कुटन्नटम् - परिपेल्लवम् 222
Kūṭaśālmaliḥ - Rohitakaḥ कूटशाल्मलिः - रोहितकः 485
Kūṭastham - Vyāghranakham कूटस्थम् - व्याघ्रनखम् 224
Kuṭherakaḥ - Tūṇiḥ कुठेरकः - तूणिः 202
Kutherakaḥ (p. 303) कुठेरकः (p. 303)
Kuṭī - Murā कुटी - मुरा 229
Kuṭilam - Tagaram कुटिलम् - तगरम् 221
Kuṭṭimaḥ - Dāḍimaḥ कुट्टिमः -दाडिमः 155
Kuṭumbakaḥ - Bhūstṛṇaḥ कुटुम्बकः - भूस्तृणः 300
Kuvalam - Saugandhikam कुवलम् - सौगन्धिकम् 371
Kuvalayam - Saugandhikam कुवलयम् - सौगन्धिकम् 371
Kuvārtikā - Lakṣmaṇā कुवार्तिका - लक्ष्मणा 36
Laghu - Lāmajjakam लघु- लामज्जकम् 241
Laghu Hemadugdhā-Udumbaraḥ (Raj.ni.) लघुहेमदुग्धा-उदुम्बरः(रा.नि.)436
Laghubrāhmī -Brāhmī (Raj. ni.) (336) लघुब्राह्मी - ब्राह्मी (रा. नि.) (336)
Laghucandanam - Kāleyakam लघुचन्दनम् - कालेयकम् 207
Laguḍaḥ - Karavīraḥ लगुडः - करवीरः 275
Laghumāmsī-Gandhamāmsī (Raj.ni.) लघुमांसी - गन्धमांसी (रा.नि.) 218

Laghupañcamūlam	लघुपञ्चमूलम्	648
Laghupatraḥ-Udumbaraḥ (Raj. ni.)	लघुपत्रः - उदुम्बरः (रा.नि.)	436
Laghupatrakaḥ - Śigruḥ	लघुपत्रकः - शिग्रुः	295
Laghupatrikā - Aśvatthī	लघुपत्रिका - अश्वत्थी	428
Laghupuṣpā - Ketakī	लघुपुष्पा - केतकी	520
Laghuudumbaraḥ-Udumbaraḥ (Raj.ni.)	लघुउदुम्बरः - उदुम्बरः (रा.नि.)	436
Laghvī - Spṛkkā (Raj. ni.)	लघ्वी - स्पृक्का (रा. नि.)	224
Lākśā (p. 239)	लाक्षा (p. 239)	
Lākśāprasādanaḥ-Paṭṭikārodhraḥ	लाक्षाप्रसादनः -पट्टिकारोध्रः	270
Lākśāvṛkśaḥ - Kśudrāmraḥ	लाक्षावृक्षः - क्षुद्राम्रः	387
Lakśmaṇā (p.36)	लक्ष्मणा (p.36)	
Lakśmīḥ - Śamī	लक्ष्मीः - शमी	442
Lakśmīḥ - Padmacāriṇī	लक्ष्मीः - पद्मचारिणी	325
Lalanā - Strī	ललना - स्त्री	615
Lalanaḥ - Priyālaḥ	ललनः -प्रियालः	423
Lalanaḥ - Rālaḥ	ललनः - रालः	250
Lalanaḥ - Sarjakaḥ (Raj. ni.)	ललनः - सर्जकः (रा. नि.)	477
Lalanāpriyaḥ - Kadambaḥ	ललनाप्रियः - कदम्बः	451
Lāmajjakam (p.241)	लामज्जकम् (p.241)	
Lambā - Kaṭukālāmbunī	लम्बा - कट्टकालाम्बुनी	63
Lambabīja - (a type of) Śreyasī (Raj. ni.)	लम्बबीजा - श्रेयसी विशेषः (रा.नि.)	163
Lambakarṇaḥ - Chāgaḥ	लम्बकर्णः - छागः	622
Lāṅgalī - Jalapippalī	लाङ्गली - जलपिप्पली	310
Lāṅgalī - Kalikārī	लाङ्गली - कलिकारी	280
Lāṅgalī - Nārikelaḥ	लाङ्गली - नारिकेलः	425
Lāṅgūlī - Kapikacchuḥ	लाङ्गूली - कपिकच्छुः	55
Laṅkā - Tripuṭah (Raj. ni.)	लङ्का - त्रिपुटः (रा. नि.)	560
Lasatphalaḥ - Khastilaḥ	लसत्फलः - खस्तिलः	567
Laśunaḥ (p. 311)	लशुनः (p. 311)	
Latā - Sārivā	लता - सारिवा	59
Latākarkaṭikā - Trapusam	लताकर्कटिका - त्रपुसम्	65
Lāṭaparṇam -Twak	लाटपर्णम् - त्वक्	145
Latārkaḥ - Palāṇḍuḥ	लतार्कः - पलाण्डुः	315
Lāvaḥ (p. 636)	लावः (p. 636)	
Lāvakaḥ - Lāvaḥ	लावकः - लावः	636
Lavam - Lāmajjakam	लवम् - लामज्जकम्	241
Lavam - Lavaṅgam	लवम् - लवङ्गम्	214
Lavaṇapañcakam	लवणपञ्चकम्	655
Lavaṇaṣaṭkam	लवणषट्कम्	658
Lavangam (p. 214)	लवङ्गम (p. 214)	
Lavaṇoktā- Jyotiṣmatī	लवणोक्ता - ज्योतिष्मती	103

Lavaṇodadhisambhavam-Sāmudram	लवणोदधिसंभवम् - सामुद्रम्	136
Laxmīḥ - Ṛddhiḥ	लक्ष्मीः -ऋद्धिः	53
Laksmīphalaḥ - Bilvaḥ	लक्ष्मीफलः - बिल्वः	39
Lekhanī - Kāśaḥ (Raj. ni.)	लेखनी - काशः (रा.नि.)	359
Lekhasārakaḥ - Śleṣmātakaḥ	लेखसारकः - श्लेष्मातकः	441
Lekhyapatraḥ - Tālaḥ	लेख्यपत्रः -तालः	421
Lelīnaḥ - Vaṭasaugandhikaḥ	लेलीनः - वटसौगन्धिकः	248
Lelitaḥ - Gandhakaḥ	लेलितः - गन्धकः	248
Lelītaḥ - Vaṭasaugandhikaḥ	लेलीतः - वटसौगन्धिकः	248
Lobhanīyā - Mahāśrāvaṇī	लोभनीया - महाश्रावणी	58
Locamarkaṭaḥ - Ajamodā	लोचमर्कटः - अजमोदा	183
Locanahitā - Cakśuṣyā	लोचनहिता - चक्षुष्या	264
Lodhraḥ (p. 267)	लोध्रः (p. 267)	
Lodhrapuṣpaḥ - Madhūkaḥ	लोध्रपुष्पः - मधूकः	406
Lohakaḥ - Pittalam	लोहकः - पित्तलम्	526
Loham - Agaru	लोहम् - अगरु	206
Loham - Kāmsyam	लोहम् - कांस्यम्	527
Loham (p. 527)	लोहम् (p. 527)	
Lohaniryāsam - Maṇḍūram	लोहनिर्यासम् - मण्डूरम्	529
Lohaśuddhikārakaḥ - Ṭaṅkaṇaḥ	लोहशुद्धिकारकः - टंकणः	134
Lohitam - Haricandanam	लोहितम् - हरिचन्दनम्	196
Lohitam - Raktacandanam	लोहितम् - रक्तचन्दनम्	193
Lohitam - Raktam	लोहितम् - रक्तम्	619
Lohitāṅgaḥ - Kampillakaḥ	लोहिताङ्गः - कम्पिल्लकः	257
Lohocchiṣṭam - Maṇḍūram	लोहोच्छिष्टम् - मण्डूरम्	529
Lohottham - Maṇḍūram	लोहोत्थम् - मण्डूरम्	529
Lolā - Kśudrāmlikā	लोला - क्षुद्राम्लिका	399
Lomakaraṇī-Māmsarohiṇī (Raj.ni.)	लोमकरणी - मांसरोहिणी (रा.नि.)	330
Loman - Roma	लोमन् - रोम	644
Lomanam - Māmsam	लोमनम् - मांसम्	618
Lomaśā - Urvāruḥ	लोमशा -उर्वारुः	65
Lomaśā - Gandhamāmsī	लोमशा - गन्धमांसी	217
Lomaśā - Kākajaṅghā	लोमशा - काकजङ्घा	287
Lomaśā - Vacā	लोमशा - वचा	125
Lomaśaḥ - Gandhamārjāraḥ	लोमशः -गन्धमार्जारः	631
Lomaśapatrikā-Jīmūtakaḥ (Raj.ni.)	लोमशपत्रिका - जीमूतकः (रा.नि.)	64
Loṇā - Kśudrāmlikā	लोणा - क्षुद्राम्लिका	399
Loṇikā - Kśudrāmlikā	लोणिका - क्षुद्राम्लिका	399
Lulāyakaḥ - Mahiṣaḥ	लुलायकः - महिषः	625
Lulāyakāntā - Mahiṣī	लुलायकान्ता - महिषी	625
Luṅgaḥ - Bījapūraḥ	लुङ्गः - बीजपूरः	396
Mācikā - Ambaṣṭhā	माचिका - अम्बष्ठा	249

Madaḍhyaḥ-Kadambaḥ (Raj. ni.) मदाढ्यः- कदम्बः (रा. नि.) 453
Madāḍhyaḥ - Tālaḥ (Raj. ni.) मदाढ्यः - तालः (रा.नि.) 421
Māḍadrumaḥ - Māḍaḥ माडद्रुमः - माडः 421
Madyagandhaḥ - Bakulaḥ मद्यगन्धः - बकुलः 511
Madagandhikā-Aśvagandhā (Raj.ni.) मदगन्धिका - अश्वगन्धा (रा.नि.)106
Māḍah (p.422) माडः (p.422)
Madahastinikā - Karañjaḥ मदहस्तिनिका - करञ्जः 461
Madakarī - Surā मदकरी - सुरा 596
Madakāriṇī - Yāvanī Yavānī मदकारिणी - यावनी यवानी 172
Madanāgrajaḥ-Kodravaḥ (Raj. ni.) मदनाग्रजः - कोद्रवः (रा.नि.) 542
Madanaḥ (p.62) मदनः (p.62)
Madanakaḥ - Dhattūraḥ मदनकः - धत्तूरः 278
Madanakam - Sikthakam मदनकम् - सिक्थकम् 250
Madanamañjarī - Jiṅgiṇī मदनमञ्जरी - जिंगिणी 272
Madanī - Kastūrikā मदनी - कस्तूरिका 208
Madanīyā - Mallikā मदनीया - मल्लिका 493
Madanodbhavā-Madhuśarkarā मदनोद्भवा - मधुशर्करा 190
Madaśauṇḍam - Jātīphalam मदशौण्डम् - जातीफलम् 211
Madayantī - Mallikā मदयन्ती - मल्लिका 493
Madyottamam - Mārdwīkam मद्योत्तमम् - मार्द्वीकम् 599
Mādhavaḥ - Asitamudgaḥ माधवः - असितमुद्गः 540
Mādhavaḥ - Madhūkaḥ माधवः -मधूकः 406
Mādhavī - Śatapuṣpā माधवी - शतपुष्पा 121
Mādhavī - Vārāhī माधवी - वाराही 326
Mādhavī - Vāsantī (Raj. ni.) माधवी - वासन्ती (रा. नि.) 499
Mādhavī - Madhuśarkarā माधवी - मधुशर्करा 189
Mādhavī - Surā माधवी - सुरा 596
Mādhavocitam - Kamkolam माधवोचितम् - कंकोलम् 213
Madhu - Mārdwīkam मधु - मार्द्वीकम् 599
Madhu (p. 591) मधु (p. 591)
Madhubhavā - Madhuśarkarā मधुभवा - मधुशर्करा 189
Madhūcchiṣṭam - Sikthakam मधूच्छिष्टम् - सिक्थकम् 249
Madhucūtaḥ - Āmraḥ मधुचूतः - आम्रः 385
Madhudhātuḥ-Hemamākśikam मधुधातुः - हेममाक्षिकम् 261
Madhugandhaḥ - Bakulaḥ मधुगन्धः - बकुलः 511
Madhujā - Mādhvīsitā मधुजा - माध्वी सिता 594
Madhujam - Sikthakam मधुजम् - सिक्थकम् 250
MadhuJambīraḥ (p. 390) मधुजम्बीरः (p. 390)
MadhuJambīraphalaḥ-Madhu Jambīraḥ मधजुम्बीरफलः - मधुजम्बीरः 390
Madhūkaḥ (p. 406) मधूकः (p. 406)
Madhukam - Sikthakam मधुकम् - सिक्थकम् 259
Madhukam - Yaṣṭīmadhu मधुकम् - यष्टीमधु 52

Madhukaphalam - Pālevatam (Raj. ni.) मधुकफलम् - पालेवतम् रा.नि.) 418
Madhukaraḥ - Bhramaraḥ मधुकरः - भ्रमरः 633
Madhukarkaṭī (p. 397) मधुकर्कटी (p. 397)
Madhukṛt - Bhramaraḥ मधुकृत् - भ्रमरः 633
Madhūkasīdhuḥ मधूकसीधुः 598
Madhūlikā - Jaladaḥ मधूलिका -जलदः 408
Madhūlikā - Klītanakam मधूलिका - क्लीतनकम् 52
Madhūlikā - Yaṣṭīmadhu मधूलिका - यष्टीमधु 52
Madhuliṭ- Bhramaraḥ मधुलिट् - भ्रमरः 633
Madhupaḥ - Bhramaraḥ मधुपः - भ्रमरः 633
Madhuparṇī - Klītanakam मधुपर्णी - क्लीतनकम् 52
Madhuparṇī - Guḍūcī मधुपर्णी - गुडूची 2
Madhuparṇī - Kāśmarī मधुपर्णी - काश्मरी 42
Madhuparṇī - Yaṣṭīmadhu मधुपर्णी - यष्टीमधु 52
Madhupīluḥ - Bṛhatpīluḥ मधुपीलुः - बृहत्पीलुः 410
Madhupuṣpaḥ-Bakulaḥ (Raj. ni.) मधुपुष्पः - बकुलः (रा. नि.) 511
Madhupuṣpaḥ - Jaladaḥ मधुपुष्पः -जलदः 408
Madhupuṣpikaḥ - Jaladaḥ मधुपुष्पिकः -जलदः 408
Madhurā - Kākolī मधुरा - काकोली 47
Madhuragaṇaḥ-Jīvanīyagaṇaḥ मधुरगणः - जीवनीयगणः 650
Madhurāgrajā - Kharjūrī मधुराग्रजा - खर्जूरी 411
Madhuraḥ - Jīvakaḥ मधुरः - जीवकः 44
Madhuraḥ - Śigruḥ (Raj. ni.) मधुरः - शिग्रुः (रा. नि.) 296
Madhuraḥ - Guḍaḥ मधुरः - गुडः 358
Madhuraḥ - Madhukarkaṭī मधुरः - मधुकर्कटी 397
Madhuraḥ - Masūraḥ मधुरः - मसूरः 550
Madhurasā - Uttarāpathikā मधुरसा -उत्तरापथिका 414
Madhurasā - Mūrvā मधुरसा- मूर्वा 5
Madhurasvaraḥ - Bhramaraḥ मधुरस्वरः - भ्रमरः 634
Madhuratrikam -Trimadhuram मधुरत्रिकम् - त्रिमधुरम् 658
Madhurikā -Miśreyā (Raj. ni.) मधुरिका - मिश्रेया (रा.नि.) 123
Madhurikā - Āsurī (Raj. ni.) मधुरिका - आसुरी (रा.नि.) 306
Madhuśarkarā (p. 188) मधुशर्करा (p. 188)
Madhuśeṣam - Sikthakam मधुशेषम् - सिक्थकम् 249
Madhuśigruḥ - Śigruḥ मधुशिग्रुः - शिग्रुः 295
Madhuśigrukaḥ -Śigruḥ (Raj. ni.) मधुशिग्रुकः - शिग्रुः (रा. नि.) 296
Madhusravā - Dīpyā मधुस्रवा - दीप्या 412
Madhusravā - Yaṣṭīmadhu मधुस्रवा - यष्टीमधु 52
Madhusravaḥ - Madhūkaḥ मधुस्रवः -मधूकः 406
Madhusravaḥ - Moraṭaḥ मधुस्रवः - मोरटः 6
Madhuṣṭhīlaḥ - Madhūkaḥ मधुष्ठीलः -मधूकः 406
Madhūtpannā - Mādhvīsitā मधूत्पन्ना - माध्वी सिता 594

Madhūtthitam - Sikthakam	मधूत्थितम् - सिक्थकम्	250
Madhuvallī - Madhukarkaṭī	मधुवल्ली - मधुकर्क्कटी	398
Madhuvṛkśaḥ - Madhūkaḥ	मधुवृक्षः - मधूकः	406
Madhuyaṣṭī - Yaṣṭīmadhu	मधुयष्टी - यष्टीमधु	52
Madhuyaṣṭikā - Yaṣṭīmadhu	मधुयष्टिका - यष्टीमधु	52
Mādhavī - Atimuktakaḥ	माधवी - अतिमुक्तकः	509
Madhvāsavaḥ	मध्वासवः	600
Mādhvī sitā (p. 594)	माध्वी सिता (p. 594)	
Madhyakeśaraḥ - Bījapūraḥ	मध्यकेशरः - बीजपूरः	396
Madhyamapañcamūlam	मध्यमपञ्चमूलम्	648
Mādikā - Vijayā	मादिका - विजया	46
Mādinī - Vijayā	मादिनी - विजया	46
Madirā - Surā	मदिरा - सुरा	596
Madirāsakhaḥ - Āmraḥ	मदिरासखः - आम्रः	385
Madotsavaḥ - Āmraḥ	मदोत्सवः - आम्रः	385
Madodbhvaḥ - Āmraḥ	मदोद्भवः - आम्रः	385
Madotkaṭam - Mārdwīkam	मदोत्कटम् - मार्द्वीकम्	599
Madhuphalaḥ - Āmraḥ	मधुफलः - आम्रः	385
Madhuśarkarā - Mādhvīsitā	मधुशर्करा - माध्वी सिता	594
Madyadruḥ - Māḍaḥ	मद्यद्रुः - माडः	422
Madyadrumaḥ - Māḍaḥ	मद्यद्रुमः - माडः	422
Madyam - Surā	मद्यं - सुरा	596
Madyāmodaḥ-Bakulaḥ (Raj. ni.)	मद्यामोदः - बकुलः (रा. नि.)	511
Madyapuṣpā-Dhātukī (Raj. ni.)	मद्यपुष्पा - धातुकी (रा. नि.)	243
Madyavāsinī - Dhātukī	मद्यवासिनी - धातुकी	243
Māgadham - Jīrakam	मागधम् - जीरकम्	157
Māgadhī - Pippalī	मागधी - पिप्पली	160
Mahā vṛkśaḥ - Bṛhatpīluḥ	महावृक्षः - बृहत्पीलुः	410
Mahābalā (p.110)	महाबला (p.110)	
Mahādāruḥ - Devadāruḥ	महादारुः - देवदारुः	27
Mahādiḥ - Karnikāraḥ	महादिः - कर्णिकारः	81
Mahāgandham - Haricandanam	महागन्धम् - हरिचन्दनम्	196
Mahājālinī - Āvartaki	महाजालिनी - आवर्तकी	74
Mahājālinī - Dhāmārgavaḥ	महाजालिनी -धामार्गवः	70
Mahājambūḥ - Jambūḥ	महाजम्बूः - जम्बूः	433
Mahākandam - Mūlakam	महाकन्दम् -मूलकम्	293
Mahākandarasonaḥ - Laśunaḥ	महाकन्दरसोनः - लशुनः	312
Mahākoṣā - Karkaṭaśṛngī	महाकोषा - कर्कटश्रृंगी	30
Mahākośātakī - Kośātakī	महाकोशातकी - कोशातकी	71
Mahākśīrā - Mahiṣī	महाक्षीरा - महिषी	625
Mahākumbhā - Kaṭphalaḥ	महाकुम्भा - कट्फलः	27
Mahāmatsyaḥ-Anyaḥ Kacchapaḥ	महामत्स्यः -अन्यः कच्छपः	630

Mahāmedā (p.45) महामेदा (p.45)
Mahāmuniḥ -Tumbaruḥ महामुनिः - तुम्बरुः 140
Mahāmūṣakaḥ (p. 631) महामूषकः (p. 631)
Mahānalaḥ (p. 367) महानलः (p. 367)
Mahāngaḥ - Mahāmūṣakaḥ महाङ्गः - महामूषकः 631
Mahānimbaḥ (p.12) महानिम्बः (p. 12)
Mahāpālevatam - Pālevatam महापालेवतम् - पालेवतम्
Mahāpārevatam - Pālevatam (Raj. ni.) महापारेवतम्-पालेवतम् (रा.नि.) 418
Mahāpāśupataḥ -Bukaḥ महापाशुपतः - बुकः 284
Mahāpatrā-Gāngerukī (Raj. ni.) महापत्रा - गांगेरुकी (रा.नि.) 112
Mahāphalā-Gāngerukī (Raj.ni.) महाफला - गांगेरुकी (रा.नि.) 112
Mahāphalā - Kaṭukālāmbunī महाफला - कटुकालाम्बुनी 63
Mahāphalā - Viśālā महाफला - विशाला 95
Rājajambuḥ - Jambūḥ राजजम्बूः - जम्बूः 433
Mahāphalā - Jambūh महाफला - जम्बूः 433
Mahāphalā - Kośātakī महाफला - कोशातकी 71
Mahāphalā - Madhukarkaṭī महाफला - मधुकर्कटी 398
Mahāphalaḥ - Bilvaḥ महाफलः - बिल्वः 39
Mahāphalaḥ - Bṛhatpīluḥ महाफलः - बृहत्पीलुः 410
Mahāpīluḥ - Bṛhatpīluḥ महापीलुः - बृहत्पीलुः 418
Mahāprarohaḥ - Plakśaḥ महाप्ररोहः - प्लक्षः 429
Mahāpuruṣadantā-Mahāśatāvarī महापुरुषदन्ता - महाशतावरी 116
Mahāraktam - Pravālam महारक्तम् - प्रवालम् 534
Mahārasam - Kāñjikam महारसम् - काञ्जिकम् 595
Mahārasam - Pāradaḥ महारसम् - पारदः 529
Mahārham - Candanam महार्हम् -चन्दनम् 191
Maharṣabhī - Kapikacchuḥ महर्षभी - कपिकच्छुः 55
Mahāsahā - Kubjakaḥ महासहा - कुब्जकः 503
Mahāsahā - Taruṇī (Raj. ni.) महासहा - तरुणी (रा. नि.) 501
Mahāsahā - Māṣaparṇī महासहा -माषपर्णी 48
Mahāśākhā-Gāngerukī (Raj.ni.) महाशाखा - गांगेरुकी (रा.नि.) 112
Mahāśāliḥ - Śāliḥ महाशालिः- शालिः 535
Mahāsamangā - Balā महासमङ्गा - बला 110
Mahāśaṇaḥ - Śaṇapuṣpī महाशणः - शणपुष्पी 75
Mahāśaraḥ - Śaraḥ (Raj. ni.) महाशरः - शरः (रा.नि.) 363
Mahāsarjah - Aśanaḥ महासर्जः - अशनः 479
Mahāśaṭhaḥ-Dhattūraḥ (Raj. ni.) महाशठः - धत्तूरः (रा. नि.) 279
Mahāskandhā - Jambūḥ महास्कन्धा - जम्बूः 433
Mahāśrāvaṇī (p.58) महाश्रावणी (p.58)
Mahāsugandhā - Gandhanākulī महासुगन्धा - गन्धनाकुली 342
Mahāsugandhaḥ महासुगन्धः 653
Mahāśvetā - Aśvakśurakaḥ महाश्वेता -अश्वक्षुरकः 323

Mahāśyāmā - Śiṁśapā	महाश्यामा - शिंशपा	473
Mahatī - Bṛhatī	महती - बृहती	35
Mahātiktakaḥ - Kirātatiktaḥ	महातिक्तः -किराततिक्तः	14
Mahaujasī - Tejasvinī	महौजसी - तेजस्विनी	102
Mahauṣadham - Laśunaḥ	महौषधम् - लशुनः	312
Mahauṣadham - Śuṇṭhī	महौषधम् - शुण्ठी	167
Mahauṣadham - Vatasanābhaḥ	महौषधम् - वत्सनाभः	667
Mahauṣadhī - Brāhmī	महौषधी- ब्राह्मी	336
Mahauṣadhī - Lakśmaṇā	महौषधी - लक्ष्मणा	36
Mahāvarṣābhūḥ - Krūraḥ	महावर्षाभूः -क्रूरः	108
Mahāvasu - Raupyam	महावसु - रौप्यम्	524
Mahāvittaḥ - Maṇḍukaviśeṣaḥ	महावित्तः - मण्डूकविशेषः	640
Mahāvrīhiḥ - Vrīhiḥ	महाव्रीहिः - व्रीहिः	538
Mahāvṛkśaḥ - Snuhī	महावृक्षः - स्नुही	88
Mahāyamalapatrakaḥ-Kovidāraḥ	महायमलपत्रकः - कोविदारः	73
Mahāyogeśvarī - Balāmoṭā	महायोगेश्वरी - बलामोटा	378
Mahendravāruṇī-Viśālā (Raj.ni.)	महेन्द्रवारुणी - विशाला (रा.नि.)	96
Maheraṇā - Śallakī	महेरणा - शल्लकी	256
Maheśvarī - Pittalam	महेश्वरी - पित्तलम्	526
Mahilā -Strī	महिला - स्त्री	615
Mahiṣaḥ (p.625)	महिषः (p.625)	
Mahiṣākśaḥ - Gugguluḥ	महिषाक्षः - गुग्गुलुः	252
Mahiṣī (p. 625)	महिषी (p. 625)	
Mahiṣī dadhi	महिषीदधि	584
Mahiṣīghṛtam	महिषीघृतम्	574
Mahiṣīmūtram	महिषीमूत्रम्	642
Mahiṣīpayaḥ	महिषीपयः	579
Mahodayā-Gāṅgerukī (Raj.ni.)	महोदया - गांगेरुकी (रा.नि.)	112
Mahoṭikā - Bṛhatī	महोटिका - बृहती	35
Mahoṭikā - Vṛntākī (Raj.ni.)	महोटिका - वृन्ताकी (रा. नि.)	37
Maireyaḥ	मैरेयः	601
Majjā (p.619)	मज्जा (p. 619)	
Mākandaḥ - Āmraḥ	माकन्दः - आम्रः	385
Makaraḥ - Mahāmatsyaviśeṣaḥ	मकरः - महामत्स्य विशेषः	628
Makarandaḥ-Kundaḥ (Raj.ni.)	मकरन्दः - कुन्दः (रा. नि.)	506
Makarandam - Padmakesaram	मकरन्दम् - पद्मकेसरम्	377
Makarandavāsaḥ-Kadambaḥ (Raj. ni.)	मकरन्दवासः - कदम्बः (रा. नि.)	452
Mākśikadhātuḥ-Hemamākśikam	माक्षिकधातुः - हेममाक्षिकम्	261
Mākśikam - Madhu	माक्षिकम् - मधु	591
Mākśīkam - Madhu	माक्षीकम् - मधु	591
Mākśīkaśarkarā-Madhuśarkarā	माक्षीकशर्करा - मधुशर्करा	189
Mākśīkaśarkarā-Mādhvīsitā	माक्षीकशर्करा - माध्वी सिता	594

Mākṡikāṡrayam - Sikthakam	माक्षिकाश्रयम् - सिक्थकम्	250
Maladrāvī - Jayapālaḥ	मलद्रावी - जयपालः	86
Mālālī - Spṛkkā	मालाली - स्पृक्का	224
Malam (p.640)	मलम् (p.640)	
Malanāṡinī - Jātipatrī	मलनाशिनी - जातिपत्री	211
Malāpahā - Cakṡuṣyā	मलापहा - चक्षुष्या	264
Mālatī - Jātī	मालती - जाती	496
Mālatī - Pāṭhā	मालती - पाठा	26
Mālatīpatrikā - Jātipatrī	मालतीपत्रिका - जातिपत्री	211
Mālatīphalam - Jātīphalam	मालतीफलम् - जातीफलम्	211
Malatīrasa sambhavaḥ-Taṅkaṇaḥ	मालतीरससंभवः - टंकणः	134
Malātṛṇaḥ - Bhūstṛṇaḥ	मालातृणः - भूस्तृणः	300
Mālavikā - Trivṛt	मालविका -त्रिवृत्	93
Malayaḥ - Padmakaḥ	मलयः - पद्मकः	242
Malayajam - Candanam	मलजयम्-चन्दनम्	191
Malayottham - Kalīyakam	मलयोत्थम् - कालीयकम्	194
Malayūḥ - Kākodumbarikā	मलयूः - काकोदुम्बरिका	438
Malinā - Kāsaghnī	मलिना - कासघ्नी	37
Malinam - Maricam	मलिनम् - मरिचम्	168
Malināṅgī - Kāsaghnī	मलिनाङ्गी - कासघ्नी	37
Mallikā - Methikā	मल्लिका - मेथिका	562
Mallikā (p. 492)	मल्लिका (p. 492)	
Mallikāpuṣpaḥ - Kuṭajaḥ	मल्लिकापुष्पः - कुटजः	131
Malodbhavam - Maṇḍūram	मलोद्भवम् - मण्डूरम्	529
Mālukāparṇaḥ - Aṡmantakaḥ	मालुकापर्णः - अश्मन्तकः	72
Mālyapuṣpī - Śaṇapuṣpī	माल्यपुष्पी - शणपुष्पी	75
Māmsajam - Medaḥ	मांसजम् - मेदः	643
Māmsalaḥ - Māṣaḥ	मांसलः - माषः	552
Māmsaliptam - Asthi	मांसलिप्तम् - अस्थि	618
Māmsam (p.618)	मांसम् (p. 618)	
Māmsamāṣā - Māṣaparṇī	मांसमाषा -माषपर्णी	48
Māmsarohā - Māmsarohiṇī	मांसरोहा - मांसरोहिणी	330
Māmsarohī-Māmsarohiṇī (Raj.ni.)	मांसरोही - मांसरोहिणी (रा.नि.)	330
Māmsarohiṇī (p. 329)	मांसरोहिणी (p. 329)	
Māmsasāraḥ - Medaḥ	मांससारः - मेदः	643
Māmsī (Jaṭāmāmsī) (Naladam) (p. 217)	मांसी (जटामांसी) (नलदम्)(p.217)	
Mānaḥṡilā (p. 245)	मनः शिला (p. 245)	
Mānavaḥ - Puruṣaḥ	मानवः - पुरुषः	615
Māṇavakam - Pālevatam	माणचकम् - पालेवतम्	418
Maṇḍā - Surā	मण्डा - सुरा	596
Mandagamanā - Mahiṣī	मन्दगमना - महिषी	625

Maṇḍaḥ	मण्डः	590
Maṇḍaḥ - Maṇḍūkaḥ	मण्डः - मण्डूकः	640
Maṇḍalapatrikā-Krūraḥ (Raj.ni.)	मण्डलपत्रिका - क्रूरः (रा.नि.)	109
Maṇḍalī- Guḍūcī	मण्डली- गुडूची	2
Maṇḍalīpātaḥ - Sarpaviśeṣaḥ	मण्डलीपातः - सर्पविशेषः	639
Maṇḍanaḥ -Atimuktakaḥ	मण्डनः - अतिमुक्तकः	509
Mandāraḥ - Rājārkaḥ	मन्दारः - राजार्कः	282
Maṇḍavyaḥ - Maṇḍūkaviśeṣaḥ	मण्डव्यः - मण्डूकविशेषः	640
Maṇḍūkaḥ (p.640)	मण्डूकः (p.640)	
Maṇḍūkaparṇaḥ - Syonākaḥ (Raj.ni.)	मण्डूकपर्णः - श्योनाकः (रा.नि.)	42
Maṇḍūkaparṇī - Suvarcalā	मण्डूकपर्णी - सुवर्चला	333
Maṇḍūkī - Brāhmī (Raj. ni.)	मण्डूकी - ब्राह्मी (रा.नि.)	337
Maṇḍūkī - Suvarcalā	मण्डूकी - सुवर्चला	333
Maṇḍūram (p. 529)	मण्डूरम् (p. 529)	
Maṅgalacchāyaḥ - Plakṣaḥ	मङ्गलच्छायः - प्लक्षः	429
Maṅgalam - Ṛddhiḥ	मङ्गलम् -ऋद्धिः	53
Māṅgalyā - Rocanā	माङ्गल्या - रोचना	203
Maṅgalyā - Śamī	मङ्गल्या - शमी	442
Maṅgalyā - Śvetavacā	मङ्गल्या - श्वेतवचा	126
Māṅgalyadarśanaḥ - Matsyaḥ	माङ्गल्यदर्शनः - मत्स्यः	626
Māṅgalyaḥ -Haritamudgaḥ	माङ्गल्यः -हरितमुद्गः	540
Maṅgalyaḥ - Pippalaḥ	मङ्गल्यः - पिप्पलः	427
Māṅgalyanāmadheyā - Jīvantī	माङ्गल्यनामधेया - जीवन्ती	49
Maṇicchidrā - Medā	मणिच्छिद्रा - मेदा	46
Maṇimantham - Saindhavam	मणिमन्थम् - सैन्धवम्	135
Maṇirāgakaram - Hiṅgulam	मणिरागकरम् - हिंगुलम्	530
Mañjarīnamraḥ - Vetasaḥ	मञ्जरीनम्रः - वेतसः	467
Mañjiṣṭhā (p.6)	मञ्जिष्ठा - (p. 6)	
Mañjukā - Mañjiṣṭhā	मञ्जुका - मञ्जिष्ठा	7
Manmathodbhavanaḥ-Rajāmraḥ	मन्मथोद्भवनः- राजाम्रः	388
Manoguptā - Manaḥśilā	मनोगुप्ता - मनःशिला	246
Manoharaḥ - Kundaḥ	मनोहरः - कुन्दः	506
Manohvā - Manaḥśilā	मनोह्वा - मनःशिला	246
Manojñā - Manaḥśilā	मनोज्ञा - मनःशिला	246
Manojñā - Karkoṭakī	मनोज्ञा - कर्कोटकी	69
Manojñya - Vandhyakarkoṭakī	मनोज्ञा - वन्ध्यकर्कोटकी	68
Manojñā - Jātī	मनोज्ञा - जाती	495
Manojñam - Jīrakam	मनोज्ञम् - जीरकम्	157
Manoramaḥ - Hamsaḥ	मनोरमः - हंसः	635
Manthaḥ	मन्थः	653
Manthanaḥ - Agnimanthaḥ	मन्थनः -अग्निमंथः	40
Manthānaḥ - Karṇikāraḥ	मन्थानः - कर्णिकारः	81

Manthanodbhavam- Navanītam	मन्थनोद्भवम् - नवनीतम्	591
Mānuṣaḥ - Puruṣaḥ	मानुषः - पुरुषः	615
Mānuṣamūtram	मानुषमूत्रम्	643
Mānuṣīpayaḥ	मानुषीपयः	580
Marakatam - Gārutmatam	मरकतम् - गारुत्मतम्	531
Marālikā - Sātalā	मरालिका - सातला	89
Maraṇam - Vatasanābhaḥ	मरणम् - वत्सनाभः	667
Mardanakam - Tailam	मर्दनकम् - तैलम्	570
Mārdwīkam (p.599)	मार्द्वीकम् (p.599)	
Maricam (p. 168)	मरिचम् (p. 168)	
Mārīcapatrakaḥ - Saralaḥ	मारीचपत्रकः - सरलः	237
Mārjāragandhikā-Mudgaparṇī	मार्जारगन्धिका -मुद्गपर्णी	49
Mārjāraḥ - Biḍālaḥ	मार्जारः - बिडालः	631
Mārjāri - Kastūrikā	मार्जारि - कस्तूरिका	208
Marjikā (p. 602)	मर्जिका (p. 602)	602
Markaṭaḥ (p. 632)	मर्कटः (p. 632)	
Markaṭapippalī - Apāmārgaḥ	मर्कटपिप्पली -अपामार्गः	100
Markatatindukaḥ-Kākatindukaḥ	मर्कटतिन्दुकः - काकतिन्दुकः	402
Markaṭī - Apāmārgaḥ	मर्कटी -अपामार्गः	100
Mārkaṭī - Kapikacchuḥ	मर्कटी - कपिकच्छुः	55
Mārkavaḥ - Bhṛṅgarājaḥ	मार्कवः -भृङ्गराजः	281
Martyaḥ - Puruṣaḥ	मर्त्यः - पुरुषः	615
Marubakaḥ - Jambīraḥ	मरुबकः - जम्बीरः	302
Marudbhavaḥ - Padmakaḥ	मरुद्भवः - पद्मकः	242
Marudbhavaḥ - Yāsaḥ	मरुद्भवः - यासः	8
Maruḥ - Jambīraḥ	मरुः - जम्बीरः	302
Marusambhavam-Cāṇākhyamūlakam	मरुसंभवम् - चाणाख्यमूलकम्	293
Mārutaḥ - Vāyuḥ	मारुतः - वायुः	616
Mārutāpahaḥ - Varuṇaḥ	मारुतापहः - वरुणः	472
Maruttakaḥ - Jambīraḥ	मरुत्तकः - जम्बीरः	302
Māṣaḥ (p. 552)	माषः (p. 552)	
Māṣaparṇī (p.48)	माषपर्णी (p.48)	
Maskaraḥ - Vaṁśaḥ	मस्करः - वंशः	364
Mastsyagandhā - Jalapippalī	मत्स्यगन्धा - जलपिप्पली	310
Mastsyaṇḍikā - Śarkarā	मस्यण्डिका -शर्करा	188
Mastyādanī - Jalapippalī	मत्स्यादनी - जलपिप्पली	310
Masūraḥ (p. 550)	मसूरः (p. 550)	
Masūravidalā - Trivṛt	मसूरविदला -त्रिवृत्	93
Mātaṅgaḥ - Hasti	मातङ्गः - हस्ति	620
Mataṅgajaḥ - Hasti	मतङ्गजः - हस्ति	620
Mātaṅgamakaraḥ-Mahāmatsyaviśeṣaḥ	मातङ्गमकरः - महामत्स्य विशेषः	628
Mātariśvā - Vāyuḥ	मातरिश्वा - वायुः	616

Mathitadadhi (583)	मथितदधि (583)	
Matibhraṁśaḥ - Mohaḥ	मतिभ्रंशः – मोहः	617
Mātṛkah - Ṛṣabhaḥ	मातृकः – ऋषभः	45
Matsyā - Potakī	मत्स्या- पोतकी	382
Matsyaḥ (p. 626)	मत्स्यः (p. 626)	
Matsyākṣī - Brāhmī (Raj. ni.)	मत्स्याक्षी – ब्राह्मी (रा.नि.)	337
Matsyākṣikā - Dūrvā	मत्स्याक्षिका – दूर्वा	368
Matsyapittā - Kaṭukā	मत्स्यपित्ता -कटुका	15
Matsyaśakalā - Kaṭukā	मत्स्यशकला -कटुका	15
Mātuḥ - Vijayā	मातुः – विजया	46
Mātuluṅgaḥ - Bījapūraḥ	मातुलुङ्गः– बीजपूरः	396
Mauktikam (p. 533)	मौक्तिकम् (p. 533)	
Mayaḥ - Uṣṭraḥ	मयः – उष्ट्रः	621
Māyāvī - Biḍālaḥ	मायावी – बिडालः	631
Mayūragrīvakam - Tuttham	मयूरग्रीवकम् – तुत्थम्	260
Mayūraḥ (p. 633)	मयूरः (p. 633)	
Mayūrajaṅghaḥ - Śyonākaḥ	मयूरजङ्घः – श्योनाकः	41
Mayūrakaḥ - Apāmārgaḥ	मयूरकः –अपामार्गः	100
Mecakam - Añjanam	मेचकम् – अञ्जनम्	262
Medā (p.45)	मेदा (p.45)	
Medaḥ (p. 643)	मेदः (p. 643)	
Medakaḥ - Surā	मेदकः – सुरा	596
Medaḥpucchaḥ - Aviḥ	मेदःपुच्छः – अविः	623
Medhāvī - Śukaḥ	मेधावी – शुकः	634
Medhāvinī - Sārikā	मेधाविनी – सारिका	634
Medhyā - Brāhmī	मेध्या – ब्राह्मी	336
Medhyā - Rocanā	मेध्या –रोचना	203
Medhyā - Śaṅkhapuṣpī	मेध्या – शंखपुष्पी	349
Medhyā-Śaṅkhapuṣpi (Raj. ni.)	मेध्या – शंखपुष्पी (रा.नि.)	349
Medhyā - Śvetavacā (Dhn.ni.)	मेध्या – श्वेतवचा (ध.नि.)	126
Medhyaḥ - Chāgaḥ	मेध्यः – छागः	622
Medomāṁsasamudbhavā-Vasā	मेदोमांससमुद्भवा – वसा	619
Meghaḥ - Mustā	मेघः – मुस्ता	15
Meghamodinī-Jambūḥ (Raj.ni.)	मेघमोदिनी – जम्बूः (रा.नि.)	434
Meghanādaḥ - Taṇḍulīyakaḥ	मेघनादः – तण्डुलीयकः	355
Meghapuṣpaḥ- Vetasaḥ	मेघपुष्पः– वेतसः	467
Meghārāvaḥ - Mayūraḥ	मेघारावः – मयूरः	633
Meṇḍhraḥ - Aviḥ	मेंढ्रः – अविः	623
Meṣaḥ - Aviḥ	मेषः – अविः	623
Meṣākṣaḥ - Cakramardaḥ	मेषाक्षः – चक्रमर्दः	277
Meṣākṣikusumaḥ-Cakramardaḥ	मेषाक्षिकुसुमः – चक्रमर्दः	277
Meṣāntrī -Vṛṣamedhā	मेषान्त्री –वृषमेधा	118

Meṣaśṛṅgī - Ajaśṛṅgī	मेषशृंगी - अजशृंगी	31
Meṣīmūtram	मेषीमूत्रम्	642
Methikā - Vanamethikā	मेथिका - वनमेथिका	563
Methikā (p. 562)	मेथिका (p. 562)	
Mīnaḥ - Matsyaḥ	मीनः - मत्स्यः	626
Mīnāṇḍī - Śarkarā	मीनाण्डी -शर्करा	188
Miśhiḥ - Miśreyā	मिशिः - मिश्रेया	122
Miśi - Māṁsī	मिशि - मांसी	217
Miśiḥ - Śatapuṣpā	मिशिः - शतपुष्पा	121
Miśraḥ - Mohaḥ	मिश्रः - मोहः	617
Miśram - Cāṇākhyamūlakam	मिश्रम् -चाणाख्यमूलकम्	293
Miśreyā (p.122)	मिश्रेया (p.122)	
Mleccham - Hiṅgulam	म्लेच्छम् - हिंगुलम्	530
Mlecchakandaḥ - Laśunaḥ	म्लेच्छकन्दः - लशुनः	312
Mlecchabhojanaḥ - Godhūmaḥ	म्लेच्छभोजनः - गोधूमः	551
Mlecchamukham - Tāmram	म्लेच्छमुखम् - ताम्रम्	524
Mocā - Nīlinī	मोचा - नीलिनी	87
Mocā - Śālmalī	मोचा - शाल्मली	481
Mocā - Kadalī	मोचा - कदली	316
Mocaniryāsaḥ-Śālmalīveṣṭakaḥ	मोचनिर्यासः -शाल्मलीवेष्टकः	481
Mocarasaḥ - Śālmalīveṣṭakaḥ	मोचरसः -शाल्मलीवेष्टकः	481
Mocasrāvaḥ - Śālmaliveṣṭakaḥ	मोचस्रावः -शाल्मलीवेष्टकः	481
Modā- Ajamodā	मोदा - अजमोदा	183
Modakī - Jiṅgiṇī	मोदकी - जिंगिणी	272
Modanī - Mallikā (Raj.ni.)	मोदनी - मल्लिका (रा. नि.)	494
Mohaḥ (p.617)	मोहः (p.617)	
Mohakārī - Māḍaḥ	मोहकारी - माडः	422
Mohanaḥ-Muṣkakaḥ (Raj.ni.)	मोहनः - मुष्ककः (रा. नि.)	483
Mokśakaḥ - Muṣkakaḥ	मोक्षकः - मुष्ककः	483
Moraṭā - Mūrvā	मोरटा - मूर्वा	5
Moraṭaḥ (p.6)	मोरटः - (p. 6)	
Moṣī - Mahāmūṣakaḥ	मोषी - महामूषकः	631
Mrakśaṇam - Tailam	म्रक्षणम् - तैलम्	570
Mṛdaṅgaphalikā - Kośātakī	मृदङ्गफलिका - कोशातकी	71
Mṛdu -Muṇḍaloham	मृदु - मुण्डलोहम्	528
Mṛdudarbhaḥ - Kuśaḥ	मृदुदर्भः - कुशः	361
Mṛduḥphalaḥ - Karīraḥ	मृदुः फलः - करीरः	448
Mṛduphalaḥ - Vikaṅkataḥ	मृदुफलः - विकंकतः	405
Mṛdupuṣpaḥ - Śirīṣaḥ	मृदुपुष्पः- शिरीषः	463
Mṛdusāram - Tūdam (Raj. ni.)	मृदुसारम् - तूदम् (रा. नि.)	417
Mṛdvīkā - Uttarāpathikā	मृद्वीका -उत्तरापथिका	414
Mṛgabhakśaḥ - Tarakśuḥ	मृगभक्षः - तरक्षुः	632

Mṛgādanī - Śve. indravāruṇī मृगादनी – इन्द्रवारुणी (श्वे.) 96
Mṛgādanī - Indravāruṇī मृगादनी – इन्द्रवारुणी 95
Mṛgadhūrtaḥ - Sṛgālaḥ मृगधूर्तः – श्रृगालः 632
Mṛgagāminī - Viḍaṅgam मृगगामिनी – विडङ्गम् 130
Mṛgaḥ - Hariṇaḥ मृगः – हरिणः 625
Mṛgairvāru - (Śve.) indravāruṇī मृगैर्वारु – इन्द्रवारुणी (श्वे.) 96
Mṛgākṣī - (Śve.) indravāruṇī मृगाक्षी – इन्द्रवारुणी (श्वे.) 96
Mṛgamadaḥ - Kastūrikā मृगमदः – कस्तूरिका 208
Mṛganābhiḥ - Kastūrikā मृगनाभिः – कस्तूरिका 208
Mṛgāṇḍajā - Kastūrikā मृगाण्डजा – कस्तूरिका 208
Mṛgāntakaḥ - Śarabhaḥ मृगान्तकः – शरभः 624
Mṛgarājaḥ - Simhaḥ मृगराजः – सिंहः 624
Mṛgāriḥ - Śigruḥ (Raj. ni.) मृगारिः – शिग्रुः (रा. नि.) 296
Mṛṇālakam - Bisam मृणालकम् – बिसम् 376
Mṛṇālam - Bisam मृणालम् – बिसम् 376
Mṛṇālam - Uśīram मृणालम् – उशीरम् 198
Mṛṇālī - Bisam मृणाली – बिसम् 376
Mṛṇālikā - Bisam मृणालिका – बिसम् 376
Mṛtajīvī - Tilakaḥ (Raj. ni.) मृतजीवी – तिलकः (रा.नि.) 514
Mṛtālakam - Saurāṣṭrī मृतालकम् – सौराष्ट्री 247
Mṛttikā - Guḍūcī मृत्तिका – गुडूची 2
Mṛtsā - Saurāṣṭrī मृत्सा – सौराष्ट्री 247
Mṛtsnā - Saurāṣṭrī मृत्स्ना – सौराष्ट्री 247
Mṛttikā - Saurāṣṭrī मृत्तिका – सौराष्ट्री 247
Mṛttikākṣāram - Mūlakam मृत्तिकाक्षारम् –मूलकम् 293
Mudgaḥ (p. 540) मुद्गः (p. 540)
Mudgaparṇī (p.48) मुद्गपर्णी (p.48)
Mudgaraḥ - Matsyabhedaḥ मुद्गरः – मत्स्यभेदः 628
Mudgaraḥ - Matsyaviśeṣaḥ मुद्गरः – मत्स्यविशेषः 627
Mukhabhaṅgaḥ - Śigruḥ मुखभङ्गः – शिग्रुः 295
Mukhadūṣakaḥ - Palāṇḍuḥ मुखदूषकः – पलाण्डुः 315
Mukhamaṇḍanakaḥ - Tilakaḥ मुखमण्डनकः – तिलकः 513
Mukhamatsyaḥ-Matsyaviśeṣaḥ मुखमत्स्यः – मत्स्यविशेषः 627
Mukhāmodaḥ - Śigruḥ मुखामोदः – शिग्रुः 296
Mukhapriyaḥ - Niṣpāvaḥ मुखप्रियः – निष्पावः 560
Mukharāgakarī - Tāmbūlī मुखरागकरी – ताम्बूली 273
Mukhaśodhyam - Twak मुखशोध्यम – त्वक 145
Mukhavācikā - Ambaṣṭhā मुखवाचिका – अम्बष्ठा 249
Mukhavāsaḥ -(Sugandha) Bhūstṛṇaḥ (Raj. ni.)
मुखवासः – (सुगंध) भूस्तृणः (रा. नि.) 300
Muktabandhanā - Vārṣikī मुक्तबन्धना – वार्षिकी 496
Muktasāram - Śuktam मुक्तसारम् – शुक्तम् 594

Mukūlakaḥ - Dantī	मुकूलकः - दन्ती	84
Makuṣṭhakaḥ (p. 548)	मकुष्ठकः (p. 548)	
Mūlakam (p. 292)	मूलकम् (p. 292)	
Mūlakaparṇī - Śigruḥ	मूलकपर्णी - शिग्रुः	295
Mūlam - Pippalīmūlam	मूलम् - पिप्पलीमूलम्	161
Mūlam - Puṣkaramūlam	मूलम् - पुष्करमूलम्	23
Muñcakaḥ -Muṣkakaḥ	मुञ्चकः - मुष्ककः	483
Muṇḍacanakaḥ - Kalāyaḥ	मुण्डचणकः - कलायः	554
Muṇḍam - Loham	मुण्डम् - लोहम्	528
Muṇḍam - Muṇḍaloham	मुण्डम् - मुण्डलोहम्	528
Muṇḍī - Mahāśrāvaṇī	मुण्डी - महाश्रावणी	58
Muṇḍitikā - Śrāvaṇī	मुण्डितिका - श्रावणी	58
Munibhaksyaḥ - Śyāmākaḥ	मुनिभक्ष्यः - श्यामाकः	545
Munibhaktaḥ - Nīvāraḥ	मुनिभक्तः - नीवारः	543
Muniḥ - Damanaḥ	मुनिः - दमनः	228
Muñjaḥ (p. 360)	मुञ्जः (p. 360)	
Murā (p. 229)	मुरा (p. 229)	
Mūrvā (p.5)	मूर्वा (p. 5)	
Mūṣakaḥ -Muṣkaka'.	मूषकः - मुष्ककः	483
Mūṣakaḥ (p. 630)	मूषकः (p. 630)	
Mūṣakāhvayā - Dravantī	मूषकाह्वया - द्रवन्ती	86
Mūṣakadweṣī - Biḍālaḥ	मूषकद्वेषी - बिडालः	631
Muṣkakaḥ (p. 483)	मुष्ककः (p. 483)	
Mustā (p.15)	मुस्ता (p. 15)	
Musṭiḥ - Mūskakaḥ	मुष्टिः - मुष्ककः	483
Muṣṭikaḥ - Śāliḥ	मुष्टिकः - शालिः	535
Mūtram (p.641)	मूत्रम् (p.641)	
Mūtraphalā - Trapusam	मूत्रफला - त्रपुसम्	65
Mūtrāṣṭakam	मूत्राष्टकम्	657
Naḍaḥ - Nalaḥ	नडः - नलः	366
Nādeyaḥ - Mustā	नादेयः - मुस्ता	15
Nādeyam - Saindhavam	नादेयम् - सैन्धवम्	135
Nādeyī - Agnimanthaḥ	नादेयी -अग्निमंथः	40
Nādeyī - Jambūḥ	नादेयी - जम्बूः	433
Nādeyī - Vetasaḥ	नादेयी - वेतसः	467
Nadī sarjaḥ - Arjunaḥ	नदीसर्जः -अर्जुनः	464
Nadīdumbarikā - Udumbaraḥ (Raj. ni.)	नदीदुम्बरिका - उदुम्बरः (रा.नि.)	436
Nāḍīhinghu (p. 139)	नाडीहि ङ्गु (p. 139)	
Nāḍikalāpaḥ - Dūrvā	नाडीकलापः - दूर्वा	368
Nadīkāntā - Kākajanghā	नदीकान्ता - काकजङ्घा	287
Nadīniṣpāvaḥ - Niṣpāvaḥ (Raj. ni.)	नदीनिष्पावः - निष्पावः (रा.नि.)	560
Nāgabalā - Gāngerukī	नागबला - गांगेरुकी	112

Nagabhid - Pāṣāṇabhedaḥ	नगभिद् - पाषाणभेदः	57
Nāgadamanī - Balāmoṭā	नागदमनी - बलामोटा	378
Nāgadamanī-Vandhyakarkoṭakī	नागदमनी - वन्ध्यकर्कोटकी	68
Nāgadantī - Śve. indravāruṇi	नागदन्ती - इन्द्रवारुणी (श्वे.)	96
Nāgagarbham - Sindūraḥ	नागगर्भम् - सिन्दूरः	246
Nāgaḥ - Hasti	नागः - हस्ति	620
Nāgaḥ - Sarpaḥ	नागः - सर्पः	639
Nāgahanuḥ - Nakham	नागहनुः - नखम्	223
Nāgāhvā - Tāmbūlī	नागाह्वा - ताम्बूली	273
Nāgajam - Sindūraḥ	नागजम् - सिन्दूरः	246
Nāgajihvā - Manaḥśilā	नागजिह्वा - मनःशिला	246
Nāgakesaram (p. 143)	नागकेसरम् (p. 143)	
Nāgakiñjalkam - Nāgakesaram	नागकिञ्जल्कम् - नागकेसरम्	143
Nāgakumārī - Guḍūcī	नागकुमारी - गुडूची	2
Nāgam - Nāgakesaram	नागम् - नागकेसरम्	143
Nāgam - Sīsakam	नागम् - सीसकम्	526
Nāgam - Vatasanābhaḥ	नागम् - वत्सनाभः	667
Nāgapuṣpam - Nāgakesaram	नागपुष्पम् - नागकेसरम्	143
Nāgaraḥ - Mustā	नागरः - मुस्ता	15
Nāgaram - Garjaram	नागरम् - गर्जरम्	314
Nāgaram - Śuṇṭhī	नागरम् - शुण्ठी	167
Nāgaraṅgaḥ - Nāraṅgaḥ	नागरङ्गः - नारङ्गः	391
Nāgāriḥ - Vandhyakarkoṭakī	नागारिः - वन्ध्यकर्कोटकी	68
Nagaśuṇḍī - Daṅgarī	नागशुण्डी - डङ्गरी	67
Nāgavallī - Tāmbūlī	नागवल्ली - ताम्बूली	273
Nāgīyakāñcanam - Nāgakesaram (Raj. ni.)	नागीयकाञ्चनम् - नागकेसरम् (रा. नि.)	143
Nahuṣam - Tagaram	नहुषम् - तगरम्	221
Nakhaḥ - Nakham	नखः - नखम्	223
Nakham (p.223)	नखम् (p.223)	
Nakhapuṣpī - Spṛkkā (Raj. ni.)	नखपुष्पी - स्पृक्का (रा. नि.)	224
Nakhī - Āmūṣikā	नखी - आमूषिका	630
Nakhī - Mūṣakaḥ	नखी - मूषकः	630
Naktacārī - Ulūkaḥ	नक्तञ्चारी - उलूकः	638
Naktamālaḥ - Karañjaḥ	नक्तमालः - करञ्जः	455
Naktancaraḥ - Gugguluḥ	नक्तञ्चरः - गुग्गुलुः	252
Naktendupuṣpikā - Kalikārī	नक्तेन्दुपुष्पिका - कलिकारी	280
Nakuleṣṭā - Gandhanākulī	नकुलेष्टा - गन्धनाकुली	342
Nākulī - Yavatiktā	नाकुली - यवतिक्ता	98
Nākulī (p. 339)	नाकुली (p. 339)	
Naladā - Māmsī	नलदा - मांसी	217
Nalaḥ (p. 366)	नलः (p. 366)	365

Nalakaḥ - Kalāyaḥ	नलकः - कलायः	554
Nalam - Raktapadmam	नलम् - रक्तपद्मम्	372
Nalī - Nalikā	नली - नलिका	216
Nalikā (p. 216)	नलिका (p. 216)	
Nālikam - Bolam	नालिकम् - बोलम्	226
Nalinam - Raktapadmam	नलिनम् - रक्तपद्मम्	372
Nalinam- Kṣudramutpalam	नलिनम् - क्षुद्रमुत्पलम्	374
Nalinī - Padminī	नलिनी - पद्मिनी	374
Nalinīruham - Bisam	नलिनीरुहम्- बिसम्	376
Nalottamaḥ - Mahānalaḥ	नलोत्तमः - महानलः	367
Namaskārī - Raktapādī	नमस्कारी - रक्तपादी	344
Nandanajam - Haricandanam	नन्दनजम् - हरिचन्दनम	196
Nandikaḥ - Tūṇiḥ	नन्दिकः - तूणिः	203
Nandikāvartaḥ-Matsyaviśeṣaḥ	नन्दिकावर्तः - मत्स्यविशेषः	627
Nandinī - Harītakī	नन्दिनी - हरीतकी	77
Nandinī - Reṇukā	नन्दिनी -रेणुका	220
Nanditaruḥ - Dhavaḥ	नन्दितरुः - धवः	522
Nandivṛkṣaḥ - Tūṇiḥ	नन्दिवृक्षः - तूणिः	202
Nandyāvartaḥ - Matsyabhedaḥ	नन्द्यावर्तः - मत्स्यभेदः	628
Nepālaḥ - Kirātatiktakaḥ	नेपालः- किराततिक्तकः	14
Nāradakandakam - Gṛñjanam	नारदकन्दकम् - गृञ्जनम्	294
Naraḥ - Puruṣaḥ	नरः - पुरुषः	615
Nāraṅgaḥ (p. 391)	नारङ्गः (p. 391)	
Nārāyanapriyam - Kāliyakam	नारायणप्रियम् - कालीयकम्	194
Nārāyaṇī - Śatāvarī (Raj. ni.)	नारायणी - शतावरी (रा.नि)	115
Nārī - Strī	नारी - स्त्री	615
Nārikelaḥ (P. 424)	नारिकेलः (P. 424)	
Nārīṣṭā - Mallikā (Raj. ni.)	नारीष्टा - मल्लिका (रा. नि.)	494
Nartakaḥ - Mayūraḥ	नर्तकः - मयूरः	633
Nartakaḥ - Nalaḥ	नर्तकः - नलः	366
Nartakī - Nalikā	नर्तकी - नलिका	216
Nāsāsamvedanaḥ - Kāṇḍīraḥ	नासासंवेदनः -काण्डीरः	309
Naṣṭasamjñakaḥ - Mohaḥ	नष्टसंज्ञकः - मोहः	617
Naṭaḥ - Nalaḥ	नटः- नलः	366
Natam - Tagaram	नतम् - तगरम्	221
Natāṅginī - Karkaṭaśṛṅgī	नताङ्गिनी - कर्कटश्रृंगी	30
Naṭī - Nalikā	नटी - नलिका	216
Navanītajam - Ghṛtam	नवनीतजम् - घृतम्	574
Navanītam (p.591)	नवनीतम् (p.591)	
Navanītodbhavam- Dadhi	नवनीतोद्भवम् - दधि	582
Navaratnāni	नवरत्नानि	661
Nemivṛkṣaḥ - Somavalkaḥ	नेमिवृक्षः - सोमवल्कः	10

Nepālī - Graiṣmī	नेपाली - ग्रैष्मी	498
Nepālikā - Manaḥśilā	नेपालिका - मनःशिला	246
Netā - Nimbaḥ	नेता - निम्बः	11
Netramīlā - Yavatiktā	नेत्रमीला - यवतिक्ता	98
Netravikārajit - Katakam	नेत्रविकारजित् - कतकम्	267
Niculaḥ - Vetasaḥ	निचुलः - वेतसः	467
Nidigdhikā - Kaṇṭakārī	निदिग्धिका - कण्टकारी	35
Nidrāriḥ - Kirātatiktaḥ	निद्रारिः - किराततिक्तः	14
Niḥsāraḥ - Śyonākaḥ (Raj. ni.)	निःसारः - श्योनाकः (रा.नि.)	41
Niḥsārā - Kadalī	निःसारा - कदली	316
Niḥśeṣaviṣanāśinī - Balāmoṭā	निःशेषविषनाशिनी - बलामोटा	378
Niḥśreṇī - Kharjūrī	निःश्रेणी - खर्जूरी	411
Nijam - Kāṃsyam	निजम् - कांस्यम्	527
Nikocakaḥ - Aṅkoṭakaḥ	निकोचकः - अङ्कोटकः	100
Nikṛntanaḥ-Vaṭasaugandhikaḥ	निकृन्तनः - वटसौगन्धिकः	248
Nikumbhā - Dantī	निकुम्भा - दन्ती	84
Nikumbhaḥ - Jayapālaḥ	निकुम्भः - जयपालः	86
Nikumbhāhvabījam-Jayapālaḥ	निकुम्भाह्वबीजम् - जयपालः	86
Nikuñjakaḥ - Vetasaḥ	निकुञ्जकः - वेतसः	467
Nīladūrva - Dūrvā	नीलदूर्वा - दूर्वा	368
Nīlaḥ - Bhramaraḥ	नीलः - भ्रमरः	633
Nīlakaṇā-Kṛṣṇajīrakaḥ (Raj.ni.)	नीलकणा - कृष्णजीरकः (रा.नि.)	158
Nīlakandam - Mūlakam	नीलकन्दम् -मूलकम्	293
Nīlakaṇṭhaḥ - Mayūraḥ	नीलकण्ठः - मयूरः	633
Nīlakapitthaḥ - Rajāmraḥ	नीलकपित्थः- राजाम्रः	388
Nīlakārakam - Śuktam	नीलकारकम् - शुक्तम्	594
Nīlakrāntā-Viṣṇukrāntā (Raj.ni.)	नीलक्रान्ता-विष्णुक्रान्ता (रा.नि.)	353
Nīlālikula samkulā - Kubjakaḥ	नीलालिकुलसंकुला - कुब्जकः	503
Nīlam - Tālīsam	नीलम् - तालीसम्	147
Nīlamañjarī - Śephālikā	नीलमञ्जरी - शेफालिका	321
Nīlamāṣaḥ - Rājamāṣaḥ	नीलमाषः - राजमाषः	542
Nīlāmbaram-Tālīsam (Raj.ni.)	नीलाम्बरम् - तालीसम् (रा.नि.)	148
Nīlāmlānaḥ-Saireyakaḥ (Raj.ni.)	नीलाम्लानः - सैरेयकः (रा.नि.)	110
Nīlapadmam - Saugandhikam	नीलपद्मम् - सौगन्धिकम्	371
Nīlapuṣpaḥ - Sinduvāraḥ	नीलपुष्पः- सिन्दुवारः	319
Nīlapuṣpī - Viṣṇukrāntā	नीलपुष्पी - विष्णुक्रान्ता	352
Nīlapuṣpī - Aśvakśurakaḥ	नीलपुष्पी -अश्वक्षुरकः	323
Nīlasāraḥ - Tindukaḥ	नीलसारः - तिन्दुकः	402
Nīlaśigruḥ - Śigruḥ (Raj. ni.)	नीलशिग्रुः - शिग्रुः (रा. नि.)	296
Nīlasindukā - Sinduvāraḥ	नीलसिन्दुका - सिन्दुवारः	319
Nīlāśmā -Rajāvartaḥ	नीलाश्मा - राजावर्तः	533
Nīlaspandā - Aśvakśurakaḥ	नीलस्पन्दा -अश्वक्षुरकः	323

Nīlavarṇā - Jambūḥ	नीलवर्णा - जम्बूः	433
Nīlavarṇam - Paruṣakaḥ	नीलवर्णम् -परुषकः	416
Nīlavṛntakam-Tūdam (Raj. ni.)	नीलवृन्तकम् - तूदम् (रा.नि.)	417
Nīlikā - Śephālīkā (Raj. ni.)	नीलिका- शेफालिका (रा. नि.)	321
Nīlikā - Nīlinī	नीलिका - नीलिनी	87
Nīlikā - Vaṅgam	नीलिका - वङ्गम्	525
Nīlinī (p.87)	नीलिनी (p.87)	
Nīlikā - Vartaloham	नीलिका - वर्तलोहम्	528
Nimbabījaḥ- Rajādanaḥ (Raj. ni.)	निम्बबीजः - राजादनः (रा.नि.)	439
Nimbaḥ (p. 11)	निम्बः (p. 11)	
Nimbarakaḥ - Mahānimbaḥ	निम्बरकः - महानिम्बः	12
Nimbatailam	निम्बतैलम्	257
Nimittakṛt - Kākaḥ	निमित्तकृत् - काकः	637
Nīpaḥ - Kadambaḥ	नीपः - कदम्बः	451
Nīrajaḥ - Kuśaḥ	नीरजः - कुशः	362
Nīram - Jalam	नीरम् - जलम्	605
Nirgandham - Barbarikam	निर्गन्धम् - बर्बरिकम्	195
Nirguṇḍī - Sinduvāraḥ	निर्गुण्डी - सिन्दुवारः	319
Nirloham - Bolam	निर्लोहम् - बोलम्	226
Nirmadhyā - Nalikā	निर्मध्या - नलिका	216
Nirmālyā - Spṛkkā	निर्माल्या - स्पृक्का	224
Nīrogaḥ	नीरोगः	660
Nirūḍhaḥ - Makuṣṭhakaḥ	निरूढः -मकुष्ठकः	548
Niryāsaḥ - Śālmaliveṣṭakaḥ	निर्यासः -शाल्मलीवेष्टकः	481
Niśā - Haridrā	निशा - हरिद्रा	20
Niśācaraḥ - Ulūkaḥ	निशाचरः - उलूकः	638
Nistrimśapatrakāḥ - Snuhī	निस्त्रिंशपत्रकः - स्नुही	88
Niṣkuṭiḥ - Elā	निष्कुटिः - एला	141
Niṣpāvaḥ (p. 561)	निष्पावः (p. 561)	
Niṣṭhuraḥ - Pittalam	निष्ठुरः - पित्तलम्	526
Nīvāraḥ (p. 544)	नीवारः (p. 544)	
Niyamanaḥ - Nimbaḥ	नियमन : निम्बः	11
Niyoddhā - Kukkuṭaḥ	नियोद्धा - कुक्कटः	636
Nṛpabadaraḥ-Badaram (Raj.ni.)	नृपबदरः - बदरम् (रा.नि.)	446
Nṛpaḥ - Rājādanaḥ	नृपः - राजादनः	439
Nṛpam - Tagaram	नृपम् - तगरम्	221
Nṛpamāṣaḥ - Rajamāṣaḥ	नृपमाषः - राजमाषः	542
Nṛpātmajaḥ - Rājāmraḥ	नृपात्मजः - राजाम्रः	388
Nṛpocitaḥ - Rājāmāṣaḥ	नृपोचितः - राजमाषः	542
Nṛpopalaḥ - Rājāvartaḥ	नृपोपलः - राजावर्तः	533
Nyagrodhā - Dravantī	न्यग्रोधा - द्रवन्ती	86
Nyagrodhaḥ - Vaṭaḥ	न्यग्रोधः - वटः	426

Nyaṅkuḥ - Hariṇaḥ	न्यङ्कुः - हरिणः	625
Odanāhvayā - Balā	ओदनाह्वया - बला	110
Odanikā -Balā	ओदनिका - बला	110
Osṭḥolpamaphalā - Bimbī	ओष्ठोपमफला - बिम्बी	76
Otuḥ - Biḍālaḥ	ओतुः - बिडालः	631
Pacampacā - Dāruharidrā	पचंपचा - दारुहरिद्रा	21
Pādam - Vyāghranakham	पादम् - व्याघ्रनखम्	223
Padmā - Bhārṅgī	पद्मा - भार्ङ्गी	24
Padmā - Padmacāriṇī	पद्मा - पद्मचारिणी	325
Padmabījam (p. 375)	पद्मबीजम् (p. 375)	
Padmacāriṇī (p. 325)	पद्मचारिणी (p. 325)	
Padmakaḥ (p. 242)	पद्मकः (p. 242)	
Padmakam - Padmabījam	पद्मकम् - पद्मबीजम्	375
Padmakandam - Padmamūlam	पद्मकन्दम् - पद्ममूलम्	377
Padmakam-Kuṣṭham (Raj. ni.)	पद्मकम् - कुष्ठम् (रा.नि.)	219
Padmakarkaṭī - Padmabījam	पद्मकर्कटी - पद्मबीजम्	375
Padmakāṣṭham-Padmakaḥ (Raj. ni.)	पद्मकाष्ठम् - पद्मकः (रा. नि.)	242
Padmakesaram (p. 377)	पद्मकेसरम् (p. 377)	
Padmākṣam - Padmabījam	पद्माक्षम् - पद्मबीजम्	375
Padmam - Kṣudramutpalam	पद्मम् - क्षुद्रमुत्पलम्	374
Padmam - Śvāsāriḥ	पद्मम् - श्वासारिः	25
Padmamūlam (p. 376)	पद्ममूलम् (p. 376)	
Padmanālam - Bisam	पद्मनालम् - बिसम्	376
Padmapatrakam-Puṣkaramūlam	पद्मपत्रकम् - पुष्करमूलम्	23
Padmarupiṇī - Vandakā	पद्मरूपिणी - वन्दका	331
Padmatantuḥ - Bisam (Raj. ni.)	पद्मतन्तुः - बिसम् (रा. नि.)	376
Padmatīrtham - Śvāsāriḥ	पद्मतीर्थम् - श्वासारिः	25
Padmavatī - Padmacāriṇī	पद्मवती -पद्मचारिणी	325
Padmavatī- Padminī	पद्मवती - पद्मिनी	374
Padmī - Hasti	पद्मी - हस्ति	620
Padminī (P. 374)	पद्मिनी (P. 374)	
Pākalam - Kuṣṭham	पाकलम् - कुष्ठम्	219
Pakṣma - Romaviśeṣaḥ	पक्ष्म - रोमविशेषः	644
Paktā - Pittam	पक्ता - पित्तम्	616
Pākyaḥ - Vrīhiḥ	पाक्यः - व्रीहिः	538
Pākyaḥ - Yavakṣāraḥ	पाक्यः -यवक्षारः	133
Pālakākhyaḥ - Niṣpāvaḥ	पालकाख्यः - निष्पावः	560
Pālakam - Śāliparṇī viśeṣaḥ	पालकम् - शालिपर्णी विशेषः	32
Palāṇḍuḥ (p. 315)	पलाण्डुः (p. 315)	
Palaṅkaṣā - Lākṣā	पलंकषा - लाक्षा	239
Palaṅkaṣaḥ - Gugguluḥ	पलंकषः - गुग्गुलुः	252
Palaśā - Śaṭhī	पलाशा - शठी	21

Palāśagandhā (p. 150)	पलाशगन्धा (p.150)	
Palāśaḥ - Kimśukaḥ	पलाशः - किंशुकः	518
Palāśakhyā - Nāḍihiṅghu	पलाशाख्या - नाडीहिगु	139
Palāśam - Tamālapatram	पलाशम् - तमालपत्रम्	146
Palāśinī - Padminī	पलाशिनी - पद्मिनी	374
Pālevatam (p. 418)	पालेवतम् (p. 418)	
Pālī - Citrakaḥ	पाली - चित्रकः	165
Pālikā - Atasī	पालिका - अतसी	565
Pālindaḥ - Kunduruḥ	पालिन्दः - कुन्दुरुः	254
Palitam - Maricam	पलितम् - मरिचम्	168
Palitam - Śaileyam	पलितम् - शैलेयम्	235
Palvalāvāsaḥ - Kacchapaḥ	पल्वलावासः - कच्छपः	630
Pāmśuḥ - Parpaṭaḥ	पांशुः - पर्पटः	17
Pāmsulaḥ - Lāvaḥ	पांसुलः - लावः	636
Pāmśulavaṇam - Audbhidam	पांशुलवणम् - औद्भिदम्	136
Pāmsavakśāram - Audbhidam	पांसवक्षारम् - औद्भिदम्	136
Pañcanakhaḥ - Vyāghraḥ	पञ्चनखः - व्याघ्रः	623
Pañcabhṛṅgam	पञ्चभृङ्गम्	648
Pañcagaṇaḥ	पञ्चगणः	657
Pañcagavyam	पञ्चगव्यम्	654
Pañcakolakam	पञ्चकोलकम्	647
Pañcaloham - Vartaloham	पञ्चलोहम् - वर्तलोहम्	52
Pañcāmṛtam	पञ्चामृतम्	654
Pancamukhaḥ - Simhaḥ	पञ्चमुखः - सिंहः	624
Pañcamuṣṭiḥ - Spṛkkā	पञ्चमुष्टिः - स्पृक्का	224
Pañcānanaḥ -Simhaḥ	पञ्चाननः - सिंहः	624
Pañcāṅgam	पञ्चाङ्गम्	656
Pañcāṅgulaḥ - Eraṇḍaḥ	पञ्चाङ्गुलः - एरण्डः	117
Pañcanimbakam	पञ्चनिम्बकम्	655
Pañcapañcamūlam	पञ्चपञ्चमूलम्	649-650
Pañcaratnāni	पञ्चरत्नानि	662
Pañcaśairīṣam	पञ्चशैरीषम्	655
Pañcasārpakam	पञ्चसार्पकम्	656
Pañcasiddhauṣadhiḥ	पञ्चसिद्धौषधिः	656
Pañcasugandhikam	पञ्चसुगन्धिकम्	652-653
Pañcasūraṇam	पञ्चसूरणम्	656
Pañcavalkalam	पञ्चवल्कलम्	647
Pañcāmlakam	पञ्चाम्लकम्	654
Punḍarīkam (p. 369)	पुण्डरीकम् (p. 369)	368
Pāṇḍavaḥ - Arjunaḥ	पाण्डवः -अर्जुनः	464
Pāṇḍukaḥ - Paṭolaḥ	पाण्डुकः - पटोलः	18
Pāṇḍupatnī - Reṇukā	पाण्डुपत्नी -रेणुका	220

Pāṇḍuphalaḥ - Paṭolaḥ	पाण्डुफलः - पटोलः	18
Pāṇḍuradrumaḥ-Kuṭajaḥ (Raj.ni.)	पाण्डुरद्रुमः - कुटजः (रा.नि.)	132
Pāṇḍurāgaḥ - Damanaḥ	पाण्डुरागः - दमनः	228
Pāṇimardakam-Karamardakam	पाणिमर्दकम् - करमर्दकम्	449
Pānīyam - Jalam	पानीयम् - जलम्	605
Paṅkajam - Kumudam	पंकजम् - कुमुदम्	373
Paṅkavāsaḥ - Karkaṭaḥ	पंकवासः - कर्कटः	640
Paṅktibījakaḥ - Karṇikāraḥ	पंक्तिबीजकः - कर्णिकारः	82
Pannagaḥ - Sarpaḥ	पन्नगः - सर्पः	639
Pāpacelikā - Pāṭhā	पापचेलिका - पाठा	26
Pāpaghnaḥ - Tilaḥ	पापघ्नः - तिलः	568
Pāpanāśinī - Śamī	पापनाशिनी - शमी	443
Parabhṛtā - Kokilā	परभृता - कोकिला	637
Parabhṛtaḥ - Kokilaḥ	परभृतः - कोकिलः	637
Pāradaḥ (p. 529)	पारदः (p.529)	
Pāradīyaḥ - Pāradaḥ	पारदीयः - पारदः	529
Parāgam -Padmakesaram (Raj. ni.)	परागम् - पद्मकेसरम् (रा. नि.)	377
Parāgapuṣpaḥ - Kadambaḥ (Raj. ni.)	परागपुष्पः - कदम्बः (रा. नि.)	452
Parapuṣṭaḥ - Āmraḥ	परपुष्टः - आम्रः	385
Parārdham	परार्धम्	653
Pāraśavam - Loham	पारशवम् - लोहम्	528
Parāśrayaḥ - Atimuktakaḥ	पराश्रयः - अतिमुक्तकः	509
Parāvaram - Paruṣakaḥ	परावरम् -परुषकः	416
Pārāvatapadī -Kākajaṅghā	पारावतपदी - काकजङ्घा	287
Pārevatam-Pālevatam (Raj.ni.)	पारेवतम् - पालेवतम् (रा. नि.)	418
Pāribhadrakaḥ- Nimbaḥ	पारिभद्रकः - निम्बः	12
Pāribhadrakam - Kuṣṭham	पारिभद्रकम् - कुष्ठम्	219
Pārijātā - Tejasvinī	पारिजाता - तेजस्विनी	102
Parimaṇḍalamalpāsthi-Paruṣakaḥ	परिमण्डलमल्पास्थि -परुषकः	416
Paripelavam - Jalamustam	परिपेलवम् - जलमुस्तम्	16
Paripellavam (p. 222)	परिपेल्लवम् (p. 222)	
Pariplavam - Paripellavam	परिप्लवम् - परिपेल्लवम्	222
Parivyādhaḥ - Karṇikāraḥ	परिव्याधः - कर्णिकारः	82
Parjanyā - Dāruharidrā	पर्जन्या - दारुहरिद्रा	21
Parṇacorakaḥ-Corakaḥ (Raj.ni.)	पर्णचोरकः - चोरकः (रा. नि.)	232
Parṇāsaḥ - Kuṭherakaḥ	पर्णासः - कुठेरकः	304
Parṇi - Pṛśniparṇī	पर्णी - पृश्निपर्णी	33
Parṇikā - (Pṛśni.) viśeṣaḥ	पर्णिका - (पृश्नि.) विशेषः	33
Parpaṭaḥ (p.17)	पर्पटः (p.17)	
Parpaṭakaḥ - Parpaṭaḥ	पर्पटकः - पर्पटः	17
Parapuṣṭā - Kokilā	परपुष्टा - कोकिला	637
Pārthaḥ - Arjunaḥ	पार्थः -अर्जुनः	464

Paruḥ - Paruṣakaḥ	परुः -परुषकः	414
Paruḥ - Vaṁśāgram	परुः - वंशाग्रम्	365
Paruṣakaḥ (p. 416)	परुषकः (p. 416)	
Paruṣam - Paruṣakaḥ	परुषम् -परुषकः	416
Parvatamocā-Girikadalī (Raj.ni.)	पर्वतमोचा - गिरिकदली (रा. नि.)	317
Pārvateyā - Jiṅgiṇī	पार्वतेया - जिंगिणी	272
Pārvatī - Atasī	पार्वती - अतसी	565
Pārvatīyā - Dhātukī	पार्वतीया - धातुकी	243
Pārvatīyaḥ - Akṣoḍaḥ	पार्वतीयः - अक्षोडः	414
Paryaṅkapādikā - Dadhipuṣpī	पर्यङ्कपादिका - दधिपुष्पी	56
Pāṣāṇabhedakaḥ (p.57)	पाषाणभेदकः (p. 57)	
Pāṣāṇagairikam - Gairikam	पाषाणगैरिकम् - गैरिकम्	262
Pāṣāṇakadalī -Kāṣṭhakadalī	पाषाणकदली - काष्ठकदली	317
Paśuḥ - Aviḥ	पशुः - अविः	623
Paśuḥ - Chāgaḥ	पशुः - छागः	622
Pāṭalā (p.43)	पाटला (p.43)	
Pāṭalam - Kattṛṇam	पाटलम् - कत्तृणम्	28
Pāṭalāpuṣpavarṇakaḥ-Padmakaḥ	पाटलापुष्पवर्णकः - पद्मकः	242
Pātālavāsinī - Tāmbūlī	पातालवासिनी - ताम्बूली	273
Pāṭaliḥ - Muṣkakaḥ (Raj. ni.)	पाटलिः - मुष्ककः (रा. नि.)	483
Pataṅgam (p. 193)	पतङ्गम् (p. 193)	
Pāṭhā (p.25)	पाठा (p.25)	
Pāṭhī - Citrakaḥ	पाठी - चित्रकः	165
Pathidrumaḥ - Somavalkaḥ	पथिद्रुमः - सोमवल्कः	10
Pāṭhikā - Pāṭhā	पाठिका - पाठा	26
Pāthīnaḥ - Citrakaḥ	पाठीनः- चित्रकः	165
Pāṭhīnaḥ - Matsyabhedaḥ	पाठीनः - मत्स्यभेदः	628
Pāṭhīnaḥ - Matsyaviśeṣaḥ	पाठीनः -मत्स्य विशेषः	628
Pāṭhīnaḥ - Matsyaḥ	पाठीनः - मत्स्यः	626
Pathyā - Harītakī	पथ्या - हरीतकी	77
Pathyaḥ - Rasaḥ	पथ्यः - रसः	619
Pathyam	पथ्यम्	660
Patrāḍhyam - Tālīsam	पत्राढ्यम् - तालीसम्	147
Patram - Tālīsam	पत्रम् - तालीसम्	147
Patram- Tamālapatram	पत्रम् - तमालपत्रम्	98
Patrāṅgam - Pataṅgam	पत्राङ्गम् - पतङ्गम्	194
Patrataṇḍulī-Yavatiktā (Raj.ni.)	पत्रतण्डुली - यवतिक्ता (रा.नि.)	98
Paṭṭarāgam - Pataṅgam	पट्टरागम् - पतङ्गम्	194
Paṭṭarañjanam - Pataṅgam	पट्टरञ्जनम् - पतङ्गम्	194
Paṭṭī - Paṭṭikārodhraḥ	पट्टी -पट्टिकारोध्रः	270
Paṭṭikārodhraḥ (p. 270)	पट्टिकारोध्रः (p. 270)	
Paṭuḥ - Kāṇḍīraḥ	पटुः -काण्डीरः	309

Pauṇḍrakaḥ - Ikśuḥ	पौण्ड्रकः - इक्षुः	357
Pauṇḍrakaḥ - Lāvaḥ	पौण्ड्रकः - लावः	636
Pauram - Kattṛṇam	पौरम् - कत्तृणम्	28
Paurarasam - Bolam	पौररसम् - बोलम्	226
Pauruṣam - Śukram	पौरुषम् - शुक्रम्	619
Pauṣkaram - Puṣkaramūlam	पौष्करम् - पुष्करमूलम्	23
Pauṣpikam - Puṣpāñjanam	पौष्पिकम् - पुष्पाञ्जनम्	266
Pāvakaḥ - Citrakaḥ	पावकः - चित्रकः	165
Pāvakam - Kusumbham	पावकम् - कुसुम्भम्	566
Pavanaḥ - Vāyuḥ	पवनः - वायुः	616
Pāvanī - Rocanā	पावनी - रोचना	203
Paviḥ - Hīrakam	पविः - हीरकम्	532
Pavitrā - Aśvatthī	पवित्रा - अश्वत्थी	428
Pavitraḥ - Damanaḥ (Raj. ni.)	पवित्रः - दमनः (रा. नि.)	228
Pavitraḥ - Śephālikā	पवित्रः - शेफालिका	321
Pavitraḥ - Tilaḥ	पवित्रः - तिलः	568
Pavitraḥ - Kuśaḥ (Raj. ni.)	पवित्रः - कुशः (रा.नि.)	362
Pavitrakaḥ - Pippalaḥ	पवित्रकः -पिप्पलः	427
Pavitram - Ghṛtam	पवित्रम् - घृतम्	574
Pavitram - Vyāghranakham	पवित्रम्- व्याघ्रनखम्	224
Payaḥ - Dugdham	पयः - दुग्धम्	577
Payaḥ - Jalam	पयः - जलम्	605
Pāyasaḥ - Śriveṣṭakaḥ	पायसः - श्रीवेष्टकः	255
Payasvalaḥ - Chāgaḥ	पयस्वलः - छागः	622
Payasvinī - Goḥ	पयस्विनी - गोः	626
Payasvinī - Mahiṣī	पयस्विनी - महिषी	625
Payasvinī - Kśīravidārī	पयस्विनी - क्षीरविदारी	54
Payasvinī - Kśīrakākolī	पयस्विनी - क्षीरकाकोली	47
Payodhijam - Samudraphenam	पयोधिजम् - समुद्रफेनम्	263
Payohetuḥ - Dadhi	पयोहेतुः - दधि	582
Peśī - Māmsī	पेशी - मांसी	217
Phalacorakaḥ - Corakaḥ	फलचोरकः - चोरकः	232
Phalaḥ - Madanaḥ	फलः - मदनः	62
Phalāmlaḥ-Amlavetasaḥ (Raj.ni.)	फलाम्लः - अम्लवेतसः (रा.नि.)	177
Phalamukhyā-Ajamodā (Raj.ni.)	फलमुख्या - अजमोदा (रा.नि.)	183
Phalapriyā - Priyaṅguḥ (Raj. ni)	फलप्रिया - प्रियङ्गुः (रा.नि.)	201
Phalapūrakaḥ - Bījapūraḥ	फलपूरकः - बीजपूरः	396
Phalapuṣpaḥ - Dīpyā	फलपुष्पः - दीप्या	412
Phalaṣāḍavaḥ - Dāḍimaḥ	फलषाडवः -दाडिमः	155
Phalaśaiśiraḥ - Badaram	फलशैशिरः - बदरम्	445
Phalasambhārī-Kākodumbarikā	फलसम्भारी - काकोदुम्बरिका	437
Phalasnehaḥ - Akśoḍaḥ	फलस्नेहः - अक्षोडः	414

Phalavalkalaḥ-Khastilavalkalaḥ	फलवल्कलः - खस्तिलवल्कलः	568
Phalacukrādi - Vṛkṡāmlam (Raj. ni.)	फलचुक्रादि- वृक्षाम्लम् (रा.नि.)	173
Phaleruhā - Kāṣṭhapāṭalā	फलेरुहा - काष्ठपाटला	44
Phalinī - Priyaṅguḥ	फलिनी - प्रियङ्गुः	201
Phalottamā - Uttarāpathikā	फलोत्तमा - उत्तरापथिका	413
Phaṇī - Jambīraḥ	फणी- जम्बीरः	302
Phanī - Sarpaḥ	फणी - सर्पः	638
Phaṇijjakaḥ - Jambīraḥ	फणिज्जकः - जम्बीरः	302
Phañjī - Bhārngī	फञ्जी - भार्ङ्गी	24
Phaṭikā - Saurāṣṭrī	फटिका -सौराष्ट्री	247
Pheravaḥ - Sṛgālaḥ	फेरवः - श्रृगालः	632
Phenā - Sātalā	फेना - सातला	89
Phenam - Samudraphenam	फेनम् - समुद्रफेनम्	263
Phenilam - Badaram	फेनिलम् - बदरम्	445
Piccaṭam - Vaṅgam	पिच्चटम् - वङ्गम्	525
Picchā - Śālmaliveṣṭakaḥ	पिच्छा -शाल्मलीवेष्टकः	481
Picchilā - Śālmalī	पिच्छिला - शाल्मली	481
Picchilabījam - Bhavam	पिच्छिलबीजम् - भवम्	401
Picchilaḥ - Ikṡuḥ (Raj. ni.)	पिच्छिलः - इक्षुः (रा. नि.)	358
Picchilaḥ - Śigruḥ (Raj. ni.)	पिच्छिलः - शिग्रुः (रा. नि.)	296
Picchilaḥ - Ślseṣmātakaḥ	पिच्छिलः - श्लेष्मातकः	441
Picumandaḥ - Nimbaḥ	पिचुमन्दः - निम्बः	12
Pikabāndhavaḥ - Āmraḥ	पिकबान्धवः - आम्रः	385
Pīluḥ (p. 409)	पीलुः (p. 409)	
Pīluparṇī - Bimbī	पीलुपर्णी - बिम्बी	76
Pilupuṣpaḥ - Moraṭaḥ	पीलुपुष्पः - मोरटः	6
Pīnaskandhaḥ - Sūkaraḥ	पीनस्कन्धः - सूकरः	624
Pīnaskandhaḥ - Mahiṣaḥ	पीनस्कन्धः - महिषः	625
Piṇḍā - Nāḍihiṅgu	पिण्डा - नाडीहिंगु	139
Piṇḍagudūcikā - Kandaguḍūcī	पिण्डगुडूचिका -कंदगुडूची	3
Piṇḍakaḥ - Turuṣkaḥ	पिण्डकः - तुरुष्कः	204
Piṇḍakam-Piṇḍamūlam (Raj.ni.)	पिण्डकम् - पिण्डमूलम् (रा.नि)	294
Piṇḍakharjūrī - Dīpyā	पिण्डखर्जूरी - दीप्या	412
Piṇḍam - Loham	पिण्डम् - लोहम्	528
Piṇḍam - Bolam	पिण्डम् - बोलम्	226
Piṇḍāmṛtā - Kandaguḍūcī	पिण्डामृता -कंदगुडूची	2
Piṇḍamūlakam-Piṇḍamūlam (Raj. ni.)	पिण्डमूलकम् -पिण्डमूलम् (रा.नि)	299
Piṇḍamūlam (Raj. ni.) (p. 294)	पिण्डमूलम् (रा.नि) (. 294)	
Piṇḍamustaḥ - Mustā	पिण्डमुस्तः - मुस्ता	15
Piṇḍaphalā - Kaṭukālāmbunī	पिण्डफला - कटुकालाम्बुनी	63
Piṇḍī - Madanaḥ	पिण्डी - मदनः	62
Piṇḍitaḥ- Turuṣkaḥ	पिण्डितः - तुरुष्कः	204

Piṇḍītakaḥ - Madanaḥ पिण्डीतकः – मदनः 62
Piṅgā - Haridrā पिङ्गा – हरिद्रा 20
Piṅgā - Rocanā पिङ्गा – रोचना 203
Piṅgaḥ - Mūṣakaḥ पिङ्गः – मूषकः 630
Piṅgaḥ - Pittalam पिङ्गः – पित्तलम् 526
Piṅgalā - Pittalam पिङ्गला – पित्तलम् 526
Piṅgalā - Rocanā पिङ्गला – रोचना 203
Piṅgalaḥ - K'sudrolūkaḥ पिङ्गलः – क्षुद्रोलूकः 638
Piṅgalaḥ - Ugrabiḍālakaḥ पिङ्गलः – उग्रबिडालकः 631
Piṅgalāk'saḥ - K'sudrolūkaḥ पिङ्गलाक्षः – क्षुद्रोलूकः 638
Piṅgalam - Turuṣkaḥ पिङ्गलम् – तुरुष्कः 204
Piṅgalam mūlam - Garjaram पिङ्गलंमूलम् – गर्जरम् 314
Piṅgam - Vālakam पिङ्गम् – वालकम् 17
Piñjaram - Haritālam पिञ्जरम् – हरितालम् 667
Piṇyākaḥ - Turuṣkaḥ पिण्याकः – तुरुष्कः 204
Pipalīmūlam (p. 161) पिप्पलीमूलम् (p. 161)
Pippalaḥ (p. 427) पिप्पलः (p. 427)
Pippalī (p.160) पिप्पली (p.160)
Pippalikā - A'svatthī पिप्पलिका – अश्वत्थी 428
Pipparī - Plak'saḥ पिप्परी – प्लक्षः 429
Pi'sācī - Gandhamāmsī पिशाची – गन्धमांसी 217
Pi'sitā - Māmsī पिशिता – मांसी 217
Pi'sitam - Māmsam पिशितम् – मांसम् 618
Pi'sunā - Spṛkkā पिशुना – स्पृक्का 224
Pi'sunam - Kumkumam पिशुनम् – कुंकुमम् 197
Pītā - Dāruharidrā पीता –दारुहरिद्रा 21
Pītā - Haridrā पीता – हरिद्रा 20
Pītā - Suvarṇakadalī पीता – सुवर्णकदली 318
Pītā Ajagandhā - Ajagandhā (Raj. ni.) पीता अजगन्धा – अजगन्धा (रा.नि.) 184
Pītabhadrakaḥ - Kiṅkirātaḥ पीतभद्रकः – किंकिरातः 511
Pītābham - Jīrakam पीताभम् – जीरकम् 157
Pītacandanam- Dāruharidrā पीतचन्दनम् – दारुहरिद्रा 21
Pītadāru - Dāruharidrā पीतदारु – दारुहरिद्रा 21
Pītadharā - Vasā पीतधरा – वसा 619
Pītadhattūrakaḥ -Dhatturaḥ (Raj. ni.) पीतधत्तूरकः –धत्तूरः (रा. नि.) 279
Pītadruḥ - Saralaḥ (Raj. ni.) पीतद्रुः – सरलः (रा. नि.) 237
Pītadruḥ - Dāruharidrā पीतद्रुः – दारुहरिद्रा 21
Pītāhvapītakā - Dāruharidrā पीताह्वपीतका – दारुहरिद्रा 21
Pītakaḥ - Kiṅkirātaḥ पीतकः– किंकिरातः 511
Pītakam - Harītālam पीतकं– हरितालम् 667
Pītakam - Kumkumam पीतकम्- कुंकुमम् 197
Pītakam - Suvarṇam पीतकम् – सुवर्णम् 523

Pītakammūlakam - Garjaram पीतकंमूलकम् - गर्जरम् 314
Pītakāṣṭham - Kālīyakam पीतकाष्ठम् - कालीयकम् 194
Pītakīlakā - Āvartakī पीतकीलका - आवर्तकी 74
Pītam - Gṛñjanam पीतम् - गृञ्जनम् 294
Pītam - Kusumbham पीतम् - कुसुम्भम् 566
Pītam (candanam) - Kālīyakam पीतं (चन्दनम्) - कालीयकम् 194
Pītamaṇḍūkaḥ-Rājamaṇḍūkaḥ (Raj.ni.) पीतमण्डूकः-राजमण्डूकः (रा.नि.)640
Pītamūlakam - Garjaram पीतमूलकम् - गर्जरम् 314
Pītanakaḥ - Āmrātakaḥ पीतनकः - आम्रातकः 388
Pītāṅgaḥ-Rājamaṇḍūkaḥ (Raj. ni.)पीताङ्गः - राजमण्डूकः (रा. नि.) 640
Pītāṅgaḥ - Śyonākaḥ (Raj. ni.) पीताङ्गः - श्योनाकः (रा.नि.) 41
Pītaprasavaḥ-Karavīraḥ (Raj. ni.) पीतप्रसवः - करवीरः (रा. नि.) 276
Pītapuṣpā - Mahābalā पीतपुष्पा - महाबला 111
Pītapuṣpā - Āḍhakī पीतपुष्पा - आढकी 549
Pītapuṣpā - Āvartakī पीतपुष्पा - आवर्तकी 74
Pītapuṣpā - Dhāmārgavaḥ पीतपुष्पा -धामार्गवः 70
Pītapuṣpaḥ - Kovidāraḥ पीतपुष्पः -कोविदारः 74
Pītaraktaḥ - Padmakaḥ पीतरक्तः - पद्मकः 242
Pītarambhā- Suvarṇakadalī पीतरम्भा - सुवर्णकदली 318
Pītasāraḥ - Aṅkoṭakaḥ पीतसारः - अङ्कोटकः 99
Pītataṇḍulaḥ - Kaṅguḥ पीततण्डुलः - कङ्गुः 546
Pītavarṇakam - Śīrṇavṛntam पीतवर्णकम् - शीर्णवृन्तम् 66
Pītavarṇam - Kāleyakam पीतवर्णम् - कालेयकम् 207
Pitayūthikā - Yūthikā पीतयूथिका - यूथिका 504
Pītikā - Śatapuṣpā पीतिका - शतपुष्पा 121
Pītikā - Haridrā पीतिका - हरिद्रा 20
Pītikā - Kūṣmāṇḍikā पीतिका- कूष्माण्डिका 68
Pītikā - Yūthikā पीतिका - यूथिका 504
Pītmudgaḥ - Kulatthaḥ पीतमुद्गः - कुलत्थः 557
Pitṛpriyaḥ-Bhṛṅgarājaḥ (Raj. ni.) पितृप्रियः - भृङ्गराजः (रा. नि.) 281
Pitṛtarpaṇaḥ - Tilaḥ पितृतर्पणः - तिलः 568
Pitryaḥ - Māṣaḥ पित्र्यः - माषः 552
Pittabheṣajam - Masūraḥ पित्तभेषजम् - मसूरः 550
Pittadrāvī - Madhu Jambīraḥ पित्तद्रावी - मधुजम्बीरः 390
Pittalam (Rītīkā) (p. 525) पित्तलम् (रीतिका) (p.525)
Pittam (p. 616) पित्तम् (p. 616)
Pitṛjottamaḥ - Māṣaḥ पितृजोत्तमः - माषः 552
Pittavallabhā - Ativiṣā पित्तवल्लभा - अतिविषा 4
Pittaprasekaḥ - Asita mudgaḥ पित्तप्रसेकः - असितमुद्गः 540
Pīvarī - Śatāvarī पीवरी - शतावरी 115
Pīyūṣamoraṭau पीयूषमोरटौ 590
Plakṣaḥ (p. 428) प्लक्षः (p. 428)

Plavagaḥ - Markaṭaḥ	प्लवगः – मर्कटः	632
Plavaḥ - Markaṭaḥ	प्लवः – मर्कटः	633
Plavakaḥ - Plakśaḥ	प्लवकः –प्लक्षः	429
Plavam - Paripellavam	प्लवम्– परिपेल्लवम्	222
Plavaṅgaḥ - Markaṭaḥ	प्लवङ्गः – मर्कटः	632
Plavaṅgamaḥ - Markaṭaḥ	प्लवङ्गमः – मर्कटः	632
Poṭagalaḥ - Nalaḥ	पोटगलः – नलः	366
Potakā - Potakī	पोतका – पोतकी	382
Potakī (p. 382)	पोतकी (p. 382)	
Paṭolaḥ (p. 18)	पटोलः (p.18)	
Prabhadraḥ - Nimbaḥ	प्रभद्रः – निम्बः	12
Prabhañjanaḥ - Vāyuḥ	प्रभञ्जनः – वायुः	616
Pracaṇḍaḥ - Karavīraḥ	प्रचण्डः – करवीरः	275
Pracībalā - Kākajaṅghā	प्रचीबला – काकजङ्घा	287
Prācīnā - Pāṭhā	प्राचीना – पाठा	26
Prācīnāmalakam (p.80)	प्राचीनामलकम् (p.80)	
Prācīnārangam-Prācīnāmalakam	प्राचीनारङ्गम् – प्राचीनामलकम्	80
Pradīpanaḥ	प्रदीपनः	665
Pragrahaḥ - Karṇikāraḥ	प्रग्रहः – कर्णिकारः	81
Prahasantī - Vāsantī	प्रहसन्ती –वासन्ती	498
Prakāśam - Kāmsyam	प्रकाशम् – कांस्यम्	527
Prakīryaḥ - Karañjaḥ	प्रकीर्यः – करञ्जः	456
Prakṛtayaḥ	प्रकृतयः	617
Pralambaḥ - Bhūstṛnaḥ	प्रलम्बः – भूस्तृणः	300
Parapuṣṭaḥ - Kokilaḥ	परपुष्टः – कोकिलः	637
Pramadā - Strī	प्रमदा – स्त्री	615
Pramodanī - Mallikā	प्रमोदनी – मल्लिका	493
Prāmśuḥ - Tālaḥ	प्रांशुः –तालः	421
Prāṇadā - Harītakī	प्राणदा – हरीतकी	77
Prāṇadaḥ - Jīvakaḥ	प्राणदः – जीवकः	44
Prāṇadam - Raktam	प्राणदम् – रक्तम्	619
Prāṇahārakam - Vatasanābhaḥ	प्राणहारक्म् – वत्सनाभः	667
Prāṇapradaḥ - Rasaḥ	प्राणप्रदः – रसः	619
Prapathyā - Harītakī	प्रपथ्या – हरीतकी	77
Prapauṇḍarīkam (p. 243)	प्रपौण्डरीकम् (p. 243)	
Prapunnāḍaḥ - Cakramardaḥ	प्रपुन्नाडः – चक्रमर्दः	277
Prapunnāṭaḥ - Cakramardaḥ	प्रपुन्नाटः – चक्रमर्दः	277
Prasādakaḥ - Śāliḥ	प्रसादकः – शालिः	535
Prasādakaḥ - Nīvāraḥ	प्रसादकः – नीवारः	544
Prasannā	प्रसन्ना	598
Prasannā - Surā	प्रसन्ना – सुरा	596
Prasaram - Elavālukam	प्रसरम् – एलवालुकम्	236

Prasāraṇī (p.114)	प्रसारणी (p.114)	
Prasrāvaḥ - Mūtram	प्रस्रावः - मूत्रम्	641
Prasravaṇam - Dugdham	प्रस्रवणम् - दुग्धम्	577
Prasūkā - Aśvā	प्रसूका - अश्वा	621
Pratānikā - Sārivā	प्रतानिका - सारिवा	59
Pratānikā - Prasāraṇī	प्रतानिका - प्रसारणी	114
Pratāpanaḥ - Rajārakaḥ	प्रतापनः - राजार्कः	282
Pratarīrkatamā - Atasī	प्रतरीर्कतमा - अतसी	565
Pratāpaḥ - Śuklārkaḥ	प्रतापः - शुक्लार्कः	283
Pratihāsaḥ - Karavīraḥ	प्रतिहासः - करवीरः	275
Pratīpadarśinī - Strī	प्रतीपदर्शिनी - स्त्री	615
Prativiṣā - Śya. Ativiṣā	प्रतिविषा -श्या.अतिविषा	4
Pratyakpuṣpī - Apāmārgaḥ	प्रत्यक्पुष्पी -अपामार्गः	100
Parākpuṣpī - Apāmārgaḥ	पराक्पुष्पी -अपामार्गः	100
Pratyakśreṇī - Dravantī	प्रत्यक्श्रेणी - द्रवन्ती	86
Pravālam (p. 533)	प्रवालम् (p. 533)	
Pravaram - Agaru	प्रवरम् - अगरु	206
Pravrajitā - Śrāvaṇī	प्रव्रजिता - श्रावणी	58
Prāvṛṣyaḥ - Kadambaḥ	प्रावृष्यः - कदम्बः	451
Priyā - Priyaṅguḥ	प्रिया - प्रियङ्गुः	201
Priyā - Vārśikī	प्रिया - वार्षिकी	496
Priyadarśanaḥ - Rajādanaḥ	प्रियदर्शनः - राजादनः	439
Priyadarśanaḥ - Śukaḥ	प्रियदर्शनः - शुकः	634
Priyaḥ - Karañjaḥ	प्रियः - करञ्जः	461
Priyakaḥ - Aśanaḥ	प्रियकः - अशनः	479
Priyālā - Drākśā	प्रियाला - द्राक्षा	413
Priyalaḥ (p. 423)	प्रियालः (p. 423)	
Priyamvadā - Jātī	प्रियंवदा - जाती	496
Priyaṅguḥ - Kaṅguḥ	प्रियङ्गुः - कङ्गुः	546
Priyaṅguḥ (p.200)	प्रियङ्गुः (p.200)	
Priyaṅkarī - Kāsaghnī	प्रियंकरी - कासघ्नी	37
Priyaśālakaḥ - Aśanaḥ	प्रियशालकः - अशनः	479
Priyavādinī - Sārikā	प्रियवादिनी - सारिका	635
Priyavallī - Priyaṅguḥ	प्रियवल्ली - प्रियङ्गुः	201
Priyajīvaḥ - Śyonākaḥ	प्रियजीवः - श्योनाकः	41
Proṣṭhī - Matsyaviśeṣaḥ	प्रोष्ठी - मत्स्य विशेषः	628
Pṛṣataḥ - Hariṇaḥ	पृषतः - हरिणः	625
Pṛśniparṇī (p.33)	पृश्निपर्णी (p.33)	
Pṛṣṭhadṛṣṭiḥ - Bhallaḥ	पृष्ठदृष्टिः- भल्लः	637
Pṛṣṭhasṛṅgakaḥ - Aviḥ	पृष्ठश्रृङ्गकः - अविः	623
Pṛṣṭiparṇī - Pṛśniparṇī	पृष्टिपर्णी - पृश्निपर्णी	33
Pṛthakparṇī - Mūrvā	पृथक्पर्णी - मूर्वा	5

Pṛthakparṇī - Pṛśniparṇī	पृथक्पर्णी – पृश्निपर्णी	33
Pṛthucchadaḥ - Akśoḍaḥ	पृथुच्छदः – अक्षोडः	414
Pṛthuḥ - Hiṅgupatrī	पृथुः – हिंगुपत्री	138
Pṛthuḥ - Masūraḥ	पृथुः – मसूरः	550
Pṛthukandakaḥ - Gunṭhaḥ	पृथुकंदकः – गुण्ठः	30
Pṛthulā - Hiṅgupatrī	पृथुला – हिंगुपत्री	138
Pṛthulaḥ - Kuśaḥ	पृथुलः – कुशः	361
Pṛthupalāśikā - Śaṭhī	पृथुपलाशिका – शठी	22
Pṛthuśimbaḥ - Śyonākaḥ	पृथुशिम्बः – श्योनाकः	41
Pṛthvī - Śwetamandāraḥ	पृथ्वी – श्वेतमन्दारः	283
Pṛthvīkā - Hiṅgupatrī	पृथ्वीका – हिंगुपत्री	138
Pṛthvīkā - Upakuñcī	पृथ्वीका – उपकुञ्ची	154
Pṛthvīkā - Bhadrailā	पृथ्वीका –भद्रैला	142
Pūgaphalam (p.213)	पूगफलम् (p.213)	
Pūjyamānakam - Jīrakam	पूज्यमानकम् – जीरकम्	157
Pulakam - Kamkuṣṭham	पुलकम् – कंकुष्ठम्	259
Pulakī - Kadambaḥ (Raj. ni.)	पुलकी – कदम्बः (रा. नि.)	453
Pulaṅgaḥ - Matsyaviśeṣaḥ	पुलङ्गः – मत्स्यविशेषः	627
Pumān - Puruṣaḥ	पुमान् – पुरुषः	615
Pumstvam - Śukram	पुंस्त्वम् – शुक्रम्	619
Punarnavā (p.106)	पुनर्नवा (p.106)	
Punḍarīkaḥ - Damanaḥ	पुण्डरीकः – दमनः	228
Punḍarīkaḥ - Vyāghraḥ	पुण्डरीकः – व्याघ्रः	623
Punḍarīkam (p.369)	पुण्डरीकम् (p.369)	
Punḍarīyakam-Prapaunḍarīkam	पुण्डरीयकम् –प्रपौण्डरीकम्	243
Punḍaryam-Prapaunḍarīkam	पुण्डर्यम् – प्रपौण्डरीकम्	243
Punḍraḥ - Ikśuḥ (Raj. ni.)	पुण्ड्रः – इक्षुः (रा.नि.)	358
Punḍraḥ - Tilakaḥ	पुण्ड्रः – तिलकः	513
Puraḥ - Gugguluḥ	पुरः – गुग्गुलुः	252
Pūrakaḥ - Bījapūraḥ	पूरकः– बीजपूरः	396
Puram - Śarīram	पुरम् – शरीरम्	615
Purāṇaghṛtam	पुराणघृतम्	576
Purīṣam - Malam	पुरीषम् – मलम्	640
Pūrṇakaḥ - Tilakaḥ	पूर्णकः – तिलकः	513
Puruṣaḥ - Moraṭaḥ	पुरुषः – मोरटः	6
Puruṣaḥ (p. 614)	पुरुषः (p. 614)	
Puṣkarādyaparṇikā - Padmacāriṇī (Raj. ni.)	पुष्कराद्यपर्णिका –पद्मचारिणी (रा.नि.)	325
Puṣkarāhvayam - Puṣkaramūlam	पुष्कराह्वयम् – पुष्करमूलम्	23
Puṣkarajaṭā - Puṣkaramūlam	पुष्करजटा – पुष्करमूलम्	23
Puṣkaram - Raktapadmam	पुष्करम् – रक्तपद्मम्	372
Puṣkariṇī-Padmacārinī (Raj. ni.)	पुष्करिणी – पद्मचारिणी (रा. नि.)	325

Puṣkaramūlam (p.23)	पुष्करमूलम् (p.23)	
Puṣpagandhā - Yūthikā	पुष्पगन्धा - यूथिका	504
Puṣpaketuḥ - Puṣpañjanam	पुष्पकेतुः - पुष्पाञ्जनम्	266
Puṣpalolupaḥ - Bhramaraḥ	पुष्पलोलुपः - भ्रमरः	633
Puṣpāñjanam (p. 265)	पुष्पाञ्जनम् (p. 265)	
Puṣparasāgaram - Śvāsāriḥ	पुष्परसागरम् - श्वासारिः	25
Puṣparasam - Madhu	पुष्परसम् - मधु	592
Puṣpāsavam - Madhu	पुष्पासवम् - मधु	592
Puṣpī - Arkaḥ	पुष्पी - अर्कः	282
Puṭā - Bhadrailā	पुटा -भद्रैला	142
Pūtadhānyaḥ - Tilaḥ	पूतधान्यः - तिलः	568
Pūtadruḥ - Kimśukaḥ	पूतद्रुः - किंशुकः	518
Puṭakinī - Padminī	पुटकिनी - पद्मिनी	374
Puṭam - Jātīphalam	पुटम् - जातीफलम्	211
Puṭam - Vyāghranakham	पुटम् - व्याघ्रनखम्	223
Pūtanā - Harītakī	पूतना - हरीतकी	77
Pūtanā- Gandhamāmsī	पूतना - गन्धमांसी	217
Pūtikaḥ - Gandhamārjaraḥ	पूतिकः -गन्धमार्जारः	631
Pūtibhṛṅgaḥ - Bhramaraḥ	पूतिभृङ्गः - भ्रमरः	634
Pūtidrumaḥ - Saralaḥ	पूतिद्रुमः - सरलः	237
Pūtigandhaḥ - Gandhakaḥ	पूतिगन्धः - गन्धकः	248
Pūtikaḥ - Karañjaḥ	पूतिकः - करञ्जः	455
Pūtikam - Malam	पूतिकम् - मलम्	640
Pūtikarṇī - Bākucī	पूतिकर्णी - बाकुची	61
Pūtikāṣṭham - Devadāruḥ	पूतिकाष्ठम् - देवदारुः	27
Pūtikāṣṭham - Saralaḥ	पूतिकाष्ठम् - सरलः	237
Pūtikeśaraḥ - Gandhamārjāraḥ	पूतिकेशरः - गन्धमार्जारः	631
Pūtimārutaḥ - Bilvaḥ	पूतिमारुतः - बिल्वः	39
Pūtimayūrikā - Ajagandhā	पूतिमयूरिका - अजगन्धा	184
Pūtimedaḥ - Irimedaḥ	पूतिमेदः - इरिमेदः	489
Pūtiphalā - Bākucī	पूतिफला - बाकुची	61
Pūtipūrakaḥ - Atasī	पूतिपूरकः - अतसी	565
Pūtirasā - Rāsnā	पूतिरसा - रास्ना	104
Putraśreṇī - Dravantī	पुत्रश्रेणी - द्रवन्ती	87
Rāgī - Aśokaḥ	रागी - अशोकः	516
Rhasvagavedhukā - Gāngerukī	ऱ्हस्वगवेधुका - गांगेरुकी	112
Rhasvaphalā - Jambūḥ (Raj. ni.)	ऱ्हस्वफला - जम्बूः (रा. नि.)	434
Raivatakam - Pālevatam	रैवतकम् - पालेवतम्	417
Rājamaṇḍūkaḥ-Maṇḍuka viśeṣaḥ	राजमण्डूकः - मण्डूकविशेषः	640
Rajā -Rajāvartaḥ	राजा - राजावर्तः	533
Rājādanaḥ (p. 439)	राजादनः (p. 439)	
Rājadriḥ - Rājāvartaḥ	राजाद्रिः- राजावर्तः	533

Rajaḥ - Parpaṭaḥ	रजः - पर्पटः	17
Rājahamsaḥ - Hamsaḥ	राजहंसः - हंसः	635
Rājajambūḥ - Jambūḥ	राजजम्बूः - जम्बूः	433
Rājakolaḥ-Badaram (Raj. ni.)	राजकोलः - बदरम् (रा. नि.)	446
Rājakśavakaḥ (p. 298)	राजक्षवकः (p. 298)	
Rājamāṣaḥ (p. 542)	राजमाषः (p. 542)	
Rājāmraḥ (p. 388)	राजाम्रः (p. 388)	
Rajanī - Haridrā	रजनी - हरिद्रा	20
Rājanyaḥ - Rājādanaḥ	राजन्यः - राजादनः	439
Rājaprastaraḥ -Rājāvartaḥ	राजप्रस्तरः - राजावर्तः	533
Rājārkaḥ (p. 282)	राजार्कः (p. 282)	
Rājasarṣapaḥ - Rajakśavakaḥ	राजसर्षपः - राजक्षवकः	299
Rajasvalaḥ - Mahiṣaḥ	रजस्वलः - महिषः	625
Rājaswarṇaḥ-Dhattūraḥ (Raj. ni.)	राजस्वर्णः - धत्तूरः (रा. नि.)	279
Rajatam - Raupyam	रजतम् - रौप्यम्	524
Rājataraṇī - Taruṇī (Raj. ni.)	राजतरणी - तरुणी (रा. नि.)	501
Rājāvartaḥ (p. 533)	राजावर्तः (p. 533)	
Rājabalā - Prasāraṇī	राजबला - प्रसारणी	114
Rājadhānyam - Śyamākaḥ	राजधान्यम् - श्यामाकः	545
Rājadhattūraḥ-Dhattūraḥ (Raj. ni.)	राजधत्तूरः - धत्तूरः (रा. नि.)	279
Rājī - Āsurī	राजी - आसुरी	306
Rājifalguḥ - Kākodumbarikā	राजिफल्गुः - काकोदुम्बरिका	437
Rājikā - Āsurī	राजिका - आसुरी	306
Rājikā - Rājakśavakaḥ	राजिका - राजक्षवकः	299
Rājīkāphalaḥ - Sarṣapaḥ	राजिकाफलः - सर्षपः	297
Rājilaḥ - Jalasarpaḥ	राजिलः - जलसर्पः	639
Rājīphalaḥ - Paṭolaḥ	राजीफलः - पटोलः	18
Rājīvaḥ - Matsyabhedaḥ	राजीवः - मत्स्यभेदः	628
Rājīvam - Raktapadmam	राजीवम् - रक्तपद्मम्	372
Rājakaserukaḥ - Mustā	राजकसेरुकः - मुस्ता	15
Rājakośātakī - Dhāmārgavaḥ	राजकोशातकी -धामार्गवः	70
Rājanāmā - Paṭolaḥ	राजनामा - पटोलः	18
Rājñī - Pittalam	राज्ञी - पित्तलम्	526
Rājaphalaḥ - Rājādanaḥ	राजफलः - राजादनः	439
Rājapīluḥ - Bṛhatpīluḥ	राजपीलुः - बृहत्पीलुः	410
Rājaputraḥ - Rājāmraḥ	राजपुत्रः - राजाम्रः	388
Rājaputrī - Jātī	राजपुत्री - जाती	496
Rājaputrī - Pittalam	राजपुत्री - पित्तलम्	526
Rājaputrī - Reṇukā	राजपुत्री -रेणुका	220
Rājarītiḥ - Pittalam	राजरीतिः - पित्तलम्	526
Rājaśukaḥ - Śukaḥ	राजशुकः - शुकः	634
Rājavṛkśaḥ - Karṇikāraḥ	राजवृक्षः - कर्णिकारः	81

Rāk'sasabhojanam - Māmsam राक्षसभोजनम् - मांसम् 618
Rak'soghnaḥ-Sarṣapaḥ(Raj. ni.) रक्षोघ्नः - सर्षपः (रा. नि.) 298
Raktā - Lāk'sā रक्ता - लाक्षा 239
Raktā - Māmsarohiṇī रक्ता - मांसरोहिणी 330
Raktā - Mañjiṣṭhā रक्ता -मञ्जिष्ठा 7
Raktā Āḍhakī - Āḍhakī रक्ताआढकी - आढकी 549
Raktabījaḥ - Dāḍimaḥ रक्तबीजः -दाडिमः 155
Raktacaṇḍakaḥ - Karavīraḥ रक्तचण्डकः - करवीरः 275
Raktacandanam (p.193) रक्तचन्दनम् (p. 193)
Raktacitraḥ-Citrakaḥ (Raj. ni.) रक्तचित्रः - चित्रकः (रा.नि.) 165
Raktacūrṇakaḥ - Kampillakaḥ रक्तचूर्णकः - कम्पिल्लकः 257
Raktadalā - Nalikā (Raj.ni.) रक्तदला - नलिका (रा.नि.) 216
Raktādhāraḥ - Twak रक्ताधारः - त्वक् 644
Raktadhātuḥ - Gairikam रक्तधातुः - गैरिकम् 262
Raktadhātukam - Tāmram रक्तधातुकम् - ताम्रम् 524
Raktadhātukartā - Rasaḥ रक्तधातुकर्ता - रसः 619
Raktagandhakam-Bolam(Raj. ni.) रक्तगन्धकम् - बोलम् (रा. नि.) 226
Raktaḥ- Ik'suḥ (Raj. ni.) रक्तः - इक्षुः (रा.नि.) 358
Raktaḥ - Sarṣapaḥ (Raj. ni.) रक्तः - सर्षपः (रा. नि.) 298
Raktaḥ - (Rakt.) Apāmārgaḥ रक्तः -(र.) अपामार्गः 101
Raktairaṇḍaḥ (p.117) रक्तैरण्डः (p.117)
Raktakaḥ - A'sokaḥ रक्तकः - अशोकः 516
Raktakaḥ - Śigruḥ रक्तकः - शिग्रुः 295
Raktakaḥ-Madhu'sigrukaḥ (Raj. ni.) रक्तकः -मधुशिग्रुकः (रा. नि.) 296
Raktakam - Tāmram रक्तकम् - ताम्रम् 524
Raktakam - Prācīnāmalakam रक्तकम् - प्राचीनामलकम् 80
Raktakāṇḍā - Krūraḥ (Raj.ni.) रक्तकाण्डा -क्रूरः (रा.नि.) 109
Raktakaravīraḥ-Karavīraḥ (Raj.ni.) रक्तकरवीरः-करवीरः (रा. नि.) 276
Raktakāṣṭham - Pataṅgam रक्तकाष्ठम् - पतङ्गम् 194
Raktam - Kumkumam रक्तम् - कुंकुमम् 197
Raktam - Pravālam रक्तम् - प्रवालम् 534
Raktam (p.619) रक्तम् (p.619)
Raktāmlānaḥ-Saireyakaḥ (Raj. ni.) रक्ताम्लानः - सैरेयकः (रा.नि.) 110
Raktamukhaḥ - Śukaḥ रक्तमुखः - शुकः 634
Raktamūlā-Raktapādī (Raj. ni.) रक्तमूला - रक्तपादी (रा. नि.) 344
Raktāṅgaḥ - Agnimanthaḥ रक्ताङ्गः -अग्निमंथः 40
Raktāṅgaḥ - Kampillakaḥ रक्ताङ्गः - कम्पिल्लकः 257
Raktāṅgī - Mañjiṣṭhā रक्ताङ्गी -मञ्जिष्ठा 7
Raktapādī (p. 344) रक्तपादी (p. 344)
Raktapadmam (p. 372) रक्तपद्मम् (p. 372)
Raktapālevatam - Pālevatam रक्तपालेवतम् - पालेवतम् 418
Raktapatrikaḥ-Krūraḥ (Raj.ni.) रक्तपत्रिकः -क्रूरः (रा.नि.) 109

Raktapatrikā-Nākulī (Raj. ni.)	रक्तपत्रिका - नाकुली (रा. नि.)	340
Raktaphalā - Bimbī	रक्तफला - बिम्बी	76
Raktaphalaḥ - Vaṭaḥ	रक्तफलः - वटः	426
Raktapitā - Rasaḥ	रक्तपिता - रसः	619
Raktapūrakam - Vṛkṣāmlam	रक्तपूरकम् - वृक्षाम्लम्	173
Raktapuṣpā - Śālmalī	रक्तपुष्पा - शाल्मली	481
Raktapuṣpaḥ - Kimśukaḥ	रक्तपुष्पः - किंशुकः	518
Raktapuṣpikā - Viṣṇukrāntā	रक्तपुष्पिका - विष्णुकान्ता	352
Raktarajaḥ - Swarṇa Gairikam	रक्तरजः - स्वर्णगैरिकम्	263
Raktareṇuḥ - Sindūraḥ	रक्तरेणुः - सिन्दूरः	246
Raktaśāliḥ - Śāliḥ	रक्तशालिः -शालिः	535
Raktasāraḥ - Khadiraḥ	रक्तसारः - खदिरः	9
Raktasāram - Raktacandanam	रक्तसारम् - रक्तचंदनम्	193
Raktasāramukhaḥ -Vrīhiḥ	रक्तसारमुखः - व्रीहिः	538
Raktasarṣapaḥ - Āsurī	रक्तसर्षपः - आसुरी	306
Raktasrāvī - Amlavetasaḥ	रक्तस्रावी - अम्लवेतसः	177
Raktavargaḥ	रक्तवर्गः	657
Raktayaṣṭī - Mañjiṣṭhā	रक्तयष्टी - मञ्जिष्ठा	7
Raktikā - Kākādanī	रक्तिका- काकादनी	290
Rālaḥ (p. 250)	रालः (p. 250)	
Rāmā - Strī	रामा - स्त्री	615
Rāmā vāmāṅghrighātakaḥ - Aśokaḥ (Raj. ni.)	रामावामाङ्घ्रिघातकः -अशोकः (रा.नि.)	516
Rāmam - Kuṣṭham	रामम् - कुष्ठम्	219
Rāmam - Tamālapatram	रामम् - तमालपत्रम्	146
Rāmaṇaḥ - Tindukaḥ	रामणः - तिन्दुकः	402
Rāmasenakaḥ - Kirātatiktakaḥ	रामसेनकः - किराततिक्तकः	14
Rāmaṭham - Hiṅgu	रामठम्- हिंगु	137
Rāmaṭhī -Nāḍīhiṅghu	रामठी - नाडीहिंगु	139
Rambhā - Kadalī	रम्भा - कदली	316
Rāmtaruṇī - Taruṇī	रामतरुणी - तरुणी -	501
Ramyā - Viśālā (Raj. ni.)	रम्या - विशाला (रा.नि.)	96
Ramyakaḥ - Mahānimbaḥ	रम्यकः - महानिम्बः	12
Raṇajit - Matsyaviśesaḥ	रणजित् - मत्स्यविशेषः	627
Raṇapriyam - Uśīram (Raj.ni.)	रणप्रियम - उशीरम् (रा.नि.)	198
Randhravamsaḥ-Vamśaḥ (Raj. ni.)	रन्ध्रवंश : - वंशः (रा.नि.)	365
Randhrī - Nalaḥ	रन्ध्री- नलः	366
Raṅgadāyakam - Kamkuṣṭham	रंगदायकम् - कंकुष्टम्	259
Raṅgam - Vaṅgam	रङ्गम - वङ्गम्	525
Raṅgamātā - Lākśā	रङ्गमाता - लाक्षा	239
Raṅgiṇī - Haridrā	रङ्गिणी - हरिद्रा	20
Rañjakam -Kānta Loham	रञ्जकम -कान्तलोहम	528

Rañjanaḥ - Kampillakaḥ	रञ्जनः - कम्पिल्लकः	257
Rañjanakaḥ-Kaṭphalaḥ (Raj. ni.)	रञ्जनकः - कट्फलः (रा.नि.)	27
Rañjanī - Nīlinī	रञ्जनी - नीलिनी	87
Rañjanī - Tāmbūlī	रञ्जनी - ताम्बूली	273
Rañjanī - Jantukārī	रञ्जनी - जन्तुकारी	324
Rañjikā - Vijayā	रञ्जिका - विजया	46
Rañjinī - Haridrā	रञ्जिनी - हरिद्रा	20
Rasā - Rāsnā	रसा - रास्ना	104
Rasā - Surā	रसा - सुरा	596
Rasā - Vācā	रसा- वाचा	616
Rāsabhaḥ - Gardabhaḥ	रासभः - गर्दभः	622
Rasāḍhyaḥ - Āmrātakaḥ	रसाढ्यः - आम्रातकः	388
Rasagarbham - Rasāñjanam	रसगर्भम् - रसाञ्जनम्	265
Rasāgryam - Rasāñjanam	रसाग्र्यम् - रसाञ्जनम्	265
Rasaḥ (p. 619)	रसः (p. 619)	
Rasajātam - Rasāñjanam	रसजातम् - रसाञ्जनम्	265
Rasālā - Drākṡā	रसाला - द्राक्षा	413
Rasālā - Marjikā	रसाला - मर्जिका	605
Rasālaḥ - Āmraḥ	रसालः - आम्रः	385
Rasālaḥ - Ikṡuḥ	रसालः - इक्षुः	357
Rasaloham - Pāradaḥ	रसलोहम् - पारदः	529
Rasam - Bolam	रसम् - बोलम्	226
Rasāmla - Amlavetasaḥ	रसाम्लः - अम्लवेतसः	177
Rasāmlam - Ṡuktam	रसाम्लम् - शुक्तम्	594
Rasanā - Rāsnā	रसना - रास्ना	104
Rasaniyāmikā-Jīvantī (Raj.ni.)	रसनियामिका - जीवन्ती (रा.नि.)	50
Rasāñjanam (p. 264)	रसाञ्जनम् (p. 264)	
Rasapākajaḥ - Guḍah	रसपाकजः - गुडः	358
Rasaphalaḥ - Nārikelaḥ	रसफलः - नारिकेलः	424
Rasapuṣpaḥ - Jaladaḥ	रसपुष्पः -जलदः	408
Rasasambhavam - Raktam	रससंभवम् - रक्तम्	619
Rasāsavaḥ	रसासवः	598,599
Rasāyanagaṇaḥ-Jīvanīyagaṇaḥ	रसायनगणः - जीवनीयगणः	650
Rasāyanasamāṡrayam-Dugdham	रसायनसमाश्रयम् - दुग्धम्	577
Rasāyanavarā - Kākamācī	रसायनवरा - काकमाची	285
Rasāyanī - Guḍūcī	रसायनी - गुडूची	2
Rasendraḥ - Pāradaḥ	रसेन्द्रः - पारदः	529
Rasikaḥ - Godhūmaḥ	रसिकः :- गोधूमः	551
Rasikaḥ - Nīvāraḥ	रसिकः - नीवारः	543
Raṡmijālam - Raupyam	रश्मिजालम् - रौप्यम्	524
Rāsnā (p.104)	रास्ना (p.104)	
Rasodbhavam - Rasāñjanam	रसोद्भवम् - रसाञ्जनम्	265

Rasonaḥ - Laśunaḥ	रसोनः - लशुनः	312
Rasottamaḥ - Mudgaḥ	रसोत्तमः -मुदगः	540
Rasottamaḥ - Pāradaḥ	रसोत्तमः- पारदः	529
Rāṣṭrikā -Bṛhatī	राष्ट्रिका - बृहती	35
Rasyā - Rāsnā	रस्या - रास्ना	104
Rasyam - Māmsam	रस्यम् - मांसम्	618
Rāṭhaḥ - Madanaḥ	राठः - मदनः	62
Rathāṅgam - Ṛddhiḥ	रथाङ्गम् -ऋद्धिः	53
Rathāṅganāmā - Cakravākaḥ	रथाङ्गनामा - चक्रवाकः	635
Rathī - Cakravākaḥ	रथी - चकवाकः	635
Rathikaḥ - Cakravākaḥ	रथिकः - चक्रवाकः	635
Ratnam - Hīrakam	रत्नम् - हीरकम्	532
Rātrijāgaraḥ - Sārameyaḥ	रात्रिजागरः - सारमेयः	632
Rauhiṇeyam - Gārutmatam	रौहिणेयम् - गारुत्मतम्	531
Raupyam (p. 523)	रौप्यम् (p. 523)	
Ravaḥ - Tindukaḥ	रवः - तिन्दुकः	402
Ravipriyaḥ-Karavīraḥ (Raj. ni.)	रविप्रियः - करवीरः (रा. नि.)	276
Raviḥ - Arkaḥ	रविः - अर्कः	282
Ṛddhiḥ (p.53)	ऋद्धिः (p.53)	
Recakaḥ- Jayapālaḥ	रेचकः - जयपालः	86
Recakam - Kamkuṣṭham	रेचकम् - कंकुष्ठम्	259
Recanaḥ - Āragvadhaḥ	रेचनः - आरग्वधः	80
Recanakaḥ - Kampillakaḥ	रेचनकः - कम्पिल्लकः	257
Recī - Kampillakaḥ	रेची - कम्पिल्लकः	257
Recī - Tilakaḥ	रेची - तिलकः	513
Recī. - Aṅkoṭakaḥ	रेची - अङ्कोटकः	99
Reṇubhūṣitaḥ - Gardabhaḥ	रेणूभूषितः - गर्दभः	622
Reṇuḥ - Parpaṭaḥ	रेणुः - पर्पटः	17
Reṇukā (Hareṇuḥ) (p.220)	रेणुका (हरेणुः) (p.220)	
Reṇukadambaḥ-Kadambaḥ (Raj. ni.)	रेणुकदम्बः-कदम्बः (रा. नि.)	452
Retaḥ - Śukram	रेतः - शुक्रम्	619
Rhāsam - Kamkuṣṭham	ऱ्हासम् - कंकुष्ठम्	259
Rhasvā - Mudgaparṇī	ऱ्हस्वा -मुदगपर्णी	49
Rhasvā - Viṣṇukrāntā	ऱ्हस्वा - विष्णुकान्ता	352
Rhasvāṅgaḥ - Jīvakaḥ	ऱ्हस्वाङ्गः - जीवकः	44
Rhasvapatrikā - Aśvatthī	ऱ्हस्वपत्रिका - अश्वत्थी	428
Rhasvaplakṣaḥ - Plakṣaḥ	ऱ्हस्वप्लक्षः - प्लक्षः	429
Rhasvapuṣpaḥ - Jaladaḥ	ऱ्हस्वपुष्पः -जलदः	408
Rhīveram - Vālakam	ऱ्हीवेरम् -वालकम्	17
Riṅgaṇī - Mudgaparṇī	रिङ्गणी - मुद्गपर्णी	49
Ripuḥ - Corakaḥ	रिपुः - चोरकः	232
Rītiḥ - Pittalam	रीतिः - पित्तलम्	526

Rītijam - Puṣpāñjanam	रीतिजम् - पुष्पाञ्जनम्	266
Rītikā - Pittalam	रीतिका - पित्तलम्	526
Rītikusumam - Puṣpāñjanam	रीतिकुसुमम् - पुष्पाञ्जनम्	266
Rītipuṣpam - Puṣpāñjanam	रीतिपुष्पम् - पुष्पाञ्जनम्	266
Ṛjuḥ - Māḍaḥ	ऋजुः - माडः	422
Rocanā (p.203)	रोचना (p.203)	
Rocanaḥ - Rohitakaḥ	रोचनः - रोहितकः	485
Rocanaḥ - Jambīraḥ	रोचनः - जम्बीरः	389
Rodhraḥ - Lodhraḥ	रोध्रः - लोध्रः	267
Rogaḥ - Kuṣṭham	रोगः - कुष्ठम्	219
Rogī	रोगी	660
Rohī - Karañjaḥ	रोही - करञ्जः	461
Rohī - Rohitakaḥ	रोही - रोहितकः	485
Rohiṇī - Harītakī	रोहिणी - हरीतकी	77
Rohiṇī - Kaṭukā	रोहिणी -कटुका	15
Rohiṣaḥ - Bhūstṛṇaḥ	रोहिषः - भूस्तृणः	300
Rohiṣakam-Kattṛṇam (Raj. ni.)	रोहिषकम् - कत्तृणम् (रा.नि)	28
Rohiṣam - Kattṛṇam	रोहिषम् - कत्तृणम्	28
Rohitaḥ - Matsyabhedaḥ	रोहितः - मत्स्यभेदः	628
Rohitaḥ - Matsyaviśeṣaḥ	रोहितः - मत्स्य विशेषः	628
Rohitaḥ - Matsayaḥ	रोहितः - मत्स्यः	626
Rohitaḥ - Matsyaviśeṣaḥ	रोहितः - मत्स्यविशेषः	627
Rohītakaḥ - Rohitakaḥ	रोहीतकः - रोहितकः	484
Rohitakaḥ (p. 485)	रोहितकः (p. 85)	
Roma (p. 644)	रोम (p. 644)	
Romabhūmiḥ - Twak	रोमभूमिः - त्वक्	644
Romakam - Audbhidam	रोमकम् - औद्भिदम्	136
Romakāntam -Kāntaloham	रोमकान्तम् -कान्तलोहम्	528
Romaphalam - Bhavam	रोमफलम् - भवम्	401
Romaśaḥ - Aviḥ	रोमशः - अविः	623
Romaśaḥ - Sūkaraḥ	रोमशः - सूकरः	624
Ṛṣabhaḥ (Vṛṣabhaḥ) (p.45)	ऋषभः (वृषभः) (p.45)	
Ṛṣiḥ - Damaḥ	ऋषिः - दमः	229
Ṛṣiputrakaḥ - Damanaḥ	ऋषिपुत्रकः - दमनः	228
Ṛṣisṛṣṭā - Ṛddhiḥ	ऋषिसृष्टा -ऋद्धिः	53
Ṛṣyagandhā - Atibalā	ऋष्यगन्धा - अतिबला	113
Ṛṣyaproktā - Atibalā	ऋष्यप्रोक्ता - अतिबला	113
Ṛṣyaproktā - Śatāvarī	ऋष्यप्रोक्ता - शतावरी	115
Rubuḥ - Raktairaṇḍaḥ	रुबुः - रक्तैरण्डः	117
Rubukaḥ - Raktairaṇḍaḥ	रुबुकः - रक्तैरण्डः	117
Rucakaḥ - Bījapuraḥ	रुचकः - बीजपूरः	396
Rucakam - Sauvarcalam	रुचकम् - सौवर्चलम्	136

Ruchiḥ - Rocanā	रुचिः - रोचना	203
Rucirā - Rocanā	रुचिरा - रोचना	203
Ruciram - Raupyam	रुचिरम् - रौप्यम्	524
Rucirañjanaḥ-Śigruḥ (Raj. ni.)	रुचिरञ्जनः - शिग्रुः (रा. नि.)	296
Rucişyam - Mūlakam	रुचिष्यम् -मूलकम्	293
Rucyam - Jīrakam	रुच्यम् - जीरकम्	157
Rucyam - Trapusam (Raj. ni.)	रुच्यम् - त्रपुसम् (रा.नि.)	65
Rudhiram - Kumkumam	रुधिरम् - कुंकुमम्	197
Rudhiram - Raktam	रुधिरम् - रक्तम्	619
Rudrapatnī - Atasī	रुद्रपत्नी - अतसी	565
Rudraretaḥ - Pāradaḥ	रुद्ररेतः - पारदः	529
Ruhā - Dūrvā	रुहा - दूर्वा	368
Ruhā - Māmsarohiṇī	रुहा - मांसरोहिणी	330
Rujā - Kuṣṭham	रुजा - कुष्ठम्	219
Rukmam - Suvarṇam	रुक्मम् - सुवर्णम्	523
Ruruḥ - Hariṇaḥ	रुरुः - हरिणः	625
Sabalam - Śāliparṇī viśeṣaḥ	सबलम् - शालिपर्णी विशेषः	32
Śābaraḥ - Śāliḥ	शाबरः -शालिः	535
Śābarakaḥ - Lodhraḥ	शाबरकः - लोध्रः	267
Śabarakandaḥ-Vārāhī (Raj. ni.)	शबरकन्दः - वाराही (रा.नि.)	327
Śabarapādapaḥ - Lodhraḥ	शबरपादपः - लोध्रः	268
Sacivaḥ - Dhattūraḥ	सचिवः - धत्तूरः (रा.नि.)	279
Sadāgatiḥ - Vāyuḥ	सदागतिः - वायुः	616
Sadāmāmsī-Māmsarohiṇī (Raj. ni.)	सदामांसी - मांसरोहिणी (रा.नि.)	330
Ṣaḍaṅgaḥ - Gokṣuraḥ	षडङ्गः - गोक्षुरः	38
Sadāphalaḥ - Udumbaraḥ	सदाफलः - उदुम्बरः	436
Sadāpuṣpaḥ - Kundaḥ	सदापुष्पः - कुन्दः	506
Sadāpuṣpī - Rājārkaḥ	सदापुष्पी - राजार्कः	282
Ṣaḍgranthā - Śaṭhī	षड्ग्रन्था - शठी	22
Ṣaḍgranthā-Śvetavacā (Dhn.ni.)	षड्ग्रन्था - श्वेतवचा (ध.नि.)	125,126
Ṣaḍgranthaḥ - Karañjaḥ	षड्ग्रन्थः - करञ्जः	461
Sādhāraṇarasāḥ	साधारणरसाः	662
Sādhugandhikaḥ - Damaḥ	साधुगन्धिकः - दमः	229
Sādhuḥ - Damaḥ	साधुः - दमः	229
Sadratnam - Hīrakam	सद्रत्नम - हीरकम्	531
Ṣaḍrasāḥ	षड्रसाः	659
Ṣaḍrasaḥ - Rasaḥ	षड्रसः - रसः	619
Śādvalam - Dūrvā	शाद्वलम् - दूर्वा	368
Sadyomaṇḍalapatrakaḥ-Krūraḥ	सद्योमण्डलपत्रकः -क्रूरः	108
Sāgaḥ (Śākaḥ) (p. 521)	सागः (शाकः) (p. 521)	
Sāgarajam malam-Samudraphenam	सागरजंमलम् - समुद्रफेनम्	263
Sāgarajam - Sāmudram	सागरजम - सामुद्रम्	136

Sahā - Taruṇī	सहा - तरुणी	501
Sahācaraḥ -Saireyakaḥ	सहचरः - सैरेयकः	109
Sahacaraḥ -Saireyakaḥ	सहाचरः - सैरेयकः	109
Sahadevā - Mahābalā	सहदेवा - महाबला	111
Sahaḥ - Nakham	सहः - नखम्	223
Sahakāraḥ - Āmraḥ	सहकारः - आम्रः	385
Sahasrāmśī - Pīluḥ	सहस्रांशी - पीलुः	409
Sahasravedhī -Hingu (Raj. ni.)	सहस्त्रवेधी - हिंगु (रा.नि.)	137
Sahasravedhī-Vṛkśāmlam (Raj. ni.)	सहस्रवेधी - वृक्षाम्लम् (रा. नि.)	177
Sahasravīryā - Dūrvā	सहस्त्रवीर्या - दूर्वा	368
Sahasravīryā - Mahāśatāvarī (p.116)	सहस्त्रवीर्या - महाशतावरी (p.116)	
Śaikharikaḥ - Apāmārgaḥ	शैखरिकः -अपामार्गः	100
Śailajāmūlam - a type of Śreyasī (Raj.ni.)	शैलजामूलम् -श्रेयसी विशेषः (रा.नि.)	163
Śaileyam - Śilājatuḥ	शैलेयम् - शिलाजतुः	266
Śaileyam (p.234)	शैलेयम् (p.234)	
Śailūṣaḥ - Bilvaḥ	शैलूषः - बिल्वः	39
Saimhalakam - Pittalam	सैंहलकम्- पित्तलम्	526
Saimhalam - Twak	सैंहलम् -त्वक्	145
Saimhalī - (a type of)Śreyasī (Raj. ni.)	सैंहली - श्रेयसी विशेषः (रा.नि.)	163
Saindhavam (p.134)	सैन्धवम् (p.134)	
Saireyaḥ -Saireyakaḥ	सैरेयः - सैरेयकः	109
Saireyakaḥ (p.109)	सैरेयकः (p.109)	
Śaivālam - Jalamustam	शैवालं - जलमुस्तम्	16
Śākaḥ - Sāgaḥ	शाकः - सागः	522
Śakalaḥ - Matsyaviśeṣaḥ	शकलः - मत्स्यविशेषः	627
Sakalam - Asthi	सकलम् - अस्थि	618
Śakalam - Padmamūlam	सकलम् - पद्ममूलम्	377
Śakalam - Twak	शकलम् -त्वक्	145
Sakalam - Kattṛaṇam	सकलम् - कत्तृणम्	28
Śākāmlam - Vṛkśāmlam	शाकाम्लम् - वृक्षाम्लम्	173
Śākāngam - Maricam (Raj. ni.)	शाकाङ्गम् - मरिचम् (रा. नि.)	168
Śākapuṣpaḥ - Karīraḥ	शाकपुष्पः - करीरः	448
Śākaśreṣṭhā - Jīvantī	शाकश्रेष्टा - जीवन्ती	49
Śakaṭākśaḥ - Dhavaḥ	शकटाक्षः - धवः	522
Śakaṭam - Śarīram	शकटम् - शरीरम्	615
Śākhākāṇḍāḥ - Snuhī	शाखाकाण्डाः - स्नुही	88
Śākhāmṛgaḥ - Markaṭaḥ	शाखामृगः - मर्कटः	632
Śākhī - Pīluḥ	शाखी - पीलुः	409
Śakrāhvāḥ - Indrayavāḥ	शक्राह्वाः - इन्द्रयवाः	131
Śakramātā - Bhārngī	शक्रमाता - भार्ङ्गी	24

Sakṡīraṡuklakaḥ - Rājādanaḥ	सक्षीरशुक्लकः -राजादनः	439
Ṡakulādanī - Jalapippalī	शकुलादनी - जलपिप्पली	310
Ṡakulādanī - Kaṭukā	शकुलादनी - कटुका	15
Ṡakulākṡikā - Dūrvā	शकुलाक्षिका - दूर्वा	368
Ṡakulī - Matsyabhedaḥ	शकुली - मत्स्यभेदः	628
Ṡākuneyaḥ - Kṡudrolūkaḥ	शाकुनेयः - क्षुद्रोलूकः	638
Ṡakunī - Matsyaḥ	शकुनी - मत्स्यः	*626*
Ṡālaḥ - Rālaḥ	शालः - रालः	250
Ṡālaḥ - Sarjakaḥ	शालः - सर्जकः	476
Ṡālāmarkaṭakam-Cāṇākhyamūlakam	शालामर्कटकम् –चाणाख्यमूलकम	293
Ṡālaniryāsaḥ - Rālaḥ	शालनिर्यासः - रालः	250
Ṡalāṭuḥ - Bilvaḥ	शलाटुः - बिल्वः	39
Salavaṇam - Vangam	सलवणम् - वङ्गम्	525
Ṡālāvṛkaḥ - Biḍālaḥ	शालावृकः - बिडालः	631
Ṡālāvṛkaḥ - Sṛgālaḥ	शालावृकः - श्रृगालः	632
Ṡāleyaḥ - Miṡreyā	शालेयः - मिश्रेया	122
Ṡāleyam - Cāṇākhyamūlakam	शालेयम् - चाणाख्यमूलकम्	293
Ṡāliḥ (p. 534)	शालिः (p. 534)	
Ṡālihotraḥ - Aṡvaḥ	शालिहोत्रः - अश्वः	621
Salilam - Jalam	सलिलम् - जलम्	605
Ṡālīnaḥ - Miṡreyā	शालीनः - मिश्रेया	122
Ṡālīnam - Padmamūlam	शालीनम् - पद्ममूलम्	377
Ṡāliparṇī (p.32)	शालिपर्णी (p.32)	
Ṡāliparṇī viṡeṣaḥ (p.32)	शालिपर्णी विशेषः (p.32)	
Ṡailuḥ - Ṡleṣmātakaḥ	शैलुः - श्लेष्मातकः	441
Ṡallakī (p. 256)	शल्लकी (p. 256)	
Ṡālmalaḥ - Ṡālmaliveṣṭakaḥ	शाल्मलः -शाल्मलीवेष्टकः	481
Ṡālmalī (p. 481)	शाल्मली (p. 481)	
Ṡālmalikaḥ - Rohitakaḥ	शाल्मलिकः - रोहितकः	485
Ṡālmalipatrakaḥ - Saptaparṇaḥ	शाल्मलिपत्रकः - सप्तपर्णः	238
Ṡālmaliveṣṭakaḥ (p.481)	शाल्मलीवेष्टकः (p.481)	
Ṡālukaḥ (p. 304)	शालुकः (p. 304)	
Ṡalūkam - Jātīphalam	शालूकम् - जातीफलम्	211
Ṡalūkam - Padmamūlam	शालूकम् - पद्ममूलम्	377
Ṡalyaḥ - Matsyabhedaḥ	शल्यः - मत्स्यभेदः	628
Ṡalyakaḥ - Madanaḥ	शल्यकः - मदनः	62
Ṡalyaparṇī - Medā	शल्यपर्णी - मेदा	46
Ṡālyodanopamaḥ - Kundaḥ	शाल्योदनोपमः - कुन्दः	506
Samagandhikam - Uṡīram	समगन्धिकम - उशीरम	198

Samakṛt - Śleṣmā समकृत् - श्लेष्मा 617
Samaṅgā - Raktapādī समङ्गा - रक्तपादी 344
Samaṅgā - Balā समङ्गा - बला 110
Samangā - Mañjiṣṭhā समङ्गा -मञ्जिष्ठा 7
Samantadugdhā - Snuhī समन्तदुग्धा - स्नुही 88
Smarādhivāsaḥ-Aśokaḥ (Raj. ni.) स्मराधिवासः - अशोकः (रा.नि.) 516
Śambarī - Dravantī शम्बरी - द्रवन्ती 86
Sambhāraḥ सम्भारः 651
Śambhuvallabham- Puṇḍarīkam शम्भुवल्लभम् -पुण्डरीकम् 370
Sandamśakaḥ - Karkaṭaḥ संदंशकः - कर्कटः 640
Sandhānam - Asthi संधानम् - अस्थि 618
Samharṣā - Jantukārī संहर्षा - जन्तुकारी 324
Śamī (p. 442) शमी (p. 442)
Samidvaraḥ - Kimśukaḥ समिद्वरः - किंशुकः 518
Śamīpatrā - Raktapādī शमीपत्रा - रक्तपादी 344
Samīraṇaḥ - Vāyuḥ समीरणः - वायुः 616
Saṅkaraḥ - Mohaḥ संकरः - मोहः 617
Sāmlā - Amlikā साम्ला - अम्लिका 398
Śampākaḥ - Karṇikāraḥ शम्पाकः - कर्णिकारः 81
Sāmrāṇijam-Pālevatam (Raj. ni.) साम्राणिजम् - पालेवतम् (रा.नि.) 418
Sāmudrajam - Pravālam सामुद्रजम् - प्रवालम् 534
Samudrakāntā -Spṛkkā (Raj. ni.) समुद्रकान्ता - स्पृक्का (रा.नि.) 224
Sāmudram (p. 136) सामुद्रम् (p. 136)
Samudrāntaḥ - Yāsaḥ समुद्रान्तः - यासः 8
Samudraphenam (p. 263) समुद्रफेनम् (p. 263)
Samudrajam - Sāmudram समुद्रजम् - सामुद्रम् 136
Samūlam - Śvāsāriḥ समूलम् - श्वासारिः 25
Samvartakaḥ - Bibhītakaḥ संवर्तकः - बिभीतकः 78
Śaṇaghaṇṭikā - Śaṇapuṣpī शणघण्टिका - शणपुष्पी 75
Śaṇapuṣpī (p. 75) शणपुष्पी (p. 75)
Sancāriṇī-Viśvagranthiḥ (Raj.ni.) संचारिणी - विश्वग्रंथिः (रा.नि.) 347
Sandhyāpuṣpā - Jātī (Raj.ni.) सन्ध्यापुष्पा - जाती (रा. नि.) 497
Śāṇḍilyaḥ - Bilvaḥ शाण्डिल्यः - बिल्वः 39
Sāndram - Mathita dadhi सान्द्रं - मथित दधि 583
Śaṅkarādiḥ - Śuklārkaḥ शङ्करादिः - शुक्लार्कः 283
Śaṅkarī - Śamī शङ्करी - शमी 442
Śaṅkhadhavalā - Yūthikā शङ्खधवला - यूथिका 504
Śaṅkhadrāvī - Madhu Jambīraḥ शंखद्रावी - मधुजम्बीरः 390
Śaṅkhaḥ - Nakham शङ्खः - नखम् 223

Śaṅkhaḥ (p. 271) शंखः (p. 271)

Śaṅkhāhvā - Śaṅkhapuṣpī शङ्खाह्वा - शंखपुष्पी 349

Śaṅkhakusumā - Śaṅkhapuṣpī शङ्खकुसुमा - शंखपुष्पी

Śaṅkhamāṃsādidrāvī - Vṛkṣāmlam (Raj. ni.) शंखमांसादिद्रावी -वृक्षाम्लम् (रा. नि.) 177

Śaṅkhapuṣpī (p. 349) शङ्खपुष्पी (p. 349)

Śaṅkhapuṣpikā - Viṣṇukrāntā शङ्खपुष्पिका -विष्णुक्रान्ता 352

Śaṅkhayūthikā - Yūthikā शङ्खयूथिका - यूथिका 504

Śaṅkhinī - Yavatiktā शङ्खिनी - यवतिक्ता 98

Śaṅkhinīphalaḥ - Śirīṣaḥ शंखिनीफलः-शिरीषः 463

Śaṅkitaḥ - Corakaḥ शंकितः - चोरकः 232

Saṅkocam - Kumkumam संकोचम् - कुंकुमम् 197

Śaṅkukarṇaḥ - Gardabhaḥ शङ्कुकर्णः - गर्दभः 622

Śaṅkuphalā - Śamī शङ्कुफला - शमी 442

Sannipātaḥ - Mohaḥ संनिपातः - मोहः 617

Sannipātahā - Kirātatiktaḥ संनिपातहा - किराततिक्तः 14

Sannyāsaḥ - Mohaḥ संन्यासः - मोहः 617

Śāntā - Reṇukā (Raj. ni.) शान्ता -रेणुका (रा.नि.) 220

Śāntā - Śamī (Raj. ni.) शान्ता - शमी (रा. नि.) 443

Śāntaḥ - Damaḥ शान्तः - दमः 229

Santarpaṇam संतर्पणम् 654

Sānujaḥ -Tumbaruḥ सानुजः - तुम्बरुः 140

Sānujam - Prapauṇḍarīkam सानुजम् - प्रपौण्डरीकम् 243

Śaphaḥ - Nakham शफः - नखम् 223

Śapharī - Matsyaviśeṣaḥ शफरी - मत्स्य विशेषः 628

Śāpitah - Śleṣmātakaḥ शापितः- श्लेष्मातकः 441

Saptacchadaḥ - Saptaparṇaḥ सप्तच्छदः - सप्तपर्णः 238

Saptadhātavaḥ सप्तधातवः 661

Saptadhātujam - Śukram सप्तधातुजम् - शुक्रम् 619

Saptalā - Graiṣmī (Raj. ni.) सप्तला - ग्रैष्मी (रा. नि.) 499

Saptalā - Sātalā सप्तला - सातला 89

Saptaparṇaḥ(p. 238) सप्तपर्णः (p. 238)

Saptaparṇī -Raktapādī (Raj. ni.) सप्तपर्णी - रक्तपादी (रा. नि.) 344

Saptiḥ - Aśvaḥ सप्तिः - अश्वः 621

Śarabhaḥ (p. 623) शरभः (p. 623)

Śāradā - Sārivā शारदा - सारिवा 59

Śāradaḥ - Mudgaḥ शारदः -मुद्गः 540

Śāradam - Puṇḍarīkam शारदम् -पुण्डरीकम् 370

Śāradī - Brāhmī (Raj. ni.) शारदी - ब्राह्मी (रा.नि.) 337

Śāradī - Jalapippalī	शारदी - जलपिप्पली	31
Śāradikaḥ - Bakulaḥ (Raj. ni.)	शारदिकः - बकुलः(रा. नि.)	511
Śaradpadmam - Puṇḍarīkam	शरद्पद्मम् -पुण्डरीकम्	370
Sāragham - Madhu	सारघम् - मधु	592
Śaraḥ (p. 363)	शरः (p. 363)	
Sārakaḥ - Jayapālaḥ	सारकः - जयपालः	86
Śārkara sīdhuḥ	शार्करसीधुः	600
Saralā - Śuklabhaṇḍī	सरला - शुक्लभण्डी	94
Saralaḥ (p. 237)	सरलः (p. 237)	
Saram - Mārdwīkam	सरम् - मार्द्वीकम्	599
Sārameyaḥ (p. 632)	सारमेयः (p. 632)	
Sāraṅgaḥ - Hariṇaḥ	सारङ्गः - हरिणः	625
Saraṇī - Prasāraṇī	सरणी - प्रसारणी	114
Sāraṇī - Prasāraṇī	सारणी - प्रसारणी	114
Śarapatraḥ - Kuśaḥ	शरपत्रः - कुशः	361
Sarasvatī - Brāhmī (Raj. ni.)	सरस्वती - ब्राह्मी (रा.नि.)	336
Sarasvatī - Suvarcalā (Raj. ni.)	सरस्वती - सुवर्चला (रा.नि.	333
Saraswatī - Vācā	सरस्वती - वाचा	616
Śārdūlaḥ - Vyāghraḥ	शार्दूलः - व्याघ्रः	623
Sārī - Sātalā	सारी - सातला	89
Sārikā (p. 634)	सारिका (p. 634)	
Śarīram (p. 615)	शरीरम् (p. 615)	
Śarīrāvaraṇam - Twak	शरीरावरणम् - त्वक्	644
Sarīsṛpaḥ - Sarpaḥ	सरीसृपः - सर्पः	638
Sāritam - Añjanam	सारितम् - अञ्जनम्	262
Sārivā (p.59)	सारिवा (p.59)	
Sarjakaḥ (p. 476)	सर्जकः (p. 476)	
Sarjarasaḥ - Rālah	सर्जरसः - रालः	250
Śarkarā (p. 188)	शर्करा (p. 188)	
Śārkaraḥ Mādhavaśca	शार्करः माधवश्च	601
Śarkarakaḥ - Madhu Jambīraḥ	शर्करकः - मधुजम्बीरः	390
Saroruhā - Padminī	सरोरुहा - पद्मिनी	375
Saroruham - Raktapadmam	सरोरुहम् - रक्तपद्मम्	372
Sarpadamanī-Vandhyakarkoṭakī	सर्पदमनी - वन्ध्यकर्कोटकी	68
Sarpadaṃṣṭrā - Ajaśṛṅgī	सर्पदंष्ट्रा -अजश्रृंगी	31
Sarpadaṇḍā -a type of Śreyasī (Raj. ni.)	सर्पदण्डा–श्रेयसी विशेषः रा.नि.)	163
Sarpādanī - Nākulī (Raj. ni.)	सर्पादनी - नाकुली (रा.नि.)	340
Sarpagandhā - Nākulī	सर्पगन्धा - नाकुली	339
Sarpaḥ (Aruṇaḥ) - Sarpaḥ	सर्पः (अरुणः) -सर्पः	639

Sarpaḥ (p. 638)	सर्पः (p. 638)	
Sarpākśī - Viṣṇukrāntā	सर्पाक्षी - विष्णुकान्ता	352
Sarpākśī - Gandhanākulī	सर्पाक्षी - गन्धनाकुली	342
Sarpasugandhā - Nākulī	सर्पसुगन्धा - नाकुली	339
Sarpiḥ - Ghṛtam	सर्पिः - घृतम्	574
Sarṣapaḥ (p. 297)	सर्षपः (p. 297)	
Sarṣapatailam	सर्षपतैलम्	571
Sarvabhūtapramardinī-Vandhyakarkoṭakī	- सर्वभूतप्रमर्दिनी-वन्ध्यकर्कोटकी	68
Sarvagranthikam-Pippalīmūlam	सर्वग्रन्थिकम् - पिप्पलीमूलम्	161
Sārvaguṇam - Audbhidam	सार्वगुणम् -औदभिदम्	136
Sarvajanapriyā - Ṛddhiḥ	सर्वजनप्रिया -ऋद्धिः	53
Sarvakśirī (p.91)	सर्वक्षीरी (p.91)	
Sarvamedaḥsamudbhavam-Asthi	सर्वमेदःसमुद्भवम् - अस्थि	618
Sarvānubhūtiḥ - Śuklabhaṇḍī	सर्वानुभूतिः - शुक्लभण्डी	94
Sarvānukāriṇī - (Pṛśni.) viśeṣaḥ	सर्वानुकारिणी -(पृश्नि.) विशेष :	33
Sarvasnehapradhanā - Vasā	सर्वस्नेहप्रधाना- वसा	619
Sarvatobhadrā - Kāśmarī	सर्वतोभद्रा - काश्मरी	42
Sarvatobhadraḥ - Nimbaḥ	सर्वतोभद्रः - निम्बः	12
Sarvauṣadhiḥ	सर्वौषधिः	652
Sasāram - Kāleyakam	ससारम् - कालेयकम्	207
Śaśī - Karpūraḥ	शशी -कर्पूरः	209
Śaśilekhā - Bākucī	शशिलेखा - बाकुची	61
Śaśivāṭikā - Punarnavā	शशिवाटिका - पुनर्नवा	107
Śaṣpam - Dūrvā	शष्पम् - दूर्वा	368
Ṣaṣṭikaḥ - Vrīhiḥ	षष्टिकः - व्रीहिः	538
Ṣaṣṭihāyanaḥ - Hasti	षष्टिहायनः - हस्ति	620
Ṣaṣṭitaṇḍulajodbhavā - Vamśarocanā (Type)	षष्टितण्डुलजोद्भवा-वंशरोचना (विशेषः)	50
Śastram - Loham	शस्त्रम् - लोहम्	528
Sasyamārī - Mahāmūṣakaḥ	सस्यमारी - महामूषकः	631
Sasyasamvarakaḥ - Sarjakaḥ	सस्यसंवरकः - सर्जकः	476
Śatadalā - Śatapatrī	शतदला - शतपत्री	507
Śatāhvā - Śatapuṣpā	शताह्वा - शतपुष्पा	121
Śatakoṭī - Hīrakam	शतकोटी - हीरकम्	532
Śātakumbham- Suvarṇam	शातकुम्भम् - सुवर्णम्	523
Sātalā (p.89)	सातला (p.89)	
Śatamūlā - Dūrvā (Raj. ni.)	शतमूला - दूर्वा (रा.नि.)	368
Śatapadī - Śatāvarī	शतपदी - शतावरी	115

Śataparvā - Vaṁśaḥ	शतपर्वा - वंशः	364
Śataparvā - Dūrvā	शतपर्वा - दूर्वा	368
Śataparvā - Kaṭukā	शतपर्वा - कटुका	15
Śatapatraḥ - Rājaśukaḥ	शतपत्रः - राजशुकः	634
Śatapatram - Raktapadmam	शतपत्रम् - रक्तपद्मम्	372
Śatapatrī (p. 507)	शतपत्री (p. 507)	
Śatapatrikā - Śatapatrī	शतपत्रिका - शतपत्री	507
Śatapuṣpā (p.121)	शतपुष्पा (p.121)	
Śataśaṅkhaḥ - Matsyaviśeṣaḥ	शतशङ्खः - मत्स्यविशेषः	627
Satataḥ - Śleṣmā	सततः - श्लेष्मा	617
Śatavallī - Dūrvā	शतवल्ली - दूर्वा	368
Śatāvarī - Mahāśatāvarī	शतावरी - महाशतावरी	116
Śatāvarī (p.115)	शतावरी (p.115)	
Śatavedhī - Amlavetasaḥ	शतवेधी - अम्लवेतसः	177
Śatavīryā - Śatāvarī (Raj. ni.)	शतवीर्या - शतावरी (रा.नि.)	115
Śatāyuḥ - Puruṣaḥ	शतायुः - पुरुषः	615
Ṣaṭcaraṇaḥ - Bhramaraḥ	षट्चरणः - भ्रमरः	633
Śaṭhaḥ - Dhattūraḥ	शठः - धत्तूरः	278
Śaṭham - Tagaram	शठम् - तगरम्	221
Śaṭhī (p.21)	शठी (p.21)	
Śaṭī - Śaṭhī	शटी - शठी	21
Satīnacchadikā - Viṣṇukrāntā	सतीनच्छदिका -विष्णुक्रान्ता	352
Satīnakaḥ - Kalāyaḥ	सतीनकः - कलायः	554
Ṣaṭkoṇam - Hīrakam	षट्कोणम् - हीरकम्	532
Sātmyam - Takram	सात्म्यम् - तक्रम्	587
Ṣaṭpadaḥ - Bhramaraḥ	षट्पदः - भ्रमरः	633
Ṣaṭpadamañjarī - Aśokaḥ	षट्पदमञ्जरी - अशोकः	516
Ṣaṭpadānandā - Vārṣikī	षट्पदानन्दा - वार्षिकी	496
Ṣaṭpadānandavardhanaḥ-Kinkirātaḥ	षट्पदानन्दवर्धनः - किंकिरातः	512
Ṣaṭpadātithiḥ - Campakaḥ	षट्पदातिथिः - चम्पकः	500
Sattukaḥ	सत्तुकः	665
Satyaḥ - Pippalaḥ	सत्यः -पिप्पलः	427
Satyakarmā - Bilvaḥ	सत्यकर्मा - बिल्वः	39
Satyanāmā - Godhūmaḥ	सत्यनामा - गोधूमः	551
Saudham - Raupyam	सौधम् - रौप्यम्	524
Saugandhikam (p. 371)	सौगन्धिकम् (p. 371)	
Saukarī - Vārāhī	सौकरी - वाराही	326
Śauktikam - Mauktikam	शौक्तिकम् - मौक्तिकम्	533
Saumanasam phalam-Jātiphalam	सौमनसंफलम् - जातीफलम्	211

Saumyā - Brāhmī	सौम्या - ब्राह्मी	336
Saumyā - Guḍūcī	सौम्या- गुडूची	2
Saumyā - Śāliparṇī	सौम्या - शालिपर्णी	32
Saumyā - Tāmbūlī	सौम्या - ताम्बूली	273
Saumyagandhā - Śatapatrī	सौम्यगन्धा - शतपत्री	507
Saumyam - Dugdham	सौम्यम् - दुग्धम्	577
Śauṇḍaḥ - Kukkuṭaḥ	शौण्डः - कुक्कुटः	636
Śauṇḍī - Pippalī	शौण्डी - पिप्पली	160
Sauparṇam - Gārutmatam	सौपर्णम् - गारुत्मतम्	
Saurabhaḥ -Tumbaruḥ	सौरभः - तुम्बरुः	140
Saurabheyī - Goḥ	सौरभेयी - गोः	626
Sauraḥ -Tumbaruḥ	सौरः - तुम्बरुः	140
Saurāṣṭraḥ - Kunduruḥ (Raj. ni.)	सौराष्ट्रः - कुन्दुरुः (रा. नि.)	254
Saurāṣṭrī (p. 247)	सौराष्ट्री (p. 247)	
Saurāṣṭrikaḥ	सौराष्ट्रिकः	666
Sauriḥ - Aśanaḥ	सौरिः - अशनः	479
Sauvarcalam (p.135)	सौवर्चलम् (p.135)	
Sauvīram - Badaram	सौवीरम् - बदरम्	445
Sauvīram (p.595)	सौवीरम् (p.595)	
Sauvīram - Añjanam	सौवीरम् - अञ्जनम्	262
Sauvīram - Kāñjikam	सौवीरम् - काञ्जिकम्	595
Sāyakaḥ - Śaraḥ	सायकः - शरः	363
Sehuṇḍaḥ - Snuhī	सेहुण्डः - स्नुही	88
Śekharī - Vandakā	शेखरी - वन्दका	331
Śeluḥ - Śleṣmātakaḥ	शेलुः - श्लेष्मातकः	441
Seluḥ - Vanamethikā	सेलुः - वनमेथिका	563
Śephālikā (p. 321)	शेफालिका (p. 321)	
Sevyā - Vāsantī	सेव्या - वासन्ती	498
Sevyaḥ - Pippalaḥ	सेव्यः -पिप्पलः	427
Sahasravedham - Śuktam	सहस्रवेधम् - शुक्तम्	594
Siddhaprayojanaḥ-Sarṣapaḥ (Raj. ni.)	सिद्धप्रयोजनः - सर्षपः (रा. नि.)	298
Sidhārthaḥ - Sarṣapaḥ	सिद्धार्थः - सर्षपः	53
Siddhī - Ṛddhiḥ	सिद्धी -ऋद्धिः	298
Sīdhugandhaḥ - Bakulaḥ	सीधुगन्धः - बकुलः	511
Śīghrā - Dantī	शीघ्रा - दन्ती	84
Śīghragaḥ - Aśvataraḥ	शीघ्रगः - अश्वतरः	622
Śīghram - Lāmajjakam	शीघ्रम् - लामज्जकम्	241
Śigrubījam - Śvetamaricam	शिग्रुबीजम - श्वेतमरिचम	168
Śigruḥ (p. 295)	शिग्रुः (p. 295)	
Śigrujam - Śvetamaricam	शिग्रुजम - श्वेतमरिचम	168

Sikatā - Śarkarā	सिकता -शर्करा	188
Śikhaṇḍī - Mayūraḥ	शिखण्डी - मयूरः	633
Śikhaṇḍī - Cūḍāmaṇiḥ	शिखण्डी - चूडामणिः	291
Śikhaṇḍī - Yūthikā	शिखण्डी - यूथिका	504
Śikharam - Lavaṅgam	शिखरम् - लवङ्गम्	214
Śikharī - Apāmārgaḥ	शिखरी -अपामार्गः	100
Śikharī - Kunduruḥ	शिखरी - कुन्दुरुः	254
Śikharī - Vandakā (Raj.ni.)	शिखरी- वन्दका (रा.नि.)	331
Śikhariṇī	शिखरिणी	651
Śikhariṇī - Graiṣmī	शिखरिणी - ग्रैष्मी	498
Śikhariṇī - Marjikā	शिखरिणी - मर्जिका	605
Śikhī - Citrakaḥ	शिखी - चित्रकः	165
Śikhī - Mayūraḥ	शिखी- मयूरः	633
Śikhī - Śitivāraḥ	शिखी - शितिवारः	56
Śikhī - Methikā	शिखी - मेथिका	562
Śikhī - Pittam	शिखी- पित्तम्	616
Śikhimodā - Ajamodā (Raj. ni.)	शिखिमोदा - अजमोदा (रा.नि.)	183
Śikhimūlam - Gṛñjanam	शिखिमूलम् - गृञ्जनम्	295
Sikthakam (p. 249)	सिक्थकम् (p. 249)	
Siktham - Sikthakam	सिक्थम् - सिक्थकम्	249
Śilā - Manaḥśilā	शिला - मनःशिला	246
Śilābhedaḥ - Pāṣāṇabhedaḥ	शिलाभेदः - पाषाणभेदः	57
Śilādadruḥ - Śaileyam	शिलादद्रुः - शैलेयम्	235
Śilagarbhajā - Pāṣāṇabhedaḥ	शिलगर्भजा - पाषाणभेदः	58
Śilājatuḥ (p. 266)	शिलाजतुः (p. 266)	
Śilāpuṣpam - Śaileyam	शिलापुष्पम् - शैलेयम्	235
Śilātmakam - Saindhavam	शिलात्मकम् - सैन्धवम्	135
Silhakaḥ - Turuṣkaḥ	सिल्हकः - तुरुष्कः	204
Śilīmukhaḥ - Bhramaraḥ	शिलीमुखः - भ्रमरः	633
Śillakaḥ - Śyonākaḥ	शिल्लकः - श्योनाकः	41
Śilodbhavam - Śaileyam	शिलोद्भवम् - शैलेयम्	235
Śilpī - Nakham	शिल्पी - नखम्	223
Sīmantinī - Strī	सीमन्तिनी - स्त्री	615
Śimbī - Mudgaparṇī	शिम्बी -मुद्गपर्णी	49
Śimhaḥ - Śigruḥ (Raj. ni.)	सिंहः - शिग्रुः (रा. नि.)	296
Simhaḥ (p. 624)	सिं हः (p.624)	
Simhaḥ-Madhuśigrukaḥ (Raj. ni.)	सिंहः -मधुशिग्रुकः (रा. नि.)	296
Simhalasthā-a type of Śreyasī (Raj. ni.)	सिंहलस्था-श्रेयसी विशेषःरा.नि.)	163
Simhamukhī - Vāsakaḥ	सिंहमुखी - वासकः	9

Simhaparṇī - Vāsakaḥ सिंहपर्णी- वासकः 9
Simhavinnā - Māṣaparṇī सिंहविन्ना - माषपर्णी 48
Simhikā - Bṛhatī सिंहिका - बृहती 35
Simhikā - Vāsakaḥ सिंहिका- वासकः 9
Śimśapā (p. 473) शिंशपा (p. 473)
Sindukah - Sinduvāraḥ सिन्दुकः - सिन्दुवारः 319
Sindhūttham - Saindhavam सिन्धूत्थम् - सैन्धवम् 135
Sindhu - Saindhavam सिन्धु - सैन्धवम् 135
Sindhujam - Saindhavam सिन्धुजम् - सैन्धवम् 135
Sindhupādapaḥ - Bījapūraḥ सिन्धुपादपः - बीजपूरः 396
Sindhupuṣpaḥ-Kadambaḥ (Raj.ni.) सिन्धुपुष्पः - कदम्बः (रा. नि.) 453
Sindhuraḥ - Hasti सिन्धुरः - हस्ति 620
Sindūraḥ (p. 246) सिन्दूरः (p. 246)
Sinduvāraḥ (p. 318) सिन्दुवारः (p. 318)
Sinduvārakaḥ - Sinduvāraḥ सिन्दुवारकः - सिन्दुवारः 319
Śiphā - Śatapuṣpā शिफा - शतपुष्पा 121
Śiraḥstham - Śukram शिरःस्थम् - शुक्रम् 619
Sīrī - Kalikārī सीरी - कलिकारी 280
Śīrī - Kuśaḥ शीरी - कुशः 362
Śirīṣaḥ (p. 462) शिरीषः (p. 462)
Śīrṇaromakam - Sthauṇeyakam शीर्णरोमकम् - स्थौणेयकम् 230
Śīrṇavṛntam (p. 66) शीर्णवृन्तम् (p. 66)
Śirovṛttam - Maricam शिरोवृत्तम् - मरिचम् 168
Śīrṣakesarakaḥ - Bakulaḥ शीर्षकेसरकः - बकुलः 511
Sīsakam (p. 526) सीसकम् (p. 526)
Śiśirā - Reṇukā (Raj. ni.) शिशिरा -रेणुका (रा. नि.) 220
Śiśiram - Sāmudram शिशिरम् - सामुद्रम् 136
Śiśupriyam - Navanītam शिशुप्रियम् - नवनीतम् 591
Sitā - Śarkarā सिता -शर्करा 188
Śītā - Atasī शीता - अतसी 565
Śītā - Tejasvinī शीता - तेजस्विनी 102
Sita Ikśuḥ - Ikśuḥ (Raj. ni.) सित (इक्षुः) - इक्षुः (रा.नि.) 358
Śītabhīruḥ - Mallikā शीतभीरुः - मल्लिका 493
Śitābhraḥ - Karpūraḥ शीताभ्र : -कर्पूरः 209
Sitābjam - Puṇḍarīkam सिताब्जम् -पुण्डरीकम् 370
Sitadhattūrakaḥ-Dhattūraḥ (Raj. ni.) सितधत्तूरकः - धत्तूरः (रा. नि.) 279
Sitādarbhaḥ - Kuśaḥ (Raj. ni.) सितदर्भः - कुशः (रा.नि.) 362
Śītaḥ - Pīluḥ शीतः - पीलुः 409
Sitahvayaḥ - Śigruḥ (Raj. ni.) सिताह्वयः - शिग्रुः (रा. नि.) 296

Śītalā - Dūrvā	शीतला - दूर्वा	368
Śītalaḥ - Campakaḥ	शीतलः - चम्पकः	500
Śītalarajaḥ - Karpūraḥ	शीतलरजः -कर्पूरः	209
Sitālarkaḥ - Śwetamandāraḥ	सितालर्कः - श्वेतमन्दारः	283
Sitālatā - Dūrvā	सितालता - दूर्वा	368
Sitam - Raupyam	सितम् - रौप्यम्	524
Śītapākī - Cūḍāmaṇiḥ	शीतपाकी - चूडामणिः	291
Śītapākī - Balā	शीतपाकी - बला	110
Sitapuṣpakaḥ - Kāśaḥ (Raj. ni.)	सितपुष्पकः - काशः (रा.नि.)	359
Sitapuṣpam - Paripellavam	सितपुष्पम् - परिपेल्लवम्	222
Sitapuṣpam - Prapauṇḍarīkam	सितपुष्पम् - प्रपौण्डरीकम्	243
Sitapuṣpī-Śaṅkhapuṣpī (Raj. ni.)	सितपुष्पी - शंखपुष्पी (रा.नि.)	349
Sitārkakaḥ - Śuklārkaḥ	सितार्ककः - शुक्लार्कः	283
Śītasahaḥ - Sinduvāraḥ	शीतसहः - सिन्दुवारः	319
Śītasamvāsā - Vāsantī	शीतसंवासा -वासन्ती	498
Sitasimhī - Lakśmaṇā	सितसिंही - लक्ष्मणा	36
Śītaśivaḥ - Miśreyā	शीतशिवः - मिश्रेया	122
Śītaśivam - Saindhavam	शीतशिवम् - सैन्धवम्	135
Śītarasikaḥ	शीतरसिकः	600
Śītavalkalaḥ - Udumbaraḥ	शीतवल्कलः - उदुम्बरः	436
Śītavallabhā - Jambūḥ	शीतवल्लभा - जम्बूः	433
Śītavīryā - Dūrvā	शीतवीर्या - दूर्वा	368
Śītavīryā - Methikā	शीतवीर्या - मेथिका	562
Śītavīryaḥ - Padmakaḥ	शीतवीर्यः - पद्मकः	242
Śītikaṇṭham - Tuttham	शितिकण्ठम् - तुत्थम्	260
Śitivaraḥ - Śitivāraḥ	शितिवरः - शितिवारः	56
Śitivāraḥ (p.46)	शितिवारः (p.46)	
Sitoccaṭā - Śvetakāmbhojī	सितोच्चटा -श्वेतकाम्भोजी	292
Sitopalā - Śarkarā	सितोपला -शर्करा	188
Śivā - Harītakī	शिवा - हरीतकी	77
Śivadwiṣṭā - Ketakī (Raj. ni.)	शिवद्विष्टा - केतकी (रा.नि.)	521
Śivaḥ - Gugguluḥ	शिवः - गुग्गुलुः	252
Śivaḥ - Bhāsaḥ	शिवः - भासः	637
Śivaḥ - Sṛgālaḥ	शिवः - श्रृगालः	632
Śivāhvaḥ -Bukaḥ	शिवाह्वः - बुकः	284
Śivam - Āmalakī	शिवम् - आमलकी	79
Śivam - Saindhavam	शिवम् - सैन्धवम्	135
Śivamallikā -Bukaḥ	शिवमल्लिका - बुकः	284
Śivāphalā - Śamī	शिवाफला - शमी	442

Śivapuṣpakaḥ - Arkaḥ (Raj. ni.)	शिवपुष्पकः - अर्कः (रा.नि.)	283
Śivaśekharaḥ -Bukaḥ	शिवशेखरः - बुकः	284
Śivāṭikā - Kākodumbarikā	शिवाटिका - काकोदुम्बरिका	437
Śivavallabhā - Śatapatrī	शिववल्लभा - शतपत्री	507
Śiveṣṭā - Dūrvā (Raj. ni.)	शिवेष्टा - दूर्वा (रा. नि.)	368
Skandhajaḥ - Vaṭaḥ	स्कन्धजः - वटः	426
Ślakṣṇam - Katakam	श्लक्ष्णम् - कतकम्	267
Ślakṣṇatwak - Aśmantakaḥ	श्लक्ष्णत्वक् - अश्मन्तकः	72
Śleṣmā (p. 617)	श्लेष्मा (p. 617)	
Śleṣmātakaḥ (p. 440)	श्लेष्मातकः (p. 440)	
Śmaśruḥ - Romaviśeṣaḥ	श्मश्रुः - रोमविशेषः	644
Snehabījaḥ - Priyālaḥ	स्नेहबीजः -प्रियालः	423
Snehaviddham - Devadāruḥ	स्नेहविद्धम् - देवदारुः	27
Snehottamam - Tailam	स्नेहोत्तमम् - तैलम्	570
Snigdhadāruḥ - Saralaḥ	स्निग्धदारुः - सरलः	237
Snigdhaparṇī - Mūrvā	स्निग्धपर्णी- मूर्वा	5
Snighdhaparṇī - Paṭolī	स्निग्धपर्णी - पटोली	19
Snuhī (p. 88)	स्नुही (p. 88)	
Snuk - Snuhī	स्नुक् - स्नुही	88
Śobhanā - Vāsantī	शोभना- वासन्ती	498
Śobhāñjanaḥ - Śigruḥ	शोभाञ्जनः - शिग्रुः	295
Śodhanam - Kamkuṣṭham	शोधनम् - कंकुष्ठम्	259
Śokanāśaḥ - Aśokaḥ	शोकनाशः - अशोकः	516
Somakṣīrī - Somavallī	सोमक्षीरी - सोमवल्ली	380
Somarajī - Bākucī	सोमराजी - बाकुची	61
Somavalkaḥ - Kaṭphalaḥ	सोमवल्कः - कट्फलः	27
Somavalkaḥ - (p. 10)	सोमवल्कः - (p. 10)	
Somavallī - Bākucī	सोमवल्ली - बाकुची	61
Somavallī (p. 380)	सोमवल्ली (p. 380)	378
Somavallī- Guḍūcī	सोमवल्ली - गुडूची	2
Somayoniḥ - Śleṣmā	सोमयोनिः - श्लेष्मा	617
Somsṛṣṭā - Kūṣmāṇḍikā	सोमसृष्टा - कूष्माण्डिका	68
Śoṇitam - Raktam	शोणितम् - रक्तम्	619
Śoṇitasambhavam - Māmsam	शोणितसंभवम् - मांसम्	618
Śoṣam - Pittam	शोषम् - पित्तम्	616
Sources of poisons of immovables	जंगम विषाश्रयाः	666
Spandanaḥ - Tindukaḥ	स्पन्दनः - तिन्दुकः	402
Sparśasankocaparṇikā-Raktapādī	स्पर्शसंकोचपर्णिका - रक्तपादी	344
Sphaṭikaḥ - Karpūraḥ	स्फटिकः -कर्पूरः	209

Sphoṭaśuktijam - Mauktikam स्फोटशुक्तिजम् - मौक्तिकम् 533
Sphūrjakaḥ - Tindukaḥ स्फूर्जकः - तिन्दुकः 402
Sphūrjanaḥ - Tindukaḥ स्फूर्जनः - तिन्दुकः 402
Sphuṭaphalaḥ-Tumbaruḥ (Raj.ni.) स्फुटफलः - तुम्बरुः (रा. नि.) 140
Spṛkka (p.224) स्पृक्का (p.224)
Śramabhañjanī - Tāmbūlī श्रमभञ्जनी - ताम्बूली 273
Sraṃsi - Pūgaphalam स्रंसि - पूगफलम् 213
Sravaḥ - Mūtram स्रवः - मूत्रम् 641
Sravaṇaḥ - Mūtram स्रवणः - मूत्रम् 641
Śrāvaṇī (p.58) श्रावणी (p.58)
Śreṣṭhā - Padmacāriṇī श्रेष्ठा - पद्मचारिणी 325
Śreṣṭhakāṣṭhaḥ -Sāgaḥ (Raj. ni.) श्रेष्ठकाष्ठः - सागः (रा.नि.) 522
Śreṣṭham - Mauktikam श्रेष्ठम् - मौक्तिकम् 533
Śreṣṭhatamaphalatrikam-Triphalā श्रेष्ठतमफलत्रिकम् - त्रिफला 645
Śreyasī - Rāsnā श्रेयसी - रास्ना 104
Śreyasī (p. 162) श्रेयसी (p. 162)
Śṛgālaḥ (p. 632) श्रृगालः (p. 632)
Śṛgālavinnā - Pṛṣniparṇī शृगालविन्ना - पृश्निपर्णी 33
Śṛgālikā - Vidāri शृगालिका -विदारी 54
Śrīketanam - Suvarṇam श्रीकेतनम् - सुवर्णम् 523
Śrīkhaṇḍam - Candanam श्रीखण्डम् -चन्दनम् 191
Śrīmad - Sindūraḥ श्रीमद् - सिन्दूरः 246
Śrīmān - Pippalaḥ श्रीमान् -पिप्पलः 427
Śrīmān - Tilakaḥ श्रीमान् - तिलकः 513
Śrīmatī - Vārṣikī श्रीमती - वार्षिकी 496
Śrīparṇī - Agnimanthaḥ श्रीपर्णी -अग्निमंथः 40
Śrīparṇī - Kāśmarī श्रीपर्णी - काश्मरी 42
Śrīparṇī - Kaṭphalaḥ श्रीपर्णी - कट्फलः 27
Śrīphalaḥ - Bilvaḥ श्रीफलः - बिल्वः 39
Śrīphalam - Āmalakī श्रीफलम् - आमलकी 79
Śrīphalikā - Nīlinī श्रीफलिका - नीलिनी 87
Śrīpuṣpam - Prapauṇḍarīkam श्रीपुष्पम् - प्रपौण्डरीकम् 243
Śrīpuṣpam - Lavaṅgam श्रीपुष्पम् - लवङ्गम् 214
Śrīvārakaḥ - Śitivāraḥ श्रीवारकः -शितिवारः 56
Śrīvāsaḥ - Śrīveṣṭakaḥ श्रीवासः - श्रीवेष्टकः 255
Śriveṣṭakaḥ (p. 254) श्रीवेष्टकः (p. 254)
Śrīvibhūṣaṇaḥ - Śaṅkhaḥ श्रीविभूषणः - शंखः 271
Śṛṅgabhedī - Guṇṭhaḥ शृङ्गभेदी - गुण्ठः 29
Śṛṅgakaḥ - Jīvakaḥ शृङ्गकः - जीवकः 44

Śṛṅgārabhūṣaṇam - Sindūraḥ शृङ्गारभूषणम् - सिन्दूरः 246
Śṛṅgāṭī - Jīvantī (Raj. ni.) शृङ्गाटी - जीवन्ती (रा.नि.) 50
Śṛṅgaveram - Śuṇṭhī श्रृङ्गवेरम् - शुण्ठी 167
Śṛṅgī - Matsyabhedaḥ श्रृङ्गी - मत्स्यभेदः 628
Śṛṅgī - Matsyaviśeṣaḥ श्रृङ्गी - मत्स्यविशेषः 627
Śṛṅgī - Vaṭaḥ श्रृङ्गी - वटः 426
Śṛṅgī (p.30) श्रृङ्गी (p.30)
Śṛṅgī - Āmrātakaḥ श्रृङ्गी - आम्रातकः 388
Śṛṅgī- Ativiṣā श्रृङ्गी - अतिविषा 4
Śṛṅgī - Karkaṭaśṛṅgī श्रृङ्गी - कर्कटश्रृंगी 30
Śṛṅgī - Mahiṣaḥ शृङ्गी - महिषः 625
Śṛṅgī - Plakṣaḥ श्रृंगी - प्लक्षः 428
Śṛṅgikaḥ श्रृङ्गिकः 664
Śṛṅgiṇī - Goḥ श्रृङ्गिणी - गोः 626
Srotojam - Añjanam स्रोतोजम् - अञ्जनम् 262
Sruvadrumaḥ-Vikaṅkataḥ (Raj.ni.) स्रुवद्रुमः - विकंकतः (रा.नि.) 405
Śravaṇaśīrṣikā - Śrāvaṇī श्रवणशीर्षिका - श्रावणी 58
Śryāhvaḥ - Śrīveṣṭakaḥ श्र्याह्वः - श्रीवेष्टकः 255
Śryāhvaḥ - Bilvaḥ श्र्याह्वः - बिल्वः 39
Stamberamaḥ - Hasti स्तम्बेरमः - हस्ति 620
Stanyaḥ - Śuklajīrakaḥ स्तन्यः - शुक्लजीरकः 157
Stanyam - Dugdham स्तन्यम् - दुग्धम् 577
Sthalapadmī-Padmacāriṇī (Raj.ni.) स्थलपद्मी - पद्मचारिणी (रा. नि.) 325
Sthalapiṇḍā - Dīpyā स्थलपिण्डा - दीप्या 412
Sthālī - Pāṭalā स्थाली - पाटला 43
Sthāpanī - Pāṭhā स्थापनी - पाठा 26
Sthauṇeyakam (p. 230) स्थौणेयकम् (p. 230)
Sthāvara viṣāṇi स्थावरविषाणि 663
Sthāvarādyam garalam-Vatsanābhaḥ स्थावराद्यं गरलं - वत्सनाभः 667
Sthaviram - Śaileyam स्थविरम् - शैलेयम् 235
Sthirā - Śāliparṇī स्थिरा - शालिपर्णी 32
Sthiraḥ - Vṛṣabhaḥ स्थिरः - वृषभः 626
Sthirakusumaḥ-Bakulaḥ (Raj.ni.) स्थिरकुसुमः - बकुलः (रा. नि.) 511
Sthirapuṣpaḥ - Tilakaḥ (Raj. ni.) स्थिरपुष्पः - तिलकः (रा.नि.) 514
Sthirasādhanakaḥ-Sinduvāraḥ (Raj. ni.) स्थिरसाधनकः-सिन्दुवारः (रा.नि.) 319
Sthirphalā - Kūṣmāṇḍikā स्थिरफला - कूष्माण्डिका 68
Sthūlā - Urvāruḥ स्थूला - उर्वारुः 65
Sthūladaṇḍaḥ - Mahānalaḥ स्थूलदण्डः - महानलः 367
Sthūladarbhaḥ - Muñjaḥ स्थूलदर्भः - मुञ्जः 360

Sthūlailā - Bhadrailā	स्थूलैला -भद्रैला	142
Sthūlajīrakaḥ - Upakuñcī	स्थूलजीरकः - उपकुञ्ची	154
Sthūlakā - Gandhapalāśī	स्थूलका - गन्धपलाशी	22
Sthūlakaṇṭākī -Bṛhatī	स्थूलकण्टाकी - बृहती	35
Sthūlanālaḥ - Mahānalaḥ	स्थूलनालः - महानलः	367
Sthūlaśaraḥ - Śaraḥ	स्थूलशरः - शरः	363
Sthūlavalkalaḥ - Pattikārodhraḥ	स्थूलवल्कलः -पट्टिकारोध्रः	270
Stokakam - Vatsanābhaḥ	स्तोकक्कम् - वत्सनाभः	667
Strī (p. 615)	स्त्री (p. 615)	615
Strī dadhi	स्त्रीदधि	585
Strīghṛtam	स्त्रीघृतम्	576
Stutyā - Saurāṣtrī	स्तुत्या - सौराष्ट्री	247
Sugandhamūlā - Gandhapalāśī	सुगन्धमूला- गन्धपलाशी	22
Śubhā - Śamī (Raj. ni.)	शुभा - शमी (रा. नि.)	443
Śubhā - Vaṃśarocanā	शुभा - वंशरोचना	150
Śubhadaḥ - Pippalaḥ	शुभदः -पिप्पलः	427
Subhagā - Suvarṇakadalī	सुभगा - सुवर्णकदली	318
Subhagā - Vārṣikī	सुभगा - वार्षिकी	496
Śubhagandham-Bolam (Raj. ni.)	शुभगन्धम् - बोलम् (रा. नि.)	226
Subhikśā - Dhātukī	सुभिक्षा - धातुकी	243
Śubhrā - Śarkarā	शुभ्रा-शर्करा	188
Śubhrā - Vaṃśarocanā	शुभ्रा - वंशरोचना	150
Śubhram - Raupyam	शुभ्रम् - रौप्यम्	524
Śubhram - Medaḥ	शुभ्रम् - मेदः	643
Śubhram - Uśīram (Raj.ni.)	शुभ्रम् - उशीरम् (रा.नि.)	199
Śubhramaricam - Śvetamaricam	शुभ्रमरिचम् - श्वेतमरिचम्	168
Śubhrapuṣpaḥ- Khastilaḥ	शुभ्रपुष्पः - खस्तिलः	568
Śubhragauraḥ - Sarṣapaḥ	शुभ्रगौरः - सर्षपः	297
Śucicīraḥ - Kuśaḥ	शुचिचीरः - कुशः	361
Śucidrumaḥ - Pippalaḥ	शुचिद्रुमः -पिप्पलः	427
Sūcikāpuṣpaḥ - Ketakī	सूचिकापुष्पः - केतकी	520
Sūcimukhaḥ - Kuśaḥ (Raj. ni.)	सूचिमुखः - कुशः (रा.नि.)	362
Sūcipatraḥ - Śitivāraḥ	सूचिपत्रः - शितिवारः	56
Sūcivaktram - Hīrakam	सूचिवक्त्रम् - हीरकम्	532
Sūcyāhvaḥ - Śitivāraḥ	सूच्याह्वः - शितिवारः	56
Sudalā - Taruṇī (Raj. ni.)	सुदला - तरुणी (रा. नि.)	501
Śuddhā - Śarkarā	शुद्धा -शर्करा	188
Śuddham - Saindhavam	शुद्धं - सैंधवम्	135
Sugandhā - Graiṣmī	सुगन्धा- ग्रैष्मी	498
Sugandhā - Nākulī	सुंगन्धा - नाकुली	339

Sugandhāḍhyā-Mallikā (Raj. ni.) सुगन्धाढ्या - मल्लिका (रा. नि.) 494
Sugandhaḥ - Caṇakaḥ सुगन्धः - चणकः 553
Sugandhaḥ - Kṛṣṇajīrakaḥ सुगन्धः - कृष्णजीरकः 158
Sugandhakesaraḥ-Śigruḥ (Raj.ni.) सुगन्धकेसरः - शिग्रुः (रा. नि.) 296
Sugandhakesaraḥ - Madhuśigrukaḥ (Raj.ni.)
सुगन्धकेशरः -मधुशिग्रुकः (रा. नि.) 296
Sugandhāmalakam सुगन्धामलकम् 652
Sugandhamūlā - Rāsnā सुगन्धमूला - रास्ना 104
Sugandhamūlā - Śaṭhī सुगन्धमूला - शठी 22
Sugandhaprasavaḥ - Śāliḥ सुगन्धप्रसवः -शालिः 535
Sugandhiḥ - Tumbaruḥ (Raj. ni.) सुगन्धिः - तुम्बरुः (रा.नि.) 140
Sugandhiḥ - Turuṣkaḥ सुगन्धिः - तुरुष्कः 204
Sugandhikam-Elavālukam (Raj.ni.) सुगन्धिकम् - एलवालुकम् (रा.नि.) 236
Sugandhikusumaḥ-Karavīraḥ (Raj.ni.) सुगन्धिकुसुमः - करवीरः (रा.नि.) 276
Sugandhimūtrapatanaḥ-Gandhamārjāraḥ सुगन्धिमूत्रपतनः-गन्धमार्जारः 631
Sugandhinī - Ketakī सुगन्धिनी - केतकी 520
Sugandhitriphalā सुगंधित्रिफला 645
Sugandhimūtra vṛṣaṇaḥ-Ugrabiḍālakaḥ सुगन्धिमूत्रवृषणः-उग्रबिडालकः 631
Śukabarham - Sthauṇeyakam शुकबर्हम् - स्थौणेयकम् 230
Śukacchadam - Sthauṇeyakam शुकच्छदम् - स्थौणेयकम् 230
Śūkaḥ (p. 633) शुकः (p. 633)
Śūkajaḥ - Yavakśāraḥ शूकजः -यवक्षारः 133
Śukanāsaḥ - Śyonākaḥ शुकनासः - श्योनाकः 41
Sukandaḥ - Palāṇḍuḥ सुकन्दः - पलाण्डुः 315
Sukāṇḍakaḥ - Kāṇḍīraḥ सुकाण्डकः -काण्डीरः 309
Śukaphalaḥ - Arkaḥ(Raj ni.) शुकफलः - अर्कः (रा. नि.) 283
Śukapriyaḥ - Śirīṣaḥ शुकप्रियः -शिरीषः 463
Śukapuṣpam - Sthauṇeyakam शुकपुष्पम् - स्थौणेयकम् 230
Sūkaraḥ (p.624) सूकरः (p.624)
Śūkarapādikā - Dadhipuṣpī शूकरपादिका - दधिपुष्पी 56
Sūkaravālakaḥ - Śāliḥ सूकरवालकः -शालिः 535
Śukataruḥ - Śirīṣaḥ शुकतरुः- शिरीषः 463
Śukavallabhaḥ - Dāḍimaḥ शुकवल्लभः -दाडिमः 155
Śukāhvayam - Jalamustam शुकाहवयम् - जलमुस्तम 16
Sukham - Ṛddhiḥ सुखम् -ऋद्धिः 53
Sukhasambhavam - Śvāsāriḥ सुखसंभवम् - श्वासारिः 25
Sukhavarcaḥ - Swarjikākśāraḥ सुखवर्चः - स्वर्जिकाक्षारः 134
Sukhodbhavā - Suvarcalā सुखोद्भवा - सुवर्चला 333
Śuklā - Śephālikā शुक्ला - शेफालिका 321
Śuklā - Kākolī शुक्ला - काकोली 47

Śuklā - Vidārī शुक्ला -विदारी 54
Śuklabhaṇḍī (p.94) शुक्लभण्डी (p.94)
Śuklaḥ - Kundaḥ शुक्लः - कुन्दः 506
Śuklaḥ - Eraṇḍaḥ शुक्लः - एरण्डः 117
Śuklājājī - Śuklajīrakaḥ शुक्लाजाजी - शुक्लजीरकः 157
Śuklajīrakaḥ (p. 157) शुक्लजीरकः (p. 157)
Śuklakandā - Ativiṣā शुक्लकन्दा - अतिविषा 4
Śuklapuṣpā - Viṣṇukrāntā शुक्लपुष्पा - विष्णुक्रान्ता 352
Śuklārkaḥ - Arkaḥ (p. 283) (Raj. ni.) शुक्लार्कः-अर्कः (p. 283) (रा. नि.)
Śuklavargaḥ शुक्लवर्गः 657
Śuklavṛkṣaḥ - Dhavaḥ (Raj.ni.) शुक्लवृक्षः - धवः (रा.नि.) 522
Śukodaram - Tālīsam शुकोदरम् - तालीसम् 147
Sukośakaḥ - Kśudrāmraḥ सुकोशकः - क्षुद्राम्रः 387
Śukram (p.619) शुक्रम् (p.619)
Sūkśmailā - Elā सूक्ष्मैला - एला 141
Sūkśmamūlā - Balāmoṭā सूक्ष्ममूला - बलामोटा 378
Sūkśmapatrā - Bṛhatpālī सूक्ष्मपत्रा - बृहत्पाली 159
Sūkśmapatrā-Śatāvarī (Raj. ni.) सूक्ष्मपत्रा - शतावरी (रा.नि.) 115
Sūkśmapatrā - Vṛddhadārukaḥ (Raj. ni.)सूक्ष्मपत्रा - वृद्धदारुकः (रा. नि.)343
Sūkśmapatrāntarā - Viṣṇukrāntā सूक्ष्मपत्रान्तरा -विष्णुक्रान्ता 352
Sūkśmavallī-Jantukārī (Raj. ni.) सूक्ष्मवल्ली - जन्तुकारी (रा. नि.) 325
Śuktā - Amlikā शुक्ता - अम्लिका 398
Śuktam (p. 594) शुक्तम् (p. 593)
Śuktiḥ - Nakham शुक्तिः - नखम् 223
Śuktikā - Amlikā शुक्तिका - अम्लिका 398
Śuktikam - Mauktikam शुक्तिकम् - मौक्तिकम् 533
Śuktiparṇaḥ - Saptaparṇaḥ शुक्तिपर्णः - सप्तपर्णः 238
Śuktisambhavam - Mauktikam शुक्तिसंभवम् - मौक्तिकम् 533
Śakulaḥ - Matsyaḥ शकुलः - मत्स्यः 626
Sukumārā - Graiṣmī सुकुमारा - ग्रैष्मी 498
Sukumārā - Spṛkkā (Raj. ni.) सुकुमारा - स्पृक्का (रा.नि.) 224
Sukumārā - Kadalī सुकुमारा - कदली 316
Sukumāraḥ - Campakaḥ सुकुमारः - चम्पकः 500
Sukumāraḥ - Śyāmākaḥ सुकुमारः - श्यामाकः 545
Sukumārakaḥ - Ikśuḥ सुकुमारकः - इक्षुः 357
Sukundraḥ - Kunduruḥ सुकुन्द्रः - कुन्दुरुः 254
Śulaharam - Śvāsāriḥ शूलहरम् - श्वासारिः 25
Śulbam - Tāmram शुल्बम् - ताम्रम् 524
Sulomā - Māmsarohiṇī (Raj. ni.) सुलोमा - मांसरोहिणी (रा.नि.) 330
Sumakarandaḥ - Kundaḥ सुमकरन्दः - कुन्दः 506

Sumanā - Jātī	सुमना - जाती	496
Sumanā - Śatapatrī	सुमना - शतपत्री	507
Sumanaḥpatrikā - Jātipatrī	सुमनःपत्रिका - जातिपत्री	211
Sumaṅgalyam - Kapaṭam	सुमङगल्यम् - कपटम्	29
Sumukhaḥ (p. 305)	सुमुखः (p. 305)	
Śunaḥ - Sārameyaḥ	शुनः - सारमेयः	632
Sunālam - Lāmajjakam	सुनालम् - लामज्जकम्	241
Sundaraḥ - Tilakaḥ (Raj. ni.)	सुन्दरः - तिलकः (रा.नि.)	514
Sundarī -Strī	सुन्दरी - स्त्री	615
Sunidrājanakaḥ - Śleṣmā	सुनिद्राजनक - श्लेष्मा	617
Sunīlaḥ - Aśanaḥ	सुनीलः - अशनः	479
Sunīlapuṣpā - Atasī	सुनीलपुष्पा - अतसी	565
Sunirghoṣā - Jiṅgiṇī	सुनिर्घोषा - जिंगिणी	272
Suniṣaṇṇakaḥ - Śitivāraḥ	सुनिषण्णकः -शितिवारः	56
Śuṇṭhaḥ - Guṇṭhaḥ	शुण्ठः - गुण्ठः	29
Śuṇṭham - Guṇṭhaḥ	शुण्टम् - गुण्ठः	29
Śuṇṭhī (p. 167)	शुण्ठी (p. 167)	
Śūnyā - Nalikā	शून्या - नलिका	216
Śūnyamadhyaḥ - Nalaḥ	शून्यमध्यः - नलः	366
Sūpadhūpanam - Hiṅgu	सूपधूपनम् - हिंगु	137
Supākyam - Biḍam	सुपाक्यम् - बिडम्	135
Suprasarā - Prasāraṇī	सुप्रसरा - प्रसारणी	114
Suparṇakaḥ - Saptaparṇaḥ	सुपर्णकः - सप्तपर्णः	238
Suparṇī - Reṇukā (Raj.ni.)	सुपर्णी -रेणुका (रा.नि.)	220
Supārśvaḥ - Plakṣaḥ	सुपार्श्वः - प्लक्षः	428
Sūpaśreṣṭhaḥ - Mudgaḥ	सूपश्रेष्ठः -मुद्गः	540
Suphalaḥ - Karṇikāraḥ	सुफलः - कर्णिकारः	82
Suphalaḥ - Āmraḥ	सुफलः - आम्रः	385
Supītam - Garjaram	सुपीतम् - गर्जरम्	314
Suprabhaḥ - Padmakaḥ	सुप्रभः - पद्मकः	242
Supraśastaḥ - Sumukhaḥ	सुप्रशस्तः -सुमुखः :	305
Supūrakaḥ - Bījapūraḥ	सुपूरकः - बीजपूरः	396
Supūraṇī - Śālmalī	सुपूरणी - शाल्मली	481
Supuṣkarā - Padmacāriṇī	सुपुष्करा - पद्मचारिणी	325
Supuṣpaḥ - Śuklārkaḥ	सुपुष्पः - शुक्लार्कः	283
Supuṣpam - Prapauṇḍarīkam	सुपुष्पम् -प्रपौण्डरीकम्	243
Supuṣpikā-Vṛddhadārukaḥ (Raj.ni.)	सुपुष्पिका - वृद्धदारुकः (रा. नि.)	343
Supuṭā - Vārṣikī	सुपुटा - वार्षिकी	495
Sūpyaḥ - Masūraḥ	सूप्यः - मसूरः	550
Surā (p. 596 597)	सुरा (p. 596 , 597)	

Surabhiḥ - Marjikā सुरभिः - मर्जिका 605
Surabhiḥ (bhī)- Surasā सुरभिः (भी)- सुरसा 301
Surabhiḥ - Campakaḥ सुरभिः - चम्पकः 500
Surabhiḥ - (Sugandha) Bhūstṛṇaḥ (Raj ni.)
सुरभिः - (सुगंध) भूस्तृणः (रा. नि.) 300
Surabhiḥ - Graiṣmī सुरभिः - ग्रैष्मी 498
Surabhiḥ - Jambūḥ सुरभिः - जम्बूः 433
Surabhiḥ - Murā सुरभिः - मुरा 229
Surabhiḥ - Śallakī सुरभिः - शल्लकी 256
Surabhipatrā - Jambūḥ सुरभिपत्रा - जम्बूः 433
Sudāruḥ - Devadāruḥ सुदारुः - देवदारुः 27
Suradāruḥ - Devadāruḥ सुरदारुः - देवदारुः 27
Suradrumaḥ - Mahānalaḥ सुरद्रुमः - महानलः 367
Śūraḥ - Śarabhaḥ शूरः - शरभः 624
Śūraḥ - Sarjakaḥ शूरः - सर्जकः 476
Surāhvam - Devadāruḥ सुराह्वम् - देवदारुः 27
Suraktakaḥ - Kśudrāmraḥ सुरक्तकः - क्षुद्राम्रः 387
Surambhikā - Suvarṇakadalī सुरम्भिका - सुवर्णकदली 318
Suramṛttikā - Saurāṣṭrī सुरमृत्तिका - सौराष्ट्री 247
Sūraṇaḥ (p. 383) सूरणः (p.383) 382
Suranālaḥ - Mahānalaḥ सुरनालः - महानलः 367
Surangakam - Patangam सुरङ्गकम् - पतङ्गम् 194
Surangī - Kākanāsā सुरङ्गी - काकनासा 289
Surangikā - Potakī सुरङ्गिका - पोतकी 382
Surapriyā - Suvarṇakadalī सुरप्रिया - सुवर्णकदली 318
Surārham - Haricandanam सुरार्हम् - हरिचन्दनम् 196
Surasā (p. 301) सुरसा (p. 301)
Surasaḥ - Bhūstṛṇaḥ (Raj. ni.) सुरसः - भूस्तृणः (रा. नि.) 300
Surasambhavā-Suvarcalā (Raj.ni.) सुरसंभवा - सुवर्चला (रा.नि.) 333
Surāṣṭrajā - Saurāṣṭrī सुराष्ट्रजा - सौराष्ट्री 247
Surāṣṭrakaḥ - Kulatthaḥ सुराष्ट्रकः - कुलत्थः 557
Surāsavaḥ सुरासवः 601
Suraṭī - Vangam सुरटी - वङ्गम् 525
Surbhījalam - Gomūtram सुरभीजलम् - गोमूत्रम् 641
Sūryāhvayaḥ - Arkaḥ सूर्याह्वयः - अर्कः 282
Śūrpaparṇī-Mudgaparṇī, Māṣaparṇī शूर्पपर्णी -मुद्गपर्णी, माषपर्णी 49
Surūpā - Vārṣikī सुरूपा - वार्षिकी 496
Suvarṇam (p. 523) सुवर्णम् (p. 523)
Sūryabhaktā - Suvarcalā सूर्यभक्ता - सुवर्चला 333

Suṣavī - Upakuñcī सुषवी - उपकुञ्ची 154
Suṣeṇaḥ - Vetasaḥ सुषेणः - वेतसः 467
Suṣeṇam - Karamardakam सुषेणम् - करमर्दकम् 449
Suṣeṇī - Trivṛt सुषेणी -त्रिवृत 93
Suṣirā - Nalikā सुषिरा - नलिका 216
Suṣiraḥ - Vamṣaḥ (Raj. ni.) सुषिरः - वंशः (रा.नि.) 365
Suśītā - Śatapatrī सुशीता - शतपत्री 507
Suśītaḥ - Plakṣaḥ सुशीतः - प्लक्षः 429
Śuṣkāśuṣkam - Samudraphenam शुष्काशुष्कम् - समुद्रफेनम् 263
Susravā - Śallakī सुस्रवा - शल्लकी 256
Suśvetā - Lakṣmaṇā सुश्वेता - लक्ष्मणा 36
Sūtaḥ - Pāradaḥ सूतः - पारदः 529
Sutīkṣṇaḥ - Śigruḥ (Raj. ni.) सुतीक्ष्णः - शिग्रुः (रा. नि.) 296
Sutiktā - Kośātakī सुतिक्ता - कोशातकी 71
Sutiktakaḥ - Nimbaḥ सुतिक्तकः - निम्बः 12
Sutiktakaḥ - Parpaṭaḥ सुतिक्तकः - पर्पटः 17
Sutittiḍī - Amlikā सुतित्तिडी - अम्लिका 398
Suturigaḥ - Nārikelaḥ सुतुङ्गः - नारिकेलः 425
Suvadaṇaḥ - Sumukhaḥ सुवदनः - सुमुखः 305
Suvahā - Gandhanākulī सुवहा - गन्धनाकुली 342
Suvaktraḥ - Sumukhaḥ सुवक्त्रः -सुमुखः 305
Suvalkalā - Atasī सुवल्कला - अतसी 565
Suvallī - Bākucī सुवल्ली - बाकुची 61
Suvallijam - Pravālam सुवल्लिजम् - प्रवालम् 534
Suvarcalā (p. 333) सुवर्चला (p. 333)
Suvarcikā - Swarjikākṣāraḥ सुवर्चिका - स्वर्जिकाक्षारः 134
Suvarcikaḥ - Swarjikākṣāraḥ सुवर्चिकः - स्वर्जिकाक्षारः 134
Suvarṇadhātū -Rājāvartaḥ सुवर्णधातू - राजावर्तः 533
Suvarṇāhvā - Yūthikā (Raj. ni.) सुवर्णाह्वा - यूथिका (रा. नि.) 504
Suvarṇakadalī (Raj. ni.) (p. 317) सुवर्णकदली (रा. नि.) (p. 317)
Suvarṇakam - Pittalam सुवर्णकम् - पित्तलम् 526
Suvarnaketakī - Ketakī सुवर्णकेतकी - केतकी 520
Suvarṇakṣīrikā - Sarvakṣīrī सुवर्णक्षीरिका -सर्वक्षीरी 91
Suvarṇalatikā - Jyotiṣmatī सुवर्णलतिका - ज्योतिष्मती 103
Suvarṇarambhā - Suvarṇakadalī सुवर्णरम्भा - सुवर्णकदली 318
Suvarṇayūthī - Yūthikā सुवर्णयूथी - यूथिका 504
Suvarvcaḥ - Swarjikākṣāraḥ सुवर्चः - स्वर्जिकाक्षारः 134
Suvāsaḥ - Kadambaḥ सुवासः - कदम्बः 451
Suvasantaḥ - Atimuktakaḥ सुवसन्तः - अतिमुक्तकः 509
Suvasantī - Vāsantī सुवसन्ती- वासन्ती 498

Suvīrajam - Añjanam	सुवीरजम् - अञ्जनम्	262
Suvirāmlam - Sauvīram	सुवीराम्लम् - सौवीरम्	595
Suvratā - Śaṭhī	सुव्रता - शठी	22
Suvrataḥ -Bukaḥ	सुव्रतः - बुकः	284
Suvarṇamocā - Suvarṇakadalī	सुवर्णमोचा - सुवर्णकदली	318
Suvarṣā - Vārṣikī	सुवर्षा - वार्षिकी	496
Suvṛttā - Śatapatrī	सुवृत्ता - शतपत्री	507
Suvṛttakaḥ - Kuśaḥ	सुवृत्तकः - कुशः	361
Suvṛttiḥ - Sūraṇaḥ	सुवृत्तिः - सूरणः	383
Suwarṇagairikam - Gairikam	सुवर्णगैरिकम् - गैरिकम्	263
Śvadaṃṣṭraḥ - Gokśuraḥ	श्वदंष्ट्रः - गोक्षुरः	38
Śvānakaḥ - Sārameyaḥ	श्वानकः - सारमेयः	632
Svaryā - Brāhmī (Raj. ni.)	स्वर्या - ब्राह्मी (रा.नि.)	337
Svaryā - Suvarcalā (Raj. ni.)	स्वर्या - सुवर्चला (रा.नि.)	333
Śvasanaḥ - Vāyuḥ	श्वसनः - वायुः	616
Śvāsāriḥ (p.25)	श्वासारिः (p.25)	
Svāsyaḥ - Sumukhaḥ	स्वास्यः -सुमुखः	305
Śvetā - Sārivā	श्वेता - सारिवा	59
Śvetā - Śarkarā	श्वेता -शर्करा	188
Śvetā - Aśvakśurakaḥ	श्वेता -अश्वक्षुरकः	323
Śvetā - Ativiṣā	श्वेता- अतिविषा	4
Śvetā - Kaṣṭhakadalī	श्वेता - काष्ठकदली	317
Śvetā (Pāṭalā) - Kāṣṭhapāṭalā	श्वेता (पाटला) - काष्ठपाटला	44
Śvetā Āḍhakī - Āḍhakī	श्वेताआढकी - आढकी	549
Śvetabṛhatī-Lakśmaṇā (Raj.ni.)	श्वेतबृहती - लक्ष्मणा (रा. नि.)	36
Śvetacāmarapuṣpaḥ- Kāśaḥ	श्वेतचामरपुष्पः - काशः	359
Śvetacandanam - Candanam	श्वेतचन्दनम् -चन्दनम्	191
Śvetadaṇḍā - Dūrvā	श्वेतदण्डा - दूर्वा	368
Śvetadrumaḥ - Varuṇaḥ	श्वेतद्रुमः - वरुणः	472
Svetadūrvā - Dūrvā	श्वेतदूर्वा - दूर्वा	368
Svetaguñjā - Śvetakāmbhoji	श्वेतगुञ्जा - श्वेतकाम्भोजी	292
Śvetaḥ - Hamsaḥ	श्वेतः - हंसः	635
Śvetaḥ - Śuklārkaḥ	श्वेतः - शुक्लार्कः	283
Śvetaḥ (Sarpaḥ) - Nāgaḥ	श्वेतः -(सर्पः) नागः	639
Śvetajalajam - Kumudam	श्वेतजलजम् - कुमुदम्	373
Śvetakaḥ - Śigruḥ	श्वेतकः - शिग्रुः	295
Śvetakam - Raupyam	श्वेतकम् - रौप्यम्	524
Śvetakāmbhojī (p. 202)	श्वेतकाम्भोजी (p. 202)	
Śvetakumbhīkā - Kāṣṭhapāṭalā	श्वेतकुम्भीका - काष्ठपाटला	44
Śvetakundaḥ - Karavīraḥ	श्वेतकुन्दः - करवीरः	275

Śvetam - Barbarikam	श्वेतम् - बर्बरिकम्	195
Śvetam - Mathita dadhi	श्वेतम् - मथित दधि	583
Śvetamaricaḥ - Śigruḥ	श्वेतमरिचः - शिग्रुः	295
Śvetamaricam (p.168)	श्वेतमरिचम् (p.168)	
Śvetamūlaḥ - Krūraḥ	श्वेतमूलः -क्रूरः	108
Śvetanāmā - Aśvakśurakaḥ	श्वेतनामा -अश्वक्षुरकः	323
Śvetapadmam - Puṇḍarīkam	श्वेतपद्मम् -पुण्डरीकम्	370
Śvetapatram-Puṇḍarīkam (Raj.ni.)	श्वेतपत्रम् -पुण्डरीकम् (रा.नि.)	370
Śvetapayaḥ - Takram	श्वेतपयः - तक्रम्	587
Śvetapingalaḥ - Simhaḥ	श्वेतपिङ्गलः - सिंहः	624
Śvetapuṣpaḥ - Karavīraḥ	श्वेतपुष्पः - करवीरः	275
Śvetapuṣpaḥ - Varuṇaḥ	श्वेतपुष्पः - वरुणः	472
Śvetapuṣpī - Aśvakśurakaḥ	श्वेतपुष्पी -अश्वक्षुरकः	323
Śvetapuṣpī - Indravāruṇī (p. 96)	श्वेतपुष्पी - इन्द्रवारुणी (p.96)	
Śvetarohitakaḥ - Rohitakaḥ	श्वेतरोहितकः - रोहितकः	485
Śvetaśāliḥ - Śāliḥ	श्वेतशालिः - शालिः	535
Śvetasāraḥ - Somavalkaḥ	श्वेतसारः - सोमवल्कः	10
Śvetaśimbaḥ - Niṣpāvaḥ	श्वेतशिम्बः - निष्पावः	560
Śvetaspandā - Aśvakśurakaḥ	श्वेतस्पंदा - अश्वक्षुरकः	323
Śvetasurasā - Śephālikā	श्वेतसुरसा - शेफालिका	321
Śvetavacā (p.126) (Raj. ni.)	श्वेतवचा (p.126) (रा. नि.)	
Śvetavārijam - Puṇḍarīkam	श्वेतवारिजम् -पुण्डरीकम्	370
Śvetpuṣpaḥ - Sinduvāraḥ	श्वेतपुष्पः - सिन्दुवारः	319
Swādukandā - Vidārī	स्वादुकन्दा -विदारी	54
Swāduḥ - Jīvakaḥ	स्वादुः - जीवकः	44
Swāduḥ - Dugdham	स्वादुः- दुग्धम्	577
Swādukaṇṭakaḥ - Gokśuraḥ	स्वादुकण्टकः - गोक्षुरः	38
Swādukaṇṭakaḥ - Vikankataḥ	स्वादुकण्टकः - विकंकतः	405
Swādumajjā - Akśoḍaḥ	स्वादुमज्जा - अक्षोडः	414
Swādumastakā - Kharjūrī	स्वादुमस्तका - खर्जूरी	411
Swādumūlam - Garjaram	स्वादुमूलम् - गर्जरम्	314
Swādupākā - Uttarāpathikā	स्वादुपाका - उत्तरापथिका	414
Swādupatraphalā - Paṭolī	स्वादुपत्रफला - पटोली	19
Swādupatraphalā (p.19)	स्वादुपत्रफला (पटोली) (p.19)	
Swāduphalā - Kośātakī	स्वादुफला - कोशातकी (रा.नि.)	72
Swāduphalā - Kadalī	स्वादुफला - कदली	316
Swāduphalā - Karkoṭakī	स्वादुफला - कर्कोटकी	69
Swādupiṇḍā - Dīpyā	स्वादुपिण्डा - दीप्या	412
Swādurasā- Mūrvā	स्वादुरसा - मूर्वा	5

Swādūṣṇaḥ - Śigruḥ (Raj. ni.) स्वादूष्णः - शिग्रुः (रा. नि.) 296
Swādutriphalā स्वादुत्रिफला 645
Swādvagaru - Agaru स्वाद्वगरु - अगरु 206
Swādvamlaḥ - Dāḍimaḥ स्वाद्वम्लः -दाडिमः 155
Swarjikā - Swarjikākṣāraḥ स्वर्जिका - स्वर्जिकाक्षारः 134
Swarjikākṣāraḥ (p.133) स्वर्जिकाक्षारः (p.133)
Swarṇabhṛṅgāraḥ - Bhṛṅgarājaḥ (Raj. ni.)
स्वर्णभृङ्गारः - भृङ्गराजः (रा. नि.) 281
Swarṇaḍugdhā - Sarvaksīrī स्वर्णदुग्धा -सर्वक्षीरी 91
Swarṇapārevatam-Pālevatam (Raj.ni.) स्वर्णपारेवतम्-पालेवतम् (रा.नि.) 418
Swarṇaphalā - Suvarṇakadalī स्वर्णफला - सुवर्णकदली 318
Swarṇapuṣpā -Kalikārī (Raj.ni.) स्वर्णपुष्पा - कलिकारी (रा. नि.) 281
Swarṇapuṣpī - Sātalā (Raj. ni.) स्वर्णपुष्पी - सातला (रा.नि.) 89
Swarṇayūthikā - Yūthikā स्वर्णयूथिका - यूथिका 504
Swastikaḥ - Śitivāraḥ स्वस्तिकः -शितिवारः 56
Swastikam-Pālevatam (Raj. ni.) स्वस्तिकम् - पालेवतम् (रा.नि.) 418
Swayamguptā - Kapikacchuḥ स्वयंगुप्ता - कपिकच्छुः 55
Śvetamandāraḥ-Arkaḥ (p.283) (Raj. ni.) श्वेतमन्दारः-अर्कः (p.283) (रा. नि.)
Śyāmā - Priyaṅguḥ श्यामा- प्रियङ्गुः 201
Śyāmā - Strī श्यामा - स्त्री 615
Śyāmā - Haridrā (Raj. ni.) श्यामा - हरिद्रा (रा.नि.) 20
Śyāmā - Padmabījam (Raj. ni.) श्यामा - पद्मबीजम् (रा. नि.) 375
Śyāmā - Pippalī श्यामा - पिप्पली 160
Śyāmā - Surasā (Raj. ni.) श्यामा- सुरसा (रा. नि.) 301
Śyāmā - Trivṛt श्यामा -त्रिवृत् 93
Śyāmaḥ - Dhattūraḥ (Raj. ni.) श्यामः - धत्तूरः (रा. नि.) 278
Śyāmaḥ - Aśanaḥ श्यामः - अशनः 479
Śyāmaḥ - Mahiṣaḥ श्यामः - महिषः 625
Śyāmaḥ - Pīluḥ श्यामः - पीलुः 409
Śyāmākaḥ (p. 545) श्यामाकः (p. 545)
Śyāmakam - Kattṛṇam श्यामकम् - कत्तृणम् 28
Śyāmakandā - Ativiṣā श्यामकन्दा - अतिविषा 4
Śyāmalacchadaḥ - Pippalaḥ श्यामलच्छदः -पिप्पलः 427
Śyāmalaḥ - Pippalaḥ श्यामलः - पिप्पलः 427
Śyāmalapṛṣṭhaḥ - Hariṇaḥ श्यामलपृष्ठः - हरिणः 625
Syāmam - Maricam श्यामम् - मरिचम् 168
Śyāmasāraḥ - Somavalkaḥ श्यामसारः - सोमवल्कः 10
Śyāmavarṇaḥ - Śirīṣaḥ श्यामवर्णः -शिरीषः 463
Śyonākaḥ (p.41) श्योनाकः (p.41)

Tāḍakā - Jimūtakaḥ	ताडका - जीमूतकः	64
Tagaram (p. 221)	तगरम् (p. 221)	
Tailabhāvinī - Jātī	तैलभाविनी - जाती	496
Tailam (p. 569)	तैलम् (p. 569)	
Tailaphalā - Atasī	तैलफला - अतसी	565
Tailaviśeṣāḥ	तैलविशेषाः	572
Takrajanma - Dadhi	तक्रजन्म- दधि	582
Takrakūrcikā	तक्रकूर्चिका	590
Takram (587)	तक्रम् (587)	
Tālaḥ (p. 421)	तालः (p. 421)	
Talāhvayam - Tālīsam (Raj. ni.)	तलाह्वयम् - तालीसम् (रा.नि.)	148
Tālam - Tālisam (Raj. ni.)	तालम् - तालीसम् (रा.नि.)	148
Tālam -Tīkṣṇa Loham	तालम् -तीक्ष्णलोहम्	528
Tālaparṇī - Miśreyā	तालपर्णी - मिश्रेया	122
Tālapatrī - Miśreyā	तालपत्री - मिश्रेया	122
Tālasambhūtā - Vaṃśarocanā (Type) (Raj. ni.)	तालसम्भूता-वंशरोचना(विशेषः) (रा.नि.)	150
Tālavṛkṣaḥ - Nārikelaḥ	तालवृक्षः - नारिकेलः	425
Tālī - Tāmalakī	ताली -तामलकी	240
Tālīsakam - Tālīsam	तालीसकम् - तालीसम्	147
Tālisam (p. 147)	तालीसम् (p. 147)	
Tālīsapatrakam - Tālīsam	तालीसपत्रकम् - तालीसम्	147
Tamakam - Tāmalakī	तमकम् -तामलकी	240
Tamālaḥ - Varuṇaḥ	तमालः - वरुणः	472
Tāmalakī (p. 240)	तामलकी (p. 240)	
Tamālam - Tāmalakī	तमालम् -तामलकी	240
Tamālapatram (p. 146)	तमालपत्रम् (p. 146)	
Tamālinī - Tāmalakī	तमालिनी -तामलकी	240
Tāmarasam - Saugandhikam	तामरसम् - सौगन्धिकम्	371
Tāmbūlavallī - Tāmbulī	ताम्बूलवल्ली - ताम्बूली	273
Tāmbūlī (p. 272)	ताम्बूली (p. 272)	
Tāmracūḍaḥ - Kukkuṭaḥ	ताम्रचूडः - कुक्कुटः	635
Tāmradhātuḥ - Gairikam	ताम्रधातुः - गैरिकम्	262
Tāmrākṣaḥ - Kokilaḥ	ताम्राक्षः - कोकिलः	637
Tāmram (p. 524)	ताम्रम् (p. 524)	
Tāmramūlī - Dhanvayāsaḥ	ताम्रमूली - धन्वयासः	7
Tāmraphalaḥ - Aṅkoṭakaḥ	ताम्रफलः - अङ्कोटकः	99
Tāmrapuṣpā - Pāṭalā	ताम्रपुष्पा - पाटला	43
Tāmrapuṣpaḥ - Kovidāraḥ	ताम्रपुष्पः - कोविदारः	73

Tāmrapuṣpī - Dhātukī तामपुष्पी - धातुकी 242
Tāmrasāram - Raktacandanam ताम्रसारम् - रक्तचंदनम 193
Tāmravarṇaḥ - Kulatthaḥ ताम्रवर्णः - कुलत्थः 557
Tāmrikā - Cūḍāmaṇiḥ ताम्रिका - चूडामणिः 291
Tandrākṛd - Vijayā तन्द्राकृद् - विजया 46
Taṇḍulaḥ - Taṇḍulīyakaḥ तण्डुलः - तण्डुलीयकः 353
Taṇḍulam - Bisam तण्डुलम् - बिसम् 376
Taṇḍulī - Viḍaṅgam तण्डुली - विडङ्गम् 130
Taṇḍulībījaḥ - Taṇḍulīyakaḥ तण्डुलीबीजः - तण्डुलीयकः 355
Taṇḍulīyaḥ - Taṇḍulīyakaḥ तण्डुलीयः - तण्डुलीयकः 355
Taṇḍulīyakaḥ (p. 355) तण्डुलीयकः (p. 355)
Taṅkaḥ - Rājāmraḥ टंकः - राजाम्रः 388
Taṅkaṇaḥ (p.134) टंकणः (p.134)
Taṅkaṇaksāraḥ - Taṅkaṇaḥ टंकणक्षारः - टंकणः 134
Tantrikā - Guḍūcī तन्त्रिका - गुडूची 2
Tanukṡīraḥ - Āmrātakaḥ तनुक्षीरः - आम्रातकः 388
Tanūruham - Roma तनूरुहम् - रोम 644
Tanvī - Hiṅgupatrī तन्वी - हिंगुपत्री 138
Tanvī - Pṛṡni. viṡeṣaḥ तन्वी - पृश्नि. विशेषः 33
Tapanaḥ - Bhallātakaḥ तपनः - भल्लातकः 259
Tapanaḥ - Ṡuklārkaḥ तपनः - शुक्लार्कः 283
Tapanīyam - Suvarṇam तपनीयम् - सुवर्णम् 523
Tāpasaḥ - Nīvāraḥ तापसः - नीवारः 543
Tāpasajam - Tamālapatram तापसजम् - तमालपत्रम् 146
Tāpasapatraḥ-Damanaḥ (Raj. ni.) तापसपत्रः - दमनः (रा. नि.) 228
Tāpasapriyaḥ - Priyālaḥ तापसप्रियः -प्रियालः 423
Tāpasapriyā - Drākṡā तापसप्रिया - द्राक्षा 413
Tāpasī - Gandhapalāṡī तापसी - गन्धपलाशी 22
Tapasvī - Damanaḥ तपस्वी - दमनः 228
Tapasvī - Vyāghraḥ तपस्वी - व्याघ्रः 623
Tapasvinī - Māmsī तपस्विनी - मांसी 217
Tāpījam - Hemamākṡikam तापीजम - हेममाक्षिकम 261
Tapodhanā - Ṡrāvaṇī तपोधना - श्रावणी 58
Taptalomaṡam - Kāsīsam तप्तलोमशम् - कासीसम 251
Taptarūpakam - Raupyam तप्तरूपकम् - रौप्यम 524
Tāpyam - Hemamākṡikam ताप्यम् - हेममाक्षिकम् 261
Tārā - Kapaṭam तारा - कपटम् 29
Tāram - Raupyam तारम् - रौप्यम 524
Tarasvī - Tarakṡuḥ तरस्वी - तरक्षुः 632

Taravaṭah - Cakramardaḥ	तरवटः - चक्रमर्दः	277
Tarkārī - Agnimanthaḥ	तर्कारी -अग्निमंथः	40
Tarakśuḥ (p. 632)	तरक्षुः (p. 632))	
Tārkśyaśailam - Rasāñjanam	ताक्ष्र्यशैलम् - रसाञ्जनम्	265
Taruḥ - Lodhraḥ	तरुः - लोध्रः	267
Taruṇaḥ - Eraṇḍaḥ	तरुणः - एरण्डः	117
Taruṇam - Kapaṭam	तरुणम् - कपटम्	29
Taruṇī - Kapaṭam	तरुणी - कपटम्	29
Taruṇī (p. 501)	तरुणी (p. 501)	
Taruruhā - Vandakā	तरुरुहा - वन्दका	331
Taskarasnāyuḥ - Kākanāsā	तस्करस्नायुः - काकनासा	289
Tavakśirī - Palāśagandhā	तवक्षीरी - पलाशगन्धा	150
Tavarājaḥ - Yavāsaśarkarā	तवराजः - यवासशर्करा	189
Tejaḥ - Śukram	तेजः - शुक्रम्	619
Tejaḥ- Majjā	तेजः - मज्जा	619
Tejanaḥ - Muñjaḥ (Raj. ni.)	तेजनः - मुञ्जः (रा.नि.)	360
Tejanī - Moraṭaḥ	तेजनी - मोरटः	6
Tejanī - Tejasvinī	तेजनी - तेजस्विनी	102
Tejasvinī (p.101)	तेजस्विनी (p.101)	
Tejavatī - Tejasvinī	तेजवती - तेजस्विनी	102
Tejohvā - Tejasvinī	तेजोह्वा - तेजस्विनी	102
Tejomayam - Pittam	तेजोमयम् - पित्तम्	616
Tīkśṇadamṣṭraḥ - Vyāghraḥ	तीक्ष्णदंष्ट्रः - व्याघ्रः	623
Tīkśṇagandhā - Āsurī	तीक्ष्णगन्धा - आसुरी	306
Tīkśṇagandhā - Śvetavacā	तीक्ष्णगन्धा - श्वेतवचा	126
Tīkśṇagandhaḥ - Śigruḥ	तीक्ष्णगन्धः - शिग्रुः	295
Tīkśṇagandhaḥ -Kunduruḥ	तीक्ष्णगन्धः - कुन्दुरुः	254
Tīkśṇakanṭakaḥ - Karīraḥ	तीक्ष्णकंटकः - करीरः	448
Tīkśṇam - Loham	तीक्ष्णम् - लोहम्	528
Tīkśṇam -Tīkśṇa Loham	तीक्ष्णम् -तीक्ष्णलोहम्	528
Tīkśṇamañjarī - Tāmbūlī	तीक्ष्णमञ्जरी - ताम्बूली	273
Tīkśṇapatraḥ -Tumbaruḥ	तीक्ष्णपत्रः - तुम्बरुः	140
Tīkśṇaphalaḥ -Tumbaruḥ	तीक्ष्णफलः - तुम्बरुः	140
Tīkśṇapuṣpā - Ketakī (Raj. ni.)	तीक्ष्णपुष्पा - केतकी (रा.नि.)	521
Tīkśṇasāraḥ - Karīraḥ	तीक्ष्णसारः - करीरः	448
Tīkśṇaśūkaḥ - Yavaḥ	तीक्ष्णशूकः - यवः	538
Tīkśṇataṇḍulā - Pippalī	तीक्ष्णतण्डुला - पिप्पली	160
Tīkśṇavalkaḥ -Tumbaruḥ	तीक्ष्णवल्कः - तुम्बरुः	140
Tiktā - Kaṭukā	तिक्ता - कटुका	15
Tiktabījā - Kaṭukālāmbunī	तिक्तबीजा - कटुकालाम्बुनी	63

Tiktadugdhā - Kśīriṇī	तिक्तदुग्धा - क्षीरिणी	90
Tiktaḥ - Kirātatiktaḥ	तित्तः - किराततित्तः	14
Tiktakandakā - Gandhapalāśī	तित्तःकन्दका - गन्धपलाशी	22
Tiktakarohiṇī - Kaṭukā	तित्तःकरोहिणी - कट्टका	15
Tiktam - Pittam	तित्तःम् - पित्तम्	616
Tiktam - Trapusam	तित्तःम् - त्रपुसम्	65
Tiktāmlā - Yavatiktā (Raj. ni.)	तित्तःाम्ला - यवतित्ता (रा.नि.)	98
Tiktaśākaḥ - Varuṇaḥ	तित्तःशाकः - वरुणः	472
Tiktataṇḍulā - Pippalī (Raj. ni.)	तित्तःतण्डुला - पिप्पली (रा.नि.)	160
Tilaḥ (p. 568)	तिलः (p. 568)	
Tilajam - Tailam	तिलजम् - तैलम्	570
Tilakaḥ - Lodhraḥ	तिलकः - लोध्रः	267
Tilakaḥ (P. 513)	तिलकः (P. 513)	
Tilakī - Śaṅkhapuṣpī	तिलकी - शंखपुष्पी	349
Tilakam - Sauvarcalam	तिलकम् - सौवर्चलम्	136
Tilaparṇakam - Candanam	तिलपर्णकम् -चन्दनम्	191
Tilasambhavam - Tailam	तिलसम्भवम् - तैलम्	570
Tilvakaḥ - Lodhraḥ	तिल्वकः - लोध्रः	267
Timiḥ - Mahāmatsyaviśeṣaḥ	तिमिः - महामत्स्य विशेषः	628
Timiṅgilagilaḥ-Mahāmatsyaviśeṣaḥ	तिमिङ्गिलगिलः - महामत्स्य विशेषः	628
Timiṅgilaḥ-Mahāmatsyaviśeṣaḥ	तिमिङ्गिलः - महामत्स्य विशेषः	628
Timiraḥ - Matsyabhedaḥ	तिमिरः - मत्स्यभेदः	628
Tintiḍīphalam - Jayapālaḥ	तिन्तिडीफलम् - जयपालः	86
Tindukaḥ (p. 401)	तिन्दुकः (p. 401)	401
Tintiḍīkā - Amlikā	तिन्तिडीका - अम्लिका	398
Ṭiṇṭukaḥ - Śyonākaḥ	टिण्टुकः - श्योनाकः	41
Tirīṭakaḥ - Lodhraḥ	तिरीटकः - लोध्रः	267
Tiryaggāmī - Karkaṭaḥ	तिर्यग्गामी - कर्कटः	640
Tiryakphalā - Jantukārī (Raj. ni.)	तिर्यक्फला - जन्तुकारी (रा. नि.)	325
Tittiḍīkam - Vṛkṣāmlam	तित्तिडीकम् - वृक्षाम्लम्	173
Tīvrā - Surasā (Raj. ni.)	तीव्रा- सुरसा (रा. नि.)	301
Tīvrā - Dūrvā	तीव्रा - दूर्वा	368
Tīvrā - Yāvanī Yavānī	तीव्रा - यावनी यवानी	172
Tīvragandhaḥ-Corakaḥ (Raj. ni.)	तीव्रगन्धः - चोरकः (रा. नि.)	232
Tīvragandhaḥ-Yawānī (Raj. ni.)	तीव्रगन्धः - यवानी (रा. नि.)	170
Toyam - Jalam	तोयम् - जलम्	605
Toyam - Vālakam	तोयम् - वालकम्	17
Toyaphalā - Urvāruḥ	तोयफला -उर्वारुः	65
Toyapippalī - Jalapippalī	तोयपिप्पली - जलपिप्पली	310
Toyavallī - Kāṇḍīraḥ	तोयवल्ली-काण्डीरः	309

Trapu - Vaṅgam	त्रपु - वङ्गम्	525
Trapukam - Vaṅgam	त्रपुकम् - वङ्गम्	525
Trapusā - Viśālā	त्रपुसा - विशाला	95
Trapusam (p.64)	त्रपुसम् (p.64)	
Trapusī - Viśālā	त्रपुसी - विशाला	95
Trāsanaḥ - Kalāyaḥ	त्रासनः - कलायः	554
Trāyamāṇā (p.96)	त्रायमाणा (p.96)	
Trāyamāṇakā - Trāyamāṇā	त्रायमाणका - त्रायमाणा	97
Trāyantī - Trāyamāṇā	त्रायन्ती - त्रायमाणा	94
Tribhaṇḍī - Śuklabhaṇḍī	त्रिभण्डी - शुक्लभण्डी	97
Tridivodbhavā - Bhadrailā	त्रिदिवोद्भवा -भद्रैला	142
Tridoṣasambhavaḥ - Mohaḥ	त्रिदोषसंभवः - मोहः	617
Trikaṇṭakaḥ - Matsyaviśeṣaḥ	त्रिकण्टकः - मत्स्यविशेषः	627
Trikaṇṭakaḥ - Gokśuraḥ	त्रिकण्टकः - गोक्षुरः	39
Trikārṣikam - Trikaṭukam	त्रिकार्षिकम् - त्रिकटुकम्	646
Trikaṭukam (p. 646)	त्रिकटुकम् (p. 646)	
Trilavaṇam	त्रिलवणम्	658
Trimadhuram	त्रिमधुरम्	658
Tripādī - Viśvagranthiḥ	त्रिपादी - विश्वग्रंथिः	347
Triparṇaḥ - Kimśukaḥ	त्रिपर्णः - किंशुकः	518
Triparṇakaḥ - Kimśukaḥ	त्रिपर्णकः - किंशुकः	518
Triparṇī - Mūrvā	त्रिपर्णी - मूर्वा	5
Triparṇī - Śāliparṇī	त्रिपर्णी - शालिपर्णी	32
Triphalā (p. 645)	त्रिफला (p. 645)	
Tripuṭā - Bhadrailā	त्रिपुटा-भद्रैला	142
Tripuṭā - Śuklabhaṇḍī	त्रिपुटा - शुक्लभण्डी	94
Tripuṭā - Vārṣikī (Raj.ni.)	त्रिपुटा - वार्षिकी (रा.नि.)	496
Tripuṭaḥ (Karaṭaḥ) (p. 560)	त्रिपुटः (करटः) (p. 560)	
Triśirā - Pāṭhā (Raj. ni.)	त्रिशिरा - पाठा (रा.नि.)	26
Trivelā - Trivṛt (Raj. ni.)	त्रिवेला -त्रिवृत (रा.नि.)	93
Trivṛntāsyaḥ - Kimśukaḥ	त्रिवृन्तास्यः - किंशुकः	518
Trivṛt - Śuklabhaṇḍī	त्रिवृत- शुक्लभण्डी	94
Trivṛt (Śyāmā) (p.92)	त्रिवृत (श्यामा) (p.92)	
Trivṛttā - Pāṭhā (Anyā)	त्रिवृत्ता - पाठा (अन्या)	26
Tṛṇabījaḥ - Śyāmākaḥ	तृणबीजः - श्यामाकः	545
Tṛṇabījottamaḥ - Śyāmākaḥ	तृणबीजोत्तमः - श्यामाकः	545
Tṛṇaketukaḥ - Vamśaḥ	तृणकेतुकः - वंशः	364
Tṛṇam - Kattṛṇam	तृणम - कत्तृणम्	28
Tṛṇapañcamūlam	तृणपञ्चमूलम्	649
Tṛṇarājaḥ - Tālaḥ	तृणराजः - तालः	421

Tṛṇaśuṇṭhaḥ - Guṇṭhaḥ तृणशुण्ठः - गुण्ठः 30
Tṛṇavālukam - Uśīram तृणवालुकम् - उशीरम् 198
Tṛṣākartā - Pittam तृषाकर्ता - पित्तम् 616
Tṛtīyam Cāturbhadrakam तृतीयं चातुर्भद्रकम् 647
Truṭiḥ -Elā त्रुटिः - एला 141
Tryambakam - Tāmram त्र्यम्बकम्- ताम्रम् 524
Tryambakaphalaḥ-Nārikelaḥ (Raj.ni.) त्र्यम्बकफलः-नारिकेलः (रा. निः) 425
Tryasrā - Śuklabhaṇḍī त्र्यस्रा - शुक्लभण्डी 94
Tryasrā - Vārṣikī त्र्यस्रा - वार्षिकी 495
Tryūṣaṇam - Trikaṭukam त्र्यूषणम् - त्रिकट्ठकम् 646
Tūdam (p. 416) तूदम् (p. 416)
Tugā - Vaṁśarocanā तुगा - वंशरोचना 150
Tugākṣīrī - Vaṁśarocanā तुगाक्षीरी - वंशरोचना 150
Tuhinaḥ - Karpūraḥ तुहिनः -कर्पूरः 209
Tūlam - Tūdam तूलम् - तूदम् 416
Tulasī - Surasā तुलसी - सुरसा 301
Tumbaruḥ (p.140) तुम्बरुः (p.140)
Tumbī - Saralaḥ (Raj. ni.) तुम्बी - सरलः (रा. नि.) 237
Tumbī - Kaṭukālāmbunī तुम्बी - कट्ठकालाम्बुनी 63
Tuṇḍī - Bimbī तुण्डी - बिम्बी 76
Tuṇḍikā - Bimbī तुण्डिका - बिम्बी 76
Tuṇḍikeraphalā - Bimbī तुण्डिकेरफला - बिम्बी 76
Tundilaphalā-Trapusam (Raj.ni.) तुन्दिलफला - त्रपुसम् (रा.नि.) 65
Tuṅgā - Śamī तुङ्गा - शमी 442
Tuṅgam -Padmakesaram तुङ्गम् - पद्मकेसरम् 377
Tuṅgī - Ajagandhā तुङ्गी - अजगन्धा 184
Tuṅginī - Mahāśatāvarī तुङ्गिनी - महाशतावरी 116
Tūṇīh (p. 202) तूणिः (p. 202)
Tūṇīkaḥ - Tūṇiḥ तूणीकः - तूणिः 202
Tūṇikaḥ - Tūṇiḥ तूणिकः - तूणिः 202
Turagaḥ - Aśvaḥ तुरगः - अश्वः 621
Turagapriyaḥ - Yavaḥ (Raj. ni.) तुरगप्रियः - यवः (रा. नि.) 539
Turagī - Aśvagandhā तुरगी - अश्वगन्धा 105
Turaṅgadweṣiṇī - Mahiṣī तुरङ्गद्वेषिणी - महिषी 625
Turaṅgaḥ - Aśvaḥ तुरङ्गः - अश्वः 621
Turaṅgamaḥ - Aśvaḥ तुरंगमः - अश्वः 621
Turuṣkaḥ - Yāvanī Yavānī तुरुष्कः- यावनी यवानी 172
Turuṣkaḥ (p. 204) तुरुष्कः (p. 204)
Tuṣāraḥ - Karpūraḥ तुषारः -कर्पूरः 209
Tuṣodakam - Sauvīram तुषोदकम -सौवीरम 595

Tuṣṭaḥ - Tindukaḥ	तुष्टः - तिन्दुकः	402
Tutthā - Elā	तुत्था- एला	141
Tutthā - Nīlinī	तुत्था - नीलिनी	87
Tutthakam - Tuttham	तुत्थकं- तुत्थम्	260
Tuttham (p. 260)	तुत्थम् (p. 260)	
Tuvarī - Āḍhakī	तुवरी - आढकी	548
Tuvarī -Saurāṣṭrī	तुवरी - सौराष्ट्री	247
Tvaṣṭā - Brāhmī	त्वष्टा - ब्राह्मी	336
Twacam - Twak	त्वचम् - त्वक्	145
Twagdoṣam -Kuṣṭham (Raj. ni.)	त्वग्दोषम् - कुष्टम् (रा.नि.)	219
Twagjam - Roma	त्वग्जम् - रोम	644
Twak (p.145)	त्वक् (p.145)	
Twak (p.643)	त्वक् (p.643)	
Twaksāraḥ - Vaṁśaḥ	त्वक्सारः - वंशः	364
Twakśīrī - Vaṁśarocanā	त्वक्क्षीरी - वंशरोचना	150
Twaksugandhā - Bhadrailā	त्वक्सुगन्धा -भद्रैला	142
Twaksugandhaḥ - Nāraṅgaḥ	त्वक्सुगन्धः - नारङ्गः	391
Twāṣṭram - Tāmram	त्वाष्ट्रम् - ताम्रम्	524
Uccaṭā - Cūḍāmaṇiḥ	उच्चटा - चूडामणिः	291
Uccaṭā - Tāmalakī (Raj. ni.)	उच्चटा -तामलकी (रा. नि.)	240
Udadhiphenam-Samudraphenam	उदधिफेनम् - समुद्रफेनम्	263
Udakam - Jalam	उदकम् - जलम्	605
Udakīryaḥ - Karañjaḥ	उदकीर्यः - करञ्जः	461
Uddālaḥ - Kodravaḥ	उद्दालः - कोद्रवः	542
Udīcyam -Vālakam	उदीच्यम् - वालकम्	17
Udumbaram - Tāmram	उदुम्बरम् - ताम्रम्	524
Udumbaraparṇī - Dantī	उदुम्बरपर्णी - दन्ती	84
Udumbaraḥ (p. 435)	उदुम्बरः (p. 435)	
Udvegam - Pūgaphalam	उद्वेगम् - पूगफलम्	213
Ugrā - Methikā	उग्रा - मेथिका	562
Ugrā - Vacā	उग्रा - वचा	125
Ugrabiḍālakaḥ - Biḍālaḥ	उग्रबिडालकः - बिडालः	631
Ugragandhā - Ajamodā (Raj. ni.)	उग्रगन्धा - अजमोदा (रा. नि.)	183
Ugragandhā - Yawānī	उग्रगन्धा - यवानी	169
Ugragandhā - Vacā	उग्रगन्धा - वचा	125
Ugraḥ - Vṛṣabhaḥ	उग्रः - वृषभः	626
Ugraḥ - Ugrabiḍālakaḥ	उग्रः- उग्रबिडालकः	631
Ugrakāṇḍaḥ - Kāṇḍiraḥ	उग्रकाण्डः -काण्डीरः	309
Ulbaṇī - Marjikā	उल्बणी - मर्जिका	605
Ūliḥ - Palāṇḍuḥ	ऊलिः - पलाण्डुः	315

Ulūkaḥ (p.638)	उलूकः (p.638)	
Ulūkajit - Kākaḥ	उलूकजित् - काकः	637
Umā - Atasī	उमा - अतसी	565
Undurukaḥ - Mūṣakaḥ	उन्दुरुकः - मूषकः	630
Unmattakaḥ - Dhattūraḥ	उन्मत्तकः - धत्तूरः	278
Upacitrā - Dantī	उपचित्रा - दन्ती	84
Upadhātavaḥ	उपधातवः	661
Upakālikā - Upakuñcī	उपकालिका - उपकुञ्ची	154
Upakulyā - Pippalī	उपकुल्या - पिप्पली	160
Upakuñcā -Upakuñcī	उपकुञ्चा - उपकुञ्ची	154
Upakuñcī (Pṛthvīkā) (p.153)	उपकुञ्ची (पृथ्वीका) (p.153)	
Upalabhedaḥ - Pāṣānabhedaḥ	उपलभेदः - पाषाणभेदः	57
Uparasāḥ	उपरसाः	662
Uparatnāni	उपरत्नानि	662
Upaviṣāṇi	उपविषाणि	667
Upavyāghraḥ - Śarabhaḥ	उपव्याघ्रः - शरभः	624
Upkuñcī - Elā (Raj. ni.)	उपकुञ्ची - एला (रा. नि.)	141
Urabhraḥ - Aviḥ	उरभ्रः - अविः	623
Uragaḥ - Sarpaḥ	उरगः - सर्पः	638
Uragam - Sīsakam	उरगम् - सीसकम्	526
Uraṇaḥ - Aviḥ	उरणः - अविः	623
Ūrdhvakaṇṭakā - Śatāvarī	ऊर्ध्वकण्टका - शतावरी	115
Ūrdhvakaṇṭikā - Mahāśatāvarī	ऊर्ध्वकण्टिका - महाशतावरी	116
Urdhwadṛk - Karkaṭaḥ	ऊर्ध्वदृक् - कर्कटः	640
Ūrṇāyuḥ - Aviḥ	ऊर्णायुः - अविः	623
Urvāruḥ (p.65)	उर्वारुः (p.65)	
Ūṣaṇā - Pippalī	ऊषणा - पिप्पली	160
Ūṣaṇam - Pippalimūlam	ऊषणम् - पिप्पलीमूलम्	161
Ūṣaṇam - Maricam	ऊषणम् - मरिचम्	168
Ūṣaram - Audbhidam	ऊषरम् - औद्भिदम्	136
Uśīram (p. 198)	उशीरम् (p. 198)	
Uṣṭraḥ (p. 621)	उष्ट्रः (p. 621)	
Uṣṭramūtram	ऊष्ट्रमूत्रम्	643
Uṣṭrī dadhi	उष्ट्री दधि	584
Uṣṭrīghṛtam	उष्ट्रीघृतम्	575
Uṣṭrīpayaḥ	उष्ट्रीपयः	579
Utkaṭā-a type of Śreyasī (Raj.ni.)	उत्कटा - श्रेयसी विशेषः (रा.नि.)	163
Utkaṭaḥ - Śaraḥ	उत्कटः - शरः	363
Utkaṭam - Twak	उत्कटम् - त्वक्	145
Utpalam - Kuṣṭham	उत्पलम् - कुष्ठम्	219

Uttānapatrakaḥ - Raktairaṇḍaḥ उत्तानपत्रकः - रक्तैरण्डः 117

Uttarāpathikā (P. 413) उत्तरापथिका (P. 413)

Utthitopataruḥ - Saralaḥ(Raj. ni.) उत्थितोपतरुः - सरलः (रा. नि.) 237

Vācā (p. 615) वाचा (p. 615)

Vacā (p.125) वचा (p.125)

Vacanī - Vācā वचनी - वाचा 616

Vādanīyaḥ - Vamśaḥ (Raj. ni.) वादनीयः - वंशः (रा.नि.) 365

Vaḍavā - Aśvā वडवा - अश्वा 621

Vadhūḥ - Spṛkkā वधूः - स्पृक्का 224

Vadhūḥ - Śaṭhī वधूः - शठी 22

Vāgūraḥ - Matsyabhedaḥ वागूरः - मत्स्यभेदः 628

Vahnipuṣpā - Dhātukī वह्निपुष्पा - धातुकी 243

Vahniśikham - Kusumbham वह्निशिखम् - कुसुम्भम् 566

Vaidehī - Pippalī (Raj. ni.) वैदेही - पिप्पली (रा.नि.) 160

Vaidyaḥ वैद्यः 660

Vaijayantikā - Agnimanthaḥ वैजयन्तिका -अग्निमंथः 40

Vaikrāntam (p. 530) वैक्रान्तम् (p. 530)

Vaikuṇṭhaḥ - Kuṭherakaḥ वैकुण्ठः - कुठेरकः 304

Vaiṇavī - Vamśarocanā वैणवी - वंशरोचना 150

Vaiparītyā Lajjāluḥ (Raj. ni.)(p.345)वैपरीत्या लज्जालुः (रा.नि.) (p.345)

Vaiśravaṇāvāsaḥ - Vaṭaḥ वैश्रवणावासः- वटः 426

Vaiśvānaraḥ - Pittam वैश्वानरः - पित्तम् 616

Vājī - Aśvaḥ वाजी - अश्वः 621

Vājigandhā - Aśvagandhā वाजिगंधा - अश्वगन्धा 105

Vājīkarī - Aśvagandhā वाजीकरी - अश्वगन्धा 105

Vājinī - Aśvā वाजिनी - अश्वा 621

Vajradamṣṭraḥ - Sūkaraḥ वज्रदंष्ट्रः - सूकरः 624

Vajrajam -Tīkṣṇa Loham वज्रजम् -तीक्ष्णलोहम् 528

Vajrakam - Vaikrāntam वज्रकम् - वैक्रान्तम् 531

Vajrakaṇṭakaḥ - Snuhī वज्रकण्टकः - स्नुही 88

Vajrakārakam - Vyāghranakham वज्रकारकम् - व्याघ्रनखम् 224

Vajraḥ - Hīrakam वज्रः- हीरकम् 531

Vajram - Vaikrāntam वज्रम् - वैक्रान्तम् 531

Vajram -Vālakam वज्रम् - वालकम् 17

Vāk- Vācā वाक् - वाचा 616

Vakrā - Karkaṭaśṛṅgī वक्रा - कर्कटश्रृंगी 30

Vakragrīvaḥ - Uṣṭraḥ वक्रग्रीवः - उष्ट्रः 621

Vakralāṅgūlaḥ - Sārameyaḥ वक्रलाङ्गूलः - सारमेयः 632

Vakram - Tagaram वक्रम् - तगरम् 221

Vaktā - Puruṣaḥ	वक्ता - पुरुषः	615
Vaktrādhivāsanaḥ - Nāraṅgaḥ	वक्त्राधिवासनः - नारङ्गः	391
Vaktraśalyā - Śvetakāmbhojī	वक्त्रशल्या -श्वेतकाम्भोजी	292
Vaktraśalyā - Kākādanī	वक्त्रशल्या - काकादनी	290
Vaktraśodhanam - Bhavam	वक्त्रशोधनम् - भवम्	401
Vaktraśodhī - Jambīraḥ	वक्त्रशोधी - जम्बीरः	389
Vākyalam - Raupyam	वाक्यलम् - रौप्यम्	524
Vālakam - Uśīram	वालकम् - उशीरम्	198
Vālakam (p.17)	वालकम् (p.17)	
Valkalaḥ - Paṭṭikārodhraḥ	वल्कलः -पट्टिकारोध्रः	270
Valkataruḥ - Pūgīvṛkśaḥ	वल्कतरुः -पूगीवृक्षः	214
Vallakī - Śallakī	वल्लकी - शल्लकी	256
Vallam -Tikśṇa Loham	वल्लम् -तीक्ष्णलोहम्	528
Vallarī - Citrakaḥ	वल्लरी - चित्रकः	165
Vallarī - Methikā	वल्लरी - मेथिका	562
Vallī - Ajamodā	वल्ली - अजमोदा	183
Vallī - Aśvakśurakaḥ	वल्ली -अश्वक्षुरकः	323
Vallījam - Maricam	वल्लीजम् - मरिचम्	168
Vallipāṣāṇasambhavam-Pravālam	वल्लीपाषाणसंभवम् - प्रवालम्	534
Vālu - Vālukam	वालु - वालुकम्	66
Vālukam - Elavālukam	वालुकम् - एलवालुकम्	236
Vālukam (p.66)	वालुकम् (p.66)	
Vāmalocanā -Strī	वामलोचना - स्त्री	615
Vamanī - Śaṇapuṣpī	वमनी - शणपुष्पी	75
Vamaśaḥ (p. 364)	वंशः (p. 364)	
Vāmī - Aśvā	वामी - अश्वा	621
Vamśgram (p. 365)	वंशाग्रम् (p. 365)	
Vamśaḥ - Iksuḥ	वंशः - इक्षुः	357
Vamśajā - Vamśarocanā	वंशजा - वंशरोचना	150
Vamśakśīrī - Vamśarocanā	वंशक्षीरी - वंशरोचना	150
Vamśāṅkuraḥ - Vamśāgram	वंशाकुरः - वंशाग्रम्	365
Vamśapatrī - Nāḍihiṅgu	वंशपत्री - नाडीहिंगु	139
Vamśarocanā (p. 150)	वंशरोचना (p. 150)	
Vāmśī - Vamśarocanā	वांशी - वंशरोचना	150
Vamśyā - Vamśarocanā	वंश्या - वंशरोचना	150
Vāmāvartā - Āvartakī	वामावर्ता - आवर्तकी	75
Vanabarbarikā-Sumukhaḥ (Raj.ni.)	वनबर्बरिका -सुमुखः (रा. नि.)	305
Vanabhūṣaṇaḥ - Kokilaḥ	वनभूषणः - कोकिलः	637
Vanacandrikā -Mallikā (Raj. ni.)	वनचंद्रिका - मल्लिका (रा. नि.)	494

Vanagoksīrajā - Vamśarocaṇā (Type) (Raj. ni.)	वनगोक्षीरजा-वंशरोचना (विशेषःरा.नि.)	150
Vanajā - Mudgaparṇī	वनजा -मुद्‌गपर्णी	49
Vanajā - Kāsaghnī	वनजा - कासघ्नी	37
Vanajā - Śephālikā	वनजा - शेफालिका	321
Vanajaḥ -Tumbaruḥ	वनजः - तुम्बरुः	140
Vanajamūrdhajā - Karkaṭasṛṅgī	वनजमूर्धजा - कर्कटशृंगी	30
Vanakhaṇḍā - Padminī	वनखण्डा - पद्मिनी	374
Vanakodravaḥ - Kodravaḥ	वनकोद्रवः - कोद्रवः	542
Vanamālikā - Graiṣmī	वनमालिका - ग्रैष्मी	498
Vanamālinī - Graiṣmī	वनमालिनी - ग्रैष्मी	498
Vanaṃālinī - Vārāhī	वनमालिनी - वाराही	326
Vanamethikā (p. 563)	वनमेथिका (p. 563)	
Vanamudgaḥ - Makuṣṭhakaḥ	वनमुद्‌गः - मकुष्ठकः	548
Vānaprasthaḥ - Madhūkaḥ	वानप्रस्थः -मधूकः	406
Vanapriyam - Twak	वनप्रियम् - त्वक्	145
Vanapuspotsavaḥ - Āmraḥ	वनपुष्पोत्सवः - आम्रः	385
Vānaraḥ - Markaṭaḥ	वानरः - मर्कटः	632
Vanarambhā-Girikadalī (Raj.ni.)	वनरम्भा - गिरिकदली (रा. नि.)	317
Vanaspatiḥ - Vaṭaḥ	वनस्पतिः - वटः	426
Vanasthā - Aśvatthī	वनस्था - अश्वत्थी	428
Vanaukaḥ - Markaṭaḥ	वनौकः - मर्कटः	632
Vanavāsī - Vārāhī (Raj. ni.)	वनवासी - वाराही (रा. नि.)	327
Vanavilāsinī - Śaṅkhapuṣpī	वनविलासिनी - शंखपुष्पी	349
Vandakā (p. 331)	वन्दका (p. 331)	
Vandākaḥ - Vandakā	वन्दाकः - वन्दका	331
Vandanīyā - Rocanā	वन्दनीया - रोचना	203
Vandhyakarkoṭakī (p.68)	वन्ध्यकर्कोटकी (p.68)	
Vandhyāputrapradā-Vandhyakarkoṭakī	वन्ध्यापुत्रप्रदा-वन्ध्यकर्कोटकी	68
Vāneyam - Jalamustam	वानेयम् - जलमुस्तम्	16
Vaṅgam (p. 525)	वङ्गम (p. 525)	
Vanhiḥ - Citrakaḥ	वह्निः - चित्रकः	165
Vanhimanthaḥ - Agnimanthaḥ	वह्निमन्थः -अग्निमंथः	40
Vanhimathanaḥ - Agnimanthaḥ	वह्निमथनः -अग्निमंथः	40
Vāṇī - Vācā	वाणी - वाचा	616
Vānīrajaḥ - Muñjaḥ (Raj. ni.)	वानीरजः - मुञ्जः (रा.नि.)	360
Vānīrajam - Kuṣṭham	वानीरजम - कुष्टम	219
Vanitā -Strī	वनिता - स्त्री	615
Vañjuladrumaḥ-Aśokaḥ (Raj.ni.)	वञ्जुलद्रुमः - अशोकः (रा.नि.)	516
Vañjulaḥ - Vetasaḥ	वञ्जुलः - वेतसः	467

Vanyadamanaḥ-Damaḥ (Raj.ni.)	वन्यदमनः- दमः (रा. नि.)	229
Vanyaḥ - Mahānalaḥ	वन्यः - महानलः	367
Vanyajīraḥ - Bṛhatpālī	वन्यजीरः - बृहत्पाली	159
Vanyam - Paripellavam	वन्यम् - परिपेल्लवम्	222
Vanyamudgaḥ - Mudgaḥ (a type)	वन्यमुद्गः -मुद्ग विशेषः	541
Vapuḥ - Śarīram	वपुः - शरीरम्	615
Vāpyam - Kuṣṭham	वाप्यम् - कुष्ठम्	219
Varā - Pāṭhā	वरा - पाठा	26
Varā - Surā	वरा - सुरा	596
Varā - Triphalā	वरा - त्रिफला	645
Varadā - Suvarcalā	वरदा - सुवर्चला	333
Varāhaḥ - Mustā	वराहः - मुस्ता	15
Varāhaḥ - Sūkaraḥ	वराहः - सूकरः	624
Varāhakandaḥ - Vārāhī (Raj. ni.)	वराहकन्दः - वाराही (रा.नि.)	327
Varāhakarṇī - Aśvagandhā	वराहकर्णी - अश्वगन्धा	105
Varāham - Hīrakam	वराहम् - हीरकम्	532
Vārāhī (p. 326)	वाराही (p. 326)	
Varakaḥ - Kṛṣṇamudgaḥ	वरकः - कृष्णमुद्गः	541
Varam - Kumkumam	वरम् - कुंकुमम्	197
Varāmlaḥ - Bījapūraḥ	वराम्लः - बीजपूरः	396
Vāraṇaḥ - Hasti	वारणः - हस्ति	620
Varāṅgam - Twak	वराङ्गम् - त्वक्	145
Varaṅgī - Araṇī	वराङ्गी - अरणी	85
Varatiktā - Pāṭhā	वरतिक्ता - पाठा	26
Varatiktaḥ - Parpaṭaḥ	वरतिक्तः - पर्पटः	17
Varavarṇinī - Haridrā	वरवर्णिनी - हरिद्रा	20
Vardhamānā - Madhukarkaṭī	वर्धमाना - मधुकर्कटी	398
Vardhamānaḥ - Eraṇḍaḥ	वर्धमानः - एरण्डः	117
Vāri - Jalam	वारि - जलम्	605
Varī - Śatāvarī	वरी - शतावरी	115
Vāri - Vālakam	वारि - वालकम्	17
Vāribhavaḥ - Śaṅkhaḥ	वारिभवः - शंखः	271
Vārisambhavam - Lavaṅgam	वारिसंभवम् - लवङ्गम्	214
Vāritaram - Uśīram (Raj. ni.)	वारितरम् - उशीरम् (रा.नि.)	199
Varmakaṇṭakaḥ - Parpaṭaḥ	वर्मकण्टकः - पर्पटः	17
Varṇabhedinī - Priyaṅguḥ	वर्णभेदिनी - प्रियङ्गुः	201
Varṇaprasādanam - Kāleyakam	वर्णप्रसादनम् - कालेयकम्	207
Varṇapūrakaḥ - Śāliḥ	वर्णपूरकः -शालिः	535
Varṇavatī - Haridrā	वर्णवती - हरिद्रा	20

Varṇavilāsinī - Haridrā	वर्णविलासिनी - हरिद्रा	20
Varṇyapuṣpakaḥ-Taruṇī (Raj.ni.)	वर्ण्यपुष्पकः - तरुणी (रा. नि.)	501
Varṣā - Kṛṣṇajīrakaḥ	वर्षा - कृष्णजीरकः	158
Varṣaketuḥ - Krūraḥ	वर्षकेतुः -क्रूरः	108
Vārṣikī - Trāyamāṇā	वार्षिकी - त्रायमाणा	97
Vārṣikī (p. 495)	वार्षिकी (p. 495)	
Vartaloham (p. 528)	वर्तलोहम् (p. 528)	
Vartakaloham - Vartaloham	वर्तकलोहम् - वर्तलोहम्	528
Vārtākī -Bṛhatī	वार्ताकी - बृहती	35
Vārtākinī - Kāsaghnī	वार्ताकिनी - कासघ्नी	37
Vartikā - Ajaśṛṅgi	वर्तिका - अजश्रृंगी	31
Vārtikā -Vṛntākī	वार्तिका - वृन्ताकी	37
Vartulaḥ - Kalāyaḥ	वर्तुलः - कलायः	554
Vartulaḥ - Guṇṭhaḥ	वर्तुलः - गुण्ठः	30
Vartulam - Gṛñjanam	वर्तुलम् - गृञ्जनम्	295
Vartuloham - Vartaloham	वर्त्तुलोहम् - वर्तलोहम्	528
Varuṇaḥ (p. 472)	वरुणः (p. 472)	
Vāruṇam - Jalam	वारुणम् - जलम्	605
Varuṇam - Jīrakam	वरुणम् - जीरकम्	157
Varuṇātmajā - Surā	वरुणात्मजा - सुरा	596
Vāruṇī - Dūrvā	वारुणी - दूर्वा	368
Vāruṇī - Śve. indravāruṇī	वारुणी - इन्द्रवारुणी (श्वे.)	96
Vāruṇī - Surā	वारुणी - सुरा	596
Vasā (p. 618)	वसा (p. 618)	
Vāsā -Vāsakaḥ	वासा - वासकः	9
Vasādanī - Śimśapā	वसादनी - शिंशपा	473
Vāsaḥ - Tamālapatram	वासः - तमालपत्रम्	146
Vāsakaḥ (p.9)	वासकः (p.9)	
Vasantadūtaḥ - Āmraḥ	वसन्तदूतः - आम्रः	386
Vasantadūtaḥ - Kokilaḥ	वसन्तदूतः - कोकिलः	637
Vasantadūtī - Pāṭalā	वसन्तदूती - पाटला	43
Vasantadūtī - Vāsantī (Raj. ni.)	वसन्तदूती - वासन्ती (रा. नि.)	499
Vāsantaḥ - Bibhītakaḥ	वासन्तः - बिभीतकः	78
Vāsantaḥ - Tilakaḥ (Raj. ni.)	वासन्तः - तिलकः (रा.नि.)	514
Vāsantaḥ - Mudgaḥ	वासन्तः -मुद्गः	540
Vasantajā - Vāsantī	वसन्तजा - वासन्ती	498
Vasantapādapaḥ - Āmraḥ	वसन्तपादपः - आम्रः	386
Vāsantī (p. 498)	वासन्ती (p. 498)	
Vasantotsavamaṇḍanam-Sindūraḥ	वसन्तोत्सवमण्डनम् - सिन्दूरः	246

Va'sirah - Rakt. Apāmārgah वशिरः -र.अपामार्गः 101
Va'sirah - Apāmārgah वशिरः -अपामार्गः 100
Vāsitā - Strī वासिता - स्त्री 615
Vasrā - Vasā वस्रा - वसा 619
Vāstikā - Vanamethikā वास्तिका - वनमेथिका 563
Vastrabhūṣaṇā - Mañjiṣṭhā वस्त्रभूषणा - मञ्जिष्ठा 7
Vastram - Tamālapatram वस्त्रम् - तमालपत्रम् 146
Vastrarañjakam - Kusumbham वस्त्ररञ्जकम् - कुसुम्भम् 566
Vasu - Ṛddhiḥ वसु -ऋद्धि 53
Vasu - Audbhidam वसु - औद्भिदम् 136
Vasuccidrā - Mahāmdeā वसुच्छिद्रा - महामेदा 46
Vasukaḥ - Asitamudgaḥ वसुकः - असितमुद्गः 540
Vasukaḥ -Bukaḥ वसुकः - बुकः 284
Vasukaḥ - Rajārkaḥ वसुकः - राजार्कः 282
Vasukam - Audbhidam वसुकम् - औद्भिदम् 136
Vasu'sreṣṭham - Raupyam वसुश्रेष्ठम् - रौप्यम् 524
Vasutarkā - Atas वसुतर्का - अतसी 565
Vātabhūtavina'sanī - Kapaṭam वातभूतविनाशनी - कपटम् 29
Vaṭah (p. 426) वटः (p. 426)
Vaṭapatrā - Mallikā (Raj. ni.) वटपत्रा - मल्लिका (रा. नि.) 494
Vaṭapatra kuṭherakaḥ-Kuṭherakaḥ वटपत्रकुठेरकः - कुठेरकः 304
Vaṭaplavaḥ - Plak'saḥ वटप्लवः -प्लक्षः 429
Vātapothaḥ - Kim'sukaḥ वातपोथः - किंशुकः 518
Vātāriḥ - Sūraṇaḥ वातारिः - सूरणः 383
Vātasāraḥ - Bilvaḥ वातसारः - बिल्वः 39
Vaṭasaugandhikaḥ (p. 248) वटसौगन्धिकः (p. 248)
Vāṭī - Balā वाटी - बला 110
Vatsādanaḥ - Vṛkaḥ वत्सादनः - वृकः 623
Vatsādanī - Guḍūcī वत्सादनी - गुडूची 2
Vatsakaḥ - Kuṭajaḥ वत्सकः - कुटजः 131
Vatsanābhaḥ वत्सनाभः 664
Vatsanābhaḥ (p.667) वत्सनाभः (p.667) 667
Vāṭyapuṣpam वाट्यपुष्पम् 653
Vāṭyapuṣpī - Atibalā वाट्यपुष्पी - अतिबला 113
Vāṭyapuṣpī - Mahābalā वाट्यपुष्पी - महाबला 111
Vāṭyāyanī - Mahābalā वाट्यायनी - महाबला 111
Vayaḥsthā - Harītakī वयःस्था - हरीतकी 77
Vayaḥsthā - Āmalakī वयःस्था - आमलकी 79
Vāyasaḥ - Kākaḥ वायसः - काकः 637
Vāyasek'sukaḥ - Kā'saḥ वायसेक्षुकः - काशः 359

Vāyasī - Kākamācī	वायसी - काकमाची	285
Vāyasolī - Kākolī	वायसोली - काकोली	47
Vayasthā - Guḍūcī	वयस्था- गुड्ची	2
Vayasthā - Kākolī	वयस्था - काकोली	47
Vayasthā - Kṣīrakākolī	वयस्था - क्षीरकाकोली	47
Vāyavālam - Gārutmatam	वायवालम् - गारुत्मतम्	531
Vāyavyā - Karañjaḥ	वायव्या - करञ्जः	462
Vāyuḥ (p.616)	वायुः (p. 616)	
Vedhamukhayā - Kastūrikā	वेधमुख्या - कस्तूरिका	208
Vedhamukhyaḥ - Karcūraḥ	वेधमुख्यः - कर्चूरः	244
Vegapūjitaḥ - Aśvataraḥ	वेगपूजितः - अश्वतरः	622
Veṇī - Jīmūtakaḥ	वेणी - जीमूतकः	64
Veṇuḥ - Vaṃśaḥ	वेणुः - वंशः	364
Veṇuniḥsvanaḥ - Ikṣuḥ	वेणुनिःस्वनः - इक्षुः	357
Veṇupatrī - Nāḍihiṅgu	वेणुपत्री - नाडीहिंगु	139
Veśavāraḥ	वेशवारः	650,651
Vetasaḥ (p. 467)	वेतसः (p. 467)	
Vetasāmlaḥ - Amlavetasaḥ	वेतसाम्लः - अम्लवेतसः	177
Vetasī - Jambūḥ	वेतसी - जम्बूः	433
Vibhāṇḍī - Āvartakī	विभाण्डी - आवर्तकी	74
Vicitraḥ - Aśokaḥ	विचित्रः - अशोकः	516
Vicitram - Śirṇavṛntam	विचित्रम् - शीर्णवृन्तम्	66
Viḍaṅgam (p.130)	विडङ्गम् (p.130)	
Vidārī (p.53)	विदारी (p.53)	
Vidārikā - Vidārī	विदारिका -विदारी	54
Vidrumalatā - Nalikā	विद्रुमलता - नलिका	216
Vidrumam - Pravālam	विद्रुमम् - प्रवालम्	534
Vidulaḥ - Vetasaḥ	विदुलः- वेतसः	467
Vidulā - Sātalā	विदुला - सातला	89
Vigandhikā - Ajagandhā	विगन्धिका - अजगन्धा	184
Vighneśavāhanaḥ-Mahāmūṣakaḥ	विघ्नेशवाहनः - महामूषकः	631
Vijayā - Balāmoṭā	विजया - बलामोटा	378
Vijayā (Bhaṅgā) (p.46)	विजया (भङ्गा) (p.46)	
Vijayā - Harītakī	विजया - हरीतकी	77
Vijayā - Mañjiṣṭhā	विजया - मञ्जिष्ठा	7
Vijayā - Śvetavacā	विजया - श्वेतवचा	126
Vikaṅkataḥ (p. 404)	विकंकतः (p. 404)	
Vikarṇam - Sthauṇeyakam	विकर्णम् - स्थौणेयकम्	230
Vikasā - Māṃsarohiṇī	विकसा - मांसरोहिणी	330

Vikasā - Mañjiṣṭhā	विकसा - मञ्जिष्ठा	7
Viksīraḥ - Arkaḥ	विक्षीरः - अर्कः	282
Vikīraṇaḥ - Arkaḥ	विकीरणः - अर्कः	282
Vikīrṇam-Sthauṇeyakam (Raj.ni.)	विकीर्णम् - स्थौणेयकम् (रा. नि.)	230
Vikrāntaḥ - Simhaḥ	विक्रान्तः - सिंहः	624
Viloḍitam - Mathita dadhi	विलोडितं - मथितदधि	583
Vimalā - Sātalā	विमला - सातला	89
Vipāṇḍuḥ - Trapusam	विपाण्डुः - त्रपुसम्	65
Vipraḥ - Pippalaḥ	विप्रः -पिप्पलः	427
Vipralambhī - Kinkirātaḥ	विप्रलम्भी - किंकिरातः	511
Viprāngī - Kaṭukā	विप्राङ्गी - कटुका	15
Vīpuṣā - Hapuṣā	विपुषा - हपुषा	128
Vīrā - Kṡīrakākolī	वीरा - क्षीरकाकोली	47
Virajapatrikā - Nākulī (Raj. ni.)	विरजपत्रिका - नाकुली (रा.नि.)	340
Vīram - Ārukam	वीरम् - आरुकम्	399
Vīram - Loham	वीरम् - लोहम्	528
Vīram - Uṡīram	वीरम् - उशीरम्	198
Vīrāmlaḥ-Amlavetasaḥ (Raj. ni.)	वीराम्लः- अम्लवेतसः (रा.नि.)	177
Vīraṇamūlakam - Uṡīram	वीरणमूलकम् - उशीरम्	198
Vīrangam - Kamkuṣṭham	विरंगम् - कंकुष्ठम्	259
Vīraṇīmūlam - Uṡīram	वीरणीमूलम् - उशीरम्	198
Vīrāntakaḥ - Arjunaḥ	वीरान्तकः -अर्जुनः	464
Virārukam -Ārukam	वीरारुकम् -आरुकम्	399
Vīrastaṇḍulaḥ-Taṇḍulīyakaḥ(Raj.ni.)	वीरस्तण्डुलः-तण्डुलीयकः (रा.नि.)	355
Vīrataram - Uṡīram	वीरतरम् - उशीरम्	198
Vīrataruḥ - Bhallātakaḥ	वीरतरुः - भल्लातकः	259
Vīravetasaḥ - Amlavetasaḥ	वीरवेतसः - अम्लवेतसः	177
Vīravetasaḥ-Amlavetasaḥ (Raj.ni.)	वीरवेतसः - अम्लवेतसः (रा.नि.)	177
Virecanaphalaḥ - Pīluḥ	विरेचनफलः - पीलुः	409
Vīrasenam - Ārukam	वीरसेनम् - आरुकम्	399
Virulaḥ - Jalasarpaḥ	विरुलः - जलसर्पः	639
Virūpā - Ativiṣā	विरूपा - अतिविषा	4
Vīryagarbhapratānaḥ - Paṭolaḥ	वीर्यगर्भप्रतानः - पटोलः	18
Vīryam - Ṡukram	वीर्यम् - शुक्रम्	619
Viṣabhadrikā - Araṇī	विषभद्रिका - अरणी	85
Viṣadā - Bṛhatī	विषदा - बृहती	35
Viṣadharaḥ - Sarpaḥ	विषधरः - सर्पः	639
Viṣaghnaḥ - Ṡephalikā	विषघ्नः - शेफालिका	321
Viṣaghnī - Haridrā	विषघ्नी - हरिद्रा	20
Viṣaghnī (Pṛṡni.) viṡeṣaḥ	विषघ्नी - (पृश्नि.) विशेषः	33

Viṣaghnī-Kāṣṭhakadalī	विषघ्नी - काष्ठकदली	317
Viṣahā - Śirīṣaḥ	विषहा - शिरीषः	463
Viśākhaḥ - Punarnavā	विशाखः - पुनर्नवा	107
Visakaṇṭakinī-Vandhyakarkoṭakī	विषकण्टकिनी - वन्ध्यकर्कोटकी	68
Viśālā (p.89)	विशाला (p.89)	
Viśalyā - Dantī	विशल्या - दन्ती	84
Viśalyā - Kalikārī	विशल्या - कलिकारी	280
Viśalyā - Guḍūcī	विशल्या - गुडूची	2
Viṣam, Viṣabhedāḥ	विषम् विषभेदाः	663
Viṣamardinī - Gandhanākulī	विषमर्दिनी - गन्धनाकुली	342
Viṣamohapraśamanī - Balāmoṭā	विषमोहप्रशमनी - बलामोटा	378
Viṣamugram - Vatasanābhaḥ	विषमुग्रम् - वत्सनाभः	667
Viṣamuṣṭikaḥ - Mahānimbaḥ	विषमुष्टिकः - महानिम्बः	12
Viṣāṇaḥ - Mahiṣaḥ	विषाणः - महिषः	625
Viṣāṇī - Āvartakī	विषाणी - आवर्तकी	75
Viṣāṇī - Karkaṭaśṛṅgī	विषाणी - कर्कटशृंगी	30
Viṣāṇī - Ṛṣabhaḥ	विषाणी - ऋषभः	45
Viṣāṇī (to be avoided)	वर्ज्यविषाणि	663-664
Viṣāṇikā -Ajaśṛṅgī	विषाणिका - अजशृंगी	31
Viṣāṇikā - Sātalā (Raj. ni.)	विषाणिका - सातला (रा.नि.)	89
Viṣapraśamanī - Karkoṭakī	विषप्रशमनी - कर्कोटकी	69
Viṣapuṣpakaḥ - Madanaḥ	विषपुष्पकः - मदनः	62
Viśāradaḥ - Bakulaḥ	विशारदः -. बकुलः	511
Visarpiṇī - Yavatikta	विसर्पिणी - यवतिक्ता	98
Viśeṣakaḥ - Tilakaḥ	विशेषकः - तिलकः	513
Viśiṣṭam - Sīsakam	विशिष्टम् - सीसकम्	526
Viṣkiraḥ - Kukkuṭaḥ	विष्किरः - कुक्कुटः	636
Viṣṇuguptam-Cāṇākhyamūlakam	विष्णुगुप्तम्- चाणाख्यमूलकम्	293
Viṣṇukrāntā (P. 352)	विष्णुक्रान्ता (P. 352)	
Viṣṇuvallabhā - Surasā (Raj. ni.)	विष्णुवल्लभा - सुरसा (रा. नि.)	301
Viśodhanī - Nīlinī	विशोधनी - नीलिनी	87
Viśokaḥ - Aśokaḥ	विशोकः - अशोकः	516
Visrā - Hapuṣā	विस्रा - हपुषा	128
Visram - Raktam	विस्रम् - रक्तम्	619
Visrgandhā - Hapuṣā	विस्रगन्धा - हपुषा	128
Viṣṭhā - Malam	विष्ठा - मलम्	640
Viśuddham - Śāliparṇī viśeṣaḥ	विशुद्धम - शालिपर्णी विशेषः	32
Viśvā - Ativiṣā	विश्वा- अतिविषा	4
Viśvabheṣajam - Śuṇṭhī	विश्वभेषजम् - शुण्ठी	167
Viśvadevā - Gāṅgerukī	विश्वदेवा - गांगेरुकी	112
Viśvagranthiḥ (p. 347)	विश्वगंथिः (p. 347)	

Viṣvaksenakāntā - Vārāhī विष्वक्सेनकान्ता - वाराही 326
Viśvam - Śuṇṭhī विश्वम् - शुण्ठी 167
Viśvarūpakam - Agaru विश्वरूपकम् - अगरु 206
Viśvauṣadham - Śuṇṭhī विश्वौषधम् - शुण्ठी 167
Viṭ - Malam विट् - मलम् 640
Vitānakaḥ- Māḍaḥ वितानकः - माडः 422
Vitunnā - Tāmalakī (Raj. ni.) वितुन्ना -तामलकी (रा. नि.) 240
Vitunnabhūtā - Tāmalakī वितुन्नभूता -तामलकी 240
Vitunnakam - Dhānyakam वितुन्नकम् - धान्यकम् 156
Valkalā - Tejasvinī वल्कला - तेजस्विनी 102
Vraṇahārakaḥ-Kadambaḥ (Raj.ni.) व्रणहारकः - कदम्बः (रा. नि.) 453
Vraṇapriyam - Uśīram व्रणप्रियम् - उशीरम् 198
Vraṇāriḥ - Bolam (Raj. ni.) व्रणारिः - बोलम् (रा.नि.) 226
Vṛddhadārukaḥ (p. 342) वृद्धदारुकः (p. 342)
Vṛddhaḥ - Vṛddhadārukaḥ वृद्धः - वृद्धदारुकः 343
Vṛddhiḥ - Ṛddhiḥ वृद्धिः -ऋद्धिः 53
Vṛddhikaram - Śukram वृद्धिकरम् - शुक्रम् 619
Vṛddham - Śaileyam वृद्धम् - शलेयम् 235
Vrīhiḥ (p. 537) व्रीहिः (p. 537)
Vṛkaḥ (p. 623) वृकः (p. 623)
Vṛkī -Pāṭhā वृकी - पाठा 26
Vṛkśādanī - Vandakā वृक्षादनी - वन्दका 331
Vṛkśakabījāni - Indrayavāḥ वृक्षकबीजानि - इन्द्रयवाः 131
Vṛkśakaḥ - Kuṭajaḥ वृक्षकः - कुटजः 131
Vṛkśāmlam (p. 173) वृक्षाम्लम् (p. 173)
Vṛkśaroham - Śvāsāriḥ वृक्षरोहम् - श्वासारिः 25
Vṛkśaruhā - Jantukārī (Raj. ni.) वृक्षरुहा - जन्तुकारी (रा. नि.) 325
Vṛkśaruhā - Vandakā वृक्षरुहा - वन्दका 331
Vṛkśaśrayī - Kśudrolūkaḥ वृक्षाश्रयी - क्षुद्रोलूकः 638
Vṛndārakaḥ - Śāliḥ वृन्दारकः - शालिः 535
Vṛntā - Vṛntākī वृन्ता - वृन्ताकी 37
Vṛntakah - Śāliḥ वृन्तकः - शालिः 535
Vṛntākī (p.37) वृन्ताकी (p.37)
Vṛṣā (Viṣā) - Dravantī वृषा - (विषा) - द्रवन्ती 86
Vṛṣabhaḥ - Ṛṣabhaḥ वृषभः - ऋषभः 45
Vṛṣabhaḥ (p. 625) वृषभः (p. 625)
Vṛṣabhākśī - Indravāruṇī वृषभाक्षी - इन्द्रवारुणी 95
Vṛṣadamśaḥ - Biḍālaḥ वृषदंशः - बिडालः 631
Vṛṣadhwaṅkśī - Mustā वृषध्वाङ्क्षी - मुस्ता 15
Vṛṣagandhā - Vṛṣamedhā वृषगन्धा -वृषमेधा 118
Vṛṣaḥ - Ṛṣabhaḥ वृषः - ऋषभः 45

Vṛṣaḥ - Vṛṣabhaḥ	वृषः - वृषभः	626
Vṛṣaḥ - Vāsakaḥ	वृषः - वासकः	9
Vṛṣākaraḥ - Māṣaḥ	वृषाकरः - माषः	552
Vṛṣamedhā (p.118)	वृषमेधा (p.118)	
Vṛṣabhī (Ṛṣabhī) - Dadhipuṣpī	वृषभी (ऋषभी) - दधिपुष्पी	56
Vṛścikālī - Ajaśṛṅgī	वृश्चिकाली -अजश्रृंगी	31
Vṛścīraḥ - Punarnavā	वृश्चीरः - पुनर्नवा	107
Vṛṣṇiḥ - Aviḥ	वृष्णिः - अविः	623
Vṛṣyakandā - Vidārī	वृष्यकन्दा -विदारी	54
Vṛṣyam - Āmalakī	वृष्यम् - आमलकी	79
Vṛṣyavallī - Vidārī	वृष्यवल्ली -विदारी	54
Vṛttā - Priyaṅguḥ	वृत्ता- प्रियङ्गुः	201
Vṛttā - Māṃsarohiṇī	वृत्ता - मांसरोहिणी	330
Vṛttabījā - Āḍhakī	वृत्तबीजा - आढकी	548
Vṛttaguṇaḥ - Guṇṭhaḥ	वृत्तगुणः - गुण्ठः	29
Vṛttaḥ - Kacchapaḥ	वृत्तः - कच्छपः	630
Vṛttakośaḥ - Jīmūtakaḥ	वृत्तकोशः - जीमूतकः	64
Vṛttamallikā - Mallikā (Raj. ni.)	वृत्तमल्लिका - मल्लिका (रा. नि.)	494
Vṛttamallikā - Śuklārkaḥ	वृत्तमल्लिका- शुक्लार्कः	283
Vṛttapuṣpā - Mallikā (Raj. ni.)	वृत्तपुष्पा - मल्लिका (रा. नि.)	494
Vṛttapuṣpaḥ - Kadambaḥ	वृत्तपुष्पः - कदम्बः	451
Vṛttapuṣpakaḥ - Kadambaḥ	वृत्तपुष्पकः - कदम्बः	452
Vyādhiḥ - Kuṣṭham	व्याधिः - कुष्ठम्	219
Vyādhighātaḥ - Karṇikāraḥ	व्याधिघातः - कर्णिकारः	81
Vyādhihā - Āragvadhaḥ	व्याधिहा - आरग्वधः	80
Vyādhiripuḥ - Karṇikāraḥ	व्याधिरिपुः - कर्णिकारः	82
Vyāghradalaḥ - Raktairaṇḍaḥ	व्याघ्रदलः - रक्तैरण्डः	117
Vyāghraḥ (p. 623)	व्याघ्रः (p. 623)	
Vyāghraḥ - Raktairaṇḍaḥ	व्याघ्रः - रक्तैरण्डः	117
Vyāghranakham (p. 223)	व्याघ्रनखम् (p. 223)	
Vyāghrapādaḥ - Vikaṅkataḥ	व्याघ्रपादः - विकंकतः	405
Vyāghratalam - Vyāghranakham	व्याघ्रतलम् - व्याघ्रनखम्	223
Vyāghrāyudham-Vyāghranakham	व्याघ्रायुधम् - व्याघ्रनखम्	223
Vyāghrī - Kaṇṭakārī	व्याघ्री -कण्टकारी	35
Vyāladaṃṣṭrakaḥ - Gokṣuraḥ	व्यालदंष्ट्रकः - गोक्षुरः	38
Vyālagandhā - Nākulī	व्यालगन्धा - नाकुली	340
Vyālaḥ - Citrakaḥ	व्यालः - चित्रकः	165
Vyālaḥ - Sarpaḥ	व्यालः - सर्पः	638
Vyālapatrā - Urvāruḥ	व्यालपत्रा -उर्वारुः	65
Vyathāntakaḥ - Karṇikāraḥ	व्यथान्तकः - कर्णिकारः	81
Vyāvartakaḥ - Cakramardaḥ	व्यावर्तकः - चक्रमर्दः	277
Vyoṣam - Trikaṭukam	व्योषम् - त्रिकटुकम्	646

Yajñāṅgaḥ - Udumbaraḥ यज्ञाङ्गः - उदुम्बरः 436
Yajñāṅgaḥ - Khadiraḥ यज्ञाङ्गः - खदिरः 10
Yājñikaḥ - Kimśukaḥ याज्ञिकः - किंशुकः 518
Yajñīyaḥ - Vikaṅkataḥ (Raj. ni.) यज्ञीयः - विकंकतः (रा.नि.) 405
Yajñiyapatrakaḥ-Kuśaḥ (Raj.ni.) यज्ञीयपत्रकः - कुशः (रा.नि.) 362
Yajñanetrī - Somvallī यज्ञनेत्री - सोमवल्ली
Yakśadhūpaḥ - Rālaḥ यक्षधूपः - रालः 250
Yakśakardamaḥ यक्षकर्दमः 653
Yakśāvāsaḥ - Vaṭaḥ (Raj. ni.) यक्षावासः - वटः(रा.नि.) 426
Yakśataruḥ - Vaṭaḥ (Raj . ni.) यक्षतरुः - वटः (रा.नि.) 426
Yamadrumaḥ-Śālmaliveṣṭakaḥ (Raj.ni.) यमद्रुमः-शाल्मलीवेष्टकः(रा.नि.)481
Yamalapatrakaḥ - Aśmantakaḥ यमलपत्रकः - अश्मन्तकः 72
Yāmuneyam - Añjanam यामुनेयम् - अञ्जनम् 262
Yāsaḥ - Dhanvayāsaḥ यासः - धन्वयासः 7
Yāsaḥ (p.8) यासः (p. 8)
Yaśaskarī - Jīvantī यशस्करी - जीवन्ती 49
Yaśaskarī - Trāyamāṇā यशस्करी - त्रायमाणा 98
Yāsaśarkarā - Yavāsaśarkarā यासशर्करा - यवासशर्करा 189
Yaṣṭī - Yaṣṭīmadhu यष्टी - यष्टीमधु 52
Yaṣṭīkam - Yaṣṭīmadhu यष्टीकम् - यष्टीमधु 52
Yaṣṭīmadhu (p.52) यष्टीमधु (p.52)
Yaṣṭyāhvam - Yaṣṭīmadhu यष्ट्याह्वम् - यष्टीमधु 52
Yavagodhūmasambhavam-Sauvīram यवगोधूमसंभवम् - सौवीरम् 59
Yavāgrajaḥ - Yawānī यवाग्रजः- यवानी 169
Yavāgrajaḥ - Yavakśāraḥ यवाग्रजः -यवक्षारः 133
Yavāgrajam - Sauvīram यवाग्रजम् - सौवीरम् 595
Yavaḥ (p. 538) यवः (p. 538)
Yavāhvaḥ - Yavakśāraḥ यवाह्वः-यवक्षारः 133
Yavajā - Vamśarocanā (Type) यवजा - वंशरोचना (विशेषः) 150
Yavajaḥ - Yavakśāraḥ यवजः -यवक्षारः 133
Yavakaḥ - Godhūmaḥ यवक :- गोधूमः 551
Yavakaḥ - Vrīhiḥ यवकः - व्रीहिः 538
Yavakśāraḥ (p.133) यवक्षारः (p.133)
Yāvanaḥ - Turuṣkaḥ यावनः - तुरुष्कः 204
Yāvanālaḥ - Jūrṇā यावनालः - जूर्णा 557
Yavaneṣṭaḥ - Palāṇḍuḥ यवनेष्टः - पलाण्डुः 315
Yavaneṣṭam - Gṛñjanam यवनेष्टम् - गृञ्जनम् 295
Yavaneṣṭam - Maricam यवनेष्टम् - मरिचम् 168
Yavaneṣṭam - Sīsakam यवनेष्टम् - सीसकम् 526
Yāvanī Yavānī (Pārasika Yavānī) (p.172)
यावनीयवानी (पारसिकयवानी) (p.172)
Yavānikā - Yawānī यवानिका - यवानी 169

Yāvanīpriyā - Tāmbūlī	यावनीप्रिया - ताम्बूली	273
Yavaphalaḥ - Vam̐śaḥ	यवफलः - वंशः	364
Yavāsakaḥ - Yāsaḥ	यवासकः - यासः	8
Yavāsaśarkarā (p. 189)	यवासशर्करा (p. 189)	
Yavasāhvaḥ - Yawānī	यवसाह्वः- यवानी	169
Yāvaśūkaḥ - Yavakśāraḥ	यावशूकः -यवक्षारः	133
Yavaśukajaḥ - Yavakśāraḥ	यवशूकजः -यवक्षारः	133
Yavasurādayaḥ	यवसुरादयः	598
Yavatiktā (p. 98)	यवतिक्ता (p. 98)	
Yavottham - Sauvīram	यवोत्थम् -सौवीरम्	595
Yavyaḥ - Yavakśāraḥ	यव्यः -यवक्षारः	133
Yawānī - Yawānikā	यवानी - यवानिका	171
Yawānī (p. 169)	यवानी (p. 169)	
Yawānikā (p.171)	यवानिका (p.171)	
Yayuḥ - Aśvaḥ	ययुः - अश्वः	621
Yugandharaḥ - Jūrṇā	युगन्धरः - जूर्णा	
Yosid - Strī	योषिद् - स्त्री	615
Yogajam - Agaru	योगजम् - अगरु	206
Yogeśvarī - Vandhyakarkoṭakī	योगेश्वरी - वन्ध्यकर्कोटकी	68
Yogī - Nāraṅgaḥ	योगी - नारङ्गः	391
Yogīraṅgaḥ - Nāraṅgaḥ (Raj.ni.)	योगीरङ्गः - नारङ्गः (रा. नि.)	392
Yogīṣṭam - Sīsakam	योगीष्टम् - सीसकम्	526
Yogyam - Ṛddhiḥ	योग्यम् - ऋद्धिः	53
Yojanavallī - Mañjiṣṭhā	योजनवल्ली - मञ्जिष्ठा	7
Yonalaḥ - Jūrṇā	योनलः - जूर्णा	557
Yoṣā -Srtī	योषा - स्त्री	615
Yugam - Ṛddhiḥ	युगम् -ऋद्धिः	53
Yuktarasā - Rāsnā	युक्तरसा - रास्ना	104
Yuktiyuktaḥ - Turuṣkaḥ	युक्तियुक्तः - तुरुष्कः	204
Yūpam - Tūdam	यूपम् - तूदम	
Yūthikā (p. 504)	यूथिका (p. 504)	
Yuvatī - Strī	युवती - स्त्री	615